THE POST ANESTHESIA CARE UNIT

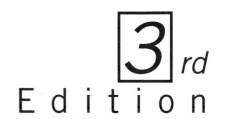
3rd Edition

THE POST ANESTHESIA CARE UNIT

A Critical Care Approach to Post Anesthesia Nursing

Cecil B. Drain, Ph.D., R.N., C.R.N.A., F.A.A.N.

Professor and Chairman, Department of Nurse Anesthesia
Virginia Commonwealth University
Medical College of Virginia Campus
Richmond, Virginia

W.B. SAUNDERS COMPANY
A Division of Harcourt Brace & Company
Philadelphia   London   Toronto   Montreal   Sydney   Tokyo

W.B. SAUNDERS COMPANY
A Division of Harcourt Brace & Company

The Curtis Center
Independence Square West
Philadelphia, Pennsylvania 19106

Library of Congress Cataloging-in-Publication Data

Drain, Cecil B.

The post anesthesia care unit: a critical care approach to post anesthesia nursing / Cecil B. Drain.—3rd ed.

p.   cm.

Rev. ed. of: The recovery room / Cecil B. Drain, Susan Shipley Christoph. 1987.

ISBN 0–7216–4571–2

1. Post anesthesia nursing.   2. Recovery rooms.   I. Drain, Cecil B.   Recovery room.   II. Title.   [DNLM: 1. Postanesthesia Nursing.   2. Postoperative Care—nursing.   3. Anesthesia Recovery Period.   4. Recovery Room—nurses' instruction.   WY 154 D759p]

RD51.3.D73 1994   617'.919—dc20

DNLM/DLC   93–8029

The Post Anesthesia Care Unit: ISBN 0–7216–4571–2
A Critical Care Approach to Post Anesthesia Nursing, 3rd edition

Last digit is the print number: 9   8   7   6   5   4   3   2   1

To my parents,
my wife Cindy, and
my children—Tim and his wife, Holly,
Steve and his wife, Christine, and Katie—
for their love, support, and understanding;

To Dan Ruth, for his patience and understanding;

To all my former colleagues in the Army Nurse Corps;

To Sue Christoph, for her support over the first two editions;

And finally, to all the post anesthesia nurses
who have made the preparation of each edition so enjoyable.

Contributors

Sandra S. Barnes, M.S., R.N., C.P.A.N.
Assistant Head Nurse, Post Anesthesia Care Unit, Northern Westchester Hospital Center, Mt. Kisco, New York

Nancy Burden, B.S., R.N., C.P.A.N.
Surgery Team Leader, Morton Plant East Lake Ambulatory Surgery, Clearwater, Florida

Susan B. Christoph, D.N.Sc., R.N.
Former Chief, Department of Nursing, Ireland U.S. Army Community Hospital, Ft. Knox, Kentucky

Kathleen A. Daly, M.S., R.N., C.C.R.N.
Instructor, Rush University College of Nursing; Clinical Nurse Specialist, Chicago, Illinois

Donna DeFazio-Quinn, B.S.N., M.B.A., R.N., C.P.A.N.
Manager, Elliot One-Day Surgery Center, Manchester, New Hampshire

Dennis M. Driscoll, Major, A.N., M.S., R.N., C.C.R.N., C.E.N.
Doctoral Student, University of Rochester Graduate School of Nursing, Rochester, New York

Sharon Farrar, B.S.N., R.N.
Operating Room and Post Anesthesia Care Unit Staff Nurse, Porter Memorial Hospital, Denver, Colorado

Anita Gurwin, B.S.N., R.N.
Post Anesthesia Care Unit Staff Nurse, Porter Memorial Hospital, Denver, Colorado

John K. Hawkins, M.H.S., R.N., C.R.N.A.
Staff C.R.N.A., Womack Army Medical Center, Fort Bragg, North Carolina

Virginia C. Hawkins, M.S.N., R.N., C.C.R.N.
Staff Nurse, Cardiac Surgery Intensive Care Unit, Cape Fear Valley Medical Center, Fayetteville, North Carolina

Linda M. Huffman, B.A., C.R.N.A.
Director of Clinical Education, Health Care Training Associates, San Antonio, Texas

Karen D. Keeler, B.S.N., R.N., C.C.R.N., C.E.N.
Manager, Emergency Department, Northern Westchester Hospital Center, Mt. Kisco, New York

Myrna E. Mamaril, M.S., R.N., C.P.A.N.
Head Nurse, Ambulatory Surgery Unit and Preadmission Testing, St. Joseph Hospital, Baltimore, Maryland

Lynda Marks, R.N.
Post Anesthesia Care Unit Staff Nurse, Porter Memorial Hospital, Denver, Colorado

Patricia A. McGaffigan, M.S., R.N.,C.
Manager, Clinical Education, Nellcor Incorporated, Groton, Massachusetts, and Hayward, California

Kathleen Millican Miller, M.S.N., R.N., C.P.A.N.
Perioperative Clinical Nurse Specialist, St. Charles Hospital, Oregon, Ohio

Carole A. Mussler, M.S., R.N.
Clinical Staff Nurse, Ireland Army Hospital, Ft. Knox, Kentucky

Denise O'Brien, B.S.N., R.N., C.P.A.N.
Educational Nurse Coordinator/Clinical Nurse III, Ambulatory Surgery Unit, Department of Operating Rooms/PACU, University of Michigan Hospitals, Ann Arbor, Michigan

Janet L. Odom, M.S., R.N., C.P.A.N.
Clinical Nurse Specialist, Surgical Services, Forrest General Hospital, Hattiesburg, Mississippi

Carolyn Zehren, R.N., C.P.A.N.
Clinical Coordinator, Wills Eye Hospital, Philadelphia, Pennsylvania

Preface

Since its initial publication in 1979, *The Recovery Room* has evolved into the standard text for post anesthesia nurses. The third edition continues this tradition, providing post anesthesia nursing with the most comprehensive coverage available under one cover. The new title, *The Post Anesthesia Care Unit: A Critical Care Approach to Post Anesthesia Nursing,* reflects the evolving professionalism of the specialty, which in 1983, under the aegis of the American Society of Post Anesthesia Nurses (ASPAN), chose the terms *post anesthesia care unit* (PACU) to designate the postoperative work area and *post anesthesia nurse* to indicate the nurse specializing in that area of patient care.

This book is organized into five major sections. Section I, "The Post Anesthesia Care Unit," focuses on the post anesthesia facilities and equipment, the specialty of post anesthesia nursing, and management and policy issues. This section has been totally rewritten by recognized leaders in post anesthesia nursing to provide the most up-to-date information in these areas for the nurse and nurse manager.

Section II deals with the physiologic considerations in the PACU. All of the chapters have been updated to reflect the current concepts in anatomy and physiology, including the most recent information available concerning the care and treatment of patients with acquired immunodeficiency syndrome (Chapter 11).

Section III, "Concepts in Anesthetic Agents," presents the reader with up-to-date pharmacologic considerations of post anesthesia care. The first chapter is completely new and presents an overview of pharmacology, including uptake and distribution, pharmacokinetic and pharmacodynamic principles, and drug-drug interactions in the PACU. Because of advances in research and applications of intravenous anesthetic agents, this content, which was presented in a single chapter in the previous edition, has been divided into two separate chapters covering opioid and nonopioid intravenous anesthetic agents. Along with this, the regional anesthesia chapter has been expanded to include the increased use of regional anesthesia in pain management.

Section IV addresses post anesthesia nursing care for the various surgical specialties. Many of the chapters in this section have been completely revised by guest authors. Chapter 20, "Assessment and Monitoring of the Post Anesthesia Patient," includes an all-new section on monitoring equipment and data interpretation. This update is especially important owing to the many technologic advances in the PACU that have occurred in the last 5 years. Chapter 21 explores the art and science of airway management, with special attention to intubation and extubation of the trachea. This addition was in response to frequent requests for more information by users of the previous edition. Also new to this text is Chapter 22, "Assessment and Management of Postoperative Pain," which includes discussions on related physiology and pharmacology.

Section V, "Special Considerations," has been revised and condensed in this edition. Two chapters are certainly worthy additions to this section: Chapter 43, "Post Anesthesia Care of the Patient with Thermal Imbalance," discusses the care of patients with hyperthermia and hypothermia, and Chapter 44 addresses the needs and care of the shock trauma patient, a topic currently receiving an exceptional amount of attention in professional meetings and literature.

The success of any multiauthored book is in large part dependent on the expertise and commitment of the contributors. The contributors to this book were invited because they are acknowledged authorities in their fields. With their help, I hope that this book will continue to inform and guide students, teachers, and clinicians in the critical care specialty of post anesthesia nursing. As in previous editions, I welcome all evaluations and suggestions for improvement.

CECIL B. DRAIN

Contents

SECTION I

The Post Anesthesia Care Unit, 1

CHAPTER 1

Space Planning and Basic Equipment Systems, 3
Linda M. Huffman, B.A., C.R.N.A.

CHAPTER 2

Post Anesthesia Nursing as a Specialty, 15
Donna DeFazio-Quinn, B.S.N., M.B.A., R.N., C.P.A.N.

CHAPTER 3

Management and Policies, 27
Janet L. Odom, M.S., R.N., C.P.A.N.

SECTION II

Physiologic Considerations in the PACU, 51

CHAPTER 4

Nervous System Anatomy and Physiology, 53

CHAPTER 5

Cardiovascular System Anatomy and Physiology, 82

CHAPTER 6

Respiratory System Anatomy and Physiology, 104

CHAPTER 7

Renal Anatomy and Physiology, 138

CHAPTER 8

Endocrine Physiology, 149

CHAPTER 9

Gastrointestinal System Anatomy and Physiology, 156

CHAPTER 10

Integumentary System Anatomy and Physiology, 165

CHAPTER 11

Immune System Physiology, 171

SECTION III

Concepts in Anesthetic Agents, 179

CHAPTER 12

Basic Principles of Pharmacology, 181

CHAPTER 13

Inhalation Anesthesia, 190

CHAPTER 14

Nonopioid Intravenous Anesthetics, 205

CHAPTER 15

Opioid Intravenous Anesthetics, 215

CHAPTER 16

Muscle Relaxants, 226

CHAPTER 17

Local Anesthetics, 245

CHAPTER 18

Regional Anesthesia, 251

SECTION IV

Nursing Care in the PACU, 259

CHAPTER 19

Assessment and Monitoring of the Post Anesthesia Patient, 261
Patricia A. McGaffigan, M.S., R.N.,C.
Susan B. Christoph, D.N.Sc., R.N.

CHAPTER 20

Care of the Post Anesthesia Patient, 289
Denise O'Brien, B.S.N., R.N., C.P.A.N.

CHAPTER 21

Assessment and Management of the Airway, 305

CHAPTER 22

Assessment and Management of Postoperative Pain, 314
Susan B. Christoph, D.N.Sc., R.N.

CHAPTER 23

Post Anesthesia Care of the Ear, Nose, Throat, Neck, and Maxillofacial Surgical Patient, 325
Lynda Marks, R.N.
Anita Gurwin, B.S.N., R.N.
Sharon Farrar, B.S.N., R.N.

CHAPTER 24

Post Anesthesia Care of the Ophthalmic Surgical Patient, 343
Carolyn Zehren, R.N., C.P.A.N.

CHAPTER 25

Post Anesthesia Care of the Thoracic Surgical Patient, 350

CHAPTER 26

Post Anesthesia Care of the Cardiac Surgical Patient, 368
Karen D. Keeler, R.N., B.S.N., C.C.R.N., C.E.N.

CHAPTER 27

Post Anesthesia Care of the Vascular Surgical Patient, 387
Kathleen A. Daly, M.S., R.N., C.C.R.N.

CHAPTER 28

Post Anesthesia Care of the Orthopedic Surgical Patient, 399
Sandra S. Barnes, M.S., R.N., C.P.A.N.

CHAPTER 29

Post Anesthesia Care of the Neurosurgical Patient, 409
John K. Hawkins, M.H.S., R.N., C.R.N.A.
Virginia C. Hawkins, M.S.N., R.N., C.C.R.N.

CHAPTER 30

Post Anesthesia Care of the Thyroid and Parathyroid Surgical Patient, 444
Susan B. Christoph, D.N.Sc., R.N.

CHAPTER 31

Post Anesthesia Care of the Gastrointestinal, Abdominal, and Anorectal Surgical Patient, 447
Denise O'Brien, B.S.N., R.N., C.P.A.N.

CHAPTER 32

Post Anesthesia Care of the Genitourinary Surgical Patient, 463
Kathleen Millican Miller, M.S.N., R.N., C.P.A.N.

CHAPTER 33

Post Anesthesia Care of the Obstetric and Gynecologic Surgical Patient, 477
Kathleen Millican Miller, M.S.N., R.N., C.P.A.N.

CHAPTER 34

Post Anesthesia Care of the Breast Surgical Patient, 484
Carole A. Mussler, M.S., R.N.

CHAPTER 35

Post Anesthesia Care of the Plastic Surgical Patient, 492
Carole A. Mussler, M.S., R.N.

CHAPTER 36

Post Anesthesia Care of the Thermally Injured Patient, 499
Dennis M. Driscoll, Major, A.N., M.S., R.N., C.C.R.N., C.E.N.

CHAPTER 37

Post Anesthesia Care of the Ambulatory Surgical Patient, 506
Nancy Burden, B.S., R.N., C.P.A.N.

SECTION V

Special Considerations, 517

CHAPTER 38

Post Anesthesia Care of the Patient with Chronic Disorders, 519

CHAPTER 39

Post Anesthesia Care of the Pediatric Patient, 534

CHAPTER 40

Post Anesthesia Care of the Geriatric Patient, 544

CHAPTER 41

Post Anesthesia Care of the Pregnant Patient, 549

CHAPTER 42

Post Anesthesia Care of the Substance Abuser, 557

CHAPTER 43

Post Anesthesia Care of the Patient with Thermal Imbalance, 563

CHAPTER 44

Post Anesthesia Care of the Shock Trauma Patient, 570
Myrna E. Mamaril, M.S., R.N., C.P.A.N.

CHAPTER 45

Cardiopulmonary Resuscitation in the Post Anesthesia Care Unit, 584

Index, 595

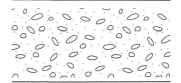

The Post Anesthesia Care Unit

Space Planning and Basic Equipment Systems

CHAPTER 1

Linda M. Huffman, B.A., C.R.N.A.

The recovery room of days past has evolved into a specialty discipline that encompasses bedside nursing and critical care expertise and is known today as the *post anesthesia care unit* (PACU). This clinical setting should be designed to promote visual observation of each patient's status, to ensure appropriate physiologic monitoring, to provide patient safety in every aspect of care, and to create an efficient and productive flow of tasks that are integral to the work of the professional nurses and support personnel employed there.

The physical structure of the PACU must be configured to help nurses prevent problems, detect problems, and appropriately treat and reverse problems as they occur. Immediate access to emergency care equipment, therefore, is essential because the mainstay of PACU nursing is the speed and effectiveness with which the staff can identify and manage common events such as upper airway obstruction, respiratory insufficiency, nausea and vomiting, cardiac compromise, aspiration, hypotension, hypertension, hypovolemia, hypervolemia, shock, dysrhythmias, respiratory distress, and cardiac failure.

In an ideal setting, the perfect PACU would be located within immediate proximity of the surgery suite; have private and public access routes; house its own mini-laboratory, blood bank, and satellite pharmacy; have an overhead radiographic imaging component conveniently located just inside the entry; have adequate space for administrative offices, restrooms, and a recreational area; and have an anesthesia call room inside its perimeter where emergency anesthesia staff could be available at all times. Monitor displays the size of big-screen television could be helpful, as would remote control operation of monitors; computer terminals at each patient station; a facsimile, modem, and information network that links all patient data into the central PACU system; and computer terminal input jacks that accept multiple cables from all patient monitors such as noninvasive blood pressure, pulse oximetry, carbon dioxide monitoring, and cardiac rhythm so that charting is automatically downloaded and displayed in the patient's data file.

However, resources are limited in the real world, and duplication of services common to other departments is simply too expensive to allow the luxury of a dedicated laboratory, radiology, and pharmacy service on the unit. Therefore, it makes sense to build new PACU units so they are located within minutes of the operating rooms and as close to needed support services as possible. A built-in x-ray machine, and a portable blood gas analysis system are affordable, and a computer-assisted drug-dispensing machine can easily dispense narcotics, thereby offsetting the cost of overtime spent on manually counting controlled drugs at the end of every shift.

Bedside documentation of vital signs is also available that permits integration of temperature, blood pressure, and pulse rate. Computer output connections (RS-232 ports) let patient monitors send data to display screens and to automated records.

To take advantage of the technology that exists and to plan now for the evolution of change during the next decade, PACU managers and other personnel are taking a more active role in planning the design, space allocation, and configurations of all aspects of these special care areas.

DESIGN

Planning Based on Human Factors Engineering

When new PACU departments are constructed and existing units are remodeled, it is beneficial to employ human factors to optimize the efficient delivery of postoperative and post anesthesia care. The study of human factors engineering involves the investigation of human and machine systems to determine what factors alter the performance of work under special conditions. The intention of this type of assessment is to resolve any problems that may develop as a result of relationships between humans and machines. By planning the design of a PACU from the standpoint of nursing care and the level of effectiveness that results from select arrangements, PACU administrators and staff members have the opportunity to do the following:

- Make the staff's contribution to work tasks as efficient as possible so that human failures are minimized.
- Make the combined nurse-machine involvement as safe as possible so that neither human failures nor product failures compromise the well-being of the nurse, the patient, or the equipment system.
- Minimize the stress that the work environment imposes on the staff as they use, operate, clean, troubleshoot, maintain, or make-ready any equipment or equipment systems that enhance the delivery of patient care.
- Limit the unnecessary demands, episodes of frustration, and extraordinary waste of energy that accelerate fatigue and lead to inattention during the work of providing total patient care.
- Increase the acceptability of a work environment, and give staff members the feeling that the design of the facility allows for efficient and appropriate work with a minimum of effort.

To apply human factors to the architectural plan, the designer of a PACU must acknowledge the needs, characteristics, capabilities, and limitations of the nursing team. The designer should make the design "fit the nursing staff" in contrast with trying to make the nursing staff "fit the design."

Human Factors and Ergonomics

The terms *ergonomics* and *human factors* are often used interchangeably in discussing the general topic of design in relation to the efficiency of work. Human factors engineers and ergonomists use the same basic information and perform the same kinds of work with respect to design. Principles of ergonomics, for example, establish how nurses interact with wall piping systems, monitors suspended on shelves, bed configurations, and lighting systems. Any aspect of the work environment that influences the expenditure of work expressed as a unit of energy over time is involved in the ergonomic and human factors plan.

Patient monitors that are positioned at eye level and tilted to improve the viewing angle produce less fatigue than similar units mounted high on the wall, requiring the nurse to expend energy constantly looking up to see the display. In another example, gas supply and vacuum outlets (on the wall) positioned too high for the nurse of average height to reach result in more energy being used by most of the staff to make and break oxygen and suction connections.

Planning Objective

The primary space planning objective in PACU design should be to seek a balanced compromise between maximizing the staff efficiency, ensuring patient safety, and maintaining adequate respect for the patients' personal needs, both physical and psychological. Foremost among any patients' needs is therapeutic care, but other needs must also be considered: a means to minimize fear in all patients, arrangements that keep noise levels at a minimum, and, in general, efforts put forth to minimize post operative pain and suffering.

For this reason, PACU units may no longer rely on standard space layout plans and must look carefully at their respective practice to estimate the actual space needed. Four feet of space on each side of a PACU bed may have been adequate in the past but may not be sufficient today. For example, if a PACU must accommodate visitors, a 24-inch-wide mechanical ventilator, and a team of one or two caregivers, all related to a single patient, there is a space problem. If the same patient develops a need for an intravenous (IV) infusion pump or a system of pumps with a controller component to be placed at the bedside and a heated warming blanket apparatus is indicated, there is simply not enough space left to perform nursing care procedures or deal with any events that require emergency patient management.

Before space can be allocated for each patient station, planners must examine the dimensions of all stand-alone equipment the staff intends to use. Common space-occupying devices in use include, but are not limited to, heat and cooling blankets and their operating systems, emergency instrument carts, mechanical ventilators, infusion pumps and controllers, additional or backup monitors, supplemental IV infusion poles, emergency resuscitation equipment, and a cardiac-assist device.

The number of beds needed in each PACU depends on the number of operative procedures performed each day, the average length of those procedures, the scope of emergency and trauma care provided, the elective scheduling pattern of surgical procedures, and the acuity of patients as determined by their preanesthetic physical status classification.

One indirect influence on PACU bed utilization depends on the size and trend in patient census in the intensive care units (ICUs). When postoperative patients require ICU admission, and that census is routinely at capacity, the number of beds in the PACU may be intentionally increased. Although it is not prudent to build more PACU beds than necessary, in the presence of acute patients and a shortage of ICU beds, operating rooms are unable to continue surgery.

Closing down an operating room to compensate for inadequate PACU space is an expensive interim solution that can be eliminated by realistic assessment of both the numbers of patients admitted to the PACU and the nature of their pre-existing and surgical conditions when they arrive for post anesthesia care. Minimum standards for space allocations are defined by the Joint Commission on Accreditation of Healthcare Organizations, (JCAHO) in its publication, "Guidelines for Post Anesthesia Care Units," available on request from the JCAHO headquarters in Chicago. Specific details about select hospital departments' design are available from the Bacon Library of the American Hospital Association in Chicago and the U.S. Public Health Service in Washington, D.C. Figure 1–1 shows the layout of a compact PACU care station with a built-in headwall of equipment. Figure 1–2 shows another layout with more space between patient beds and patient monitors positioned at eye level.

SPACE CONFIGURATIONS

Routine Access and Emergency Evacuation

Although a disaster requiring emergency evacuation of patients and staff members is rare, it continues to be a critical consideration in terms of both location of the unit and the

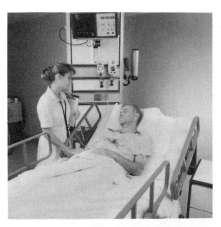

FIGURE 1–1. A modern built-in headwall system that incorporates gas supply, vacuum, mercury blood pressure manometer, and patient monitor into one space-saving design. (Courtesy of Ohmeda, Madison, WI.)

layout of the floor plan. Entry routes should be logical to permit rapid transfer of a critically ill patient with multiple devices in use and the anesthesia and surgical staff that accompany the patient. When possible, avoid use of irregular pathways, curved or angular geometric designs, irregular elevations, narrow doorways, and any barriers or interruptions that delay traffic flow. A confusing and inconvenient access route from the operating room to the PACU and back to the operating room, if needed, may mean the difference between a desirable and an undesirable outcome.

Signage requirements should be addressed at the same time that the physical layout is considered. Bed identification signs should be designated logically, using numbers or letters of the alphabet to denote each location. Signs help define an appropriate design but they do not compensate for a convoluted layout.

The general principals that apply to entryway planning and design suggest that a prudent planning team would

- Provide two or more entries so there will always be an alternative exit route.
- Locate entryways so that internal and external traffic patterns are as short and convenient as possible.
- Create an appropriate service area entrance so that deliveries of supplies to utility rooms do not have to travel the same pathway as patients-in-transit to or from the operating room or to and from other patient care areas.
- Allow for adequate external threshold space to safely accommodate the expected traffic

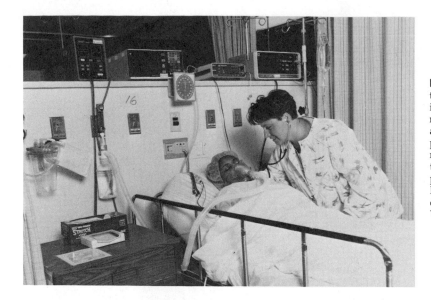

FIGURE 1–2. A modern care station that has centrally piped oxygen, medical air, and vacuum wall outlets; a nurse call system; electrical outlets; and an eye-level stationary shelf supporting stand-alone monitors for noninvasive blood pressure and end-tidal carbon dioxide determinations, pulse oximetry, invasive pressure lines, and aneroid sphygmomanometry. (Courtesy of Medical College of Virginia Hospitals, Richmond, VA.)

of staff members, beds and stretchers, and equipment on wheels.

- Provide safe access when using swinging doors.
- Provide sufficient clearance in all entryways to manipulate furniture, equipment, wheelchairs, and boxes of supplies to avoid conflicts between entering and exiting traffic.
- Allow for a similarly appropriate internal threshold space to avoid obstruction to traffic flow when manipulating beds or equipment being moved into the unit.
- Provide adequate lighting for both the external and the internal entry spaces to accommodate adequate visualization of floor surfaces during evening and night shifts.
- Provide for appropriate communications systems, such as an intercom for nurses, and computer interface connectors at the bedside and the nurses' station to accommodate the facility's use of medical information hardware and software.

Other Special Considerations

Isolation Room. Although universal precautions are the standard of care for all patients, it is unacceptable to assume that these measures alone offer an adequate means of preventing transmission of organisms from one patient to another in an open care area. In patients with tuberculosis, airborne transfer of bacteria must be minimized using isolation procedures consistently. Patients with incompetent immune

systems, from any cause, benefit from reverse isolation in a private room setting to minimize their potentially fatal contact with contamination from other patients or staff members. In addition, patients who present to the operating room and subsequently to the PACU with purulent discharge should be isolated as a means of minimizing the exposure of infection to others who have had recent surgical procedures.

Based on the number of procedures identified as "infected" in each respective surgical suite, the PACU should have at least one isolation room. This area should be enclosed, properly piped for medical gases and vacuum, equipped with a complete physiologic monitoring system, and permit visual observation of the patient at all times. In instances when isolation rooms have been temporarily converted to other uses, such as a lounge area, office space, or storage space, it is important to verify the integrity of the wall-supply gas and vacuum outlets before returning this space to a patient care area.

Regardless of the need for isolation or the presence of an isolation room, soiled linen, dressings, and garments should be properly contained and placed in appropriate receptacles without making contact with surfaces of monitors, furniture, shelves, or the floor.

Utility Area. A clean-up area should be conveniently located and serve as a depository for soiled linen, refuse, and reusable instruments or devices that need to be cleaned, decontaminated, rinsed, and wrapped before being transferred to central supply for sterilization.

Storage Space. Equipment that should be stored in the unit and available at all times includes, but is not limited to, multiple stretchers, one or more volume ventilators, a resuscitation cart or cabinet on wheels with a defibrillator and adult and pediatric paddles; one full E-size of oxygen as a reserve supply; one or more full E-size cylinders of oxygen for transport use; an appropriate regulator and oxygen delivery hose with a self-inflating non-rebreathing bag, such as the Ambu and Hope resuscitators; infusion pumps and controllers; a 12-lead electrocardiogram machine; warming blanket; transducer systems for invasive monitoring; and radiant heat warmer.

Shelves and Bracket Systems. Properly secured shelves at the head of each patient station allow storage of select supplies and equipment, and, under the proper conditions, may hold monitoring components. When a shelf is used to support any monitor or other medical device, the specification of load limit of the shelf should be verified to ensure that the weight of the monitor does not exceed the capability of the shelf to support it.

Flooring Materials. The floor should be constructed of a material that is easily cleaned, is resistant to abrasion, will endure harsh detergents, and will not cause incidental "slip and fall" accidents. It is not necessary to use antistatic materials, but the static charge on stretcher wheels makes them prone to attracting dust and debris, so they need periodic cleaning.

New synthetic floor coverings, including carpet, are available and may be used to help minimize noise. However, if these flooring materials are considered, a "spot test" using tincture of benzoin, coffee, and blood to demonstrate actual stain resistance and cleaning effectiveness is recommended prior to purchases.

Fire Extinguishers. Fire-fighting equipment should be present at all times, and staff members should be trained in the proper use of fire extinguishers. Instructions on what to do in case of fire and a fire evacuation plan for both patients and staff should be included in the regular education conferences.

Subsystems of the Overall Design

Hospital architects and industrial designers rarely create new designs for subsystems such as the electrical power supply, heat and air conditioning, information management, and lighting, plumbing, and gas supply. Instead, they typically search for subsystems, components, and products that meet the needs of the staff, are effective in performance, and conform to the budget plan. Once subsystems are identified, it is important for the PACU staff to examine each one carefully to ensure that they are adequate and appropriate to the scope of nursing care delivered in the unit.

The following planning steps are suggested before any subsystem is specified or incorporated into the design:

- Determine the operational and cost constraints placed on the subsystem by the work being performed.
- Make a detailed analysis of the operational and functional requirements for the subsystem itself, even though a general specification plan may have already been prepared.
- Determine which work functions should be performed by an automated device and which should be performed as a manual task. Establish specifications for both types of functions. Examine routine tasks that may be performed with automation, and apply them accordingly.
- Identify the equipment, displays, controls, furnishings, and other support items that are generally available "off the shelf" to avoid the cost of customized accessories.
- Develop a traffic analysis to describe how each subsystem will probably be used. Are there enough electrical outlets for general surgical patients but not enough for complicated thoracic procedures? A mock-up drawing is useful to test if the specification written is realistic for a particular unit's case mix.

Will the Design Really Work?

The design process in general should always start with the user at the task level and work outward, step by step. The following are typical steps in a task analysis:

- Determine who the user or users will be: a nurse, a technician, a nurse's aide, or a unit secretary. Then determine what functions the user has to perform, individually or in conjunction with others.
- Determine how each user will perform the functions he or she is responsible for and what tools, equipment, components, connections, and furnishing each will probably have to use.
- Re-evaluate the immediate "use space" required by the staff and their related devices and tools. Then examine again the

interrelationships among several use spaces, such as multiple beds, placed side by side. Check to determine if necessary communications and traffic flow are optimized.

- Select information systems, displays, controls, consoles, light fixtures, writing surfaces, and even chairs that fit the human point of view and ensure that each person has the maximum opportunity to perform whatever task he or she is assigned as efficiently as possible.
- Examine the environmental conditions surrounding each patient care station and nursing space to minimize the possibility that excessive noise, vibration, extreme temperature, or poor ventilation may degrade the nurse's performance, cause annoyance, or affect his or her health and safety.

Throughout each of these planning phases, continue to evaluate, test, and re-examine the specifications to develop a balance between the staff members, the space, and the hardware priorities. The ultimate success of the physical structure depends on how well staff members perform their work, which is a combination of their skill plus the physical and psychological interactions with the environment where they work. Try not to assume that because certain layout plans, equipment configurations, and subsystems have traditionally been designed in a certain way, they have been successful in the past. If nursing advisors and collaborators can remain sensitive to the possibilities of improvement in work performance and reduction in energy expended, the needs of nurses and patients in PACU can be met as the first priority and still accommodate design criteria.

Because this stage of evaluation is the most important part of any structural design, ask the architect to show you scale models of the unit as it is intended to function. This effort permits realistic evaluation to be made about the physical space and the procedures to be performed there. Avoid the mistake of believing that a three-dimensional work environment can be evaluated by looking at drawings alone. Nurses and patients live, think, act, and work in three-dimensional environments, and therefore it is necessary to confirm that a proposed space and its human-to-equipment interface allows efficient performance of tasks.

Any PACU design for new construction or a remodeling project must adapt to the staff and the patients. Although nursing groups are known to be adaptable to their environmental

constraints, they pay a considerable penalty in fatigue, impaired performance, and physical and psychological stress when they are called on to do multiple sophisticated tasks in a poorly designed unit. It is most important to evaluate any design system from the standpoint of its performance rather than its appearance. Many PACUs with impressive configurations of equipment and furniture are attractive to look at but difficult to endure.

Power Outlets. A sufficient number of electrical outlets should be located at each patient care station. They may be incorporated into a headwall design or be strategically placed to accommodate the available area. Numerous outlets are needed to allow easy access to connect ancillary equipment to power and to prevent power cords from being draped near or across traffic areas.

All outlets must be properly grounded, and isolation circuit breakers must be installed to meet or exceed the electrical safety standards incorporated into the specific building codes for each respective hospital facility.

Provisions for access to the emergency power generating system are needed at every patient station to permit uninterrupted care in the event of a power failure. One 220-volt isolated line with an appropriate outlet and cord adapters is needed to power x-ray equipment.

Air Conditioning. Adjustable heating, cooling, and humidification controls and systems are required to ensure comfortable conditions for the patients and the staff. Specifications for complete air exchange at least 12 to 15 times per hour, endorsed by the plant engineering department, should be checked regularly and maintained in keeping with the air quality protocol applied in the facility.

Plumbing. Multiple sinks with foot controls for handwashing are appropriate for the PACU and should be conveniently located near patient care areas. Disposable towels packaged in germicidal solution should be provided at each work station when an adequate number of sinks are not available or when staff members are temporarily unable to leave the bedside.

Wall-Supply Oxygen. The presence of a piped medical gas, installed within the wall, is common in U.S. hospitals, both in newly constructed and remodeled PACUs. However, having a piped-in oxygen supply does not alleviate the need to have a reserve oxygen cylinder present in the PACU that is set up and ready to deliver oxygen within a moment's notice. The reserve system is necessary to supplement oxygen to a patient in the presence of an oxygen wall-supply failure. Additional cylinders of oxygen are needed for supplemental oxygen delivery during transportation.

The bulk oxygen storage plant is typically located outside the facility itself and is connected to a pipeline network of distribution channels within the ceiling and walls. The terminal outlet mounted behind the head of the bed at most patient care stations is connected to a flexible hose that is detachable. Connections between the flexible hoses and the patient complete the system. Figure 1–3 shows a typical oxygen flowmeter, as used in the PACU.

Most accidents involving oxygen delivery systems result from alterations or faulty repairs made by unauthorized or untrained personnel. However, the most common failure of oxygen delivery systems is known to result from failure to check the system prior to the admission of a patient. Always verify that the flow of oxygen is present, that the "float" moves freely within the flow tube, and that all connections are leak-tight before the patient's appearance in the unit.

Flow Rate of Oxygen. Modern flowmeters depend on the fact that when a gas passes through an orifice, there is a difference of pressure between the two sides. The fall in pressure is proportional to the flow rate of the gas and inversely proportional to the diameter of the orifice. If the orifice is of a fixed size, the pres-

sure difference across it will be proportional to the gas flow through it. Conversely, if the pressure difference is kept constant, such as that pressure required to lift a bobbin in a flow tube, the gas flow rate will vary with the diameter of the orifice. The resistance to flow of an orifice also varies with the density of the gas flowing through it. This means a flowmeter calibrated for one gas will not be accurate for another.

Some oxygen flowmeters are designed with a tapered bore so that the higher the float is lifted, the wider is the gap between the side of the bobbin and the wall of the tube. This variable gap, or "annulus," is the orifice. The float has a special shape, and it rotates freely in the middle of the gas stream and normally does not touch the walls of the tube.

Misuse of Flowmeters. If the oxygen flow tube is not vertical, the shape of the annulus becomes asymmetrical, and at certain flow rates there is a significant variation in the relationship between the orifice and the flow tube, resulting in inaccurate flow. If the flowmeter tube is further tilted, the float may actually touch the tube and the resulting friction may cause even less flow, even though the float is visibly located higher up into the tube. Therefore, on wall and cylinder supply oxygen sources, it is appropriate to keep the flowmeter tube in the vertical position at all times.

The float may also stick to the side of the tube as a result of static electricity, particularly in very dry atmospheres. This is one reason why the ambient relative humidity in PACU is maintained at 50 percent minimum. Particles of dirt on the float or on the inner wall of the flow tube can change the effective diameter of the annulus, causing the oxygen flow rate to be inaccurate. A float that is "sticking" to the sides of the tube should be replaced by a backup oxygen flowmeter and immediately sent for repair.

Flowmeters are precision devices that need to be handled with respect. The interior has a valve and a valve seat that control flow to ensure the desired concentration. When turning off a flow control, close it but do not tighten it.

Calibration and Maintenance of Flowmeters. Flowmeter tubes are individually calibrated with their floats and tubes assembled at a specific temperature and pressure. Floats and tubes that are calibrated as one single unit should be repaired as one single unit. Floats and tubes should not be interchanged. Flowmeters with ball floats instead of rotating bobbins may be less prone to stick to the sides of

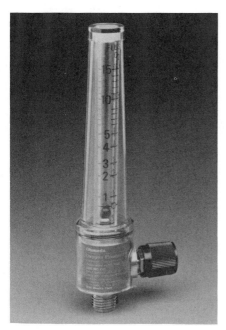

FIGURE 1–3. An oxygen flowmeter with a ball flow indicator and a therapeutic range of 1 to 15 L/min. (Courtesy of Ohmeda, Madison, WI.)

the tube when influenced by dirt and static electricity. The tube and float should be regularly dismantled and cleaned by a properly trained technician.

Wall Vacuum System. Prior to the anticipated arrival of a patient, it is important to ensure that there is adequate vacuum supply, that all suction apparatus connections are properly made, and that the system is in working order before the patient appears. The ability to immediately suction a patient's airway is a life-saving maneuver that cannot be delayed while the apparatus is being set up and tested.

In addition, it is inappropriate to operate a suction system that is not equipped with an adjustable vacuum regulator. Because the vacuum supply fluctuates based on the hospital-wide demand, there are times when the vacuum supply varies.

A vacuum of approximately 200 mm Hg below standard atmospheric pressure (760 mm Hg) should be maintained at the vacuum outlets. The flow rate of ambient air at each suction system is about 40 L per min. There should be at least three outlets per patient care station to accommodate three types of therapeutic suction: oral and tracheal, gastrointestinal, and thoracic. Figure 1–4 shows the adjustable control vacuum regulator. Figure 1–5 is an example of an intermittent-to-continuous suction regulator.

Lighting. The overall lighting intensity should be high to provide appropriate determination of skin color and subtle movements or changes but not be dazzling to the patient. A reserve spotlight is usually for special procedures such as a venous cutdown or a regional block.

Instruments. A selection of laryngoscopy instruments should be available, checked for proper operation at the start of each day, and include a full range of infant to adult sizes in both curved-blade and straight-blade styles. The most commonly used curved laryngoscope is the MacIntosh or a modification of this blade. The most commonly used straight blade is the Miller series of laryngoscopes. In reusable laryngoscopes, the entire range of blades is detachable and interchangeable, and one handle may also be used for all blades. Disposable laryngoscopes often are one-piece devices intended for a single patient use.

The electrical system of the laryngoscope is battery powered, and a small bulb is positioned at the end of the blade. The bulb makes

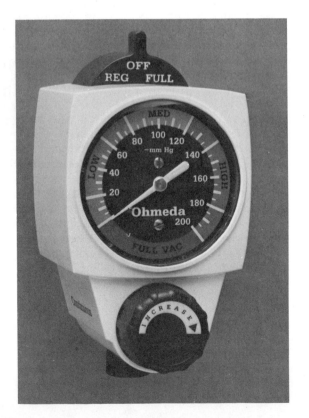

FIGURE 1–4. An adjustable suction regulator that allows precise control of the vacuum applied to oral or tracheal suctioning procedures. (Courtesy of Ohmeda, Madison, WI.)

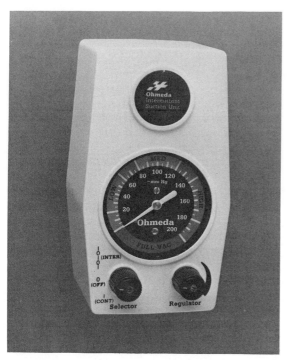

FIGURE 1–5. An intermittent suction regulator that provides user control and easy-to-read ranges of low, medium, and high vacuum. (Courtesy of Ohmeda, Madison, WI.)

contact with a core of metal inside the socket. When a bulb fails to "light," the cause is often related to the position of the bulb against its contacts. When a light is markedly dim, weak battery power is suspected.

Laryngoscope bulbs have a long life and, unless they are mishandled, offer excellent reliability. Often, good bulbs are inappropriately discarded when a laryngoscope fails to light. Because the most frequent cause of light failure stems from the bulb's position in the blade, it is important to open a laryngoscope gently. It needs to make contact only in its right-angled or open position. Do not jerk the blade up to meet the handle, because this may damage the wire connections between the bulb and the battery. When replacing the batteries in the handle, ensure that the spiral spring is still in the base of the battery compartment. Leak-proof batteries should be used.

Table 1–1 is a brief summary of the most common instruments and supplies used in airway management.

Fiberoptic Laryngoscopy. A fiberoptic laryngoscope should be present in the PACU and in working order to minimize delay when an emergency intubation is required or tracheal tube replacement is needed. When a patient's history includes a difficult laryngoscopy, an anatomic airway abnormality, or any condition that might compromise the success of using a rigid laryngoscope, the fiberoptic laryngoscopy system should be placed in readiness near the patient's care station.

The object of the fiberoptic laryngoscopy system is to transmit light from a powerful external light source through a flexible instrument that can pass easily through a series of curvatures in the airway and transmit an image of that area through the eyepiece. The light source is electrically powered and contains a brighter lamp than does the traditional laryngoscope.

The pathways through which the light (and the image) pass consist of bundles of fine glass fibers. Each fiber has a central glass core surrounded by another thin layer of glass. The light passing down the fiber is internally repeated. Fiberoptic bundles tolerate being flexed to acute angles, but they do not tolerate being twisted, pinched, or knocked against a rigid surface. These maneuvers are known to break the longitudinally arranged fibers and distort or eliminate the image.

The fiberoptic laryngoscope has four parts: an optical bundle, light guides, a channel for suction, and a channel for the passage of instruments such as a biopsy forceps. At the end of the optical bundle, a lens focuses the image on the ends of the fibers and relays the image to the eyepiece. Near the eyepiece there is a connection for the vacuum.

STANDARDS AND PATIENT MONITORING

Standards are not new to health care, particularly in terms of equipment systems, patient monitoring, nursing practice, and patient care.

Table 1–1. INSTRUMENTS AND SUPPLIES USED IN TRACHEAL INTUBATION AND AIRWAY MANAGEMENT

Oral airways—infant to adult sizes
Tracheal tubes—infant to adult sizes
Laryngoscopes—with adult and pediatric blades
Topical anesthetic spray
Magill's tracheal tube–introducing forceps
Syringe for tracheal cuff inflation
Tongue depressors
Scissors
Mouth or bite block
Suction catheters—all sizes
Yankauer or tonsil-style suction tip
Stethoscope
Tape to secure tube
Analgesic ointment and lubricating jelly

In the United States there are more than 400 organizations that write standards for performance and safety. These societies are standards-specific organizations such as the American National Standards Institute (ANSI) and the American Society of Testing and Materials (ASTM), trade associations, and professional organizations. All of these organizations collectively make up the standards-writing community.

A *standard* is defined as a rule established by authority, expertise, custom, or general consensus as a model or example to be followed. This definition applies to social and technical standards. For example, standards for nursing practice were established by the American Nurses Association. Practice Standards for the PACU have been set forth by American Society of Post Anesthesia Nurses, the American Association of Nurse Anesthetists, and the American Society of Anesthesiologists to define the minimum level of care expected.

Standards are based on theory, experience, science, principles of practice, and the philosophy of professions who share responsibility for post anesthesia care. These standards act as a social standard, providing the clinician with a level of expectation and a framework within which to operate. In addition, they serve to guide society to the quality of behavior to expect. Standards are not law unless they are specifically incorporated into documents called *practice acts* that govern nursing and medicine or become implied law based on court precedence.

Technical standards, such as those developed by ANSI and ASTM, perform the same basic function as standards of practice do— they create order out of disorder. Standards for safety and performance of patient monitors, for example, are developed by representatives of practice, manufacturing, government, academic, and consumer groups focused on monitoring safety.

In its public information booklet, "Standards Make the Pieces Fit," ASTM describes the following four levels of standards based on the degree of consensus needed for their development and use:

- A company standard is one in which consensus is among the employees of an organization, that is, the standard applied in one hospital or established by one manufacturer.
- An industry standard, typically developed by a trade association, also has consensus among its members. Here the word *industry* has a broad definition and may refer to professional associations or manufacturers when they deal with similar issues.
- Government standards reflect many degrees of consensus. A government agency may adopt standards developed by private organizations or may assign persons in a given department of government to write a standard. Standards of weight, measure, and environment are examples of government action.
- A full-consensus standard is developed by representatives of all sectors that have interest in its use. Full-consensus standards are the most comprehensively sound and credible of the four categories and often are the basis for commercial and regulatory policies. Standards for the performance and safety of medical devices and systems used in respiratory care, anesthesia, and monitoring are examples of full-consensus standards.

Table 1–2 contains a list of organizations that prepare standards specifications for medical devices used in respiratory and anesthesia care.

Success Through Standardization

The purpose of setting a standard is to define and specify minimum performance and safety. Whenever two standards exist, the one that requires a higher level of performance always applies.

Standardizing any function, procedure, equipment, or policy recognizes and respects change, allows for newer and better methods and technology to upgrade an existing standard, and by definition is always evolving into a better or higher level of quality.

Because temperature, pulse, respiration, blood pressure, oxygen saturation, and carbon dioxide monitoring offers nurses and physicians a way to prevent, detect, diagnose, and treat problems and then evaluate the results, monitoring is indeed the cornerstone of post anesthesia patient care.

If instruments, devices, components, and monitors are all the same, it is still necessary to recognize that products and procedures must adapt to the people who use them or need them for their care. Not all people work in the same physical layout, but they all must work to administer the care required. Not all people need or want the same configuration in vital

Table 1–2. STANDARDS WRITING ORGANIZATIONS THAT DEFINE SAFETY AND PERFORMANCE OF MEDICAL DEVICES USED IN POST ANESTHESIA CARE

International Organization for Standardization (ISO) is the specialized international agency for standardization, comprising the national standardizing bodies of more than 80 countries. The results of ISO's work are published as International Standards. ISO covers standardization in all fields except electrical and electronic engineering.

International Electrotechnical Commission (IEC) is the organization responsible for international standardization in the electrical and electronics fields. It is presently composed of 42 national committees that collectively represent some 80% of the world's population.

American National Standards Institute (ANSI) coordinates the voluntary development of standards to ensure that they meet national needs, do not significantly overlap or conflict with each other, and are produced without unnecessary duplication of effort. ANSI is the U.S. member of ISO and IEC.

American Society for Testing and Materials (ASTM) is a management system for the development of standards and the promotion of related technical knowledge. The Society was one of the five originators of ANSI. ASTM standards are voluntary consensus documents developed by more than 29,000 members from around the world.

Underwriter's Laboratories, Inc. (UL) is an independent organization devoted to testing for public safety. It was established to maintain and operate laboratories for the examination and testing (for safety) of devices, systems, and materials. Its goal is to reduce and prevent loss of life and property from fire, crime, and casualty.

Compressed Gas Association, Inc. (CGA) is active primarily in the fields of safety and technical specifications pertaining to the compressed gas and related product/service industries. The Association collaborates with ANSI and ASTM, as well as others.

The Association for the Advancement of Medical Instrumentation (AAMI) is a nonprofit international association of clinical practitioners, engineers, hospital personnel, educators, researchers, and industry/government representatives who are furthering advances in medical instruments, devices, and systems and their use.

National Fire Protection Association (NFPA) is an organization whose representatives include clinicians, scientists, engineers, and technical experts. Initially recognized for their work in defining requirements for electrical safety and combustible anesthetics in the operating room, their work has expanded to include the use of inhalation anesthetics, nonflammable medical gases, bulk and cylinder oxygen supply systems, and test specifications for anesthesia machines following adjustment, modification, or repairs.

signs monitors, for any number of reasons. And also, not all of the rooms, work stations, or beds are the same.

Short-term and long-term measurement and monitoring needs frequently change from one patient to the next and from one measurement to the next.

Monitors and Memory

Continuous monitoring serves two functions: it allows clinicians to follow "wellness" when the measurements are normal, and it documents abnormal conditions that permit decision making without delay.

Trends of information made available by memory features in monitoring systems allow clinicians to see what happened in the past, observe what is happening in the present, and determine how a change may affect a patient's future. This capability enables nurses to make appropriate decisions in the shortest period.

Vital signs monitors that have temperature, pulse, and blood pressure integrated so that all the information can be printed on the same recorded strip allow users to see the memory

trend of the past and document any sudden change, without dividing their attention between patient care and charting duties. These advantages are most appropriate for the PACU where vital signs must be repeatedly monitored and documented in a timely fashion.

One vital signs monitor, the Press-Mate shown in Figure 1–6, is well suited to the PACU because the microprocessor is "smart" enough to look for defined, valid, and credible pulse readings over a brief time span. If readings are not credible and present due to hypothermia, hypovolemia, or increased perfusion, the processor looks a little harder to find valid pulses or oscillations so it can take a proper blood pressure measurement. As a result, changes in physiology violate alarms; subtle patient movement does not. And, if the patient moves significantly or the alarms are indeed violated, the printer produces an oscillometric profile, a graphic illustration that demonstrates the following:

● If the oscillometric profile is rounded and bell shaped, the reading is good, and one can act on the information provided without any delay.

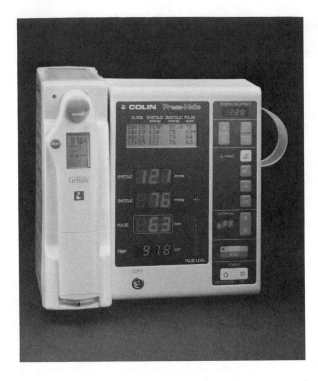

FIGURE 1–6. The Press-Mate noninvasive blood pressure (NIBP) monitor. The first integrated tympanic thermometer, pulse, and NIBP vital sign monitor that prints out all parameters on one record. An RS-232 interface port allows this monitor to transfer data to the hospital's information system. (Courtesy of COLIN MEDICAL INSTRUMENTS CORP., San Antonio, TX.)

• If the oscillometric profile has an irregular shape and part of the bell curve is not present, one can determine the need to take the blood pressure again without question.

Error Messages. Monitors should talk to nurses in their own language, not in numeric codes or acronyms. Monitors that display real English words increase the nurse's confidence, guide the nurse when troubleshooting, save time, and make operation easy for any staff member.

If monitoring is indeed the foundation of patient safety, the primary requirement of any monitor is to provide appropriate information. That means that all the information should be in one place (a central display panel) and available for nursing observation at all times.

Because every PACU nurse makes responsible decisions about when to act on the data displayed by any monitor and when to disregard them, error messages need to be immediately recognizable and simply defined.

Disabling Alarms. Sometimes nurses need silence to sort out what is going on. But nurses have been trapped by silencing an alarm, then forgetting to "rearm" their electronic "observer" to help them look out for the next crisis. Nurses, physicians, hospitals, and lawyers know the value of "alarms attended" and "alarms ignored." Therefore, it is inappropriate to permanently silence alarms in PACU. To minimize nuisance alarms, adjust the alarm setpoints to fit the specific needs of each patient. This effort takes seconds and offers the reward of "adequate warning" when the patient's status abruptly changes.

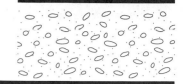

CHAPTER 2

Post Anesthesia Nursing as a Specialty

Donna DeFazio-Quinn, B.S.N., M.B.A., R.N., C.P.A.N.

Recognition of post anesthesia nursing as a critical care specialty has been well established. This past decade has been witness to a number of significant factors that have influenced the practice of post anesthesia nursing. Among these are the emphasis on cost containment in health care, the aging and the increased acuity level of our population, and the impact of human immunodeficiency viral infection.

The emphasis on cost containment has stimulated the regionalization of health care and the development of tertiary care centers in major cities while primary care has increasingly moved to ambulatory settings. As a consequence, post anesthesia nursing is being practiced in a variety of settings, from the physician's office to post anesthesia care centers to highly specialized post anesthesia care units (PACUs) in dedicated medical centers such as eye and heart institutes. At the same time, in an effort to contain costs, many community hospitals have increased the use of the PACU for special procedures such as electroconvulsive therapy (ECT), elective cardioversion, and endoscopic examination. In addition, the PACU is being used for services such as pain clinics, preoperative holding areas (for both inpatients and outpatients), and overflow units when intensive care unit beds are full. Although some of these changes seem to create less than optimal conditions for patient care, it is imperative that all health care practitioners collaborate creatively to meet the challenges of the rapidly changing health care environment. PACUs have the unique opportunity to be innovative and creative in implementing methods to meet these changes.

The increasingly competitive business environment for health care, as well as technologic advances, has significantly increased the use of ambulatory surgical settings. Consequently, the acuity of inpatients has greatly increased. In addition, the increasing age of the population in the United States means many surgical patients are presenting with a number of concomitant chronic problems, such as chronic obstructive lung disease, diabetes mellitus, and chronic heart conditions. The provision of quality care in the PACU requires a strong, knowledgeable leader with excellent skills and a highly skilled nursing staff. In addition to the promotion and support of the nursing staff, attention must be paid to the organizational and operational structure of the unit.

In an effort to define the role of the post anesthesia nurse, the American Society of Post Anesthesia Nurses (ASPAN) has published a formal Scope of Practice document (Table 2–1), which addresses the core, dimensions, boundaries, and intersections of post anesthesia nursing practice.

ORGANIZATIONAL STRUCTURE

One person should be ultimately responsible for the management of the PACU. Typically, this person holds the title of nurse manager, director, supervisor, clinical leader, or head nurse. For the purpose of clarity, we will refer to this person as the *nurse manager*. The nurse manager is responsible for the administrative control of the PACU and may report directly to the surgical or the anesthesia service, depending on the institution's organizational structure.

The medical director of the PACU should be the chief of anesthesiology. In large institutions, if it is not possible for the chief of anesthesiology to fill this role because of other required duties, he or she may appoint a designee to this position. The medical director works closely with the nurse manager to develop policies and procedures and to assist with continuing education activities for the nursing staff. He or she may also be involved in the development and implementation of

Table 2–1. SCOPE OF PRACTICE: POST ANESTHESIA NURSING

The American Society of Post Anesthesia Nurses (ASPAN), the professional organization for the specialty of post anesthesia nursing, is responsible for defining and establishing the scope of post anesthesia nursing. In doing so, ASPAN recognizes the role of the American Nurses Association (ANA) in defining the scope of practice for the nursing profession as a whole.

ASPAN supports the ANA Social Policy Statement. This statement charges specialty nursing organizations with defining their individual scope of practice and identifying the characteristics within their unique specialty area.

ASPAN's Scope of Practice document uses the same framework as the ANA's Social Policy Statement: core, dimensions, boundaries, and intersections.

The *core* of post anesthesia nursing addresses the essence of post anesthesia practice, the environment in which it occurs, and the consumers.

The *dimensions* specify those roles, behaviors, and processes inherent in post anesthesia practice and identify those characteristics unique to the specialty.

The *boundaries* of post anesthesia nursing are described as both internal and external limits with sufficient flexibility and resilience to change in response to societal needs and demands.

The *intersections* describe the interface of post anesthesia nursing with other professional groups for the improvement of health care. Post anesthesia nursing is distinguished at the intersections by its unique knowledge, environment, and focus.

During the last decade, evolving professional and societal demands have necessitated a statement clarifying the scope of post anesthesia nursing practice. Given rapid changes in health care delivery trends and technologies, the task of defining this scope is complex. This document allows for flexibility in response to emerging issues and technologies in health care delivery and the practice of post anesthesia nursing.

CORE

The Scope of Post Anesthesia Nursing Practice involves the assessment, diagnosis, treatment, and evaluation of perceived, actual, or potential physical or psychosocial problems that may result from the intrusion of anesthetic agents and techniques.

The environment includes but is not limited to

- PACUs
- Ambulatory care settings
- Special procedures (cardioversion, ECT, radiology, etc.)
- Dental offices
- Labor and delivery suites

Our unique knowledge base regarding anesthetic agents and techniques, the physiologic and psychological bodily responses to these intrusions, vulnerability of patients subjected to anesthesia, and medical interventions requiring anesthesia is coupled with all the principles of medical-surgical nursing. Basic life-sustaining needs are of the highest priority, and constant vigilance is required because the post anesthesia needs of the patients are neither minimal nor episodic.

DIMENSIONS

Post anesthesia nursing is multidimensional. These dimensions comprise the responsibilities, functions, roles, and skills that involve a specific body of knowledge and are manifested through post anesthesia nursing processes and behaviors.

Characteristics unique to post anesthesia practice are

- *Preanesthesia phase*—The nursing roles focus on preparing patients both physically and emotionally for their experience. Interviewing and assessment techniques are used to identify potential or actual problems that may result.
- *Post anesthesia Phase I*—The nursing roles during this phase focus on providing a transition from a totally anesthetized state to one requiring less acute interventions.
- *Post anesthesia Phase II*—The nursing roles in this phase focus on preparing

Table 2–1. SCOPE OF PRACTICE: POST ANESTHESIA NURSING *Continued*

the patients to care for themselves or to be cared for in an extended care facility.

Nursing roles include those of patient care, research, administration, management, education, consultation, and advocacy. The specialty practice of post anesthesia nursing is defined through the implementation of specific role functions that are delineated in documents such as ASPAN's Core Curriculum for Post Anesthesia Nursing Practice and ASPAN's Standards of Post Anesthesia Nursing Practice.

Post anesthesia nursing practice is systematic in nature and includes nursing process, decision making, analytic and scientific thinking, and inquiry.

Professional behaviors inherent in post anesthesia practice are the acquisition and application of a specialized body of knowledge and skills, accountability and responsibility, communication, autonomy, and collaborative relationships with others. Certification in post anesthesia nursing, as recognized by ASPAN, validates the defined body of knowledge for post anesthesia nursing practice.

BOUNDARIES

The Scope of Post Anesthesia Nursing Practice has both external and internal boundaries. The external boundaries include legislation/regulation, societal demands for expedient quality care, economic climate, and health care delivery trends. Individual state nurse practice acts are examples of legal boundaries used to provide the basis for interpretation of safe nursing practice. Rules and regulations that evolve from these acts are used as guidelines by state boards of nursing to issue licenses and ensure the public safety.

Examples of the legislative/regulatory factors are federal and state health codes, the Joint Commission for Accreditation of Healthcare Organizations, and mandated reporting requirements. Health care delivery trends, such as increased number of ambulatory care centers and patient participation in health maintenance organizations and preferred provider organizations, influence

the demand for post anesthesia services in a variety of settings.

The internal boundaries include those forces that fall within the practice of professional nursing. Specific internal boundaries include ANA guidelines for practice, such as the Social Policy statement or the Code for Nurses, Risk Management guidelines, quality assurance monitoring activities, and institutional and departmental policies and procedures. ASPAN Position Statements and Core Curriculum define boundaries unique to post anesthesia nursing practice.

INTERSECTIONS

ASPAN interacts with a variety of professional organizations for the common purpose of improving health care through education, administration, consultation, and collaboration in practice, research, and policy making. Within these roles, post anesthesia nurses communicate, network, and share resources, information, research, technology, and expertise. This is done to address common concerns such as bioethical issues, humanism, biopsychosocial needs of patients, trends, management of patient care, and alternative care modalities.

ASPAN intersects with other professional groups within the domain of nursing such as the ANA, the National League for Nursing, the American Association of Critical Care Nurses, the American Association of Nurse Anesthetists, and the Association of Operating Room Nurses. ASPAN also maintains an official liaison relationship with the American Society of Anesthesiologists, the American College of Surgeons, and the National Federation of Specialty Nursing Organizations. Intersection is not limited to these groups, however, and may occur with any group as appropriate.

These health care professions interact with a common overall mission: the unique knowledge, environment, and focus that post anesthesia nursing uses to influence the process and outcomes at these intersections.

The intent of this document is to conceptualize practice and provide education to practitioners, educators, researchers, and administrators, and to inform other health

Table continued on following page

Table 2–1. SCOPE OF PRACTICE: POST ANESTHESIA NURSING *Continued*

professionals, legislators, and the public about the participation in and contribution to health care by post anesthesia nursing. Through articulation of the elements of care, dimensions, boundaries, and intersections, the Post Anesthesia Nursing Scope of Practice documents define the specialty practice of post anesthesia nursing.

References

American Nurses' Association: Code for Nurses with Interpretive Statements. Kansas City, MO, ANA, 1985.
American Nurses' Association: Nursing: A Social Policy Statement. ANA Publication No. NP-63 20 M. Kansas City, MO, ANA Publishing, 1980.

continuous quality improvement activities in the unit. It is essential that the PACU nurse manager and the medical director of the unit maintain a good working relationship. In this manner, areas of concern can be addressed in a collaborative, productive fashion.

STAFFING

Nurse Manager

The nurse manager of the PACU is responsible for planning, organizing, implementing, and evaluating the activities of both the nursing staff and the patient care functions. In addition, he or she is responsible for staff scheduling, assignments, performance evaluation, counseling, and hiring and firing; educational program coordination (including the development and implementation of a unit-specific orientation program); and the unit budget formulation and monitoring. The nurse manager is also responsible for developing and implementing both standards of care and the unit's quality improvement program. He or she maintains responsibility for evaluating and monitoring the effectiveness of the quality improvement program as well.

The PACU nurse manager needs to possess skills in time management, decision making, organization, financial management, communication, interpersonal relations, and conflict resolution. In addition, he or she should have the ability to negotiate and collaborate with other departments and health care team members. The nurse manager should also project a positive nursing image.

The nurse manager of the PACU should have a strong medical-surgical and post anesthesia background, preferably with critical care experience. He or she should also have previous management experience. The nurse man-

ager should have, at minimum, a baccalaureate degree in nursing and, preferably, a master's degree in nursing or another health-related field, with emphasis on administration and business. A minimum of 5 years of experience in acute care nursing, with at least two of those years being in the PACU, is desirable. The nurse manager should also be certified in post anesthesia nursing (CPAN) and be actively involved in ASPAN to ensure that the unit is informed about the latest professional developments.

Selection of Nurses

The most important ingredient in a successful PACU is a well-educated, highly skilled, flexible nursing staff. The registered nurse must have not only a solid background in physiology, pathophysiology, and surgical procedures but also an understanding of medicine, pediatrics, geriatrics, and critical care. In addition, nurses must be thoroughly familiar with the pharmacodynamics of anesthesia and analgesia.

Selection of nursing personnel for the PACU is of the utmost importance. Qualifications for PACU nursing personnel should be established by the nurse manager in conjunction with the clinical specialist. These qualifications should be written and used in all employment proceedings. This practice tends to preclude, or at least minimize, subsequent problems such as job dissatisfaction, unsatisfactory work performance, and staff turnover. It also helps ensure a smoothly functioning PACU.

The following characteristics should be considered in establishing selection criteria. The nurse considering employment in the PACU should have an interest in post anesthesia nursing. He or she should be committed to providing high-quality, individualized patient care.

The nurse should have the ability to form good working relationships with all members of the health care team as well as to be a positive team player. The PACU nurse should be capable of making intelligent, independent decisions and initiating appropriate action as necessary. He or she should be willing to accept the responsibility that accompanies working in a critical care unit. The ability to be flexible is of the utmost importance for nurses working in the PACU.

The nurse seeking employment in the PACU should also express an interest in and ability to learn the scientific principles and theory underlying patient care, as well as the technologic aspects of post anesthesia nursing. The person should be in good health, dependable, and motivated and should express an intention to stay at least 1 year in the PACU after completing the unit orientation. The orientation and training of a PACU nurse requires significant time, energy, and money. Temporary assignment to the PACU is not worthwhile, except as a student learning experience.

There are some professional qualifications for the nurse manager to consider when hiring for the PACU. It is recommended that the candidate be baccalaureate prepared. At least 1 year of general medical-surgical nursing is required, and critical care experience is suggested. The ability to coordinate care being rendered by a variety of health team members is a necessary skill, and the ability to function effectively in a crisis situation is essential.

Certification in basic cardiac life support (BCLS) and advanced cardiac life support (ACLS) should be required of all nurses working in the PACU. Application of BCLS in the PACU or ambulatory surgical unit helps sustain a patient in crisis until ACLS techniques can be instituted. ACLS includes training in arrhythmia recognition, intravenous infusion, blood gas interpretation, defibrillation, intubation, and emergency drug administration. If the PACU nurse responds quickly and efficiently during crisis situations, the patient's chances of survival increase.

Certification by one of the professional nursing associations (Table 2–2) demonstrates commitment to professional excellence and should be considered positively when selecting PACU nurses. Ideally, candidates for PACU positions who have attained a CPAN credential should be given preference when hiring is done. Commitments to other professional nursing organizations should also help the candidate to be considered for a PACU position.

Table 2–2. CERTIFICATION BY PROFESSIONAL NURSING ASSOCIATIONS

Professional Association	Credential
American Nurses Association	Medical-surgical certification
American Association of Critical Care Nurses	CCRN
American Society of Post Anesthesia Nurses	CPAN
Association of Operating Room Nurses	CNOR
Emergency Nurses Association	CEN

Nursing Personnel

Assignment of nursing personnel to the PACU should be permanent, and staff members should not be routinely rotated to other units. At least one registered professional nurse should be assigned for every 2.5 beds. Higher nurse-to-patient ratios are necessary for units that consistently deal with critical patients, such as those who have undergone open heart, thoracic, neurologic, and multiple trauma procedures. Optimal patient care is the goal of the unit. To accomplish this, continuous professional nursing judgment is required. Therefore, ideally, only registered professional nurses should be assigned patient care. Minimal numbers of ancillary personnel should be assigned to the unit to support the registered nurses.

Each PACU should have a registered nurse functioning in the position of clinical nurse specialist (CNS). This person may hold a title such as clinical leader, education coordinator, clinical expert, or preceptor. The CNS's role encompasses many spectra, including education, direct patient care, quality improvement, research, and consultation.

The role of education is filled by providing or arranging for continuing education of all PACU nursing staff. Support for continuing education activities increases satisfaction within the work environment, promotes stability of staff and, in turn, decreases turnover in the PACU. PACU nurses take pride in their competence to deliver safe patient care. Opportunities to broaden and expand the PACU nurse's knowledge base should be fostered.

Direct patient care is provided by working individually with staff members to ensure the necessary training, support, and guidance that will eventually enable the nurse to function in an efficient and competent manner. This process allows for consistent teaching and evaluation on an individual level. In addition, the CNS becomes involved in ensuring the clinical competencies of each PACU nurse as required by the Joint Commission on Accreditation of Healthcare Organizations.

The CNS role should include involvement in quality improvement activities of the PACU. The CNS can play an important part in development of an effective monitoring and evaluation program. He or she is instrumental in implementing corrective action to improve deficiencies.

Research activities should be ongoing in the PACU. Research can serve to strengthen the identity of post anesthesia nursing as a specialty. The CNS can be invaluable in assisting staff members to develop and implement a research project.

The CNS is also the resource person for clinical problem solving and dissemination of information of an advanced nature. In addition, the CNS can ensure that standards of practice are being implemented consistently throughout the organization. As a liaison, the CNS can work closely with units outside the PACU that are involved in recovering patients. These areas would include labor and delivery, endoscopic, or special procedure units.

The role of the CNS is an important one. Through skill and expertise, the CNS can offer support and encouragement to staff members, thereby promoting satisfaction and teamwork in the PACU. These factors ultimately lead to continued individual and professional growth among team members.

Licensed practical or vocational nurses (LPNs or LVNs) assigned to the PACU are restricted in their role. It is necessary that a registered nurse be the primary nursing care provider in the PACU, thereby limiting the role of the practical nurse in the PACU setting to one that does not allow the person to function to his or her fullest capacity. It is therefore recommended that practical nurses not be employed in the PACU. If the unit does have LPNs or LVNs, one role they could fill would be to assist in the transport of patients from the PACU to the nursing unit. Orderlies and nurse's aides could be assigned to the unit to perform technical tasks that would be helpful to the nurse. These include tasks such as restocking supplies, assisting with transfer of patients, and running errands to the laboratory, central supply, or other locations.

A skilled secretary-clerk is a definite asset to the PACU. A person adept at handling and redirecting the numerous phone calls to the PACU and proficient in clerical duties makes the job of the PACU nurse much easier. The proficient secretary can assist the unit by being the liaison to family members. Providing frequent updates on the status of the patient helps reassure family members that the surgery is progressing as planned.

Staffing Patterns

Ideally, staffing patterns are developed based on the acuity of the patients cared for in the PACU. A number of patient classification systems have been proposed for use in the PACU that may be used to develop an acuity-based staffing system. The reader is referred to reference 27 at the end of this chapter for additional information regarding patient acuity in the PACU.

The staffing pattern developed for the PACU must include consideration for the length of patient stay, the type of surgical procedures performed, the type of anesthesia administered, and the patient population served. In addition, the skill level of the staff must be considered. According to the 1992 ASPAN Standards of Post Anesthesia Nursing Practice (see reference 28 at end of chapter), two licensed nurses, one of whom is a registered nurse, should be present whenever a patient is recovered in a Phase I or II unit. Institutions unable to meet this ASPAN standard must have a policy outlining the manner in which services are provided in their PACU and delineating how direct access to emergency assistance is accomplished. Other creative means to meet this standard include recovering the patient in an area where additional staff are present, such as the intensive care unit, or assigning the operating room staff nurse to remain available during the recovery process.

BASIC STAFF ORIENTATION PROGRAM

The orientation program for the PACU should be designed to specifically meet the needs of the nurse working in the PACU. The program should include formal lectures and discussions as well as informal demonstrations and supervised practice. Each nurse being oriented to the PACU should have an individually assigned preceptor. The preceptor works closely with the orientee to ensure that the person's needs are met and deficiencies are promptly addressed. In addition, anesthesiologists, surgeons, the CNS, and other nurses in the PACU should be involved in the orientation program. Lectures should be geared toward the specific needs of the orientee.

The orientation program should be structured to include objectives, content, and resources. It should also include the method used to evaluate the orientee's progress. The orientee should be provided with materials that clearly delineate the structure of the orientation program. There should be no question in anyone's mind as to what is expected of the orientee.

Objectives should be clearly stated, and methods for evaluating the achievement of the objectives should be clearly outlined. A notebook containing the objectives, resources, evaluation forms, pertinent PACU policies and procedures, and other valuable resources should be given to each orientee. The notebook should be carefully reviewed with each orientee. A clear understanding of objectives and expectations in the beginning avoids problems in the long term.

Content of the Orientation Program

The content of the PACU orientation program should include at least the following topics. Additional material, as appropriate to the practice setting, should also be included.

I. Review of the anatomy and physiology of the cardiorespiratory system
   A. Pathophysiologic processes of the cardiorespiratory system
   B. Factors altering circulatory or respiratory function following surgery and anesthesia
      1. Position
      2. Type of incision
      3. Medication
      4. Blood loss and replacement; intake and output
      5. Anesthetic agent(s) used
      6. Type of operative procedure
   C. Monitoring techniques
      1. Hemodynamic monitoring
      2. Pulse oximetry
   D. Cardiac dysrhythmias
   E. Airway maintenance, equipment, and techniques
      1. Techniques to maintain a patent airway
      2. Administration of oxygen
      3. Use of suction equipment
   F. Ventilatory support, equipment, and procedures
   G. Cardiorespiratory arrest and its management
      1. Use of monitor-defibrillator
      2. Emergency medications
   H. Treatment of hypotension or hypertension
   I. Interpretation of laboratory values
   J. Identification and treatment of malignant hyperthermia
II. Review of other physiologic considerations in the PACU
   A. Neurologic system
   B. Musculoskeletal system
   C. Genitourinary system
      1. Fluid and electrolyte balance
      2. Fluid and electrolyte imbalance
   D. Gastrointestinal system
   E. Integumentary system
   F. Pediatric-adolescent physiology
   G. Geriatric physiology
   H. Physiology of pregnancy
III. Anesthesia
   A. General concepts
      1. Induction
      2. Emergence
   B. Administration and properties of selected agents (include all agents routinely used in the institution)
      1. Intravenous agents
      2. Muscle relaxants
      3. Conduction anesthesia
      4. Reversal agents
   C. Nursing implications
IV. Care of the PACU patient
   A. Physical assessment of the postoperative patient
   B. General PACU care
      1. Psychological considerations
         a. Anxiety
         b. Coping responses
      2. The stir-up regimen
      3. Intravenous therapy and blood transfusion
      4. Infection control
         a. Universal precautions
         b. Occupational Safety and Health Administration regulations
      5. General comfort and safety measures
   C. Specific care required following surgical procedures
      1. Ear, nose, and throat surgery
      2. Ocular surgery
      3. Cardiothoracic surgery
      4. Neurosurgery
      5. Orthopedic surgery
      6. Genitourinary surgery
      7. Gastrointestinal surgery

8. Gynecologic and obstetric surgery
9. Plastic surgery
10. Vascular surgery
11. Special considerations for the pediatric-adolescent patient
12. Special procedures, such as ECT and pain blocks
  D. Postoperative medications
   1. Pain control medications (intravenous, intramuscular, oral, epidural, patient-controlled analgesia)
   2. Antiemetics
   3. Others (antihypertensives, antiarrhythmics)
  E. Patient teaching
   1. Preprocedure
   2. Postprocedure
  F. Department specifics
   1. Layout
   2. Policies and procedures
   3. Preparation of patient units

The length of the orientation program should be tailored to meet the individual needs and prior experience of the orientees. Consideration should be given to the expectations placed on the orientees. Will they be expected to perform in a "call" situation at the conclusion of the orientation period, or will an experienced PACU nurse be working with them for an indefinite period? It is suggested that the orientation period be at least 3 months for nurses without previous PACU experience. During this time, the orientee should work full time. An experienced PACU nurse should complete a 6-week orientation program before being placed in the position of functioning without special supervision.

Regardless of the orientation period, it is essential that careful communication be maintained among the nurse manager, the orientee, and the preceptor. There should be an ongoing evaluation by the nurse manager and preceptor and a formalized (written) evaluation at the end of the orientation period. The orientee should understand clearly the expectations as set forth by the PACU nurse manager.

DEVELOPMENT OF EXPERTISE

Expertise in nursing involves the overlapping of three basic components of nursing: knowledge, skill, and experience (Fig. 2–1). Mastering any one or two of these components will never equate with expertise. The expert nurse uses a complex linkage of knowledge, experience, skill, clue identification, "gut feel-

ings," logic, and intuition as the problem-solving or the nursing process is worked through. As the nurse gains knowledge and experience through formal and informal programs, nursing intuition begins to develop. Intuition may be thought of as identifying a deviation from the expected, or the feeling that "something just doesn't seem right." Over time, with experience and practice, the nurse will become proficient. The accumulation of knowledge, along with the chance to practice the skills acquired, will lead to competence.

Once the nurse finishes the formal PACU orientation program, he or she should work continuously on improving background theory and skills. This may be accomplished by active participation in on-the-job training, nursing in-service programs presented on the unit, outside reading, membership in ASPAN and other state and local professional nursing organizations, and attendance at both in-house and outside-sponsored seminars and educational offerings. Constant review of basic knowledge and procedures is essential. Keeping abreast of new scientific information and innovations is necessary to ensure quality care. It is essential that the budget for the unit include funds to pay for sending nurses to important educational and information-sharing meetings. An investment made to stimulate the professional development of the nursing staff will be directly reflected in the level of nursing care provided to the patient.

STRESS AND BURNOUT IN THE POST ANESTHESIA NURSE

Stress is a word often too familiar to the PACU nurse. It can be defined as the nonspecific response of the body to any demand, whether it be caused by or results in a pleasant or an unpleasant condition.

The Stress Syndrome

The stress syndrome is, basically, a physiologic response by the endocrine system to external or internal psychological stimuli (stressors). In some ways, stress is purported to have a positive influence on the quality of life, but if it is not controlled, it can become deleterious to a person's health. Hans Selye, a Canadian physiologist, first introduced the concept that in response to various stressors, the adrenal cortex is activated, producing an increase in cortisol secretion. As the body is stressed, the

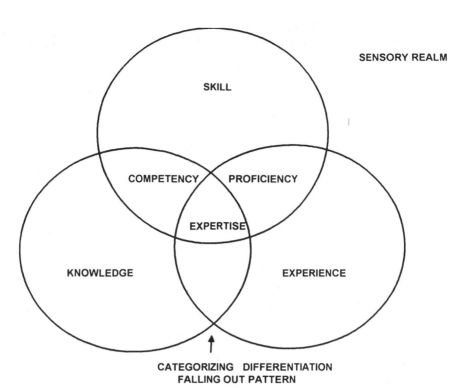

FIGURE 2-1. Model showing development of nursing expertise.

level of secretions from the adrenal cortex become elevated. If the level of stress is not reduced, tissue changes can occur. For a stimulus to produce a stress reaction, harm does not need to occur but need only be anticipated.

Stress can take the form of being either positive or negative, that is, good or bad. The body responds to good or bad stress in essentially the same physiologic manner. The difference between the two responses is the body's ability to relax after encountering the stress. Left untreated, stress can act as a negative force that, in turn, can lead to physical ailments. There are many adaptive methods available to assist people dealing with stress. The real challenge, however, is successfully employing these adaptive measures.

The body's response to stress is an activation of both the pituitary-cortical and the pituitary-medullary axes. When a stressor is applied, the brain determines that the stimulus is a threat to the preservation of the organism, and the hypothalamus is activated. This, in turn, produces corticotropin-releasing hormones that trigger the release of adrenocorticotropic hormone (ACTH) and beta-endorphins. ACTH then activates the adrenal cortex to secrete cortisol and aldosterone. This will influence blood glucose levels, metabolism, blood volume, and the immune system. The beta-endorphins affect mood, learning, and pain perception, whereas the hypothalamic stimulus activates the adrenal medulla, causing it to secrete the catecholamines epinephrine and norepinephrine. The catecholamine stimulation results in physiologic changes that cause an increase in heart rate, blood pressure, and body metabolism. This physiologic and behavioral response is sometimes referred to as the *fight or flight response*. When this response is evoked, the body automatically prepares for the ensuing stressor.

If the person perceives the response as positive, the body returns to its normal state. The heart rate decreases and blood pressure and body metabolism return to normal. If, however, the person perceives the stress as negative, the body is unable to return to a relaxed state. Continued negative stress can lead to physical problems such as hypertension, ulcers, and heart conditions.

Selye's general adaptation syndrome is a three-stage biologic process in response to a stressor. The three stages are alarm reaction, resistance, and exhaustion.

In the first stage, *alarm reaction*, the body makes a biochemical response in an effort to mobilize defensive forces. During the alarm reaction, the body either becomes overwhelmed and dies or enters a second stage called *resistance*.

During resistance, the body continues its biochemical response. If appropriate adjustments are not made, the person can enter the third stage, called *exhaustion.* It is in this third stage that tissue damage can and does occur. Disorders such as migraine headache, colitis, indigestion, insomnia, depression, hypersensitivity reactions, cardiac dysrhythmias and palpitations, and reactive hypoglycemia can occur if the physiologic response to stress is allowed to continue. Over time, continued stress can lead to burnout.

Developing the ability to deal with daily stressors is essential, but before beginning to deal with daily stress, one must first be able to recognize it. Stress can manifest itself differently in each person. Being able to recognize your own individual response to stress is essential. Learning to recognize the individual message your body is sending you is a first step. Do you feel tightness in your chest? heart palpitations? a nervous feeling in your gut? something click in your head? Being able to recognize stress early will be of benefit in the long term. Learning to recognize your body's reaction to stress early is important, because with early detection stress is easier to manage.

Stress in the PACU

Behavioral symptoms of stress are exhibited in a number of ways (Table 2–3). These include behaviors such as temper outbursts, restlessness, impatience, forgetfulness, boredom, mood swings, and difficulty concentrating. When several people in the PACU exhibit symptoms of burnout, the unit will be faced with problems such as low morale, interpersonal conflict, decreased productivity, and lack of teamwork.

In the PACU, burnout may result from the lack of positive feedback received from patients who do not remember the nurse who took care of them. The PACU nurse rarely has the opportunity to see the positive results of care unless postoperative visits are a part of the PACU routine. Positive reinforcement by peers as well as the manager(s) aids in building self-esteem

Table 2–4. CAUSES OF STRESS IN THE PACU

Understaffing	Working overtime
Critical patients	Lack of sleep
Changes in policies	Additional responsibilities

for the PACU nurse. PACU nurses must learn to take care of themselves as well as they care for their patients. We as caregivers must be able to care for ourselves first if we are to remain productive.

PACU nurses are susceptible to burnout because they experience many of the same frustrations as other nurses. In actuality, the incidence of burnout in the PACU is very low. The reasons for this have not been fully explained, but it would seem that the regular hours as well as the social support gleaned from the close relationships developed with the entire surgical team assist in the prevention of burnout.

When stress is a factor, how does one deal with it at work, at home, and in everyday life? The nurse manager plays an important role when dealing with a staff that is overworked, understaffed, and stressed for any number of reasons. The manager must be able to offer support and guidance to nursing staff members so that they will be better able to deal with the numerous stressful situations they face every day.

The manager should reassure staff members that their concerns are legitimate (when they are). Listening to staff concerns with an active ear can also assist the staff nurse to deal with his or her own frustrations. Sometimes, just being able to vent concerns will help the situation. Managers should offer possible solutions to problems.

Stress in the PACU can be caused by a number of factors (Table 2–4). Understaffing, critical patients, changes in policies, working overtime, lack of sleep, and additional responsibilities all contribute to stress. How does the PACU nurse deal with the continuous evolution of change in the workplace? The PACU nurse must first recognize that there is a problem. Once this has been accomplished, there are three possible directions the nurse can take: (1) to totally eliminate the stress, (2) to resist or minimize it, or (3) to accept the stress.

Eliminating the stress sometimes seems like the best way to go. You eliminate the stressor; therefore, you do not have to face the problem. However, total elimination of the stress factor is not always possible. In circumstances in

Table 2–3. BEHAVIORAL SYMPTOMS OF STRESS

Temper outbursts	Boredom
Restlessness	Mood swings
Impatience	Difficulty concentrating
Forgetfulness	

which the stress can be totally removed, you may be faced with undesirable consequences as a result of the elimination. For example, if working with a certain physician causes you a great deal of stress, it may be possible for you to switch assignments with another PACU nurse. The two of you may be able to come to an agreement that you will care for all of Dr. X's patients if he or she cares for all of Dr. Y's. You alone must weigh the consequences of always caring for Dr. X's patients. On the other hand, if the consequence is of no concern to you, then eliminating the stressor through this option is the way to achieve your ultimate goal of avoiding Dr. Y.

The second approach is to minimize the stress element. Is there some way of reducing the stress factor so that its effect on you becomes minimal? Does accepting the responsibility to preceptor yet another staff nurse push you over the edge? It may be that you are already in the process of orienting two new staff members. As much as you enjoy this, you may have to decline. The level of energy required to be a preceptor is high. In this instance, refusing the assignment may be the alternative to choose. When making choices that ultimately affect your well-being, guilt should not be the deciding factor. Nurses tend to feel guilty when they make unpopular decisions. Overcoming the feeling of guilt is essential if true acceptance of the decision is expected.

Another part of reducing stress is to set priorities. Being able to look at your current responsibilities and honestly assess what is important to accomplish at this particular time is a necessary step in reducing stress. Whenever possible, avoid procrastinating about tasks that you dislike but must be completed. Sometimes, getting the "dislikes" out of the way first will allow you to thoroughly enjoy the work that remains.

The third approach to dealing with stress is to accept it. Some stress factors cannot be alleviated and must be accepted. These include realities such as divorce, death, or resignation of a favorite peer or manager. Although these events are difficult to manage, accepting them and moving ahead is one way to handle the stress. By managing the stressors that cannot be eliminated, you will be able to achieve the goal of final acceptance.

PACU nurses must take time out to reward themselves and to set aside time for their personal needs. Too often nurses are absorbed in everyday activities and are too quick to give helpful advice to others yet neglect to follow their own advice. Set aside 30 minutes three times a week for exercise. No one says that nurses need to be world-class athletes, but a brisk 30-minute walk three times a week is certainly in order.

Take time to work on your favorite hobby or craft. Engage in an activity you enjoy, such as sports, cross-stitching, or sewing. Set aside some time to read that current best seller you have been saving. Relaxation is an important element necessary to successfully reduce stress. Take time out to enjoy your free time. Do not fill every spare moment with work. It may be that the best way to relax is to just do nothing.

Activities such as bicycling, hiking, and swimming are also ways to reduce stress. When the body is physically fit, it is better able to handle stress. Nurses should also eat well and get plenty of rest. Nutrition plays an important part in maintaining a healthy lifestyle; avoidance of sugar, salt, caffeine, and alcohol is important. Eating well is essential for health maintenance, which, in turn, will assist the body in dealing with stress. Rest is vital for the rejuvenation of body cells.

Managing stress is important for the PACU nurse. Once you have identified the stressors in your life, you need to consciously respond to them. Take a moment to relax and "regroup." Eliminating, minimizing, and accepting the different stressors allow you the opportunity to experience a more productive and enjoyable life.

CONCLUSION

What makes post anesthesia nurses so special? It is our ability to blend expert clinical knowledge that is based on experience, education, and collegial sharing with caring practices that come from within and from being a nurse. It is this special ability to provide the highest level of quality care with the minimal amount of resources that gives PACU nurses pride.

The specialty of post anesthesia nursing is a little more than a decade in age. Post anesthesia nurses have expanded their roles to include all phases of post anesthesia care, from preadmission to discharge. The future will bring even more challenges for our specialty as we face reforms in health care delivery. It is the ability of the PACU nurse to be flexible enough to handle whatever situation he or she is faced with in a competent and efficient manner that will allow the specialty of post anesthesia nursing to survive. The "specialness" of post anesthesia nursing will continue to develop and flourish as each individual nurse strives to gain that special expertise prevalent in PACUs across the country.

References

1. Albrecht, T., and Halsey, J.: Supporting the staff nurse under stress. Nurs. Manage., 22:60–64, 1991.
2. Allen, A. (ed.): Core Curriculum For Post Anesthesia Nursing Practice. 2nd ed. Philadelphia, W. B. Saunders, 1991.
3. Allen, A.: Strategies for surviving stress in the PACU. J Post Anesth. Nurs., 1:85–86, 1986.
4. Barton, A.: Conflict resolution by nurse managers. Nurs. Manage., 22(5):83–86, 1991.
5. Bass, L.: Motivation strategies: A new twist. Nurs. Manage., 22(2):24–26, 1991.
6. Blacharski, C.: Quality improvement in nursing: Implementation of a comprehensive program using cost-effective automation. Milit. Med., 156:666–670, 1991.
7. Cornwall, S.: Opting out of burn-out. Nurs. Times, 87(20):34–35, 1991.
8. Cramer, C.: Primary nursing in post anesthesia practice. J Post Anesth. Nurs., 1:121–126, 1986.
9. Evans, S.: Critical care nursing: The ordinary is extraordinary. Heart Lung, 20:21A–32A, 1991.
10. Frost, E. (ed.): Post Anesthesia Care Unit. 2nd ed. St. Louis, C. V. Mosby, 1990.
11. Grainger, R.: Managing stress. Am. J. Nurs., 91:15–16, 1991.
12. Hildman, T.: Daily hassles cause burnout. J. Nurs. Admin., 21(9):44-A5, 1991.
13. Kramer, M., and Schmalenberg, C.: Job satisfaction and retention. Nursing 91, 21:51–55, 1991.
14. Litwack, K.: Career development for the PACU Nurse. Curr. Rev. Post Anesth. Care Nurs., 11(8):57–64, 1989.
15. Loveridge, C.: Lessons in excellence for nurse administrators. Nurs. Manage., 22(5):46A7, 1991.
16. Luczun, M.: Stress management techniques for PACU practitioners. Curr. Rev. Post Anesth. Care Nurs., 11(6):43A7, 1989.
17. Muller, P.: Change, conflict and coping. J. Post Anesth. Nurs., 7:54–55, 1992.
18. Muller, P.: Innovation: The nurse manager's critical skill: I. The people process. J. Post Anesth. Nurs., 1:140–143, 1986.
19. Muller, P.: Leadership versus management: A matter of focus. J. Post Anesth. Nurs., 6:361–363, 1991.
20. Muller, P.: Today's manager: Surviving or thriving. J. Post Anesth. Nurs., 4:118–120, 1989.
21. Murray, S.: Patient assessment in the PACU: A critical care approach. J. Post Anesth. Nurs., 4:232–238, 1989.
22. O'Brien, D.: What makes us so special? J. Post Anesth. Nurs., 6:88–89, 1991.
23. Quinn, C., and Quinn, J.: Why post anesthesia nurses like their jobs. J. Post Anesth. Nurs., 2:95–97, 1987.
24. Reynolds, N., and Blatchley, M.: Staffing options in the post anesthesia care unit. J. Post Anesth. Nurs., 1:260–264, 1986.
25. Schneider, M.: Nursing administration of the PACU. J. Post Anesth. Nurs., 3:123–126, 1988.
26. Simon, S.: A self-instructional program on stress management. J. Post Anesth. Nurs., 4:239–246, 1989.
27. Spadaccia, K.: Nursing requirements in the PACU. Curr. Rev. Recovery Room Nurs., 15(8):114–l20, 1986.
28. Standards of Post Anesthesia Nursing Practice—1992. Richmond, American Society of Post Anesthesia Nurses, 1992.
29. Starfield, V.: Perioperative education: Changing to meet short-stay needs. J. Post Anesth. Nurs., 2:74–75, 1987.
30. Trobaugh, M.: Preceptorship: A quality issue in the PACU. J. Post Anesth. Nurs., 5:321–322, 1989.
31. Vaughn, G.: Workaholism: Learning self-care to prevent burnout. AORN J., 26:873–877, 1992.
32. Wigley, E.: Advanced cardiac life support: A PACU perspective. J. Post Anesth. Nurs., 4:228–231, 1989.

CHAPTER 3

Management and Policies

Janet L. Odom, M.S., R.N., C.P.A.N.

All management procedures and policies of the post anesthesia care unit (PACU) should be established through joint efforts of the PACU staff, the nurse manager, and the medical director of the unit. These should be written and readily available to all staff working in the PACU and all physicians who use the area for post anesthesia care of their patients.

Policies are guidelines that give direction and have been approved by the administration of the institution. Procedures specify the way a policy is to be implemented and are either managerial in scope or specific to clinical nursing methods. The PACU policies and procedures should be reviewed periodically so that appropriate changes can be made when necessary. Policies and procedures must always reflect the actual practice of the unit.

Changes in the clinical situation of the hospital and advances in science and technology make revision of policies and procedures a continuous challenge. Some suggested areas that often require a written policy for the PACU are noted in Table 3–1. Policies and procedures must be tailored to meet the individual unit's needs.

PURPOSE OF THE PACU

The PACU is designed and staffed to provide intensive observation and care of patients following a procedure for which an anesthetic agent has been required. Criteria for admission to the PACU should be clearly outlined, and exceptions to the policy should be specifically delineated.

Of special concern, owing to the effects on staffing and utilization of PACU beds, is use of the PACU as a place to perform special procedures or to observe patients who have undergone special procedures, such as cardiac catheterization, arteriography or other specialized radiologic tests, and electroshock therapy. Specific policies and procedures should address any of these special procedures performed in the unit.

Many large hospitals have PACUs in various parts of the hospital, for example, labor and delivery, freestanding ambulatory, and endoscopy units. Other areas such as intensive care units and the radiology and emergency departments frequently administer intravenous conscious sedation and then monitor those patients. Open heart surgical patients are frequently taken to a specific unit for recovery. The most important concern in these instances is that all post anesthesia patients in the hospital receive consistent care. In other words, the post anesthesia care delivered to the patient must meet the same standards in all areas that deliver the care. Management in the Phase I PACU as the expert must take the initiative to see that consistent care is delivered.

STAFF

Nursing staff should consist of registered professional nurses to provide direct patient care (see Chapter 2). Each unit also should have a clinical nurse specialist to provide for orientation and educational needs and to offer expertise in direct care of the patients. The clinical nurse specialist also functions in research and consultative roles. Licensed vocational or practical nurses may be employed in the area to assist the professional nurse, but they must be supervised by a registered nurse at all times. Some units use licensed vocational or practical nurses as members of the transport team.

Student nurses should not be used to staff the PACU. Students are assigned to the PACU primarily to observe. Any patient care delivered by student nurses should be accomplished only under the direct supervision of a permanent staff nurse. No private duty or "float" nurses should be used to staff the PACU.

SHARED GOVERNANCE

Many units are using a participative type of management. It is well documented that nurses want to be treated as professionals and desire autonomy and participation. A concept used by many hospitals to meet these needs is that of shared governance. In this form of management, the PACU nurse assumes more authority and responsibility and shares management skills with peers. The overall structure is that of self-management, with the staff involved in the decision-making processes that affect nursing practice and management.

Committees are set up that address the needs of the unit, the employees, and the patients. Usually, a nursing practice committee is in charge of any decisions about policies and procedures or practice issues; a quality improvement committee is in charge of quality improvement in the unit; and an educational committee is responsible for meeting the educational needs of the unit. Other unit-specific committees that have been used are equipment supply, budget and finance, communications, and statistics.

The nurse manager becomes a facilitator and a resource person for the staff. Most nurse managers retain responsibilities such as employee evaluations, interviews, and liaison with administration or physicians. The challenge for the nurse manager within this system of management is to maintain a vision and impart that vision to the staff.

SELF-SCHEDULING

One option for scheduling of staff is a system that is totally coordinated by the staff nurses. This is another method that recognizes professional nurses as capable of making crucial decisions about their practice. The schedule is developed and implemented by nurses and other staff in the unit. Advantages include decreased amount of time spent by the nurse manager on scheduling, increased team building by the staff, increased job satisfaction and autonomy of the staff, and decreased staff turnover.

PATIENT CLASSIFICATION

Most PACUs have some type of patient classification system (PCS). The most accurate

Table 3–1. SUGGESTED POLICIES AND PROCEDURES FOR THE PACU

Purpose and Structure of the Unit
　Unit philosophy of nursing
　Unit goals and objectives
　Patient population (scope of service)
　Admission and discharge criteria
　Admission and discharge procedures
　Staffing protocols
　Hours of operation

Job Descriptions
　Lines of authority
　Medical director
　Nurse manager
　Clinical nurse specialist
　Staff nurses
　Nursing assistants
　Unit clerk

Nursing Procedures
　All specific procedures
　Protocols
　Emergencies and code situations

Special Procedures, Equipment, and Supplies

Maintenance and Safety
　Electrical safety
　Control of radioactive materials
　Role of biomedical engineers
　Internal disaster plan
　External disaster plan

Infection Control
　Universal precautions
　Respiratory (acid-fast) isolation
　Unit exposure control plan
　OSHA regulations
　Traffic control
　Visitors
　Attire

Laboratory Procedures

Physician's Orders
　Standing orders
　Intravenous medications
　Intravenous fluids
　Blood or blood component transfusions

Staff Education
　Orientation
　Continuing education
　Basic life-support programs and certification
　Advanced life-support programs and certification
　Certification of specialty skills

Quality Improvement
　Unit monitors
　Unit-based continuous quality improvement plan

OSHA = Occupational Safety and Health Administration.

PCSs seem to be those that base the patient classification on length of stay in the PACU and intensity of the care required. The PCS can be used to justify staffing and charges for the PACU stay. For example, a patient with a classification of 1 has a lower charge than a patient with a classification of 3.

Developing a PCS for the PACU is difficult at best. There are many variables that must be considered; for example, the length of stay of each patient varies, the acuity of one patient can change within a short period, and patient populations can range from pediatric to geriatric and from minor to extensive surgical procedures.

There are several PCSs in the literature. One example of a PCS is included in Table 3–2, in which five classes of care are described. Each patient is classified at discharge by the patient's primary nurse during the PACU stay.

Advantages of a PCS include a more accurate assessment of the nursing time and energy required by each patient. This, in turn, allows a manager to estimate staffing requirements based on the next day's schedule. Other advantages may include knowledge of the peak workload each day and patient charges reflecting not only the length of stay but also the intensity of care required. PACU nurses also feel that the type of workload experienced in the PACU is acknowledged and that management is responsive to the staffing needs.

VISITORS

Visiting may be allowed if staffing and the physical structure of the unit permit. Traditionally, family visitation in the PACU has not been allowed. The restrictions have been due to lack of privacy, the acuity of the patients, and the fast turnover that is common to PACU patients. However, nurses are beginning to discuss the value of allowing visitation in the PACU. The catalyst behind the change has been, in part, the extended PACU stays many patients now require. For example, some patients may have a prolonged stay in the PACU while waiting for critical care or telemetry beds. As the incidence of morning admissions increases, the incidence of extended PACU

Table 3–2. POST ANESTHESIA CARE UNIT CLASSIFICATION SYSTEM

Class	Description
I: one nurse to four patients	Patient who has had either local or no anesthetic requiring minimal observation
II: one nurse to three patients	No airway Vital signs every 15 min Continuous assessment of patient and monitoring of dressing intravenous monitoring Outpatient discharge teaching
III: one nurse to two patients	All of class II (exception: outpatient discharge teaching if patient is an inpatient) and one or more of the following: Vital signs every 15 min Neurologic signs assessment Drainage tube monitoring Spinal anesthesia without complication Administration of medications Laboratory studies and calling physician with results Blood administration only Dressing change
IV: one nurse to one patient	Requires high-level nursing involvement; includes more frequent or intensive class III activities Child younger than 12 years of age Management of airway Administration of blood and blood products Treatment of hypotension or hypertension Frequent medication administration Frequent assessment
V: two or more nurses for a period	Requires intense critical care nursing involvement Ventilator-assisted patient Invasive pressure monitoring Arterial blood gas determinations Management of complication: bleeding, shock, respiratory complications, complications requiring return to surgery Combative, confused, and/or restlessness requiring more than one nurse

Courtesy of Forrest General Hospital, Hattiesburg, MS.

stays also increases owing to lack of bed availability postoperatively. In some hospitals, the PACU is used to help with emergency department overflow.

The nursing care in the PACU has historically concentrated on the patient. However, family members also require nursing interventions. Because of this need, many PACUs are adapting critical care unit visiting policies, which may include a 5-minute visit each hour (or a 20-minute visit every 4 hours). Other criteria may include a limit of two family members at one time and visitation changes if warranted by the unit needs or patient condition. Privacy of other PACU patients must also be a priority.

Other situations in which visitation may be permitted include the following:

1. Death of the patient may be imminent.
2. The patient must return to surgery.
3. The patient is a child whose physical and emotional well-being may depend on the calming effect of the parent's presence.
4. The patient's well-being depends on the presence of a significant other. Patients in this category include the mentally retarded, the mentally ill, or persons with profound sensory deficits.
5. The patient requires a translator owing to language differences.

PATIENT RECORDS

A post anesthesia record should be kept on every patient admitted to the PACU. An example of a post anesthesia record is shown in Figures 3–1 and 3–2. The format may be modified to meet the needs dictated by specific procedures. Anecdotal notes should detail admission observations. The assessment, planning, and implementation phases of the nursing process should be documented as well as an evaluation of how the patient responded to the care provided. A discharge summary should also be included.

Patient records in some institutions are fully computerized. The computerized record may begin in the preoperative phase and follow the patient to the PACU. One advantage of a computerized patient record is that it is a valuable time-saver for nurses. Disadvantages may include the cost of installation and education and the time required to orient the staff to the system.

DISCHARGE OF THE PATIENT FROM THE PACU

Written criteria for discharge of the patient from the PACU must be available and should include (1) when the patient has regained consciousness and is oriented to time and place (provided he or she was oriented to time and place preoperatively); (2) when the airway is clear and the danger of vomiting and aspiration is past; and (3) when circulatory and respiratory vital signs are stabilized. Criteria for discharge of a patient from the PACU vary depending on the type of unit or the location to which the patient will be going from the PACU, the anesthetic technique used, and the physiologic status of the patient. Ultimately, the physician is in charge of the patient's discharge from the PACU. Predetermined criteria can be applied if the criteria have been approved by the physician staff.

Use of a numeric scoring system that assesses the patient's recovery from anesthesia is common. Many institutions have incorporated the post anesthesia recovery score as criteria for discharge (Table 3–3). This scoring system was introduced by Aldrete and Kroulik in 1970. The policy of the unit determines the appropriate score for discharge from the PACU. In most institutions, a patient with a score lower than 8 would require an evaluation by the anesthesia provider and surgeon and possible disposition to a special care or critical care unit. A maximum score of 10 would indicate that the patient is in optimal condition to return to the nursing unit or to be discharged to home.

Color is probably the most difficult entity to assess with any reliability, and some PACUs have elected to delete this parameter from the score or to substitute a pulse oximetry reading for the score. Currently, there is a lack of research to substantiate the substitution of a pulse oximetry reading for color or the use of a numeric scoring system as the only criterion in the discharge of the patient. Clinical assessment must also be used in determining a patient's readiness for discharge from the PACU. This scoring system does not include detailed observations such as urinary output, bleeding or other drainage, changing requirements for hemodynamic support, low arterial oxygen saturation levels, and temperature trends that should be considered when determining readiness for discharge.

No specific time required for the PACU stay can be stated, because patient conditions vary

FORREST GENERAL HOSPITAL
POST ANESTHESIA CARE UNIT RECORD

POST ANESTHESIA RECOVERY SCORE	MINUTES				
	in	30	60	90	out
Activity					
Able to move 4 extremities voluntarily or on command = 2					
Able to move 2 extremities voluntarily or on command = 1					
Able to move 0 extremities voluntarily or on command = 0					
Respiration					
Able to deep breath and cough freely = 2					
Dyspnea or limited breathing = 1					
Apneic = 0					
Circulation					
BP ± 20 of Preanesthetic level = 2					
BP ± 20-50 of Preanesthetic level = 1					
BP ± 50 of Preanesthetic level = 0					
Consciousness					
Fully Awake = 2					
Arousable on calling = 1					
Not Responding = 0					
Color					
Pink Normal = 2					
Pale Dusky Blotchy Jaundiced Other = 1					
Cyanosis = 0					
TOTAL					

Pre-op B.P. _____

Allergies:

Airway: On Adm.

Jawthrust _____

Chin Hold _____

Endotracheal _____

Oral Airway _____

Mask Oxygen _____

Nasal Oxygen _____

Trach _____

T-Tube _____

Nasal Airway _____

Ventilator Settings _____

Addressograph

Time In _____ Time Out _____

Accompanied by _____

Type of anesthesia _____

Surgical Procedure:

PULSE - RESPIRATION - BLOOD PRESSURE

240 220 200 180 160 140 120 100 80 60 40 20

O₂ Sat.
CVP

CODES: ⊥ A-line T B.P.   V Manual or ∧ NBP   Pulse • Resp. o   Siderails: Yes No   Restraints: Yes No

A-LINE _____

INTAKE

I.V. Running _____
Total
I.V. in Surgery _____

BLood in Surgery _____

BLood in PACU _____

TOTAL IV FLUIDS
Given in PACU _____

RN Signature _____

Foley Cath. _____
Supra pubic _____
Ureteral _____

OUTPUT
Urinary
In OR _____
Urinary
In PACU _____

Voided _____
Total _____

Levine _____

Hemovac:

Drains:

MEDICATIONS AND TREATMENTS

	AMT.	ROUTE	TIME
Demerol			
Morphine			
Phenergan			
Droperidol			

FIGURE 3–1. Post anesthesia care record, page 1. (Courtesy of Forrest General Hospital, Hattiesburg, MS.)

with surgical procedure, anesthesia used, use of analgesics, and patient response. Professional judgment is required to determine when the patient is ready for discharge from the PACU. A complete, accurate report from the PACU nurse to the nurse who will be responsible for the care of the patient is required.

When ambulatory surgical patients are dis-

DATE	TIME	DESCRIPTIVE NOTES (Sign Each Entry)	DATE	TIME	DESCRIPTIVE NOTES (Sign Each Entry)

DIAGNOSIS (Circle number of any diagnosis made)	GOAL	Goal Achieved YES	NO
1 Alteration in neurological status			
2 Alteration in comfort level			
3 Alteration in emotional status			
4 Alteration in circulation			
5 Alteration in fluid volume			
6 Alteration in mobility			
7 Alteration in respiratory function			
8 Alteration in skin integrity			
9 Alteration in temperature			
10 Alteration in elimination			
11 Alteration in gastrointestinal function			
12 Potential for injury			
13 Potential for bleeding			
14 Other			

FGH ·215003

STANDARD OFFICE SUPPLY - HATTIESBURG

FIGURE 3–2. Post anesthesia care record, page 2. (Courtesy of Forrest General Hospital, Hattiesburg, MS.)

charged to home, other criteria should be assessed. These criteria may include the following:

Control of pain is acceptable to the patient.
Nausea is controlled.
Patient is tolerating oral fluids.
Patient is ambulating in a manner consistent with the procedure and previous ability.

A responsible adult is present to accompany the patient.

Some PACUs require the patient to void before discharge to home. Home care instructions should have been written and taught to the patient and responsible adult, both of whom have verbalized an understanding of the in-

Table 3–3. POST ANESTHESIA RECOVERY SCORE (PARS)

Activity
0 = Unable to lift head or move extremities voluntarily or on command
1 = Moves two extremities voluntarily or on command and can lift head
2 = Able to move four extremities voluntarily or on command. Can lift head and has controlled movement. *Exceptions:* patients with a prolonged IV block such as bupivacaine (Marcaine) may not move an affected extremity for as long as 18 hours; patients who were immobile preoperatively

Respiration
0 = Apneic; condition necessitates ventilator or assisted respiration
1 = Labored or limited respirations. Breathes by self but has shallow, slow respirations. May have an oral airway
2 = Can take a deep breath and cough well; has normal respiratory rate and depth

Circulation
0 = Has abnormally high or low blood pressure: BP 50 mm Hg of preanesthetic level
1 = BP 20–50 mm Hg of preanesthetic level
2 = Stable BP and pulse. BP 20 mm Hg of preanesthetic level (minimum 90 mm Hg systolic). *Exception:* Patient may be released by anesthesia provider after drug therapy

Neurologic Status
0 = Not responding or responding only to painful stimuli
1 = Responds to verbal stimuli but drifts off to sleep easily
2 = Awake and alert; oriented to time, place, and person. *Note:* After ketamine anesthesia, the patient must have no nystagmus when released

Color
0 = Cyanotic, dusky
1 = Pale, blotchy
2 = Pink

IV = intravenous; BP = blood pressure.
Modified from Aldrete, J., and Kroulik, D.: A post anesthestic recovery score. Anesth. Analg., *49*:924–933, 1970.

structions. Emergency and routine phone numbers should be included with the instructions.

Patients should receive a follow-up visit by the anesthesia provider and be released as appropriate. In instances in which the nursing staff of the PACU is appropriately educated, a policy may be in effect that defines discharge criteria and allows the nurse to discharge the patient. Discharge criteria should be developed that meet appropriate standards but are individualized to each PACU.

STANDARDS OF CARE

Standards of post anesthesia nursing practice have been published and are available from the American Society of Post Anesthesia Nurses (ASPAN) (see Appendix). These standards have been devised to stand alone or to be used in conjunction with other health care standards, and they provide a basic framework for nurses practicing in all phases of post anesthesia care. A copy of these standards may be obtained by writing the ASPAN National Office, 11512 Allecingie Parkway, Richmond, Virginia 23235.

All preanesthesia, post anesthesia, and ambulatory surgical nurses should be familiar with these standards of practice, and a copy should be available on each unit. The PACU may develop its own standards specific to the hospital using the ASPAN standards as a reference or may adopt the ASPAN standards for use. If the ASPAN standards are adopted by the PACU, they must be adopted in their entirety or a policy has to be added noting any exceptions. Whenever standards are written, they have to be attainable and must reflect the actual practice delivered.

Nurses must possess a minimum standard of knowledge and ability. Standards are objective and are the same for all persons. This is the reason that an inexperienced nurse in the PACU will be held to the same standard as an experienced nurse. Standards are commonly used today in legal proceedings to measure the care a patient received. The ASPAN standards have already been used in court proceedings, and many medical malpractice attorneys have a copy of the ASPAN *Standards of Post Anesthesia Nursing Practice* in their libraries.

INFECTION CONTROL

Infection control has always been of importance in the perioperative process. It is even more significant now with the advent of multidrug-resistant tuberculosis (MDR-TB), the human immunodeficiency virus (HIV), and continued concerns with the hepatitis B (HBV) and hepatitis C viruses (HCV).

Tuberculosis

TB is a communicable disease spread through droplets of bacteria in the air released when an infected person coughs, sneezes, or expectorates. TB has been about 98 percent curable since the 1950s owing to drug therapy. TB rates, however, have risen steadily since 1984, largely related to the HIV outbreak. Once infected with TB, HIV-infected persons quickly progress to an active state of the disease.

A newer and deadlier form of MDR-TB has become more common. This form of TB does not respond to the traditional treatments that are available. MDR-TB developed initially in patients who were noncompliant in taking their medication. It has in turn spread to non-infected persons.

The Centers for Disease Control and Prevention (CDC) has recommended the following to health care settings:

1. Early identification and preventive treatment for those who have active TB and are at high risk for active TB.
2. Ventilation in the facility should be considered and designed so that air flows from clean areas to less clean areas.
3. Supplemental approaches can include high-efficiency filtration, germicidal ultraviolet irradiation, and disposable particulate respirators (PRs) to be worn by those caring for patients suspected of having TB. These PRs should also be worn by those performing procedures that are likely to produce bursts of droplet nuclei, such as bronchoscopy and endotracheal suctioning.
4. Any patient suspected or known to have active TB should be placed in respiratory isolation in a private room.

Blood-Borne Diseases

The CDC has documented 32 cases of HIV transmitted in the work setting to health care workers, including 12 nurses. HBV is transmitted more easily: more than 8000 health care workers contract HBV each year, and more than 200 die. The Occupational Health and Safety Administration (OSHA) mandates that employers offer health care workers HBV vaccine free of charge. HCV, which is associated with a high risk for chronic liver disease, is a growing threat to nurses. No vaccine is currently available.

Prevention is the key to control of the blood-borne pathogens. Prevention of transmission includes three important elements: universal precautions, protective barriers, and sharps management.

In 1987, the CDC recommended that universal precautions be applied to all patients. With *universal precautions,* blood and certain body fluids are considered potentially infectious for HIV, HBV, and other blood-borne pathogens. The *protective gear* used depends on the type of patient contact or procedure. Gloves are worn anytime it is anticipated that exposure to blood or body fluids will occur. Gloves should be changed and hands washed after each patient contact. If the procedure is likely to produce droplets or splashes of body fluid, appropriate gear would include gowns or aprons and protective eye wear and mask or face shield. Mouthpieces or artificial ventilation devices should be used instead of mouth-to-mouth resuscitation. *Used needles* should not be bent, broken, or otherwise manipulated. Needles are recapped only if necessary (e.g., for incremental doses of intravenous narcotics in the PACU), and a one-handed method is used to resheathe the needle. New needle designs are being developed, and the use of improved safety features is increasing. Used needles and syringes should be placed in a puncture-resistant container immediately after use.

If an exposure occurs, there are several steps that should be taken. The first step should be to decontaminate immediately with soap and water for the skin or a rinse with saline or water for the eyes, nose, or mouth. The exposure should then be reported as soon as the area is disinfected. A baseline HIV test is recommended, with a follow-up at 6 weeks, 12 weeks, and 6 months as well as frequent physical examinations when possible. A prophylaxis for HIV, such as zidovudine (AZT), should be considered and ongoing counseling support used.

OSHA: Final Rule

OSHA released guidelines regulating occupational exposure to blood-borne pathogens on December 6, 1991. See Table 3–4 for a list of OSHA requirements that should be addressed by PACU policies.

Table 3–4. SUGGESTED PACU POLICIES BASED ON OSHA REQUIREMENTS
Exposure control plan
Engineering and work practice controls
Handling of specimen and blood containers
Biohazard labeling
Needle use and disposal
Personal protective equipment
Housekeeping
Hepatitis B vaccination
Postexposure evaluation and follow-up
Employee training

OSHA = Occupational Safety and Health Administration.

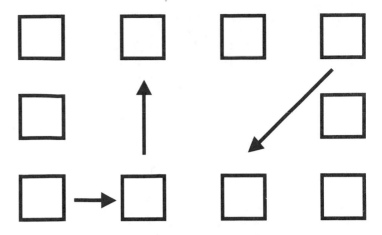

FIGURE 3-3. Quality improvement demarcated intermittent interaction model. (From Moran M., and Johnson, J.: Quality improvement: The nurse's role. In Dienemann, J. [ed]: Continuous Quality Improvement in Nursing. Washington, DC, American Nurses Publishing, 1992.)

QUALITY IMPROVEMENT

Each PACU should have a planned quality improvement program. Quality improvement programs differ from the quality assurance (QA) programs of the past in that the emphasis on inspection has changed to an emphasis on continuous improvement. Continuous quality improvement (CQI) is based on overall improvement of the system and includes the consumer in that process. A consumer is any person who uses output at any point in the system. Examples include the patient receiving care in the PACU or the PACU nurse who receives supplies from a central materials supply location.

The Joint Commission on Accreditation of Healthcare Organizations has established standards that focus on the role of the nursing staff in quality improvement. Every nurse is responsible for CQI. The result is that effective CQI will have a positive impact on the process and outcome of care. Patient care problems can be prevented, or basic operating procedures or systems can be changed and improved.

One of the aspects of CQI is interdisciplinary participation in these activities. The common focus is on quality patient care or service. Departmental boundaries fade with a common focus on the patient. Figure 3-3 illustrates the way that QA was practiced in the past. Each department had its own QA plan developed with occasional interdepartmental and interdisciplinary participation. Figure 3-4 represents CQI as it must be practiced now, with no boundaries between departments and disciplines. The focus is on improved patient care.

CQI incorporates and uses QA but broadens its scope. Monitoring and evaluation are still a part of the process. Expansions include the role of leadership in improving quality, the scope of assessment from strictly clinical to other systems and processes that affect patients, and the focus on the processes, and not performance, of individual staff members.

Forrest General Hospital in Hattiesburg, Mississippi, formed an ad hoc task force (known as the quality improvement team) to study the consistency of care for the PACU patient. This team crossed departmental lines and had a representative from every area in the hospital caring for any type of PACU patient, from intravenous conscious sedation to general anesthesia. Standards, policies and procedures, and CQI activities in all departments were studied. The outcome was consistent post anesthesia care for all patients throughout the hospital. Evaluation is in progress, with results to be monitored.

Other examples of CQI studies might include reducing the time it takes for the pharmacy to

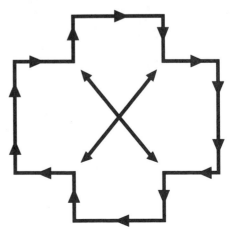

FIGURE 3-4. Quality improvement seamless continuous interaction model. (From Moran, M., and Johnson, J.: Quality improvement: The nurse's role. In Dienemann, J. [ed]: Continuous Quality Improvement in Nursing. Washington, DC, American Nurses Publishing, 1992.)

respond to PACU needs, improving the system to decrease the length of time patients remain in the PACU waiting for beds, changing staffing patterns in the PACU or ambulatory care areas to meet patient care needs, or writing a patient education program for all outpatients discharged with a venous access device to ensure that all patients receive the same quality education.

SUMMARY

This chapter has focused on the management of a PACU and an ambulatory care setting involved in post anesthesia care. Important policies and management techniques were discussed, along with aspects of infection control and quality improvement.

References

1. Aldrete, J., and Kroulik, D.: A post anesthetic recovery score. Anesth. Analg., 49:924–933, 1970.
2. Allen, J.: Patient classification in the post anesthesia care unit. J. Post Anesth. Nurs., 5:228–238, 1990.
3. Cormier, S., Pickett, S., and Gallagher, J.: Comparison of nurses' and family members' perceived needs during post anesthesia care unit visits. J. Post Anesth. Nurs., 7:387–391, 1992.
4. Dienemann, J. (ed.): Continuous Quality Improvement in Nursing. Washington, D.C., American Nurses Publishing, 1992.
5. Dooley, S., Castro, K., Hutton, M., et al.: Guidelines for preventing the transmission of tuberculosis in health care settings, with special focus on HIV-related issues. MMWR, 39(RR-17):1–29, 1990.
6. Fields, F.: PACU visiting policies. J. Post Anesth. Nurs., 4:85–89, 1989.
7. Frost, E. (ed.): Post Anesthesia Care Unit. 2nd ed. St. Louis, C.V. Mosby, 1990.
8. Gay, C.: The development of a post anesthesia record incorporating the nursing process. J. Post Anesth. Nurs., 5:85–90, 1990.
9. Gerberding, J. L., Luce, J., Stamm, W., et al.: HIV and the Health Care Worker. Research Triangle Park, NC, Glaxo, 1992.
10. Griffin, D.: A tool to develop standards of quality care in PACUs. J. Post Anesth. Nurs., 4:99–102, 1989.
11. Guinn, J.: Shared governance. Today's OR Nurse, 11(2):10–12, 1989.
12. Jackson-Frankl, K.: Quality assurance and quality improvement: A PACU focus. J. Post Anesth. Nurs., 6:402–408, 1991.
13. Jacobsen, W. (ed.): Manual of Post Anesthesia Care. Philadelphia, W.B. Saunders, 1992.
14. Joint Commission on Accreditation of Healthcare Organizations: Transitions: From QA to CQI. Oakbrook Terrace, IL, JCAHO, 1991.
15. Kahl, K., and Preston, B.: Use of care levels in the post anesthesia care setting. J. Post Anesth. Nurs., 5:91–95, 1990.
16. Korttila, K.: Practical discharge criteria for the 1990s: Assessing home readiness. Anesthesiol. Rev. 18(Suppl 1):23–27, 1991.
17. Litwack, K.: Post Anesthesia Care Nursing. St. Louis, C.V. Mosby, 1991.
18. Occupational Safety and Health Administration: 29 CFR 1910.1030: Occupational Exposure to Blood-Borne Pathogens: Final Rule. (56 FR 64175, December 6, 1991.). Washington, D.C., OSHA, 1991.
19. Poole, E.: The visiting needs of critically ill patients and their families. J. Post Anesth. Nurs., 7:377–386, 1992.
20. Ringl, K., and Dotson, L.: Self-scheduling for professional nurses. Nurs. Manage., 20(2):42–44, 1989.
21. Summers, S.: Using nursing diagnosis to document nursing care in the post anesthesia care unit. J. Post Anesth. Nurs., 4:306–311, 1989.
22. Van De Linder, J.: Hepatitis B: The disease, the risk, the answer. J. Post Anesth. Nurs., 4:416–419, 1989.
23. Van Slyck, A.: A systems approach to the management of nursing services: II. Patient classification system. Nurs. Manage., 22(4):23–25, 1991.
24. Vender, J., and Spiess, B. (eds.): Post Anesthesia Care. Philadelphia, W.B. Saunders, 1992.
25. Willock, M.: Post anesthesia care unit administration and staffing. Anesthesiol. Clin. North Am., 8:223–233, 1990.

Standards of Post Anesthesia Nursing Practice and Selected Resources*

Table 3–1A. STANDARD I: PATIENT RIGHTS AND ETHICS

Standard: Post anesthesia nursing practice is based on philosophic and ethical concepts that recognize and maintain the autonomy, dignity and worth of individuals.

Rationale: Each individual has dignity and worth, deserves respect and recognition, and has the right to quality health care services. Patient and family have the right to explore health care alternatives and to make choices regarding their care. Consideration of social and economic status, culture, personal attributes and the nature of the health care problem must be given when working with patient, family and community.

Structure Criteria	Process Criteria	Outcome Criteria
1. A written statement of the philosophy, goals and objectives of post anesthesia nursing exists that reflects the mission statement of the organization.	1. Philosophy, goals, and objectives are incorporated into nursing practice.	1. Nursing practice reflects the organization's philosophy, goals, and objectives.
2. A mechanism exists for identifying and resolving ethical dilemmas through a separate and/or collaborative process.	2. Nursing staff utilize the appropriate methods to identify and resolve ethical dilemmas.	2. Issues are addressed in an ethical manner.
3. Written policies are designed to protect patients' rights.	3. Nursing staff participate in the development of departmental policies and procedures. Departmental policies and procedures are implemented, monitored and evaluated.	3. All policies and procedures are congruent with the **Patient's Bill of Rights** and the **Code for Nurses**.
4. Job descriptions, policies and procedures exist to support the nurses' role as a patient advocate.	4. Nursing staff assure that the patient has the information needed to make decisions about his/her health care. Nursing staff support the patient's right to make independent decisions.	4. Individual's autonomy, dignity and worth are maintained.
5. A process exists to provide continuing education on moral, ethical, and legal issues.	5. Nursing staff participate in ongoing education relative to moral, ethical and legal issues.	5. Nursing practice reflects an understanding of moral, ethical, and legal issues as evidenced by adherence to the **Code for Nurses**, the **Patient's Bill of Rights**, and appropriate legislation.

*From American Society of Post Anesthesia Nursing Practice 1992. Richmond, VA, ASPAN, 1992.

Table 3-2A. STANDARD II: ENVIRONMENT

Standard: Post anesthesia nursing practice promotes and maintains a safe, comfortable and therapeutic environment for patients, staff and visitors.

Rationale: The intrusion of anesthesia and surgery has significant impact on motor and sensory functions that necessitates a safe, supportive environment. Individuals may be exposed to infectious organisms, hazardous materials and other environmental risk factors.

Structure Criteria	Process Criteria	Outcome Criteria

1. Written policies and procedures related to fire, safety, infection control and CPR include:
  a. Personnel and visitor dress code is determined by proximity and frequency of access to Operating Rooms.
  b. Waste gas levels are monitored in Phase I per OSHA requirements established for Operating Rooms.
  c. Patients requiring isolation are provided with a private room.
  d. CPR review is annual, with renewal every two years.
	1. Staff follow established policies and procedures.	1. Individuals are not exposed to unsafe conditions and are not exposed to infectious organisms.
		
		  c. Care meets the same standards of practice wherever the care is provided in the health care organization.

2. A system exists to assure appropriate emergency drugs, equipment and supplies are present, readily available and checked at regular intervals.	2. Emergency drugs, equipment and supplies are checked at regular intervals to assure they are current and adequate to meet the needs of the patient population.	2. Documentation reflects regular inspections and availability of emergency drugs, equipment, and supplies.

3. A mechanism exists for identifying, obtaining and evaluating appropriate space, supplies and equipment.
  a. Phase I is in close proximity to where anesthesia is administered.
  b. Phase I and Phase II are separate and distinct areas.
  c. In Phase I, preoperative patients are not present when patients are recovering from anesthesia.
	3. Nursing staff identify, obtain, and evaluate utilization of space, patient care, supplies and equipment.	3. Supplies and equipment needed for patient care are available to meet the needs of patients and staff.

4. Orientation and on-going training programs include, but are not limited to, fire safety, patient and staff safety and infection control.	4. Staff participate in fire safety, patient and staff safety, and infection control programs at least annually.	4. Staff demonstrate knowledge about fire safety, patient and staff safety and infection control.
5. A mechanism exists to identify, prevent and/or correct hazards within the work environment.	5. Staff report and document hazardous situations and intervene as appropriate.	5. Hazardous situations are identified and corrective actions are taken.
6. Nursing staff is involved in planning environmental and/or program changes that affect the work/care environment.	6. Nursing staff identify needed environmental services and space and make appropriate recommendations/changes.	6. Adequate support services are available, e.g., environmental services and transportation services. Adequate space exists to assure patient privacy and to perform patient care and administrative activities.

7. A mechanism exists to provide safe transportation of patients.	7. Professional nurses determine mode, number, and skill level of accompanying personnel based on patient needs.
	  a. Transportation from a free standing facility to a full service hospital will be utilized in emergency situations.
	  b. Professional nurse (Phase II) assures the availability of safe transport of the patient to his/her home.
		7. Patients are transported without incident.

Table 3-3A. STANDARD III: PERSONNEL MANAGEMENT

Standard: A sufficient number of qualified nursing staff with demonstrated competency in the provision of nursing care during all phases of post anesthesia are available to meet the individual needs of patients and families.

Rationale: Nursing is a unique and separate discipline that contributes positively to the patient's health and wellness. Nursing care in post anesthesia settings is directed toward provision of direct patient care, supervision of care given by others, health teaching and patient advocacy. The expertise of professional registered nurses is necessary to implement and supervise the care provided to patients in all post anesthesia settings.

Structure Criteria	Process Criteria	Outcome Criteria
1. Written job descriptions for each category of staff clearly define the lines of authority, role and functions of the position consistent with the state nurse practice act and other applicable regulatory agencies.	1. Staff function within assigned job performance descriptions.	1. Staff have the appropriate qualifications and skills required for their position.
2. A mechanism exists to assure that staff performance is reviewed and documented on an ongoing basis.	2. Staff receive regularly scheduled performance appraisals that are competency based. Progress will be monitored by the staff member or manager.	2. Appraisals occur at least annually. Areas for improvement and growth are documented and needed changes in practice occur.
3. Policies reflect professional nurses supervise all nursing care provided.	3. A professional nurse is present at all times to provide direct care and/or supervision.	3. Records and staffing patterns reflect that adequate professional nurses are present to supervise care delivered by staff.
4. A mechanism exists to assure adequate numbers and appropriate skill levels of personnel to provide the required nursing care.	4. Staffing is based on patient acuity, census, and physical facility. Two licensed nurses, one of whom is an RN, are present whenever a patient is recovering in Phase I and/or Phase II. Patient–staff ratios will vary according to patient classification.	4. Determined staffing needs are met.
5. A written plan for orientation and ongoing continuing education exists to assure and improve competency.	5. All staff participate in orientation and ongoing education programs.	5. a. New staff members demonstrate competency in the performance of responsibilities as defined in the job description. b. Nursing staff members demonstrate the competencies annually. c. Staff members performing direct patient care successfully complete the national cognitive and skills examinations in accordance with the standards of the American Heart Association for BLS Rescuer—C (or the equivalent).
6. Written guidelines for professional nurses practicing in expanded roles describe the type and level of practice they provide.	6. Professional nurses in expanded roles practice within written guidelines/job descriptions.	6. Credentialing files are current for practitioners in expanded roles and include initial credentialing, annual performance reviews, and proof of current credentials.

Table 3–4A. STANDARD IV: CONTINUOUS QUALITY IMPROVEMENT

Standard: Post anesthesia nursing practice is monitored and evaluated on an ongoing basis. Identified problems are resolved in order to assure the quality and appropriateness of patient care.

Rationale: Evaluation of the quality of patient care through examination of the clinical practice of nurses is one way to fulfill the profession's obligation to ensure that consumers are provided excellence in care.

Structure Criteria	Process Criteria	Outcome Criteria
1. Established and organized quality improvement activities identify issues, implement resolutions, and evaluate outcomes through continuous monitoring systems.	1. The program includes monitoring and evaluation of the care provided, the process of care, and the desired outcome.	1. Documentation reflects an ongoing quality improvement program and incorporation of findings into practice.
2. A mechanism exists to assure integration of post anesthesia quality improvement activities into the overall organizational program.	2. The post anesthesia quality improvement process encourages a multidisciplinary approach, providing information to the appropriate committee.	2. a. Written reports of quality improvement activities are available and forwarded to the organizational program. b. Quality improvement programs lead to the identification of research priorities.
3. The quality improvement program includes a written plan to monitor and evaluate staff competency.	3. Specified indicators are identified, monitored, and evaluated by staff annually.	3. Documentation reflects changes in staff competency programs based on quality improvement findings.
4. The quality improvement program includes a mechanism to obtain patient/family input regarding the quality of care.	4. Patient/family satisfaction is measured at intervals.	4. Patient and family concerns are resolved and re-evaluated as appropriate.
5. The quality improvement program includes evaluation of the environment to assure compliance with safety and infection control policies.	5. Staff participate in an ongoing quality improvement program to evaluate the environment and its impact on patients and staff.	5. Activities result in changes in the environment to improve care and safety.

Table 3–5A. STANDARD V: RESEARCH

Standard: Post anesthesia nurses participate in research designed to improve patient care by initiating and conducting studies, utilizing results and incorporating findings into practice.

Rationale: Each professional has accountability for continuing development and refinement of knowledge in the post anesthesia field through development of new and creative approaches to practice, use of relevant research findings and participation in research. The professional nurse assumes responsibility for this at a level appropriate to his/her educational and experiential knowledge base.

Structure Criteria	Process Criteria	Outcome Criteria
1. The philosophy of nursing includes research as an integral part of professional nursing practice. A process exists to facilitate incorporation of research findings into post anesthesia care practice.	1. Professional nurses read and evaluate research, and apply valid findings in the practice setting.	1. Validated research findings are incorporated into nursing practice and formally disseminated to peers and colleagues.
2. Written policies protect patient and staff rights in the conduct of research activities.	2. Research is conducted according to organizational policies.	2. Rights of all research participants and staff are protected throughout the research process.
3. A mechanism exists within nursing to encourage and foster nursing staff participation in research projects.	3. a. Nursing staff participate in formal/informal research including problem identification, data collection, analysis, and interpretation. b. Nursing staff collaborate with colleagues in other disciplines who engage in research in the practice setting.	3. Nursing staff participate in research activities that occur within the practice setting.
4. A mechanism exists for the nursing department to participate in reviewing, evaluating, and recommending approval of all clinical studies that involve or affect nursing practice.	4. Nursing staff participate actively in reviewing, evaluating and recommending approval of all clinical studies that involve or affect nursing practice.	4. Nursing staff are aware of research done in the post anesthesia setting and are involved as appropriate.

Table 3–6A. STANDARD VI: INTERDISCIPLINARY COLLABORATION

Standard: Nursing personnel facilitate continuity of care by assuring that the needs of patients and families are recognized and addressed through coordination with other health team members within the health care system and the community.

Rationale: Post anesthesia practice involves multiple disciplines. The professional nurse is responsible for coordination of patient care through collaboration with those disciplines.

Structure Criteria	Process Criteria	Outcome Criteria
1. A mechanism exists to facilitate multidisciplinary plans of care, including the development of a scope of practice for each care area.	1. The professional nurse collaborates with other health team members.	1. Documentation will reflect a multidisciplinary approach to patient care.
2. Written guidelines exist to assure appropriate referral.	2. The professional nurse provides referral for follow-up care.	2. Documentation reflects appropriate referrals.
3. A mechanism exists to assess and meet the educational needs in the health care facility and the community.	3. The professional nurse participates in the planning, implementation and evaluation of multidisciplinary educational activities.	3. Documentation reflects provision of programs.
4. The health care facility provides the opportunity for nurses to participate on multidisciplinary committees addressing patient care.	4. The professional nurse serves on committees within the health care system, contributing nursing expertise to the decision-making process.	4. Minutes of committee meetings reflect the involvement of the professional nurse.
5. A mechanism exists to involve professional nurses in evaluating and selecting new health care technology and information systems.	5. Professional nurses obtain and maintain knowledge of current health care technology and information systems which relate to their practice.	5. Professional nurses evaluate and select new technology and information systems.
6. A mechanism exists to provide a post anesthesia clinical practicum in facilities where clinical learning opportunities are available for the professional nursing student.	6. Post anesthesia nurses collaborate with nursing educators to assist in developing curricula.	6. Post anesthesia care settings provide clinical learning experiences for nursing education programs.

Table 3–7A. STANDARD VII: ASSESSMENT

Standard: Post anesthesia nursing practice includes the systematic and continuous assessment of the patient's condition. The nurse assures that the data are collected, documented, and communicated. The professional nurse analyzes the data to determine appropriate nursing interventions.

Rationale: Assessment and data collection provide a clinical and legal basis for nursing actions and accountability.

Structure Criteria	Process Criteria	Outcome Criteria
1. Specific admission protocols and guidelines are identified for all post anesthesia care settings. These guidelines will address general, local and regional anesthesia, special procedures, preanesthesia, infectious and critical care patients.	1. The professional nurse assures that all admissions are identified as appropriate and evaluated based on written guidelines.	1. Inappropriate admissions are identified through Quality Improvement program (e.g., Occurrence Screens).
2. Unit policies define the components and frequency of nursing assessment.	2. The professional nurse performs the initial assessments and assures a systematic and pertinent collection of data. (See Resource 14).	2. Assessment and data analysis are documented and based on reliable data and are consistent with accepted practice.
3. A mechanism exists to set patient care priorities based on the uniqueness of each patient.	3. The professional nurse differentiates the severity of patient problems and prioritizes patient care, designating an appropriate acuity level.	3. Appropriate personnel deliver patient care.
4. A mechanism exists to assure that assessment data are available to all appropriate health care providers.	4. The professional nurse reviews available patient care documentation, revises the data as appropriate and shares information with other health care team members.	4. Writen evidence of nursing assessment is available for every patient. Usage of Nursing Diagnosis is at the discretion of individual units.

41

Table 3–8A. STANDARD VIII:PLANNING AND IMPLEMENTATION

Standard: The professional nurse designs and coordinates the implementation of a plan of care to achieve optimal patient outcomes.

Rationale: The nursing plan of care documents the patient's response to nursing interventions which are directed toward promotion, maintenance and restoration. The plan guides each nurse to intervene in a manner congruent with the patient's needs and goals and provides outcome criteria for measurement of patient progress. Professional nurses can contribute effectively to the formulation of a multidisciplinary treatment plan and collaborative therapeutic interventions.

Structure Criteria	Process Criteria	Outcome Criteria
1. A mechanism exists to facilitate the formulation of multidisciplinary treatment plan.	1. The nurse collaborates with the patient, family, and other health care providers to establish a plan of care.	1. Documentation reflects collaboration with the patient, family, and other health care providers. In PACU Phase II, the postdischarge plan is provided to the patient/family.
2. A mechanism exists for standardized and/or individualized plans to be recorded, communicated to others and/or revised. Plans of care can take many forms including management protocols, standing orders, nursing care plan and standards of care.	2. The professional nurse develops the plans for nursing care reflecting current and acceptable nursing practice and research. The plans are developed with and communicated to the patient, significant others and the health care team as appropriate. The plans for nursing care describe a systematic method for achieving the goal of post anesthesia nursing care.	2. Plans reflect nursing care as an ongoing process.
3. Written guidelines provide for dependent and independent nursing functions. These guidelines are consistent with state licensure, established standards, and organizational policy.	3. The professional nurse initiates the appropriate nursing interventions identified in the guidelines of plan of care.	3. Documentation reflects interventions based on established guidelines and plan of care.
4. A mechanism exists for nursing follow-up to promote continuity of care and evaluation of patient care in the PACU, Phase I or Phase II.	4. The professional nurse conducts follow-up visits/calls based on availability of resources and patient needs.	4. Documentation reflects compliance with post discharge plan of care and follow up as needed.

Table 3–9A. STANDARD IX: EVALUATION

Standard: The professional nurse continuously measures the patient's progress toward the desired outcomes and revises the plan of care and interventions as necessary.

Rationale: Evaluation of the health status of the patient is done to determine the effectiveness of nursing interventions so that the plan of care may be continued, or altered.

Structure Criteria	Process Criteria	Outcome Criteria
1. Written guidelines are established by patient care evaluation to assure that nursing actions are analyzed and evaluated.	1. When interventions are not effective, the professional nurse revises the plan of care.	1. Documentation reflects current data are recorded and used to measure progress toward goal achievement.
2. A mechanism exists for consultation to assist the nurse in evaluating the effectiveness of interventions.	2. The professional nurse consults and/or collaborates with peers, physicians and other resources when evaluating the effectiveness of interventions.	2. Consultation is documented as appropriate.
3. Written guidelines are established for discharge of the patient from Phase I and II.	3. Nursing staff utilize guidelines for discharge. (See Resource 14).	3. Documentation reflects that the patient was appropriately discharged.

Table 3–10A. STANDARD X: ADVANCED CARDIAC LIFE SUPPORT (ACLS)

Standard: Post anesthesia nursing practice involves autonomous decision-making and implementation of interventions in a crisis situation. ACLS certification or the equivalent is a necessary component to support this aspect of practice in Phase I.

Rationale: Post anesthesia care units are, by their nature, critical care units. The patient is in a very vulnerable stage of the perioperative course during the immediate post anesthesia period. Professional nurses with specific education, experience and knowledge about the post operative period can recognize and help manage anesthesia, surgery and medically related complications.

Structure Criteria	Process Criteria	Outcome Criteria
1. A job description for the professional nurse in Phase I includes a requirement of ACLS certification or the equivalent educational process.	1. Professional nursing staff obtain ACLS certification or the equivalent within one year of employment.	1. Staff demonstrates knowledge and skills about responses to emergency or critical situations.
2. A mechanism exists for the provision of the educational requirements for ACLS or the equivalent educational process.	2. Professional nursing staff participate, on a biannual basis in ACLS certification course or the equivalent educational process. (See Resource 16.)*	2. Adequate opportunity for education exists.
3. Policies and procedures, standing orders and protocols direct the professional nurses' practice to respond to crisis situations.	3. Professional nursing practice in Phase I reflects knowledge and skills obtained via ACLS or the equivalent educational process.	3. Policies and procedures are congruent with skill levels.

*Excludes hands-on intubation experience.

Table 3–11A. STANDARD XI: PAIN MANAGEMENT

Standard: Post anesthesia nursing practice utilizes established modalities of pain management to assist the patient toward optimal comfort.

Rationale: Current techniques and practices related to surgery, anesthesia, or other procedures have the potential to cause altered comfort levels. It is within the scope of this specialty to create an environment directed toward the management of these needs.

Structure Criteria	Process Criteria	Outcome Criteria
1. Written policies and procedures are developed by nurses, in conjunction with anesthesiologists and physicians, which outline specific guidelines for care of the patient receiving analgesia via established modalities.	1. a. Nursing staff participate in development of policies and procedures. The policies and procedures conform to the scope of nursing practice established by the state nurse practice act and professional nursing organizations.	1. a. Written policies and procedures are available in the patient care area and their use is reflected in the care delivered.
	b. An environment as specified in Standard II and personnel requirements as specified in Standard III are provided.	b. Patients receive care that meets the same standards of practice wherever and by whomever the care is provided within the health care organization.
2. A mechanism exists to provide the knowledge of anatomy and physiology, pharmacology, and complications related to pain management modalities.	2. Nursing staff participate in orientation and ongoing education relative to the management of pain.	2. Nursing staff periodically demonstrate and document competence and knowledge of pain management modalities.

Table 3–12A. RESOURCE 5: RECOMMENDED EQUIPMENT FOR PHASE I PACU

The following is the recommended list of equipment for Phase I PACU, including bed space:

1. One and one half beds will be available in the PACU for every one operating room. Two beds will be available in the PACU for every one operating room when dealing with short, simple procedures on relatively healthy patients.
2. Each patient care unit will be equipped with the following:
   a. various means of oxygen delivery
   b. constant and intermittent suction
   c. means to monitor blood pressure
   d. adjustable lighting
   e. capacity to ensure patient privacy
   f. one EKG monitor per patient
   g. one pulse oximeter per patient
3. Monitors for arterial, central venous and/or pulmonary artery pressures for those patients requiring these measures will be available.
4. A means to monitor patient temperature will be available. A method to warm the patient with low temperature will also be available. Supplies to handle a malignant hyperthermia crisis must also be available. These supplies should include:
   a. means to deliver 100 percent oxygen
   b. dantrolene
   c. mannitol
   d. bicarbonate
   e. cool IV fluids or cooling blanket
5. At least one ventilator will be maintained in PACU at all times. A suffecent number of ventilators will be available to care for any post anesthesia patient who requires one. A bag-valve mask, adult and pediatric, must be in the PACU and easily accessible at all times.
6. Portable oxygen, suction and cardiac monitoring equipment will be available for those patients requiring such equipment during transport.
7. A method of calling for assistance in emergency situations shall be provided.
8. An emergency cart will be in the PACU at all times.
   a. supplies necessary for insertion of arterial line, central venous lines and pulmonary artery catheters easily accessible
   b. IV pole
9. Stock medications should include the following:
   a. antibiotics
   b. medication for control of blood pressure, heart rate and respiratory drugs
   c. antiemetics
   d. anesthesia reversal agents
   e. analgesics, narcotic and non-narcotic
   f. muscle relaxants
   g. steroids
   h. sedatives
10. Intravenous supplies shall include:
    a. various types of solutions
    b. various types of intravenous catheters
    c. various type of IV tubing
    d. IV dressing supplies per hospital protocol
    e. at least one IV infusion control device
11. Patient restraints will be available to use per hospital policy
12. Stock supplies should include:
    a. dressings
    b. facial tissues
    c. gloves
    d. bedpans and urinals
    e. syringes and needles
    f. emesis basin
    g. patient linens
    h. alcohol swabs
    i. ice bags
    j. tongue blades
    k. irrigation trays
    l. Foley insertion supplies
    m. eye protection, such as goggles
13. A means to safely transport patients from Phase I PACU will be available.

Table 3–12A. RESOURCE 5: RECOMMENDED EQUIPMENT FOR PHASE I PACU *Continued*

Recommended Equipment for Phase II PACU
The following is the recommended list of equipment for Phase II PACU:

1. Each patient care unit will be equipped with the following:
   a. means to deliver oxygen
   b. constant and intermittent suction
   c. means to monitor blood pressure
   d. adjustable lighting
   e. capacity to ensure patient privacy
   f. means of monitoring patient temperature
2. An EKG and pulse oximeter will be readily available for use in Phase II PACU.
3. A bag-valve mask, adult and pediatric, must be easily accessible at all times.
4. A means to monitor patient temperature will be available. Supplies to handle a malignant hyperthermia crisis must be easily accessible. These supplies should include:
   a. means to deliver 100 percent oxygen
   b. Dantrolene
   c. Mannitol
   d. Bicarbonate
   e. cool IV fluids or cooling blanket
5. A method of calling for assistance in emergency situations should be provided.
6. An emergency cart will be in the Phase II PACU at all times and should include the following:
   a. endotracheal blade light handle
   b. various endotracheal blades
   c. various size endotracheal tubes
   d. oral and nasal airways
   e. these shall also include pediatric sizes
7. A defibrillator with adult and pediatric paddles must be readily available.
8. Stock medications should include the following:
   a. antibiotics
   b. antiemetics
   c. anesthesia reversal agents
   d. analgesics, narcotic and non-narcotic
9. Intravenous supplies shall include:
   a. various types of solutions
   b. various types of intravenous catheters
   c. various types of IV tubing
   d. IV dressing supplies per hospital protocol
10. Stock supplies should include:
    a. dressings
    b. facial tissues
    c. gloves
    d. bedpans and urinals
    e. syringes and needles
    f. emesis basin
    g. patient linens
    h. alcohol swabs/wipes
    i. ice bags
    j. tongue blades
    k. Foley insertion supplies
11. A means to safely transport patients from Phase II PACU will be available.

Table 3–13A. RESOURCE 10: PATIENT CLASSIFICATION

Preprocedural
A professional registered nurse assesses the patient and develops a plan of care designed to meet the patient's preprocedural needs.

Phase I

Class 1:3   One nurse to three patients who are awake, stable and uncomplicated

Class 1:2   One nurse to two patients who are
      a. unconscious, stable without artificial airway and over 9 years of age
      b. awake, stable, 11 and under years of age and with family or support staff present

Class 1:1   One nurse to one patient
      a. at the time of admission
      b. requiring mechanical life support and/or artificial airway
      c. any unconscious patient 9 and under years of age
      d. a second nurse must be available to assist as necessary

Phase II

Class 1:5   One nurse to five patients
      a. over 5 years of age who are ready for discharge
      b. 5 and under years of age and ready for discharge who have family present

Class 1:4   One nurse to four patients
      a. over 5 years of age, awake and stable
      b. 5 and under years of age, awake and stable with family present

Class 1:3   One nurse to three patients
      a. over 5 years within 1/2 hour of procedure/discharge from Phase I
      b. 5 and under years of age within 1/2 hour of procedure/discharge from Phase I with family present

Class 1:2   One nurse to two patients
      a. 5 and under years of age without family or support staff present
      b. initial admission of patient post procedure

Class 1:1   One nurse to one patient
      a. unstable patient of any age requiring transfer

Staffing is based on patient acuity, census and physical facility. Two licensed nurses, one of whom is an RN, are present whenever a patient is recovering in Phase I and/or Phase II.

Table 3–14A. RESOURCE 14: DATA REQUIRED FOR INITIAL, ONGOING AND DISCHARGE ASSESSMENT

Phase I

Assessment factors include but not limited to:
1. Relevant preoperative status including: electrocardiogram vital signs, radiology findings, laboratory values, oxygen saturation, allergies, disabilities, substance abuse, physical or mental impairments, mobility limitations, prostheses (including hearing aids) and in the pediatric patient, birth history, development stages and parent/child interactions.
2. Anesthesia technique (general, regional, local) effect of preoperative medication.
3. Anesthesia agents, muscle relaxant, narcotics and reversal agents used.
4. Length of time anesthesia administered, time reversal agents given.
5. Type of surgical procedure.
6. Estimated fluid/blood loss and replacement.
7. Complications occurring during anesthesia course, treatment initiated response and emotional status on arrival to the operating or procedure room.

Initial Assessment: Phase I
Initial assessment to include documentation of:
1. Vital signs
   a. airway patent, respiratory rate and competency, breath sounds, type of artificial airway, mechanical ventilator settings and oxygen saturations
   b. blood pressure: cuff or arterial line
   c. pulse: apical, peripheral
   d. temperature: oral, rectal, axillary, digital through dermal sensor, tympanic
2. Level of consciousness
3. Pressure readings: central venous, arterial blood, pulmonary artery wedge and intracranial pressure if indicated
4. Position of patient
5. Condition and color of skin
6. Patient safety needs
7. Neurovascular: peripheral pulses and sensation of extremity (ies) as applicable
8. Condition of dressings
9. Condition of suture line, if dressing absent
10. Type, patency and securement of drainage tubes, catheters and receptacle
11. Amount and type of drainage
12. Muscular response and strength
13. Pupillary response as indicated
14. Fluid therapy, location of lines, condition of IV site and securement and amount of solution infusing (including blood)
15. Level of physical and emotional support
16. Numerical score if used

Ongoing Assessment: Phase I
Ongoing assessment should include, but not be limited to the following:
1. Monitor, maintain and/or improve respiratory function
2. Monitor, maintain and/or improve circulatory function
3. Promote and maintain physical and emotional comfort
4. Monitor surgical site
5. Interpret and document data obtained during assessment
6. Document nursing action and/or intervention with outcome
7. Notify patient care unit of any needed equipment
8. Include parent/legal guardian in care of patient as indicated
9. Notify patient care unit when patient is ready for discharge from PACU and provide report of all operating and PACU significant happenings

Discharge Assessment: Phase I
Data collected and recorded to evaluate the patient's status for discharge:
1. Airway patency, respiratory function and oxygen saturation
2. Stability of vital signs, including temperature
3. Level of consciousness and muscular strength
4. Mobility
5. Patency of tubes, catheters, drains, intravenous lines
6. Skin color and condition
7. Condition of dressing and/or surgical site
8. Intake and output
9. Comfort
10. Anxiety
11. Child-parent/significant others interactions

Table continued on following page

Table 3–14A. RESOURCE 14: DATA REQUIRED FOR INITIAL, ONGOING AND DISCHARGE ASSESSMENT *Continued*

Phase II

Initial Assessment: Phase II

Initial assessment to include documentation of:
1. Vital signs
    a. respiratory rate, competency
    b. blood pressure
    c. pulse
    d. temperature
2. Level of consciousness
3. Position of patient
4. Patient safety needs
5. Condition and color of skin
6. Neurovascular assessment as applicable
7. Condition of dressings, drains and tubes as applicable
8. Muscular response and strength
9. Fluid therapy, location of lines, condition of IV sites and securement, type and amount of fluid infusing
10. Level of physical and emotional comfort
11. Numerical score if used

Ongoing Assessment: Phase II

Ongoing patient care and assessment should include but not be limited to the following:
1. Identification of patient and name family normally uses
2. Receiving report from PACU Phase I nurse
3. Monitor, maintain and/or improve respiratory function
4. Monitor, maintain and/or improve circulatory function
5. Promote and maintain physical and emotional comfort
6. Monitor surgical site
7. Interpret and document data obtained during assessment
8. Administer analgesics as necessary, record results
9. Administer other medication as ordered, record results
10. Provide maximum degree of privacy
11. Provide for safety
12. Provide for confidentiality of information and records
13. Encourage fluids by mouth
14. Ambulate with assistance
15. Position patient gradually from supine to Fowler's position
16. Ask patient to urinate prior to discharge
17. Review discharge planning with patient, family/significant others or legal guardian as appropriate; provide written home care instructions
18. Provide follow-up for extended care as indicated: next day follow-up phone call is recommended to evaluate status

Discharge Assessment: Phase II

Current assessment data are collected and recorded to evaluate the patient's status for discharge to home:
1. Adequate respiratory function
2. Stability of vital signs, including temperature
3. Level of consciousness and muscular strength
4. Ability to ambulate consistent with developmental age level
5. Ability to swallow oral fluids, cough or demonstrate gag reflex
6. Ability to retain oral fluid
7. Skin color and condition
8. Pain minimal
9. Adequate neurovascular status of operative extremity
10. Patient and home care provider understands all home instructions
11. Written discharge instructions given to patient/family
12. Concur with prearrangements for safe transportation home
13. Provide additional resource to contact if any problems arise

Table 3–15A. RESOURCE 16: ACLS AND EQUIVALENT TESTING

In accordance to standard X, ACLS or the equivalent is a necessary component to support PACU nursing practice in Phase I.

The guideline which follows should be used in developing a program for your institution should they choose not to utilize the defined ACLS. Competence in this area must be documented and verified by the use of written tests and return demonstrations with use of algorithms.

Guidelines for ACLS Equivalent Program

1. Identification of life threatening dysrhythmias
   a. bradycardia
   b. electromechanical dissociation
   c. ventricular tachycardia
   d. ventricular fibrillation
   e. asystole
   f. heart blocks
2. Pharmacologic therapy of life threatening dysrhythmias
   a. mechanism of action
   b. indications
   c. recommended dosage
   d. route of administration
   e. complications
   f. drugs to be included:
      1. Sodium bicarbonate
      2. Epinephrine
      3. Atropine
      4. Lidocaine
      5. Procainamide
      6. Calcium chloride
      7. Bretylium tosylate
      8. Oxygen
      9. Verapamil
      10. Morphine
      11. Norepinephrine
      12. Dopamine
      13. Dobutamine
      14. Isoproterenol
      15. Digoxin
      16. Sodium nitroprusside
      17. Nitroglycerin
      18. Beta blockers
3. Defibrillation and cardioversion therapy
   a. indications
   b. precautions
   c. technique

Physiologic Considerations in the PACU

Nervous System Anatomy and Physiology

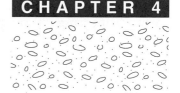

The nervous system is affected not only by surgery carried out on it directly but also by regional and general anesthetics. Hence, most patients in the post anesthesia care unit (PACU) are experiencing some alteration in central nervous system (CNS) function. Consequently, it is important for the PACU nurse to have an understanding of some of the basic anatomic and physiologic principles that are operative in the CNS.

Definitions

Afferent: carrying sensory impulses toward the brain.

Autoregulation: an alteration in the diameter of the resistance vessels to maintain a constant perfusion pressure during changes in blood flow.

Cistern: a reservoir or cavity.

Commissure: white or gray matter that crosses over in the midline and connects one side of the brain or spinal cord with the other side.

Decussate: commonly refers to crossing of parts.

Dorsal: posterior.

Efferent: carrying motor impulses away from the brain.

Estrus: the cycle of changes in the female genital tract produced as a result of ovarian hormonal activity.

Inferior: beneath; also used to indicate the lower portion of an anatomic part.

Lower motor neurons: neurons of the spine and cranium that directly innervate the muscles (e.g., those found in the anterior horns or anterior roots of the gray matter of the spinal cord).

Metabolic regulation: a change in blood flow in response to the metabolic requirements of tissues.

Neuroglia: the supporting structure of nervous tissue, consisting of a fine web of tissue made up of modified ectodermal elements. It encloses branched cells known as neuroglia or glia cells but lacks nerve fibers itself. It performs less specialized functions of the nerve network.

Plexus: a network of nerves.

Postural reflexes: reflexes that are basically proprioceptive, being concerned with the position of the head in relation to the trunk and with adjustments of the extremities and eyes to the position of the head.

Proprioception: the awareness of posture, movement, and changes in equilibrium.

Ramus (rami): the primary division of a nerve.

Righting reflexes: reflexes that maintain the head in an upright position in relation to the environment, through use of the eyes, inner ears, and muscles of the neck and trunk.

Upper motor neurons: neurons in the brain and spinal cord that activate the motor system (e.g., the descending fibers of the pyramidal and extrapyramidal tracts).

Ventral: anterior.

THE CENTRAL NERVOUS SYSTEM

The CNS is composed of the brain and spinal cord and is exceedingly complex, both anatomically and physiologically. None of the structures in the CNS function in an isolated manner. Neural activity at any level of the CNS always modifies or is modified by influences from other parts of the system. This accounts for the unique nature and extreme complexity of the CNS, much of which remains to be clearly understood.

The Brain

The human brain serves both structurally and functionally as the primary center for control and regulation of all nervous system functions. As such, it is the highest level of control and integration of sensory and motor information in the entire body.

The *brain (encephalon)* is divided into three

large areas based on its embryonic development: (1) the *forebrain (prosencephalon)* contains the *telencephalon (cerebrum)* with its hemispheres, and the *diencephalon;* (2) the *midbrain (mesencephalon)* contains the *cerebral peduncles,* the *corpora quadrigemina,* and the *cerebral aqueduct;* and (3) the *hindbrain (rhombencephalon)* consists of the *medulla oblongata,* the *pons,* the *cerebellum,* and the *fourth ventricle.*

The Forebrain

The telencephalon (cerebrum)

The cerebrum is the largest part of the brain. It fills the entire upper portion of the cranial cavity and consists of billions of neurons that synapse to form a complex network of neural pathways.

The cerebrum consists of two hemispheres interconnected only by a large band of white fiber tracts known as the *corpus callosum.* Each hemisphere is further subdivided into four lobes corresponding in name to the overlying bones of the cranium. These are the *frontal, parietal, temporal,* and *occipital lobes* (Fig. 4–1). Both hemispheres consist of an *external cortex* of gray matter, the underlying *white matter tracts,* and the *basal ganglia (cerebral nuclei).* Each hemisphere also contains a *lateral ventricle,* which is an elongated cavity concerned with the formation and circulation of cerebrospinal fluid (CSF).

The cerebral cortex

The cerebral cortex has an elaborate mantle of *gray matter* and is the most highly integrated area in the nervous system. It is arranged in a series of folds dipping down into the underlying regions. These folds greatly expand the surface area of the gray matter within the limited confines of the skull. Each fold is known as a *convolution* or *gyrus.* Deeper grooves exist between these convolutions. A shallow one is known as a *sulcus,* whereas a deeper one is known as a *fissure.*

The cerebral hemispheres are separated from each other by the *longitudinal fissure* anteroposteriorly. The *transverse fissure* separates the cerebrum from the cerebellum beneath it.

Each hemisphere has three sulci between the lobes. The *central sulcus* (also known as the *fissure of Rolando*) separates the frontal and parietal lobes. The *lateral sulcus* (the fissure of Sylvius) lies between the frontal and parietal lobes above and the temporal lobe below. The small

parieto-occipital sulcus is located between its corresponding lobes (Figs. 4–1 and 4–2).

The *white matter* of the cerebrum is situated below the cortex and is composed of three main groups of myelinated nerve fibers arranged in related bundles or tracts. The *commissural fibers* transmit impulses between the hemispheres. The largest of these is the corpus callosum. The *projection fibers* ascend and descend to transmit impulses from one level of the CNS to another. A notable example is the internal capsule that surrounds most of the basal ganglia and connects the thalamus and the cerebral cortex. Finally, the *association fibers* disseminate impulses from one part of the cortex to another within the same hemisphere.

The basal ganglia (cerebral nuclei)

A cerebral nucleus is a group of neuron cell bodies lying within the CNS. Four of these deep-lying masses of gray matter are located within the white matter of each hemisphere and are collectively known as the *basal ganglia* (Fig. 4–3). These are the *caudate nucleus,* the *lentiform nucleus* (divided into the putamen and the globus pallidus), the *amygdala,* and the *claustrum.* Together, they exert a steadying influence on muscle activity. Along with that portion of the internal capsule that lies between them, the caudate and lentiform nuclei compose the *corpus striatum,* the most significant functional unit of the basal ganglia. The basal ganglia are an important part of the extrapyramidal motor pathway connecting nuclei with each other, with the cortex, and with the spinal cord. The ganglia also connect with areas in the hindbrain (the red nucleus and the substantia nigra) to assist in carrying out their role in smoothing and coordinating muscle movements. Disturbances in these ganglia result in tremor, rigidity, and loss of expressive and walking movements, as seen in *Parkinson's syndrome.*

Functional aspects of the cerebrum

Nearly every portion of the cerebral cortex is connected with subcortical centers, and there are no areas in the cortex that are exclusively motor (expressive) or exclusively sensory (receptive) in nature. However, there are some regions that are primarily concerned with the expressive phase of cortical functioning and others that are primarily receptive in nature. The activities of these areas are integrated by association fibers that compose the remainder of the cerebral cortex. Association fibers play

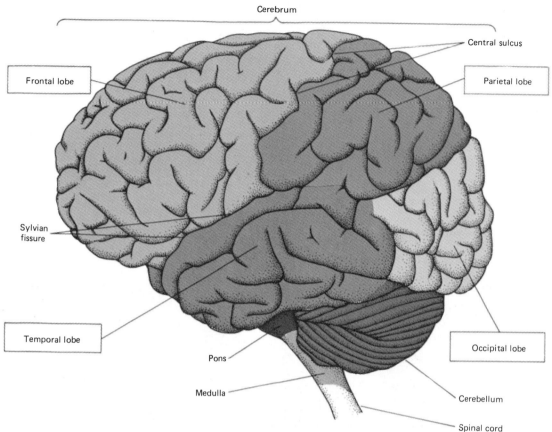

FIGURE 4–1. Left lateral view of the brain, showing the principal divisions of the brain and the four major lobes of the cerebrum. (From Guyton, A. C.: Basic Neuroscience: Anatomy and Physiology. 2nd ed. Philadelphia, W. B. Saunders, 1991, p. 12.)

important roles in complex intellectual and emotional processes.

Motor areas

There is no single area of motor control within the brain, because the integration and control of muscle activity are dependent on the harmonious activities of several areas, including the cerebral cortex, the basal ganglia, and the cerebellum.

The Primary Motor Area. The primary motor area of the cerebral cortex is located in the precentral gyrus of the frontal lobe, just anterior to the central sulcus, and is concerned mainly with the voluntary initiation of finely controlled movements, such as those of the hands, fingers, lips, tongue, and vocal cords. Skeletal muscles responsible for these discrete movements are largely represented by neurons in the motor cortex. Muscles of the arms, legs, and trunk are served by a comparatively small group of neurons, so that this part of the motor

cortex controls larger groups of muscles and produces grosser movements (Fig. 4–4).

The axons of the pyramidal cell bodies in the primary motor area descend through the internal capsule, midbrain, and pons to the medulla, where most of them decussate, or cross, to the opposite side and continue down into the spinal cord, where they are known as the *crossed pyramidal* or *lateral corticospinal tracts.* Fibers that have not crossed are known as the *uncrossed pyramidal* or *ventral corticospinal tracts.* Most of these fibers eventually decussate at lower levels within the cord. Pyramidal cell axons also connect within the brain with the basal ganglia, the brain stem, and the cerebellum. All of the complex connections of the pyramidal cells play important roles in the overall coordination and control of skeletal muscle activity.

The Premotor Area. The premotor area of each hemisphere is located in the cortex immediately anterior to the precentral gyrus in the frontal lobe. On the whole, it is concerned with movement of the opposite side of the body, especially with control and coordination of

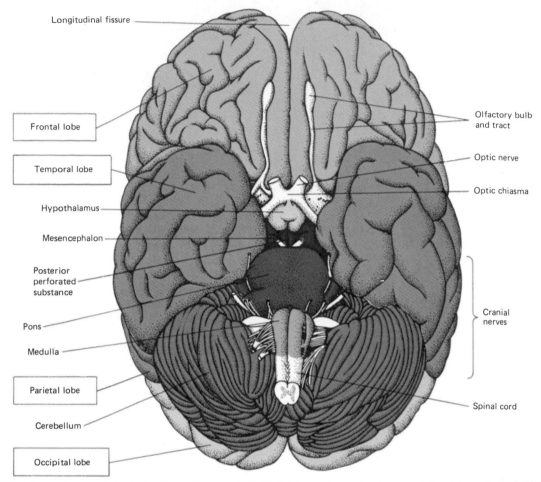

FIGURE 4–2. Basal view of the brain. (From Guyton, A. C.: Basic Neuroscience: Anatomy and Physiology. 2nd ed. Philadelphia, W. B. Saunders, 1991, p. 13.)

skilled movements of a complex nature. In addition to its subcortical connections with the primary motor area, its neurons also have direct connections with the basal ganglia and related nuclei in the brain stem, for example, the reticular formation. Many of the axons from these subcortical centers cross to the opposite side before descending as *extrapyramidal tracts* in the spinal cord. Collectively, the connections from the premotor area to these related nuclei make up the extrapyramidal system, which coordinates gross skeletal muscle activities that are largely automatic in nature. Examples are postural adjustments, chewing, swallowing, gesticulating, and associated movements that accompany voluntary activities. Certain portions of the extrapyramidal tract also have an inhibitory effect on spontaneous movements initiated by the cerebral cortex. They serve to prevent tremors and rigidity. Complete structural and functional separation of the pyramidal and extrapyramidal systems is impossible,

because they are so closely connected in the harmonious work of executing complex coordinated movements (see Fig. 4–3).

Of interest to the PACU nurse is that drugs used to produce neuroleptanesthesia may cause extrapyramidal reactions. More specifically, the neuroleptics such as the phenothiazines, of which chlorpromazine (Thorazine) is the prototypal drug, and the butyrophenones, as typified by droperidol (Inapsine) and haloperidol (Haldol), are known to produce extrapyramidal reactions. There are four types of extrapyramidal reaction: drug-induced parkinsonism, akathisia, acute dystonic reactions, and tardive dyskinesia.

Drug-induced parkinsonism, which can occur from 1 to 5 days after the administration of the neuroleptic drug, is typified by a generalized slowing of automatic and spontaneous movements (bradykinesia), with a masklike facial expression and a reduction in arm movements. The most noticeable signs of the drug-induced

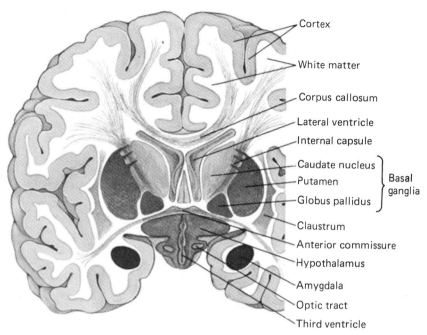

FIGURE 4–3. A coronal section of the cerebrum in front of the thalamus, showing especially the basal ganglia. (From Guyton, A. C.: Basic Neuroscience: Anatomy and Physiology. 2nd ed. Philadelphia, W. B. Saunders, 1991, p. 17.)

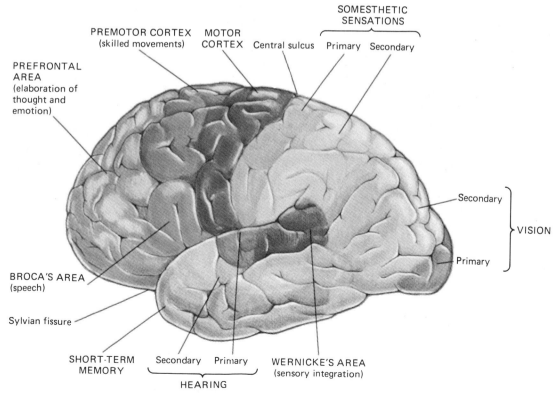

FIGURE 4–4. The functional areas of the cerebral cortex. (From Guyton, A. C.: Basic Neuroscience: Anatomy and Physiology. 2nd ed. Philadelphia, W. B. Saunders, 1991, p. 16.)

parkinsonism syndrome are rigidity and oscillatory tremor at rest. Treatment is with antiparkinsonian agents, such as levodopa (Larodopa), trihexyphenidyl (Artane), and benztropine (Cogentin).

Akathisia, which can occur 5 to 60 days after the administration of a neuroleptic drug, is a term that refers to a subjective feeling of restlessness accompanied by a need on the part of the patient to move about and to pace back and forth. Treatment requires a reduction in the dosage of the responsible drug.

Acute dystonic reactions may occur after the administration of some psychotropic drugs and are characterized by torsion spasms such as facial grimacing and torticollis. These reactions are occasionally seen when a phenothiazine is first administered and are associated with oculogyric crises. Acute dystonic reactions may be mistaken for hysterical reactions or seizures and may usually be reversed by anticholinergic antiparkinsonian drugs such as benztropine or trihexyphenidyl.

Tardive dyskinesia is a late-appearing neurologic syndrome that is characterized by stereotypic, involuntary, rapid, and rhythmically repetitive movements, such as continual chewing movements, and darting movements of the tongue. Treatment is not always satisfactory, because antiparkinsonian drugs sometimes exacerbate tardive dyskinesia. Tardive dyskinesia often persists despite discontinuation of the responsible drug.

Two important structural aspects of the premotor area are worth noting for those caring for neurosurgical patients. First, the fibers from both the primary motor and the premotor areas are funneled through the narrow *internal capsule* as they descend to lower areas of the CNS. This is significant because the internal capsule is a frequent site of cerebrovascular accidents. Second, lesions within one side of the internal capsule result in paralysis of the skeletal muscles on the opposite side of the body, owing to the crossing of fibers within the medulla.

The Motor Speech Area. The motor speech area is only one point in the complicated network required to form spoken and written words. It lies at the base of the motor area and slightly anterior to it in the inferior frontal gyrus and is also known as *Broca's area* (see Fig. 4–4). In right-handed people (the majority of the population), the language and speech areas are usually located in the left hemisphere. In those who are left handed, these areas may lie within the right or the left hemisphere.

The Prefrontal Area. The prefrontal area of the frontal lobe lies anterior to the premotor area. It has extensive connections with other cortical areas and is believed to play an important role in complex intellectual activities, such as mathematic and philosophic reasoning, abstract and creative thinking, learning, judgment and volition, and social, moral, and ethical values. The prefrontal area also influences certain autonomic functions of the body through the conduction of impulses directly or indirectly through the thalamus to the hypothalamus, which makes possible certain physiologic responses to feelings such as anger, fear, and lust.

Sensory areas

Sensory information from one side of the body is received by the *general sensory* (or *somesthetic*) *area* of the opposite hemisphere. It is located in the parietal lobe in the area of the postcentral gyrus. Crude sensations of pain, temperature, and touch can be experienced at the level of the thalamus, but true discrimination of these sensations is a function of the parietal cortex. The activities of the general sensory area allow for proprioception; for the recognition of the size, shape, and texture of objects; and for the comparison of stimuli as to intensity and location.

The *auditory area* lies in the cortex of the superior temporal lobe. Each hemisphere receives impulses from both ears. The *visual area* is located in the posterior occipital lobe, where extremely complex transformations in the signals conveyed by the optic nerve occur. The right occipital cortex receives impulses from the right half of each eye, and the left occipital cortex receives impulses from the left half of each eye. It is believed that the *olfactory area* (sense of smell) is located in the medial temporal lobe and that the *gustatory area* (sense of taste) is located nearby at the base of the postcentral gyrus.

Association areas

Large areas of the cortex remain for which no discrete function is known. They are referred to as *association areas*. They play a major role in the integration of the sensory and motor phases of cortical function by providing complex connections between them.

The limbic system

The principal structural and functional units of the limbic system are the two rings of limbic cortex and a number of related subcortical nuclei, the anterior thalamic nuclei, and portions of the basal nuclei (Fig. 4–5). The terms *limbic system*, *limbic lobe*, and *rhinencephalon* are often used interchangeably. In general, the limbic system is concerned with a wide variety of autonomic somatosensory and somatomotor responses, especially those involved with emotional states and other behavioral responses. It is within the limbic system that the benzodiazepine and opiate receptors have been identified (see Chapters 14 and 15).

The limbic system, acting in close concert with the hypothalamus, can evoke a wide variety of autonomic responses, including changes in heart rate, blood pressure, and respiratory rate. It plays an intimate role in the genesis of emotional states, particularly anxiety, fear, and aggression. Stimulation of the limbic system also evokes complex motor responses directly related to feeding behavior. It has been demonstrated that the limbic system has major relationships with the reticular formation of the brain stem and is presumed to have a role in the alerting or arousal process. It is also implicated in the hypothalamic regulation of pituitary activity. It may be associated somehow with the memory process for recent events as well. In addition, it is intimately concerned with complex phenomena such as the control of various biologic rhythms, sexual behavior, and motivation.

The diencephalon

The second major division of the forebrain is the diencephalon (Fig. 4–6). It consists of the thalamus, the epithalamus, the subthalamus, and the hypothalamus. The diencephalon also contains the third ventricle and is almost completely covered by the cerebral hemispheres. This portion of the brain has a primary role in sleep, emotion, thermoregulation, autonomic activity, and endocrine control of ongoing behavioral patterns.

The *thalamus* consists of right and left egg-shaped masses that make up the greatest bulk of the diencephalon and form the lateral wall of the third ventricle. Each thalamus serves as a relay center for all incoming sensory stimuli except taste and smell. These impulses are then grouped and transmitted to the appropriate area of the cerebral cortex. Because of its interconnections with the hypothalamus, the limbic

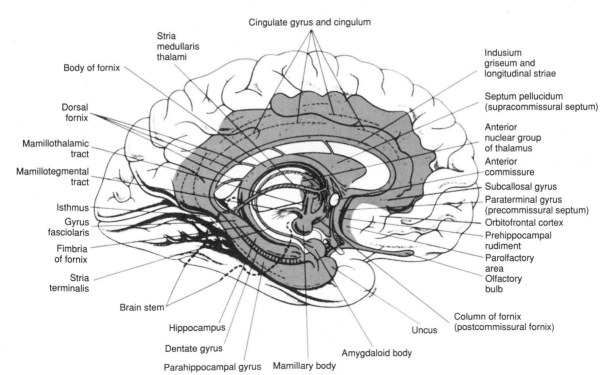

FIGURE 4–5. Anatomy of the limbic system illustrated by the shaded areas of the figure. (From Warwick, R., and Williams, P. L.: Gray's Anatomy. 35th Br. ed. Philadelphia, W. B. Saunders, 1973, p. 930.)

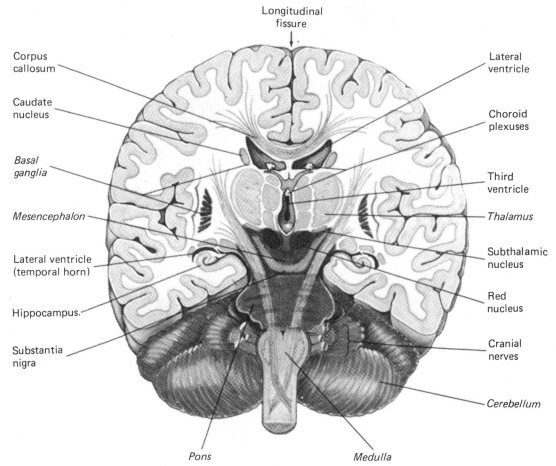

FIGURE 4–6. A coronal view of the cerebrum looking from anterior backward. This section was made immediately anterior to the lower brain stem and through the middle of the thalamus. (From Guyton, A. C.: Basic Neuroscience: Anatomy and Physiology. 2nd ed. Philadelphia, W. B. Saunders, 1991, p. 20.)

system, and the frontal, temporal, and parietal lobes, this structure is also integrally involved with emotional activities, instinctive responses, and attentive processes.

The *epithalamus* contains the pineal body (or gland), which is known to secrete melatonin. Melatonin inhibits gonadal development and regulates estrus. Its most important function is to slow maturation. It is believed that melatonin has its greatest effect on brain tissue rather than on the gonads themselves.

Situated below the thalamus and above the midbrain, the *subthalamus* serves as a correlation center for the optic and vestibular impulses. Stimulation of centers in or around the subthalamic nuclei produce the excitation of appropriate patterns of action in the brain stem and spinal cord, which results in rhythmic motions of forward progression necessary in the act of walking. Damage to the subthalamic nuclei on one side is known to cause violent in-

voluntary movements on the limbs of the opposite side of the body, brought about by contractions of their proximal muscles.

The *hypothalamus* is a group of bilateral nuclei that forms the floor and part of the lateral walls of the *third ventricle*. Extremely complex in function, it has extensive connections with the autonomic nervous system as well as with other parts of the CNS. It also influences the endocrine system by virtue of direct and indirect connections with the pituitary gland and the release of its own hormones. In association with these other structures, it participates in the regulation of appetite, water balance, carbohydrate and fat metabolism, growth, sexual maturity, body temperature, pulse rate, blood pressure, sleep, and aspects of emotional behavior. Because of the connection of the hypothalamus with the thalamus and cerebral cortex, it is possible for emotions to influence visceral responses on certain occasions.

The Midbrain

The midbrain, or mesencephalon, is a short, narrow segment of nervous tissue connecting the forebrain with the hindbrain (Fig. 4–7). The midbrain is vital as a conduction pathway and as a reflex control center. Passing through the center of the midbrain is the *cerebral aqueduct*, a narrow canal that serves to connect the third ventricle of the diencephalon with the fourth ventricle of the hindbrain for the circulation of CSF.

The *cerebral peduncles* are located in the anterior portion of the midbrain and consist of multiple projection fibers that connect the cerebral cortex with other structures in the brain stem. Their dorsal aspect (the *tegmentum*) contains the motor nuclei of the oculomotor, trigeminal, and trochlear nerves. The ventral aspect contains the *red nucleus*, a part of the reticular formation, and the origin of a portion of the extrapyramidal system.

The *corpora quadrigemina* is a group of cells divided in the midline and transversely to form four distinct areas, or *colliculi*. The inferior colliculi are vital components of the auditory pathway and are responsible for complex

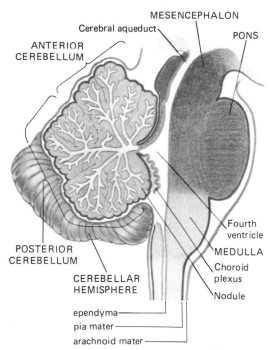

FIGURE 4–8. Relationship of the cerebellum to the brain stem. (From Guyton, A. C.: Basic Neuroscience: Anatomy and Physiology. 2nd ed. Philadelphia, W. B. Saunders, 1991, p. 30.)

acoustic reflexes. The superior colliculi are optic reflex centers.

The centers for postural and righting reflexes are found in the midbrain. The dorsal, or posterior, portion of the midbrain is concerned with visual and auditory reflexes, such as movement of the eyes in accordance with changes in head position, the pupillary light reflex, and turning the head in the direction of a noise. Key structures of the reticular formation also originate in this area. Also, cranial nerves III (oculomotor) and IV (trochlear) originate in the ventral aspect of the midbrain.

The Hindbrain

The hindbrain, or rhombencephalon, consists of the pons, the medulla oblongata, the cerebellum, and the fourth ventricle (Fig. 4–8).

The pons

Lying in front of the fourth ventricle and separating it from the cerebellum, the pons is literally the bridge between the midbrain and the medulla oblongata. It receives many ascending and descending fibers en route to other points in the CNS. It also contains the motor and sensory nuclei of cranial nerves V

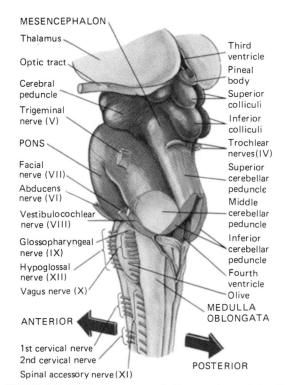

FIGURE 4–7. The brain stem, including portions of the diencephalon, the midbrain, and the hindbrain. (From Guyton, A. C.: Basic Neuroscience: Anatomy and Physiology. 2nd ed. Philadelphia, W. B. Saunders, 1991, p. 26.)

(trigeminal), VI (abducens), VII (facial), and VIII (acoustic). The pontine nuclei of the pons are composed of gray matter. White fiber tracts connect the medulla below with the cerebrum above. These are the so-called *corticospinal tracts.* White fiber (*corticobulbar*) tracts also connect the cerebellum with the pons. The roof of the pons contains a portion of the reticular formation, and the lower pons assists in the regulation of respiration.

The medulla oblongata

The medulla oblongata is an expanded continuation of the spinal cord and is located between the foramen magnum and the pons. It is anatomically complex and not usually amenable to surgery. Many of the white fiber tracts between the brain and spinal cord decussate as they pass through the medulla. Centers for many complex reflexes are located in the medulla oblongata and include those for swallowing, vomiting, coughing, and sneezing. The originating nuclei of cranial nerves IX (glossopharyngeal), X (vagus), XI (accessory), and XII (hypoglossal) are found in the medulla oblongata (Table 4–1 and Fig. 4–7). Because of this, the medulla plays an essential role in the regulation of cardiac, respiratory, and vasomotor reflexes. Injuries to the medulla, such as those accompanying basal skull fracture, often prove fatal.

The cerebellum

Having two hemispheres and a constricted central portion, the cerebellum overlaps the pons and the medulla oblongata dorsally and is located just below the occipital lobes of the cerebrum. It is separated from the cerebrum by the tentorium above it and has a bilayered cortex composed of gray matter. Beneath the gray matter are white fiber tracts that extend like branches of a tree to all parts of the cortex. Deep within the white matter are masses of gray matter called the *cerebellar nuclei.* These connect the cerebellar hemispheres with each other and with areas in the cerebrum, the hindbrain, and the spinal cord.

The cerebellum has no sensory function and does not initiate movement as the cerebrum does. Functionally, it does coordinate muscle tone and voluntary movements through important connections via the spinal cord with the proprioceptor endings in skeletal muscles, tendons, and joints. In addition, the cerebellum is involved in reflexes necessary for the maintenance of equilibrium and posture, through its connections with the vestibular apparatus of the inner ear. The cerebellum also receives optic and acoustic information, but the anatomic pathways involved have not yet been discerned.

Damage to the cerebellum does not result in paralysis or sensory loss. The outcome of damage depends on which portion of the structure is involved. Damage to one part may result in loss of balance, nystagmus, and a reeling gait (cerebellar ataxia). Damage to another area may cause disturbances in the postural reflexes. Posterior lobe disturbances result in changes in voluntary movements such as discrepancies in force, direction, and range of movements, lack of precision in movements, and, possibly, intention tremors.

The fourth ventricle

The fourth ventricle is a diamond-shaped space between the cerebellum posteriorly and the pons and medulla oblongata anteriorly; it contains CSF.

The Brain Stem

There is some disagreement among authors as to what structures collectively constitute the brain stem. All agree that it includes the *midbrain,* the *pons,* and the *medulla oblongata.* Some believe that the *diencephalon* rightly belongs in the group also. Whichever grouping is used, all functions of each structure within it may be considered to be basic activities of the brain stem. All of the cranial nerves are attached to the brain stem (if the diencephalon is included), with the exception of the olfactory nerve and the spinal portion of the accessory nerve.

The reticular formation

The reticular formation lies within the brain stem (including the diencephalon). An important function of the reticular formation is its action as an intermediary between the upper and lower motor neurons of the extrapyramidal system. In this way it facilitates or augments reflex activity as well as voluntary movements. Its motor neurons can be excitatory or inhibitory in action. For example, by inhibiting extensor muscles, it facilitates the action of flexor muscles.

Every pathway that carries information to the brain also contributes afferent fibers to the reticular formation, so that it is kept well informed about conditions of both the outside

Table 4–1. CRANIAL NERVES AND THEIR FUNCTIONS

Number	Name	Type	Function
I	Olfactory	Sensory	Smell
II	Optic	Sensory	Vision
III	Oculomotor	Mixed—mainly motor	Motion of eye up, in, and down Raising of eyelid Constriction of pupil Accommodation of pupil to distance Proprioceptive impulses
IV	Trochlear	Mixed—mainly motor	Motion of eye down and out Proprioceptive impulses

V	Trigeminal:
	  Ophthalmic branch
	  Maxillary branch
	  Mandibular branch
		Mixed	Motor: muscles of mastication
			Sensory: face, nose, mouth
			Proprioceptive impulses from teeth sockets and
			  jaw muscles

VI	Abducens	Mixed—mainly motor	Outward motion of eye Proprioception from eye muscles

VII	Facial	Mixed—mostly motor; some
		  sensory and autonomic
			Motor: movement of facial muscles, ear, nose, and
			  neck
			Sensory: taste, anterior two thirds of tongue
			Autonomic: secretion of saliva, tears

VIII	Acoustic:
	  Cochlear branch
	  Vestibular branch
		Sensory	Cochlear: hearing
			Vestibular: maintenance of equilibrium and
			  posturing of head

IX	Glossopharyngeal	Mixed—motor, sensory, and
		  autonomic
			Motor: muscles of swallowing
			Sensory: taste, posterior third of tongue; sensation
			  from pharynx
			Autonomic: impulses to parotid glands; decrease
			  blood pressure and pulse

X	Vagus	Mixed—motor, sensory, and
		  autonomic
			Motor, sensory, and autonomic: information to
			  and from larynx, pharynx, trachea, esophagus,
			  heart, and abdominal viscera

XI	Spinal accessory	Mixed—mostly motor	Cranial portion: motor and sensory information to
			  and from voluntary muscles of pharynx, larynx,
			  and palate (swallowing)
			Spinal portion: motor information to
			  sternocleidomastoid and trapezius muscles
			May form components of cardiac branches of
			  vagus

XII	Hypoglossal	Mixed—mostly motor	Motor and sensory information to/from tongue muscles Position sense

world and the internal organs. Efferent impulses leaving the reticular formation travel to the cerebral cortex and to the spinal cord. By virtue of its location in and connections with the brain stem and diencephalon, it participates integrally in their activities.

Another important function of the reticular formation is the activation and regulation of those brain activities related to attention-arousal and consciousness. For this reason, it is often referred to as the *reticular activating system* (RAS).

Damage to the reticular formation results in greatly decreased levels of consciousness. When the cerebral cortex is isolated from the RAS by disease or injury of the upper portion of the midbrain, decerebrate rigidity occurs. This abnormal posturing results from the dom-inant effect of the extensor muscles and a lack of inhibition from opposing motor neurons and flexor muscles. This rigidity is accompanied by a profoundly reduced level of consciousness.

Protection of the Brain

The brain is protected by the cranial bones, the meninges, and the CSF (Figs. 4–9 and 4–10).

The cranial bones

There are eight cranial bones that encase the brain, supporting it and protecting it from most ordinary bumps and jarring. In the adult, immovable fibrous joints, or sutures, fuse these bones together to form the rigid walls of the

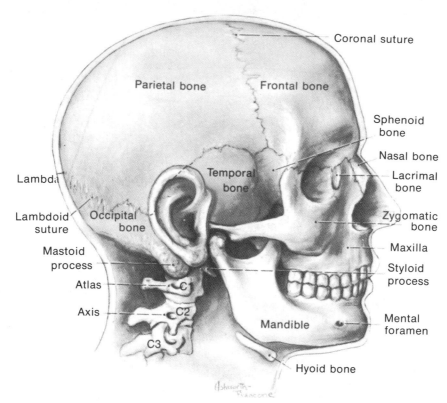

FIGURE 4–9. Lateral view of the skull showing the relationship of the skull and cervical vertebrae to the face. (From Jacob, S. W., Francone, C. A., and Lossow, W. J.: Structure and Function in Man. 5th ed. Philadelphia, W. B. Saunders, 1982, p. 123.)

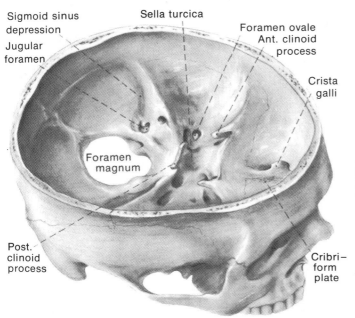

FIGURE 4–10. Interior of the cranial cavity. (From Jacob, S. W., Francone, C. A., and Lossow, W. J.: Structure and Function in Man. 5th ed. Philadelphia, W. B. Saunders, 1982, p. 123.)

box known as the *cranium.* The base of the cranium is both thicker and stronger than its roof or walls.

The bones of the cranium are the frontal, right and left parietal, occipital, sphenoid, ethmoid, and right and left temporal bones. The frontal bone forms the anterior roof of the skull and the forehead. Within the frontal bone are the frontal sinuses, which communicate with the nasal cavities. The parietal bones form much of the top and sides of the cranium. The occipital bone forms the back and a large portion of the base of the skull. The two temporal bones are complicated and form part of the sides and a part of the base of the skull. Their inner surfaces are not as smooth and regular as the bones previously mentioned. Parts of the temporal bones articulate with the condyles of the lower jaw, and air cells in the mastoid portions of the temporal bones communicate with the middle ear. The sphenoid bone occupies a central portion of the floor of the skull. It alone articulates with each of the other cranial bones. Its middle portion contains the sphenoid sinuses, which open into the nasal cavity. The upper portion of the sphenoid bone has a marked saddlelike depression, the sella turcica, which holds the pituitary gland. The ethmoid bone is light and has a spongy structure. It is located between the orbital cavities. It is a cribriform plate that forms the roof of the nasal cavity and part of the base of the cranium. The ethmoid sinuses open into the nasal cavities.

Several features of the cranial bones are particularly noteworthy for the PACU nurse. Among these are the fact that the air cells in the mastoid portion of the temporal bone may become infected secondary to otitis media or following surgery on the middle or inner ear. This mastoiditis may cause severe complications if it extends through the thin plate of bone that separates it from the cranial meninges. Another point of interest is that surgical access to the pituitary gland is commonly accomplished through the sphenoid bone via the nostrils; one example is transsphenoidal hypophysectomy. Finally, nasal suctioning is absolutely contraindicated in the cranial surgery patient because of the danger of perforating the cribriform plate of the ethmoid bone, which would result in leakage of CSF and would permit direct access to the brain by infectious organisms.

There is one main opening at the base of the skull, called the *foramen magnum.* It marks the point at which the brain stem changes structure and becomes identified inferiorly as the spinal cord. Many smaller openings in the skull allow the cranial nerves and some blood vessels to pass through it to and from the face, the jaw, and the neck. The atlas of the vertebral column (the first cervical vertebra) supports the skull and forms a moveable joint with the occipital bone.

The meninges

The meninges (Fig. 4–11) are three fibrous membranes between the skull and the brain and between the vertebral column and the spinal cord. The outer membrane is the dura mater, the inner one is the pia mater, and between them lies the arachnoid mater.

The Dura Mater. The dura mater is a shiny, tough, inelastic membrane that envelops and supports the brain and spinal cord and, by various folds, separates parts of the brain into adjoining compartments. The portion within the skull differs from the dura of the spinal cord in three ways. First, the cranial dura is firmly attached to the skull. The spinal dura has no attachment to the vertebrae. Second, the cranial dura consists of two layers: It not only covers the brain (meningeal dura) but also lines the interior of the skull bones (periosteal dura). Third, the two layers of the cranial dura are in contact with each other in some places but separate in others where the inner layer dips inward to form the protective partitions between parts of the brain. Also, the spaces or channels formed by these separations of dural layers are filled with venous blood leaving the brain and are called *cranial venous sinuses,* an elaborate network unique to the brain (Fig. 4–12; see also Fig. 4–11).

There are three major partitioning folds of the meningeal dura. The falx cerebri separates the right and left hemispheres of the cerebrum. The tentorium cerebelli supports and separates the occipital lobes of the cerebrum from the cerebellum. The falx cerebelli separates the two cerebellar hemispheres. The tentorium separates the posterior cranial chamber from the remainder of the cranial cavity and serves as a line of demarcation for describing the site of a surgical procedure or a lesion as either supratentorial or infratentorial.

Encased between the two dural layers are two major groups of venous channels draining blood from the brain. None of these vascular channels possesses valves, and their walls are extremely thin owing to the absence of muscular tissue. The superior-posterior group consists of one paired and four unpaired sinuses. The anterior-inferior group consists of four paired sinuses and one plexus. The sinuses function to drain venous blood into the internal

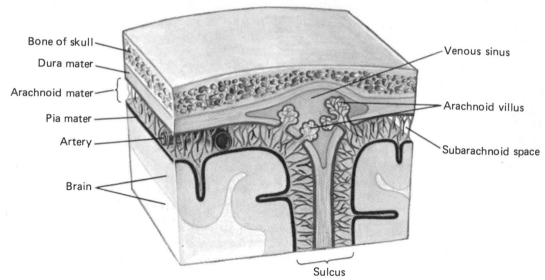

FIGURE 4–11. An expanded view of the meninges covering a section of the brain. Note also the venous sinus with arachnoid villi protruding into it. (From Guyton, A. C.: Basic Neuroscience: Anatomy and Physiology. 2nd ed. Philadelphia, W. B. Saunders, 1991, p. 37.)

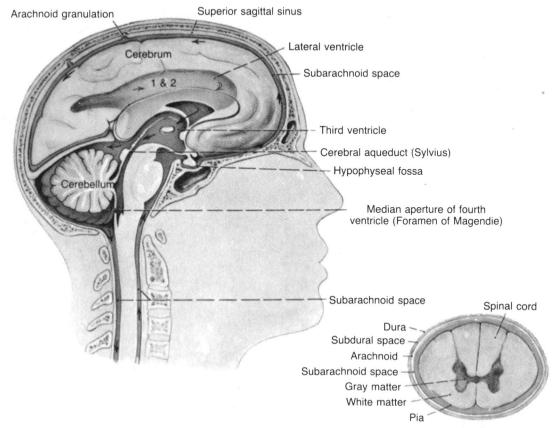

FIGURE 4–12. Circulation of cerebrospinal fluid in the brain and the spinal cord. Note the superior sagittal sinus. (From Jacob, S. W., Francone, C. A., and Lossow, W. J.: Structure and Function in Man. 5th ed. Philadelphia, W. B. Saunders, 1982, p. 262.)

jugular veins, which are the principal vessels responsible for the return of the blood from the brain to the heart (Fig. 4–13).

The Arachnoid. The arachnoid is a fine membrane between the dura mater and the pia mater. Between the arachnoid and the dura is the subdural space, a noncommunicating space filled with CSF. The cerebral blood vessels traversing this space have little supporting structure, making them particularly vulnerable to insult at this point.

The arachnoid forms a type of roof over the pia mater, to which it is joined by a network of trabeculae in the subarachnoid space. It does not follow the depressions of the surface architecture. The arachnoid sends small, tuftlike extensions through the meningeal layer of the dura into the cranial venous sinuses. These are called the *arachnoid granulations* or *arachnoid villi.* The arachnoid villi serve as a pathway for the return of CSF to the venous blood system. Subarachnoid CSF is most abundant in the grooves between the gyri, particularly at the base of the brain, where the more freely communicating compartments form six subarachnoid cisternae, or reservoirs.

The Pia Mater. The inner layer of the meninges, the pia mater, is a fine membrane rich in

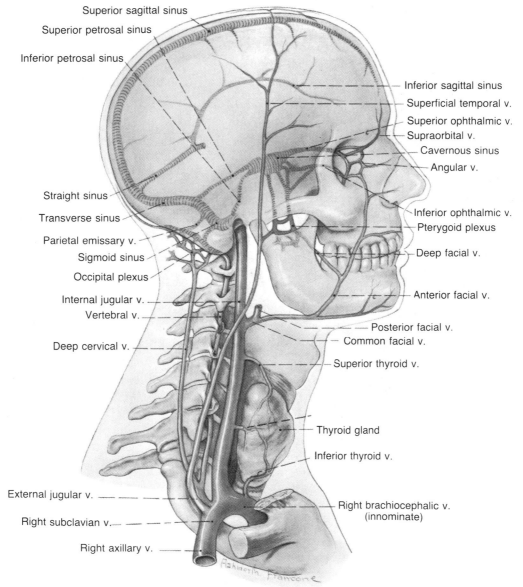

FIGURE 4–13. Venous drainage of the brain, head, and neck. (From Jacob, S. W., Francone, C. A., and Lossow, W. J.: Structure and Function in Man. 5th ed. Philadelphia, W. B. Saunders, 1982, p. 406.)

blood (choroid) plexuses and mesothelial cells. It is closely associated with the arachnoid and covers the brain intimately, following the invaginations and convolutions of the brain surface. The veins of the brain lie between thread-like trabeculae in the subarachnoid space. Branches of the cortical arteries in the subarachnoid space are carried with the pia mater and enter the brain substance itself (Fig. 4–14).

The cerebrospinal fluid system

The CSF is a clear, colorless, watery fluid with a specific gravity of 1.007. A principal function of this fluid is to act as a cushion for the brain. Because both brain tissue and CSF have essentially the same specific gravity, the brain literally floats within the skull. CSF also serves as a medium for the exchange of nutrients and waste products between the blood stream and the cells of the CNS.

CSF is found within the ventricles of the brain, in the cisterns surrounding it, and in the subarachnoid spaces of both the brain and the spinal cord (Figs. 4–15 and 4–16). Largest of the cisterns is the *cisterna magna,* located beneath and behind the cerebellum.

Although some CSF is formed by filtration through capillary walls throughout the brain's vascular bed, its primary site of formation is in the choroid plexuses within the ventricles. This is achieved by a system of secretion and diffusion. The choroid plexuses are highly vascular, tufted structures composed of many small granular pouches that project into the ventri-

cles of the brain. CSF is formed continuously and is reabsorbed at a rate of approximately 750 ml per day. The net pressure of the CSF is regulated, in part, by a balance between formation and reabsorption.

The four ventricles of the brain communicate directly with each other. The first and second (lateral) ventricles are elongated cavities that lie within the cerebral hemispheres. The third ventricle is a slitlike cavity beneath and between the two lateral ventricles. The fourth ventricle is a diamond-shaped space between the cerebellum posteriorly and the pons and medulla oblongata anteriorly.

The circulation of CSF is as follows: Each lateral ventricle contains a large choroid plexus that forms CSF. From the lateral ventricles, the fluid passes through an interventricular foramen (foramen of Monro) into the third ventricle. Together with the additional fluid formed there, the CSF travels posteriorly through the cerebral aqueduct (aqueduct of Sylvius) into the fourth ventricle, where more fluid is produced. The combined CSF volumes then pass through three openings leading from the fourth ventricle to the cranial subarachnoid space of the cisterna magna. These openings are the two lateral foramina of Luschka and the medial foramen of Magendie. From the cisterna magna, CSF flows freely within the entire subarachnoid space of the brain and spinal cord.

The main route of reabsorption of excess CSF is through the arachnoid villi that project from the subarachnoid spaces into the venous sinuses of the brain, particularly those of the su-

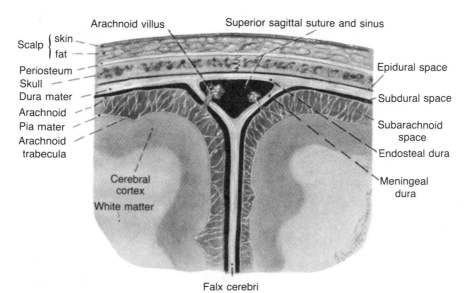

FIGURE 4–14. Coronal section of the skull, brain, meninges, and superior sagittal sinus. (From Jacob, S. W., Francone, C. A., and Lossow, W. J.: Structure and Function in Man. 5th ed. Philadelphia, W. B. Saunders, 1982, p. 263.)

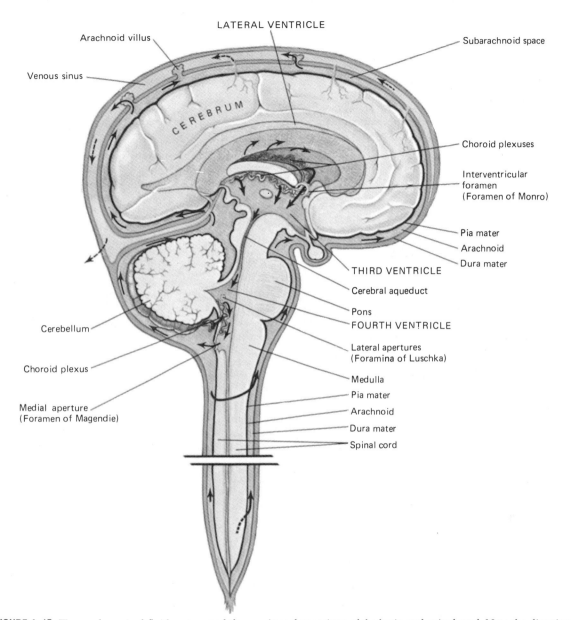

FIGURE 4–15. The cerebrospinal fluid system and the meningeal coverings of the brain and spinal cord. Note the directions of flow of cerebrospinal fluid indicated by the *arrows*. (From Guyton, A. C.: Basic Neuroscience: Anatomy and Physiology. 2nd ed. Philadelphia, W. B. Saunders, 1991, p. 36.)

perior sagittal sinus. The arachnoid villi provide highly permeable regions that allow free passage of CSF, including protein molecules and some small particulate matter contained within it. It is believed that the process of osmosis is mainly responsible for the reabsorption of the fluid.

Blood-brain and blood-CSF barriers of the CNS

Throughout the body, the constancy of the composition of the extracellular fluid is main-

tained by multiple homeostatic mechanisms. Because of the exquisite sensitivity of the neurons in the CNS, additional mechanisms are necessary to prevent the far-reaching consequences that even minor fluctuations in their chemical environment would cause. In health, the unique blood-brain and blood-CSF barriers present in most regions of the CNS have evolved to accomplish this task. The development of the blood-brain barrier occurs gradually during the first several years of childhood.

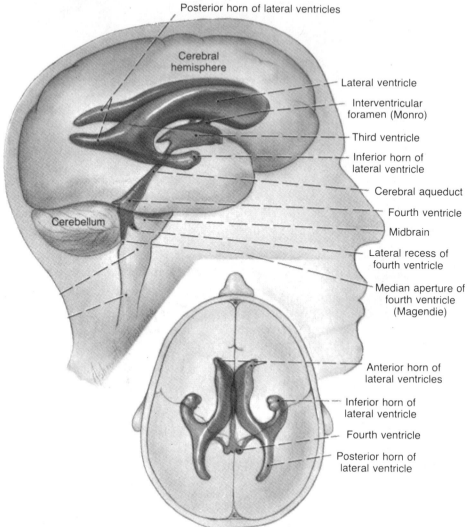

FIGURE 4–16. The ventricular system, lateral and superior views. (From Jacob, S. W., Francone, C. A., and Lossow, W. J.: Structure and Function in Man. 5th ed. Philadelphia, W. B. Saunders, 1982, p. 261.)

The site of the blood-brain barrier is *not* at the surface of the neurons themselves. Rather, it is located between the plasma within the capillaries and the extracellular space of the brain. It is generally believed that the exchange of many physiologically important substances within the capillaries of the CNS is slowed or practically prohibited by several anatomic factors rather than by any single factor alone. It is also likely that these structures form a sequence of morphologic barriers acting in concert to prevent the rapid transport of substances from the blood to the nervous tissue. These include the tight intercellular junctions between the epithelial cells of the capillaries that appear to effectively reduce permeability. There is also a substantial basement membrane surrounding the capillaries and an external membrane provided by the end-feet of the astrocytes between the neurons and the capillaries. These appear to have a major role in retarding or preventing the passage of foreign substances into the brain tissue.

Despite the uncertainty as to the ultimate site of the blood-brain barrier, it has been firmly established that the rapidity with which substances penetrate brain tissue is inversely related to their molecular size and directly related to their lipid solubility. Only water, carbon dioxide, and oxygen cross the blood-brain barrier rapidly and readily, whereas glucose crosses more slowly and by a facilitated transport mechanism. Water-soluble compounds, electrolytes, and protein molecules generally cross slowly. Most general anesthetics effectively cross the blood-brain barrier because of their high lipid solubility.

Of critical importance clinically is the fact that the effectiveness of the blocking mechanism of the blood-brain barrier may break down in areas of the brain that are infected, traumatized, or irradiated or that contain tumors. As effective as the blood-brain barrier is, no substance is completely excluded from reaching the central neurons. Instead, it is the *rate* of transport of substances through the barrier that is of major significance in maintaining the constancy of the internal environment of the brain.

There are a limited number of structures in the brain that have unique capillaries and that are not restricted by the blood-brain barrier. These organs appear to function as chemoreceptors and, as such, must be in intimate contact with the chemical substances within the blood. The posterior pituitary gland is one of these structures. The blood-CSF barrier is located at the choroid plexus. As in the case of the blood-brain barrier, the rate of transport of substances across the blood-CSF barrier is controlled by molecular size and lipid solubility.

The routes whereby substances leave the CSF are different from those by which they enter. They may leave rapidly via the arachnoid villi, regardless of their molecular size or lipid solubility. Alternatively, the bulk circulation of the CSF throughout the brain enhances the direct removal of certain lipid-soluble substances across the blood-brain barrier.

Arterial Blood Supply to the Brain

The entire arterial blood supply to the brain, with the exception of a small amount that flows in the anterior spinal artery to the medulla, is carried through the neck by four vessels: the two *vertebral arteries* and the two *carotid arteries* (Figs. 4–17 and 4–18).

The two vertebral arteries supply the posterior portion of the brain. They ascend in the neck through the transverse foramina on each side of the cervical vertebrae, enter the skull through the foramen magnum, and anastomose near the pons to form the *basilar artery* of the hindbrain. A relatively small volume of the total blood flow to the brain is carried by the vertebral or basilar artery. The *circle of Willis*, in turn, is formed by the union of the basilar artery and the two internal carotid arteries. Before they join the circle of Willis, these arteries send essential branches to the brain stem, cerebellum, and falx cerebelli.

The circle of Willis is a ring of blood vessels that surrounds the optic chiasm and the pituitary stalk. Three pairs of large arterial vessels that supply the cerebral cortex originate from the circle of Willis: the anterior, the middle, and the posterior cerebral arteries. Each pair of arteries supplies specific areas of the brain: (1) the *anterior cerebral arteries* supply about half of the frontal and parietal lobes, including much of the corpus callosum: (2) the *middle cerebral arteries* perfuse most of the lateral surfaces of the hemispheres and send off branches to the corpus striatum and the internal capsule; and (3) the *posterior cerebral arteries* supply the occipital lobes and the remaining portions of the temporal lobes that are not supplied by the middle cerebral arteries.

Intracranial Pressure Dynamics

Intracranial pressure (ICP) is that pressure exerted against the skull by its contents: CSF, blood, and brain. The volumes of these contents may fluctuate slightly, but, despite variations, the total volume and ICP remain nearly constant. Compensatory mechanisms account for this stability in the overall ICP.

In health, the CSF pressure system is a dynamic one, allowing the pressure to vary only slightly by means of a compensatory mechanism that shunts CSF into the spinal subarachnoid space. The spinal dura covers the cord loosely and does not adhere to the vertebrae, which allows it to expand, whereas the cranial dura cannot. When CSF pressure becomes too great within the cranium, owing to an increase in volume of any of its contents, CSF is shunted out of the cranium, decreasing cranial volume and CSF pressure. In addition, CSF may be absorbed at an increased rate, which further aids in maintaining normal pressure.

Autoregulation of cerebral blood volume is another compensatory mechanism responsible for maintaining cerebral perfusion pressure (CPP) at a constant level. It is an alteration in the diameter of the resistance vessels aimed at maintaining a constant perfusion pressure during changes in blood flow. When autoregulation is intact, vasodilatation occurs in response to moderate degrees of hypercapnia, hypoxia, hyperthermia, and increased ICP. The normal ICP ranges from 4 to 15 mm Hg. Normal CPP is 80 to 90 mm Hg.

Under normal conditions, CPP and resultant blood flow are determined by the difference between the inflow and the outflow pressures. Inflow pressures are represented by the mean systemic arterial pressure (MSAP), and under

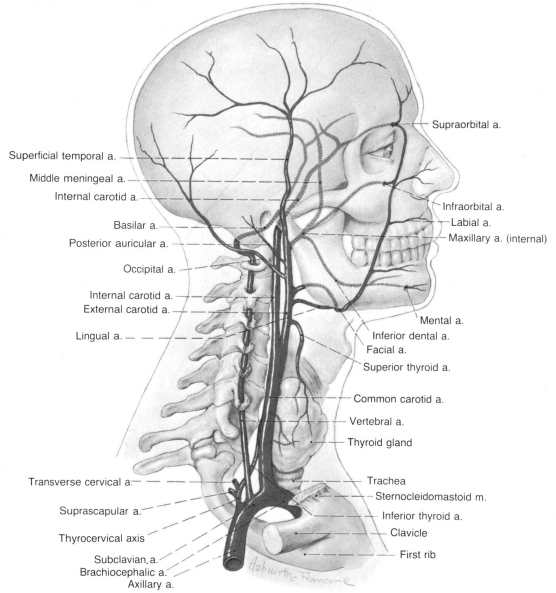

FIGURE 4–17. Arterial supply to the neck and head. (From Guyton, A. C.: Basic Neuroscience: Anatomy and Physiology. 2nd ed. Philadelphia, W. B. Saunders, 1991, p. 405.)

normal conditions the mean outflow pressure is equivalent to the mean venous pressure. In situations in which ICP is greater than venous pressure,

$$CPP = MSAP - ICP$$

It is readily apparent that any increase in ICP or reduction in MSAP will reduce CPP and the resulting cerebral blood flow.

Autoregulation is capable of maintaining a constant CPP only until the finite limit of CSF compensation is reached (Fig. 4–19). The spinal subarachnoid space is capable of holding only a limited amount of fluid and, despite its inability to hold any additional displaced fluid, autoregulation continues. In this event, autoregulation ceases to be beneficial or effective in preventing further increases in ICP.

The Spinal Cord

Protection of the Spinal Cord

The bones of the spine

The spine is composed of a series of irregular bony vertebrae "stacked" one atop the other to

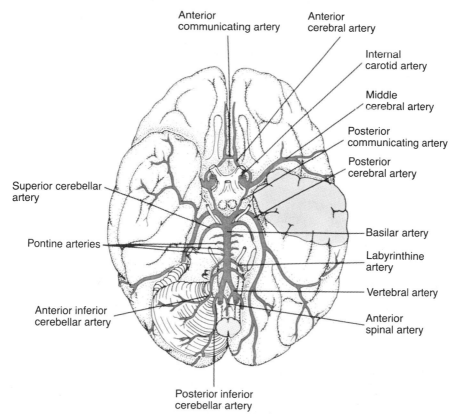

FIGURE 4–18. Major arteries as seen on the base of the brain. (From Burt, A. M.: Textbook of Neuroanatomy. Philadelphia, W. B. Saunders, 1993, p. 179.)

form a strong but flexible column. They are joined by a series of ligaments and intervening cartilages and have two primary functions. Together these structures support the head and trunk. The spine also protects the spinal cord and its 31 pairs of spinal nerve roots by encasing them in a long canal formed by openings in the center of each vertebra. This vertebral canal extends the entire length of the spine and conforms to the various spinal curvatures as well as to the variations in size of the spinal cord itself.

There are 7 cervical, 12 thoracic, and 5 lumbar vertebrae. In the adult, the sacrum consists of five vertebrae fused to form one bone. Similarly, the coccyx results from the fusion of four or five rudimentary vertebrae.

Despite variations in their structure, all but

two vertebrae share certain anatomic and functional aspects. With the exception of C1 and C2, all have a solid drum-shaped *body* anteriorly that serves as the weight-bearing segment. The posterior segment of the vertebra is called the *arch*, and each one consists of two pedicles, two laminae, and seven processes (four articular, two transverse, and one spinous). Projecting from the upper part of the body of each vertebra is a pair of short, thick *pedicles*. The concavities above and below the pedicles are the four *intervertebral notches*. When the vertebrae are articulated, the notches in each adjacent pair of bones form the oval *intervertebral foramina*, which communicate with the vertebral canal and transmit the spinal nerves and blood vessels.

Arising from the pedicles are two broad

FIGURE 4–19. CSF shunting and autoregulation as effective compensatory mechanisms. ICP = intracranial pressure; CPP = cerebral perfusion pressure; CSF = cerebrospinal fluid.

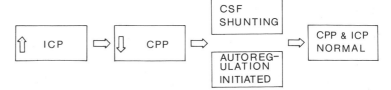

plates of bone, the *laminae*, which meet and fuse at the midline posteriorly to form an arch. Projecting backward and downward from this junction is the *spinous process*, a knobby projection easily palpated under the skin of the back. Lateral to the laminae, near their junction with the pedicles, are paired *articular processes*, which facilitate movement of the vertebral column. The two superior processes of each vertebra articulate with the inferior processes of the vertebra immediately above it. The small surfaces where they articulate are called *facets*. The *transverse processes* are located somewhat anterior to the junction of the pedicles and the laminae. They are between the superior and inferior articular processes. These and the spinous processes provide sites for the attachment of muscles and ligaments. The hollow opening formed by the body of the vertebra and the arch is termed the *vertebral foramen*, a protected space through which the spinal cord passes.

Between each of the vertebrae and atop the sacrum is an *intervertebral disk* composed of compressible, tough, fibrous cartilage concentrically arranged around a soft, pulpy substance called the *nucleus pulposus.* Each disk acts as a cushionlike shock absorber between the vertebrae. When the intervertebral disk is ruptured, the soft nucleus pulposus may protrude into the vertebral canal, where it can exert pressure on a spinal nerve root, causing disturbances in motor and sensory functions. This herniated nucleus pulposus may require surgical excision through a laminectomy, if the herniation is severe enough.

Many important variations exist among the regional vertebrae. For example, the first cervical vertebra, or *atlas*, is ring shaped and supports the cranium. It has no body or spinous process and allows for nodding motion of the head. The second cervical vertebra, or *axis*, is most striking because of the *odontoid process,* or *dens*, that arises perpendicularly to articulate with the atlas and allows rotation of the head. The cervical spine as a whole is extremely mobile and is therefore particularly susceptible to acceleration-deceleration and torsion injuries that hyperflex or hyperextend the neck. Also, the spinal cord is relatively large in this area and therefore sustains damage fairly easily after injury to the cervical spine (Fig. 4–20).

The 12 thoracic vertebrae increase in size as they approach the lumbar area. They are distinctive in that they have facets on their transverse processes and bodies for articulation with the ribs. The thoracic spine is fixed by the ribs, but the lumbar spine is not. This creates a vulnerability that is responsible for an increased incidence of fracture-dislocation at T12, L1, and L2. These injuries are typically found in motor vehicle accident victims who had been wearing lap seatbelts without shoulder restraints.

The five lumbar vertebrae are large and massive because of their prominent role in weight bearing. They have no transverse foramina. The sacrum, with its five fused vertebrae, is large, triangular, and wedge shaped. It forms the posterior wall of the pelvis and articulates with L5, the coccyx, and the iliac portions of the hips. The triangular coccyx is formed by four small segments of bone, the most rudimentary part of the vertebral column.

The spinal meninges

In addition to the bony vertebral column, the spinal cord is covered and protected by the continuous downward projection of the three meninges that perform the same protective function for the brain. The dura mater is the outermost membrane, a strong but loose and expandable sheath of dense, fibrous connective tissue that ends in a blind sac at the end of the second or third segment of the sacrum and protects the cord and the spinal nerve roots as they leave the cord. The dura does not extend beyond the intervertebral foramina. In contrast with the cranial dura, the spinal dura is not attached to the surrounding bone, consists of only one layer, and does not send partitions into the fissures of the cord.

The *epidural space* is located between the outer surface of the dura and the bones of the vertebral canal. It contains a quantity of loose areolar connective tissue and a plexus of veins. The *subdural space* is a potential space that lies below the inner surface of the dura and the arachnoid membrane. It contains only a limited amount of CSF.

The middle meningeal layer is the arachnoid membrane. Thin, delicate, and nonvascular, it is continuous with the cranial arachnoid and follows the spinal dura to the end of the dural sac. For the most part, the dura and arachnoid are unconnected, although they are in contact with each other.

The arachnoid is attached to the pia mater by delicate filaments of connective tissue. The considerable space between these two meningeal layers is called the *subarachnoid space.* It is continuous with that of the cranium and is largest at the lower end of the spinal canal, where it encloses the masses of nerves that form the cauda equina. The spinal subarachnoid space contains an abundant amount of CSF and is capable of expansion to the point of

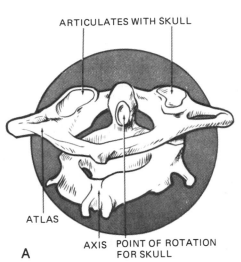

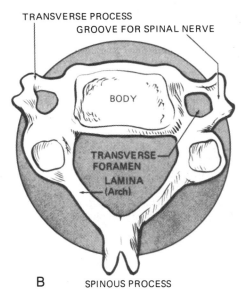

FIGURE 4–20. Types of vertebrae. *A*, cervical vertebrae. *B*, atlas and axis. (Adapted from Synder, M., and Jackle, M.: Neurologic Problems: A Critical Care Nursing Focus. Bowie, MD, Robert J. Brady, 1981.)

completely filling the entire space included in the dura mater. It plays a vital role in the regulation of ICP by allowing for the shunting of CSF away from the cranium. When spinal anesthesia is used, the local anesthetic agent is deposited into the subarachnoid space. Because the CSF in the subarachnoid space bathes the spinal nerves before they exit, the local anesthetic effectively blocks spinal nerve conduction.

The third and innermost meningeal layer of the spine is the delicate pia mater. Although it is continuous with the cranial pia mater, it is less vascular, thicker, and denser in structure than the pia mater of the brain. The pia mater intimately invests the entire surface of the cord and, at the point where the cord terminates, it contracts and continues down as a long, slender filament (central ligament) through the center of the bundle of nerves of the cauda equina and anchors the cord at the base of the coccyx.

Lumbar Puncture. The examination of CSF and determination of CSF pressure are frequently of great value in the diagnosis of neurologic and neurosurgical conditions. The collection of CSF is ordinarily accomplished through the insertion of a long spinal needle between L3 and L4 or L4 and L5, through the dura and arachnoid into the subarachnoid space. Because the spinal cord in adults ends at the level of the disk between L1 and L2, there is minimal danger of injuring the cord through this procedure. In children, the spinal cord may extend below L3 so that the subarachnoid space is usually safely entered in the areas between L4 and L5. In both adults and children, flexion of the spine raises the cord superiorly somewhat farther, minimizing the risk of damage to the cord. Because the most superior points of the iliac crests are at the level of the upper border of the spine of L4, they are used as anatomic reference points in selecting the site for lumbar puncture.

Structure and Function of the Spinal Cord and the Spinal Nerve Roots

It is in the spinal cord that the lowest level of the functional integration of information in the CNS takes place. Here information is received in the form of afferent (sensory) nerve impulses from the periphery of the body. This information may be acted on locally within the cord but more often is relayed to higher brain centers for additional processing and modification, resulting in sophisticated and elaborate motor (efferent) responses. A discussion of the spinal cord involves primarily the consideration of its function as a relay system for both afferent and efferent impulses.

The spinal cord is the elongated, slightly ovoid mass of central nervous tissue that occupies the upper two thirds of the vertebral canal. In the adult, it is approximately 45 cm (17 in.) long, although this varies somewhat from individual to individual depending on the length of the trunk. The cord is actually an inferior extension of the medulla oblongata and begins at the level of the foramen magnum of the occipital bone. From there it continues downward to the upper level of the body of L2, where it narrows to a sharp tip called the *conus medullaris*. From the end of the conus, an extension of the pia mater known as the *filum terminale* continues to the first segment of the coccyx, where it attaches (Fig. 4–21).

The small central canal of the spinal cord contains CSF. This cavity extends the entire length of the cord and communicates above directly with the fourth ventricle of the medulla oblongata.

The spinal cord (Fig. 4–22) is composed of 31 horizontal segments of varying lengths. There are 8 cervical, 12 thoracic, 5 lumbar, 5 sacral, and 1 coccygeal segment, each with a corresponding pair of spinal nerves attached.

During the growth of the fetus and young child, the spinal cord does not continue to lengthen as the vertebral column lengthens. Consequently, the cord segments, from which spinal nerves originate, are displaced upward from their corresponding vertebrae. This discrepancy becomes greater with each downward segment. For example, the cervical and thoracic nerve roots take an almost horizontal course as they leave the spinal cord and emerge through the intervertebral foramina. The lumbar and sacral nerve roots, however, are extremely long and take an oblique, downward course before finally emerging from their

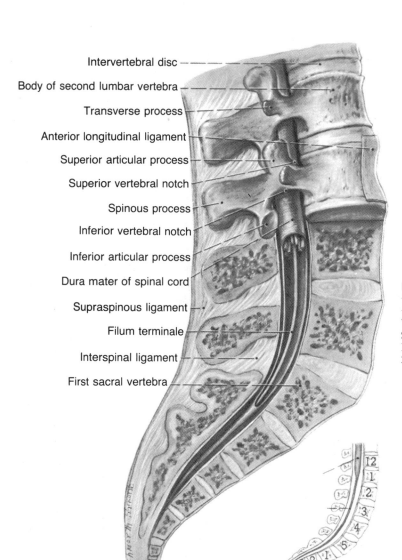

Intervertebral disc
Body of second lumbar vertebra
Transverse process
Anterior longitudinal ligament
Superior articular process
Superior vertebral notch
Spinous process
Inferior vertebral notch
Inferior articular process
Dura mater of spinal cord
Supraspinous ligament
Filum terminale
Interspinal ligament
First sacral vertebra

FIGURE 4–21. Vertebral column showing the structure of vertebrae, filum terminale, termination of dura mater. (From Jacob, S. W., Francone, C. A., and Lossow, W. J.: Structure and Function in Man. 5th ed. Philadelphia, W. B. Saunders, 1982, p. 264.)

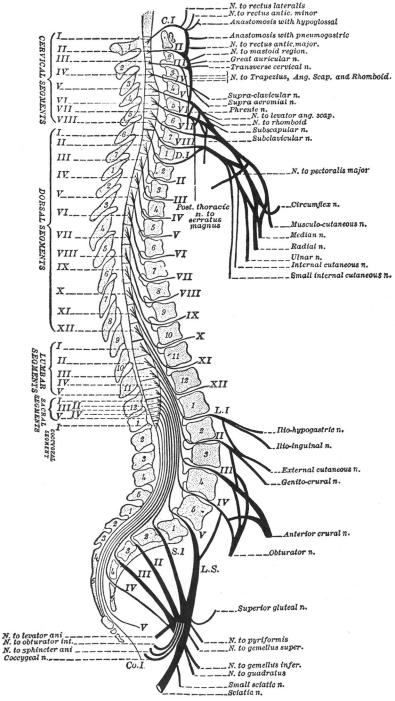

FIGURE 4–22. Relationship of the segments of the spinal cord and their nerve roots to the bodies and spinous processes of the vertebrae. (From Anson, B. J., and McVay, C. B.: Surgical Anatomy. 5th ed. Philadelphia, W. B. Saunders, 1971, p. 934.)

appropriate lumbar or sacral intervertebral foramina. The large bundle of nerves lying within the inferior vertebral canal is called the *cauda equina* for its resemblance to a horse's tail (see Fig. 4–22). Several longitudinal grooves divide the spinal cord into regions. The deepest of these grooves is the anterior median fissure. Opposite this, on the posterior surface of the cord, is the posterior median fissure. These divide the cord into symmetric right and left halves that are joined in the central midportion (Fig. 4–23).

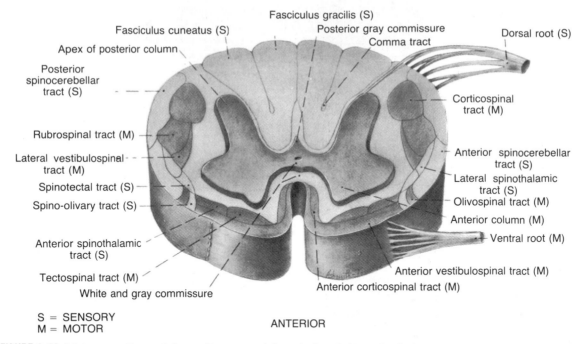

FIGURE 4–23. Major ascending and descending tracts of the spinal cord. (From Jacob, S. W., Francone, C. A., and Lossow, W. J.: Structure and Function in Man. 5th ed. Philadelphia, W. B. Saunders, 1982, p. 268.)

Like the brain, the spinal cord is composed of areas of gray matter and areas of white matter. Unlike their locations in the brain, the gray matter of the cord is situated deep in its center, whereas the white matter is on the surface. The gray matter of the cord is composed of large masses of nerve cell bodies, along with dendrites of association and efferent neurons, and unmyelinated axons, all embedded in a framework of neuroglia cells. It is also rich in blood vessels. The gray matter has two main functions: (1) synapses within the gray matter relay signals between the periphery and the brain, sometimes via the white matter of the cord; and (2) nuclei in the gray matter also function as centers for all spinal reflexes, and even integrate some motor activities within the cord itself (such as the "knee-jerk" stretch reflex).

The white matter of the cord completely invests the gray matter. It consists primarily of long myelinated axons in a network of neuroglia and blood vessels. Its fibers are arranged into bundles called *tracts, columns,* or *pathways* that pass up and down, linking various segments of the cord and connecting the spinal cord with the brain, thus integrating and coordinating sensory and motor functions to or from any level of the CNS.

When viewed in cross section, the gray mat-

ter of the cord looks like the letter H, two crescent-shaped halves joined together by the gray commissure surrounded by white matter. For descriptive purposes, the four segments of the H, are referred to as right and left anterior (ventral) and posterior (dorsal) horns. The *anterior motor (efferent) neurons* lie within the anterior (ventral) gray horns and send fibers through the spinal nerves to the skeletal muscle. The nerve cell bodies making up the posterior (dorsal) gray horns receive sensory (afferent) signals from the periphery via the spinal nerve roots. The lateral gray horns project from the intermediate portion of the H. The nerve cells in these horns (called *preganglionic autonomic neurons*) give rise to fibers that lead to the autonomic nervous system.

The white matter of each half of the cord is divided into three columns (or funiculi): the ventral, the lateral, and the dorsal. Each column is subdivided into tracts, which are large bundles of nerve fibers that are arranged in functional groups. The ascending or sensory projection tracts transmit impulses to the brain, and the descending or motor projection tracts transmit impulses away from the brain to various levels of the spinal cord. Some short tracts travel up or down the cord for only a few segments of the cord. These propriospinal (association or intersegmental) tracts connect and integrate separate cord segments of gray matter with one another and, consequently, have important roles in the completion of various spinal reflexes.

There are 31 pairs of symmetrically arranged spinal nerves. Each nerve contains several types of fibers and arises from the spinal cord by two roots: a posterior (dorsal) and an anterior (ventral) root (Fig. 4–24). The axons that make up the fibers in the anterior roots originate from the cell bodies and dendrites in the anterior and lateral gray horns. The *anterior (ventral) root* is the *motor root,* conveying impulses from the CNS to the skeletal muscles. The *posterior (dorsal) root* is known as the *sensory root.* Sensory fibers originate in the *posterior root ganglia* of the spinal nerves. Each ganglion is an oval enlargement of the root lying just medial to the intervertebral foramen and contains the accumulated cell bodies of the axons making up the sensory fibers. One branch of the ganglion extends into the posterior gray horn of the cord. The other branch is distributed to both visceral and somatic organs and mediates afferent impulses to the CNS. The cutaneous (skin) area innervated by a single posterior root is called a *dermatome.* Knowledge of dermatome levels is useful clinically in determining the level of anesthesia after spinal or regional anesthesia (see Chapter 18).

The lateral gray horns of the spinal cord give rise to fibers that lead into the autonomic nervous system controlling many of the internal (visceral) organs. Sympathetic fibers from the thoracic and lumbar cord segments are distributed throughout the body to the viscera, blood vessels, glands, and smooth muscle. Parasympathetic fibers, present in the middle three sacral nerves, innervate the pelvic and abdominal viscera. Hence, the ventral (anterior) root of the spinal nerve is often referred to as the *motor root,* although it is also responsible for the preganglionic output of the autonomic nervous system.

The anterior and posterior roots extend to the intervertebral foramen corresponding to their spinal cord segment of origin. As they reach the foramen, the two roots unite to form a single mixed spinal nerve containing both motor and sensory fibers. As the nerve emerges from the foramen, it gives off a small meningeal branch that turns back through the same foramen to innervate the spinal cord membranes, blood vessels, intervertebral ligaments, and spinal joint surfaces. The spinal nerve then branches into two divisions that are called *rami.* Each ramus contains fibers from both roots.

The posterior rami supply the skin and the longitudinal muscles of the back. The larger anterior rami supply the anterior and lateral portions of the trunk and all of the structures of the extremities. However, the anterior rami (except those of the 11 thoracic nerves) do not go directly to their destinations. Instead, they are first rearranged without intervening synapses to form intricate networks of nerve fibers called *plexuses.*

There are five major plexuses: cervical, brachial, lumbar, sacral, and pudendal. Peripheral nerves emerge from each plexus and are named according to the region that they supply.

The cervical plexus is composed of the first four cervical spinal nerves. The phrenic nerve is the most important branch of the cervical plexus, because it supplies motor impulses to the diaphragm. Any injury to the spinal cord above the origin of the phrenic nerve (C4) will result in paralysis of the diaphragm and death. Selective anesthesia of the brachial or pudendal plexuses is often used in regional anesthesia. By depositing the local anesthetic at or near the brachial plexus, the musculocutaneous, median, ulnar, and radial nerves can be anesthetized, allowing painless surgery from the elbow to the fingers. The pudendal nerve, which supplies motor and sensory fibers to the perineum, can be anesthetized by a pudendal plexus block. This type of nerve block is effective in relieving some of the pain of childbirth. Among the nerves given off by the lumbar plexus are the ilioinguinal, genitofemoral, obturator, and femoral nerves. Among those given off by the sacral plexus are the superior and the inferior gluteal nerves.

Anterior rami from the thoracic area do not form a plexus but lead instead to the skin of the thorax and to the intercostal muscles directly. The thoracic and upper lumbar spinal nerves also give rise to white rami (visceral efferent branches), or preganglionic autonomic nerve fibers. Parts of this ramus join the spinal nerves to the sympathetic trunk. The gray ramus is present in all spinal nerves.

The term *final common pathway* is often seen in the literature. It refers to the motor neurons in the anterior gray horns. All excitatory or inhibitory impulses controlling movement, from the cerebral cortex to the proprioceptors, influence the motor neurons of the anterior horn either directly or indirectly. Thus, all neural impulses arising in receptors, as well as in the brain and spinal cord, must ultimately converge in this area before movement of skeletal muscle can be integrated. Hence, the term final common pathway.

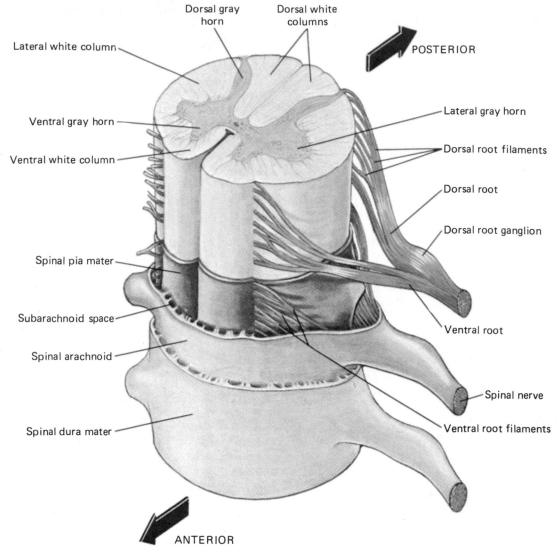

FIGURE 4–24. Structure of the spinal cord and its connections with the spinal nerves by way of the dorsal and ventral spinal roots. Note also the spinal pia mater, spinal arachnoid, and spinal dura mater, which are known as the meninges, or coverings of the spinal cord. (From Guyton, A. C.: Basic Neuroscience: Anatomy and Physiology. 2nd ed. Philadelphia, W. B. Saunders, 1991, p. 33.)

Vascular Network of the Spinal Cord

The spinal cord derives its rich arterial blood supply from the vertebral arteries and from a series of spinal arteries that enter the cord at successive levels. Segmentally, the spinal arteries that enter the intervertebral foramina are given off by the intercostal vessels and by the lateral sacral, iliolumbar, inferior thyroid, and vertebral arteries.

The venous supply inside and outside the entire length of the vertebral canal is derived from a series of venous plexuses that anastomose with each other and end in intervertebral veins. The intervertebral veins leave the cord through the intervertebral foramina with the spinal nerves.

THE AUTONOMIC NERVOUS SYSTEM

The autonomic nervous system is made up of the sympathetic and parasympathetic nervous systems. These two divisions of the autonomic nervous system function to regulate and control the visceral functions of the body. In their regulation and control function, they usually work in opposition of each other.

The Sympathetic Nervous System

The sympathetic nervous system originates from the thoracolumbar (T1 to L2) segments of the spinal cord. This system is mainly excitatory in physiologic function. Because the sympathetic nervous system involves the cardiovascular system and cardiovascular drugs, it is discussed in detail in Chapter 5.

The Parasympathetic Nervous System

The parasympathetic nervous system basically functions as an inhibitor of the sympathetic nervous system. It originates in the cranium via cranial nerves III, V, VII, IX, and X. Cranial nerve X, or the vagus nerve, is the most important nerve because it carries about 75 percent of the parasympathetic nerve impulses. The parasympathetic nervous system also originates in the sacral portion of the spinal cord. Consequently, the parasympathetic nervous system uses the craniosacral outflow tracts. Because of the pharmacologic implications of the parasympathetic nervous system, it is discussed in detail in Chapters 5 and 16.

References

1. Barash, P., Cullen, B. and Stoelting, R.: Clinical Anesthesia. 2nd ed. Philadelphia, J. B. Lippincott, 1992.
2. Bates, B.: A Guide to Physical Examination and History Taking. 5th ed. Philadelphia, J. B. Lippincott, 1991.
3. Campkin, T. and Turner, J.: Neurosurgical Anesthesia and Intensive Care. 2nd ed. New York, Butterworth-Heinemann, 1987.
4. Chusid, J.: Correlative Neuroanatomy and Functional Neurology. 19th ed. Los Altos, CA, Lange Medical Publications, 1985.
5. Conway-Rutkowski, B.: Carini and Owens Neurological and Neurosurgical Nursing. 8th ed. St. Louis, C. V. Mosby, 1982.
6. Cottrell, J., and Turndorf, H.: Anesthesia and Neurosurgery. 2nd ed. St. Louis, Mosby-Year Book, 1986.
7. Cucchiara, R., and Michenfelder, J. (eds.): Clinical Neuroanesthesia. New York, Churchill Livingstone, 1990.
8. Ganong, W.: Review of Medical Physiology. 15th ed. Los Altos, CA, Appleton & Lange Medical Publications, 1991.
9. Guyton, A. C.: Textbook of Medical Physiology. 8th ed. Philadelphia, W. B. Saunders, 1991.
10. Hanlon, K.: Description and use of intracranial pressure monitoring. Heart Lung, 5:277, 1976.
11. Marshall, S. B., Marshall, L. F., Vos, H. R., and Chestnut, R. M.: Neuroscience Critical Care: Pathophysiology and Patient Management. Philadelphia, W. B. Saunders, 1990.
12. Miller, R. (ed.): Anesthesia. 3rd ed. New York, Churchill Livingstone, 1990.
13. Nauta, W., and Feirtag, M.: The organization of the brain. Sci. Am., 241(3):88–111, 1979.
14. Netter, F.: The CIBA Collection of Medical Illustrations. Vol. 1: The Nervous System. Summit, NJ, CIBA Pharmaceutical, 1972.
15. Solomon, E., and Davis, P.: Human Anatomy and Physiology. Philadelphia, W. B. Saunders, 1983.
16. Stoelting, R.: Pharmacology and Physiology in Anesthetic Practice. 2nd ed. Philadelphia, J. B. Lippincott, 1991.
17. Tortora, G., and Anagnostakos, G.: Principles of Anatomy and Physiology. 6th ed. New York, Harper & Row, 1990.
18. Waugaman, W. (ed.): Principles and Practice of Nurse Anesthesia. 2nd ed. Norwalk, CT, Appleton & Lange, 1992.
19. Williams, P., Warwick, R., Dyson, M., et al. (eds.): Gray's Anatomy. 37th ed. New York, Churchill Livingstone, 1989.

Cardiovascular System Anatomy and Physiology

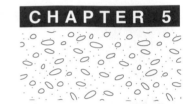

Many drugs used for anesthesia depend on the cardiovascular system to produce their effects. Many of the same drugs also have effects on the cardiovascular system. It is therefore imperative for the post anesthesia care unit (PACU) nurse to understand the physiologic principles relating to the cardiovascular status of the patient who has received an anesthetic.

The basic anatomy of certain structures of the cardiovascular system is not covered completely in this chapter, because basic nursing texts provide ample material on this subject.

Definitions

Adrenergic: a term describing nerve fibers that liberate norepinephrine.

Afterload: the impedance to left-ventricular ejection. The afterload is expressed as total peripheral resistance (TPR).

Angina pectoris: chest pain caused by myocardial ischemia.

Arrhythmia: an abnormal rhythm of the heart, also referred to as dysrhythmia.

Arteriosclerosis: degenerative changes in the arterial walls resulting in thickening and loss of elasticity.

Automaticity: the ability of the cardiac pacemaker cells to undergo depolarization spontaneously.

Bathmotropic: affecting the response of cardiac muscle (or any tissue) to stimuli.

Bigeminy: a premature beat along with a normal heart beat.

Bradycardia: a heart rate of 60 beats per min or less.

Cardiac arrest: ventricular standstill.

Cardiac index: a "corrected" cardiac output used to compare that of patients with different body sizes. The cardiac index (CI) equals the cardiac output (CO) divided by the body surface area (BSA).

Cardiac output: the amount of blood pumped to the peripheral circulation per minute.

Cholinergic: a term describing nerve fibers that liberate acetylcholine.

Chronotropic: affecting the rate of the heart.

Conduction: implies movement of cardiac impulses through specialized conduction systems of the heart that facilitate coordinated contraction of the heart.

Cor pulmonale: pulmonary hypertension due to obstruction of the pulmonary circulation, causing right-ventricular hypertrophy.

Cyanosis: bluish discoloration, seen especially on the skin and mucous membranes, due to a reduced amount of oxygen in the hemoglobin.

Diastole: the period of relaxation of the heart, especially of the ventricles.

Dromotropic: affecting the conductivity of a nerve fiber, especially the cardiac nerve fibers.

Ectopic: located away from a normal position; in the heart, a beat arising from a focus outside the sinus node.

Ectopic pacemaker: focus of ectopic pacemaker is demonstrated as premature contractions of the heart that occur between normal beats.

Electrolyte: an ionic substance found in the blood.

Embolism: a blood clot or other substance, such as lipid material, in the blood stream.

Excitability: the ability of cardiac cells to respond to a stimulus by depolarizing.

Fibrillation: an ineffectual quiver of the atria or ventricles.

Flutter: a condition, usually atrial, in which the atria contract 200 to 400 beats per min.

Heart block (complete): a condition that results when conduction is blocked by a lesion at any level in the atrioventricular junction.

Hypertension: persistently elevated blood pressure.

Hypervolemia: an abnormally large amount of blood in the circulatory system.

Infarction: a necrotic area due to an obstruction of a vessel.

Inotropic: affecting the force of contraction of muscle fibers, especially those of the heart.

Ischemia: local tissue hypoxia due to decreased blood flow.

Leukocytosis: increased number of white blood cells—a white blood cell count higher than 10,000 per mm^3.

Leukopenia: decreased number of white blood cells—a white blood cell count lower than 5000 per mm^3.

Murmur: an abnormal heart sound heard during systole, diastole, or both.

Myocardium: the muscular middle layer of the heart between the inner endocardium and the outer epicardium.

Normotensive: having a normal blood pressure.

Occlusion: an obstruction of a blood vessel by a clot or foreign substance.

Pacemaker: the area in which the cardiac rate commences, normally at the sinoatrial node.

Palpitation: an abnormal rate, rhythm, or fluttering of the heart experienced by the patient.

Paroxysmal tachycardia: a period of rapid heart beats that begins and ends abruptly.

Pericarditis: an inflammation of the pericardium.

Peripheral resistance: resistance to blood flow in the microcirculation.

Polycythemia: an excessive number of red blood cells, which is reflected in an abnormally high hematocrit level.

Pre-excitation syndrome: when the atrial impulse bypasses the atrioventricular node to produce early excitation of the ventricle.

Preload: the left-ventricular end-diastolic volume (LVEDV).

Pulse deficit: the difference between the apical and radial pulses.

Re-entry (circus movement): re-excitation of cardiac tissue by the return of the same cardiac impulse using a circuitous pathway.

Syncope: fainting, giddiness, and momentary unconsciousness, usually caused by cerebral anoxia.

Systole: the period of contraction of the heart, especially the ventricles.

Thrombosis: the formation of a clot (thrombus) inside a blood vessel or a chamber of the heart.

THE HEART

The Cardiac Cycle

The *heart* is a four-chambered mass of muscle that pulsates rhythmically, pumping blood into the circulatory system. The chambers of the heart are the atria and the ventricles. The atria, which are pathways for blood into the ventricles, are thin-walled, have myocardial muscle, and are divided into the right and left atria by a partition. During each cardiac cycle, approximately 70 percent of the blood flows from the great veins through the atria and into the ventricles before the atria contract. The other 30 percent is pumped into the ventricles when the atria contract. On contraction of the right atrium, the pressure in the heart is 4 to 6 mm Hg. The contraction of the left atrium produces a pressure of 6 to 8 mm Hg.

Three pressure elevations are produced by the atria, as depicted on the atrial pressure curve. They are termed the *a, c,* and *v waves* (Fig. 5–1). The a wave is a result of atrial contraction. The c wave is produced by both the bulging of atrioventricular (AV) valves and the pulling of the atrial muscle when the ventricles contract. The v wave occurs near the end of the ventricular contraction as the amount of blood in the atria slowly increases and the AV valves close.

The ventricles receive blood from the atria and then act as pumps to move blood through the circulatory system. During the initial third of diastole, the AV valves open and blood rushes into the ventricles. This is referred to as the period of *rapid filling* of the ventricles. The middle third of diastole is referred to as *diastasis,* during which a small amount of blood moves into the ventricles. It is during the final third of diastole that the atria contract and the other 30 percent of the ventricles fills. As the ventricles contract, the AV valves contract and then close, thereby preventing blood from flowing into the ventricles from the atria.

As the ventricles begin to contract during systole, the pressure inside the ventricles increases but no emptying of the ventricles occurs. During this time, referred to as the period of *isometric contraction,* the AV valves are closed. As the right-ventricular pressure rises above 8 mm Hg and the left-ventricular pressure exceeds 80 mm Hg, the valves open to allow the blood to leave the ventricles. This period, termed the *period of ejection,* consumes the first three quarters of systole. The remaining fourth quarter is referred to as *protodiastole,* when almost no blood leaves the ventricles yet the ventricular muscle remains contracted. The ventricles then relax, and the pressure in the large arteries pushes blood back toward the ventricles, which forces the aortic and pulmonary valves to close. This is the period of *isometric relaxation.*

At the end of diastole, each ventricle usually contains approximately 120 ml of blood. This is

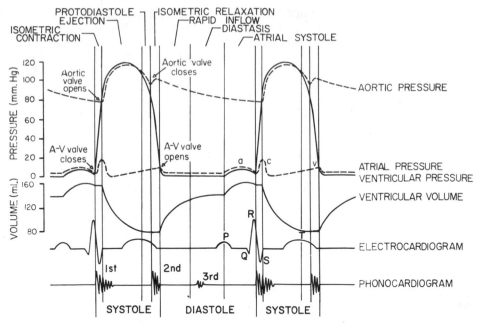

FIGURE 5–1. The events of the cardiac cycle, showing changes in left atrial pressure, left ventricular pressure, aortic pressure, ventricular volume, the electrocardiogram, and the phonocardiogram. (From Guyton, A. C.: Textbook of Medical Physiology. 8th ed. Philadelphia, W. B. Saunders, 1991, p. 102.)

the *end-diastolic volume*. During systole, each ventricle ejects 70 ml of blood, which is the *stroke volume*. The blood that remains in the ventricle at the end of systole is *end-systolic volume* and amounts to approximately 50 ml.

Cardiac Output

Cardiac output is the amount of blood ejected from the left or right ventricle in 1 minute. In the normal adult with a heart rate of 70 beats per min, the cardiac output is approximately 4900 ml. This estimate can be derived by taking the rate of 70 times the stroke volume of 70 ml. "User friendly," sophisticated equipment is now available that makes it possible to monitor a patient's cardiac output in the PACU. The information derived from serial measurements of the cardiac output can be helpful in the assessment of the general status of the cardiovascular system as well as in the determination of the appropriate amount and type of fluid therapy for the patient.

The cardiac output is measured by a variety of techniques. Kaplan suggests that the thermodilution method, employing the Swan-Ganz catheter, is the clinical method of choice. To facilitate a higher degree of reproducibility, Kaplan recommends a technique of standardization in which the injectate temperature and volume, as well as the speed of injection,

should be carefully controlled and duplicated. The most reproducible results have been obtained using injections of 10 ml of cold (1 to 2°C) 5 percent dextrose in water. It should be remembered that the thermodilution technique measures right-sided cardiac outputs. Hence, patients with intracardiac shunts usually have unreliable measurements of their cardiac output when the thermodilution technique is used.

Other methods of calculating the cardiac output are the Fick and Stewart techniques. The *Fick technique* involves calculations of the amount of blood required to carry oxygen taken up from the alveoli per unit of time. This technique is said to be accurate within a 10 percent margin of error. In the *Stewart technique*, a known quantity of dye is injected and its concentration measured after the dye is dispersed per unit of time.

Cardiac output can be influenced by *venous return*. As the *Frank-Starling law* of the heart states, "The heart pumps all the blood that it receives so that damming of the blood does not occur." If the heart receives an extra amount of blood from the veins (↑ preload), the cardiac muscle becomes stretched, and the stretched muscle will contract with an increased force to pump the extra blood out of the heart. If the heart receives less blood than normal (↓ preload), according to the Frank-Starling law of the heart, it will contract with less force. This concept is important to the PACU nurse. For example, if a patient is receiving mechanical ventilation and his or her lungs are being overinflated by too much positive end-expiratory pressure, the venous return to the heart will be impeded by the increased pressure on the inferior vena cava, and this will cause a decrease in the blood pressure. The blood pressure is derived from the following interacting factors: the force of the heart, the peripheral resistance, the volume of blood, the viscosity of blood, and the elasticity of the arteries. Thus, it can be seen that cardiac output plays a major role in the maintenance of a normal blood pressure.

Arterial Blood Pressure

The *arterial blood pressure* consists of the systolic and diastolic arterial pressures. The *systolic blood pressure* is the highest pressure that occurs within an artery during each contraction of the heart. The *diastolic blood pressure* is the lowest pressure that occurs within an artery during each contraction of the heart. The *mean arterial pressure* is the average pressure that pushes blood through the systemic circulatory system. Methods of assessment and monitoring of the arterial blood pressure in the PACU are discussed in Chapter 19.

Some factors that affect the arterial blood pressure are the vasomotor center, the renal system, vascular resistance, the endocrine system, and chemical regulation. The *vasomotor center*, located in the pons and the medulla, has the greatest control over the circulation. This center picks up impulses from all over the body and transmits them down the spinal cord and through vasoconstrictor fibers to most vessels of the body. These impulses may be excitatory or inhibitory. One type of pressoreceptor that sends impulses to the vasomotor center is the *baroreceptor*. The baroceptors are located in the walls of the major thoracic and neck arteries, in particular the arch of the aorta. When these vessels are stretched by an increased blood pressure, they send inhibitory impulses to the vasomotor center, which will result in a lowering of the blood pressure. The aortic and carotid bodies located in the bifurcation of the carotid arteries and along the aortic arch, when stimulated by a low PaO_2, can increase systemic pressure.

The renal regulation of arterial pressure occurs through the renin-angiotensin-aldosterone mechanism (discussed in Chapter 7).

The *vascular resistance* of the systemic vascular system can alter systemic pressure. As the total cross-sectional area of an artery decreases, the systemic vascular resistance increases. Therefore, as the blood flows out of the aorta, a decrease in the arterial pressure in each portion of the systemic circulation is directly proportional to the amount of vascular resistance. This principle is the reason that the arterial pressure in the aorta is much higher than the pressure in the arterioles, which have a small cross-sectional area.

The nervous system, when stimulated by exercise or stress, elevates the arterial pressure via sympathetic vasoconstrictor fibers throughout the body.

When the radial artery is to be cannulated for direct monitoring of blood pressure and sampling of arterial blood gases in the PACU, an *Allen test* should be performed. This test is used to assess the risk of hand ischemia if occlusion of the cannulated vessel should occur. The Allen test is performed by having the patient make a tight fist, which will partially exsanguinate the hand. The nurse then occludes both the radial and the ulnar arteries with digital pressure. The patient is asked to open his or her hand, and the compressed radial artery is then released. Blushing of the palm (postischemic hyperemia) should be observed. After about a minute, the test should be repeated on the same hand with the nurse now releasing the ulnar artery while continuing to compress the radial artery. If the release of pressure over the ulnar artery does not lead to postischemic hyperemia, the contralateral artery should be similarly evaluated. The results of the Allen test should be reported as "refill time" for each artery.

The Valves of the Heart

The *semilunar valves* are the aortic and pulmonary valves. They consist of three symmetric valve cusps, which can open to the full diameter of the ring yet provide a perfect seal when closed. During diastole, they prevent backflow from the aorta and pulmonary arteries into the ventricles.

The *AV valves* are the tricuspid and mitral valves. These valves prevent blood from flowing back into the atria from the ventricles during systole.

Attached to the valves are the *chordae tendineae*, which are attached to the papillary muscles, which in turn are attached to the endocardium of the ventricles. When the ventricles contract, so do the papillary muscles, pulling the valves toward the ventricles to prevent bulging of the valves into the atria (Fig. 5–2).

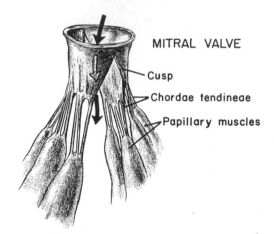

FIGURE 5–2. The mitral valve and its attachments. (From Guyton, A. C.: Textbook of Medical Physiology. 8th ed. Philadelphia, W. B. Saunders, 1991, p. 103.)

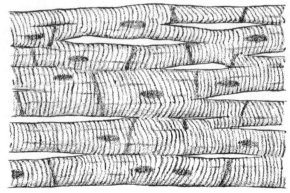

FIGURE 5–3. The "syncytial" nature of cardiac muscle. (From Guyton, A. C.: Textbook of Medical Physiology. 8th ed. Philadelphia, W. B. Saunders, 1991, p. 99.)

The Heart Muscle

The heart muscle is composed of three major muscle types: atrial muscle, ventricular muscle, and excitatory and conductive muscle fibers. The atrial and ventricular muscles act much like skeletal muscles. The excitatory and conductive muscles function primarily as an excitatory system for the heart and a transmission system for conduction of impulses throughout the heart.

The cardiac muscle fibers are arranged in a latticework—they divide and then rejoin. The constriction of the cardiac muscle fibers facilitates action potential transmission. The muscle is striated, and the myofibrils contain *myosin* and *actin filaments.* Cardiac muscle cells are separated by *intercalated disks,* which are actually the cardiac cell membranes that separate the cardiac muscle cells from one another. The intercalated disks do not hinder conductivity or ionic transport between cardiac muscle cells to any great extent. When the cardiac muscle is stimulated, the action potential spreads to excite all the muscles. This is referred to as a *functional syncytium* (Fig. 5–3). It can be divided into *atrial* and *ventricular syncytia,* which are separated by fibrous tissue. However, an impulse can be transmitted throughout the atrial syncytium and then via the *AV bundle* to the ventricular syncytium. The "all-or-none" principle is in effect: when one atrial muscle fiber is stimulated, all the atrial muscle fibers will react if the action potential is met. This principle applies to the entire ventricular syncytium as well.

The main properties of cardiac muscle are excitability (bathmotropism), contractility (ino-

tropism), rhythmicity and rate (chronotropism), and conductivity (dromotropism.) When cardiac muscle is excited, its action potential is reached and the muscle will contract. Certain chemical factors alter the excitability and contractility of cardiac muscle (Table 5–1).

Conduction of Impulses

The heart not only has a special system for generating rhythmic impulses but this system is able to conduct these impulses throughout the heart. This system for providing rhythmicity and conductivity consists of the sinoatrial (SA) node, the AV node, the AV bundle, and the Purkinje fibers (Fig. 5–4). The *SA node* is situated at the posterior wall of the right atrium and just below the opening of the superior vena cava. The SA node generates impulses by self-excitation, which is produced by the interaction of sodium and potassium ions. The SA node provides a rhythmic excitation approximately 72 times per min in the adult at rest. The action potential then spreads throughout the atria to the AV node.

Table 5–1. CHEMICAL FACTORS THAT AFFECT CARDIAC MUSCLE EXCITABILITY AND CONTRACTILITY

Causing Increase
High pH
Alkalosis
High calcium concentration

Causing Decrease
High potassium concentration
High lactic acid concentration
Acidosis

The *AV node* is located at the base of the wall between the atria. Its primary function is to delay the transmission of the impulses to the ventricles. This allows time for the atria to empty before the ventricles contract. The impulses then travel through the *AV bundle,* sometimes referred to as the *bundle of His.* The AV node is able to discharge impulses 40 to 60 times per min if not stimulated by an outside source.

The *Purkinje fibers* originate at the AV node, form the AV bundle, divide into the right and left bundle branches, and spread downward around the ventricles. The Purkinje fibers can transmit the action potential rapidly, thus allowing immediate transmission of the cardiac impulse throughout the ventricles. The Purkinje fibers are able to discharge impulses between 15 and 40 times per min if not stimulated by an outside source.

The parasympathetic nerve endings are distributed mostly at the SA and AV nodes, over the atria, and, to a lesser extent, over the ventricles. If stimulated, they produce a decrease in the rate of rhythm of the SA node and slow the excitability at the AV node. The sympathetic nerves are distributed at the SA and AV nodes and all over the heart, especially the ventricles. Sympathetic stimulation increases the SA node rate of discharge, increases cardiac excitability, and increases the force of contraction.

The Coronary Circulation

The coronary arteries furnish the heart with its blood supply. The main coronary arteries are on the surface of the heart, but smaller arteries penetrate the heart muscle to provide it with nutrients. The inner surface of the heart derives its nutrition directly from the blood in its chambers.

The coronary arteries originate at two orifices just above the aortic valve. The right coronary artery descends by the right atrium and ventricle and usually terminates as the posterior descending coronary artery. The left coronary artery is usually about 1 cm in length and divides into the anterior descending and the circumflex arteries. The anterior descending artery usually terminates at the apex of the heart, anastomosing with the posterior descending artery. The anterior descending artery supplies part of the left ventricle, the apex of the heart, and most of the interventricular septum.

The left circumflex artery descends posteriorly and inferiorly down to and terminates in

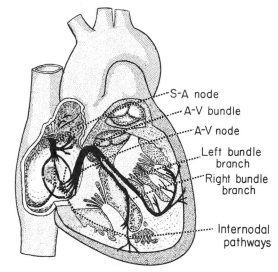

FIGURE 5–4. The sinoatrial node and the Purkinje system of the heart. (From Guyton, A. C.: Textbook of Medical Physiology. 6th ed. Philadelphia, W. B. Saunders, 1981, p. 165.)

the left marginal artery or communicates with the posterior descending coronary artery. Venous drainage is by superficial and deep circuits. The superficial veins empty into either the coronary sinus or the anterior cardiac veins, both of which drain into the right atrium. The deep veins drain into the thebesian or sinusoidal channels.

The regulation of coronary blood flow is determined primarily by the oxygen tension of the cardiac tissues. The most powerful vasodilator of the coronary circulation is hypoxemia. Other factors that may affect coronary blood flow are carbon dioxide, lactate, pyruvate, and potassium, all of which are released from the cardiac muscle. *Coronary artery steal* occurs when there is a significant reduction in collateral perfusion of the myocardium due to an increase in blood flow to a portion of the myocardium that is normally perfused. More specifically, drug-induced vasodilatation of normal coronary arterioles can then divert or steal blood flow from potentially ischemic areas of the myocardium being perfused by the vessels that have increased resistance (atherosclerotic vessels). Coronary artery steal can occur when arteriolar-vasodilating drugs, such as nitroprusside and isoflurane (Forane), are administered. This situation is especially likely to occur in "steal-prone" people. Steal-prone people constitute about 23 percent of the patients with coronary artery disease, especially those patients who have significant stenosis and occlusions to one or more coronary arteries.

Stimulation of the parasympathetic nervous

system causes an indirect decrease in coronary blood flow. Direct stimulation is slight, owing to the sparse amount of parasympathetic nerve fibers to the coronary arteries. The sympathetic nervous system serves to increase coronary blood flow both directly (as a result of the action of acetylcholine and norepinephrine) and indirectly (caused by a change in the activity level of the heart). The coronary arteries have both alpha and beta receptors in their walls (see section on adrenergic and cholinergic receptors).

Because so much cardiac disease involves the coronary arteries, the anesthetic risk increases in patients with cardiac disease. A functional classification of cardiac patients is based on their ability to perform physical activities (Table 5–2). Patients who are classes III and IV represent a significant risk for surgery and anesthesia and should be completely monitored when they receive care in the PACU.

Effect of Anesthesia on the Heart

Research now demonstrates that cardiac dysrhythmias are observed in about 60 percent of all patients undergoing anesthesia. The inhalation anesthestics, such as halothane, enflurane, and isoflurane, can evoke nodal rhythms or increase ventricular automaticity, or both. They also slow the rate of SA node discharge and prolong the bundle of His–Purkinje and ventricular conduction times. Along with these changes in rhythm, alterations in the balance of the autonomic nervous system between the

Table 5–2. FUNCTIONAL CLASSIFICATION OF CARDIAC PATIENTS

Class I: No limitation. Ordinary physical activity does not cause undue fatigue, dyspnea, palpitation, or angina

Class II: Slight limitation of physical activity. Such patients will be comfortable at rest. Ordinary physical activity will result in fatigue, palpitation, dyspnea, or angina

Class III: Marked limitation of physical activity. Less than ordinary activity will lead to symptoms. Patients are comfortable at rest

Class IV: Inability to carry on any physical activity without discomfort. Symptoms of congestive failure or angina will be present even at rest. With any physical activity, increased discomfort is experienced

Reproduced with permission. Perloff, J. K.: The clinical manifestations of cardiac failure in adults. HOSPITAL PRACTICE, 5:43, 1970.

parasympathetic and sympathetic systems due to drugs such as anticholinergics and catecholamines or to light anesthesia can initiate cardiac dysrhythmias. Hence, in the immediate postoperative period, there is a likelihood of cardiac dysrhythmias due to light anesthesia during emergence or from the administration of drugs that alter sympathetic activity. Consequently, continuous monitoring of cardiac rate and rhythm is mandated in the PACU.

Myocardial Infarction

Acute myocardial infarction is a frequently encountered medical emergency that can occur in the PACU. The objectives in the management of a patient with an acute myocardial infarction are to relieve pain, control complications, salvage ischemic myocardium, and return the patient to a productive life. The diagnosis of a myocardial infarction is based on clinical findings, and therapy should be instituted immediately when it is suspected. (Cardiopulmonary resuscitation is discussed in Chapter 45.) An electrocardiogram performed in the PACU may reveal an injury pattern, but a normal electrocardiogram certainly does not exclude a diagnosis of myocardial infarction.

Physical assessment of a patient with a suspected myocardial infarction may include the following subjective findings: (1) pain or pressure, which is usually substernal but may be manifested in the neck, shoulder, jaws, arms, or other areas; (2) nausea; (3) vomiting; (4) diaphoresis; (5) dyspnea; and (6) syncope. The onset of pain may occur with activity but may also occur at rest. The duration may be prolonged, from 30 minutes to several hours. Objective findings may include hypotension, pallor, and anxiety. The blood pressure, pulse, and heart sounds may be normal in the patient who is experiencing an acute myocardial infarction. On auscultation of the chest, the abnormal cardiac findings may include atrial gallop, ventricular gallop, paradoxical second heart sound (S_2), friction rub, and abnormal precordial pulsations.

The electrocardiographic pattern may vary according to the location and extent of the infarction, but myocardial damage may occur without changes in the electrocardiogram. Some typical features of a transmural infarction are acute ST-segment elevation in leads reflecting the area of injury, abnormal Q waves, and T-wave inversion.

The laboratory data usually reflect an elevated sedimentation rate and white blood cell count. The enzymes serum glutamic-oxaloac-etic transaminase, lactic dehydrogenase (LDH), and creatine phosphokinase (CPK) may be elevated. Results of enzymatic studies in the patient with acute myocardial infarction do not indicate a specific cause, because other conditions and disease states may affect these enzymes. LDH and CPK isoenzyme studies may be necessary to differentiate the various disease abnormalities. Intramuscular injections may significantly elevate the level of CPK and therefore should be avoided. Along with this, surgical procedures that involve major trauma to muscle cause an increase in the CPK level postoperatively. Because of the increase in the CPK level associated with surgical trauma, the PACU nurse should use good judgment when evaluating enzyme studies in patients in whom acute myocardial infarction is suspected.

Research studies have demonstrated that patients who have had a myocardial infarction within 6 months before surgery will have a recurrence rate of 54.5 percent for a myocardial infarction that could occur during or after the surgical procedure. If the myocardial infarction occurred between 6 months and 2 years before surgery, the rate of recurrence of infarction is between 20 and 25 percent; in between the second and third years, the incidence of reinfarction is about 5 percent. Most studies indicate that 3 years after the original myocardial infarction, the recurrence rate is about 1 percent, which equals the normal rate of myocardial infarction in the general population. Hence, the chance of a patient's having an acute myocardial infarction in the PACU can be considered significant. This is especially true for PACU patients who have had a myocardial infarction within the last 3 years or who have a documented myocardial infarction risk factor, such as angina, hypertension, and diabetes, or for those with some combination of the above factors.

PACU Nursing Care

The PACU nurse should be constantly alert for complications such as anxiety, arrhythmias, shock, left-ventricular failure, and pulmonary and systemic embolisms. Pain and apprehension may be relieved by morphine sulfate or meperidine hydrochloride (Demerol). Oxygen should be administered by nasal prongs, because a face mask may increase the patient's apprehension. Continuous cardiac monitoring should be instituted, and the patient should be kept in a quiet area. Drugs such as atropine,

lidocaine, digitalis, quinidine, sodium nitroprusside (SNP), phentolamine, and nitroglycerin should be available. A machine for countershock should be immediately available. Fluid therapy and urine output should be monitored completely to prevent fluid overload. A Swan-Ganz catheter or central venous pressure (CVP) monitor may be used to determine fluid replacement in patients with reduced intravascular volume and hypotension (see discussion of CVP catheters in the following section). There is no such thing as a benign myocardial infarction—all patients with a diagnosed myocardial infarction require constant, competent nursing care.

The Central Venous Pressure Monitor

The CVP monitor enhances the assessment of venous return and hypovolemia. More specifically, the CVP monitor assesses the adequacy of central venous return, blood volume, and right-ventricular function. The actual pressure reading obtained from this monitor is a reflection of the pressure in the great veins when blood returns to the heart.

The left-ventricular end-diastolic pressure (LVEDP) serves as a good indicator of left-ventricular preload. Given that a patient has a good ejection fraction, the CVP measurement serves as an approximate value for the LVEDP. However, it should be remembered that the CVP has limited value in assessing left-ventricular hemodynamics.

In the immediate postoperative setting, the CVP remains an excellent parameter to indicate the adequacy of blood volume. In the hypovolemic state, the CVP is decreased. The administration of appropriate fluids and blood to expand the intravascular space increases the CVP toward the patient's baseline reading. In the clinical setting, there is no absolute, predetermined normal value for a CVP reading. The best use of this particular monitoring mode is to gather serial measurements to assess the patient's cardiovascular performance. See Chapter 19 for a complete discussion of the CVP monitor.

The Pulmonary Artery Catheter

The pulmonary artery catheter monitors the central venous, pulmonary artery, and pulmonary capillary wedge pressures. This balloon-tipped catheter with four or five ports is discussed in detail in Chapter 19.

In the immediate postoperative period, the pulmonary artery catheter is usually used for patients with clinical shock, compromised ventricular function, and severe cardiac or pulmonary disease. Along with this, patients who have had extensive surgical procedures or major cardiovascular surgery can benefit from this monitor. Accurate monitoring of left- and right-sided preload along with the rapid determination of cardiac output makes this monitor an excellent parameter to determine mechanical and pharmacologic therapy, with the intended outcome of enhanced cardiac performance and tissue perfusion.

THE CIRCULATORY SYSTEM
The Red Blood Cell

The normal red blood cell is in the form of a biconcave disk, which can change its shape to move through the microcirculation. The major function of the red blood cell is the transport of oxygen to the tissue cells; it is also an important factor in carbon dioxide transport. The red blood cell is responsible for approximately 70 percent of the buffering power of whole blood in maintaining acid–base balance.

Red blood cells are produced by the bone marrow. The normal rate of production is sufficient to form about 1250 ml of new blood per month. This is also the normal rate of destruction. The average life span of a red blood cell is 120 days. The *hematocrit* is the percentage of red blood cells in the blood. The optimal range in adults is between 30 and 42 percent. When the hematocrit is reduced to lower than 30 percent, a steep decline in oxygen-carrying capacity ensues. In addition, when the hematocrit rises higher than 55 percent, a decline in oxygen-carrying capacity will occur, because the increase in blood viscosity causes increased work for the heart and decreased cardiac output. The normal amount of *hemoglobin* in the red blood cell ranges from 10 to 13.5 g. Indeed, it is the amount and type of hemoglobin that determine the oxygen-carrying capacity. Recent evidence indicates that the cutoff value for risk of reduced oxygen-carrying capacity and blood volume is a hemoglobin level of 9 g, a hematocrit of 27 percent, or both. Transfusion with blood or blood products to raise the level of hemoglobin should be strongly considered for any patient with values lower than the cutoff values.

The White Blood Cell

White blood cells, or leukocytes, are the body's major defense against infection. The two primary types of circulating leukocytes are polymorphonuclear leukocytes (PMNs) and lymphocytes. The role of the PMNs in combating infection is to migrate to the infectious site in large numbers and phagocytize the invading microbe. The role of the lymphocytes is to mediate immunoglobulin production and act in the delayed hypersensitivity in the type IV reaction (see Chapter 11). When evaluating the white blood cell count, the number of PMNs should be focused on. When the PMN level is lower than 1000 per mm³, there is an increased incidence of infections. Post anesthesia patients with a PMN level of 500 to 100 per mm³ are at great risk of infection. Some of the major clinical situations that cause a reduction in PMNs (leukopenia) are viral infections, including human immunodeficiency virus, and cancer chemotherapy.

The Blood Platelets

Normal hemostasis requires a proper interaction between blood vessels, platelets, and coagulation proteins. Any dysfunction in any one of the three components has a profound effect on hemostasis. Basically, when a tissue injury occurs, the vessel wall will vasoconstrict and activate the extrinsic pathway for coagulation proteins. Platelet adhesion and aggregation occur along with the activation of the intrinsic and extrinsic pathways for the coagulation proteins. The result of this interaction is a hemostatic plug.

Clinical evaluation for proper coagulation focuses on four tests: bleeding time (BT), platelet count (PC), prothrombin time (PT), and partial thromboplastin time (PTT). The BT and PC are tests to evaluate platelet function, and the PT and PTT are tests to evaluate the coagulation system.

There seems to be a correlation between a prolongation of the BT and surgically related hemorrhage. The normal BT is between 2 and 9 minutes. The test results are considered abnormal when the BT is longer than 12 minutes. The template procedure should be used when the BT is performed, because it is more sensitive than older methods. The normal platelet count is between 200,000 and 450,000 per mm³. More specifically, the patient will usually tolerate surgery and the post anesthesia phase quite well in regard to hemostasis with a platelet count of 100,000 per mm³ or higher. Patients with a platelet count of 50,000 to 100,000 per mm³ may experience ecchymoses due to tissue trauma. If the platelet count is lower than

50,000 per mm³, many alterations in bleeding may occur. These patients require constant evaluation and therapy in the postoperative period.

The PTT is a test that evaluates the intrinsic and common coagulation pathways of the coagulation system. It is most commonly used to monitor heparin therapy. Normal results are considered to be 25 to 32 seconds, depending on the reagent used. Abnormal results are considered to be longer than 35 seconds. The PT examines the extrinsic coagulation system. This test is used to evaluate oral anticoagulant therapy. Normal results are based on laboratory control for interpretation. Usually, the control is normal in patients with an appropriately functioning extrinsic coagulation system. When the value is more than 3 seconds above the control, the test results are considered to be abnormal.

Postoperative bleeding can occur when the patient's preoperative or intraoperative coagulation studies were abnormal. Bleeding tendencies are enhanced by the presence of postoperative hypertension. In addition, when there is a lack of hemostasis at the suture line or extensive surgical tissue trauma, the likelihood of postoperative bleeding is increased. Finally, the use of antibiotics intraoperatively and postoperatively can also increase bleeding tendencies. Therefore, the PACU nurse should evaluate the patient's preoperative and intraoperative coagulation studies and examine the surgical incision for bleeding during the initial assessment of the patient. Certainly, the postoperative trauma patient who has undergone extensive surgical trauma should be constantly monitored for bleeding tendencies, especially if the patient received intraoperative antibiotics. If the patient is receiving anticoagulant therapy, continued monitoring of the anticoagulant activity is mandated. Finally, in the patient in whom a bleeding tendency has been demonstrated, maintenance of a normal arterial blood pressure must be ensured.

The Blood Vessels

The circulatory system can be divided into the *systemic* and the *pulmonary circulation.* The systemic or peripheral circulation is made up of arteries, arterioles, capillaries, venules, and veins.

The walls of the blood vessels, except the capillaries, are composed of three distinct coats: the tunica adventitia, the tunica media, and the tunica intima. The outer layer, the tunica adventitia, consists of white fibrous connective tissue, which gives strength to and limits the distensibility of the vessel. The vasa vasorum, which supplies nourishment to the larger vessels, is in this layer. The middle layer, the tunica media, consists of mostly circularly arranged smooth muscle fibers and yellow elastic fibers. The innermost layer, the tunica intima, is a fine transparent lining that serves to reduce resistance to the flow of blood. The valves of the veins are formed by the foldings of this layer. The capillaries consist of a single layer of squamous epithelial cells, which is a continuation of tunica intima.

The arteries are characterized by elasticity and extensibility. The veins have a poorly developed tunica media and, therefore, are much less muscular and elastic than arteries.

The Microcirculation

Microcirculation is the flow of blood in the finer vessels of the body. It involves the arterioles, capillaries, and venules. The arteries subdivide to the last segment of the arterial system, the arteriole. The *arteriole* consists of a single layer of smooth muscle in the shape of a tube to conduct blood to the capillaries. As the arterioles approach the capillaries, they lack the coating of smooth muscle and are termed *metarterioles.* At the point at which the capillaries originate from the metarterioles, a smooth muscle fiber, the *precapillary sphincter,* encircles the capillary. At the other end of the capillary is the *venule,* which is larger but has a much weaker muscular coat than the arteriole.

The capillaries are usually no more than 8 μ in diameter, which is barely large enough for corpuscles to pass through in single file. Blood moves through the capillaries in intermittent flow, caused by the contraction and relaxation of the smooth muscle of the metarterioles and the precapillary sphincter. This motion is termed *vasomotion.* The metarterioles and precapillary sphincter open and close in response to oxygen concentration in the tissues—a form of local autoregulation.

The microcirculation serves three major functions: (1) transcapillary exchange of nutrients and fluids; (2) maintenance of blood pressure and volume flow; and (3) return of blood to the heart and regulation of active blood volume.

ADRENERGIC AND CHOLINERGIC RECEPTORS

The cardiovascular system and the concept of adrenergic and cholinergic receptors are closely related. It is important for the PACU nurse to have an understanding of the pharmacodynamics of these receptors.

Functional Anatomy: The Mediators

Cholinergic is a term used to describe the nerve endings that liberate acetylcholine. The cholinergic neurotransmitter, acetylcholine, is present in all preganglionic parasympathetic fibers, all preganglionic sympathetic fibers, all postganglionic parasympathetic fibers, and all somatic motor neurons. Two exceptions to the general rule are postganglionic sympathetic fibers to the sweat glands and to the vasculature of skeletal muscle. These are considered sympathetic anatomically but cholinergic in terms of their neurotransmitter; that is, they release acetylcholine as their neurotransmitter.

The term *adrenergic* is used to describe nerves that release norepinephrine as their neurotransmitter. Epinephrine may be present in the adrenergic fibers in small quantities, usually representing less than 5 percent of the total amount of both epinephrine and norepinephrine. The adrenergic fibers are the postganglionic sympathetic fibers, with the exception of the postganglionic sympathetic fibers to the sweat glands and to the efferent fibers to the skeletal muscle (Table 5–3).

The adrenal medulla should be considered separately, in that it is innervated by a preganglionic sympathetic fiber liberating the neurotransmitter acetylcholine; yet, the postganglionic portion is the adrenal medulla, which behaves much like a postganglionic sympathetic fiber. The adrenal medulla is therefore stimulated by acetylcholine, which causes the release of both epinephrine and norepinephrine from its chromaffin cells. As opposed to the usual finding of a preponderance of norepinephrine at the postganglionic nerve fiber terminals, the distribution in the adrenal medulla is 80 percent epinephrine and 20 percent norepinephrine. Therefore, the neurotransmitter of the adrenal medulla is epinephrine.

Cholinergic Neurotransmitter: Biochemistry

The neurotransmitter acetylcholine is synthesized from choline and acetate through the enzymatic activity of choline acetylase to form acetylcholine (Table 5–4); it is then stored in vesicles. When acetylcholine is released from a preganglionic fiber, it may then act on the membrane of the preganglionic fiber with a positive feedback mechanism, enhancing the release of acetylcholine. The calcium ion facilitates this additional release of acetylcholine. This process is referred to as *excitation-secretion coupling* through calcium.

Adrenergic Neurotransmitter: Biochemistry

The adrenergic neurotransmitter, epinephrine, begins in the body as phenylalanine. This is hydroxylated to tyrosine, which is again hydroxylated to form L-dopa, an amino acid. This process is probably the weakest step in the biosynthetic chain and may be a possible site of action of an autonomic drug. A soluble enzyme, L-dopa decarboxylase, acts on L-dopa to form dopamine, which, in turn, is synthesized to norepinephrine. In the adrenal medulla, norepinephrine may be methylated in the cell to form the final product, epinephrine. This reaction is catalyzed by the enzyme phenylethanolamine-N-methyltransferase (see Table 5–4).

The storage site of norepinephrine in the adrenergic nerves appears to be in the intracellular granules. It is difficult to deplete the total content of norepinephrine through continued nerve stimulation, but through continuous chronic drug administration, a clinical hypotensive state may occur owing to the decreased sympathetic vasomotor tone.

The mechanism of release of norepinephrine from the adrenergic fibers and epinephrine from the adrenal medulla appears to be that of reverse pinocytosis. (Pinocytosis is a mechanism by which the membrane engulfs substances in the extracellular fluid.) Under the influence of the appropriate stimuli, an opening is created through which the soluble con-

---

Table 5–3. CHOLINERGIC AND ADRENERGIC NERVES

Mediator: Acetylcholine—Cholinergic Nerves
Effects:
  All preganglionic parasympathetic fibers
  All preganglionic sympathetic fibers
  All postganglionic parasympathetic fibers
  All somatic motor neurons
  Postganglionic sympathetic fibers to sweat glands
  Postganglionic sympathetic vasodilator fibers
    innervating skeletal muscle vasculature

Mediator: Nonepinephrine—Adrenergic Nerves
Effects:
  All postganglionic sympathetic fibers (except those to
    sweat glands and efferent fibers to skeletal muscle)

Adapted from Drain, C. B.: Current concepts on the pharymacodynamics of adrenergic and cholinergic receptors. AANA J., 44:272–280, 1976.

Table 5–4. SYNTHESIS OF NEUROTRANSMITTERS

Cholinergic

$$\text{Choline + Acetate} \xrightarrow{\text{Choline acetylase}} \text{Acetylcholine}$$

Adrenergic

$$\text{Phenylalanine} \longrightarrow \text{Tyrosine} \xrightarrow{\text{Tyrosine hydrolase}} \text{L-dopa}$$

$$\xrightarrow{\text{L-dopa decarboxylase}} \text{Dopamine} \xrightarrow{\text{Dopamine beta oxidase}}$$

$$\text{Norepinephrine} \xrightarrow{\text{Phenylethanolamine-N-methyltransferase}} \text{Epinephrine}$$

From Drain, C. B.: Current concepts on the pharmacodynamics of adrenergic and cholinergic receptors. AANA J., 44:272–280, 1976.

tents of a portion of the storage granules are released. The major means of inactivation of norepinephrine is through a mechanism known as *uptake*, in which the released neurotransmitter is recaptured into the neuronal system by the neuron that released it or by neurons adjacent to it and, in some instances, by neurons associated with tissues some distance from the original site of release.

The norepinephrine that is not recaptured is metabolized eventually to vanillylmandelic acid. Epinephrine also undergoes a number of steps in its biodegradation to vanillylmandelic acid. An increase in vanillylmandelic acid concentration in the urine is useful in the diagnosis of conditions such as pheochromocytoma and neuroblastoma (Fig. 5–5).

When a patient is receiving a drug that is a

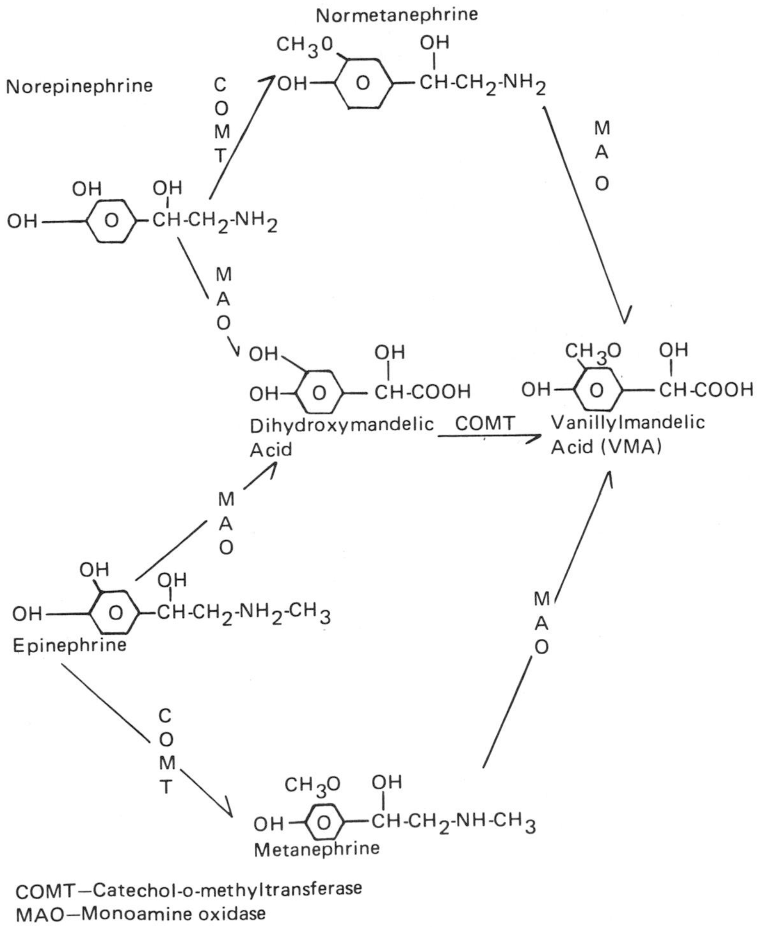

FIGURE 5–5. Metabolism of epinephrine and norepinephrine. (From Drain, C. B.: Current concepts on the pharmacodynamics of adrenergic and cholinergic receptors. AANA J., 44[3]:272, 1976.)

COMT—Catechol-o-methyltransferase
MAO—Monoamine oxidase

monoamine oxidase inhibitor, such as isocar-boxazid (Marplan), pargyline (Eutonyl), phe-nelzine sulfate (Nardil), or tranylcypromine (Parnate), a buildup of epinephrine or norepi-nephrine can occur, leading to sympathetic hy-peractivity. This is especially likely to occur when substances or drugs such as tyramine or indirect-acting vasopressors such as ephedrine are administered.

Cholinergic Receptors

The pharmacologic and physiologic actions of acetylcholine are apparently mediated by its combination with specific cholinergic recep-tors. The actions of acetylcholine and drugs that mimic acetylcholine are mediated through two types of cholinergic receptors: *nicotinic* and *muscarinic*. (For a complete discussion of the cholinergic receptors, see Chapter 16.)

When the nicotinic receptors are stimulated, the following responses are observed:

1. Stimulation of autonomic ganglia—both parasympathetic and sympathetic.
2. Stimulation of the adrenal medulla, result-ing in the release of both epinephrine and norepinephrine.
3. Stimulation of skeletal muscle at the motor end-plate.

The muscarinic responses elicited by muscar-ine as well as acetylcholine are the following:

1. Stimulation or inhibition of smooth muscle in various organs or tissues.
2. Stimulation of exocrine glands.
3. Slowing of cardiac conduction.
4. Decrease in myocardial contractile force.

Nicotinic responses in terms of antagonism can be blocked by drugs such as ganglionic or neuromuscular blocking agents, or both, whereas muscarinic responses are blocked by the class of drugs best typified by atropine.

Muscarine is a specific agonist at muscarinic receptors, whereas nicotine is a specific agonist at nicotinic receptors; however, acetylcholine is capable of stimulating both receptor types (Ta-ble 5–5).

There is a series of compounds specific in their ability to combine with acetylcholinester-ase and inhibit its activity through competitive inhibition. The prototype compounds in this category are neostigmine (Prostigmin), physo-stigmine salicylate (Antilirium), pyridostig-mine (Regonol, Mestinon), and edrophonium (Tensilon, Enlon).

Belladonna alkaloids such as atropine have ad-verse effects that are peculiar to the PACU phase of the surgical experience. More specifi-cally, belladonna alkaloids that cross the blood-brain barrier can cause disorientation, violent behavior, or somnolence. Physostigmine sali-cylate, an anticholinesterase that is capable of penetrating the blood-brain barrier, has been shown to be useful in reversing the adverse effects of belladonna alkaloids on the central nervous system. Physostigmine salicylate is also useful in reversing the disorientation or somnolence caused by drugs such as diaze-pam, the phenothiazines, the tricyclic antide-pressants, the antiparkinsonian drugs, pro-methazine, droperidol, and, in some instances, halothane. Patients in the PACU who may ben-efit from treatment with physostigmine are those who have received a belladonna alkaloid or neuroleptic type of agent either preopera-tively or intraoperatively, who have demon-strated disorientation or restlessness or both for more than 30 minutes after anesthesia, and who are difficult to arouse over an appropriate period. Patients who demonstrate any one of these dysfunctions qualify for treatment and can be given 1-mg increments of physostig-mine intravenously at 15-minute intervals until they are conscious and oriented to time, place, and person. Once treatment has begun, the PACU nurse should monitor the blood pres-sure and pulse immediately before and 5 min-utes after the administration of physostigmine. Also, some patients may experience side effects from physostigmine, such as nausea, pallor, sweating, and bradycardia. Because glycopyr-rolate (Robinul) does not cross the blood-brain barrier, it is especially helpful in treating the side effects of physostigmine. Finally, patients who have been treated with physostigmine probably should remain in the PACU for about 1 hour after the administration of the anticho-linesterase.

Adrenergic Receptors

The stimulation of the sympathetic nervous system can be both inhibitory and excitatory, which has caused considerable confusion. Originally, theories were postulated that this phenomenon dealt with the release of two dif-ferent compounds. It was later discovered that the variation in the effects of stimulation is re-lated not to the differences in chemical release

Table 5–5. CHOLINERGIC RECEPTORS

Organ Stimulated by Cholinergic Agonist	Response	Type of Cholinergic Receptor Response
Heart		
SA node	Negative chronotropic effect	Muscarinic
Atria	Decreased contractility and increased conduction velocity	Muscarinic
AV node and conduction system	Decrease in conduction velocity—AV block	Muscarinic
Eye		
Sphincter muscle of the iris	Contraction (miosis)	Muscarinic
Lung		
Bronchial muscle	Contraction	Muscarinic
Bronchial glands	Stimulation	Muscarinic
Exocrine Glands		
Salivary glands	Profuse, watery secretion	Muscarinic
Lacrimal glands	Secretion	Muscarinic
Nasopharyngeal glands	Secretion	Muscarinic
Adrenal Medulla	Catecholamine secretion	Nicotinic
Autonomic Ganglia	Ganglion stimulation	Nicotinic Muscarinic
Skeletal Muscle		
Motor end-plate	Stimulation	Nicotinic (motor end-plate receptor)

From Drain, C. B.: Current concepts on the pharmacodynamics of adrenergic and cholinergic receptors. AANA J., 44:272–280, 1976.

but rather to a difference in the receptors' responses to the transmitter.

The adrenergic receptors, which respond to catecholamines, can be subdivided into three main types: the dopaminergic, the alpha, and the beta. The *dopaminergic receptors* are primarily in the central nervous system and the mesenteric and renal blood vessels. The agonist for these receptors is dopamine. The *alpha receptors* can be further divided into alpha₁ and alpha₂ receptors. The postsynaptic alpha₁ receptors are excitatory in action, except in the intestine. Stimulation of the alpha₁ receptors causes smooth muscle contraction, which results in a vasoconstriction or pressor response. Hence, the alpha₁ receptor is activated by the release of norepinephrine, and this released norepinephrine also activates the presynaptic alpha₂ receptors to inhibit the further release of norepinephrine. Thus, the alpha₁ receptor is activated by the release of norepinephrine, and the released norepinephrine in turn stimulates the alpha₂ receptor, producing inhibition of the release of norepinephrine, resulting in a negative feedback loop (Fig. 5–6).

It is believed that the drug clonidine (Catapres) stimulates the alpha₂ receptors, which lowers the sympathetic outflow of norepinephrine and ultimately leads to a hypotensive effect. In addition to lowering catecholamine levels, clonidine can reduce the plasma renin

activity. This antihypertensive drug enjoys a significant degree of popularity, but it can have a negative impact on the patient in the PACU. More specifically, the "clonidine withdrawal syndrome" has been reported when the drug has been stopped abruptly. The sequelae of the syndrome resemble pheochromocytoma in that shortly after the withdrawal of the clonidine,

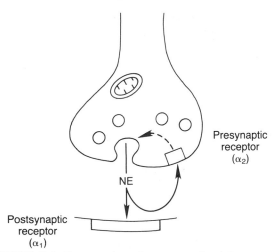

FIGURE 5–6. Presynaptic and postsynaptic alpha receptors at the ending of a norepinephrine-secreting neuron. (Adapted from Ganong, W. F.: Review of Medical Physiology. 12th ed. Palo Alto, Lange Medical Publications, 1985, p. 76).

the patient can experience hypertension, tachycardia, and increased blood levels of catecholamines. Treatment of this syndrome usually involves a reinstitution of the clonidine therapy and alpha-adrenergic blocking agents, such as phentolamine.

Stimulation of the *beta receptor* causes vascular smooth muscle relaxation, which then leads to a decrease in blood pressure through a decrease in peripheral resistance. The beta receptor can be divided into two types: *beta₁* and *beta₂*. Beta₁-subtype receptors are found in all cardiac tissue except the coronary vasculature and are responsible for characteristic effects noted after stimulation of the heart by epinephrine, including (1) increase in heart rate, (2) increase in contractile force, (3) increase in conduction velocity, and (4) shortening of the refractory period. Beta₁-subtype receptors mediate effects elicited by catecholamines (Table 5–6).

The physiology of the beta receptor has many implications for the care of the PACU patient. Once the beta receptor has been activated by "first messengers," which are endogenous catecholamines or exogenous beta agonists such as isoproterenol, certain biochemical events occur (Fig. 5–7). The enzyme adenylate cyclase, which is located on the plasma membrane, is stimulated by beta-receptor activation. Then, within the cell, adenosine triphosphate (ATP) is broken down to 3′,5′-adenosine monophosphate (cyclic AMP). The cyclic AMP is then released into the cytoplasm of the cell and acts to modulate cellular activities. Hence, the cyclic AMP is considered to be the "second messenger." Cyclic AMP is inactivated to 5-AMP by the enzyme phosphodiesterase.

Clinically, isoproterenol or terbutaline may be administered to increase the cyclic AMP levels in the beta₂ receptors in the bronchial airways with the intended result of bronchodilatation. Another way to increase the cyclic AMP levels is to inhibit the action of phosphodiesterase. Caffeine and the methylxanthines, such as aminophylline, are inhibitors of the enzyme

Table 5–6. ADRENERGIC RECEPTORS

Response	Type of Adrenergic Receptor
Heart	
Positive inotropic effect	Beta₁
Positive chronotropic effect	Beta₁
Cardiac arrhythmias	Beta₁
Positive dromotropic effect	Beta₁
Vascular	
Arterial and arteriolar constriction	Alpha₁
Coronary artery constriction	Alpha₁
Coronary artery dilatation	Beta₁
Arteriolar relaxation	Beta₂
Gastrointestinal Tract	
Intestinal relaxation	Alpha₁, beta₁
Sphincter contraction (usually)	Alpha₁
Urinary Bladder	
Bladder relaxation (detrusor)	Beta₂
Bladder contraction (trigone and sphincter)	Alpha₁
Eye	
Contraction (mydriasis)	Alpha₁
Ciliary muscle of iris	Beta₂
Metabolic	
Liver glycogenolysis (hyperglycemia)	Alpha₁, beta₂
Muscle glycogenolysis	Beta₁
Lipolysis	Beta₁
Oxygen consumption (increases)	Beta₁, beta₂
Other Smooth Muscle	
Bronchial (relaxation)	Beta₂
Spleen (contraction)	Alpha₁
Ureter (contraction)	Alpha₁
Uterus (contraction)	Alpha₁
Uterus (relaxation)—nonpregnant condition	Beta₂

Adapted from Drain, C. B.: Current concepts on the pharmacodynamics of adrenergic and cholinergic receptors. AANA J., 44:272–280, 1976.

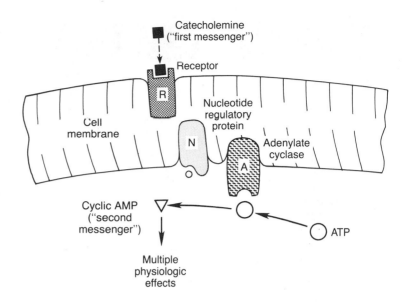

FIGURE 5-7. Catecholamine ("first messenger") binds to the beta-receptor protein, which activates the enzyme adenylate cyclase via the nucleotide regulatory protein, which binds guanosine monophosphate. Via adenylate cyclase, ATP is broken down to cylic AMP. The cyclic AMP, or "second messenger," then activates protein kinase, which ultimately produces a variety of physiologic effects. (Adapted from Catt, K. J., Harwood, J. P., Clayton, R. N., et al.: Regulation of peptide hormone receptors and gonadal steroidogenesis. Recent Prog. Horm. Res., 36:557–662, 1980.)

phosphodiesterase and can be used alone or in combination (for synergistic effects) with the beta agonists to produce the desired bronchodilatation in the patient. It should be remembered that other catecholamine effects are produced by the increase in cyclic AMP levels. Consequently, even though aminophylline is considered a bronchodilator, it does increase the myocardial contractility and heart rate of the patient, thus mandating the PACU nurse to monitor both respiratory and cardiac function when methylxanthines are administered.

The coronary arteries contain alpha$_1$ and beta$_1$ receptors and, therefore, also have the ability to vasoconstrict and vasodilate (see Table 5–6). The endogenous catecholamines, norepinephrine and epinephrine, are capable of stimulating both the alpha and the beta receptors.

Site of Action of Autonomic Drugs

Methyldopa (Aldomet) (the alpha-methylated analogue of L-dopa) is an antihypertensive drug. Methyldopa reduces the sympathetic nerve stimulation through the production of a selective agonist, alpha methylnorepinephrine.

Guanethidine has the ability to prevent nerve stimulation, thus inhibiting norepinephrine release. Guanethidine interferes with the storage of norepinephrine and, if given chronically, results in a decrease in the amount of norepinephrine stored in adrenergic nerves. Reserpine also shares this latter action with guanethidine. Thus, chronic use of guanethidine and reserpine results in a relative deple-

tion of the norepinephrine content from sympathetic nerves (Table 5–7).

Recently, the *calcium channel blockers* have been found to have considerable value in the treatment of supraventricular tachycardias, angina pectoris, and myocardial infarction. The prototype calcium channel blockers are verapamil (Isoptin), nifedipine (Procardia, Adalat), and diltiazem (Cardizem). All three drugs depress calcium entry into conduction tissue and cardiac muscle, which results in a depression of conduction leading to a reduction of the circus movements. These calcium entry blockers produce hypotension by different mechanisms: nifedipine, like SNP, decreases the systemic vascular resistance with a compensatory tachycardia, and verapamil and diltiazem lower the cardiac output by exerting a negative dromotropic effect. The effects of the calcium channel blockers may be enhanced by inhalation anesthesia agents such as halothane. Consequently, in the PACU, patients who received an inhalation anesthetic and are being treated with a calcium channel blocker may experience some hypotension. Hence, the PACU nurse should vigorously monitor the cardiovascular parameters of these patients and report any confirmed hypotension to the attending physician.

Dopamine is a naturally occurring biochemical catecholamine precursor of norepinephrine. It exerts a positive inotropic effect and a minimal chronotropic effect on the heart. Therefore, the contractility of the heart is increased without changing the afterload (total peripheral resistance), which leads to an increase in cardiac output. The increase is in the systolic and pulse pressures, with virtually no effect on the diastolic pressure. Dopamine is not associated

Table 5–7. DRUGS THAT INTERFERE WITH SPECIFIC STEPS IN THE PROCESS OF CHEMICAL (NEUROHUMORAL) TRANSMISSION

	Adrenergic Nerves	Cholinergic Nerves
Synthesis of the mediator	Methyldopa	Hemicholinium
Storage of the mediator	Reserpine	—
Release of the mediator	Guanethidine	Botulinus toxin
Combination of the mediator with its receptor	Phenoxybenzamine (alpha receptor)	Atropine (muscarinic)
	Propranolol (beta receptors)	Nicotine (nicotinic)
Enzymatic destruction of the mediator	Pyrogallol (COMT inhibitor) Tranylcypromine (MAO inhibitor)	Physostigmine (cholinesterase inhibitor)
Prevention of inactivation of the mediator (blocks the uptake)	Cocaine	—
Repolarization of the postsynaptic membrane (persistent depolarization)	—	Succinylcholine

MAO = monoamine oxidase; COMT = catechol-O-methyl transferase.
From Drain, C. B.: Current concepts on the pharmacodynamics of adrenergic and cholinergic receptors. AANA J., 44:272–280, 1976.

with tachyarrhythmias and produces less of an increase in myocardial oxygen consumption than does isoproterenol. Blood flow to peripheral vascular beds may decrease while mesenteric flow increases. One of the major reasons for the increase in the use of dopamine clinically is its dilatation of the renal vasculature. This action is secondary to the inotropic effect and decreased peripheral resistance. Therefore, the glomerular filtration rate is increased along with the renal blood flow and sodium excretion.

Dobutamine (Dobutrex) is synthetically derived from the catecholamine isoproterenol. Consequently, it produces a positive inotropic effect with specificity to the beta$_1$ receptors, resulting in an increase in cardiac output with minimal effects on blood pressure, heart rate, and systemic vascular resistance. The drug is usually administered intravenously in a dose range of 2 to 10 µg per kg per min and is especially useful for patients recovering from cardiopulmonary bypass surgery. Dobutamine is sometimes combined with a vasodilator to reduce afterload in an effort to optimize the cardiac output.

Hypotension Therapy

Hypotension in the immediate postoperative period is of great concern, and it deserves the prompt attention of the PACU nurse. When hypotension is detected in the post anesthesia patient, the nurse should first reaffirm the measurements. An incorrectly placed or sized blood pressure cuff or malfunction of the stethoscope can yield incorrect measurements (see

Chapter 19). If an arterial catheter transducer system is being used, it should be appropriately zeroed and calibrated and the air bubbles should be removed to ensure that artificially low readings are not observed. Also, if the patient is hypothermic or receiving alpha-adrenergic agonists, such as phenylephrine (Neo-Synephrine), he or she may have low blood pressures in the radial and brachial arteries, whereas the central blood pressure will be higher. This difference is because of the peripheral vasoconstriction produced by the alpha-adrenergic drugs.

If the hypotension is confirmed, hypovolemia should be considered as a possible cause. The clinical signs of hypotension due to hypovolemia include cold, pale, clammy, or diaphoretic skin; rapid, thready pulse; shallow, rapid respirations; disorientation, restlessness, or anxiety; decreased CVP; and oliguria. The nursing assessment of the hypotensive patient should include an inspection of the dressings for excessive bleeding and the evaluation of the clinical signs of hypovolemia. If the patient's circulating blood volume is reduced by more than 15 to 20 percent, hypotension can ensue. This usually happens when the patient has not received appropriate fluid volume replacement intraoperatively. Other factors in the development of postoperative hypovolemia are ongoing internal or external hemorrhage, sweating, insensible losses, and "third-space" losses. Third-space losses occur when there is an exudation of fluid into the tissues. Other causes of hypotension include a high alveolar-inflating pressure when a patient is receiving mechanical ventilation, ventricular dysfunction, myocardial ischemia, and cardiac dysrhythmias. If the hypotension is 30 percent below preoperative baseline blood pressure readings, or one or more of the clinical signs of hypovolemia is present, the attending physician should be notified.

Usual therapy for hypotension in the PACU includes the administration of a high fractional concentration of oxygen, fluid infusion, reversal of residual anesthetic depressant effects, repositioning of the patient to facilitate venous return, reduction in ventilator airway pressures, and administration of vasopressors or anticholinergics or both, such as glycopyrrolate or atropine, as indicated. More specifically, the first line of defense is to return the patient to normovolemia and, in this instance, administer a bolus of crystalloid solution of about 300 to 500 ml. The anticholinergics are indicated if sinus bradycardia accompanies the hypotension. The vasopressors exert their effect either directly or indirectly. The direct-acting vasopressor exerts its effect directly on the receptor. Conversely, the pharmacologic action of an indirect vasopressor facilitates the release of norepinephrine from its storage vesicles (primarily the terminal sympathetic nerve fibers), which stimulates the adrenergic receptor to achieve the desired effect. Therefore, a direct-acting vasopressor is probably necessary to achieve a response in patients who are depleted of catecholamines by drugs such as reserpine and guanethidine (Table 5–8).

Another area of consideration when selecting a vasopressor is the cardiotonic action desired. Metaraminol (Aramine), by its action of norepinephrine release, causes improved cardiac function as a result of its beta-receptor activity. Conversely, phenylephrine and methoxamine (Vasoxyl) possess little or no cardiac effect and exert a pressor action by pure alpha stimulation. The alpha-adrenergic agonists are useful especially for patients that have received a "high" spinal or epidural anesthetic. High levels of regional anesthetics are associated with peripheral vasodilatation and bradycardia due to a sympathetic blockade. Consequently, an alpha-adrenergic agonist produces peripheral vascular vasoconstriction, or a mixed-action alpha and beta) drug such as ephedrine can be administered.

A new category of drugs to combat hypotension is the cardiac inotropic agents. This class of drugs produces positive inotropic and vasodilating effects and can be considered to be related to digitalis in regard to pharmacologic effects. The major pharmacologic actions of these drugs include increased cardiac output and decreased LVEDP. These drugs are of benefit for the short-term management of congestive heart failure, especially in patients with congestive heart failure who do not respond adequately to digitalis, diuretics, or vasodilators. Along with this, the inotropic agents may be valuable in the treatment of cardiogenic shock. This class of drugs can be considered as an alternative to catecholamines for the treatment of low cardiac output in the postoperative period. Drugs in this category include amrinone (Inocor) and milrinone. As with other vasopressors, when inotropic agents are administered, constant monitoring of the patient's vital signs is warranted.

Hypertension Therapy

A hypertensive emergency may occur in the PACU. The patient may arrive in a hypertensive state or become hypertensive during the post anesthesia phase. If the diastolic blood pressure rises to about 120 to 140 mm Hg and the patient complains of headache and blurred vision and has papilledema along with disorientation, the physician should be notified immediately.

Before any intervention can be instituted, the cause of the postoperative hypertension must be determined. First, the evaluation should focus on the equipment being used to determine the blood pressure because it may not be functioning correctly. For example, the blood pressure cuff may be too narrow, the transducer may not be calibrated correctly, or there may be transducer overshoot. Next, the evaluation should focus on pre-existing diseases. More specifically, the patient may have essential hypertension, and the blood pressure readings may be "normal" for that patient.

Table 5–8. ADRENERGIC DRUGS ACCORDING TO ACTION

Generic Name	Trade Name
Direct-Acting Adrenergic Amines	
Epinephrine	Adrenalin
Norepinephrine	Levophed
Dopamine	Intropin
Dobutamine	Dobutrex
Isoproterenol	Isuprel
Methoxamine	Vasoxyl
Phenylephrine	Neosynephrine
Indirect-Acting Adrenergic Amines	
Metaraminol	Aramine
Mephentermine	Wyamine
Ephedrine	Ephedrine

Increased sympathetic nervous system activity causes postoperative hypertension. More specifically, pain, stimulation by an endotracheal tube, bladder distention, and pre-eclampsia are some of the clinical phenomena that may lead to hypertension. Postoperative pain should be assessed, because it can cause a significant degree of hypertension. Pain can be eliminated as a causative factor by determining if adequate analgesia exists. If the patient is experiencing a significant amount of pain, an analgesic should be administered immediately. In addition, if the hypertension is due to acute anxiety, the use of sedatives may dramatically reduce the blood pressure. Hypoxemia along with hypercarbia due to hypoventilation is also a common cause of postoperative hypertension. Hence, during the evaluation of the patient, the patient's rate and depth of ventilation should be assessed. If the patient is experiencing hypoventilation, prompt use of the stir-up regimen is mandated. Another assessment tool to use in the evaluation of postoperative hypertension is the amount and degree of hypothermia. More specifically, if the patient is shivering, an accompanying increase in blood pressure will be seen. Prompt interventions to increase the patient's core temperature that will reduce shivering is warranted (see Chapter 43). Assessment of the patient's fluid volume status should be made to determine if he or she is hypervolemic, because fluid overload can cause postoperative hypertension. Also, if the patient has acute pulmonary edema due to hypertensive heart disease, correction of the pulmonary edema usually reduces the blood pressure to acceptable limits. Certainly, a determination should be made to see if a hypertensive emergency exists—if it does, treatment must be started promptly.

If pharmacologic antihypertensive therapy is deemed necessary by the physician, the drugs listed in Table 5–9 usually are instituted. For severe postoperative hypertension, SNP is probably the drug of choice. While the SNP is being prepared, nifedipine (Adalat, Procardia) can be given sublingually. Nifedipine reduces the blood pressure and enhances coronary blood flow, especially in the presence of ischemic heart disease. Also, the use of nifedipine may preclude the use of a central venous catheter that is required when SNP is given. To give nifedipine sublingually, puncture a 10-mg capsule with a pin in several places and squeeze the contents under the tongue. Should SNP be required, the dose is 0.25 to 0.5 μg per kg per min. Once the patient is stabilized, hydralazine 5 to 10 mg and propranolol 0.2 to 0.5 mg may be given in repeated doses intravenously to wean the patient off SNP. Propranolol should be titrated to maintain the heart rate at about 100 beats per min. Other beta blockers, such as labetalol, metoprolol, and esmolol, may be used intravenously. Esmolol may be the drug of choice because of its short duration of action and rapid onset. The hydralazine can be given as intravenous boluses every 20 to 30 minutes to keep the patient normotensive. Because these drugs are extremely potent and have their own complications, they are discussed briefly in the following sections.

Diazoxide (Hyperstat)

Diazoxide is avidly bound to and inactivated by serum proteins and thus must be given as a rapid (within 15 seconds) intravenous bolus of 3 to 5 mg per kg every 5 minutes. After three bolus administrations, if the desired response is still not obtained, use of SNP should be considered. This is the major disadvantage of diazoxide as compared with SNP: diazoxide cannot be titrated in accordance with the patient's response. The onset of action of this drug is within 3 to 5 minutes, and its duration is between 5 and 12 hours. Its action is immediate and is achieved through its direct vasodilating effects. Because it has more effect on the resistance vessels than the capacitance vessels, it decreases the afterload and has no effect on the preload. It is usually advantageous to concurrently administer a loop diuretic, such as furosemide (40 to 80 mg intravenously), especially if the patient is edematous as a result of either cardiac or renal failure.

Sodium Nitroprusside (Nipride)

A compound of unusual chemical structure, SNP is immediately effective in all cases of severe hypertensive crises, including those resistant to diazoxide. Its action is thought to result from the peripheral arteriolar dilatory effect of the drug. Because it can lower blood pressure rapidly, it requires careful intravenous administration with constant bedside arterial pressure monitoring. The drug is extremely light sensitive and must be administered through bottles and tubing that are wrapped and protected from the light. Only fresh solutions should be used. Solutions that are more than 4 hours old should be discarded because they may form thiocyanates. Treatment is started with a solution of 250 ml of 5 percent dextrose in water and 50 mg of SNP (200 μg per ml), using an infusion pump to ensure a precise

Table 5–9. DRUGS USED TO TREAT HYPERTENSIVE CRISIS

Drug*	Route	Initial Dose	Onset of Action (min)	Duration of Action	Comment
Diazoxide (Hyperstat)	IV	3–5 mg/kg slow bolus	3–5	5–12 hr	
Sodium nitroprusside (Nipride, Nitropress)	IV	0.25–0.5 μg/kg/min	1–2	<5 min	Titrate dose for desired effect
Nitroglycerin (Tridil, Nitrol IV, Nitrostat IV)	IV	0.25–3 μg/kg/min	2–5	<5 min	
Phentolamine (Regitine)	IV	5–15 mg bolus; 200–400 mg/L infusion	Immediate	<15 min	Titrate dose for desired effect
Hydralazine (Apresoline)	IV	5–10 mg	15–20	4–6 hr	Given slowly when IV
	IM	10–40 mg	30		
Trimethaphan camsylate (Arfonad)	IV	10–20 μg/kg/min	1	2–4 min	
Propranolol (Inderal, Ipran)	IV	0.1–0.5 mg slowly, up to 2 mg	10	4–6 hr	May repeat dose
Esmolol (Brevibloc)	IV	50–300 μg/kg/min	5	20 min	Avoid concentration >10 mg/ml
Labetalol (Normodyne, Trandate)	IV	0.25 mg/kg	10	4–6 hr	Give slowly
Nifedipine (Procardia, Adalat)	SIV	10 mg	3	7 hr	SIV dose while preparing nitroglycerin
	IV	10 mg (slow)	5–10		
Verapamil (Calan, Isoptin)	IV	2.5–5 mg	2–5	4–6 hr	

*Listed by generic name, with trade name in parentheses.
IV = intravenous; IM = intramuscular; SIV = Slow intravenous infusion.

flow rate. A dose of 1 to 2 μg per kg per min usually produces a prompt decrease in blood pressure, which will return to control levels within 5 minutes after the drug is stopped. Acute postoperative hypertension can be treated with a one-time single intravenous injection of 50 to 100 μg of SNP. The onset of action of this drug is 1 or 2 minutes, and its duration of action is 2 to 5 minutes. Because of its unique chemical structure, cyanide is released into the blood stream when the drug is used. The cyanide is quickly converted to thiocyanate by the liver. Thiocyanate toxicity (fatigue, nausea, anorexia, muscle spasms, and disorientation) may result from prolonged use or from high dosages; therefore, monitoring of serum thiocyanate levels is advised when the drug is used longer than 24 hours. Toxic symptoms appear with serum thiocyanate levels of 5 to 10 mg per dl, and the compound can be rapidly removed by peritoneal dialysis. As with diazoxide, once blood pressure has been brought to control levels, concomitant use of an oral medication such as guanethidine or methyldopa allows the gradual tapering and discontinuance of SNP.

Phentolamine (Regitine)

Phentolamine mesylate, an alpha-receptor blocker, is specifically indicated for managing hypertensive crises associated with increased circulating catecholamines. These crises may result from pheochromocytoma or the sudden release of tissue catecholamine stores caused by certain drugs or foods containing tyramine in patients receiving monoamine oxidase (MAO) inhibitors (pargyline derivatives, primarily Eutonyl). The antipressor effect of a single intravenous injection is short lived, usually lasting less than 15 minutes. Therefore, it is desirable to administer phentolamine by intravenous infusion (200 to 400 g per L), titrating the dosage to achieve the desired pressure level after the blood pressure has been controlled initially by a rapid intravenous dose of 2 to 15 mg. Because the drug blocks only alpha receptors, beta-mediated effects of the circulating catecholamine on the heart must be controlled with the specific beta blocker, propranolol hydrochloride.

With rare exception, these three drugs (diazoxide, SNP, and phentolamine) can be considered the mainstays of modern therapy in acute hypertensive crises. The other drugs discussed here should be considered second-line drugs. Their primary disadvantages include slower onset of action, rapid development of tachyphylaxis, and marked central nervous system depressant effects. In most instances, they should be used to supplement and initiate long-term control once the acute crisis is resolved by the primary drugs.

Hydralazine (Apresoline)

Hydralazine is not effective in hypertensive encephalopathy complicating acute or chronic glomerulonephropathy; it is used in encephalopathy that has chronic essential hypertension as an underlying cause. Blood pressure is reduced through vasodilatation, which reduces vascular resistance. This results in a marked increase in cardiac output and heart rate that can aggravate underlying angina and cardiac failure. The determining factor in this situation is the net change in myocardial oxygen consumption achieved by lowering the elevated afterload. On the other hand, a decrease in blood pressure produced by hydralazine is not accompanied by a commensurate decrease in renal blood flow, so it is especially suited for managing hypertensive emergencies associated with renal insufficiency. The initial intravenous dose of 5 to 10 mg should be given. The onset of action of this drug is 15 to 20 minutes, and the duration is about 4 to 6 hours. Alternatively, the drug dosage may be increase in 5-mg increments up to 20 mg. The maintenance dose depends on patient response but is generally 5 to 10 mg intravenously every 4 to 6 hours.

Trimethaphan Camsylate (Arfonad)

Trimethaphan is a ganglionic vasodepressor that blocks both the sympathetic and parasympathetic systems at the autonomic ganglia. The effect is primarily orthostatic; therefore, large doses must be employed to reduce blood pressure in supine patients. The head of the bed should be elevated (reverse Trendelenburg), if possible, to augment the antipressor action. The dose of this drug is 10 to 20 µg per kg per min. The onset of action is about 1 minute, and the duration of action is 2 to 4 minutes. The 500-mg ampule of trimethaphan is mixed in 250 ml of normal saline, which results in a strength of 2 mg per ml. Complications of such ganglionic blockade include atony of the bowel and bladder and paralytic ileus, especially when the drug is used longer than 24 hours. Because of the commensurate decrease in the glomerular filtration rate when the blood pressure is lowered by the use of this agent, it is not recommended for use in patients for whom renal insufficiency complicates the hypertensive crisis. Its major disadvantage is that it rapidly loses effectiveness after 24 to 72 hours and another agent must be substituted. Use of the drug requires extremely close monitoring by the PACU nurse.

Nitroglycerin

Nitroglycerin is a potent vasodilator that produces relaxation of both arterial and venous smooth muscles. The pharmacologic effects of nitroglycerin are mainly on the venous circulation. It produces an increase in venous capacitance, which leads to a reduction in venous return and a decrease in right atrial and pulmonary capillary wedge pressures. Therefore, the main effect of nitroglycerin is a reduction in the preload. Also, the myocardial oxygen demand is decreased owing to the decrease in myocardial wall tension.

Intravenous nitroglycerin may be indicated to treat myocardial ischemia, to control hypertension, to relieve angina pectoris, and to produce vasodilatation for patients in severe congestive heart failure.

When intravenous nitroglycerin is administered in the PACU, an automated infusion pump should be used. The usual dosage is between 0.25 and 3 µg per kg per min. The onset of action for this drug is 2 to 5 minutes, and the duration of action is between 3 and 5 minutes. The patient should be continuously monitored for hypotension. Should hypotension occur, an alpha agonist, such as methoxamine, may be used to ensure that the patient's coronary perfusion pressure is maintained. *Nitroglycerin migrates into plastic*; hence, the PACU nurse should periodically change the plastic tubing on the automated infusion pump and also ensure that only glass bottles are used for dilution.

Propranolol (Inderal, Ipran)

Propranolol is the prototype beta-blocking drug; consequently, all drugs in this class are compared with propranolol. This drug is known to be nonselective, because it blocks both beta$_1$ and beta$_2$ receptors. After administration of this drug, decreased heart rate, contractility, and cardiac output occur. It can be administered in single intravenous doses of 0.1 to 0.5 mg, with a maximum dose of about 2 mg.

Esmolol (Brevibloc)

Esmolol is a cardioselective, ultrashort-acting, beta-blocking agent with a rapid onset and short duration of action. Because it is cardioselective, esmolol does not appear to affect bronchial or vascular tone at the doses required to reduce the heart rate. This drug has also been shown to blunt the response to endotracheal intubation and can be effective in treating postoperative hypertension. In the treatment of postoperative hypertension, a loading dose of 500 µg per kg should be administered over a 1-minute period. Then, a continuous infusion of 50 to 300 µg per kg per min should be started. The peak response of esmolol occurs in 5 minutes, with a duration of action of about 20 minutes.

Labetalol (Normodyne, Trandate)

Labetalol is a drug that possesses antagonist activity at both the alpha and beta receptors. Given intravenously, it is about seven times more potent on the beta receptors than on the alpha receptors. More specifically, this drug is an $alpha_1$ antagonist and has antagonist activities on both the $beta_1$ and $beta_2$ receptors. For treatment of postoperative hypertension, a loading dose of 0.25 mg per kg should be administered over a 2-minute period. After this, intravenous titration to effect should be done at 10-minute intervals to a total of 300 mg. If a continuous infusion is required, a dose of 2 mg per min can be used.

Metoprolol (Lopressor)

Metoprolol is a beta blocker that can be used in patients with reactive and obstructive lung disease. This is because this drug selectively blocks the $beta_1$ effects and, consequently, blocks the inotropic and chronotropic responses. This selective beta-adrenergic effect is dose related; at high doses, both $beta_1$ and $beta_2$ receptors become blocked and airway resistance may increase. For treatment of postoperative hypertension, an intravenous dose of 2 to 5 mg should be used.

References

1. Litwick, K. (ed.): Core Curriculum for Post Anesthesia Nursing Practice. 3rd ed. Philadelphia, W. B. Saunders, 1994.
2. Alspach, J.: Core Curriculum for Critical Care Nursing. 4th ed. Philadelphia, W. B. Saunders, 1991.
3. Barash, P., Cullen, B. and Stoelting, R.: Clinical Anesthesia. 2nd ed. Philadelphia, J. B. Lippincott, 1992.
4. Benumof, J., and Saidman, L. (eds.): Anesthesia and Perioperative Complications. St. Louis, Mosby-Year Book, 1992.
5. Cullen, D. J.: Recovery room management of the surgical patient. Curr. Rev. Recovery Room Nurses, 3(19):146–151, 1981.
6. Drain, C.: Current concepts on the pharmacodynamics of adrenergic and cholinergic receptors. AANA J., 44:272–280, 1976.
7. Gilman, A., Rall, T., Nies, A., et al. (eds.): Goodman and Gilman's The Pharmacological Basis of Therapeutics. 8th ed. New York, Pergamon Press, 1990.
8. Guyton, A. C.: Textbook of Medical Physiology. 8th ed. Philadelphia, W. B. Saunders, 1991.
9. Kaplan, J.: Cardiac Anesthesia. 2nd ed. Orlando, Grune & Stratton, 1987.
10. Lake, C.: Clinical Monitoring. Philadelphia, W. B. Saunders, 1990.
11. Martin, D., and Hensley, F.: The Practice of Cardiac Anesthesia. Boston, Little, Brown, 1990.
12. Messick, J.: Allen's test—neither positive nor negative. Anesthesiology, 54:523, 1981.
13. Miller, R.: Anesthesia. 3rd ed. New York, Churchill Livingstone, 1990.
14. Orkin, L., and Cooperman, L.: Complications in Anesthesiology. Philadelphia, J. B. Lippincott, 1983.
15. Reves, J.: Myocardial Ischemia and Perioperative Infarction. Anesthesiol. Clin. North Am., 6(3), 1988 (entire issue).
16. Prys-Roberts, C.: Anaesthetic considerations for the patient with coronary artery disease. Br. J. Anaesth., 61(1):85–96, 1988.
17. Stoelting, R.: Pharmacology and Physiology in Anesthetic Practice. Philadelphia, J. B. Lippincott, 1989.
18. Stoelting, R., and Miller, R.: Basics of Anesthesia. 2nd ed. New York, Churchill Livingstone, 1991.
19. Thomas, S.: Manual of Cardiac Anesthesia. 2nd ed. New York, Churchill Livingstone, 1991.
20. Waugaman, W., Foster, S., and Rigor, B. (eds.): Principles and Practice of Nurse Anesthesia. 2nd ed. Norwalk, CT, Appleton and Lange, 1992.
21. Wood, M., and Wood, A. (eds.): Drugs and Anesthesia: Pharmacology for Anesthesiologists. 2nd ed. Baltimore, Williams & Wilkins, 1990.

Respiratory System Anatomy and Physiology

The inhalation anesthetic agents depress respiratory function. They also depend largely on the respiratory system for their removal during emergence from anesthesia. The other anesthetic agents, such as intravenous agents, also depress respiration. Much of the morbidity and mortality that occurs in the post anesthesia care unit (PACU) can be attributed to an alteration in lung mechanics and a dysfunction in airway dynamics. In fact, it is postulated that 70 to 80 percent of the morbidity and mortality occurring in the PACU is associated with some form of respiratory dysfunction. Consequently, a detailed discussion of the many facets of respiratory anatomy and physiology is presented in this chapter. If the PACU nurse incorporates this information into nursing practice, care of the surgical patient in the immediate postoperative period will be enhanced.

Definitions

Acidemia: lower than normal blood pH (increased hydrogen ion concentration).

Acidosis: the process leading to an increase in hydrogen ion concentration in the blood.

Adventitious sounds: abnormal noises that may be heard superimposed on the patient's breath sounds.

Alkalemia: higher than normal blood pH (decreased hydrogen ion concentration).

Alkalosis: the process leading to a decrease in hydrogen ion concentration in the blood.

Apnea: the absence of breathing.

Apneustic breathing: prolonged inspiratory efforts interrupted by occasional expirations.

Atelectasis: collapse of the alveoli.

Bradypnea: respiratory rate in the adult that is lower than 8 breaths per min.

Bronchiectasis: dilatation of the bronchi.

Bronchospasm: constriction of the bronchial airways due to an increase in smooth muscle tone in the airways.

Cheyne-Stokes respirations: periods of apnea alternating with rhythmic, shallow, progressively deeper and then shallower respirations that are associated with brain damage, heart or kidney failure, or drug overdose.

Compliance (lung): a measure of distensibility of the lungs; the amount of change in volume per change in pressure across the lung.

Cyanosis: a sign of poor oxygen transport, characterized by a bluish discoloration of the skin produced when more than 5 g of hemoglobin per dl of arterial blood is in the deoxygenated, or reduced, state.

Dyspnea: a patient's perception of shortness of breath.

Epistaxis: hemorrhage from the nose.

F_{IO_2}: fractional inspired concentration of oxygen.

Hypercapnia: increased tension of carbon dioxide (P_{CO_2}) in the blood.

Hyperoxemia: increased tension of oxygen (P_{O_2}) in the blood.

Hyperpnea: increased rate of respirations.

Hyperventilation: overventilation of the alveoli in relation to the amount of carbon dioxide produced by the body.

Hypocapnia: decreased tension of carbon dioxide (P_{CO_2}) in the blood.

Hypoventilation: underventilation of the alveoli in relation to the amount of carbon dioxide produced by the body.

Hypoxemia: decreased tension of oxygen (P_{O_2}) in the blood.

Hypoxia: inadequate tissue oxygen levels.

Kussmaul respirations: rapid, deep respirations associated with diabetic ketoacidosis.

Methemoglobin: hemoglobin that has the iron atom in the ferric state.

Minute ventilation ($\dot{V}_E$): the volume of air expired during a period of 1 minute.

Orthopnea: severe dyspnea relieved when the patient elevates his or her head and chest.

Oxyhemoglobin: hemoglobin that is fully oxygenated.

Paroxysmal nocturnal dyspnea (PND): a sudden onset of severe dyspnea when the patient is lying down.

Partial pressure: the pressure exerted by each individual gas when mixed in a container with other gases.

PEEP: positive end-expiratory pressure.

Polycythemia: increased number of red blood cells in the blood.

Rales: short, discontinuous, explosive adventitious sounds, usually called *crackles.*

Reduced hemoglobin: hemoglobin in the deoxy state (not fully saturated with oxygen).

Respiration: the process by which oxygen and carbon dioxide are exchanged between the outside atmosphere and the cells in the body.

Rhonchi: continuous musical adventitious sounds.

Torr: units of the Torricelli scale, the classic mercury scale, which is used to express the same value as mm Hg.

Ventilation: the mechanical movement of air in and out of the lungs.

Wheeze: a high-pitched, sibilant rhonchus usually produced on expiration.

RESPIRATORY SYSTEM ANATOMY

The Nose

The nose, which is the first area in which inhaled air is filtered (Fig. 6–1), is lined with ciliated epithelium. Cilia move mucus and particles of foreign matter to the pharynx to be expectorated or swallowed (Fig. 6–2). Other functions of the nose include humidification and warming of the inhaled air and the olfactory function of smell.

Many times during anesthesia dry gases are administered. These gases dry the mucous membranes and slow the action of the cilia. The administration of moist gases in the PACU by various humidification and mist therapy devices keeps this physiologic filter system viable.

A tracheostomy precludes the functions of the nose, and it is important that proper tracheostomy care, including the administration of humidified oxygen, be instituted.

The blood supply to the nose is provided by the internal and external maxillary arteries, which are derived from the external carotid artery, and by branches of the internal carotid arteries. The venous plexus of the nasal mucosa is drained into the common facial vein, the anterior facial vein, the exterior jugular vein, or the ophthalmic vein. A highly vascular plexus of vessels is located in the mucosa of the anterior nasal septum. This plexus is referred to as *Kiesselbach's plexus* or *Little's area.* In most instances, this area is the source of epistaxis.

Epistaxis may occur in the PACU following

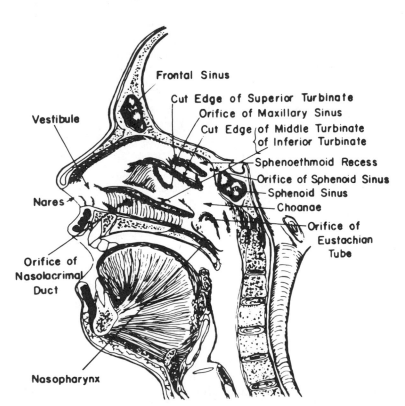

FIGURE 6–1. Sagittal section through the nose. (From Lough, M., Boat, T., and Doershuk, C. F.: The nose. Respir. Care, *20*[9]:844, 1975.)

Frontal Sinus

Cut Edge of Superior Turbinate
Orifice of Maxillary Sinus
Cut Edge of Middle Turbinate
of Inferior Turbinate

Vestibule

Sphenoethmoid Recess
Orifice of Sphenoid Sinus
Sphenoid Sinus
Choanae

Nares

Orifice of
Eustachian
Tube

Orifice of
Nasolacrimal
Duct

Nasopharynx

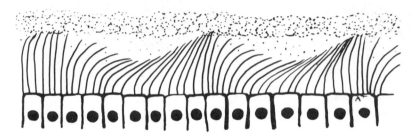

FIGURE 6–2. Mucus blanket of the nasal airways. The outer (gel-like) layer rests on the tips of the beating cilia, and the inner (water) layer bathes the cilia. Particles are trapped on the sticky outer blanket and carried posteriorly into the nasopharynx by the organized beating of cilia. (From Lough, M., Boat, T., and Doershuk, C. F.: The nose. Respir. Care, *20*[9]:845, 1975.)

trauma to the nasal veins from nasotracheal tubes or to nasal airways during anesthesia. If epistaxis occurs, prompt action should be taken to prevent aspiration of blood into the lungs. The patient should be positioned with his or her head up and flexed forward toward the chest. Cold compresses applied to the bridge of the nose and neck may be effective in slowing or stopping the bleeding. If the bleeding is profuse, the oral cavity should be suctioned carefully and the attending physician notified. A nasal pack or cautery with silver nitrate or electrical current may be necessary to stop the bleeding.

The Pharynx

The pharynx originates at the posterior aspect of the nasal cavities. It is called the *nasopharynx* until it reaches the soft palate, where it becomes the *oropharynx*. The oropharynx extends to the level of the hyoid bone, where it becomes the laryngeal pharynx, which extends caudally to below the hyoid bone.

The Larynx

The larynx, or voice box (Fig. 6–3), is situated anterior to the third, fourth, and fifth cervical vertebrae in the adult male. It is situated higher in women and children. Nine cartilages held together by ligaments and intertwined with many small muscles constitute the larynx. The thyroid cartilage, the largest, is V-shaped; its protruding prominence is commonly referred to as the *Adam's apple*. The thyroid cartilage is attached to the hyoid bone by the hyothyroid membrane and to the cricoid cartilage. The cricoid cartilage is situated below the thyroid cartilage and forms a ring anteriorly. It is in the shape of a signet ring. The "signet" lies posteriorly as a quadrilateral lamina joined in front by a thin arch. The inner surface of the cricoid cartilage is lined with a mucous membrane. In children younger than 10 years of age, the cricoid cartilage is the smallest opening to the bronchi of the lungs.

The epiglottis, a cartilage of the larynx, is an important landmark for tracheal intubation that serves to deflect foreign objects away from the trachea. This cartilage is leaf shaped and projects outward above the thyroid cartilage over the entrance to the trachea. The lower portion is attached to the thyroid lamina, and the anterior surface is attached to the hyoid bone and thereby to the base of the tongue. The valleys on either side of the glossoepiglottic fold are termed the *valleculae*.

The arytenoid cartilages are paired and articulate with the lamina of the cricoid through the articular surface on the base of the arytenoid. The anterior angle of the arytenoid cartilage projects forward to form the vocal process. The medial surface of the cartilage is covered by a mucous membrane to form the lateral portion of the rima glottis, the split between the vocal cords. The rima glottis is completed anteriorly by the thyroid cartilage and posteriorly by the cricoid cartilage.

The corniculate cartilages are two small nodules lying at the apex of the arytenoid. The cuneiform cartilage is a flake of cartilage within the margin of the aryepiglottic folds. It probably serves to stiffen the folds.

The larynx has nine membranes and extrinsic or intrinsic ligaments. Extrinsic ligaments connect the thyroid cartilage and the epiglottis with the hyoid bone and the cricoid cartilage with the trachea. Intrinsic ligaments connect the cartilages of the larynx with each other.

The fissure between the vocal folds, or true cords, is termed the *rima glottidis* or *glottis*. In the adult, this opening between the vocal cords is the narrowest part of the laryngeal cavity. Any obstruction in this area leads to death by suffocation if not promptly relieved. The rima glottidis divides the laryngeal cavity into two main compartments: (1) the upper portion is the vestibule, which extends from the laryngeal outlet to the vocal cords and includes the laryngeal sinus, sometimes referred to as the *middle compartment*; and (2) the lower compartment,

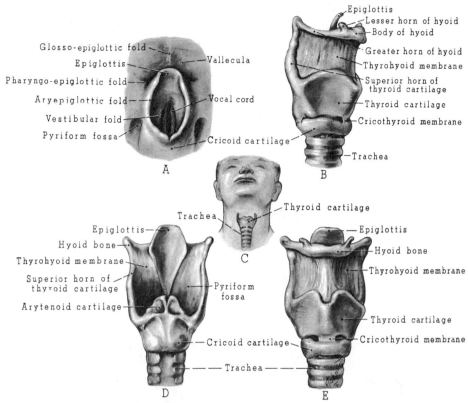

FIGURE 6–3. The larynx as viewed from above *(A)* and the side *(B)* in relation to the head and neck *(C)*, from behind *(D)*, and from the front *(E)*. *(A* through *E* from Jacob, S. W., Francone, C. A., and Lossow, W. J.: Structure and Function in Man. 5th ed. Philadelphia, W. B. Saunders, 1982, p. 447.)

which extends from the vocal cords to the lower border of the cricoid cartilage and thereafter is continuous with the trachea.

The muscles of the larynx are also either intrinsic or extrinsic. The intrinsic muscles control the movements of the laryngeal framework. They open the cords on inspiration, close the cords and the laryngeal inlet during swallowing, and alter the tension of the cords during speech. The extrinsic muscles are involved in the movements of the larynx as a whole, such as in swallowing.

The nerve supply to the larynx is from the superior and recurrent laryngeal nerves of the vagus. The superior laryngeal nerve passes deep to both the internal and the external carotid arteries and divides into a small external branch that supplies the cricothyroid muscles that tense the vocal ligaments. The larger internal branch pierces the thyrohyoid membrane to provide sensory fibers to the mucosa of both sides of the epiglottis and the larynx above the cords.

The recurrent laryngeal nerve on the right side exits from the vagus as it crosses the right subclavian artery and ascends to the larynx in the groove between the trachea and esophagus (Fig. 6–4). Once it reaches the neck, it assumes the same relationships as on the right. This nerve provides the motor function to the intrinsic muscles of the larynx, with the exception of the cricothyroid. It also provides sensory function to the laryngeal mucosa below the vocal cords.

Laryngospasm, a spasm of the laryngeal muscle tissue, may be complete, when there is complete closure of the vocal cords, or incomplete, when the vocal cords are partially closed. Patients experiencing partial or complete airway obstruction, such as laryngospasm, usually have a paradoxical, rocking motion of the chest wall. This motion can be misinterpreted as normal abdominal breathing. Hence, the PACU nurse should *always* auscultate the patient's lungs to determine the degree of ventilation and not rely on just a visual assessment of the motion of the chest.

When a laryngospasm occurs in the PACU, prompt emergency treatment is necessary to save the patient's life. The PACU nurse should have someone on the PACU staff summon the anesthetist or anesthesiologist when laryngo-

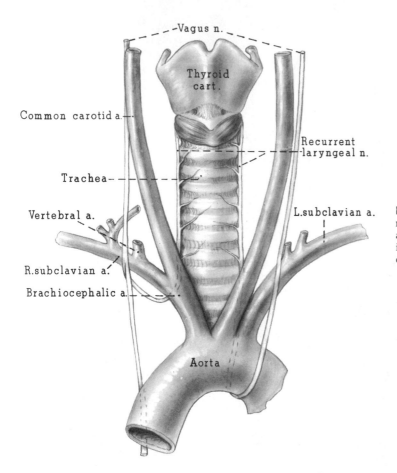

FIGURE 6–4. Course of recurrent laryngeal nerve. (From Jacob, S. W., Francone, C. A., and Lossow, W. J.: Structure and Function in Man. 5th ed. Philadelphia, W. B. Saunders, 1982, p. 292.)

spasm is suspected. Treatment consists of mask ventilation using *sustained moderate pressure* on the reservoir bag. This maneuver usually helps overcome the partial laryngospasm. Complete laryngospasm not relieved by positive pressure within at least 1 minute requires more aggressive treatment. Intravenous (0.5 mg per kg) or intramuscular (1 mg per kg) succinylcholine may be administered to relax the smooth muscle of the larynx. Endotracheal intubation may be necessary. The nurse must remember that ventilation of the patient should be continued until *complete* respiratory functioning has returned.

The Trachea

The *trachea* is a musculomembranous tube surrounded by 16 to 20 incomplete cartilaginous rings. These C-shaped rings prevent the collapse of the trachea, thereby maintaining free passage of air. The trachea is lined by ciliated columnar epithelium, which aids in the removal of foreign material.

The area at the distal end of the trachea at the point of bifurcation into the right and left main stem bronchi is called the *carina* (Fig. 6–5). The carina contains sensitive pressoreceptors, which on stimulation (i.e., an endotracheal tube) cause the patient to cough and "buck." The angle created at the point of bifurcation into the right and left main stem bronchi is clinically significant to the PACU nurse. This angle varies according to the age and gender of the person (Table 6–1). The angle at the right main stem bronchus is smaller than the angle at the left main stem bronchus. Foreign material can easily enter the right main stem bronchus at this point. Endotracheal tubes, if advanced too far, usually enter the right main stem bronchus, occluding the left main stem bronchus. Thus, the left lung cannot be ventilated. Signs of this complication include decreased or absent breath sounds in the left side of the chest, tachycardia, and uneven expansion of the chest on inspiration and expiration.

The Bronchi and Lungs

Each primary bronchus supplies a number of lobar bronchi (Fig. 6–6). Humans have an up-

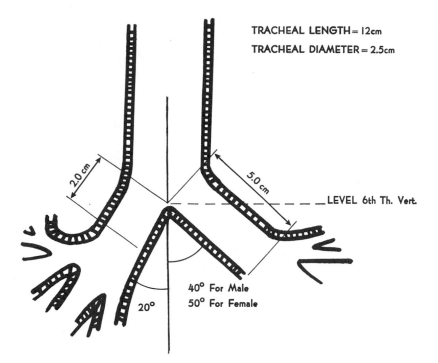

FIGURE 6–5. Bifurcation of the trachea into the main stem bronchi. (From Collins, V. J.: Principles of Anesthesiology. 2nd ed. Philadelphia, Lea & Febiger, 1976, p. 351.)

per, middle, and lower lobe bronchus on the right and only an upper and lower lobe bronchus on the left. Within each pulmonary lobe, a lobar (secondary) bronchus soon divides into tertiary branches remarkably constant as to their number and distribution within the lobe. The segment of a lobe aerated by a tertiary bronchus is usually well delineated from adjoining segments by complete planes of connective tissue. These areas of the lung are well defined; therefore, pulmonary diseases may be limited to a particular segment or segments of a lobe.

The bronchi bifurcate 22 or 23 times from the main stem bronchus to the terminal bronchi. These bronchi have connective tissue and cartilaginous support. The terminal bronchi branch to the bronchioles with a diameter of 1 mm or smaller and lack cartilaginous support. Bronchioles have thin, highly elastic walls composed of smooth muscle, which is arranged circularly. When the circular smooth muscle is

contracted, the bronchiolar lumen is constricted. This circular smooth muscle is innervated by the parasympathetic nervous system (vagus nerve), which causes constriction, and the sympathetic nervous system, which causes dilatation. The patency of the terminal bronchioles, therefore, is determined by the tonus of the muscle produced by a balance between the two components of the nervous system. Bronchospasm occurs when the smooth muscles constrict or experience spasm, ultimately leading to airway obstruction.

The terminal bronchioles divide into the respiratory bronchioles in which actual gas exchange first occurs. The respiratory bronchioles bifurcate to form alveolar ducts, and these, in turn, terminate in spherical enclosures called the *alveolar sac*. The sacs enclose a small but variable number of terminal alveoli.

The number of alveoli in an average adult's lungs is estimated to be about 750 million. The surface area available for gas exchange is approximately 125 m^2. Alveoli are shaped like soap bubbles in a glass. The interalveolar septum has a supporting latticework composed of elastic collagenous and reticular fibers. The capillaries are incorporated into and supported by the fibrous lattice. The capillary networks in the lungs are the richest in the body.

The lungs receive unoxygenated blood from the left and right pulmonary arteries, which originate from the right ventricle of the heart. The divisions of the pulmonary artery tend to

Table 6–1. VARIATIONS OF BRONCHIAL BIFURCATION ANGLES IN ADULTS AND CHILDREN

	Right Bronchus (degrees)	Left Bronchus (degrees)
Newborn	10–35	30–65
Adult male	20	40
Adult female	19	51

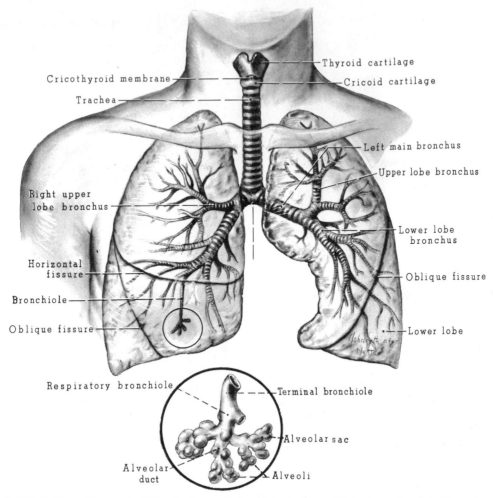

FIGURE 6–6. Distribution of bronchi within the lungs. Enlarged *inset* shows detail of an alveolus. (From Jacob, S. W., Francone, C. A., and Lossow, W. J.: Structure and Function in Man. 5th ed. Philadelphia, W. B. Saunders, 1982, p. 452.)

follow the bifurcations of the airway. Typically, two pulmonary veins exit from each lung and all four veins empty separately into the left atrium. The blood arriving in the rich pulmonary capillary network from the pulmonary arteries provides for the metabolic needs of the pulmonary parenchyma. Other portions of the lungs, such as the conducting vessels and airways, require their own private circulation. The bronchial arteries, which arise from the aorta, provide the oxygenated blood to the lung tissue. The blood of the bronchial arteries returns to the heart by way of the pulmonary veins.

Each lung is contained in a thin, elastic membranous sac called the *visceral pleura,* which is adherent to the external surface of the lung. Another membrane, the parietal pleura, lines the chest wall. These two membranes normally are quite close to each other. A few milliliters of viscous fluid is secreted between them to provide lubrication. The visceral pleura continuously absorbs this fluid.

RESPIRATORY SYSTEM PHYSIOLOGY

Lung Volumes and Capacities

Care of the PACU patient is based largely on knowledge of the physiology and pathophysiology of the respiratory system. Dysfunction in lung volumes and capacities that occur in the postoperative patient is the compelling reason for instituting the stir-up regimen in the PACU. Accordingly, the physiology of the lung volumes and capacities as well as lung mechanics will be described in detail. Table 6–2 provides the definition and normal value for each lung volume and capacity. As shown in Table 6–2

Table 6–2. LUNG VOLUMES AND CAPACITIES

Terminology	Definition	Normal Male*	Normal Female*
Tidal volume (V_T)	Volume of air inspired or expired at each breath	660 (230)	550 (160)
Inspiratory reserve volume (IRV)	Maximum volume of air that can be inspired after a normal inspiration	2240 —	1480 —
Expiratory reserve volume (ERV)	Maximum volume of air that can be expired after a normal expiration	1240 (410)	730 (300)
Residual volume (RV)	Volume of air remaining in the lungs after a maximum expiration	2100 (520)	1570 (380)
Vital capacity (VC)	Maximum volume of air that can be expired after a maximum inspiration	4130 (750)	2760 (540)
Total lung capacity (TLC)	The total volume of air contained in the lungs at maximum inspiration	6230 (830)	4330 (620)
Inspiratory capacity (IC)	The maximum volume of air that can be inspired after a normal expiration	2900 —	2030 —
Functional residual capacity (FRC)	The volume of gas remaining in the lungs after a normal expiration	3330 (680)	2300 (490)

Adapted from Wylie, W. B., and Churchill-Davidson, H. C., eds.: A Practice of Anaesthesia. 4th ed. London, Lloyd-Luke Medical Books, 1978. Reproduced by permission of Edward Arnold (Publishers) Limited.
*Data are mean values, with the standard in milliliters deviation in parentheses.

and Figure 6–7, a lung capacity comprises two or more lung volumes.

The Lung Volumes

The *tidal volume* (V_T) represents the amount of air moved into or out of the lungs during a normal ventilatory excursion. It is an important lung volume to monitor when the patient is receiving ventilatory support. Because the V_T measurement is highly variable, it is not an extremely helpful parameter in pulmonary function tests. Clinically, the V_T can be estimated at 7 ml per kg. For example, a man weighing 70 kg has a V_T of approximately 490 ml ($7 \times 70 = 490$).

The *expiratory reserve volume* (ERV) is the maximum amount of air that can be expired from the resting position following a normal spontaneous expiration. The ERV reflects muscle strength, thoracic mobility, and a balance of forces that determine the resting position of the lungs and chest wall following a normal expiration. It is a lung volume that is usually decreased in patients who are morbidly obese (see Chapter 38). It is also a lung volume that is decreased in the immediate postoperative period in patients who have had an upper abdominal or thoracic operation.

The *residual volume* (RV) is the volume of air that remains in the lungs at the end of a maximum expiration. This lung volume represents the balance of forces of the lung elastic forces and thoracic muscle strength. Patients who did not have their skeletal muscle relaxant ade-

quately reversed at the end of the anesthetic may experience an elevated RV, because they are unable to generate enough muscle strength to force all the air out of their lungs. As the RV increases, more air will remain in the lungs, so

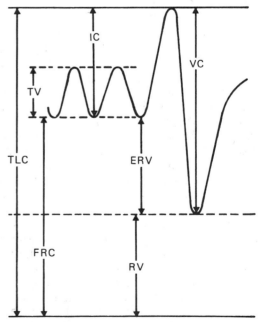

FIGURE 6–7. Graphic representation of normal lung volumes and capacities. TLC = total lung capacity; TV = tidal volume; FRC = functional residual capacity; IC = inspiratory capacity; ERV = expiratory reserve volume; RV = residual volume; VC = vital capacity. (From Drain, C.: The anesthetic management of the patient: A broad view of the anesthetic considerations necessary regarding the respiratory system. AANA J., 50[2]:192–201, 1982.)

that it will not participate adequately in gas exchange and will become dead-space air. As the dead-space volume of air increases, it can impinge on the V_T, and hypoxemia can ensue. The importance of the RV is that it allows for continuous gas exchange throughout the entire breathing cycle by providing air to most of the alveoli, and it aerates the blood between breaths. Consequently, the RV prevents wide fluctuations in oxygen and carbon dioxide concentrations during inspiration and expiration.

The *inspiratory reserve volume* (IRV) reflects a balance of the lung elastic forces, muscle strength, and thoracic mobility. It is the maximum volume of air that can be inspired at the end of a normal spontaneous inspiration. Physiologically, the IRV is available to meet increased metabolic demand at a time of excess physical exertion. It assists in moving a larger volume of air into the alveoli through each ventilatory cycle to increase the overall performance and efficiency of the respiratory system.

The Lung Capacities

The *inspiratory capacity* (IC) is the maximum volume of air that can be inspired from the resting expiratory position. The IC is the sum of the V_T and the IRV.

The *functional residual capacity* (FRC) represents the previously mentioned resting position. The FRC is the volume of air remaining in the lungs at the end of a normal expiration when no respiratory muscle forces are applied. At FRC, the mechanical forces of the lung and thorax are at rest and no air flow is present. This particular lung capacity is of great importance to the PACU nurse when intensive nursing care is rendered to the patient recovering from anesthesia, because the FRC is usually reduced in patients recovering from anesthesia. That is the reason why breathing maneuvers such as the sustained maximum inspiration (SMI) are instituted in the PACU—to raise the FRC (see section on lung mechanics). The FRC represents the sum of the ERV and the RV. A severe increase in the FRC is often associated with pulmonary distention, which is technically a state of hyperinflation of the lung. This state of hyperinflation can be caused by two abnormal conditions: airway obstruction and loss of elasticity. Airway obstruction is exemplified by an episode of acute bronchial asthma; a loss of lung elasticity is usually associated with emphysema. A severe decrease in FRC is associated with pulmonary fibrosis

and can be the sequela of postoperative atelectasis.

The *vital capacity* (VC) is the amount of air that can be expired following the deepest possible inspiration. It is the sum of the V_T, the ERV, and the IRV. The VC measures many factors that simultaneously affect ventilation, including activity of respiratory centers, motor nerves, and respiratory muscles, as well as thoracic maximum, airway and tissue resistance, and lung volume.

The *total lung capacity* (TLC) is simply the total amount of air in the lung at a maximum inspiration. The TLC is the sum of the VC and the RV.

The TLC, FRC, and RV are difficult to measure clinically, because they include a gas volume that cannot be exhaled. Therefore, the measurements require sophisticated pulmonary function testing equipment using gas dilution techniques or plethysmography. As will be seen, measurements of lung volumes and capacities are useful in the evaluation of lung function.

Lung Mechanics

Mechanical Features of the Lungs

Mechanical forces of the respiratory system actually determine the lung volumes and capacities. To understand how these lung volumes and capacities are determined and how they are affected by anesthesia and surgery, the PACU nurse should become familiar with the "balance of forces" concept of the respiratory system (see section on the combined mechanical properties of the lungs and chest wall). The PACU stir-up regimen is designed to increase the postoperative patient's lung volumes and capacities by enhancing the mechanical forces of the respiratory system.

The lungs and chest wall are viscoelastic structures, one within the other. Because they are elastic, the lungs always want to collapse or recoil to a smaller position. Therefore, as can be seen in the pressure-volume (P-V) curve of the lungs alone (Fig. 6–8), below RV the lungs are collapsed and no pressure is transmitted across the lungs (i.e., there is no transpulmonary pressure). When the lungs are inflated to a volume halfway between RV and TLC, the lungs seek to recoil or collapse back to the resting position at or actually below RV; this is reflected by an increase in transpulmonary pressure. When the lungs are fully inflated at TLC, a maximum transpulmonary pressure is

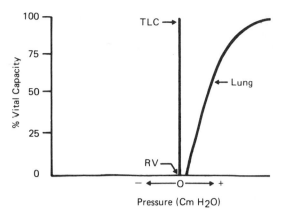

FIGURE 6–8. Static deflation pressure-volume curve for the lung. The positive pressures represent pressures tending to decrease lung volume. TLC = total lung capacity; RV = residual volume. (From Drain C.: The anesthetic management of the patient: A broad view of the anesthetic considerations necessary regarding the respiratory system. AANA J., *50*[2]:192–201, 1982.)

also exhibited. By analogy, when a balloon is completely deflated, the pressure measured at the mouth of the balloon is zero. When the balloon is partially inflated, the pressure increases as the elastic forces of the balloon try to make the balloon recoil to its resting position. If the balloon is maximally inflated, the elastic recoil of the balloon is greater, as is the pressure measured at the mouth of the balloon.

Pulmonary Hysteresis

Inflation and deflation paths of the P-V curve of the lung are not aligned on top of each other (Fig. 6–9). The path of deformation (inspiration) to TLC is different from the path followed when the force is withdrawn (expiration) from TLC to RV. This phenomenon is known as *pulmonary hysteresis*. The factors that contribute to pulmonary hysteresis are (1) properties of the tissue elements (a minor factor); (2) recruitment of lung units; and (3) the surface tension phenomenon (surfactant).

Elastic Properties of the Lung. The elastic properties of the lung tissue contribute only a small part to the phenomenon of hysteresis.

Recruitment of Lung Units. Recruitment of lung units has an important part in pulmonary hysteresis. To understand recruitment of lung units, the nurse must be familiar with the concept of *airway closure*. In the lung, there is an apex-to-base gradient of alveolar size (Fig. 6–10). This gradient occurs because of the weight of the lung, which tends to "pull" the lung toward its base. As a result, the pleural pressure is more negative at the apex than at the base of the lung. Ultimately, at low lung volumes, the alveoli at the apex are *inflated more* than the alveoli at the base. At the base of the lungs, some alveoli are closed to ventilation because the weight of the lungs in that area causes the pleural pressure to become positive. Airways open only when their critical opening pressure is achieved during inflation, and the lung units peripheral to them are recruited to participate in volume exchange. This is called *radial traction* or a *tethering effect* on airways. An analogy of a nylon stocking may aid in explaining this concept: when no traction is applied to the nylon stocking, the holes in the stocking are small. As traction is applied to the stocking from all sides, each nylon filament pulls on the others, which will spread apart all the other filaments, and the holes in the stocking will enlarge. Similarly, as one airway opens, it produces radial traction on the next airway and pulls the next airway open; in other words, it recruits airways to open. The volume of air in the alveoli behind the closed airways is termed the *closing volume* (CV). The CV plus the RV is termed the *closing capacity* (CC). The CC normally occurs below the FRC (see Fig. 6–21).

During the early emergence phase of anesthesia, patients usually have low lung volumes, which can lead to airway closure. Consequently, a postoperative breathing maneuver having a maximum alveolar inflating pressure, a long alveolar inflating time, and high alveolar inflating volume, such as the *SMI* or *yawn maneuver*, should facilitate the maximum recruitment of lung units. With the recruitment of lung units, the FRC could be raised out of the closing volume range, and, ultimately, there would be a reduction in hypoxemia.

Surface Tension Phenomenon. The surface tension phenomenon basically has to do with the action of surfactant on lung tissue. Surfactant is a phospholipid rich in lecithin that is produced by the type II alveolar cells. Surfactant lines the alveolus as a thin, surface-active film. This film has a physiologic action of reducing the surface tension of the alveoli and terminal respiratory airways. If the surfactant were not present, the surface tension would be fixed and greater pressure would be required to keep the alveolus open. As a result, small alveoli would empty into larger ones, atelectasis would regularly occur at low lung volumes, and large expanding pressures would be required to reopen collapsed lung units. Surfactant is also an important factor in alveolar inflation, because it provides uniformity in the inflation of lung units. In these ways, surfactant helps impart stability to alveoli in the normal

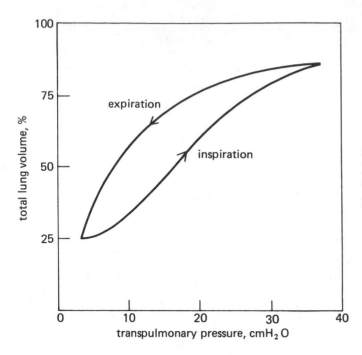

FIGURE 6–9. The inflation and deflation paths of the pressure-volume curve of the lungs. (From Levitzky, M.: Pulmonary Physiology. 3rd ed. New York, McGraw-Hill, 1991, p. 21; reprinted with permission of McGraw-Hill.)

lung. In addition to playing a major role in pulmonary hysteresis, surfactant also contributes to lung recoil and reduces the workload of breathing.

Lung Compliance

Several other terms relating to the P-V curve of the lung deserve attention. One is *lung compliance* (C_L), which is defined as the change in volume for a given change in pressure, or the pressure required to maintain a given volume of inflation. The normal value for C_L is 0.1 L per cm H_2O.

$$C_L = \frac{\Delta V}{\Delta P}$$

C_L is a measure of the distensibility of the lungs during breathing. According to convention, C_L means the slope on the static deflation portion of the P-V curve over the V_T range. Therefore, it can be said that C_L is the slope of the P-V curve, and it may remain unchanged even if there are marked changes in lung elastic properties resulting in a shift of the P-V curve to the left or right. Hence, when the compliance of the lung is measured clinically, it is done over the V_T range, during deflation. Measuring the C_L over any other portion of the P-V curve may result in an inaccurate reading as compared with normal. Lung elastic recoil (Pst_L) is the pressure exerted by the lung (transpulmonary pressure) because of its tendency to recoil or collapse to a smaller resting state. At low lung volumes, the Pst_L is low, and at high lung volumes, the Pst_L is high. This elastic retractive force (Pst_L) is the result of the overall structural elements of the lung combined with the lung surface tension forces. As mentioned earlier, the C_L represents the slope of the P-V curve, and the Pst_L represents the points along the P-V curve. Changes in C_L and Pst_L have dramatic implications in the alteration in lung volumes

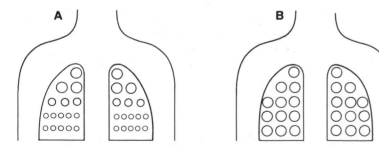

FIGURE 6–10. Alveolar size from apex to base of lungs, as a subject inhales from residual volume *(A)* to total lung capacity *(B)*.

that occurs in the immediate postoperative period (see section on postoperative lung volumes).

The Pulmonary Time Constant

The pulmonary time constant is similar to the half-life used to assess the pharmacokinetic activity of drugs. A time constant represents the amount of time required for flow to decrease by a rate equal to one half the initial flow. A time constant equals the resistance multiplied by the compliance. Therefore, the time required to reach each time constant is dependent on the individual values of resistance and compliance. Under normal conditions, the decrease in flow at the first time constant is about 37 percent of the initial flow, or about 63 percent of the total volume added or removed from the lungs. The first time constant represents the time required to remove or add 63 percent of the total volume of air in the lungs. The decrease in flow rate at the second time constant is about 14 percent, and the percent volume of air added or removed from the lungs is 86 percent. The decrease in flow at the third time constant is 5 percent, with a corresponding 95 percent volume added or removed. Hence, the higher the time constant, the more air that is removed or added to the lungs.

The clinical implications of time constants are extremely important in the care of PACU patients who have received an inhalation anesthetic. Patients who have increased airway resistance or increased C_L, or both, experience a prolonged time necessary for filling and emptying of the lungs. The lung units in this situation are referred to as "slow lung units." The type of patient with slow lung units usually has chronic obstructive pulmonary disease. Patients with a significant amount of increased secretions also have some slow lung units. Consequently, patients who have slow lung units usually experience a *slow emergence* from inhalation anesthesia. Patients with a low C_L, such as patients with pulmonary fibrosis, have "fast lung units." Hence, these patients can fill or empty their lungs rather rapidly and experience a *rapid emergence* from inhalation anesthesia.

Mechanical Features of the Chest Wall

Because of the elastic properties of the chest wall, it always springs out or recoils outward, seeking larger resting volume. The resting volume of the lungs alone is below RV, and the resting volume of the chest wall is about 60 percent of the VC.

Action of the chest wall can be illustrated by the analogy of a wire screen attached around a balloon. The wire screen tends to spring outward, so at lower balloon volumes the screen pulls the balloon open. Measuring the pressure at the mouth of the balloon would reflect a negative number. At about 60 percent of the total capacity of the balloon, the screen no longer tends to spring outward. At that point, the addition of air causes the screen to push down on the balloon, reflecting a positive pressure at the mouth of the balloon. The screen around the balloon can be likened to the chest wall. As shown in Figure 6–11, it is clear that at lower lung volumes the chest wall is inclined to recoil outward, creating a negative pressure, and at about 60 percent of the VC the chest wall starts to push down on the lungs, creating a positive pressure. The result of the interplay between the chest wall's strong tendency to spring outward and the lung's strong tendency to recoil inward is the subatmospheric pleural pressure.

Pleural pressure can become positive during a cough or other forced expiratory maneuvers. Pneumothorax can occur when the chest wall is opened or when air is injected into the pleural cavity. When this occurs, the lungs collapse because they naturally recoil to a smaller position; the ribs flare outward, because of their natural inclination to recoil outward.

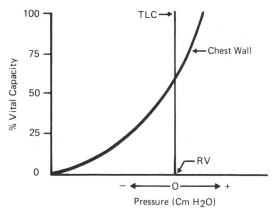

FIGURE 6–11. The pressure-volume curve of the chest wall during deflation going from TLC to RV. Positive pressures of the chest wall represent pressures tending to decrease lung size, and the negative pressures represent the pressure tending to increase lung volume because of the outward recoil tendency of the chest wall at about 60 percent of the vital capacity or less. TLC = total lung capacity; RV = residual volume. (From Drain, C.: The anesthetic management of the patient: A broad view of the anesthetic considerations necessary regarding the respiratory system. AANA J., 50[2]:192–201, 1982.)

Clinically, when a patient has a pneumothorax, inspection may reveal that the ribs on the affected side protrude.

There are two types of pneumothorax: open (simple) and closed (tension). *Simple pneumothorax* occurs when there is air flow into the pleural space that results in a positive pleural pressure. The lungs collapse because their recoil pressure is not counterbalanced by the negative pleural pressure. Treatment for a pneumothorax can be conservative or more aggressive, depending on the type and amount of pneumothorax. Aggressive treatment consists of the insertion of chest tubes into the pleural space to re-create the negative pleural pressure. This maneuver re-establishes normal ventilatory excursions. In most instances, the air leak between the lung and the pleural space will seal after the chest tubes have been removed. If air continues to flow into the intrapleural space but cannot escape, the intrapleural pressure will continually increase with each succeeding inspiration. Like a one-way valve, pressure increases and a *tension pneumothorax* develops. In a brief period, as the intrapleural pressure increases, the affected lung is compressed and puts a great amount of pressure on the mediastinum. Hypoxemia and a reduction in cardiac output result, and if treatment is not instituted immediately, the patient may die. Treatment consists of immediate evacuation of the excess air from the intrapleural space either by chest tubes or by a large-bore needle. A tension pneumothorax is truly a medical emergency.

Combined Mechanical Properties of the Lungs and Chest Wall

The combined P-V characteristics of the lung and the chest wall have many implications for the PACU nurse. The combined P-V curve is the algebraic sum of the individual P-V curves of the lung and chest wall. When no muscle forces are applied to the respiratory system, the FRC is determined by a balance of elastic forces between the lung and the chest wall (Fig. 6–12). Any pathophysiologic or pharmacologic process that affects the elasticity of either the lung or the chest wall affects the FRC.

Alterations in the Balance of Pulmonary Forces in the PACU Patient

During the induction of anesthesia, the shape of the P-V curve of the chest wall is altered. This agent-independent phenomenon is probably the result of loss of chest wall elasticity. Thus, the P-V curve of the chest wall of a pa-

tient with normal lung function is shifted to the right, the balance of forces occurs sooner, and the FRC decreases (Fig. 6–13). This shift to the right has an impact on the P-V curve of the lung: it also shifts to the right, and secondary changes occur in the lung. More specifically, the changes consist of an increase in lung recoil ($\uparrow Pst_L$) and a decrease in C_L ($\downarrow C_L$). Ultimately, the lung becomes stiffer and the FRC decreases and may drop into the closing capacity range. Hence, during tidal ventilation, some airways are closed to ventilation, and ventilation-perfusion mismatching occurs ($\downarrow \dot{V}_A/\dot{Q}_C$), which ultimately leads to hypoxemia. Research indicates that this phenomenon plus sighless breathing patterns in the PACU can cause patients to experience hypoxemia in the recovery phase of the anesthetic (see section on postoperative lung volumes).

Pulmonary Circulation

The basic functions of the pulmonary circulation are exchanging gas, providing a reservoir for the left ventricle, furnishing nutrition, and protecting the lungs.

Gas Exchange. The major aspects of gas exchange are discussed in the section on blood gas transport, but because of the implications for PACU nursing care, the concepts of transit time and pulmonary vascular resistance are presented here.

Of the 5 L of blood that flows through the lungs every minute, only 70 to 200 ml is active in gas exchange at any one time. The time it takes a red blood cell to cross the pulmonary capillary bed is 0.75 second, yet it takes the red blood cell only 0.25 second to become saturated with oxygen, that is, until all the oxygen-bonding sites on the hemoglobin molecule are occupied. Because the transit time is 0.75 second and the saturation time is only 0.25 second, the body has a tremendous back-up of 0.5 second for hemoglobin saturation with oxygen. If the red blood cells move across the pulmonary capillary bed at an accelerated pace (decreased transit time), the amount of time available for oxygen to saturate the red blood cells is decreased; but during stress or exercise, the complete saturation of the hemoglobin can still be accomplished because the transit time of a red blood cell rarely decreases below 0.25 second.

However, this is not true for patients with interstitial fibrosis who have a thickened respiratory exchange membrane. They may have a normal PaO_2 at rest, but exercise or exertion of surgery increases the cardiac output and de-

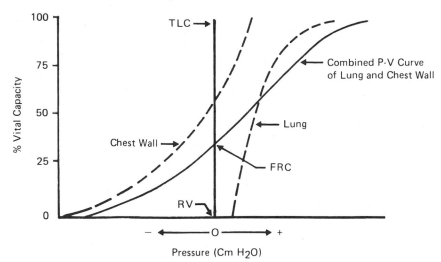

FIGURE 6–12. The combined P-V curves of the lungs and chest wall. The individual P-V curves of the lungs and chest wall are represented by *dashed lines.* They are transposed from the static deflation P-V curves of the lungs (see Fig. 6–8) and chest wall (see Fig. 6–11). The combined P-V curve is the algebraic sum of the deflation curves of the lungs and chest wall. In the combined P-V curve, it can be seen that the FRC is determined by the balance of elastic forces of the lungs and chest wall when no respiratory muscles are applied. P-V = pressure-volume; TLC = total lung capacity; RV = residual volume; FRC = functional residual capacity. (From Drain, C.: The anesthetic management of the patient: A broad view of the anesthetic considerations necessary regarding the respiratory system. AANA J., *50*[2]:192–201, 1982.)

creases the red blood cell transit time. Therefore, the hemoglobin will not become completely saturated during its passage through the pulmonary capillary bed. This phenomenon occurs because more time is needed for oxygen to pass through the diseased membrane. For these patients, the lower limit for complete saturation may be 0.5 second, not 0.25 second. Hence, patients with disorders of the respiratory exchange membrane can demon-

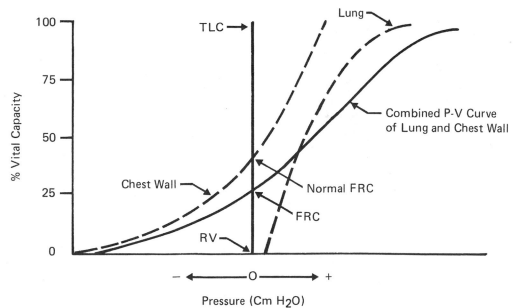

FIGURE 6–13. P-V curve representing the lung mechanics of a patient in the immediate postoperative period who has undergone an upper abdominal or thoracic surgical procedure. This patient has a loss of chest wall elastic recoil causing the lungs to become less compliant. Consequently, the combined P-V curve shifts to the right, leading to a decline in FRC because the balance of forces occurs at lower lung volumes. P-V = pressure-volume; FRC = functional residual capacity; TLC = total lung capacity; RV = residual volume. (From Drain, C.: The anesthetic management of the patient: A broad view of the anesthetic considerations necessary regarding the respiratory system. AANA J., *50*[2]:192–201, 1982.)

strate a lower oxygen saturation (SaO_2) on the pulse oximeter when they experience any exertion that could decrease red blood cell transit time. Clinically, this phenomenon is sometimes called *desaturation on exercise*. Therefore, in the PACU, patients suspected of having this problem should be given low-flow oxygen and closely monitored for desaturation via a pulse oximeter. Because of the possibility of desaturation, the low-flow oxygen should not be discontinued until the patient stabilizes, which may include continued administration after the patient is discharged from the PACU. Measures should be started to reduce the extrinsic factors, such as stress, elevated body temperature, and anxiety, which increase the cardiac output.

The pulmonary and systemic circulations have the same pump—the heart. The pulmonary system receives the same cardiac output as the systemic circulation—approximately 5 L per min. The pulmonary circulation, compared with the systemic circulation, is a low-pressure system, with low resistance to flow, having distensible vessels with extremely thin walls and a small amount of smooth muscle. Many stimuli affect *pulmonary vascular resistance*. Probably the most potent vasoconstrictor of the lung is alveolar hypoxia. Research indicates that *neuroendothelial bodies*, which respond to a low PaO_2, may exist close to the pulmonary vascular bed. Also, the neuroendothelial bodies may liberate prostaglandins or histamine, or both, when alveolar hypoxia is present. Pulmonary vascular resistance does not seem to be affected by the volatile anesthetics such as halothane, enflurane, and isoflurane. However, nitrous oxide can increase pulmonary vascular resistance, especially in patients with preexisting pulmonary hypertension. Neonates who may or may not have pre-existing pulmonary hypertension are prone to develop increased pulmonary vascular resistance when nitrous oxide is administered. If a PACU patient is prone to develop increased pulmonary vascular resistance, the effect of nitrous oxide on pulmonary vascular resistance will almost be dissipated due to the rapid excretion from the lungs of nitrous oxide because of its low blood-gas coefficient.

In the postoperative period, if a patient experiences atelectasis in some portion of the lungs, the PaO_2 in that particular area of the lungs will be reduced. As a result, the neuroendothelial bodies are stimulated to produce increased pulmonary vascular resistance in that area of the lungs. Eventually, the blood is redirected or shunted to areas of the lungs that are adequately ventilated. Because of this, the SaO_2 in a patient with atelectasis may indicate hypoxemia (<90 percent). After about 5 to 10 minutes, the SaO_2 may be slightly improved because of the increased pulmonary vascular resistance in the area of atelectasis. Therefore, the PACU nurse should continue to use an aggressive stir-up regimen on a patient with atelectasis, even though the patient's SaO_2 values indicate a slight improvement.

Reservoir for the Left Ventricle. In regard to their functioning as a reservoir for the left ventricle, the pulmonary veins are considered to be an extension of the left ventricle.

Nutrition. The pulmonary circulation can be divided into the bronchial circulation and the actual pulmonary circulation. The bronchial circulation carries nutrients and oxygen down to the respiratory bronchioles in the lungs. The bronchial circulation empties its deoxygenated blood via the pulmonary veins to the left heart. The pulmonary circulation carries nutrients to the respiratory bronchioles and the alveoli.

Protection. The role of the lungs in protection is vital for the preservation of the human organism. For example, on the surface of the pulmonary epithelium are invaginations called *caveoli*. Bradykinin and angiotensin I are enzymatically converted on the surface of the caveoli. Ninety percent of the bradykinin is deactivated in the caveoli during each pass through the lungs, and angiotensin I is converted to angiotensin II by angiotensin-converting enzyme in the lungs. In the presence of hypoxia, the conversion of angiotensin I to angiotensin II is inhibited. Also, in the hypoxemic state, less than 10 percent of the bradykinin is deactivated by the lungs. In the hypoxemic state, the liberated bradykinin then becomes prostaglandins. Interestingly, the inappropriate levels of prostaglandins due to hypoxemia in the chronic state are thought to produce the clubbing of the fingers in patients who experience long-standing chronic hypoxemia. Finally, the pulmonary epithelium also deactivates norepinephrine and serotonin. Serotonin plays an important part in platelet aggregation. Increased levels of serotonin due to decreased lung function caused by hypoxia or lung disease lead to a high risk of developing a venous thrombus. The implications for PACU care are that patients who are immobile and hypoxemic (SaO_2 <90 percent) should be monitored for pulmonary and systemic thromboemboli.

Water Balance in the Lung

The alveoli stay dry by a combination of pressures and lymph flow (Fig. 6–14). The

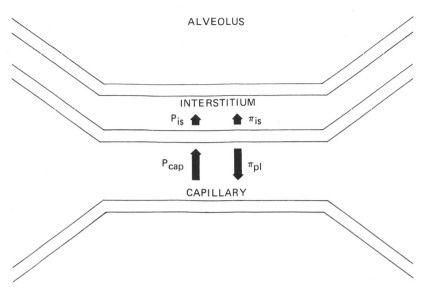

FIGURE 6–14. Illustration of the factors that affect the movement of fluid from the pulmonary capillaries. P_{cap} = capillary hydrostatic pressure; P_{is} = interstitial hydrostatic pressure (assumed to be negative); π_{pl} = plasma colloid pressure; π_{is} = interstitial colloid osmotic pressure. (From Levitzky, M.: Pulmonary Physiology. 3rd ed. New York, McGraw-Hill, 1991, p. 102; reprinted with permission of McGraw-Hill.)

forces tending to push fluid out of the pulmonary capillaries are the *capillary hydrostatic pressure* (P_{cap}) minus the *interstitial fluid hydrostatic pressure* (P_{is}). The forces tending to pull fluid into the pulmonary capillaries are the *colloid osmotic pressure of the proteins in the plasma of the pulmonary capillaries* (π_{pl}) minus the *colloid osmotic pressure of the proteins in the interstitial fluid* (π_{is}). The Starling equation describes the movement of fluid across the capillary endothelium:

$$Q_f = K_f \left(P_{cap} - P_{is}\right) - \sigma_f \left(\pi_{pl} - \pi_{is}\right)$$

where

Q_f = net flow of fluid
K_f = capillary filtration coefficient. This describes the permeability characteristics of the membrane to fluids.
σ_f = is the reflection coefficient. This describes the ability of the membrane to prevent extravasation of solute particles.

Thus, the membrane is permeable to fluid, and in normal circumstances, σ_f is equal to 1.0 in the equation.

Substituting normal values into the Starling equation,

$$Q_f = K_f \left[10 \text{ torr} - (-3 \text{ torr})\right]$$
$$- \sigma_f \left(25 \text{ torr} - 19 \text{ torr}\right)$$

where K_f and σ_f are dropped out of the equa-

tion because they are considered normal and do not affect the outcome of the example; therefore,

$$Q_f = (13 \text{ torr}) - (6 \text{ torr})$$
$$Q_f = +7 \text{ torr}$$

Thus, the pressure favors flow out of the capillaries to the interstitium of the alveolar wall tracts through the interstitial space to the perivascular and peribronchial spaces to facilitate transport of the fluid to the lymph nodes. Hence, there is a net pressure of +7 torr pushing fluid to the interstitial space. The lymph flow draining the lungs is about 20 ml per hr in rate of flow. Thus, the lungs depend on a continuous net fluid flux to remain in a consistently "dry" state.

Pulmonary edema, defined as increased total lung water, is associated with dysfunction of any parameter of the Starling equation. Examples of conditions that produce an overwhelming amount of fluid to be drained by the lymphatic system are elevated pulmonary capillary pressure (due to left-sided heart failure), decreased capillary colloid osmotic pressure (due to hypoproteinemia or overadministration of intravenous solutions), and extravasation of fluid through the pulmonary capillary membrane (due to adult respiratory distress syndrome). The earliest form of pulmonary edema is characterized by engorgement of the peribronchial and perivascular spaces and is known as *interstitial edema*. If interstitial edema is allowed to continue, alveolar pulmonary edema develops.

Pulmonary edema is difficult to assess in the early stages. As the fluid volume increases in the interstitium that surrounds the blood vessels and airways, reflex bronchospasm may occur. A chest radiograph at this time would reveal Kerley's B lines, denoting fluid in the interstitium. Once the lymphatics become completely overwhelmed, fluid will enter the alveoli. In the beginning of this pathophysiologic process, fine crackles are heard on auscultation. As pulmonary edema progresses into the alveoli, coarse crackles are heard, especially at the base of the lungs. Owing to the direct stimulation of the J-receptors in the interstitium, the patient has a tachypneic ventilatory pattern. Initial arterial blood gas values demonstrate a low Pa_{O_2} and Pa_{CO_2}. As the pulmonary edema progresses, the Pa_{CO_2} increases because hyperventilation (tachypnea) is not able to counterbalance the rise in the carbon dioxide in the blood. Finally, when the pulmonary edema becomes fulminant, the sputum becomes frothy and blood tinged.

Treatment of pulmonary edema is based on the Starling equation. If edema is cardiogenic, the focus of the treatment is to lower the hydrostatic pressures within the capillaries. Noncardiogenic pulmonary edema is usually treated with the infusion of albumin to increase the osmotic forces. Diuretics and dialysis also may be used in noncardiogenic edema in an effort to lower the vascular pressures. Positive end-expiratory or continuous positive airway pressure is used with high oxygen concentrations to correct the hypoxemia.

Blood Gas Transport

Respiration is the gas exchange between cellular levels in the body and the external environment. There are three phases of respiration: (1) *ventilation*, the phase of moving air in and out of the lungs; (2) *transportation*, which includes diffusion of gases in and out of the blood in both pulmonary and systemic capillaries, reactions of carbon dioxide and oxygen in the blood, and circulation of blood between the lungs and the tissue cells; and (3) *gas exchange*, in which oxygen is utilized and carbon dioxide is produced. Blood gas transport is the important link in carrying gas to or from the cell.

At sea level the barometric pressure is 760 torr. Air contains approximately 21 percent oxygen, which exerts a partial pressure of 159 torr. As described by Dalton's law of partial pressure, the total pressure of a given volume of a gas mixture is equal to the sum of the separate or partial pressures that each gas would exert if that gas alone occupied the entire volume. Therefore, the total pressure is equal to the sum of the partial pressures of the major gases in the atmosphere. For example:

$$P_{TOTAL} = P_{N_2} + P_{O_2}$$

where P_{TOTAL} = total atmospheric pressure and P_{N_2} = partial pressure of nitrogen. If the actual numeric quantities are then substituted into the formula,

$$760 \text{ torr} = 601 \text{ torr} + 159 \text{ torr}$$

Expressed in percentages, 100 percent (total atmospheric pressure) is equal to 79.07 percent (nitrogen) plus 20.93 percent (oxygen). Thus, nitrogen is 601 torr (0.7907 × 760) and oxygen is 159 torr (0.2093 × 760). In the lower airways, water vapor exerts a pressure that can be accounted for by Dalton's law. At the body temperature of 37°C, the water vapor pressure in the lower airways is 47 torr. Because the water vapor pressure affects the partial pressures of both nitrogen and oxygen, it is subtracted from the atmospheric pressure of 760 torr, which results in a pressure of 713 torr (760 torr − 47 torr = 713 torr). To determine the P_{O_2} in the lower airways, the percent oxygen (20.93) is multiplied by 713 torr, with a resultant P_{O_2} of 149.2 torr. The respiratory exchange ratio can be used to understand how the alveolar partial pressure of oxygen is determined. This ratio represents carbon dioxide production divided by oxygen consumption. The normal respiratory exchange ratio is 0.8. Theoretically then, *for every 10 torr of carbon dioxide that is added to the alveolus, 12 torr of oxygen is displaced.* Therefore, with no respiratory pathophysiology present, if the Pa_{CO_2} is 40 torr, then 48 torr of oxygen will be removed from the alveolus. Where

$$4 \times 10 = 40 \text{ torr (carbon dioxide)}$$

so

$$4 \times 12 = 48 \text{ torr (oxygen)}$$

This results in a Pa_{O_2} of 101 torr (149 torr − 48 torr = 101 torr). This is called the *12–10 concept* and is very helpful in assessing arterial blood gas determinations in the PACU (see section on causes of hypoxemia).

As oxygen diffuses across the pulmonary

membrane, the PO_2 is further decreased to 95 torr by a venous admixture. This effect occurs because of vascular shunts that normally redirect 1 or 2 percent of the total cardiac output either to nonaerated areas in the lungs themselves or directly through the heart, bypassing the lungs.

Oxygen Transport

Oxygen is carried in the blood in two forms: in combination with hemoglobin or in simple solution. About 98 percent of oxygen transported from the lungs to the cells is carried in combination with hemoglobin in the red blood cell; it is a reversible chemical combination. The remaining 2 percent is dissolved in the plasma and in the cytoplasm of the red blood cell. The amount of oxygen transported in both forms is directly proportional to the PO_2.

When the blood passes through the lungs, it does not normally become completely saturated with oxygen. Usually, the hemoglobin becomes about 97 percent saturated. When hemoglobin is saturated with oxygen, it is called *oxyhemoglobin*.

Normally, the oxygen content of the arterial blood is 19.8 ml per dl of blood. This total oxygen content in the arterial blood (CaO_2) is equal to the oxygen-carrying capacity of hemoglobin, which is 1.34 times the number of grams of hemoglobin. That number divided by 100 is the oxygen content carried by the hemoglobin. To determine the total amount of oxygen in the blood, the oxygen content that is dissolved in the plasma must be added to the oxygen content of the hemoglobin. The amount of oxygen dissolved in the plasma is determined by multiplying the PaO_2 by the solubility coefficient for oxygen in plasma, which is 0.003.

Therefore, the equation for the total oxygen content in the blood is:

$$CaO_2 = \frac{(Hb \times 1.34 \times \% \text{ Hb saturation})}{100} + (PaO_2 \times 0.003)$$

where Hb = hemoglobin. If the normal values of Hb = 15 g, percent Hb saturation = 97, and PaO_2 = 95 torr are substituted into the equation:

$$CaO_2 = \frac{(15 \times 1.34 \times 97)}{100} + (95 \times 0.003)$$

$$CaO_2 = 19.497 + 0.285$$

$$CaO_2 = 19.782 \text{ ml of oxygen per dl of blood}$$

It must be remembered that oxygen content is different from oxygen partial pressures. *Content* refers only to the amount of oxygen carried by the blood, not to its partial pressure (PO_2).

In the lungs, venous blood is oxygenated or arterialized. The oxygen bond with hemoglobin is loose and reversible. The bond is also PO_2 dependent; that is, the higher the PaO_2, the more oxygen saturation of the hemoglobin. However, the hemoglobin cannot be supersaturated, because when all the bonding sites on the hemoglobin molecule are occupied by oxygen, no matter how much more oxygen is presented to the hemoglobin, it will not be able to bond to the hemoglobin.

The *oxygen-hemoglobin dissociation curve* relates the percentage of oxygen saturation of hemoglobin to the PaO_2 value. Note in Figure 6–15 that the curve is sigmoid in shape with a very steep portion between the 10- and 50-torr PaO_2 range, with a leveling off above 70 torr. The flat portion of the curve indicates the capacity to oxygenate most of the hemoglobin despite wide variations in the PO_2 (70 to 98 torr). This flat portion of the curve can be referred to as the *association portion* of the curve, and it corresponds to the external respiration that is taking place in the lungs. The steep portion of the curve indicates the capacity to unload large amounts of oxygen in response to small tissue PO_2 changes. This part of the curve is called the *dissociation portion* of the oxygen-hemoglobin dissociation curve.

As discussed, the normal oxygen content at the association portion of the curve is about 19.8 ml of oxygen per dl of blood. At the venous dissociation portion of the curve, the content of oxygen is 15.2 ml of oxygen per dl of blood. The following formula is used to derive the content of oxygen in the mixed venous blood ($C\bar{v}O_2$):

$$C\bar{v}O_2 = \frac{(Hb \times 1.34 \times \% \text{ Hb saturation})}{100} + (P\bar{v}O_2 \times 0.003)$$

Substituting normal values for mixed venous blood of Hb = 15 g, percent Hb saturation = 75, and $P\bar{v}O_2$ = 40 into the formula:

$$C\bar{v}O_2 = \frac{(15 \times 1.34 \times 75)}{100} + (40 \times 0.003)$$

$$C\bar{v}O_2 = 15.08 + 0.12$$

$$C\bar{v}O_2 = 15.20 \text{ ml of oxygen per dl of blood}$$

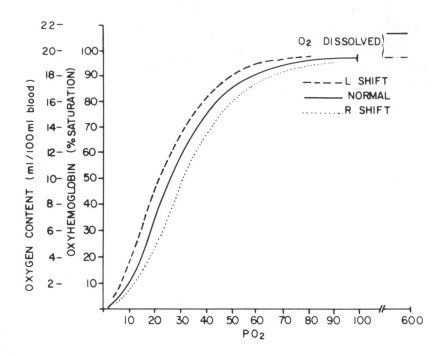

FIGURE 6–15. Oxyhemoglobin dissociation curve. (From Guenter, C., and Welch, M.: Pulmonary Medicine. Philadelphia, J. B. Lippincott, 1977, p. 151.)

Therefore, in this example the net delivery of oxygen to the tissues is 4.6 ml of oxygen per dl of blood (19.8 − 15.2 = 4.6).

Factors Affecting Oxygen Transport

The association portion of the oxygen-hemoglobin dissociation curve is not necessarily a fixed line determined solely by the PaO_2. The height and the slope of the curve are dependent on many factors, including pH and temperature. Generally, a decrease in pH (an increase in hydrogen ions) or an increase in body temperature causes a shift of the curve to the right, which leads to a decrease in the height and slope of the curve. Ultimately, there will be less saturation (loading) of the hemoglobin for a given PaO_2. Hence, patients who have a low pH or high temperature, or both, will probably benefit from a higher fraction of inspired oxygen (FIO_2) than normal to facilitate an appropriate level of saturation of their hemoglobin. However, before changes in the FIO_2 are made, arterial blood gas determinations should be analyzed.

At the dissociation portion of the oxygen-hemoglobin dissociation curve, the same is true. It is not a fixed line, because it also changes position in response to physiologic processes. At the tissue level, metabolically active tissues produce more carbon dioxide and more acid (↓ pH) and have an elevated temperature. All these products of metabolism

shift the curve to the right. The curve shifts far more in response to physiologic processes in the dissociation portion than in the association part. Metabolically active tissues produce more carbon dioxide and need more oxygen. The effect of carbon dioxide on the curve is closely related to the fact that deoxyhemoglobin binds hydrogen ions more actively than does oxyhemoglobin. As a result, at the tissue level, increased carbon dioxide decreases the affinity of hemoglobin for oxygen. Thus, the dissociation portion of the curve is shifted to the right and more oxygen is given to the tissue. This effect of carbon dioxide on oxygen transport is called the *Bohr effect*.

2,3-Diphosphoglycerate (2,3-DPG) regulates the release of oxygen to the tissue. It is a glycolytic intermediary metabolite that is more concentrated in the red blood cell than anywhere else in the body. High concentrations of 2,3-DPG shift the oxyhemoglobin dissociation curve to the right, making oxygen more available to the tissues. Lower concentrations of 2,3-DPG cause a shift of the curve to the left, ultimately leading to the release of less oxygen to the tissues. The clinical implications of these observations involve the administration of outdated whole blood. Whole blood stored longer than 21 days has low levels of 2,3-DPG. Therefore, if outdated blood were administered to a patient, the tissues would not receive an appropriate amount of oxygen due to the shift to the left of the oxygen-hemoglobin dissociation curve.

Pulse Oximetry and the Oxygen Dissociation Curve

Oxygen delivered to the tissues is determined by the cardiac output and the CaO_2. Most of the oxygen is bound to the hemoglobin, and the percentage of the oxygen bound to the hemoglobin is expressed as the SaO_2. The amount of oxygen that is dissolved in simple solution in the arterial blood is the PaO_2. A gradient is set from the lung to the tissues in regard to oxygen delivery, and that is represented by the oxygen dissociation curve. A normal curve, without any shifts left or right, is determined by the $PaCO_2$, pH, body temperature, and hemoglobin and 2,3-DPG levels. A normal curve is therefore set at values of $PaCO_2$ of 40 torr, pH of 7.4, temperature of 37°C, and hemoglobin of 15 g per dl. Using the oxygen dissociation curve (see Fig. 6–15), the PaO_2 can be determined by the SaO_2 reading on the pulse oximeter. For example, an SaO_2 of 90 percent corresponds to a PaO_2 of 60 torr. Looking at the curve, below an SaO_2 of 90 percent, the PaO_2 drops rapidly (the dissociation portion of the curve). Clinically, an SaO_2 of 90 percent can be considered to be hypoxemia, and severe hypoxemia occurs when the PaO_2 is less than 40 torr or the SaO_2 is 75 percent.

Carbon Dioxide Transport

The transport of carbon dioxide begins within each cell in the body. Carbon dioxide is a main by-product of the energy-supplying mechanisms of the cell. Approximately 200 ml per min of carbon dioxide is produced within the body at rest. Carbon dioxide is 20 times more soluble in water than oxygen; therefore, it traverses the fluid compartments of the body rapidly. The intracellular partial pressure of carbon dioxide is 46 torr. A 1-torr gradient exists between the cell and the interstitial fluid. Carbon dioxide will diffuse out of the cell to the interstitial fluid and have a new partial pressure of 45 torr. When the tissue capillary blood enters the venules, the partial pressure of the carbon dioxide is 45 torr.

Carbon dioxide is transported in the blood in three forms: (1) physically dissolved in solution, (2) as carbaminohemoglobin, and (3) as bicarbonate ions.

Carbon Dioxide in Simple Solution. About 10 percent of the total amount of carbon dioxide transported in the body is physically dissolved in solution.

Carbaminohemoglobin. Approximately 30 percent of carbon dioxide is transported as car-*baminohemoglobin*, a chemical combination of carbon dioxide and hemoglobin that is reversible because the binding point on the hemoglobin is on the amino groups and is a very loose bond. This chemical bonding of carbon dioxide with hemoglobin can be graphically described by the use of the *carbon dioxide dissociation curve*. There are two differences between the carbon dioxide dissociation curve (Fig. 6–16) and the oxygen-hemoglobin dissociation curve. First, over the normal operating range of blood PCO_2 from 47 (venous) to 40 (arterial) torr, the slope of the carbon dioxide dissociation curve is nearly linear and not sigmoid like the oxygen-hemoglobin dissociation curve. Second, the total carbon dioxide content is about twice the total oxygen content. Oxygen has a definite effect on carbon dioxide transport. On the upper curve, or venous portion of the carbon dioxide curve, note that the point for the $PvCO_2$ is 47 and the PvO_2 is 40. On the lower curve, or arterial carbon dioxide curve, observe the points for the $PaCO_2$ of 40 torr and the PaO_2 of 100 torr. Notice how the venous carbon dioxide curve is shifted to the left and is above the arterial curve. This description is the effect of oxygen on carbon dioxide transport, or the *Haldane effect*. In terms of physiologic significance, the Haldane effect plays a more important role in gas transport than does the Bohr effect. Specifically, in the lungs, the binding of oxygen with hemoglobin tends to displace carbon dioxide from the hemoglobin (oxyhemoglobin is more acidic than deoxyhemoglobin). At the tissue level, oxygen is removed from the hemoglobin (due to a pressure gradient), reducing the acidity of the hemoglobin and enabling it to bind more carbon dioxide. In fact, because the hemoglobin is in the reduced state (deoxygenated), the hemoglobin can carry 6 volumes percent more carbon dioxide than the amount of carbon dioxide that could be carried by oxyhemoglobin.

Bicarbonate. Sixty-five percent of carbon dioxide is transported as bicarbonate, which is the product of the reaction of carbon dioxide with water. When the carbon dioxide and water join, they form carbonic acid. Almost all the carbonic acid dissociates to bicarbonate and hydrogen ions, as seen in the following equation:

$$CO_2 + H_2O \xrightarrow{\text{Carbonic anhydrase}} H_2CO_3 \rightarrow H^+ + HCO_3$$

This reaction occurs mostly within the red

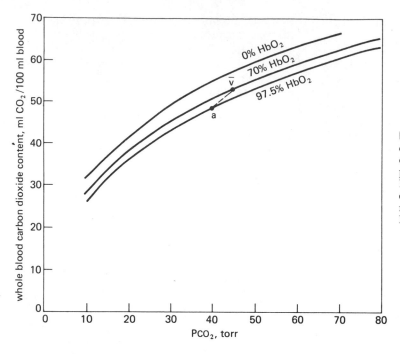

FIGURE 6–16. Carbon dioxide dissociation curves for whole blood at 37°C at different oxyhemoglobin saturations. a = arterial point; v̄ = mixed venous point. (From Levitzky, M.: Pulmonary Physiology. 3rd ed. New York, McGraw-Hill, 1991, p. 149; reprinted with permission of McGraw-Hill.)

blood cells, because carbonic anhydrase accelerates the hydration of carbon dioxide to carbonic acid 220 to 300 times faster than if carbon dioxide and water were joined without this enzymatic catalyst.

When the bicarbonate produced in this reaction in the red blood cells exceeds the bicarbonate ion level in the plasma, it will diffuse out of the cell. The positively charged hydrogen ion tends to remain within the red blood cell and is buffered by hemoglobin. Because of

ionic imbalance, chloride, a negatively charged ion that is abundant in the plasma, diffuses into the red blood cell to maintain electrical balance. This movement is referred to as the *chloride shift*. Because of the increase in osmotically active particles within the cell, water from the plasma diffuses into the red blood cell. This process explains why the red blood cells in the venous side of the circulation are slightly larger than the arterial red blood cells (Fig. 6–17).

As the venous blood enters the pulmonary

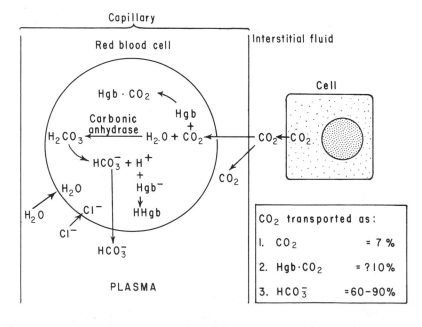

FIGURE 6–17. Transport of carbon dioxide in the blood. (From Jacob, S. W., and Francone C. A.: Structure and Function in Man. 3rd ed. Philadelphia, W. B. Saunders, 1974, p. 410.)

capillaries, the carbon dioxide in simple solution freely diffuses to the alveoli. The carbaminohemoglobin reverses to free the carbon dioxide, which diffuses across the alveoli and is then expired. The hydrogen and the bicarbonate combine to form carbonic acid, which is rapidly broken down by carbonic anhydrase to form carbon dioxide and water. The carbon dioxide then diffuses through the alveoli and is expired.

Not all carbon dioxide is eliminated by pulmonary ventilation. Other buffer systems that remove excess carbon dioxide are acid–base buffers and urinary excretion by the kidneys. The respiratory system can adjust to rapid fluctuations in carbon dioxide, whereas the kidneys may require hours to restore a normal carbon dioxide tension.

Acid–Base Relationships

A buffer is a substance that causes a lesser change in hydrogen ion concentration to occur in a solution, on addition of an acid or base, than would have occurred had the buffer not been present. The buffers can respond in seconds to fluctuations in carbon dioxide tension. Buffers include the carbonic acid–bicarbonate system, the proteinate–protein system, and the hemoglobinate–hemoglobin system.

The pH is a measure of alkalinity or acidity and is dependent on the concentration of hydrogen ions. Acidic solutions have more hydrogen ions, and alkaline solutions have fewer hydrogen ions. The pH is described in logarithmic form. Acid solutions have a greater amount of hydrogen ions and a lower pH (which would indicate acidity). If, on the other hand, the hydrogen ion concentration is low, then the pH is high, indicating alkalinity. The pH range is from 1 to 14, with 7 being equilibrium (pK). The normal pH in extracellular fluid is 7.35 to 7.45, which is slightly alkaline.

The normal bicarbonate level in the extracellular fluid is 24 mEq. *Base excess* is used to describe alkalosis or acidosis. If a positive base excess number is noted, this indicates more base in the extracellular fluid. If a negative number is reported, the base is being used to neutralize the acid to a point of encroaching on the amount of available base, which is demonstrated by a negative value for the base excess (acidosis).

Respiratory Acid–Base Imbalances

Respiratory acidosis is characterized by a Pa_{CO_2} above the normal range of 36 to 44 torr. All other primary processes tending to cause acidosis are metabolic. Some common causes of carbon dioxide retention and respiratory acidosis are summarized in Table 6–3.

Respiratory alkalosis is characterized by a reduced Pa_{CO_2}. Hyperventilation frequently causes this disorder. Common causes of excessive carbon dioxide elimination and respiratory alkalosis are summarized in Table 6–4.

In respiratory alkalosis or acidosis, a linear exchange takes place between the carbon dioxide and bicarbonate concentrations, which is summarized as follows:

1. In acute respiratory acidosis, bicarbonate

Table 6–4. COMMON CAUSES OF EXCESSIVE CARBON DIOXIDE ELIMINATION AND RESPIRATORY ALKALOSIS (HYPERVENTILATION)

Normal Lungs
Anxiety
Fever
Drugs (aspirin)
Central nervous system lesions
Endotoxemia

Abnormal Lungs
Pneumonia
Diffuse infiltrative pulmonary disease (early)
Acute bronchial asthma (early)
Pulmonary vascular disease
Congestive heart failure (early)

Table 6–3. COMMON CAUSES OF CARBON DIOXIDE RETENTION AND RESPIRATORY ACIDOSIS (HYPOVENTILATION)

Normal Lungs
Anesthesia
Sedative drugs (overdose)
Neuromuscular disease
  Poliomyelitis
  Myasthenia gravis
  Guillain-Barré syndrome
Obesity (pickwickian syndrome)
Brain damage
Cardiac arrest
Pneumothorax
Pulmonary edema
Bronchospasm
Laryngospasm

Abnormal Lungs
Chronic obstructive pulmonary disease (chronic bronchitis, asthma, and emphysema)
Diffuse infiltration pulmonary disease (advanced)
Kyphoscoliosis (severe)

concentration is approximately 1 mEq per L for each 10-torr change in $PaCO_2$.

2. In chronic respiratory acidosis, the change in actual bicarbonate concentration is approximately 2 mEq per L for each 10-torr change in $PaCO_2$.

3. The change in actual bicarbonate concentration with a chronic change in $PaCO_2$ above the range of 40 torr change is approximately 4 mEq per L for each 10-torr change in $PaCO_2$. This rule holds true for 1 or 2 days after the onset of the disorder because of the slow renal buffer system.

Another rule of thumb to determine if the acid–base disorder is entirely respiratory in origin is that an acute increase in $PaCO_2$ by 10 torr produces a corresponding decrease in pH by 0.07 pH units. In chronic hypercapnia, each increase in $PaCO_2$ by 10 torr results in a corresponding decrease in pH by 0.03 pH units. $PaCO_2$ and pH changes that deviate significantly from these standards suggest that the acid–base disorder is not completely respiratory in origin. For example, if a patient recovering from a spinal anesthetic in the PACU has blood gases (room air) of PaO_2 = 92 torr, $PaCO_2$ = 30 torr, and pH = 7.47 as compared with preoperative arterial blood gas values (room air) of PaO_2 = 80 torr, $PaCO_2$ = 40 torr, and pH = 7.40, the rule of thumb can be applied. Because the $PaCO_2$ decreased by 10 torr and the pH increased by 0.07 pH units, it is clear that the patient is experiencing *respiratory* alkalosis, not a metabolic disorder. Further, using the 12–10 concept, it can be determined that this patient is probably suffering from acute hyperventilation. This is because the $PaCO_2$ decreased by 10, so the PaO_2 should increase by 12, or from 80 to 92 torr.

Metabolic Acid–Base Imbalances

Metabolic acidosis usually results when there is an increase in nonvolatile acids or a loss of bases from the body. The usual result is a deficit in buffer, base excess, and bicarbonate. Because acidosis stimulates respiration, the $PaCO_2$ will usually decrease. The magnitude of the ventilatory response usually serves to differentiate between acute and chronic metabolic acidosis. Some of the common causes of metabolic acidosis are summarized in Table 6–5.

Metabolic alkalosis is produced by an excessive elimination of nonvolatile acids (such as in vomiting, gastric aspiration, and hypokalemic alkalosis) or by an increase in bases (such as in alkali administration or hypochloremic alka-

Table 6–5. COMMON CAUSES OF METABOLIC ACIDOSIS

Increased nonvolatile acids
Diabetes mellitus
Uremia
Severe exercise
Hypoxia
Shock
Idiopathic
Methyl alcohol ingestion (formic acid)
Aspirin ingestion (salicylic acid)
Excessive loss of bases (usually $NaCO_3$ from lower gastrointestinal tract)
Severe diarrhea (e.g., cholera, diarrhea in infants)
Fistulas (e.g., pancreatic, biliary)

losis caused by some diuretics). A summary of blood gas discrepancies in each condition is provided in Table 6–6.

Matching of Ventilation to Perfusion

Distribution of Ventilation

There is a gravity-dependent gradient of pleural pressure in the upright lung at resting lung volumes. The weight of the lung tends to pull the lung tissue toward the base of the lung. As a result, the intrapleural pressure is more negative at the apex of the lung as compared with the intrapleural pressure at the base and over the V_T range (the alveoli at the apex being more fully inflated as compared with the alveoli at the base). Consequently, the alveoli at the base have a greater capacity for volume change during inspiration, whereas the alveoli at the apex are already "stretched" or distended. In a normal subject who breathes out to RV and then inspires in small steps, the initial inspired air (a small portion) goes to the apex and the base remains completely underventilated. After a certain lung volume is attained, the base of the lung will receive almost all of the air because of the capacity of the alveoli at the base of the lung for volume

Table 6–6. SUMMARY OF BLOOD GAS DISCREPANCIES IN ACIDOSIS AND ALKALOSIS

Condition	HCO_3^-	PCO_2	pH
Metabolic acidosis	↓	↓	↓
Respiratory acidosis	↑	↑	↓
Metabolic alkalosis	↑	↑	↑
Respiratory alkalosis	↓	↓	↑

change. Therefore, because of the mechanical properties of the lung, the greatest volume change during inspiration from RV to TLC occurs near the base of the lungs.

Distribution of Perfusion

There is a gravity-dependent gradient for perfusion in the lungs, with approximately 80 to 90 percent of the blood flow occurring from the middle portion to an area near the base of the lungs. Therefore, the blood flow per unit of lung volume increases down the lung from the apex to the base.

Matching

Matching of alveolar ventilation ($\dot{V}_A$) to perfusion ($\dot{Q}_C$) is defined in terms of a certain volume of alveolar gas that is required to arterialize a given volume of mixed venous blood. The normal alveolar ventilation ratio is:

$$\frac{\dot{V}_A}{\dot{Q}_C} = \frac{4000 \text{ ml/min}}{5000 \text{ ml/min}} = 0.8$$

If blood and gas were matched equally throughout the lung, the $\dot{V}_A/\dot{Q}_C$ would be 1.0. However, in the normal lung, the matching of ventilation to perfusion is not proportional, which results in varying $\dot{V}_A/\dot{Q}_C$ throughout the lung. More specifically, at the apex, ventilation is high as opposed to perfusion, and perfusion is higher than ventilation at the base of the lung. Finally, if all the $\dot{V}_A/\dot{Q}_C$ relationships were added together, the mean ratio would be 0.8.

Causes of Hypoxemia

Hypoventilation

The Pa_{O_2} and Pa_{CO_2} are determined by the balance between the addition of oxygen and the removal of carbon dioxide by the alveolar ventilation and the removal of oxygen and the addition of carbon dioxide by the pulmonary capillary blood flow. If the alveolar ventilation is decreased (with no other lung pathologic changes present), the Pa_{O_2} will decrease and the Pa_{CO_2} will increase. In fact, the Pa_{O_2} will decrease almost proportionally to the increase in the Pa_{CO_2}. Recall the calculations made in the 12–10 concept. At any specific inspired oxygen tension, a 10-torr increase in the Pa_{CO_2} causes an approximate 12-torr decrease in the

arterial oxygen tension. For example, if the normal Pa_{CO_2} is equal to 40 torr and the Pa_{O_2} is equal to 95 torr and the patient's alveolar ventilation decreases owing to narcotics given in the PACU, the Pa_{CO_2} will increase to 60 torr. The new Pa_{O_2} should be 71 torr (change of 20 torr in the Pa_{CO_2}, so 12 + 12 = 24 − 95 = 71). Therefore, when one is assessing blood gas data and the 12–10 relationship is determined to be present, hypoventilation should be suspected. Remember, the 12–10 relationship does not have to be exact, but if the numbers are close to the 12–10 relationship, hypoventilation is the probable cause. An increased F_{IO_2} will affect the 12–10 relationship. However, most patients in the PACU receive low-flow oxygen therapy and, therefore, the F_{IO_2} is usually between 25 and 50 percent. Consequently, if the values seem to change proportionally, hypoventilation can still be suspected. Hypoventilation is the most common cause of hypoxemia in the PACU. Nursing interventions should include administration of a higher F_{IO_2} via low-flow oxygen therapy, stimulation of the patient, use of an aggressive stir-up regimen, and possible pharmacologic reversal of narcotics or muscle relaxants.

Ventilation/Perfusion Mismatching

If the 12–10 relationship is not present during the analysis of the arterial blood gases, ($\dot{V}_A/\dot{Q}_C$) mismatching is probably the cause. However, it is difficult to determine if the mismatching problem is the result of increased or decreased $\dot{V}_A/\dot{Q}_C$. As seen in Figure 6–18, *normal $\dot{V}_A/\dot{Q}_C$* exists when there is appropriate matching of ventilation to perfusion. *Decreased $\dot{V}_A/\dot{Q}_C$* occurs when the matching ventilation is reduced as compared with perfusion of the alveoli, and *increased $\dot{V}_A/\dot{Q}_C$* is caused by increased ventilation as compared with perfusion.

Decreased Ventilation to Perfusion ($\downarrow \dot{V}_A/\dot{Q}_C$). Reduced ventilation as compared with perfusion may be caused by excessive secretions or partial bronchospasm. When atelectasis or airway closure occurs, intrapulmonary shunting results. In these situations, oxygen cannot diffuse properly across to the pulmonary capillary blood. In decreased $\dot{V}_A/\dot{Q}_C$, some oxygen diffuses across from the alveoli to the pulmonary capillary blood. Thus, the alveolar-arterial oxygen difference ($P_{AO_2} - Pa_{O_2}$) will be slightly reduced. If there is a large gradient in the $P_{AO_2} - Pa_{O_2}$, intrapulmonary shunting is probably present. For a patient breathing room air, the normal $P_{AO_2} - Pa_{O_2}$ is

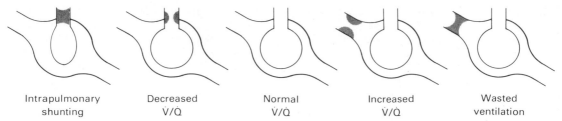

| Intrapulmonary shunting | Decreased $\dot{V}/\dot{Q}$ | Normal $\dot{V}/\dot{Q}$ | Increased $\dot{V}/\dot{Q}$ | Wasted ventilation |

FIGURE 6–18. Graphic representation of normal and abnormal matching of ventilation ($\dot{V}_A$) to perfusion ($\dot{Q}_C$). (From Harper, R.: A Guide to Respiratory Care: Physiology and Clinical Applications. Philadelphia, J. B. Lippincott, 1981, p. 98.)

between 5 and 15 torr. When a patient is breathing oxygen at a FIO_2 of 0.5 (50 percent), the $PAO_2 - PaO_2$ should be about 50 torr. A gradient greatly in excess of 50 torr suggests $\dot{V}_A/\dot{Q}_C$ mismatching. The focus of the nursing interventions to improve decreased $\dot{V}_A/\dot{Q}_C$ is on airway clearance, reinflation of alveoli, and enhanced patency of the airways. The newly advocated stir-up regimen of turn, cascade cough, and SMI should improve the decreased $\dot{V}_A/\dot{Q}_C$. Percussion or vibration, or both, may also need to be instituted to facilitate secretion clearance. Also, if partial bronchospasm (expiratory wheeze) is suspected, the attending physician should be consulted about instituting appropriate bronchodilator therapy.

At this point, a clarification of terms used to describe decreased $\dot{V}_A/\dot{Q}_C$ and shunt is in order. Basically, *intrapulmonary shunts* result in the mixing of venous blood that has not been properly oxygenated into the arterial blood (pulmonary vein). *Anatomic shunts*, which occur normally, are attributed to the 2 or 3 percent of the cardiac output that bypasses the lungs. The shunted, unoxygenated venous blood comes mainly from the bronchial circulation, which empties into the pulmonary veins, and from the thebesian vessels that drain the myocardium into the left heart. Intrapulmonary shunts occur when mixed venous blood does not become oxygenated when it passes by underventilated, unventilated, or collapsed alveoli. *Absolute intrapulmonary shunts*, sometimes called *true shunts*, are associated with totally unventilated or collapsed alveoli. *Shuntlike intrapulmonary shunts* are the areas of low $\dot{V}_A/\dot{Q}_C$ in which blood draining the partially obstructed alveoli has a lower arterial oxygen content than the alveolar capillary units that are well matched. As a result, the presence of anatomic shunts is normal. Abnormal shunts can be classified as physiologic shunts. *Physiologic shunts* are made up of the anatomic shunts plus *intrapulmonary shunts* (absolute and shuntlike intrapulmonary shunts).

Increased Ventilation to Perfusion. According to Figure 6–19, when the circulation to the individual alveolocapillary unit is compromised, there is an excess of ventilation as compared with perfusion. If the flow of blood in the pulmonary capillary is partially obstructed, increased $\dot{V}_A/\dot{Q}_C$ results. If the flow of blood is completely obstructed, such as by a pulmonary embolus, only ventilation continues, producing wasted or dead space. Wasted ventilation is the total amount of inspired gas that does not contribute to carbon dioxide removal; it is also known as *physiologic dead space* ($V_D$physio). $V_D$physio is that volume of each breath that is inhaled but does not reach functioning terminal respiratory units. $V_D$physio has two components: alveolar and anatomic dead space. *Alveolar dead space* ($V_D$alv), as depicted in Figure 6–19, is that volume of air contributed by all those terminal respiratory units that are overventilated relative to their perfusion. *Anatomic dead space* ($V_D$anat) consists of the volume of air in the conducting airways that does not participate in gas exchange. This category includes all air down to the respiratory bronchioles. The following formula depicts $V_D$physio:

$$V_D\text{physio} = V_D\text{alv} + V_D\text{anat}$$

Normally, $V_D$physio consists mainly of $V_D$anat, with the $V_D$alv component being minute. That is why the normal $V_D$physio volume in milliliters is approximately equal to the weight of a person in pounds. For example, a person weighing 150 lb has a $V_D$physio of 150 ml. When alveoli become overventilated as compared with perfused, the $V_D$alv increases, which in turn increases the $V_D$physio.

The amount of $V_D$physio can be determined by the Bohr equation. Clinically, the Bohr equation is commonly referred to as the V_D/V_T. The ratio of dead space (V_D) to V_T can be used to determine whether the obstruction to pulmonary capillary blood flow is partial ($\dot{V}_A/\dot{Q}_C$) or complete (wasted ventilation). The V_D/V_T can be derived from the following equation:

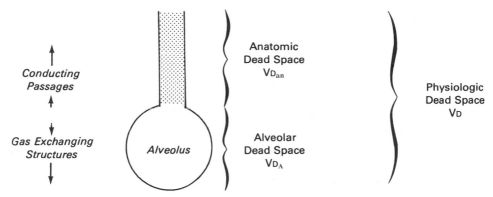

FIGURE 6–19. Graphic representation of dead space. The physiologic dead space represents the sum of the anatomic dead space in the conducting passages *(shaded area)* and alveolar dead space in the alveoli *(circle)*. (From Harper, R.: A Guide to Respiratory Care: Physiology and Clinical Applications. Philadelphia, J. B. Lippincott, 1981, p. 48.)

$$\frac{V_D}{V_T} = \frac{Pa_{CO_2} - P_{ECO_2}}{Pa_{CO_2}}$$

where the Pa_{CO_2} is the arterial carbon dioxide partial pressure and the P_{ECO_2} is the partial pressure of the expired carbon dioxide. The V_D/V_T ratio is normally 0.3. If the V_D/V_T increases to 0.6, more than half of the V_T is dead space. Most patients can double their minute ventilation ($\dot{V}_E$), but beyond that amount the effort is too exhausting, and a V_D/V_T ratio of more than 0.6 usually mandates that the patient's ventilation be assisted mechanically.

Implications for PACU Care

In the early postoperative period (including the transport of the patient from the operating room to the PACU), the patient should be considered to have a reduced FRC and hypoventilation and to experience some ventilation-perfusion mismatch. All these factors lead to a reduction in arterial oxygenation as reflected by a low Sa_{O_2} and Pa_{O_2}. Research now demonstrates that hypoxemia exists during transport to the PACU. Consequently, all patients should receive supplemental oxygenation during transport to the PACU and certainly throughout their stay there. In addition, because these respiratory alterations occur in almost all patients recovering from anesthesia, pulse oximetry should be used on each patient during transport and in the PACU.

REGULATION OF BREATHING

In the past, medullary control of breathing was thought to be a function of reciprocal in-

hibition between the inspiratory and expiratory centers. Research now indicates a more discrete regulatory process occurring at two levels: the sensors and the controllers. Patients with altered regulation and control of breathing present a significant challenge to the PACU nurse. Also, anesthesia, surgery, and medications administered in the PACU can have a profound impact on the patient's regulatory processes of breathing.

The Sensors

Peripheral Chemoreceptors. The carotid and aortic bodies are the peripheral chemoreceptors and are located at the bifurcation of the common carotid arteries and at the arch of the aorta, respectively. The carotid and aortic bodies are responsible for the immediate increase in ventilation due to lack of oxygen. These peripheral chemoreceptors are made up of highly vascular tissue and glomus cells. The carotid and aortic bodies monitor only the Pa_{O_2}, not the Ca_{O_2} of the hemoglobin. Therefore, the receptors are not stimulated in conditions such as anemia and carbon monoxide and cyanide poisoning.

The carotid bodies are much more important physiologically than the aortic bodies. The carotid bodies respond, in order of degree of response, to low Pa_{O_2}, high Pa_{CO_2}, and low pH. The carotid bodies respond to a low Pa_{O_2}, and the response is augmented by a high Pa_{CO_2}, a low pH, or both. The physiologic responses to the stimulation of the carotid sinus are hyperpnea, bradycardia, and hypotension. The aortic bodies, on the other hand, respond to a low Pa_{O_2} and high Pa_{CO_2} but not to pH. The results of stimulation of the aortic bodies are hyperpnea, tachycardia, and hypertension.

The carotid and aortic bodies mainly respond to a low PaO_2. This response is commonly referred to as the *hypoxic* or *secondary drive*. The impulse activity in these chemoreceptors begins at a PaO_2 of about 500 torr. A rapid increase in impulses occurs at a PaO_2 lower than 100 torr. The impulses are greatly increased as the PaO_2 falls below 60 torr. Below 30 torr, the impulse activity from the chemoreceptors decreases owing to direct oxygen deficit in the glomus cells. In addition, these peripheral arterial chemoreceptors are stimulated by low arterial blood pressure and increased sympathetic activity.

Central Chemoreceptors. The central chemoreceptors lie near the ventral surface of the medulla. Specifically, these chemosensitive areas are near the choroid plexus (venous blood) and next to the cerebrospinal fluid (CSF). The central chemoreceptors respond *indirectly* to carbon dioxide. This is because the blood-brain barrier allows lipid-soluble substances, such as carbon dioxide, oxygen, and water, to cross the barrier, whereas water-soluble substances, such as sodium, potassium, hydrogen ion, and bicarbonate, pass through the membrane at a *very slow rate*. Bicarbonate requires active transport to cross the barrier. Therefore, carbon dioxide enters the CSF and is hydrated to form carbonic acid. The carbonic acid rapidly dissociates to form hydrogen ion and bicarbonate. The hydrogen ion concentration in the CSF parallels the arterial PCO_2. Actually, it is the hydrogen ion concentration that stimulates ventilation via hydrogen receptors located in the central chemoreceptor area. In summary, carbon dioxide has little direct effect on the stimulation of the receptors in the central chemoreceptor area but does have a *potent indirect effect*. This indirect effect is due to the inability of hydrogen ions to easily cross the blood-brain barrier. For this reason, changes in hydrogen ion concentration in the blood have considerably less effect in stimulating the chemoreceptor area than do changes in carbon dioxide. Consequently, the central chemoreceptor area precisely controls ventilation and therefore the $PaCO_2$. For that reason, *the index to the adequacy of ventilation is the $PaCO_2$*.

Bicarbonate is the only major buffer in the CSF. The pH of the CSF is a result of the ratio between bicarbonate and carbon dioxide in the CSF. Carbon dioxide is freely diffusible in and out of the CSF via the blood-brain barrier. However, bicarbonate is not freely diffusible and requires active or passive transport to enter or leave the CSF. When an acute increase in the $PaCO_2$ occurs, carbon dioxide enters the CSF

and is hydrated, and hydrogen ions and bicarbonate are formed. The hydrogen ion stimulates the chemoreceptors, and the bicarbonate decreases the pH of the CSF. The resultant hyperpnea lowers the blood $PaCO_2$, creating a gradient favoring the diffusion of carbon dioxide out of the CSF. The blood $PaCO_2$ and pH will be corrected immediately, but the pH in the CSF requires some time to re-establish a normal carbon dioxide–bicarbonate level owing to the poor diffusibility of bicarbonate. This is usually not a problem for the person with normal respiratory function. However, for the patient with chronic carbon dioxide retention (chronic hypercapnia) who is hyperventilated to a "normal" $PaCO_2$ of 40 torr, serious deleterious effects may occur. Patients with a chronically elevated $PaCO_2$ have a higher amount of carbon dioxide and bicarbonate in the CSF, but the ratio is maintained in a chronic situation. In this instance, the patient will be breathing at a higher *set point*. That is, instead of being maintained at 40 torr, the normal $PaCO_2$ for this patient might be maintained at 46 torr, and near-normal sensitivity to changes in the $PaCO_2$ would be present. If this patient were aggressively ventilated in the PACU with the goal of lowering the $PaCO_2$ to 40 torr, significant negative repercussions could occur. With a lower $PaCO_2$ the carbon dioxide in the CSF diffuses out and the bicarbonate remains, owing to its inability to diffuse out of the CSF. Thus, an excess of bicarbonate as compared with carbon dioxide (↑ bicarbonate pool) exists in the CSF, causing the primary stimulus to ventilation to *cease*. Because the patient was hyperventilated, the $PaCO_2$ decreases and the PAO_2 increases (because of the 12–10 concept; see section on blood gas transport). Therefore, the secondary (hypoxic) drive may also become extinguished so that this patient will have no effective drive for ventilation. If patients with chronic hypercapnia are acutely hyperventilated, they must be monitored for apnea once the accelerated ventilation is discontinued. It is more appropriate to maintain the $PaCO_2$ at the level that is normal for that patient to avoid an apneic situation. Thus, for the patient with chronic carbon dioxide retention who is emerging from anesthesia, an overaggressive stir-up regimen (hyperventilation) should be avoided. The patient should perform the SMI at normal intervals, and the arterial blood gas values should be closely monitored.

In some patients with chronic carbon dioxide retention (chronic hypercapnia), the sensitivity to hydrogen ions via the carbon dioxide may be effectively decreased to the point at which the primary stimulus to ventilation becomes the low PaO_2 at the carotid and aortic bodies. The low PaO_2 becomes an effective stimulus to ventilation, especially when the $PaCO_2$ is elevated. The high $PaCO_2$ augments the response to the low PaO_2 by the peripheral chemoreceptors. For this reason, the patient is breathing via his or her hypoxic drive. Because the carotid bodies are the major peripheral chemoreceptors, patients using the hypoxic drive may also experience bradycardia and hypotension. For that reason, patients with abnormally high preoperative $PaCO_2$ values who have bradycardia and hypotension should be suspected of using the hypoxic drive as their primary drive to ventilation. In the PACU, patients suspected of primarily using this drive should be monitored closely and given oxygen to attain adequate oxygen content (a hemoglobin saturation of between 80 and 90 percent). The primary goal is to keep patients oxygenated without extinguishing their main control of ventilation. High-flow techniques using a Venturi mask that works on the Venturi principle to ensure precise FIO_2 values (i.e., 24 to 50 percent) can be used with these patients.

The Response to Carbon Dioxide. Carbon dioxide is the primary stimulus to ventilation. The carbon dioxide response test is used to assess the ventilatory response to carbon dioxide. In this test, the subject inhales carbon dioxide mixtures (with the PaO_2 held constant) so that the inspired PCO_2 gradually increases. Normally, the $\dot{V}E$ increases linearly as the PCO_2 increases (Fig. 6–20). Some disease states and drugs cause the carbon dioxide response curve to shift to the left or the right. If the curve shifts to the left, the subject is more responsive to carbon dioxide. Factors such as thyroid toxicosis, aggressive personality, salicylates, and

ketosis shift the curve to the left. A decreased ventilatory response to carbon dioxide occurs when the curve is shifted to the right. This is called a *blunted response*. Patients who have a blunted response to carbon dioxide require intensive PACU nursing care. The ventilatory response to an increased concentration of inspired carbon dioxide is blunted by hypothyroidism, mental depression, aging, general anesthetics, barbiturates, and narcotics. Many patients in the PACU either have these conditions or have received these drugs intraoperatively. This blunted response to carbon dioxide is one of the main justifications for giving supplemental oxygen to all patients emerging from anesthesia in the PACU. It is also the rationale behind the need for critical PACU nursing care that includes frequent assessment and interventions such as the stir-up regimen to prevent respiratory depression.

Upper Airways Receptors. There are receptors located in the nose that are sensitive to mechanical stimulation and chemical agents and have afferent pathways via the trigeminal and olfactory nerves. Activation of these receptors can cause apnea, bradycardia, and, most commonly, a sneeze. When a patient is to be intubated nasally, the PACU nurse should monitor for bradycardia and apnea and be prepared for necessary interventions. Atropine or glycopyrrolate (Robinul) may be required for their vagolytic effect; succinylcholine may facilitate the intubation. Finally, to provide positive-pressure ventilation, a bag-valve-mask system should be immediately available should apnea occur.

Receptors located in the epipharynx are sensitive to mechanical stimulation. Their activation is associated with the *sniff* or *aspiration reflex*. Mechanical stimulation of these receptors causes deep inspiration, bronchodilatation, and hypertension. This is a protective reflex allowing material in the epipharynx to be brought down to the pharynx, clearing the nasal airways. In the larynx are irritant receptors that respond to both mechanical and chemical stimulation. Afferent pathways from these receptors travel along the internal branch of the superior laryngeal nerve. Stimulation invokes many responses, including coughing, slow deep-breathing, apnea, bronchoconstriction, and hypertension. In addition, the trachea possesses irritant receptors. Stimulation of these receptors can cause responses such as coughing, bronchoconstriction, and hypertension.

During any procedure that involves the intubation of the trachea, the PACU nurse should be prepared to assess the appropriate cardio-

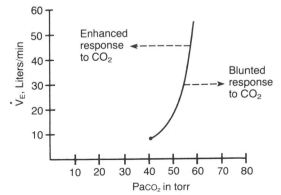

FIGURE 6–20. Carbon dioxide response curve (see text for details). (From Traver, G. [ed.]: Respiratory Nursing: The Science and the Art. New York: John Wiley & Sons, 1982. Reprinted by permission of John Wiley & Sons, Inc.)

respiratory parameters and implement nursing care as required.

Lung Receptors. *Pulmonary stretch receptors* (PSR) lie within the smooth muscle of the small airways. These receptors are activated by marked distention or deflation (atelectasis) of the lungs. On marked inflation of the lungs, the activation of the PSR leads to a slowing of inspiratory frequency owing to an increase in expiratory time. Bronchodilatation and tachycardia also may result from activation of these receptors. The PSRs are thought to be part of the *Hering-Breuer reflex.* The low threshold for the PSR is present for approximately the first 3 months of life; after that the threshold is high throughout adulthood. Hence, for the adult, the Hering-Breuer reflex is not important in the control of ventilation except in the anesthetized state. When an adult is under general anesthesia and ventilated with prolonged maximum lung inflations, a prolonged expiratory time can result owing to activation of the PSR.

Of great interest in regard to the pathogenesis of asthma are the *irritant receptors* that lie between the airway epithelial cells. These receptors respond to chemical irritants, such as histamine, and mechanical irritants, such as small particles and aerosols that irritate the pulmonary epithelium. The irritant receptors are mediated by vagal afferent fibers, and, on receptor stimulation, bronchoconstriction and hyperpnea occur. It is suggested that the pathogenesis of asthma revolves around the sequence of histamine release, which stimulates the irritant receptors and ultimately leads to bronchoconstriction mediated via the vagus nerve.

The J, or *juxtapulmonary capillary, receptors* are located in the wall of the pulmonary capillaries. Like the irritant receptors, J-receptors' afferent impulses are transmitted to the central nervous system by the vagus nerve. Normal stimuli of the J-receptors include pneumonia, pulmonary congestion, and increased interstitial fluid pressure. Stimulation of these receptors by interstitial or pulmonary edema results in tachypnea, bradycardia, and hypotension. Therefore, when assessing patients who are at risk for developing pulmonary edema, the nurse should always evaluate the rate of ventilation. Knowing that interstitial edema usually precedes pulmonary edema, and that increased interstitial congestion stimulates the J-receptors, the nurse should consider a rapid, shallow breathing pattern to be a danger signal and report it to the attending physician.

Located in the walls of the large systemic arteries, especially in the aortic and carotid sinuses, are *stretch receptors* called *baroreceptors.* These receptors help to control the systemic blood pressure. They also affect ventilation. When the systemic blood pressure increases, a reflex hypoventilation will occur owing to stimulation of the baroreceptors. On the other hand, a low systemic blood pressure causes the baroreceptors to produce a reflex hyperventilation. Hence, if a patient in the PACU experiences a significant amount of hypertension or hypotension, a reflex ventilatory response will usually occur owing to the stimulation of the baroreceptors in the large systemic arteries.

The Controllers

The controllers of breathing are located in the central nervous system. They are composed of two functionally and anatomically separate components. Voluntary breathing is controlled in the cortex of the brain. Automatic breathing is controlled by structures within the brain stem. The spinal cord functions to integrate the output of the brain stem and the cortex. The cortex can override the other controllers of breathing if voluntary control is desired. Examples of voluntary control include voluntary hyperventilation and breath-holding.

The Brain Stem. Located bilaterally in the upper pons is the *pneumotaxic center.* This center functions to fine-tune the respiratory pattern by modulating the activity of the apneustic center and regulating the respiratory system's response to stimuli such as hypercarbia, hypoxia, and lung inflation. Near the pontomedullary border lies the *apneustic center.* This center is probably the site of the inspiratory cutoff switch that terminates inspiration. In fact, apneusis, which consists of prolonged inspirations with occasional expirations, results when the apneustic center has been deactivated. Consequently, the apneustic center is also a fine-tuner of the rhythm of breathing.

Located in the medullary center, above the spinal cord, are two groups of neurons: the *dorsal respiratory group* (DRG) and the *ventral respiratory group* (VRG). The DRG is composed of inspiratory neurons and is the initial intracranial processing site for many reflexes affecting breathing. It is probably the site of origin of the rhythmic respiratory drive. The DRG sends motor fibers via the phrenic nerve to the diaphragm. It sends inspiratory fibers to the VRG, which is also part of the medullary center. However, the VRG does not send fibers to the DRG; therefore, the reciprocal inhibition theory of the regulation of breathing seems unlikely. The VRG is made up of both inspiratory and expiratory cells. The VRG neurons are driven by the cells of the DRG and, therefore, respiratory rhythmicity and the processing of sensory inputs do not occur initially within the VRG. The major function of the VRG is to project impulses to distant sites and drive either spinal respiratory motor neurons (primary intercostal and abdominal) or the auxiliary muscles of breathing innervated by the vagus nerve.

The DRG receives information from almost all the chemoreceptors, the baroreceptors, and the other sensors in the lung. In turn, the DRG generates a breathing rhythm that is fine-tuned by the apneustic center (inspiratory cutoff switch) and the pneumotaxic center. The inspiratory motor impulses are sent to the diaphragm and to the VRG. The VRG then drives spinal respiratory neurons (innervating the intercostal and abdominal muscles) or the auxiliary muscles of respiration innervated by the vagus nerve. Again, the cerebral cortex can override these centers if voluntary control of breathing is desired. Also, the vagus nerve has a profound effect on many aspects of the control of breathing, because the afferent pathways of the vagus nerve from the stretch, J-, and irritant receptors serve to modulate the rhythm of breathing. Thus, any dysfunction that includes transection of the vagi results in irregular breathing patterns, depending on the level of dysfunction (pons or medulla).

POSTOPERATIVE LUNG VOLUMES

Postoperative pulmonary complications are the most common single cause of morbidity and mortality in the postoperative period. The reported incidence of postoperative pulmonary complications ranges from 4.5 to 76 percent.

Patients with Abnormal Pulmonary Function

When patients undergo anesthesia and surgery, certain risk factors predispose them to develop postoperative pulmonary complications. Patients at the highest risk are those with pre-existing pulmonary problems with abnormal pulmonary function before surgery. The other major risk factors associated with postoperative pulmonary complications are chronic cigarette smoking, obesity, and advanced age.

Pre-existing Pulmonary Disease. Patients with pre-existing pulmonary disease can have clinical or subclinical manifestations of their disease state. Consequently, preoperative pul-

monary function tests are valuable in assessing the presence or absence of pulmonary pathophysiology as well as in determining operative risk. *Obstructive lung disease* (i.e., asthma, emphysema, and chronic bronchitis), the most common category of lung disease, can be assessed by flow-volume measurements. Burrows and associates suggest that a maximum voluntary ventilation that is less than 50 percent of what is predicted, a maximum expiratory flow rate below 220 L per min, or a forced expiratory volume in 1 second below 1.5 L indicates an increased operative risk for pulmonary complications. These flow-volume measurements are valuable predictors of the patient's ability to generate an adequate cough, which is a pulmonary defense mechanism rendered ineffective in the immediate postoperative period by anesthesia and surgery. Consequently, these patients require vigorous, informed nursing care in the immediate postoperative period. Priorities of nursing care should include frequent use of the stir-up regimen of turn, cascade cough, and SMI, along with the use of appropriate nursing interventions designed to enhance secretion clearance, which ensures airway patency.

Patients with *restrictive lung disease* (i.e., pulmonary fibrosis and morbid obesity) represent a significant risk for postoperative pulmonary complications when their pulmonary function test reveals a VC or a diffusion capacity of less than 50 percent of predicted values, or exercise arterial blood gas values that demonstrate slight hypoxemia on exertion. In the PACU, these patients require a vigorous stir-up regimen with attention to tissue oxygenation via monitoring for hypoxemia. This is needed because during the surgical experience and in the PACU, physiologic stress can occur. One of the major products of physiologic stress is an increase in cardiovascular parameters, which reduces the transit time of the red blood cells across the respiratory gas exchange membrane. Because of the pathologic changes in the respiratory membrane, patients with restrictive lung disease can desaturate on exertion, such as in the stress reaction.

Cigarette Smoking. Chronic cigarette smoking has been shown to increase the incidence of postoperative pulmonary complications. Morton suggests that patients smoking only 10 cigarettes a day have a sixfold increase in pulmonary morbidity in the postoperative period. The incidence of pulmonary embolism is higher in the smoker because of increased coagulability produced by chronic cigarette smoking. The ciliated epithelium of the lungs is damaged by chronic cigarette smoking. This damage can cause some blockage of the mucociliary transport system, finally resulting in bronchiolar obstruction, infection, and atelectasis. Patients who smoke should be encouraged to stop smoking for *at least 2 weeks* before surgery to allow the mucociliary transport system to return to a nearly normal level of function. The focus of nursing care for the active chronic cigarette smoker should be similar to the interventions discussed for the patient with obstructive lung disease.

Obesity. The markedly overweight patient has a significant chance of developing postoperative pulmonary complications. This is due to the altered lung volumes and capacities caused by the excess adipose tissue. Expansion of the lungs is hindered by an enlarged abdomen, which elevates the diaphragm and adds weight on the chest wall, thereby hindering the outward recoil of the chest wall. This leads to a decreased thoracic wall compliance and, ultimately, a reduced FRC. Finally, these complications result in hypoxemia from increased airway closure and $\dot{V}_A/\dot{Q}_C$ abnormalities (see Chapter 38). The goal of nursing interventions in the PACU is to prevent further airway closure. Thus, a vigorous stir-up regimen, including early ambulation, should help prevent further reduction in the FRC. That measure reduces the amount of airway closure, alleviates the hypoxemia, and ultimately improves the outcome of the patient.

Advanced Age. Patients of advanced age (older than 70 years of age), have a slightly higher risk of developing postoperative pulmonary complications. A greater decrease in the FRC following surgery in patients of advanced age has been demonstrated. Because the closing volume increases with age, significant airway closure can occur during tidal ventilation postoperatively. Although advanced age is not associated with the same degree of risk as the factors previously discussed, it can increase the danger of the other risk factors. However, patients of advanced age should receive a vigorous stir-up regimen in the PACU if only because of the alterations in their lung mechanics.

Physiology of Postoperative Pulmonary Nursing Care

Because of the change in the mechanical properties of the lungs and chest wall, patients emerging from anesthesia experience a decrease in their lung volumes and capacities

(Fig. 6–21). This is especially true of the patient who has undergone a thoracic or upper abdominal surgical procedure. In the PACU, a further reduction in lung volumes and capacities may be seen. The major factor contributing to this reduction in lung volumes in the postoperative patient is a shallow, monotonous, *sighless* breathing pattern that is caused by general inhalation anesthesia, pain, and narcotics. Sighless ventilation may result in an uneven distribution of surfactant and a loss of stability of the small airways and alveoli, which can then lead to alveolar collapse and, ultimately, to atelectasis. Normally, adults breathe regularly and rhythmically, spontaneously performing a maximum inspiration that is held for about 3 seconds at the peak of inspiration. This physiologic process, or SMI, is commonly referred to as a *sigh* or a *yawn*.

In normal lungs, the closing volume is less than the resting lung volume (i.e., the FRC), and airways remain open during tidal breathing. In the immediate postoperative period, patients who have a sighless, monotonous, low V_T ventilatory pattern usually have a reduced FRC. When the FRC plus V_T is within the closing volume range, the airways leading to dependent lung zones may be effectively closed throughout tidal breathing (Fig. 6–22). Inspired

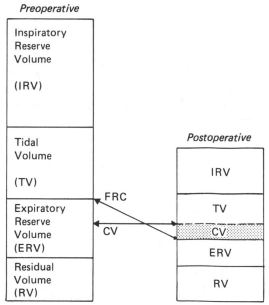

FIGURE 6–21. Graphic comparison of preoperative lung volumes to the probable lung volumes in the immediate postoperative period in a patient who has undergone an upper abdominal surgical procedure. FRC = functional residual capacity; CV = closing volume. (From Drain, C.: Post anesthesia lung volumes in surgical patients. AANA J., *49*[3]:261–268, 1981.)

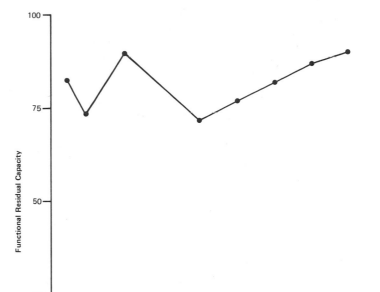

FIGURE 6–22. Composite curve of the mean values of the functional residual capacity in the postoperative period. (From Drain, C.: Post anesthesia lung volumes in surgical patients. AANA J., *49*[3]:261–268, 1981.)

gas is then distributed mainly to the upper or nondependent lung zones. Perfusion continues to follow the normal gradient, with higher flows to the dependent areas of the lung.

In the immediate postoperative period, as airway closure occurs, gas is trapped behind closed airways. This sequestered air can become absorbed and the alveoli then become airless (atelectasis). The atelectasis, as it becomes more widespread, leads to a decrease in ventilation as compared with perfusion (low $\dot{V}_A/\dot{Q}_C$), which results in a widening of the $P_{AO_2} - P_{aO_2}$ and, ultimately, to hypoxemia. In addition, atelectatic areas in the lung provide an excellent culture medium in which pneumonia can develop.

Various investigators have demonstrated a decrease in lung volumes in the postoperative period. Patients who have undergone an upper abdominal surgical procedure experience an immediate decrease in the FRC from hour 1 to hour 2 postoperatively (see Fig. 6–21). The FRC then seems to return to near the baseline value by about the fourth postoperative hour. A second subsequent decrease in the FRC is then seen after hour 4, and baseline values are not restored until 5 days postoperatively. A possible explanation of the "peaks and valleys" in the FRC during the postoperative period may

be that the first reduction in the FRC is associated with anesthesia and the latter reduction may be due to pain. General inhalation anesthesia and pain can dampen the physiologic sigh mechanism. Consequently, all patients who have undergone a surgical procedure, especially those who have their incision sites near the thorax or diaphragm, should be strongly encouraged to perform the SMI maneuver both in the PACU and on the surgical unit. The incentive spirometer, a device designed to encourage the patient with positive feedback to perform the SMI maneuver, can be used by the patient on the surgical unit.

OXYGEN ADMINISTRATION IN THE PACU

Administration of oxygen to the patient in the PACU is an important facet in the emergence phase of anesthesia. Oxygen is given to the PACU patient primarily because of the blunted or depressed response to carbon dioxide and low lung volumes. It is especially important that the patient who has received a general or spinal anesthetic be given supplemental oxygen during the recovery phase of anesthesia. The methods of oxygen administration are summarized in Chapter 20 (see Fig. 20–1).

PACU Nursing Care

A patent airway must be maintained throughout the administration of oxygen. The patient should be encouraged to cascade cough, perform the SMI, and change positions according to the stir-up regimen discussed in this chapter and in Chapter 20. If a nasal catheter is used, the catheter should be removed every 6 hours to be cleaned and reinserted into the other nostril. Also, the nasal mucosa should be inspected periodically for dryness when a nasal catheter or prongs are used. Oxygen given in the dry gas form can cause drying and irritation of the mucosa, impair the ciliary action, and thicken secretions; therefore, oxygen should always be administered with humidity.

It is imperative for the PACU nurse to receive a report from the anesthesiologist or anesthetist or both as to the patient's preoperative pulmonary status. It is especially important to ascertain if the patient has a history of chronically retaining carbon dioxide, as occurs in chronic obstructive pulmonary disease. As described in this chapter, the patient with carbon dioxide retention who is receiving oxygen in the PACU should be monitored carefully for any signs of hypoventilation, confusion, or becoming semicomatose. If any of these signs appear, the surgeon and anethesiologist or anesthetist should be notified immediately.

Oxygen Toxicity

When excessive concentrations of inspired oxygen (>60 percent) are administered to patients for a prolonged period, the eyes, lungs, and central nervous system can be damaged.

Eyes. Premature infants who have a high PaO_2 longer than 24 hours are at risk for developing *retrolental fibroplasia*, which is caused by vasoconstriction of the blood vessels of the retina as a result of high oxygen concentrations in the blood. It presents in an acute form as vascular retinopathy occurring at the developing edge of blood vessels in the premature infant's eye. This is followed by perivascular exudation, tissue hyperplasia, and scar tissue that exerts traction on the retina, leading to retinal detachment and destruction of the infant's vision. Research indicates that the incidence of acute retrolental fibroplasia is inversely proportional to birth weight. Most of the clinical research indicates that to minimize the risk of development of retrolental fibroplasia, the infant's PaO_2 should be maintained between 60 and 90 torr. The PACU nurse should use his or her best informed judgment when caring for these infants. As with the adult, the infant who needs a high inspired oxygen concentration to provide adequate oxygenation should not be denied oxygen because of fear of complications.

Lungs. Concentrations of oxygen higher than 60 percent damage the lungs within 3 or 4 days. A 100 percent oxygen concentration administered for 24 to 48 hours also causes pulmonary damage, the signs of which are manifested by type II cell dysfunction in the lung. The type II cells secrete surfactant, and the lack of surfactant in the alveoli leads to alveolar collapse. The hyperoxic environment also stops the ciliary action in the lungs. The early symptoms of this disorder include cough, nasal congestion, sore throat, reduced VC, tracheobronchitis, and substernal discomfort. The early signs of airway irritation may appear when a patient has received 80 to 100 percent oxygen continuously for 8 hours or longer. The lung appears to tolerate oxygen concentrations lower than 40 percent indefinitely.

Central Nervous System. Headache is an early indicator of oxygen toxicity. As oxygen toxicity continues to develop, the patient will demonstrate some confusion. When a patient is receiving a high concentration of oxygen and has these signs and symptoms, the attending physician should be notified. Convulsions usually are not seen in the PACU but may occur when oxygen is delivered in above-normal atmospheric pressure, such as in hyperbaric oxygen chambers.

References

1. Barash, P., Cullen, B., and Stoelting, R.: Clinical Anesthesia. 2nd ed. Philadelphia, J. B. Lippincott, 1992.
2. Barnes, P., Baraniuk, J., and Belvisi, M.: Neuropeptides in the respiratory tract. Am. Rev. Respir. Dis., 144:1187–1198, 1991.
3. Berels, D., and Marz, M.: SaO_2 monitoring in the postanesthesia care unit. J. Post Anesth. Nurs., 6(6):394–401, 1991.
4. Blosser, S., and Rock, P.: Asthma and chronic obstructive lung disease. In Breslow, M., Miller, C., and Rogers, M. (eds.): Perioperative Management. St. Louis, C. V. Mosby, 1990, pp. 259–280.
5. Burrows, B., Knudson, R., Quan, S., et al.: Respiratory Disorders: A Pathophysiologic Approach. 2nd ed. Chicago, Year Book Medical, 1983.
6. Butterworth, J.: Atlas of Procedures in Anesthesia and Critical Care. Philadelphia, W. B. Saunders, 1992.
7. Coe, A., Sarginson, R., Smith, M., et al.: Pain following thoracotomy. Anaesthesia, 46:918–921, 1991.

8. Drain, C.: Comparison of two inspiratory maneuvers on increasing lung volumes in postoperative upper abdominal surgical patients. AANA J., *52*:379–388, 1984.
9. Drain, C.: Managing postoperative pain . . . it's a matter of sighs. Nursing, *14*(8):52–55, 1984.
10. Drain, C.: Post anesthesia lung volumes in surgical patients. AANA J., *49*:261–268, 1981.
11. Drain, C.: The anesthetic management of the patient: A broad view of the anesthetic consideration necessary regarding the respiratory system. AANA J., *50*:192–201, 1982.
12. Flynn, J.: Oxygen and retrolental fibroplasia: Update and challenge. Anesthesiology, *60*(5):397–399, 1984.
13. Frost, E.: Preanesthetic assessment of the patient with respiratory disease. Anesthesiol. Clin. North Am., *8*:657–676, 1990.
14. Guyton, A.: Textbook of Medical Physiology. 8th ed. Philadelphia, W. B. Saunders, 1991.
15. Harper, R.: A Guide to Respiratory Care: Physiology and Clinical Applications. Philadelphia, J. B. Lippincott, 1981.
16. Hoffman, C., Nakamoto, D., Okal, R., et al.: Effect of transport time and FIO_2 on SpO_2 during transport from the OR to the PACU. Nurse Anesth., *2*(3):119–125, 1991.
17. Jacobsen, W. K., Lobo, D. P., Cole, D. J., et al. (eds.): Manual of Post Anesthesia Care. Philadelphia, W. B. Saunders, 1992.
18. Kaplan, J.: Thoracic Anesthesia. 2nd ed. New York, Churchill Livingstone, 1991.
19. Katz, J., Benumof, J., and Kadis, L. (eds.): Anesthesia and Uncommon Diseases. 3rd ed. Philadelphia, W. B. Saunders, 1990.
20. Levitzky, M.: Pulmonary Physiology. 3rd ed. New York, McGraw-Hill, 1991.
21. Longnecker, D. E., and Murphy, F. L. (eds.): Dripps/Eckenhoff/Vandam Introduction to Anesthesia: Principles of Safe Practice. 8th ed. Philadelphia, W. B. Saunders, 1992.
22. Miller, R. (ed.): Anesthesia. 3rd ed. New York, Churchill Livingstone, 1990.
23. Murray, J.: The Normal Lung. 2nd ed. Philadelphia, W. B. Saunders, 1986.
24. Newton, N.: Supplementary oxygen—potential for disaster. Anaesthesia, *46*:905–906, 1991.
25. Shapiro, B.: Clinical Applications of Blood Gases. 4th ed. Chicago, Year Book Medical, 1988.
26. Snyder, J., and Pinsky, M.: Oxygen Transport in the Critically Ill. Chicago, Year Book Medical, 1987.
27. Taylor, L., and Stephens, D.: Arterial blood gases: Clinical application. J. Post Anesth. Nurs., *5*(4):264–272, 1990.
28. Traver, G. (ed.): Respiratory Nursing: The Science and the Art. New York, John Wiley & Sons, 1982.
29. Waugaman, W., Foster, S. D., and Rigor, B. (eds.): Principles and Practice of Nurse Anesthesia. 2nd ed. Norwalk, CT, Appleton & Lange, 1992.

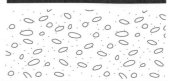

CHAPTER 7

Renal Anatomy and Physiology

Most of the drugs used in anesthesia are excreted unchanged or as a metabolic by-product by the kidneys. Homeostasis is maintained by proper kidney function, because the kidneys regulate the balance of acid–base, electrolyte, and fluid volumes and remove waste materials and toxic substances from the body.

Kidney function is sometimes difficult to assess in the post anesthesia care unit (PACU), especially in the uncatheterized patient. In patients who do have urinary catheters in place after surgery, assessment of kidney function should be part of the PACU nursing care. It is important to understand renal anatomy and physiology so that total PACU nursing care can be rendered to the patient.

Definitions

Acetonuria: the appearance of acetone in the urine. It is present when excessive fats are consumed or when an inadequate amount of carbohydrates is metabolized.

Albuminuria: the presence of protein in the urine, also referred to as proteinuria. Albumin is the most common protein found in the urine. This condition is usually indicative of malfunction in glomerular filtration.

Azotemia: the presence of nitrogenous products in the blood, usually because of decreased kidney function.

Cystitis: an inflammation of the bladder.

Dysuria: painful or difficult urination.

Enuresis: involuntary discharge of urine.

Glycosuria: the presence of glucose in the urine.

Hematuria: the presence of blood in the urine.

Nephritis: inflammation of the kidney; called Bright's disease.

Nephrosis: degeneration of the kidney without the occurrence of inflammation.

Oliguria: a decrease in the normal amount of urine formation.

Pyelitis: an inflammation of the renal pelvis and calices.

Stricture: an abnormal narrowing; in the urinary tract, a narrowing of the ureter or urethra.

Uremia: the toxic condition usually caused by renal insufficiency and retention of nitrogenous substances in the blood.

Urinary incontinence: the inability to retain urine in the bladder.

Urinary retention: failure to expel urine from the bladder.

ANATOMY OF THE KIDNEYS

The kidneys are two bean-shaped organs in the retroperitoneal spaces near the upper lumbar area. The right kidney is at a slightly lower level than the left. Each kidney weighs approximately 150 g. The notched portion of the kidney is called the *hilum,* and it is here that the ureter, the renal vein, and the renal artery enter the kidney (Fig. 7–1).

The ureter opens into a large cavity called the *pelvis.* From the pelvis, two to five *major calices* project deeper into the kidney. The major calices branch out to form six to ten *minor calices.* The ends of the minor calices are capped by the *renal papillae.*

The *medulla* is the inner portion of the kidney. It is made up of several *pyramids,* which correspond to the number of minor calices. The base of the pyramid projects toward the outer portion of the kidney, which is termed the *cortex.* The apex of the pyramid forms the papillae, which cap each minor calix.

Blood is supplied to the kidney by the *renal artery.* The rate of blood flow through both kidneys of a man weighing 70 kg is about 1200 ml per min, or about 21 percent of the cardiac output. As the renal artery enters the kidney at the hilum, it divides into the interlobar arteries in the medulla; then, as they enter the cortex, they divide into the *arciform (arcuate) arteries.* The afferent arteries project from the interlobar arteries and go to the nephron, where they di-

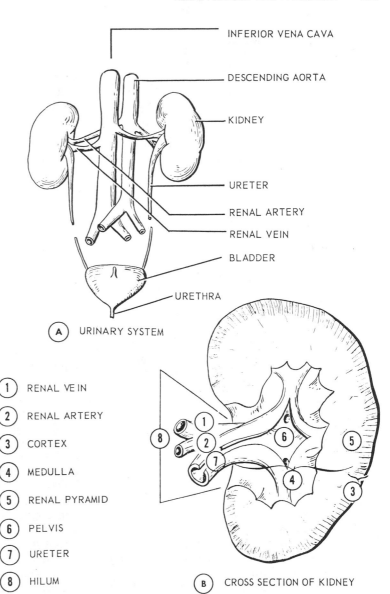

FIGURE 7–1. Anatomy of the renal and urinary systems.

A URINARY SYSTEM

INFERIOR VENA CAVA

DESCENDING AORTA

KIDNEY

URETER

RENAL ARTERY

RENAL VEIN

BLADDER

URETHRA

1 RENAL VEIN
2 RENAL ARTERY
3 CORTEX
4 MEDULLA
5 RENAL PYRAMID
6 PELVIS
7 URETER
8 HILUM

B CROSS SECTION OF KIDNEY

vide into capillaries. The capillaries form the efferent arterioles, which then divide to form the *peritubular capillaries,* which help supply the nephron, a portion of the tubular capillaries, and the vasa recta, which descend around the loop of Henle, in the case of juxtamedullary nephrons. These nephrons, which are close to the renal medulla, have a long, extended loop of Henle that dips deep into the medulla. They then return to the venules, as do the tubular capillaries (Figs. 7–2 and 7–3).

The *nephron* is the functional unit of the kidney. The two kidneys contain approximately 2.4 million nephrons. Each nephron can be divided into three major portions: the renal corpuscle, the renal tubule, and the collecting ducts. The blood enters the afferent arteriole

and goes into the glomerulus in the cortex. It consists of a network of 50 parallel capillaries encased in Bowman's capsule. This structural component is the renal capsule.

The renal tubules begin in Bowman's capsule. A pressure gradient forces fluid to leave the glomerulus and enter Bowman's capsule. The fluid then flows into the proximal tubule, which is still in the cortex of the kidney, and then into the loop of Henle. The loop of Henle is at first thick-walled but becomes thin-walled at the distal segment in the medulla of the kidney. The fluid then flows into the distal tubule, located in the cortex of the kidney, and passes into the collecting ducts, which go from the cortex to the medulla where they form papillary ducts (ducts of Bellini) and into the renal

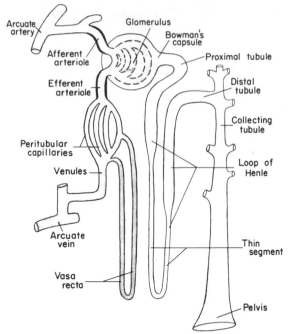

FIGURE 7–2. The functional nephron. (From Guyton, A. C.: Textbook of Medical Physiology. 8th ed. Philadelphia, W. B. Saunders, 1991, p. 212.)

pelvis by way of the renal calices. It is at this point that the fluid in the renal pelvis is termed *urine*.

RENAL PHYSIOLOGY

The constituents of urine are formed by filtration, reabsorption, and secretion. *Filtration* occurs as the blood passes through the glomerulus. The force of filtration is a pressure gradient pushing fluid through the glomerular membrane. Approximately 180 L of water every 24 hours is filtered out of plasma with other substances (Table 7–1). Blood cells and colloidal substances are usually retained in the blood, because they are too large to pass through the epithelium. The presence of red blood cells or protein in the urine is usually indicative of some pathologic process occurring in the kidney.

Reabsorption occurs in the proximal and distal tubules. Approximately 99 percent of the water is reabsorbed. Many substances in the water are reabsorbed by active or passive transport. Active transport requires energy for movement of the substance across the membrane. Passive transport can be regarded as simple diffusion that is devoid of energy.

Substances such as glucose, amino acids, sodium, potassium, calcium, and magnesium, which are important constituents of body fluids, are almost entirely reabsorbed. Certain substances are reabsorbed in limited quantities and consequently appear in the urine in considerable amounts. Some of these substances are urea, creatinine, and the phosphates.

The last mechanism in the formation of urine is *secretion*. Various substances, including hydrogen and potassium ions, are secreted directly into the tubular fluid through the epithelial cells lining the renal tubules.

REGULATION OF KIDNEY FUNCTION

The formation of urine and the retention of substances needed for proper body function are aided by three physiologic mechanisms: the countercurrent mechanism, autoregulation, and hormone control.

Countercurrent Mechanism. The countercurrent mechanism is used by the kidneys to concentrate urine. This mechanism is aided by the anatomic arrangement of the loops of Henle of the juxtamedullary nephrons, which go deep into the medulla, and the peritubular capillaries, called the *vasa recta*. The osmolality of the interstitial fluid increases as it moves more deeply into the medulla; this greater osmolality results in active transport of solutes into the interstitial fluid. This countercurrent mechanism is useful when the body needs to excrete a large amount of waste products and yet reabsorb the normal amount of solutes. This is also true when the water in the body needs to be conserved, as in conditions of inadequate water supply. Therefore, water is conserved while waste products are eliminated.

Autoregulation. Autoregulation helps to keep the glomerular filtration at a near-normal rate, despite fluctuations in arterial pressure. In fact, within the blood pressure range of 60 to 160 torr, there is little change in either renal plasma flow or glomerular filtration rate. Consequently, as the arterial pressure increases, the sympathetic innervation to the afferent arterioles causes constriction, keeping the glomerular filtration rate constant. The reverse is also true. When the arterial pressure is low, dilatation of the afferent arterioles serves to keep the glomerular filtration rate constant.

Hormone Control. The antidiuretic hormone (ADH) is secreted by the posterior pituitary gland. The secretion of this hormone is influenced by plasma osmolality. If hypertonicity of the blood occurs, ADH is secreted and water is retained by the kidneys. If the blood is hypo-

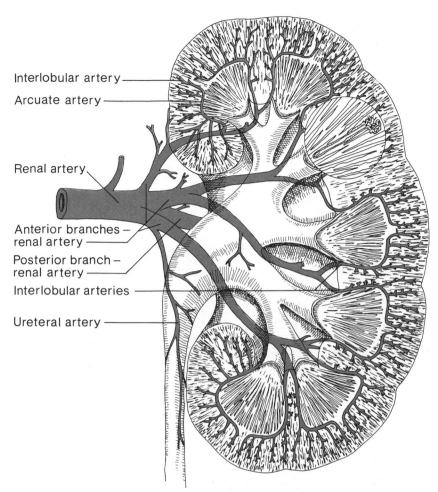

FIGURE 7–3. Arterial supply to the kidney. Soon after entering the hilum of the kidney, the renal artery divides into several anterior and posterior branches. The branches divide into interlobar arteries, which course between the medullary pyramids. The interlobar arteries then give off the arcuate arteries, which course between the cortex and the medulla. From this arcuate complex arise the interlobar arteries, which give off the afferent arterioles to the glomeruli. (From Wilson, R. F.: Principles of Critical Care. Kalamazoo, MI, The Upjohn Company, 1976.)

Table 7–1. MEASURE OF REABSORPTION BY THE KIDNEY

Substance	Filtered (mEq/24 hr/170 L)	Reabsorbed (mEq/24 hr/169 L)	Excreted (mEq/24 hr/45 L)
Sodium	24,500	24,350	150
Chloride	17,800	17,700	150
Bicarbonate	4,900	4,900	1
Potassium	700	600	24
Glucose	780	780	0
Urea	870	460	410
Creatinine	12	0	12
Uric acid	50	45	5

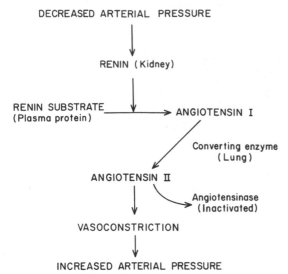

DECREASED ARTERIAL PRESSURE

↓

RENIN (Kidney)

↓

RENIN SUBSTRATE ————→ ANGIOTENSIN I
(Plasma protein)

Converting enzyme
(Lung)

ANGIOTENSIN II

↓   Angiotensinase
              (Inactivated)

VASOCONSTRICTION

↓

INCREASED ARTERIAL PRESSURE

FIGURE 7–4. The renin-angiotensin-vasoconstrictor mechanism for arterial pressure control. (From Guyton, A. C.: Textbook of Medical Physiology. 8th ed. Philadelphia, W. B. Saunders, 1991, p. 288.)

tonic, less ADH is formed and the kidneys release water. This hormone acts on the distal tubule and collecting tubules by altering their permeability to water.

The *juxtaglomerular apparatus* is located just before the glomerulus. If the sodium concentration is low, if the pressure in the afferent arteriole is low, or if a reduced glomerular filtration rate or increased sympathetic stimulation exists, an enzyme, renin, will be released from the juxtaglomerular cells.

Renin probably plays an important role in conserving sodium in hypotensive states and controlling fluid volume excretion. Renin, when released in the blood, catalyzes the splitting of angiotensin I from a renin substrate. As angiotensin I passes through the lungs, it is converted to angiotensin II (Fig. 7–4). *Angiotensin II* is a highly effective pressor agent and a major stimulus to the secretion of aldosterone. *Aldosterone*, a mineralocorticoid, appears to act on the distal tubule and the thick segment of the ascending loop of Henle. When secreted, it controls the reabsorption of some of the sodium and water. Because the renin-angiotensin system causes this reabsorption of water and sodium, it plays a role in the control of arterial blood pressure.

RENAL ROLE IN REGULATION OF BODY HOMEOSTASIS

The kidneys play a role in regulation of body fluids. For the most part, they determine the

adjustment of blood volume, extracellular fluid volume, and osmolality of the extracellular fluids, electrolytes, and ions; they remove waste products and toxic substances; and they maintain the acid–base balance.

The kidneys regulate blood volume in the following manner: When the circulating blood volume is excessive, the cardiac output and arterial pressure increase, causing stimulation of volume receptors located in the left and right atria and the baroreceptors located in the carotid, aortic, and pulmonary regions. The net effect is an increase in urine formation, returning blood volume to a normal range. Aldosterone and ADH also have a role in improving the economy of blood volume and electrolytes.

If the patient is hypovolemic, the kidney will conserve fluid and thus return the blood volume to normal limits.

The normal intake of water into the body in 24 hours is 2500 ml. Of this, 1200 ml is ingested liquids and 1000 ml is water in solid food. The remaining 300 ml is water derived from oxidation of food in the tissue cells. Table 7–2 shows the avenues by which water is lost in a 24-hour period.

The extracellular fluid volume is controlled by the kidneys as they control the blood volume. The relative ratio of the extracellular fluid volume to blood volume depends on the physical properties of the circulation and of the interstitial spaces, including their compliances and their dynamics.

The kidney maintains the osmolality of the extracellular fluid mainly by regulating the extracellular sodium concentration. Extracellular sodium controls 90 to 95 percent of the effective osmotic pressure of extracellular fluid.

The kidneys also control the extracellular concentration of other electrolytes, such as potassium, calcium, magnesium, and phosphate ions.

COMPONENTS OF URINE

The end product of excretion by the kidneys is urine, which is 95 percent water and 5 per-

Table 7–2. AVERAGE WATER LOSS PER 24 HOURS AT AVERAGE TEMPERATURE AND HUMIDITY

Route	Amount (ml)
Through the skin	500
Through the lungs	350
Through the kidneys	1500
Through the feces	150

Table 7–3. PRINCIPAL CONSTITUENTS OF URINE

Constituents	Amount (g/L)
Organic	
Urea	20–300
Uric acid	0.6–0.75
Creatinine	1.5
Others	2.6
Inorganic	
Sodium chloride	9.0
Potassium chloride	2.5
Sulfuric acid	1.8
Phosphoric acid	1.8
Ammonia	0.5–15
Calcium	0.2
Magnesium	0.2

cent solids. The solids, which account for approximately 60 g per L of urine, are listed in Table 7–3. *Urea* is derived mostly from the catabolism of amino acids. *Creatinine* is thought to be derived from creatine, a nitrogenous substance found in muscle tissue. Because it is not reabsorbed by the tubular mechanism of the kidney, creatinine is a good indicator of kidney function. Creatinine and sulfates are considered nonthreshold substances because they are excreted in their entirety. *Uric acid* is an end product of purine metabolism, formed from purines ingested as food and from those formed in the body.

High-threshold substances are almost entirely reabsorbed in the kidney. They are an important portion of the blood and are excreted only if they are in an excess concentration. Some of the high-threshold substances are glucose, potassium, calcium, and magnesium. Low-threshold substances, such as urea, uric acid, and phosphates, are only minimally reabsorbed by the kidney.

In considering the substances found in urine, it is useful to know the characteristics of normal urine. Normal urine should be amber in color, owing to the pigment urochrome, and it should also be clear and transparent. It usually is acidic, with a pH of about 6, owing to the presence of sodium acid phosphate. The specific gravity is between 1.003 and 1.025. The volume of urine excreted every 24 hours is about 1500 ml.

ACID–BASE BALANCE

The kidneys play a major role in acid–base balance. Although they are the most powerful acid–base regulators, they require several hours to 1 day to return the hydrogen ion concentration to a normal range. The buffer systems (bicarbonate, phosphate, and protein) can react within a fraction of a second to alterations in hydrogen ion concentration. In contrast, the respiratory system usually takes 1 to 3 minutes to react.

The pH is a negative logarithmic expression of the hydrogen ion concentration in the body fluids (see Chapter 6). Bicarbonate and carbon dioxide are also factors. The bicarbonate is mainly under renal control and the carbon dioxide is under respiratory control, and because there is approximately 20 times more bicarbonate than carbon dioxide in the plasma, a 20-to-1 ratio exists. Thus, any change in the 20-to-1 ratio affects the pH. Any change that negates the functioning of the kidneys or the rest of the body may affect the bicarbonate portion of the ratio and is a metabolic problem. Conversely, any change in the function of the lungs, which usually affects the carbon dioxide portion of the ratio, is a respiratory problem.

If, for example, a large amount of a bicarbonate solution were rapidly infused into a patient and his or her ventilation did not change (PCO_2 stays constant), the result would be a higher value for the bicarbonate and no change in the PCO_2. The net result would be a higher pH, which would constitute alkalosis, in this case termed *metabolic alkalosis*. On the other hand, if an acid were infused, the ratio would become smaller and the pH would fall, indicating acidosis, which would be termed *metabolic acidosis*.

Respiratory acidosis occurs when the PCO_2 is increased, as in acute hypoventilation, for example. The pH will be lowered because the ratio will become smaller. Conversely, if the patient hyperventilates, the PCO_2 will drop and the ratio will rise, thus increasing the pH and producing *respiratory alkalosis*.

The kidneys regulate pH by increasing or decreasing the bicarbonate ion concentration in the body fluid. This is done by a complex series of reactions, which begins with hydrogen ions being secreted into the tubular fluid. Carbon dioxide, an end product of tubular cell metabolism, combines with water to form carbonic acid (H_2CO_3). The carbonic acid dissociates to form hydrogen (H^+) and bicarbonate (HCO_3). The hydrogen ion is taken by active transport to the renal tubule and usually exchanges in the tubule with sodium. By active transport the sodium moves to the extracellular fluid, where it combines with the bicarbonate that was reabsorbed into the extracellular fluid to form sodium bicarbonate ($NaHCO_3$). In the tubules, the hydrogen ion that was actively transported to the tubule combines with the filtrate bicarbonate to form carbonic acid. The carbonic acid dissociates to form carbon dioxide and water. The carbon dioxide is reabsorbed into the extracellular fluid and eventually excreted by the lungs, while the water is excreted as part of the urine.

The kidneys correct alkalosis by decreasing the bicarbonate in the extracellular fluid. This occurs because fewer hydrogen ions enter the tubules, owing to a low carbon dioxide concentration, and there is a high bicarbonate concentration in the tubules. The bicarbonate cannot be reabsorbed without first combining with the hydrogen; therefore, the excess bicarbonate ions are lost to the urine as are other positive ions such as sodium and hydrogen. Cellular potassium may exchange with the sodium instead of the cellular hydrogen to conserve the hydrogen, which may help return the pH to normal limits.

Renal correction of acidosis is done by increasing the amount of bicarbonate in the extracellular fluid. There is an excess of hydrogen ions as compared with the bicarbonate filtration into the tubules. The excess hydrogen ions are secreted into the tubules, where they combine with the phosphate or the ammonia buffer systems. The sodium ions in the tubules move by active transport to the extracellular fluid and combine with the bicarbonate ion to form sodium bicarbonate, which helps correct the acidosis. The urine is acidic because the kidney is excreting the excess hydrogen ions.

DIURETIC THERAPY IN THE PACU

In the PACU, diuretics are commonly used to reduce brain size and intracranial pressure, to treat hypervolemia, to prevent oliguria, or to help in diagnosing the cause of the oliguria. The major side effects of diuretic therapy are related to the contraction of the extracellular fluid volume and the alterations in potassium concentrations. Diuretics are categorized according to their site of action on renal tubules and their mechanism of altering the secretion of urine. The major categories of diuretics are osmotic diuretics, thiazide diuretics, potassium-sparing diuretics, loop diuretics, aldosterone antagonists, and carbonic anhydrase inhibitors. Because the use of diuretics is so important in the PACU, a brief review of the major types of diuretics will be presented.

Osmotic Diuretics. Osmotic diuretics are used to evaluate the cause of oliguria, to reduce intracranial pressure and brain size, and to protect the kidneys against the development of acute renal failure. Urea is an effective osmotic diuretic; however, this drug does have some disadvantages that limit its use as compared with mannitol. The major disadvantage of urea is that it causes a significant amount of rebound increase in intracranial pressure and a high incidence of venous thrombosis. Mannitol, a six-carbon sugar, is the prototype of the osmotic diuretics. This high-molecular-weight drug, when given intravenously, increases the plasma osmolality, with a resulting expansion of the intravascular volume by means of drawing fluid from the intracellular space into the extracellular space. In the kidneys, mannitol's osmotic effect on the tubules leads to a diuretic effect. The major concern with mannitol therapy is an increased extracellular fluid volume. This can be of grave consequence in patients with impending pulmonary edema. Hence, the PACU nurse should frequently assess the pulmonary parameters in patients receiving mannitol in whom pulmonary edema is a possibility. An early sign of pulmonary edema is wheezing. Wheezing is usually indicative of interstitial edema. If wheezing is detected in a nonasthmatic patient, the attending physician should be notified immediately. As the edema formation progresses, wet basilar rales or crackles may be heard during auscultation of the chest. The crackles become coarser as the pulmonary edema worsens.

Thiazide Diuretics. Thiazide diuretics are mainly used in the treatment of hypertension, edema, and diabetes insipidus. These diuretics are secreted in the proximal convoluted tubule and have their major effect in the loop of Henle, where chloride reabsorption is inhibited. This results in diluting defects and increased distal delivery of salt and water. Patients on long-term thiazide diuretic therapy can experience increased urinary losses of water, sodium, chloride, and potassium and some loss of bicarbonate. Hence, these patients are particularly susceptible to hypochloremic, hypokalemic metabolic alkalosis. Some of the common thiazide diuretics are chlorothiazide (Diuril), benzthiazide (Exna), and hydrochlorothiazide (Esidrix, Hydrodiuril, Oretic).

The most common untoward effect of thiazide diuretics is hypokalemia. Hypokalemia, which is a reduced serum potassium level, can cause paralytic ileus, severe weakness or flaccid paralysis, hypotension, atrial and ventricular dysrhythmias, and potentiation of digitalis toxicity. If it is determined that treatment for hypokalemia should be instituted, intravenous potassium replacement may be given in the PACU. If the infusion rates of the potassium replacement exceed 40 mEq per hr or if the concentration of potassium in the individual intravenous container is greater than 40 mEq per L, continuous electrocardiographic (ECG) monitoring should be instituted to detect any dysrhythmias. Also, if potassium chloride is added to solutions in flexible plastic bags in the PACU, the nurse should ensure that it is properly mixed in the infusion solution to prevent the patient's receiving an inadvertent bolus of potassium chloride. Other untoward side effects of thiazide diuretics are dermatitis, bone marrow depression, and reduced liver function.

Potassium-Sparing Diuretics. This class of diuretics acts on the distal convoluted tubule. The product of their actions is an increased urinary output without potassium loss. The most popular potassium-sparing diuretics include triamterene (Dyrenium) and amiloride (Midamor). A fixed-dose combination of triamterene and hydrochlorothiazide, which is marketed under the trade name of Dyazide, can also be considered to be in this category of diuretics. The major side effect of this class of diuretics is hyperkalemia, which can occur because of excess usage along with overusage of potassium supplementation. The symptoms of hyperkalemia include muscular weakness, conduction defects, ventricular dysrhythmias, and ileus. To reduce the effects of hyperkalemia, calcium gluconate or calcium chloride may be administered. Also, to reduce the high potassium levels, sodium bicarbonate, glucose, or insulin and glucose may be given.

Loop Diuretics. The loop diuretics, of which ethacrynic acid (Edecrin), bumetanide (Bumex), and furosemide (Lasix) are the prototype drugs, are used primarily in the treatment of pulmonary edema and general edema and in the diagnosis of acute renal failure. The loop diuretics are secreted into the tubule and have their major action on the medullary concentrating segment where chloride transport is inhibited. Consequently, the concentrating and diluting mechanisms of the kidneys are interfered with, which results in the production of isotonic urine. In addition, because of the increased delivery of salt with these drugs, potassium secretion is increased. Hence, the major problems with these drugs are in the realm of deafness (caused by ethacrynic acid), hepatic dysfunction, hypokalemia, alkalosis, extracellular fluid volume contraction, and electrolyte imbalance. Owing to their high potency and their ability to act rapidly, loop diuretics are usually the diuretic of choice, when indicated, for the patient in the PACU. The two major concerns when one of these drugs is administered are hypokalemia and hypovolemia. The effects and treatment of hypokalemia were discussed in the section on thiazide diuretics. The objective findings that indicate hypovolemia (contraction of the extracellular fluid volume) are hypotension, tachycardia, and low right- and left-ventricular filling pressures. Treatment can include repositioning the patient with the legs elevated or the administration of intravenous salt-containing solutions, or both.

Aldosterone Antagonists. Drugs in this category, of which spironolactone (Aldactone) is the prototype drug, act on the aldosterone receptors in the conducting ducts. Spironolactone acts to antagonize the effects of aldosterone. Aldosterone enhances the reabsorption of sodium and chloride and increases the excretion of potassium in the renal tubules. Consequently, when spironolactone is administered there is a reduction in sodium and chloride reabsorption and a decrease in potassium excretion. Because of this decrease in potassium excretion in the conducting ducts, hyperkalemia, especially when renal dysfunction is present, is a serious side effect of the drug. Spironolactone is indicated for patients with fluid overload due to cirrhosis of the liver, nephrotic syndrome, and congestive heart failure.

Carbonic Anhydrase Inhibitors. Drugs in this class bind to the carbonic anhydrase enzyme in the proximal renal tubules. The outcome is to inhibit the actions of carbonic anhydrase, which results in the diminished excretion of hydrogen ions and increased excretion of bicarbonate with an ionic exchange with potassium and sodium. The net result is a diuresis of alkaline urine. The prototype drug in this category is acetazolamide (Diamox). This drug is indicated for the reduction of intraocular pressure and the management of seizures. If this drug is administered to a patient with chronic obstructive pulmonary disease, careful monitoring of the patient's rate of ventilation and Pa_{CO_2} is mandated. This is because excessive bicarbonate is lost in the urine, and hypercarbia can result, which can ultimately lead to central nervous system (CNS) depression.

EFFECTS OF ANESTHESIA ON RENAL FUNCTION

In patients with normal renal function who receive general inhalation anesthesia, some depression of renal function occurs. This is because all of the general anesthetics depress functions such as glomerular filtration rate, renal blood flow, and urinary flow. The depression in renal function is the result of direct and indirect effects of the general anesthetic agents. In regard to the vascular effects, during general anesthesia the renal blood flow may be depressed owing to renal vasoconstriction or systemic hypotension, or both. Of interest is that droperidol, the tranquilizer component of Innovar, has the smallest effect on the changes in renal function. It should be stated that, in most instances, the renal depression due to the anesthetic agents is completely reversible at the end of the operative procedure.

Patients who are anesthetized in lighter planes of anesthesia may experience some manifestations of the stress response. One of the hormones that is released in response to a stressor is ADH. This hormone is the most important regulator of urine volume. When ADH is released, it promotes an increase in tubular reabsorption of water, which results in a decrease in urine volume and an increase in urine concentration. Other biochemical products of the stress response, namely epinephrine, norepinephrine, and the renin-angiotensin system, also affect the renal system. More specifically, when these amines are liberated, renal blood flow is decreased. Because some patients can undergo a stress response under anesthesia, it is important for the PACU nurse to monitor renal function during the emergent phase of the anesthesia. It is not uncommon for patients who have undergone major abdominal or thoracic surgery to experience some diuresis during the immediate postoperative period. Hence, urine volume and concentration should be monitored in all patients who (1) have undergone a major surgical procedure, (2) have received general anesthesia for more than 2 hours, (3) have a compromised cardiovascular or renal system, or both, and (4) have had a significant blood volume replacement during the preoperative or intraoperative phase of the anesthetic experience.

EFFECTS OF DRUGS IN PATIENTS WITH COMPROMISED RENAL FUNCTION

Patients with severe renal disease usually have anemia, body fluid relocation, abnormal cell membrane activity, and alterations in blood albumin and electrolytes. In addition, these patients are usually debilitated and, if in the uremic state, CNS depression is usually present. Drugs that are not metabolized in the body and are therefore excreted unchanged by the kidneys should be avoided in patients with severe renal disease. Hence, the long-acting barbiturates barbital and phenobarbital and the skeletal muscle relaxants decamethonium and gallamine, along with digoxin and lanatoside C, should be avoided in these patients. Because about half of the administered dose of the belladonna alkaloids atropine and hyoscyamine is excreted unchanged, the dosage should be modified depending on the degree of severity of the renal impairment. When CNS depression is present in the patient with renal impairment, the actions of narcotics are intensified and prolonged. Along with this, diazepam, which has a 24-hour half-life, is probably not a good choice because of its additive effect on the CNS depression. In patients with mild to moderate renal dysfunction, all inhalation anesthetics except methoxyflurane and possibly enflurane can be used in the usual clinical dose range. Because thiopental depends on redistribution for the termination of its action, it may be used in patients with renal impairment. However, the sleeping time is increased in proportion to the degree of uremia. Along with this, the skeletal muscle relaxants succinylcholine, curare, and pancuronium are also acceptable for use in the patient with compromised kidney function. Neuroleptanalgesia, which derives from the combination of a narcotic and a tranquilizer, when achieved with nitrous oxide and oxygen, is an acceptable technique for the uremic patient. If a patient has received Innovar, which is the prototype neuroleptanalgesic drug, the PACU nurse should monitor the patient for prolonged depressant effects of the drug. More specifically, the tranquilizer component of Innovar, droperidol, has a very long half-life; therefore, its prolonged effects, coupled with CNS depression from the uremia, may cause the patient to be slow to arouse in the immediate postoperative emergence phase. Consequently, airway patency and the cardiovascular parameters should be monitored closely for an extended period when droperidol has been administered to the patient in either the preoperative or the intraoperative phase of the anesthetic experience.

RENAL SHUTDOWN OR FAILURE

Acute renal failure can occur in the PACU owing to a variety of reasons such as hemorrhage and circulatory failure from trauma or extensive surgery, acute glomerulonephritis, vascular occlusions, or toxicity from drugs.

The most common cause of acute renal failure is acute tubular necrosis. Oliguria produces the clinical setting in which renal cell necrosis may develop. Persistent oliguria, less than 25 ml of urine per hour for more than 2 hours, constitutes a medical emergency, and the surgeon should be notified immediately. The urine volume may be abnormally high in conditions in which the glomerular filtration rate is reduced to the point of renal failure, and the increased urine volume represents a supplemental failure of tubular function. In patients with mild to moderate renal dysfunction, enflurane may potentially cause nephrotoxicity. This is because enflurane is metabolized to inorganic fluoride. However, clinical studies have not been able to demonstrate this possibility. Nephrotoxicity is characterized by polyuria and azotemia. Therefore, the accurate and continuous measurement of urine volume is essential in the postoperative nursing care of the patient with suspected renal failure.

Creatinine clearance is a laboratory test that provides an excellent index to measure the quantity of glomerular filtrate. Creatinine is a component of urine not reabsorbed by tubular mechanisms. Hence, every milliliter of glomerular filtrate should contain precisely the same quantity of creatinine as 1 ml of plasma.

Measurement of *urinary sodium* yields information about sodium absorption. The *urine plasma osmolar ratio* provides an index of water reabsorption in the collecting tubules and is an excellent measurement of tubular function. The quality rather than the quantity of the urine provides useful information about the renal state of the patient (Fig. 7–5).

PACU NURSING CARE

PACU nursing care centers on recognition and care of the patient in impending renal failure. Urinary output should be monitored by an indwelling urethral catheter. This monitoring provides moment-to-moment information concerning urine output and its constituents that can be measured. Modern collecting devices provide a closed system between the catheter and a graduated measuring flask that can be emptied from the bottom without disconnecting the catheter. In this way, the danger of

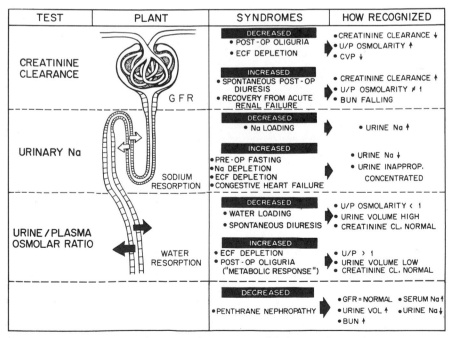

TEST	PLANT	SYNDROMES	HOW RECOGNIZED
CREATININE CLEARANCE	GFR	**DECREASED** • POST-OP OLIGURIA • ECF DEPLETION	• CREATININE CLEARANCE ↓ • U/P OSMOLARITY ↑ • CVP ↓
		INCREASED • SPONTANEOUS POST-OP DIURESIS • RECOVERY FROM ACUTE RENAL FAILURE	• CREATININE CLEARANCE ↑ • U/P OSMOLARITY ≠ ↑ • BUN FALLING
URINARY Na	SODIUM RESORPTION	**DECREASED** • Na LOADING	• URINE Na ↑
		INCREASED • PRE-OP FASTING • Na DEPLETION • ECF DEPLETION • CONGESTIVE HEART FAILURE	• URINE Na ↓ • URINE INAPPROP. CONCENTRATED
URINE/PLASMA OSMOLAR RATIO	WATER RESORPTION	**DECREASED** • WATER LOADING • SPONTANEOUS DIURESIS	• U/P OSMOLARITY < ↑ • URINE VOLUME HIGH • CREATININE CL. NORMAL
		INCREASED • ECF DEPLETION • POST-OP OLIGURIA ("METABOLIC RESPONSE")	• U/P > ↑ • URINE VOLUME LOW • CREATININE CL. NORMAL
		DECREASED • PENTHRANE NEPHROPATHY	• GFR = NORMAL • SERUM Na ↑ • URINE VOL ↑ • URINE Na ↓ • BUN ↑

FIGURE 7–5. Alterations in renal function that result from a normal kidney acting to correct or preserve an abnormal internal environment. The quantity and quality of urine are appropriate for preserving the entire organism, but alterations, if uncorrected, may result in renal damage. GFR = glomerular filtration rate; ECF = extracellular fluid; U/P = urine/plasma; CVP = central venous pressure; BUN = blood urea nitrogen; CL = clearance; VOL = volume. (From Kinney, J. M., Egdahl, R. H., and Zuidema, G. D.: Manual of Preoperative and Postoperative Care. 2nd ed. Philadelphia, W. B. Saunders, 1971, p. 244.)

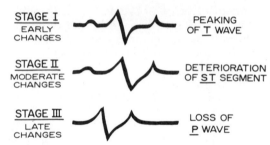

STAGE I EARLY CHANGES		PEAKING OF <u>T</u> WAVE
STAGE II MODERATE CHANGES		DETERIORATION OF <u>ST</u> SEGMENT
STAGE III LATE CHANGES		LOSS OF <u>P</u> WAVE

FIGURE 7–6. Stages of electrocardiographic evidence of hyperkalemia. (From Kinney, J. M., Egdahl, R. H., and Zuidema, G. D.: Manual of Preoperative and Postoperative Care. 2nd ed. Philadelphia, W. B. Saunders, 1971, p. 256.)

gross contamination is minimized while the necessary monitoring facility is still provided.

Continuous ECG monitoring should be done because the patient in acute renal failure probably has hyperkalemia, which can lead to cardiac arrest. The ECG changes indicative of hyperkalemia are initially high-peaked T waves and depressed S-T segments. Subsequent disappearance of T waves, heart block, and diastolic cardiac arrest occur with increasing levels of potassium (Fig. 7–6).

Osmotic diuretics, such as mannitol, or one of the loop diuretics, such as ethacrynic acid and furosemide, may be used in the treatment of tubular necrosis. A central venous pressure monitor may be inserted to measure blood volume. If renal failure continues, dialytic therapy will probably be necessary.

References

1. Guyton, A.: Textbook of Medical Physiology. 8th ed. Philadelphia, W. B. Saunders, 1991.
2. Katz, J., Benumof, J., and Kadis, L.: Anesthesia and Uncommon Diseases. 3rd ed. Philadelphia: W. B. Saunders, 1989.
3. Miller, R.: Anesthesia. 3rd ed. New York, Churchill Livingstone, 1990.
4. Stoelting, R.: Pharmacology and Physiology in Anesthetic Practice. 2nd ed. Philadelphia, J. B. Lippincott, 1991.
5. Walsh, P. C., Retik, A. B., Stamey, T. A., et al. (eds.): Campbell's Urology. 6th ed. Philadelphia, W. B. Saunders, 1992.
6. Waugaman, W., Foster, S., and Rigor, B. (eds.): Principles and Practice of Nurse Anesthesia. 2nd ed. Norwalk, CT, Appleton & Lange, 1992.
7. Wood, M., and Wood, A.: Drugs and Anesthesia: Pharmacology for Anesthesiologists. Baltimore, Williams & Wilkins, 1990.

CHAPTER 8

Endocrine Physiology

The essence of physiology is regulation and control. Physiologic functions of the body are regulated by two major controls: the nervous system and the endocrine system. Many interrelationships exist between the endocrine and the nervous systems. Dysfunction of the endocrine system is associated with overproduction or underproduction of a single hormone or multiple hormones. This dysfunction may be the primary reason for surgery, or it may coexist in patients requiring surgery on other organ systems. To ensure the provision of appropriate nursing interventions for the patient with endocrine dysfunction, the post anesthesia care unit (PACU) nurse must understand the physiology and pathophysiology of the endocrine system.

Definitions

Endocrine gland: a group of hormone-secreting and -excreting cells.

Gluconeogenesis: the conversion of amino acids into glucose.

Glycogenesis: the deposition of glycogen in the liver.

Hormone: a biochemical substance secreted by a specific endocrine gland and transported in the blood to distant points in the body to regulate rates of physiologic processes.

Lipolysis: the mobilization of deposited fat.

Releasing factor (RF): a hormone of unknown chemical structure secreted by the hypothalamus.

Releasing hormone (RH): a hormone secreted from the hypothalamus.

Stress: a chemical or physical disturbance in the cells or tissues produced by a change either in the external environment or within the body that requires a response to counteract the disturbance.

Target organ: a gland whose activities are regulated by tropic hormones.

Tropic hormone: a hormone that regulates the blood level of a specific hormone secreted from another endocrine gland.

MEDIATORS OF THE ENDOCRINE SYSTEM—THE HORMONES

A hormone is a biochemical substance synthesized in an endocrine gland and secreted into body fluids to regulate or control physiologic processes in other cells of the body. Biochemically, hormones are either proteins (or derivatives of proteins or amino acids) or steroids.

Protein hormones, such as the releasing hormones, catecholamines, and parathormone, fit the *fixed-receptor model* of hormone action. In this model, the stimulating hormone, called the *first messenger*, combines with a specific receptor for that hormone on the surface of the target cell. This hormone-receptor combination activates the enzyme adenylate cyclase in the membrane. That portion of the adenylate cyclase that is exposed to the cytoplasm causes the immediate conversion of cytoplasmic adenosine triphosphate into cyclic adenosine monophosphate (AMP). The cyclic AMP then acts as a *second messenger* and initiates any number of cellular functions.

In the *mobile receptor model*, a steroid hormone, because of its lipid solubility, passes through the cell membrane into the cytoplasm, where it binds with a specific receptor protein. The combined receptor protein–hormone either diffuses or is transported through the nuclear membrane, transferring the steroid hormone to a smaller protein. In the nucleus, the hormone activates specific genes to form the *messenger ribonucleic acid* (RNA). The messenger RNA then passes out of the nucleus into the cytoplasm, where it promotes the translation process in the ribosomes to form new proteins. Hormones that fit the fixed-receptor model produce an almost instantaneous response on the part of the target organ. In contrast, because of their action on the genes to cause protein synthesis, when the steroid hormones are secreted there is a characteristic delay in the initiation of hormone response that varies from minutes to days.

PHYSIOLOGY OF THE ENDOCRINE GLANDS

The Pituitary Gland

The pituitary gland rests in the sella turcica of the sphenoid bone at the base of the brain. This gland is divided into the anterior and posterior lobes. Because of its glandular nature, the anterior lobe is called the *adenohypophysis*; the posterior lobe, which is an outgrowth of a part of the nervous system—the hypothalamus—is called the *neurohypophysis*. The pituitary gland receives its arterial blood supply from two paired systems of vessels: (1) the right and left superior hypophyseal arteries from above, and (2) the right and left inferior hypophyseal arteries from below. However, the anterior lobe receives no arterial blood supply. Instead, its entire blood supply is derived from the hypophyseal portal veins. This rich capillary system facilitates the rapid discharge of releasing hormones that have target cells in the anterior hypophysis.

Although the pituitary gland is called the *master gland,* it is actually regulated by other endocrine glands and by the nervous system. The secretion of the hormones of the anterior hypophysis is primarily influenced and controlled by the higher centers in the hypothalamus. Releasing hormones are secreted by the hypothalamic nuclei through the infundibular tract to the portal venous system of the pituitary gland to their respective target cells of the adenohypophysis. Consequently, the hypothalamus brings about fine regulation of the action of the anterior pituitary, and still higher nervous centers apparently further modulate the production of the releasing factors. Hence, the many influences coming into the brain and central nervous system impinge on the anterior pituitary gland either to enhance or to dampen its activity.

Hormonal control of the pituitary involves certain feedback systems. For example, corticotropin-releasing hormone stimulates the production and release of adrenocorticotropin (ACTH). The increased concentration of ACTH causes the hypothalamus to decrease its production of corticotropin-releasing hormone, which in turn reduces ACTH production, ultimately reducing the blood level of ACTH.

Therefore, when exogenous corticoids are administered chronically, ACTH secretion decreases and the adrenal cortex atrophies. On the other hand, the removal of endogenous corticoids by a bilateral adrenalectomy can result in a tumor of the pituitary gland owing to the absence of the feedback depression of the corticotropin-releasing hormone.

The posterior lobe of the pituitary gland has an abundant nerve supply. Nerve cell bodies in the posterior lobe produce two neurosecretions (antidiuretic hormone [ADH] and oxytocin), which are stored as granules at the site of the nerve cell bodies. When the hypothalamus detects a need for either neurohypophyseal hormone, nerve impulses are sent to the posterior lobe and the hormone is released by granules into the neighboring capillaries. Consequently, the hormonal function of the posterior lobe is under direct nervous system regulation.

Hormones of the Adenohypophysis

Growth Hormone, or Somatotropin. This hormone is unique because it has no target gland to stimulate but acts on all tissues of the body. Its primary functions are to maintain blood glucose levels and to regulate the growth of the skeleton. Growth hormone conserves blood glucose by increasing fat metabolism for energy. It enhances the active transport of amino acids into cells, increases the rate of protein synthesis, and promotes cell division. In addition, growth hormone enhances the formation of somatomedin, which acts directly on cartilage and bone to promote their growth. The active secretion of growth hormone is regulated in the hypothalamus via growth hormone–releasing hormone. Stimuli such as hypoglycemia, exercise, and trauma cause the hypothalamus to secrete growth hormone–releasing hormone, which is transported to the anterior lobe of the pituitary gland and released into the blood. Secretion of growth hormone can be inhibited by somatostatin, also referred to as *growth hormone–inhibiting hormone*, secreted by the hypothalamus and the delta cells of the pancreas.

Hyposecretion of the growth hormone before puberty leads to *dwarfism,* or failure to grow. After puberty, growth hormone hypofunction may result in the condition known as *Simmonds' disease.* This disease is characterized by premature senility, weakness, emaciation, mental lethargy, and wrinkled, dry skin. *Giantism* is the result of growth hormone hyperfunction before puberty. After puberty, when the epiphyses of the long bones have closed, growth hormone hyperfunction leads to *acromegaly*. In this disease, the face, hands, and feet become enlarged. Patients with acromegaly are prone to airway obstruction owing to their protruding lower jaw and enlarged tongue. Hence, in the PACU, constant vigilance as to the respiratory status of these patients is essential.

Thyroid-Stimulating Hormone (TSH), or Thyrotropin. The follicular cells of the thyroid are the target for TSH. This hormone promotes the growth and secretory activity of the thyroid gland. Production of TSH is regulated in a reciprocal fashion by the blood levels of thyroid hormone and the formation of *thyrotropin-releasing hormone* in the hypothalamus.

Adrenocorticotropin (ACTH). ACTH promotes glucocorticoid, mineralocorticoid, and androgenic steroid production and secretion by the adrenal cortex. This hormone is released in response to stimuli such as pain, hypoglycemia, hypoxia, bacterial toxins, hyperthermia, hypothermia, and physiologic stress. More specifically, the hypothalamus monitors for these various stressors, and on excitation *corticotropin-releasing hormone (CRH)* is secreted, which stimulates ACTH secretion from the adenohypophysis. Levels of adrenocortical hormones in the blood regulate secretion of ACTH by a hypothalamic feedback mechanism.

Gonadotropic Hormones. Gonadotropic hormones regulate the growth, development, and function of the ovaries and testes. The gonadotropic hormones are the *follicle-stimulating hormone* and the *luteinizing hormone*. Secretion of the gonadotropic hormones is stimulated by *gonadotropin-releasing hormone* and secreted by the hypothalamus.

Lactogenic Hormone, or Prolactin. Prolactin stimulates post-partum lactation. Unlike other pituitary hormones, the hypothalamic control of prolactin secretion is predominantly inhibitory.

Melanocyte-Stimulating Hormone. Melanocyte-stimulating hormone exerts its effect on the melanin granules in pigmented skin.

Hormones of the Neurohypophysis

Antidiuretic Hormone, or Vasopressin. During normal activities of daily living, ADH is secreted in small amounts into the blood stream to promote reabsorption of water by the renal tubules, which leads to a decreased excretion of water by the kidneys. When ADH is secreted in large quantities, vasoconstriction of the smooth muscles occurs, which ultimately elevates the blood pressure. The pressor effects of ADH are produced only by large doses that are not in the usual physiologic range. The secretion of ADH is regulated by several feedback loops, one of which involves plasma osmolality. Within the hypothalamus are *osmoreceptors*, whose function is to secrete ADH when plasma osmolarity is increased. On the other hand, dilution of plasma inhibits ADH secretion. The second feedback loop or major stimulus of ADH secretion is the *volume* or *stretch receptors* located in the left atrium. These receptors are activated when the extracellular fluid volume is increased, and, when this happens, ADH secretion is inhibited. The *baroreceptors*, which are located in the carotid sinus and aortic arch, are the receptors for the third feedback loop. A decrease in the arterial blood pressure stimulates the baroreceptors, which in turn stimulate a release of ADH. Both the stretch receptors and the baroreceptors transmit their neuronal input to the brain by way of the vagus nerve.

Lack of ADH leads to a condition called *diabetes insipidus*. This condition is characterized by the output of a large volume of dilute, sugar-free urine.

Oxytocin. Oxytocin produces contraction of uterine muscle at the end of gestation and has a role in milk excretion, that is, in stimulating the contraction of the surrounding myoepithelial cells of the mammary glands.

Pituitary Dysfunction

Hyperfunction rarely involves more than one endocrine gland. On the other hand, hypofunction does usually involve more than one endocrine gland, although instances of isolated deficiencies have been reported. A common cause of pituitary hypofunction is compression of glandular cells by the expansion of a functional or nonfunctional tumor. In this situation, an excess of one hormone may coexist with a deficiency of another.

The Pineal Gland

The pineal gland is situated in the diencephalon just above the roof of the midbrain. This gland is considered an intricate and highly sensitive biologic clock, because the secretory activity of the pineal gland is greatest at night. The pineal gland secretes melatonin, which affects the size and secretory activity of the ovaries and other organs. The production and release of melatonin are regulated by the sympathetic nervous system. In fact, the pineal gland is considered a neuroendocrine transducer because it converts nervous system input into a hormonal output.

The Thyroid Gland

The thyroid gland is located in the anterior middle portion of the neck immediately below the larynx. The gland consists of two lobes that are attached by a strip of tissue called the *isthmus*. Structurally, this gland is made up of tiny sacs called *follicles*. Each follicle is formed by a single layer of epithelial cells surrounding a cavity that contains a secretory product known as *colloid*. This colloid fluid consists mainly of a glycoprotein-iodine complex called *thyroglobulin*.

On stimulation by TSH, thyroid hormones are produced in the following steps: (1) iodide trapping, (2) oxidation and iodination, (3) storage of the hormones in the colloid as part of the thyroglobulin molecules, and (4) proteolysis (which can be inhibited by iodide) and release of the hormones. The two hormones released from the thyroid gland are triiodothyronine (T_3) and thyroxine (T_4). T_4 represents more than 95 percent of the circulating thyroid hormone and is considered to be relatively inactive physiologically as compared with T_3. Consequently, although T_3 has a relatively low concentration, it passes out of the blood stream faster than T_4, has a more rapid action, and is probably the major biologically active thyroid hormone. After these hormones are secreted by the thyroid gland, they are transported to all parts of the body by means of plasma proteins in the form of protein-bound iodinated compounds. Hence, the laboratory test for *protein-bound iodine* is useful in determining the amount of circulating thyroid hormone in the blood.

T_3 and T_4 regulate the metabolic activities of the body. More specifically, they regulate the rate of cellular oxidation. Along with this, they are essential for the normal growth and development of the body. Other metabolic activities that are influenced by T_3 and T_4 are the promotion of protein synthesis and breakdown, increase of glucose absorption and utilization, facilitation of gluconeogenesis, and maintenance of fluid and electrolyte balance. The thyroid hormones are also involved in a feedback mechanism. The concentration of T_3 and T_4 in the blood regulates the secretion of TSH by the anterior pituitary gland. TSH regulates the growth and secretory activity of the thyroid gland.

The thyroid gland also secretes *thyrocalcitonin*, or *calcitonin*, to maintain the proper level of calcium in the blood. More specifically, calcitonin decreases the serum concentration of calcium by counteracting the effects of parathormone and inhibiting the resorption of calcium from the bones.

The Parathyroid Glands

The parathyroid glands are located on the posterior portion of the thyroid gland. In most instances there is one parathyroid gland on each of the four poles of the thyroid gland. The parathyroid glands release a polypeptide hormone called *parathormone*. This hormone is the principal regulator of the calcium concentration in the body. Parathormone is released into the circulation by a negative feedback mechanism that is dependent on the serum concentration of calcium. Hence, a high serum concentration of calcium suppresses the synthesis and release of parathormone and a low serum calcium concentration stimulates the release of the hormone. Normal serum calcium concentrations depend on the regulatory mechanisms, which include parathormone, calcitonin, phosphorus, magnesium, and vitamin D. In fact, the serum calcium concentration is maintained by these regulatory mechanisms within narrow and constant limits. The normal serum calcium level is 9 to 10.3 mg per dl for men and 8.9 to 10.2 mg per dl for women. Serum levels of calcium expressed in milliequivalents per liter are one half the value given in milligrams per deciliter.

Parathormone influences the rate at which calcium is transported across membranes in the bone, the gastrointestinal tract, and the kidneys. More specifically, calcium release from bone is facilitated by parathormone-induced stimulation of osteoclastic activity. The absorption of calcium by the gastrointestinal tract is enhanced by the parathormone-induced synthesis of vitamin D. Parathormone activates the synthesis of vitamin D, which leads to increased tubular reabsorption of calcium and enhanced renal tubular clearance of phosphorus. This results in more calcium entering the circulation.

The Adrenal Glands

The adrenal glands are located on the apex of each kidney. Each gland consists of an outer portion called the *cortex* and an inner portion called the *medulla*. The medulla is responsible for the secretion of catecholamines (see Chapter 5). The preganglionic fibers of the sympathetic nervous system provide the stimulation that facilitates the liberation of the catecholamines by the medullary cells. The cortex makes up the bulk of the adrenal gland and is responsible for the secretion of the *steroids*. The cortex is divided anatomically and physiologically into three zones: the *zona glomerulosa*, the *zona fasciculata*, and the inner *zona reticularis*. These are the sites of secretion of the three major steroid hormones: the *mineralocorticoids*, the *glucocorticoids*, and the *androgens*, respectively.

The mineralocorticoids are responsible for the maintenance of fluid and electrolyte balance. Aldosterone is, physiologically, the most important mineralocorticoid. The basic action of aldosterone is to promote the reabsorption of sodium by stimulating cellular sodium pumps in the target tissue. Overall, aldosterone causes increased tubular reabsorption of sodium and excretion of potassium. This decreases urinary excretion of sodium and chloride and increases urinary secretion of potassium, consequently expanding the extracellular fluid compartment. Aldosterone secretion is increased by ACTH, a depletion in sodium, and an increase in potassium. The secretion of aldosterone is also regulated by the *renin-angiotensin system*. Thus, when the blood supply to the kidneys is low, the juxtaglomerular cells are stimulated to release *renin*. Renin, which is an enzyme, enters the blood and converts the plasma protein *angiotensinogen* to *angiotensin I*. In the lungs and elsewhere, angiotensin I is converted enzymatically to the physiologically active form, *angiotensin II*. One of the basic actions of angiotensin II is to stimulate the adrenal cortex to secrete aldosterone. Thus, aldosterone secretion is regulated by the blood pressure and volume, and, because it causes retention of sodium and a rise in blood pressure, aldosterone also acts as a feedback mechanism to shut off the further release of renin.

The glucocorticoids are secreted in the zona fasciculata. *Cortisol (hydrocortisone)* constitutes about 95 percent of the total glucocorticoid activity, with *corticosterone* and *cortisone* making up the remaining 5 percent. These hormones function to preserve the carbohydrate reserves of the body. They do this by promoting gluconeogenesis, glycogenesis, lipolysis, and oxidation of fat in the liver. Because they conserve carbohydrate, these hormones serve as functional antagonists to insulin. Finally, these hormones possess an excellent anti-inflammatory action. The major regulator of their secretion is ACTH, which is secreted by cells in the anterior pituitary gland. ACTH is, in turn, modulated by CRH, which is secreted by the hypothalamus. Cortisol serves as a negative feedback mechanism to inhibit both ACTH and CRH production. Physical and mental stress stimulate the release of CRH from the hypothalamus. Hence, in addition to the catecholamines, cortisol and ACTH are considered to be the major stress hormones.

The *androgens*, or sex hormones, are actively involved in the preadolescent growth spurt and the appearance of axillary and pubic hair.

The Pancreas

Islet of Langerhans cells are scattered throughout the pancreas. There are three islet cell types—*alpha*, *beta*, and *delta*—which secrete *glucagon*, *insulin*, and *somatostatin*, respectively. Glucagon has several functions that are diametrically opposed to those of insulin. Glucagon is commonly referred to as *hyperglycemic factor*, and its most important function is to increase the blood glucose level. This increased glucose level in the blood is due to the effects of glucagon on glucose metabolism, that is, glycogenolysis (in the liver) and increased gluconeogenesis. When the blood glucose concentration decreases lower than 70 mg per dl, the alpha cells secrete glucagon to protect against hypoglycemia. Along with this, amino acids enhance the secretion of glucagon. In this instance, the glucagon helps prevent the hypoglycemia that can result, because amino acids stimulate insulin release, which tends to reduce the blood glucose concentration. The secretion of glucagon appears to be inhibited by the release of somatostatin from the delta cells of the pancreas, and, because it is a polypeptide, glucagon is rapidly destroyed by proteolytic enzymes.

Insulin is a protein secreted by the beta cells of the islets of Langerhans in response to elevated levels of blood glucose. Its secretion is inhibited by low blood glucose levels and somatostatin. In addition, insulin secretion can be inhibited by epinephrine, glucocorticoids, and thyroxine. When insulin is secreted by the beta cells, a metabolic state favoring the storage of nutrients is set into action. These physiologic actions include (1) retention of glucose by the liver, (2) slowing of hepatic glucose release, (3) increase in uptake of glucose by muscle (stored as glycogen) and adipose tissue (stored as triglycerides), (4) translocation of amino acids and neutral fats into muscle and adipose tissue, and (5) retardation of lipolysis and proteolysis. Hence, insulin seems to "open the door" of most of the cell membranes of the body to facilitate the movement of glucose, amino acids, and fatty acids into the cells. *Diabetes mellitus,* which is a disease involving the synthesis, storage, and release of insulin, is discussed in detail in Chapter 38.

The Gonads

The hormone *testosterone* is produced in the interstitial cells of the testes. The synthesis and secretion of this hormone are regulated by luteinizing hormone, which is secreted by the anterior pituitary gland. Testosterone regulates the development and maintenance of the male secondary sexual characteristics as well as produces some metabolic effects on bone and skeletal muscle. Another action of this hormone is the modulation of male behavior by limbic system stimulation. *Estrogen,* another gonadal hormone, is secreted by the ovarian follicles in response to the follicle-stimulating hormone and the luteinizing hormone of the anterior pituitary gland and is responsible for the development and maintenance of the secondary sexual characteristics in the female. Estrogen, along with progesterone, which is produced by the cells of the corpus luteum, plays an important role in the menstrual cycle.

SELECTED SYNDROMES AND DISEASES ASSOCIATED WITH THE ENDOCRINE SYSTEM

Hypoadrenocorticism

A reduction in function of the hormones associated with the pituitary-adrenal axis can develop as a result of (1) the destruction of the adrenal cortex by degenerative disease, neoplastic growth, or hemorrhage; (2) a deficiency of ACTH; or (3) a prolonged administration of corticosteroid drugs. *Primary adrenal insufficiency* (*Addison's disease*) results from destruction of the adrenal cortex. At present, most cases of Addison's disease are caused by idiopathic atrophy that is probably the result of an autoimmune disease. Other causes include tuberculosis, histoplasmosis, bilateral hemorrhage due to anticoagulation therapy, surgical removal of the adrenal glands, tumor chemo-

therapy, metastasis to the adrenal glands, and sepsis.

A deficiency of ACTH is associated with *panhypopituitarism.* Patients who have been administered frequent "bursts" of exogenous steroid preparations such as prednisone can experience a suppression of their output of endogenous corticosteroids because of augmentation of the feedback mechanism to the anterior pituitary gland. Concern about the development of hypoadrenocorticism should be shown in the case of any patient who has received 20 mg of prednisone per day for more than 2 weeks in the preceding 12 months (although authors vary on dosage and length of time). The recovery of the normal function of the pituitary-adrenal axis may require as long as 12 months following the discontinuation of steroid therapy. Patients who are even remotely suspected of having hypoadrenocorticism are usually administered steroids preoperatively, intraoperatively, and postoperatively.

The reason for this perioperative steroid coverage is that infection, injury, operation, or other stressors activate the pituitary-adrenal axis. If this axis is suppressed (i.e., hypoadrenocorticism), *acute adrenal insufficiency (addisonian crisis)* can develop. This is a life-threatening situation requiring prompt action by the PACU nurse. Clinical manifestations of the addisonian crisis include dehydration, nausea and vomiting, muscular weakness, and hypotension, which are followed by fever, marked flaccidity of the extremities, hyponatremia, hyperkalemia, azotemia, and shock. Therefore, the PACU nurse should monitor patients who are even remotely likely to develop the addisonian crisis. If some of the signs and symptoms appear, the attending physician should be notified immediately. The severely ill patient must be treated while the diagnosis is being confirmed. Two to 4 mg of dexamethasone is usually administered intravenously along with intravenous therapy of 5 percent dextrose in normal saline. Dexamethasone is the drug of choice because it does not interfere with the diagnostic tests and yet does provide the needed glucocorticoid. If dexamethasone is not available, it would be advantageous to administer a single 100-mg dose of hydrocortisone intravenously to obtain both the glucocorticoid and the mineralocorticoid activity. This can be followed by 50 to 100 mg of hydrocortisone administered parenterally every 6 hours. During the administration of the treatment, the PACU nurse should continuously monitor the patient's cardiorespiratory status.

Syndrome of Inappropriate Secretion of ADH

The syndrome of inappropriate secretion of antidiuretic hormone (SIADH) occurs when there is a continued secretion of ADH in the presence of serum hypo-osmolality. More specifically, there is a failure in the feedback loops that regulate ADH secretion and inhibition. Usually, both dilution and expansion of the blood volume serves to stimulate a suppression of the release of ADH. However, in SIADH, the feedback loops do not respond appropriately to the osmolar or volume change, and a pathologic positive feedback loop continues, resulting in continued production of ADH.

When hemorrhage and trauma occur during a surgical procedure, ADH secretion is appropriately elevated, and in this situation SIADH can be induced as a result of overzealous fluid administration. Because of the urinary sodium loss occurring along with the water retention, the *syndrome of acute water intoxication* may be seen in the PACU. The symptoms of water intoxication derive from increased brain water, inoperative sodium pump, and hyponatremia. The symptoms begin with headache, muscular weakness, anorexia, nausea, and vomiting and progress to confusion, hostility, disorientation, uncooperativeness, drowsiness, and terminal convulsions or coma. These symptoms usually do not occur if the serum sodium level is higher than 120 mEq per L. Therefore, in patients who have experienced major vascular surgery, trauma, or hemorrhage, the PACU nurse should assess frequently for the symptoms of SIADH and notify the attending phy-

sician if the symptoms become evident. The focus of treatment for SIADH is fluid restriction, diuresis with mannitol or furosemide, and administration of sodium chloride. Along with this, the PACU nurse should frequently assess the neurologic signs and cardiorespiratory status of the patient with SIADH and measure and record accurately the intake and output of all fluids.

References

1. Benumof, J., and Saidman, L.: Anesthesia and Perioperative Complications. St. Louis, Mosby-Year Book, 1992.
2. Brown, B.: Anesthesia and the Patient with Endocrine Disease. Philadelphia, F. A. Davis, 1980.
3. Degroot, L. J.: Endocrinology. 2nd ed. Philadelphia, W. B. Saunders, 1989.
4. Greenspan, F., and Forsham, P.: Basic and Clinical Endocrinology. 3rd ed. Los Altos, Lange Medical, 1990.
5. Guyton, A.: Textbook of Medical Physiology. 8th ed. Philadelphia, W. B. Saunders, 1991.
6. Kubo W., and Grant, M.: The syndrome of inappropriate secretion of antidiuretic hormone. Heart Lung, 7(3):469–476, 1979.
7. Longnecker, D. E., and Murphy, F. L. (eds.): Dripps/Eckenhoff/Vandam Introduction to Anesthesia: Principles of Safe Practice. 8th ed. Philadelphia, W. B. Saunders, 1992.
8. Miller, R.: Anesthesia. 3rd ed. New York, Churchill Livingstone, 1990.
9. Roizen, M. F.: Diseases of the endocrine system. *In* Katz, J., Benumof, J., and Kadis, L.: Anesthesia and Uncommon Diseases. 3rd ed. Philadelphia, W. B. Saunders, 1990, pp. 245–292.
10. Stoelting, R.: Pharmacology and Physiology in Anesthetic Practice. 2nd ed. Philadelphia: J. B. Lippincott, 1991.
11. Stoelting, R., and Dierdorf, S.: Anesthesia and Co-Existing Disease. 3rd ed. New York, Churchill Livingstone, 1993.

Gastrointestinal System Anatomy and Physiology

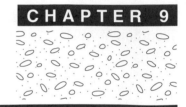

Because so many surgical procedures involve the gastrointestinal tract, it is important for the post anesthesia care unit (PACU) nurse to understand some functions of the organs of this system. This chapter discusses the overall function of each organ and the possible postoperative complications that may involve the gastrointestinal tract.

Definitions

Achalasia: a condition in which the lower esophageal sphincter fails to relax during the swallowing mechanism and food transmission from the esophagus to the stomach is impeded or prevented. This condition is also called *megaesophagus*.

Achlorhydria (hypochlorhydria): a condition in which hydrochloric acid is not secreted by the stomach.

Biliary: pertaining to the gallbladder and bile ducts.

Cholelithiasis: the presence of a common bile duct stone. Also called *chronic cholangitis.*

Chyme: food that has become mixed with the secretions of the stomach and is passed down the gut.

Deglutition: the act of swallowing.

Diarrhea: rapid movement of fecal matter through the large intestine.

Enteric system: the gastrointestinal tract.

Gastritis: inflammation of the gastric mucosa.

Lithotripsy: a procedure for treating upper urinary tract stones.

Nausea: conscious recognition of subconscious excitation in an area of the medulla closely related to the vomiting center.

Oxyntic glands: gastric glands that secrete hydrochloric acid, pepsinogen, intrinsic factor, and mucus.

Pancreatitis: inflammation of the pancreas.

Peptic ulcer: an excoriated area of the mucosa caused by the digestive action of gastric acid; frequently located in the first few centimeters of the duodenum.

Pyrosis: heartburn, of which gastroesophageal reflux is usually the cause.

Vomiting: a method for the gastrointestinal tract to rid itself of its contents when almost any part of the upper gastrointestinal tract becomes overirritated, distended, or excitable. The physical act of vomiting results when the muscles of the diaphragm and abdomen contract so that the gastric contents can be expelled.

THE ESOPHAGUS

The esophagus is a muscular tube extending from the pharynx to the stomach (Fig. 9–1). It is located behind the trachea and in front of the thoracic aorta and traverses the diaphragm to enter the esophagogastric junction, sometimes referred to as the *cardia.* Approximately 5 cm above the junction with the stomach is the gastroesophageal sphincter, which functions to prevent the reflux of stomach contents into the esophagus. The resting pressure is normally about 30 torr. This pressure is maintained by the vagus nerve as well as the nervous system. Ordinarily, the sphincter remains constricted except in the act of swallowing. Anticholinergic drugs, such as atropine, and pregnancy decrease the resting pressure of the lower esophagus. Drugs that increase the lower esophageal pressure include metoclopramide (Reglan) and antacids. Another factor preventing reflux of gastric contents into the esophagus is physiologic compression by intra-abdominal pressure on the esophagus just below the diaphragm. This mechanism is referred to as a *flutter valve closure.* The main function of the esophagus is to conduct ingested material to the stomach. The innervation of the esophagus appears to originate from the vagus.

Disorders of the Esophagus

Esophageal achalasia, a disease of unknown origin, is characterized by an absence of peri-

This is especially important if the surgery was performed on an emergency basis when the patient had a full stomach.

THE STOMACH

The stomach can be anatomically divided into three sections: the fundus, the body, and the pyloric portion (Fig. 9–2). The *fundus* is the dome of the stomach, where peptic juice is secreted. The *body* is the middle portion of the stomach and is lined with parietal cells that secrete hydrochloric acid. The pH of the solution as secreted is approximately 0.8, which is extremely acidic. The total gastric secretion on a 24-hour basis is about 2 L. This volume normally has a pH of about 1 to 3.5. Histamine has a major role in hydrochloric acid production by the parietal cells in the stomach. This is an effect mediated by histamine$_2$ (H$_2$) receptors, vagal stimulation, and the hormone gastrin. Activation on any one of these receptors potentiates the response of the other to stimulation. Blockade of the activated receptor produces a reduction in acid response because the potentiating effect of the stimulation is reduced. The third portion of the stomach is the *pyloric portion*, sometimes called the *pyloric antrum.* Here, a thick, viscous mucus and the hormone gastrin are secreted. At the end of the antrum is the pylorus, an opening surrounded by a strong band of sphincter muscle that controls the amount of gastric contents entering the duodenum.

The *vagus nerve* (parasympathetic nervous system) provides the nerve supply to the stomach. When the vagus is stimulated, it causes increased motility of the stomach and the secretion of acid, pepsin, and gastrin. Thus, a vagotomy is sometimes performed during gastric surgery to decrease gastric motility and acid production. However, it should be stated that the H$_2$ receptor is a major pathway for stimuli of acid secretion.

Nervous and hormonal stimulation have profound effects on gastric volume and pH. More specifically, stimulation of the parasympathetic nervous system causes increased gastric secretion, and stimulation of the sympathetic nervous system causes decreased gastric secretion. Consequently, pain and fear, which activate the sympathetic nervous system, decrease gastric emptying. In addition, the administration of opioids and active labor prolong gastric emptying. Food, depending on the type and amount, passes through the stomach at a variable rate. For example, foods rich in

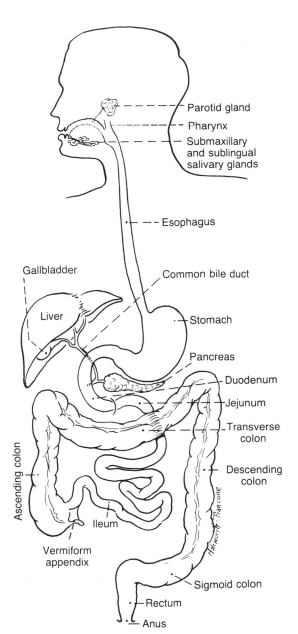

FIGURE 9–1. The digestive system and its associated structures. (From Jacob, S. W. and Francone, C.: Elements of Anatomy and Physiology. 2nd ed. Philadelphia: W.B. Saunders, 1989, p. 243.)

stalsis in the esophagus and by constriction of the cardiac sphincter. The patient with this disorder usually has hypermotility and diffuse spasms of the esophagus.

Hiatal hernia can occur where the esophagus traverses the diaphragm. Ultimately, a lower esophageal stricture may occur that can cause symptoms such as heartburn, pain, and vomiting. Patients with a hiatal hernia require constant observation for active and passive vomiting during the emergent phase of anesthesia.

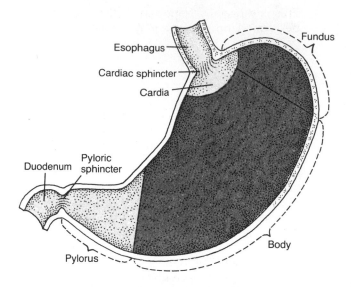

FIGURE 9–2. Anatomy of the stomach. (From Ignatavicius, D. D., and Bayne, M. V.: Medical-Surgical Nursing: A Nursing Process Approach. Philadelphia, W. B. Saunders, 1991, p. 1222.)

carbohydrates pass through the stomach in a few hours, whereas proteins exit more slowly. The emptying time for fats is the slowest. Fluids, on the other hand, pass through the stomach rather rapidly. In fact, 90 percent of 750 ml of ingested saline exits the stomach within 30 minutes. Also, 150 ml of fluids, taken 1 or 2 hours before induction of anesthesia, stimulates peristalsis and facilitates gastric emptying. Consequently, the small "sips" of water taken with the preoperative oral medications may, in fact, contribute to lower intraoperative and postoperative gastric volumes. Finally, a prolonged period of fasting does not completely ensure that the stomach is completely empty of fluids or food.

Effect of Pregnancy on Gastric Motility and Secretions

During pregnancy, many alterations occur as a result of the enlarged uterus and altered hormonal state. Because of the enlarged uterus, the stomach and intestine are moved cephalad and the axis of the stomach is shifted to a more horizontal position. The gastric emptying time is increased in women who are at least 34 weeks pregnant. In regard to the gastric volume and pH, there does not seem to be any difference between pregnant and nonpregnant states. Consequently, pregnant patients who have been NPO for elective surgery do not present any additional risk of aspiration pneumonitis than do nonpregnant patients. However, research does suggest that pregnant patients who have pyrosis (heartburn) may be at greater risk for regurgitation and subsequent

development of aspiration pneumonitis. In addition, if intramuscular narcotics are given during labor, there will be a substantial delay in gastric emptying time. Epidural anesthesia with local anesthetics does not seem to have an effect on gastric volume or pH; however, if narcotics are introduced into the epidural space, a delay in gastric emptying will occur.

Vomiting and Regurgitation

Vomiting and regurgitation with subsequent aspiration of gastric contents into the airways and lungs are an important cause of morbidity and mortality in the PACU. Various reports have indicated that there is a 4 to 27 percent risk of this phenomenon occurring. Patients with a gastric pH lower than 2.5 and a gastric volume of more than 25 ml are at high risk of serious pulmonary complications should they experience vomiting and regurgitation with subsequent aspiration.

Various methods of increasing the pH and decreasing the volume of the gastric contents can be used. Anticholinergic agents, such as atropine and glycopyrrolate, inhibit the production of gastric juice, but only to a highly variable degree. These drugs also have side effects of tachycardia, reduced gastric sphincter tone, and delayed gastric emptying. Antacid prophylaxis with the administration of oral antacids has had mixed success, because the subsequent aspiration of the antacid particles, which are nonabsorbable, can have devastating effects on the lungs. The oral antacid sodium citrate (Bicitra) has become popular because it has soluble particles that produce less severe hypoxia and lung abnormalities if aspirated. This drug has been used with great success in patients who require cesarean section.

H_2 receptor–blocking drugs have met with some success in the treatment of gastric hypersecretory states. Cimetidine (Tagamet) is an H_2 receptor–blocking agent that is used as a premedication regimen to control gastric acid production before the induction of anesthesia. The length of action of this drug is 3 hours, with a peak action of about 60 to 90 minutes. Cimetidine does not change the lower esophageal pressure, the rate of gastric emptying, or the volume of gastric juice. Cimetidine can cause a dose-related neuropsychiatric disturbance that is characterized by confusion, slurred speech, hallucinations, delirium, and coma. These symptoms dissipate once the blood level of cimetidine is reduced to 1.5 μg per ml or lower. Because cimetidine inhibits the metabolism of any drug that is biotransformed by the cytochrome P-450 microsomal enzyme system in the liver, drugs such as propranolol, metoprolol, lidocaine, bupivacaine, diazepam, midazolam, theophylline, and warfarin are potentiated when given in conjunction with cimetidine. Hence, cimetidine can prolong the length of action of these drugs.

Ranitidine (Zantac) is an H_2 receptor–blocking agent that is gaining wide popularity as a premedication. By virtue of its H_2 receptor–blocking actions, ranitidine inhibits gastric secretion in response to acetylcholine, histamine, and gastrin. It is more potent than cimetidine, and it is administered in about half the dose of cimetidine, with a peak of 90 minutes and a length of action of about 10 hours. This drug is usually given orally about 1 hour before anesthesia. The usual dose is 150 mg. Ranitidine has a small, clinically insignificant effect on the cytochrome P-450 system. Two new H_2-receptor antagonists, famotidine and nizatidine, have been introduced into clinical practice. These drugs are similar to cimetidine and ranitidine. Unlike cimetidine, neither drug binds to the cytochrome P-450 system and, hence, does not interfere with the hepatic metabolism of other drugs.

Metoclopramide (Reglan) is a drug that is often included in the premedication regimen. This drug is a dopamine antagonist that increases the lower esophageal sphincter pressure; speeds gastric emptying, thereby reducing the gastric volume; and prevents or alleviates nausea and vomiting. Metoclopramide can be given orally in a 10 mg-dose as part of a premedication regimen. It also can be given intravenously at 0.15 mg per kg to produce its antiemetic properties. Metoclopramide has minimal side effects.

A problem every PACU nurse should watch for is *regurgitation after anesthesia*. When a patient is under the influence of a general anesthetic, the swallowing mechanism is abolished. Foodstuffs or fluids can be passively or actively vomited. The vomitus may then be aspirated into the trachea and lungs. In some instances, this type of aspiration is called *Mendelson's syndrome*. Inspiring vomitus can lead to *aspiration pneumonia*. It can occur during the induction of anesthesia, during the operation, or in the immediate PACU phase as the patient emerges from anesthesia.

If a patient begins vomiting, he or she should be placed in a head-down position and given oxygen immediately. The purpose of the head-down position is to allow fluid to flow AWAY from the lungs and not INTO the lungs. Consequently, if at all possible, the patient should be placed in this position if aspiration is suspected. Fluid should be suctioned rapidly while administration of oxygen continues. If the patient's airway is obstructed by large particles, finger or forceps should be used to clear the debris and then oxygen should be administered. The physician or anesthetist should be notified immediately.

Further treatment may include intubation and instillation of a weak solution of bicarbonate or saline through the endotracheal tube to aid in the neutralization of acidic gastric fluid in the respiratory tract. Steroids and antibiotics may also be administered.

A patient recovering from a general anesthetic should be assessed for possible *passive regurgitation,* especially if the patient was not intubated during surgery. Clinical signs include dyspnea, cyanosis of varying degrees, and tachycardia. On auscultation of the lungs, abnormal sounds are usually heard. If the assessment indicates the possibility of this syndrome, oxygen should be administered and the physician notified at once.

Patients who had a "full stomach" at induction of anesthesia, who have had intestinal or emergency surgery, or who have a suspected hiatal hernia have a higher incidence of this syndrome. The best treatment is prevention. These patients should have a complete return of consciousness before the endotracheal tube is removed. If the endotracheal tube is to be removed in the PACU, the patient should be placed in a lateral position with the head down. Oxygen should be administered, and suction should be available for immediate use before the extubation is performed.

THE INTESTINE

The *duodenum,* which is a part of the small intestine, arises at the pylorus of the stomach and ends at the duodenojejunal junction. The duodenum is divided into four segments: superior, descending, transverse, and ascending. The common bile duct and the main pancreatic duct empty into the descending duodenum. The main function of the stomach and the first portion of the duodenum is to alter the form of food and to supply enzymes for digestion.

The *jejunum* begins at the descending duodenum at the duodenojejunal angle. It constitutes the first two fifths of the small intestine, and the ileum occupies the distal three fifths of the small intestine. The mesentery, which contains blood vessels, nerves, lymphatics, lymph nodes, and fat, stabilizes the small bowel and prevents it from twisting and constricting its blood supply.

The digestive glands secrete large quantities of water to aid in the digestive process. It has been estimated that between 5 and 10 L of water enters the small intestine and only about 500 ml leaves the ileum and enters the colon. Among the important materials absorbed from the small intestine are sodium, bicarbonate, chloride, calcium, iron, carbohydrates, fats, and amino acids.

Sodium is absorbed by the small intestine at a rate of 25 to 35 g per day. This accounts for approximately 14 percent of all the sodium in the body. When a patient is experiencing extreme diarrhea, sodium can be depleted to a lethal level within a few hours.

THE COLON AND RECTUM

At the end of the small intestine is the *ileocecal valve,* which functions to prevent backflow of fecal material from the colon into the small intestine.

The colon is divided anatomically into the cecum, ascending colon, transverse colon, and descending and sigmoid colon. The functions of the colon are the absorption of water and electrolytes, which occurs principally in the proximal half of the colon, and the storage of fecal material, which occurs in the distal colon. The contents of the cecum are mainly liquid, as compared with the solid material contained in the sigmoid colon. Therefore, if a patient has had a colostomy, it is important to know from which portion of the colon the stoma originates, so as to determine if the excreted fecal

material has the normal amount of water content.

Of surgical importance is the *appendix,* which arises from the cecum at its inferior tip. It represents a special type of intestinal obstruction when it becomes inflamed owing to hyperplasia of submucosal lymphoid follicles, fecaliths, foreign bodies, or tumors.

The rectum functions entirely as an excretory canal and has no digestive function. It begins anatomically at the distal end of the sigmoid colon and ends at the anus. It is tubular and has two layers. The innermost layer is the lumen of the intestinal tract, and the outermost layer is skeletal muscle of the pelvic floor. The muscle is innervated by the parasympathetic nervous system.

THE ANUS

The anus is the termination of the alimentary canal. It is encircled by striated muscle and innervated by somatic sympathetic and parasympathetic fibers. Owing to the parasympathetic innervation of the rectum and anus, parasympathetic stimulation may occur during a rectal examination or surgical procedure. This parasympathetic reflex can also occur when a patient is recovering from a general anesthetic. If a physician deems it necessary to perform a rectal examination, the PACU nurse should be prepared to monitor the patient for bradycardia and laryngospasm, because they may result from stimulation of the anus and rectum.

THE LIVER

The importance of the liver is generally underestimated. In Chinese medicine, the liver is considered the most important organ of the body. It is one of the basic homeostatic organs, because it maintains the consistency of the blood on a minute-to-minute basis.

The liver is located in the right upper quadrant of the abdomen. It has a dual blood supply, consisting of the hepatic artery and the portal vein. Both carry oxygen and nutrients to the liver for assimilation. The *sinusoids,* which surround the hepatocytes (liver cells), empty into a venous system that eventually forms the hepatic vein and empties into the inferior vena cava. About 1400 ml of blood per min flows through the liver; this amount is about 30 percent of the cardiac output. The hepatocytes absorb nutrients from the portal venous blood;

store and release proteins, lipids, and carbohydrates; excrete bile salts; synthesize plasma proteins, glucose, cholesterol, and fatty acids; and metabolize exogenous and endogenous compounds. Along with this, hepatocytes have alpha$_1$-, alpha$_2$-, and beta$_2$-adrenergic receptors on their plasma membrane. The preponderance of adrenergic receptors seems to be alpha$_1$, and on stimulation of these receptors, an increase in intracellular calcium ions has been demonstrated.

The liver is the body's most important storage organ. It is able to absorb glucose in the form of glycogen, and it maintains a normal glucose concentration in the body. The liver also stores amino acids, iron, and vitamins. The liver can store up to 400 ml of blood in the sinusoids. If a person loses an appreciable amount of blood, the liver can release stored blood into the circulation to replace that which was lost.

The liver performs many vital physiologic functions that have a significant impact on the pharmacologic actions of many of the drugs used in the perioperative period. More specifically, the liver performs biotransformation of drugs by the cytochrome P-450 microsomal enzyme system. Consequently, knowledge of bilirubin metabolism, protein synthesis, and drug biotransformation is of critical importance to the PACU nurse.

Bilirubin Metabolism. Bilirubin is made from one of the by-products of red blood cell hemolysis—hemoglobin. The reticuloendothelial system converts hemoglobin to unconjugated bilirubin. The bilirubin is transported to the liver via serum albumin. In the liver, the bilirubin is then removed from the albumin and is conjugated with glucuronic acid. Conjugated bilirubin is highly water soluble and easily excreted in the urine. The other type of bilirubin, which is unconjugated, is lipid soluble and not excreted in the urine. Conditions such as sickle cell disease, thalassemia minor, drug-induced hemolysis, and breakdown of red blood cells following massive transfusions can cause an increase in unconjugated bilirubin levels. This eventually leads to an increase in bilirubin production. *Jaundice,* a yellowish tint to the body tissues, can be caused by a high concentration of bilirubin in the extracellular fluids. Consequently, diseases that are considered prehepatic cause an increase in unconjugated bilirubin and eventually lead to what is known as *hemolytic jaundice. Obstructive jaundice* occurs when the outflow of bile is blocked by an obstruction such as gallstones, stricture, and compression from external

masses. In this instance, the conjugated bilirubin level increases in the serum. The third type of jaundice, *toxic jaundice,* usually follows damage to the liver cells. Use of chloroform can cause this type of jaundice, as can use of carbon tetrachloride.

Protein Synthesis. The liver is responsible for the synthesis of most of the proteins found in the plasma. Albumin is the most notable of the plasma proteins synthesized by the liver. Albumin synthesis is regulated by the state of nutrition; therefore, a nutritional deficit results in reduced albumin production. Because many drugs used in anesthesia are protein bound, a reduction in the albumin level can have a significant impact on the pharmacologic action of the drugs. Because the protein-binding sites are reduced, the unbound fraction of the drug is increased, which ultimately leads to an increased sensitivity to the drug or a prolonged action. This is particularly true for the highly protein–bound barbiturates. Hence, in the PACU, hyponatremic patients who have received thiopental intraoperatively should be closely monitored for respiratory and cardiovascular depression due to the prolonged action of the ultra–short-acting barbiturate. The liver also synthesizes the enzyme pseudocholinesterase (plasma cholinesterase). This protein is the principal enzyme in the metabolism of succinylcholine and the ester-type local anesthetics. Succinylcholine, which is the principal depolarizing skeletal muscle relaxant in use, demonstrates an inverse correlation between duration of action and pseudocholinesterase levels. Therefore, any patient with suspected liver dysfunction who has received succinylcholine intraoperatively should be closely monitored for respiratory depression in the immediate postoperative period. Finally, the liver produces a large proportion of the protein substances used in coagulation.

Drug Biotransformation. The enzymes required for oxidation and conjugation in the liver are referred to as the *microsomal enzymes.* These enzymes are part of the cytochrome P-450 microsomal system. Exposure to certain drugs, including barbiturates and some anesthetics, can lead to an increase in the microsomal enzymes. This process is commonly called *enzyme induction.* When enzyme induction occurs, the result is an increase in the rate of drug biotransformation. Patients with severe liver disease may have reduced microsomal activity in the liver. Hence, drugs such as thiopental, diazepam, and meperidine have a prolonged action owing to a decreased rate of drug biotransformation by the microsomal enzymes. Consequently, patients with severe hepatic disease should be closely monitored for respiratory and cardiovascular depression in the PACU phase of their anesthetic experience.

Acute Hepatic Failure

Acute hepatic failure is a rare syndrome that may be seen if the patient has undergone a period of severe hypotension (40 mm Hg systolic) during anesthesia. Because of the hypotension, the liver cells die and the patient appears lethargic and drowsy postoperatively. Persistent oliguria, which leads to anuria within 24 to 48 hours, is the cardinal symptom of this syndrome. The signs of liver damage ensue and include headache, anorexia, malaise, vomiting, and pyrexia. The syndrome progresses to persistent vomiting and, by the end of the first week, jaundice may be present. The final stages of this disease are marked by delirium, coma, and death.

Treatment of this syndrome is entirely symptomatic and includes maintenance of fluid and electrolyte balance, treatment of the anuria, and a high carbohydrate diet.

THE GALLBLADDER

The gallbladder is a thin-walled, pear-shaped organ attached to the inferior surface of the liver (Fig. 9–3). It is 7 to 10 cm long and 3 to 5 cm wide. It has a capacity of 30 to 60 ml of fluid. Anatomically, it is divided into the *fundus*, the distal tip; the *corpus* (body), the middle body portion; the *infundibulum*, a pouchlike structure; and the *neck*, which leads to the cystic duct. The cystic duct joins the common hepatic duct to form the common bile duct. The common bile duct and the main pancreatic duct of Wirsung usually join at the choledochoduodenal junction, which is a passageway through the duodenal wall. The muscle of the choledochoduodenal junction is the *sphincter of Oddi*, which regulates the flow of bile into the duodenum. Many common narcotic analgesics can produce spasm of the sphincter of Oddi and the duodenum and can increase the pressure in the biliary tree.

Cholelithiasis is a common occurrence in patients with chronic gallbladder disease. As many as 20 million people suffer from some form of cholelithiasis. Gallstones are composed of cholesterol, which is almost insoluble in pure water. The causes of gallstones include

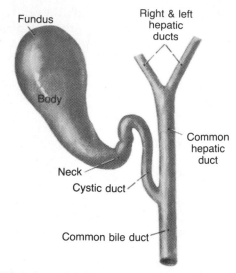

FIGURE 9–3. Gallbladder showing right and left hepatic ducts coming from the liver, common hepatic duct, cystic duct, and common bile duct. (From Jacob, S., Francone, C., and Lossow, W. J.: Structure and Function in Man. 5th ed. Philadelphia, W. B. Saunders, 1982, p. 495.)

too much cholesterol in the bile, chronic inflammation of the epithelium, too much absorption of bile acids from the bile, and too much absorption of water from the bile. A new surgical procedure called *biliary lithotripsy* offers distinct advantages over cholecystectomy. The advantages include no surgical incision, less pain, a shorter postoperative period, and a reduction in costs to the patient. Consequently, the patient has a 50 percent reduction in postoperative pulmonary complications because of this new procedure. Formerly, a cholecystectomy was performed, and that procedure was associated with a 50 percent reduction in the vital capacity on the first postoperative day. In fact, in the immediate postoperative period, the total lung capacity, vital capacity, and functional residual capacity all tend to decrease, causing a closure of the small airways and atelectasis. With the advent of biliary lithotripsy, the gallstones are broken into small fragments, with the patient receiving either local anesthesia and sedation or general anesthesia. Complications of this procedure are associated with the type of anesthetic technique and its inherent complications and from the shock wave therapy used during the procedure. The most common problems from this procedure include nausea, vomiting, abdominal pain, hemoptysis, and diarrhea. PACU care for a patient recovering from biliary lithotripsy should include the normal post anesthesia care of an upper abdominal surgical patient (see Chapter 31).

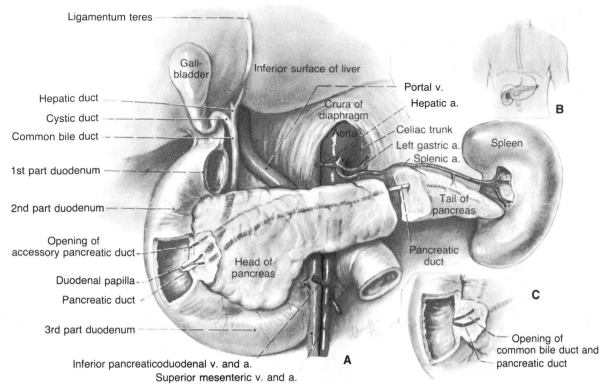

FIGURE 9–4. *A*, relationship of the pancreas to the duodenum, showing the pancreatic and bile ducts joining at the duodenal papilla. A section has been removed from the pancreas to expose the pancreatic duct. *B*, anatomic position of the pancreas. *C*, common variation. (*A* through *C* from Jacob, S. W., Francone, C. A., and Lossow, W. J.: Structure and Function in Man. 5th ed. Philadelphia, W. B. Saunders, 1982, p. 491.)

THE PANCREAS

The pancreas is situated in the upper abdomen behind the stomach. It is a slender organ that consists of a head, a body, and a tail (Fig. 9–4). Its main duct, through which pass the pancreatic enzymes, runs the entire length of the gland and opens into the duodenum along with the common bile duct. Scattered throughout the pancreas are small clusters of cells called the *islets of Langerhans.* They are responsible for the production and secretion of hormones that they empty directly into the blood stream; therefore, the islets of Langerhans are considered an endocrine gland. Three types of cells are found in the islets of Langerhans: alpha, beta, and delta. The alpha cells are associated with the production of the hormone *glucagon,* and the beta cells are associated with *insulin.* The physiologic significance of the delta cells has not been determined.

Insulin is secreted in response to an increase in the concentration of glucose. The secretion of insulin is inhibited when a low concentration of glucose exists. Glucagon is frequently called *hyperglycemic factor* because it causes hyperglycemia by stimulating the breakdown of liver glycogen with consequent release of glucose into the circulation. It also stimulates gluconeogenesis, which is the formation of glucose from noncarbohydrate sources.

The pancreas excretes juice for digesting all three major types of food: carbohydrates, fats, and proteins. The pancreatic juice also contains large amounts of bicarbonate ions, which help neutralize the acidic chyme as it passes into the duodenum from the stomach.

Pancreatitis

Acute pancreatitis is a serious complication of surgery on the biliary tract. It can occur as a result of common duct exploration during gallbladder surgery. Acute postoperative pancreatitis should be suspected if there is excessive pain, vomiting, fever, tachycardia, persistent ileus, or jaundice. The PACU nurse should be aware of these symptoms, which, if detected, should be reported to the surgeon. Treatment of this disorder may include nasogastric suction, anticholinergic drugs, antibiotics, and replacement of fluids and electrolytes.

THE SPLEEN

Because of its anatomic location, not its physiologic functions, the spleen will be discussed here (see Chapter 31).

The spleen is an oval organ located in the upper left quadrant of the abdominal cavity. Its physiologic functions include the filtering of blood and foreign material, hematopoiesis, and, in some instances, the production of lymphocytes and antibodies.

The spleen is a highly vascular organ, and approximately 350 L of blood normally flows through it daily. The spleen acts as a reservoir of blood. It can store so many red blood cells that splenic contraction can cause the hematocrit of the systemic blood to increase as much as 3 or 4 percent.

Normal health is possible after splenectomy, because other tissues can assume the functions the spleen normally performs. Splenectomy is usually performed for the cure or alleviation of hematologic disease or because of its traumatic rupture. Because the spleen is friable and vascular, blood loss from a splenectomy can be high. It is important, therefore, for the PACU nurse to assess the blood loss as well as the cardiovascular status of the patient during the recovery phase.

References

1. Barash, P., Cullen, B. and Stoelting, R.: Clinical Anesthesia. 2nd ed. Philadelphia, J. B. Lippincott, 1992.
2. Conklin, K.: Maternal physiological adaptations during gestation, labor, and the puerperium. Semin. Anesth., 10(4):221–234, 1991.
3. Guyton, A.: Textbook of Medical Physiology. 8th ed. Philadelphia, W. B. Saunders, 1991.
4. Hiley, M., and Giesecke, A.: The patient with a full stomach. Semin. Anesth., 9(3):204–210, 1990.
5. Jacobs, B., Swift, C., Dubow, H., et al.: Time required for oral ranitidine to decrease gastric fluid acidity. Anesth. Analg., 73:787–789, 1991.
6. Katz, J., Benumof, J., and Kadis, L.: Anesthesia and Uncommon Diseases. 3rd ed. Philadelphia, W. B. Saunders, 1990.
7. Miller, R. (ed.): Anesthesia. 3rd ed. New York, Churchill Livingstone, 1990.
8. Palmer, A., Waugaman, W., Conklin, K., et al.: Does the administration of oral bicitrate before elective cesarean section affect the incidence of nausea and vomiting in the parturient? Nurse Anesth., 2(3):126–133, 1991.
9. Roberts, A.: Post anesthesia care of the biliary lithotripsy patient. J. Post Anesth. Nurs., 56:392–396, 1990.
10. Sabiston, D. (ed.): Textbook of Surgery: The Biological Basis of Modern Surgical Practice. 14th ed. Philadelphia, W. B. Saunders, 1990.
11. Stoelting, R.: Pharmacology and Physiology in Anesthetic Practice. 2nd ed. Philadelphia: J. B. Lippincott, 1991.
12. Vila, P.: Acid aspiration prophylaxis in morbidly obese patients: Famotidine versus ranitidine. Anaesthesia, 46:967–969, 1991.
13. Waugaman, W., Foster, S. D., and Rigor, B. (eds.): Principles and Practice of Nurse Anesthesia. 2nd ed. Norwalk, CT, Appleton & Lange, 1992.
14. Wood, M., and Wood, A.: Drugs and Anesthesia: Pharmacology for Anesthesiologists. 2nd ed. Baltimore: Williams & Wilkins, 1990.

Integumentary System Anatomy and Physiology

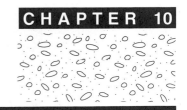

The integumentary system performs many functions that influence the nursing interventions in the post anesthesia care unit (PACU). Aseptic technique, intravenous cannulation, and care of the burn patient are discussed in this chapter because of their involvement with the integumentary system.

INTEGUMENTARY SYSTEM ANATOMY

The skin, or integument, provides a boundary between the internal and external environments of the body. The surface area covered by the skin is about 1.8 m² in the average male and 1.6 m² in the average female and accounts for 15 percent of the total body weight. It is divided into two major layers: the *epidermis* and the *dermis*, which includes the hypodermis.

The Epidermis

The epidermis consists of stratified squamous epithelium and has no blood vessels. The cells of the innermost, or basal, layer (stratum basale or stratum germinativum) of the epidermis are constantly dividing and producing cells of the outer layers. Basal cell cancer develops from this layer. The prickly layer, or *stratum spinosum,* located immediately above the basal layer, consists of cells that are connected by intercellular bridges. It is from this layer that squamous cell cancer arises (Fig. 10-1).

The granular layer, or *stratum granulosum,* contains three or four layers of cells. Squamous epithelial cells are converted in this layer into hard material by a process called *cornification.* The next layer, the *stratum lucidum,* develops only on the palms of the hands and the soles of the feet. The outermost epidermal layer, called the *horny layer,* or *stratum corneum,* is composed of dead cells, keratin, surface lipids, and dirt. Dead cells are shed at a fairly constant rate by a process called *desquamation.* The epidermis also has keratinizing and glandular appendages. Keratinizing appendages comprise the hair and the nails, and glandular appendages include the sweat, scent, and sebaceous glands.

The Dermis

The dermis, or corium, lies below the epidermis and consists of collagenous, elastic, and reticular fibers. It also contains blood vessels, nerves, lymphatics, and smooth muscle.

The Hypodermis

The hypodermis functions as a shock absorber and heat insulator. Located under the dermis, it is made up of fat, smooth muscle, and areolar tissue.

INTEGUMENTARY FUNCTIONS

The skin has many important functions, the most important of which is to act as a barrier between the internal and external environments. In addition, it plays an important part in body temperature and fluid regulation, excretion, secretion, vitamin D production, sensation, appearance, and many other functions that have yet to be identified.

Thermoregulation

Skin, subcutaneous tissue, and fat in the subcutaneous tissue provide heat insulation for the body. Heat is lost from the body to the surroundings by radiation, conduction, convection, and evaporation (Fig. 10–2). Radiation of heat from the body accounts for about 60 percent of the total heat loss. In this mechanism, heat is lost in the form of infrared heat waves. Conduction of heat to objects represents about 3 percent of the total heat loss, whereas con-

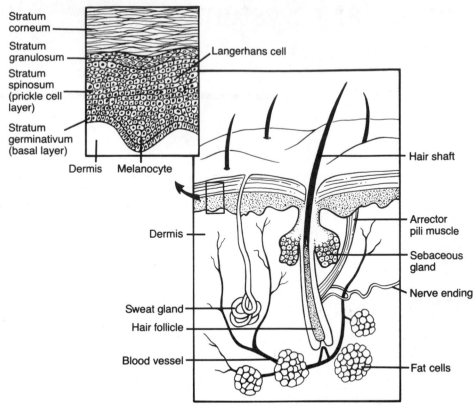

FIGURE 10–1. Layers of the epidermis. (From Monahan, F. D., Drake, T., and Neighbors, M.: Nursing Care of Adults. Philadelphia, W. B. Saunders, 1994, p. 156.)

duction of heat to the air represents about 15 percent of the total heat loss. When water is carried away from the skin by air currents, convection of heat occurs. Evaporation constitutes about 22 percent of the heat loss. Even when a person is not sweating, water still evaporates from the skin and the lungs. This insensible loss is about 600 ml per day.

The skin regulates body temperature by conserving heat in a cold environment. Sweating can lower the body temperature in hot environments. The sweat glands are innervated by the sympathetic and parasympathetic nervous systems. When the anterior hypothalamus in the preoptic area is stimulated by excess heat, im-

pulses are sent from this area by way of the autonomic pathways to the spinal cord. From the spinal cord through the sympathetic outflow tracts, the impulses go to the skin all over the body. The sweat glands are innervated by sympathetic nerve fibers. However, in these specific fibers, the neurotransmitter is acetylcholine. Consequently, these fibers are actually sympathetic cholinergic nerve fibers and are stimulated by epinephrine or norepinephrine.

The sweat gland consists of two portions: a deep subdermal coiled portion that secretes the sweat and a duct portion that conducts the sweat to the skin. Sweat has a pH of 3.8 to 6.5 and contains sodium, chloride, potassium, cal-

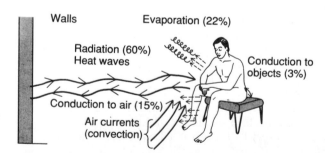

FIGURE 10–2. Major mechanisms of heat loss from the body. (From Guyton, A.: Textbook of Medical Physiology. 8th ed. Philadelphia: W. B. Saunders, 1991, p. 799).

cium, and lactic acid as well as urea. Therefore, sweating is an act of excretion as well as secretion.

Protection

The skin protects the body from injurious physical, chemical, electrical, thermal, or biologic stimuli. Of particular importance to the PACU nurse is the presence of bacteria on the skin that may cause sepsis when a patient's skin barrier is broken. Normal flora of the skin include gram-positive cocci and rods. Diphtheroids are also widely distributed on the skin, especially in moist areas. The normal pH of the skin is 4 to 6, from lactic acid and amino acid residues of keratinization.

When intact, the skin stops pathogenic organisms from entering the body and at the same time prevents the loss of *water, electrolytes*, and *proteins* to the external environment. Once the skin is broken, for example, by surgical incision or venipuncture, the barrier between the internal and external environments is broken. This is why aseptic technique is important whenever opening of the skin is anticipated or has occurred.

IMPORTANCE OF ASEPTIC TECHNIQUE

Because all skin has pathogenic organisms on it, skin can never be sterile. Precautions should be taken to reduce the number of pathogenic organisms that may be introduced into a wound. Handwashing technique is most important. This should be accomplished before care is given to the patient. A good mechanical scrub with a skin antiseptic, such as a soap containing iodine, should be done.

The surgical wound site should be kept clean, and the dressings should remain sterile. If there is any question about sterility because of excess bleeding, fluid, or physical contamination, the dressing should be changed. Special precautions to reduce the introduction of pathogenic organisms should be taken with patients who are prone to infection. This includes patients who are obese, anemic, or debilitated; those with vascular insufficiency, chronic obstructive pulmonary disease, and diabetes mellitus; and those with an immune deficiency, including patients who are on chemotherapy or chronic steroid therapy or who have acquired immunodeficiency syndrome. Aseptic technique in wound care of these patients should include the wearing of a surgical mask and the use of sterile gloves and drapes.

Universal Precautions in the PACU

The Centers for Disease Control (CDC) developed the "Universal Precautions for Prevention of Transmission of the Human Immunodeficiency Virus (HIV) and Hepatitis B Virus (HBV) in Healthcare Settings," which is summarized in Table 10–1. The Occupational Health and Safety Administration's universal standards are presented in Table 10–2 and serve to supplement the CDC precautions.

Sterile Technique for Intravenous Therapy

Establishing an intravenous infusion should be accomplished with sterile technique. The

Table 10–1. UNIVERSAL PRECAUTIONS

1. All needles, blades, and sharp instruments should be handled to prevent accidental injuries, and all should be considered potentially infected. Disposable sharp items should be placed in puncture-resistant containers located as close as practical to the area in which they are used. Needles should not be recapped, bent, broken, or removed from disposable syringes before placing them in appropriate disposable containers.
2. Gloves should be worn when touching mucous membranes or open skin of all patients. When the possibility exists of exposure to blood, body fluids, or items soiled with these, gloves should be used. With some procedures, such as endoscopy when aerosolization or splashes of blood or secretions are likely to occur, masks, eye coverings, and gowns are indicated. Gloves and body coverings should be removed and disposed of properly after patient contact.
3. Frequent handwashing, especially after contact with patients and after removal of gloves, should be encouraged. If hands are accidentally contaminated with blood or other body fluids, they should be washed as soon as possible.
4. Ventilation devices for resuscitation should be available at appropriate locations to prevent the need for emergency mouth-to-mouth resuscitation.
5. Health care workers who have exudative lesions or weeping dermatitis should not participate in direct patient care activities until the condition resolves.

From Berry, A. J.: Infection hazards for the anesthesiologist. Clin. Anesth. Updates, 2:10, 1991.

Table 10–2. OSHA UNIVERSAL STANDARDS OVERVIEW (TAKEN FROM 29 CFR PART 1910)

Infection Control Plan

• Employers need to identify in writing all tasks, procedures, and role descriptions that carry the potential exposure.

• Employers must develop a written Infection Control Plan that includes a schedule and method of implementation for each category of the standards.

• An Infection Control Plan must be completed within 120 days of the effective date of the final standards.

• The Infection Control Plan must be updated and reviewed as tasks and procedures are added or changed.

Engineering and Work Practice Controls

• Protective equipment must be available in appropriate sizes. It must be removed immediately after leaving the work area, or upon contamination, and placed in a designated receptacle for disposal, washing or disinfection.

• Hands should be washed after contact with blood or other potential pathogens and after removal of protective gloves.

• Contaminated needles should not be bent, broken or otherwise manipulated.

• Eating, drinking, applying cosmetics or handling of contact lenses should be prohibited in areas of potential exposure.

• All laboratory specimens should be handled in a fashion that minimizes splashing or spraying.

Protective Equipment

• Personal protective clothing and equipment should be easily accessible, in the appropriate sizes, and replaced or repaired when necessary.

• Gloves should be worn when handling blood or infectious materials or when handling items or surfaces soiled by blood or other pathogens.

• Masks and eye protection should be worn whenever splashes, spray or aerosols of blood may occur.

• Gowns, warm-up jackets, or similar clothing should be worn if there is a potential for soiling clothes or skin contact.

• The protective barrier selected should be appropriate for the procedure being performed and the anticipated occupational exposure.

• The decision not to use protective clothing and equipment rests with the employee and not the employer.

Housekeeping

• A written schedule for cleaning and disinfecting all anesthesia equipment and work surfaces is required, as well as prompt cleaning and disinfecting at the end of a treatment or whenever contamination occurs.

• Laboratory specimens to be transported should be placed in color-coded, leakproof bags with an appropriate label.

• Disposal of infectious waste should be in accordance with all federal, state, and local regulations.

• Sharps should be disposed of in impermeable, puncture-resistant containers that are accessible to the staff; sharps containers should be labeled and precautions taken to prevent overfilling of the receptacles.

• Laundry, contaminated with blood or other infectious materials, must be placed in labeled or color-coded leakproof bags.

Hepatitis B Vaccination and Postexposure Followup

• Employers must make the HBV vaccination available to all staff members who have occupational exposure to blood or other potential pathogens one or more times per month.

• Postexposure followup and reporting of all staff with an occupational exposure to HBV are required.

• HBV antibody testing should be made available to employees prior to deciding whether or not to receive the vaccination; if testing indicates that an employee has immunity to HBV, the employer is not required to offer the vaccine.

• Following an occupational exposure, the employer should provide medical evaluation and followup care to the employee.

• Permission for antigen or antibody testing of the source patient's blood should be obtained if possible to determine HBV and HIV infection status.

• An employee with an occupational exposure should be tested as soon as possible for the determination of HIV and HBV status.

Communication of Hazards to Employees

• Labels or other forms of warning should be placed on containers of infectious waste, refrigerators that are used to store blood, and containers used to transport laboratory specimens.

• Employee training about the hazards associated with blood and other infectious materials and the protective measures required to minimize the risk of exposure should be accomplished within 150 days of the effective date of the final standards.

• Employee training and inservice education are required for all new employees and annually thereafter.

• Employee training should include epidemiology, symptomatology, modes of transmission of diseases, and work practice controls instituted to prevent contamination.

• Employee training records should be maintained for 5 years.

• Medical records should be maintained on each employee who receives the hepatitis B vaccine or who experiences an occupational exposure; medical records must be maintained for the duration of employment plus 30 years.

HBV = hepatitis B virus; HIV = human immunodeficiency virus.

Reprinted with permission. Fay, M. F.: Anesthesia: Employee health safety. Anesth. Today, 2(4):6, 1991. CoMed Communications, Philadelphia, PA, pubs.

site chosen for cannula (needle) placement should be prepared in a suitable fashion. An excellent method uses 1 percent iodine in 70 percent isopropyl alcohol. After at least 30 seconds of drying time, the iodine solution should be washed off with 70 percent isopropyl alcohol. Both agents should be applied with friction, working from the center of the field to the periphery. An iodophor skin preparation may be substituted in patients with sensitive skin but should not be washed off with alcohol, because its antibacterial action may depend in part on the sustained release of free iodine. In the rare instance in which iodine preparations cannot be tolerated at all, vigorous, prolonged (more than 1 minute) washing with 70 percent isopropyl alcohol is acceptable.

After the intravenous administration route is established, the cannula (needle) should be securely anchored to prevent irritating to-and-fro motion and to avoid potential transport of cutaneous bacteria into the puncture wound. Although evidence is not conclusive, additional protection from infectious complications may follow topical antimicrobial applications to the infusion site. Because studies have demonstrated that antibiotic ointments may actually favor the selective growth of fungi, the use of topical antiseptic iodophor ointment should be considered. The intravenous site should be covered with a sterile dressing.

Burn Injuries

The care of the postoperative burn patient can be most challenging to the PACU nurse. These patients usually present a complex array of pathophysiologic difficulties, from deranged fluid and electrolyte balance, respiratory complications, and disrupted temperature regulation to psychological disturbances. A burn, no matter how small, represents a total body assault.

Infection is the most common and the most dreaded complication following a burn injury; therefore, aseptic skin care is of primary importance. Nursing care of the patient with a burn injury is complex; the reader is referred to Chapter 36 for discussion of specific pathophysiologic processes, assessment, and nursing interventions for the burn patient in the PACU.

The four main types of burn injuries include cold, chemical, electrical, and thermal. A *cold* injury is trauma caused by exposure to cold. Conditions such as frostbite, chilblain, immersion foot, and trench foot are the result. *Frostbite* results from the crystallization of tissue fluids in the skin or subcutaneous tissue. *Chilblain* results from exposure to cold temperatures above freezing associated with high humidity. *Immersion foot* occurs when the skin of the foot is exposed to water that is below 50°F for a long period.

Chemical burns are produced by caustic agents, either acid or base. They are devastating because, without appropriate emergency treatment, these agents continue to cause destruction of fascia, fat, muscle, and bone.

Electrical burns, which result from direct contact with electrical voltage, are deceiving in appearance. Although only the entrance and exit wounds may be visible, massive damage is often sustained as the high-energy sources follow conductive muscle and nerves. Damage may require amputation of extremities. Thermal injury often occurs in addition to the electrical burn from the heat of arcing currents or ignited clothing.

The most common type of burn injury is the *thermal burn*, caused by excessive heat. Metabolic derangement and problems in maintaining thermal control develop. Unless otherwise indicated, this discussion will cover thermal burns. The terms *partial-thickness, deep-dermal,* and *full-thickness* are commonly used to classify burn injuries. The terms *first degree, second degree, third degree,* and sometimes *fourth degree burns* are based on the characteristics and surface appearance of the burn wound.

A *partial-thickness burn* heals without grafting. This is when only part of the skin has been damaged or destroyed but enough epithelial cells remain in the skin to provide new epidermis, which includes hair follicles and sweat glands. The partial-thickness burn can also be referred to as a first- or second-degree burn. Partial-thickness burns can be divided into three categories: (1) *superficial burns,* in which there is partial skin loss but no dermal death and, therefore, no slough forms; (2) *intermediate partial-thickness burn,* characterized typically by healing from the level of the hair follicles; and (3) *deep partial-thickness burn,* which heals typically from the level of the sweat ducts.

A *deep-dermal burn* is a partial-thickness burn that can heal without grafting. However, if it is complicated by infection or mechanical trauma, it is likely to be converted into a full-thickness burn.

Full-thickness burns cause destruction of all the skin. No viable epithelial elements are present, and there may be destruction of the subcutaneous tissue, muscles, and bones. The wound must be grafted, as the skin does not regenerate. The full-thickness burn is equivalent to the third-degree burn. Destruction of the full-thickness burn extending to the structures underneath the skin to include the bone is called a *fourth-degree burn*.

References

1. Barash, P., Cullen, B., and Stoelting, R.: Clinical Anesthesia. 2nd ed. Philadelphia, J. B. Lippincott, 1992.
2. Benumof, J., and Saidman, L.: Anesthesia and Perioperative Complications. St. Louis, Mosby-Year Book, 1992.
3. Centers for Disease Control: Universal precautions for prevention of transmission of the human immunodeficiency virus (HIV) and hepatitis B virus (HBV) in healthcare settings. Atlanta, Centers for Disease Control, 1989.
4. Guyton, A.: Textbook of Medical Physiology. 8th ed. Philadelphia, W. B. Saunders, 1991.
5. Katz, J., Benumof, J., and Kadis, L.: Anesthesia and Uncommon Diseases. 3rd ed. Philadelphia, W. B. Saunders, 1990.
6. Longnecker, D. E., and Murphy, F. L. (eds.): Dripps/ Eckenhoff/Vandam Introduction to Anesthesia: Principles of Safe Practice. 8th ed. Philadelphia, W. B. Saunders, 1992.
7. Miller, R. (ed.): Anesthesia. 3rd ed. New York, Churchill Livingstone, 1990.
8. Sabiston, D. (ed.): Textbook of Surgery: The Biological Basis of Modern Surgical Practice. 14th ed. Philadelphia, W. B. Saunders, 1990.
9. Waugaman, W., Foster, S., and Rigor, B.: Principles and Practice of Nurse Anesthesia, 2nd ed. Norwalk, CT: Appleton & Lange, 1992.

Immune System Physiology

Over the past two decades, there has been a virtual explosion of information about the immune system. Diseases whose causes were believed to be based in one of the other physiologic systems are now found, as a result of medical research, to have their basis in the immune system. For example, myasthenia gravis was once thought to be a neuromuscular disease; however, research has demonstrated the origin of the disease to be in the immune system. Today, post anesthesia care unit (PACU) nurses must deal with patients who are immunosuppressed or experiencing a hypersensitivity reaction, or who have immune diseases such as acquired immunodeficiency syndrome (AIDS). An informed appreciation of the physiology and pathophysiology of the immune system is essential for the appropriate PACU care of the surgical patient.

Definitions

Acquired immunity: the ability of the human body to develop an extremely powerful specific immunity against most invading agents.

Active acquired immunity: immunity that develops when a person comes into direct contact with a pathogen either by contracting the disease produced by the pathogen or by being vaccinated against the disease.

Antibody: a globulin molecule with the potential to attack agents that are foreign to the host.

Antigen: a protein, large polysaccharide, or large lipoprotein complex that stimulates the process of acquired immunity.

B lymphocytes or bursa-dependent cells: immunocompetent lymphocytes that are named for the preprocessing that occurs in the bursa of Fabricius of birds and is responsible for humoral immunity.

Cellular or cell-mediated immunity: a type of acquired immunity that uses sensitized lymphocytes as the primary defense.

Clone: a group of cells that originate from a single parent cell.

Hapten: a substance that has a low molecular weight and combines with an antigenic substance to elicit an immune response.

Humoral immunity: a type of acquired immunity that uses antibodies as the primary defense.

Immunodeficiency disease: immunosuppression that results from a deficiency of a single humoral antibody group or from a combined deficiency of both the T- and B-cell systems.

Immunosuppression: a state of nonresponsiveness of the immune system to antigenic challenge.

Immunity: the ability of the human body to resist almost all types of organisms or toxins that can damage tissues and organs.

Innate immunity: general processes in the human body, other than those of acquired immunity, that are responsible for protection against organisms and toxins.

Lymphopenia: decreased function of the lymphoid organs.

Passive acquired immunity: immunity resulting when a person receives immune cells or immune serum produced by someone else.

Phagocytosis: the envelopment and digestion of bacteria or other foreign substances.

Sensitized lymphocytes: lymphocytes that are made competent by processing to facilitate their immunologic activity, such as their attachment to and destruction of a foreign agent.

Stem cells: an unspecialized cell that gives rise to specific specialized cells such as T and B lymphocytes.

T lymphocytes: sensitized lymphocytes that are responsible for cellular immunity.

PHYSICAL AND CHEMICAL BARRIERS

The body's *first line of immunologic defense* is the mechanical barrier provided by the epithelial surface. Some parts of the epithelium have extensions from their surface, such as the cilia and the mucus in the respiratory system. These extensions provide not only an additional physical barrier to the entrance of foreign substances but also an efficient removal system. In the stomach, hydrochloric acid, which is thought to have bactericidal action, is secreted. As an additional defense, the skin produces chemicals that inactivate bacteria. The surfaces of the boundary tissues also have specific defenses in the form of secretory antibodies. Consequently, surgical incisions, intravenous cannulation, and many other invasive procedures can cause major breaks in the first line of defense. Hence, the PACU nurse should use good aseptic or sterile technique to prevent an overwhelming bacterial invasion through the boundary tissues.

INNATE IMMUNITY

Innate or nonspecific immunity is the body's *second line of immunologic defense* against foreign material. In this type of immunity, activation occurs during each exposure to an invading substance. Recognition does occur at the level of distinguishing between self and nonself; however, the mechanisms of innate immunity cannot identify the specific invader.

Phagocytosis is the primary mechanism of innate immunity. The cells in the body that carry out the phagocytic functions of innate immunity are *monocytes*, which are *macrophages,* and *neutrophils (polymorphonuclear leukocytes)*, which are *microphages*. The phagocytes' overall immunologic functions are to localize the antigen and to destroy, inactivate, or process it for handling by other components of the immune system. The process of phagocytosis can be enhanced by the combination of an antigen with a plasma protein called *opsonin*, a substance associated with the immune system. Finally, phagocytosis gives transitory protection to the body so that it will not be overwhelmed by foreign materials before the immune system (acquired immunity) is activated.

ACQUIRED IMMUNITY

Acquired or adaptive immunity is the body's *third line of immunologic defense*. It is mediated by the capability of specific antibodies or sensitized lymphocytes to recognize and to react to antigens from the offending agent. Two closely allied types of acquired immune mechanisms occur in the body: *humoral immunity* and *cellular (cell-mediated) immunity*.

Humoral Immunity

Humoral immunity is conferred by circulating antibodies found in the globulin fraction of blood proteins and are therefore referred to as *immunoglobulins (Ig)*. The processing that is involved to produce the immunoglobulin begins with the lymphocytic stem cells in the bone marrow. These stem cells, being incapable of forming antibodies, make pre-B lymphocytes that are taken up by the lymph nodes and processed in the as yet unidentified "bursa-equivalent" tissue to become mature immunocompetent B lymphocytes. These processed B lymphocytes are then released into the blood, where they become entrapped in the lymphoid tissue. On stimulation by an antigen, the B lymphocyte specific for that antigen enlarges, divides, and differentiates into plasma cells having specificity for that antigen. The plasma cells then produce and secrete an antibody or sensitized lymphocyte. During their first exposure to the antigen, lymphocytes from one specific type of lymphoid tissue form *clones*. The clones are responsive only to the antigen responsible for their initial development. On their second stimulation by the same antigen, the clones proliferate rapidly, leading to the formation of a large amount of antibody. Some cells in this clone mature to form plasma cells, whereas other cells of the clone become B lymphocyte memory cells. When the immune system responds to the first presentation of the antigen, the immune system will "remember" the antigen by means of the B lymphocyte memory cell. The immune system can remember the antigen for years. In other words, on the first stimulation by an antigen, the plasma cells produce antibodies (immunoglobulins) as their *primary response*. The primary response is usually evident about 4 to 10 days after the initial exposure to the antigen. On the second stimulation by the same antigen, a *second response* occurs. This secondary response, in which a massive amount of antibody specific to the antigen is produced within 1 or 2 days, lasts for months. The secondary response is more rapid, stronger, and more persistent than the primary response. This is because of the memory cells and clones that are produced by the initial exposure to the antigen. If the T lymphocytes are activated by the same antigen, the T-lymphocyte helper cells will enhance the response of the B lymphocytes. Therefore, because of this cooperative effort, the total number of lymphocytes in the lymphoid tissue increases markedly. On second exposure to an antigen, the same plasma cell can produce the particular antibody needed and can convert from one type of antibody secretion to another as needed. Once the specific antibodies from the plasma cells are no longer needed, further production of the antibodies is suppressed by the antibodies themselves or by *T-lymphocyte suppressor cells* (Fig. 11–1).

The immunoglobulins are large proteins with specific structural arrangements of polypeptide chains with specific amino acid sequences. The immunoglobulins are divided into five primary classes based on structural arrangements: IgA, IgD, IgE, IgG, and IgM.

IgA is a small molecule that constitutes about 15 percent of the total immunoglobulins and is present in most body secretions. This antibody activates complement through the alternate properdin pathway. Along with this, secretory immunity is mediated by IgA. The secretory antibodies are found on the mucosal surfaces of the oral cavity, the lungs, and the intestinal and urogenital tracts, as well as in mammary

secretions. This secretory IgA differs from other antibodies in that it has a protein molecule, called a *secretory piece*, attached to it. *Secretory IgA* is effective against viruses and some bacteria.

IgD constitutes about 1 percent of the total immunoglobulins. The exact function of IgD is unknown. However, this immunoglobulin may be involved with the differentiation of the B lymphocytes, and a relationship has been suggested between IgD and antibody activity directed toward insulin, penicillin, milk proteins, diphtheria toxoid, thyroid antigens, and the products of abnormal tissue growth.

IgE is present in minute quantities (about 0.002 percent of total serum immunoglobulins) and is associated with type I immediate hypersensitivity reaction.

IgG is the smallest antibody, and it constitutes about 75 percent of the total plasma antibodies. It is the only antibody that can cross the placental barrier, thus conferring passive

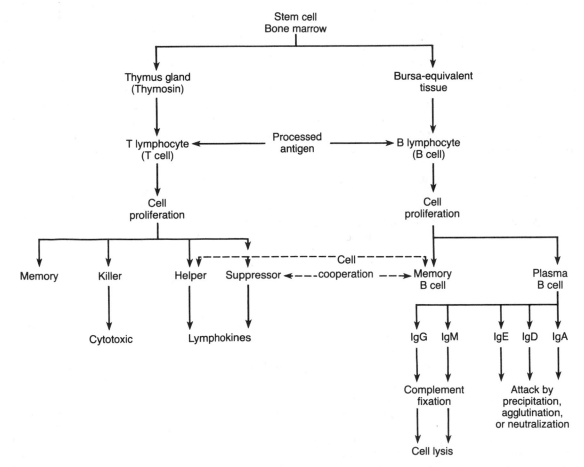

FIGURE 11–1. Schematic overview of the humoral and cellular immunologic pathways and the resulting effector substances or mechanisms of activity.

immunity to the fetus. IgG is the primary antibody involved in the secondary response. It is active against many blood-borne infectious agents such as bacteria, viruses, parasites, and some fungi.

IgM is the largest antibody, and it constitutes about 10 percent of plasma antibody. It is the main antibody involved in the primary antibody response, and IgM will fix complement.

Antibodies, once secreted by the plasma cells, protect the body against invading agents by three mechanisms of action: (1) attacking the antigen; (2) activating of the complement system, which results in cell lysis; and (3) activating the immediate hypersensitivity reaction, which localizes the invader and may negate its virulence. More specifically, antibodies can inactivate the invading antigen by precipitation, agglutination, neutralization, or complement fixation. *Precipitation* occurs when an insoluble antibody forms a complex with a soluble antigen (such as tetanus toxin) and the resulting antigen-antibody complex becomes insoluble and precipitates. When antigens are bound together and react with an antibody, *agglutinated aggregates* occur. *Neutralization* is achieved when antibodies cover the toxic sites of an antigenic agent or when antibodies counteract toxins released by bacteria. Rarely are the potent antibodies able to attack a cell membrane directly and cause lysis. However, one of the powerful effects of the binding of the antigen-antibody complex is the activation of *complement*, which serves to amplify this interaction. More specifically, when IgG or IgM binds to an antigen, the complement system is activated, and a cascade system of nine different enzyme precursors (C1 through C9) reacts sequentially. The final result of the activation of the complement system is puncture of the antigen's cell membrane (cell lysis), causing rupture of its cellular agents.

Cellular Immunity

Cellular immunity is the second type of specific immunity, and it utilizes *T lymphocytes* and *macrophages.* Some specific functions of the cellular immunity system are protection against most viruses, slow-acting bacteria, and fungal infections; mediation of cutaneous delayed hypersensitivity reactions; rejection of foreign grafts; and immunologic surveillance.

The T lymphocytes, like the B lymphocytes, originate from primitive stem cells and go through stages of maturation (see Fig. 11–1). Once the immature lymphocyte leaves the bone marrow, it migrates to the thymus gland, where it is acted on by the hormone *thymosin.* The T lymphocyte then becomes mature and immunocompetent. Thus, they are thymus-dependent, or T, lymphocytes. These mature T lymphocytes can circulate in the blood and lymph, or they may come to rest in the inner cortex of the lymph nodes, where they may form subgroups of T lymphocytes.

These T lymphocytes function overall in the immune system by serving in regulatory, effector, and cytotoxic capacities. The *regulatory T lymphocytes* are the *helper* or *suppressor T lymphocytes.* These lymphocytes amplify or suppress responses of other T lymphocytes or responses of B lymphocytes. The helper T lymphocytes produce a soluble factor that is required, in some instances, for antibody formation by B lymphocytes. This helper action is most important for IgE and IgG production. The underproduction of helper cells is associated with AIDS. The suppressor T lymphocytes appear to regulate or to suppress the activity of B lymphocytes in the production of antibodies. Evidence indicates that the suppressor T lymphocytes can become pathologically active against helper T lymphocytes and other aspects of cellular immunity. For this reason, these suppressor T lymphocytes may have a role in immune tolerance and in the development of autoimmune disease, such as *myasthenia gravis.* *Effector T lymphocytes* are probably responsible for the delayed hypersensitivity reactions, the rejection of foreign tissue grafts and tumors, and the elimination of viral-infected cells. Effector T lymphocytes have antigen receptors on their surfaces that are significant in the initiation of cellular immunity. When an antigen enters the body, it undergoes processing by the phagocytes. The antigen then travels to the regional lymph node, which drains the area of antigen invasion. In this lymph node, the T lymphocyte recognizes the antigen, binds to the antigen, and proliferates. The T lymphocyte becomes sensitized when it comes into contact with the antigen. In addition, memory T lymphocytes result from this interaction. Hence, on a second exposure to the antigen, a more intense, efficient, and rapid cellular immunity will result. This contact also results in the release of lymphokines by the T lymphocyte. Some of the lymphokines are (1) *chemotactic factor,* which recruits phagocytes into the area; (2) *migration inhibitory factor,* which prevents the migration of phagocytes away from the area; (3) *transfer factor,* which induces noncommitted T lymphocytes to form T lymphocytes of the same antigen-specific clone as the original cells;

(4) *lymphotoxin*, which is a nonspecific cellular toxin; and (5) *interferon*, which inhibits the replication of viruses.

The direct cellular cytotoxicity that is mediated by cellular immunity involves *cytotoxic lymphocytes*, or *killer cells*, and *macrophages*. The role of these cytotoxic T lymphocytes is not well established; however, they are believed to be involved in nonspecific killing of viruses, rejection of allografts, and immune surveillance of malignant diseases.

HYPERSENSITIVITY REACTIONS

The immune system serves mainly to protect a person from harmful substances. However, in some instances, the activation of the immune system can cause many deleterious effects; this is termed *allergic response* or *hypersensitivity reaction*. Briefly, this response represents a magnified or inappropriate reaction by the host to an antigenic substance, and it can result in an immunologic disease. Hypersensitivity reactions are divided into four major categories and are called *type I* through *type IV hypersensitivity reactions* (Table 11–1).

Type I Hypersensitivity Reaction (Anaphylactic, Immediate)

Type I hypersensitivity reaction occurs in persons who were previously sensitized to a specific antigen. The antibodies formed against that antigen are of the IgE classification. The term *reagins* is used to describe these IgE antibodies. Reaginic antibodies bind to mast cells

in tissues surrounding the blood vessels and to blood basophils. When the previously sensitized host is re-exposed to the same antigen, the antigen reacts with the *reaginic antibody* that is attached to the cell, and there is an immediate swelling and then rupture of the basophil or mast cell, resulting in a release of chemical mediators into the local environment. These chemical mediators include (1) *histamine*, which causes local vasodilatation and increased permeability of the capillaries; (2) *slow-reacting substance of anaphylaxis*, which causes prolonged contraction of some smooth muscle, such as that of the bronchi; (3) *chemotactic factor*, which draws neutrophils and macrophages into the area of the antigen-antibody reaction; and (4) *lysosomal enzymes*, which elicit a local inflammatory reaction. These chemical mediators act on the "shock organs," such as the mucosa, skin, bronchi, and heart. The resulting clinical manifestations of the type I reaction include urticaria, allergic rhinitis, allergic asthma, and, in severe cases, systemic anaphylaxis.

Type II Hypersensitivity Reaction (Cytotoxic)

In the type II hypersensitivity reaction, the antigen and the antibody complex react, causing injury to the cell membrane or to a surface tissue by direct destruction by antibody of cellular elements. The antibodies involved in the type II reaction are either IgG or IgM, and the reaction is enhanced by complement. *Hemolytic anemia* is an example of a type II reaction that affects the red blood cells. For example, when penicillin is absorbed on the red blood cell

Table 11–1. CATEGORIES OF HYPERSENSITIVITY REACTIONS

Type	Mechanism	Outcome	Reaction Time	Examples
I (anaphylactic)	Antigen-IgE reaction at surface of mast cells and basophils	Release of mediators	Immediate	Asthma Hay fever Systemic anaphylaxis
II (cytotoxic)	Binding of IgM or IgG with antigens on surface of cell; enhanced by complement fixation	Cell lysis and tissue damage	Variable	Hemolytic anemia Goodpasture's disease
III (arthus)	Microprecipitation of immune complex formed by antigen and IgM or IgG; enhanced by complement fixation	Tissue damage and release of vasoactive substances	4–18 hr	Serum sickness Farmer's lung Allergic alveolitis Glomerulonephritis SLE
IV (delayed)	Direct interaction of antigen with sensitized T lymphocytes	Release of mediators and tissue damage	24–48 hr	Contact dermatitis Tuberculosis

SLE = systemic lupus erythematosus.

membrane, the interaction of antipenicillin antibody, penicillin, and complement causes a reaction that results in the lysis of red blood cells.

Type III Hypersensitivity Reaction (Arthus)

The type III hypersensitivity reaction involves the formation of immune complexes of antigen and antibody (IgG or IgM). These immune complexes precipitate in and around small vessels and damage the target tissue by activating complement. Also involved in this process is an inflammatory reaction that is initiated by the gathering of inflammatory cells and the release of vasoactive amines from platelets. As this process continues, polymorphonuclear leukocytes phagocytize the immune complexes, causing inflammation and necrosis of the blood vessels and surrounding tissue owing to the release of lysosomal enzymes. *Serum sickness* and *systemic lupus erythematosus* are clinical examples of type III hypersensitivity reactions.

Type IV Hypersensitivity Reaction (Delayed or Cell Mediated)

Type IV hypersensitivity reaction is the only hypersensitivity reaction that does *not* involve antibodies. In the type IV reaction, the exposure to an antigen and the subsequent binding of the antigen with antigen-specific reactive T lymphocytes initiates the production of lymphokines from the T lymphocytes, with tissue damage as the end result. The antigen responsible for the type IV reaction can be bacterial, fungal, protozoan, or viral. *Contact dermatitis, allograft rejection,* and *delayed response in tuberculin skin tests* are examples of delayed hypersensitivity reactions.

IMMUNOSUPPRESSION

With the advent of organ transplantation, patients can and do arrive in the PACU in an immunosuppressed state. Consequently, it is important for the PACU nurse to have a basic knowledge of the forms of immunosuppression and the appropriate nursing care measures that can be implemented for the immunosuppressed patient.

Forms of Immunosuppression

The nonresponsive state of the immune system may be due to a natural tolerance to self-antigens, to a pathologic state, or to induced immunosuppression. Researchers are attempting to understand immunosuppression by artificially manipulating the immune system to produce a natural tolerance to self-antigens. Pathologic states such as lymphoma and leukemia are examples of the second form of immunosuppression, in which the immune system becomes unresponsive owing to the pathologic changes in the immunocompetent cells. Induced immunosuppression can be accomplished by the administration of an antigen, antisera or antibody, or hormones and cytotoxic drugs, by radiation, and by surgery. For the most part, induced immunosuppression is used for tissue and organ transplants.

For patients suffering from allergies, the administration of low-dose antigen, in some instances, provides relief from the antigen-antibody reaction. This *desensitizing* process produces antibodies that block the interaction between the antigen and the antibody-producing cells. Another method of providing tolerance to self-antigens is by the administration of antisera or antibody in an attempt to coat the antigenic sites. The object is to prevent immunocompetent cells from combining with the antigen. This method of immunosuppression is 100 percent effective in preventing Rh sensitization and, ultimately, *erythroblastosis fetalis.* Corticosteroids produce immunosuppression by reducing the amount of T and B lymphocytes circulating in the blood, blocking lymphokine release, and decreasing the number of monocytes. Cytotoxic drugs are used in the treatment of cancer and autoimmune diseases. The most popular drugs are azathioprine and cyclophosphamide. These drugs suppress immune system function by killing unstimulated lymphocytes. X-irradiation suppresses most of the immunocompetent cells by the induction of a profound lymphopenia. Surgical removal of the thymus gland, spleen, or lymph nodes may alter the immune response by removing tissue needed for the maturation of both the cellular and the humoral immune systems.

PACU Care of the Immunosuppressed Patient

The major responsibilities of the PACU nurse caring for the immunosuppressed patient are prevention of and early diagnosis and treatment of infection. Opinions differ in regard to placement of the nonleukopenic patient in protective isolation. However, if the peripheral leukocyte count is less than 2000 cells per mm³, the patient probably will benefit from protective isolation. Before the patient is admitted to the PACU, sources of cross-contamination should be eliminated. Blood pressure cuffs and other equipment that are to be used directly on the patient should be cleaned and disinfected with appropriate solutions. Aseptic technique should be adhered to at all times. In addition, needle puncture sites and surgical wounds should be cleaned and dressed with appropriate cleaners and ointments. If Foley catheters are used, open skin should be monitored closely for the beginning signs of infection. Immunosuppressed patients may not demonstrate the classic symptoms of infection. The temperature of the immunosuppressed patient should be closely monitored, and if it rises above 38°C, the attending physician should be notified immediately. The use of rectal thermometers should be avoided because they can cause mucosal injury and contamination.

References

1. Chaffee, E., and Lytle, I.: Basic Physiology and Anatomy. 4th ed. Philadelphia, J. B. Lippincott, 1980.
2. Fruth, R.: Anaphylaxis and drug reactions: Guidelines for detection and care. Heart Lung, 9(4):662–664, 1980.
3. Ganong, W.: Review of Medical Physiology. 15th ed. Los Altos, Lange, 1990.
4. Gorringe-Moore, R.: Immunology and the lung. *In* Traver, G. (ed.): Respiratory Nursing: The Science and the Art. New York, John Wiley & Sons, 1982, pp. 232–250.
5. Groenwald, S.: Physiology of the immune system. Heart Lung, 9(4):645–650, 1980.
6. Guyton, A.: Textbook of Medical Physiology. 8th ed. Philadelphia, W. B. Saunders, 1991.
7. Jocius, M.: Immunohematology and transfusion reaction. AANA J., 50(1):42–48, 1982.
8. Murray, J.: The Normal Lung. 2nd ed. Philadelphia, W. B. Saunders, 1986.
9. Rana, A., and Luskin, A.: Immunosuppression, autoimmunity, and hypersensitivity. Heart Lung, 9(4):651–657, 1980.
10. Stites, D., Stobo, J., Fudenberg, A., et al.: Basic and Clinical Immunology. Los Altos, Lange, 1984.
11. Vance, D.: Interferon. J. Post Anesth. Nurs., 2(1):43–44, 1987.
12. Waugaman, W., Foster, S. and Rigor, B.: Principles and Practice of Nurse Anesthesia. 2nd ed., Norwalk, CT, Appleton & Lange, 1992.

Concepts in Anesthetic Agents

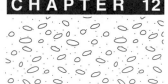

CHAPTER 12

Basic Principles of Pharmacology

Because of the increasing use of new and more potent drugs administered in the perioperative period, an overview of the basic principles of pharmacology is presented in this section. The specific pharmacology of drugs related to post anesthesia care unit (PACU) care is discussed in the physiology chapters in Section II along with the chapters dealing with anesthetic agents and adjuncts in this section. It is believed that the pharmacology of the individual drugs can be best understood in relation to the functions of the physiologic system that is most impacted by the particular drug or classification of drugs.

The final portion of this chapter provides an overview of drug interactions between anesthetic and nonanesthetic drugs. These concepts are discussed in detail because they are increasingly relevant to the PACU nurse. With the growth of interest in the fields of drug interaction, drug surveillance, and clinical pharmacology, knowledge of drug-drug interactions in anesthesia and post anesthesia care should become an exceedingly meaningful and useful tool in the delivery of nursing care to the PACU patient.

DRUG RESPONSES

Drugs are administered by a certain route of administration at a certain dosage with the expectation of achieving a desired response. Many factors affect the time of onset, the intensity, and the duration of action of a particular drug. The PACU nurse must become aware of the basic principles of drug interaction with the biologic system. Hence, a review of the basic concepts of drug responses is presented, with particular emphasis on the patient in the PACU.

Definitions

Additive or synergistic effect: occurs when a second drug with properties similar to the first is added, and the result is greater than the algebraic sum of effects of the two individual drugs.

Cross-tolerance: occurs when two drugs with similar actions are given to a patient who has developed tolerance to that category of drugs (i.e., narcotics). The amount of each individual drug must be increased to achieve the desired effect. An example of cross-tolerance is a heroin addict receiving high-dose narcotics in the PACU to maintain minimal analgesia.

Efficacy of a drug: refers to the maximum effect that can be produced by a drug.

Hyperreactivity: occurs when a person reacts abnormally to an unusually low dose of a drug. For example, patients with Addison's disease, myxedema, or dystrophia myotonica exhibit hyperreactivity to unusually low doses of the barbiturates.

Hypersensitivity (anaphylaxis): refers to a drug-induced antigen-antibody reaction. The particular hypersensitivity reaction can be either a type I immediate (anaphylactic) or a type IV delayed reaction. Hypersensitivity reactions can occur with succinylcholine, with antibiotics, and with many other drugs that are administered in the PACU (see Chapter 11).

Hyporeactivity: indicates that a person requires excessively large doses of a drug to obtain a therapeutic or desired effect.

Metareactivity: when a drug produces unusual side effects unrelated to the dosage strength. Metareactivity is also referred to as an *idiosyncratic reaction*. An example of metareactivity is the occurrence of skeletal muscle pain and increased intraocular pressure when succinylcholine is administered.

Potency of a drug: refers to the dose required of a particular drug to produce an effect similar to another drug.

Tachyphylaxis: occurs when a drug tolerance occurs acutely. An example of tachyphylaxis is when succinylcholine is administered by intravenous drip. Over time, a higher drip rate will be needed to achieve the required response.

Tolerance: a type of hyporeactivity that is acquired during chronic exposure to a drug in which unusually large doses are required to reach a desired effect. A prime example is a person who has become addicted to narcotics and who requires larger than normal doses to elicit the desired therapeutic response.

Dose-Response Relationships

The response of a drug in changing a physiologic state may be either a quantal response or a graded response. The *quantal response* is the final intended response, such as sleep, that is intended to be produced by the drug. The quantal data are usually plotted on a dose-response curve of log-dose distribution. The dose of the drug is plotted against the frequency of response to the drug. The *median effective dose* is the ED_{50} and represents the point on the slope of the curve when 50 percent of the subjects report a quantal response to the drug. The *therapeutic index* represents the relative safety of a drug and is the ratio between the toxic dose (TD_{50}) and the ED_{50}. The *margin of safety* is another way to measure the safety of a drug. It is the ratio between the time when 5 percent of the subjects experience toxic effects (TD_5) and the dose at which 95 percent of them experience the quantal or desired response (ED_{95}).

The *graded response* is that at which multiple evaluations of the response of the drug are made. A continuous scale is used that ranges from no response to maximum response. An example of graded response criteria is the train-of-four (see Chapter 16) that is used to measure the response to muscle relaxants. Usually, the percentage of skeletal muscle function represents the percentage of occupancy of the receptors by the drug being evaluated.

Pharmacokinetic Actions

Pharmacokinetics comprises the absorption, distribution, and elimination of a drug in the body. Consequently, pharmacokinetics can be viewed as what the body does to a drug.

The pharmacokinetic models for the distribution of drugs are based on either a physiologic or a compartmental model. The physiologic model for drug distribution quantifies a drug according to its distribution in various anatomic and physiologic compartments. For example, parameters such as tissue mass, blood volume and flow, partition coefficients, diffusion, and active transport mechanisms are con-

sidered in identifying the distribution of a drug. An example of the physiologic model is seen when distribution of the anesthetic drug thiopental is described. After thiopental is injected intravenously, it goes through various anatomic and physiologic organ systems. By redistribution from the brain, the drug is dissipated and, consequently, its anesthetic actions are terminated. Because of the difficulty in obtaining human data for the physiologic model of drug distribution, this model is rarely used.

The compartmental model has replaced the physiologic model for determining drug distribution. This model mathematically predicts a drug's concentration in blood or plasma. A compartment represents a theoretical space. A mathematical model can be used to describe the pharmacokinetics of the disposition of a drug. A two-compartment model is usually used to depict a central compartment and a peripheral compartment. The *central compartment* includes plasma and blood cells and highly perfused tissues such as the heart, lungs, brain, liver, and kidneys. The *peripheral compartment* represents all other fluids and tissues in the body. Using this two-compartment model, a drug can be introduced into the central compartment, move into the peripheral compartment, and then return to the central compartment where removal from the body occurs. The two-compartment model is constructed using the serum concentration versus time and is called the *plasma concentration curve*. From this curve, the distribution and elimination half-times of the drug can be determined using logarithms. The resulting curve (Fig. 12–1) can be divided into two phases: the distribution (alpha) phase and the elimination (beta) phase.

Elimination clearance quantifies the ability of the body to remove the drug. The major mechanisms for eliminating a drug from the body are hepatic clearance and renal clearance. The half-life ($T\frac{1}{2}$) of a drug is the time at which 50 percent of the total amount of the drug has been eliminated from the body. The elimination half-life ($T\frac{1}{2}_\beta$) is the time when the plasma concentration is at 50 percent of the elimination phase; it is directly proportional to the volume distribution of the drug and inversely proportional to the drug clearance. Consequently, when the $T\frac{1}{2}_\beta$ for a particular drug is known, a large initial dose called a *loading dose* of a drug can be given to achieve a therapeutic concentration. The drug can then be given by infusion or in multiple doses at calculated intervals, based on the $T\frac{1}{2}_\beta$, to produce a steady-state plasma concentration. In addition, the time necessary for

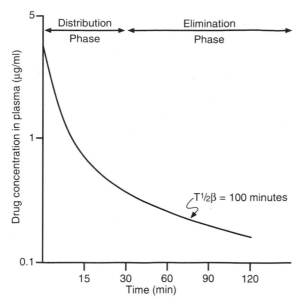

FIGURE 12–1. Concentrations of a drug that is administered intravenously plotted on a logarithmic scale over time.

elimination of a particular dose of a drug can be predicted by the $T\frac{1}{2}_\beta$. Usually, 95 percent of the drug can be eliminated in five half-lives.

Systemic Absorption by Routes of Administration

Oral Route of Administration. When a drug is administered orally, it is absorbed in the small intestine, which has a large surface area. A drug must be lipid soluble to cross the gastrointestinal lining. After such absorption, the drug passes to the liver by way of the portal veins before it can enter the systemic circulation. The liver extracts and metabolizes some of the drug, a process termed the *first-pass hepatic effect.* The drugs that are particularly subject to this effect are lidocaine and propranolol, which is why these drugs are administered in much higher doses orally than when they are given intravenously.

Oral administration of drugs in the PACU has some distinct disadvantages. For example, nausea and vomiting may occur, which reduces the amount of the drug available for absorption by the small intestine. Also, because the gastric volume and pH are altered either by preoperative drugs or anesthesia and surgery, the absorption process can be affected.

Sublingual Route of Administration. The sublingual route of administration has several important advantages over the oral route. This is because the sublingual route bypasses the

first-pass hepatic effect. This route can be particularly favorable in the PACU for drugs such as nifedipine and nitroglycerin.

Subcutaneous and Intramuscular Routes of Administration. These routes of administration require simple diffusion from the site of injection into the systemic circulation. Consequently, they do not provide a reliable rate of systemic absorption. This is particularly true in the PACU when patients are hypothermic, hypotensive, and usually have some peripheral vasoconstriction. In addition, if a hypothermic patient in the PACU is administered a drug either subcutaneously or intramuscularly, the drug probably will not produce the desired effects. However, when the patient is rewarmed, a significant amount of the drug can be rapidly liberated from the injection site, causing a large concentration of the drug in the systemic circulation. This can be dangerous when narcotics are administered.

Intravenous Route of Administration. This route of administration facilitates the delivery of a desired concentration of a drug in a rapid and precise fashion. In the PACU, because patients generally experience a certain amount of hypothermia, hypotension, delirium, and unconsciousness, the intravenous route is most acceptable route for administration of drugs.

Removal of Drugs from the Systemic Circulation

The principal ways drugs are cleared from the systemic circulation are by the hepatic, biliary, and renal systems. The hepatic system has a high blood flow and can extract many lipid-soluble drugs from the systemic circulation. In the liver, drugs undergo biotransformation and become pharmacologically inactive. Enzyme induction or a decrease in protein binding enhances the hepatic clearance of some drugs (see Chapter 9). After they have been metabolized in the liver, drugs can be transported to the biliary system for excretion. Also, some drugs, such as the glucuronides, are actively transported to the bile and excreted in an inactive form.

The kidneys secrete many water-soluble drugs in their unchanged form. Renal excretion of drugs is dependent on the major physiologic processes that occur in the kidneys: glomerular filtration, active tubular secretion, and passive tubular reabsorption. Appropriate renal function is needed to facilitate many of the drugs administered in the perioperative period. Consequently, if there is a concern about renal function, a creatinine clearance or serum creatinine level should be obtained because these laboratory tests correlate well with renal drug elimination.

Effects of Physiologic Dysfunction on Pharmacologic Action

Renal Disease. Kidney disease reduces the effectiveness of drug clearance. Indirectly, it also reduces hepatic clearance with a resultant production of exaggerated effects and a prolongation in the action of the drugs that experience a reduction in renal clearance. In renal drug clearance, the laboratory test of creatinine clearance, which measures glomerular filtration (see Chapter 7), can be used to predict the degree of a drug's renal clearance. Anesthetic drugs, such as d-tubocurarine (curare) and gallamine (Flaxedil), are excreted by the kidney mostly unchanged. In anephric patients or patients with severe kidney disease, the elimination clearance is decreased and the $T\frac{1}{2}_\beta$ increased, prolonging the effects of the drugs, especially when they are administered at particular dosing intervals. However, a single dose of these nondepolarizing neuromuscular blocking agents is usually unaffected in the anephric patient.

Hepatic Disease. Patients with hepatic diseases such as cirrhosis and ascites may have difficulty in clearing some anesthetic drugs from their body. Liver function testing is unreliable in predicting the level of impairment in hepatic clearance. Any patient with documented liver disease should be considered at risk for decreased clearance of drugs. Therefore, in patients with documented hepatic disease, all drugs administered in the PACU should be titrated to desired effect to gain an appropriate pharmacologic outcome.

Cardiovascular Disease. Cardiovascular diseases that cause a reduction in tissue perfusion have a significant impact on drug distribution and clearance. For example, when lidocaine is administered to patients with congestive heart failure, the dose should be reduced by one half because of changes in volume distribution and clearance. Postoperative cardiopulmonary bypass patients can experience a hemodilution of drugs. However, this change in the central compartment is transitory because the plasma drug concentration is compensated in the peripheral tissue compartment.

DRUG-DRUG INTERACTIONS

When a patient is simultaneously receiving two or more drugs, the drugs may or may not interact to cause a toxic reaction. Patients are often given drugs other than the ones associated with anesthesia and surgery. Thus, in these patients, the potential for a drug-drug interaction is present (Table 12–1). These interactions are divided into two broad categories: pharmacokinetic and pharmacodynamic.

Pharmacokinetic Interactions

Interactions of a second drug that produces alterations in absorption, distribution, metabolism, or excretion of the first drug are known as *pharmacokinetic interactions*. Hence, when one drug alters any pharmacokinetic parameter of another, with a resultant alteration in the concentration of the drug at the receptor site, a pharmacokinetic interaction has taken place. In other words, the absorption, distribution, or elimination of the drug concentration at the receptor site is changed, which results in an altered pharmacologic response from the person.

Absorption

The absorption of one drug may be enhanced or inhibited by another drug. With the addition of epinephrine to solutions of local anesthetics, the absorption of the anesthetic is prolonged through the vasoconstrictive action of epinephrine. The local vasoconstriction produced by epinephrine delays the systemic absorption of the local anesthetic, and, ultimately, the effect of the local anesthetic is prolonged. When a patient has been administered a preoperative aluminum-containing antacid and then is administered tetracycline in the late postoperative period, absorption of the tetracycline will be reduced.

Distribution

Pharmaceutical incompatibility is one type of pharmacokinetic distribution interaction. This situation occurs, for example, when one drug reacts chemically with another. In this situation, when one drug (e.g., aspirin) displaces another drug (e.g., phenytoin) from plasma protein-binding sites, the blood concentration of the free drug will be increased, which may result in toxic blood levels. Or, when a large dose of thiopental is administered to an obese

Table 12–1. DRUG-DRUG OR DRUG-INDUCED INTERACTIONS IN THE PACU

Drug(s)	Interact(s) with	Result	Mechanism
Antihypertensive Drugs			
Reserpine	Inhalation anesthetics	Hypotension	Inhibits the synthesis and storage of norepinephrine in the sympathetic nerve endings
Diuretics	Halothane	Hypotension	Reduced extracellular sodium and water, which is compensated for by vasoconstriction. Halothane dilates the constricted vascular beds
Propranolol	Lidocaine	Enhanced negative inotropic effect	Propranolol reduces liver blood flow and lidocaine clearance
Lidocaine Procainamide Bretylium Phenytoin Digitalis Quinidine Disopyramide Propranolol	d-Tubocurarine	Increased duration of neuromuscular blockade	Synergistic effect
Digitalis	Succinylcholine	Arrhythmias	Direct effect, or due to the hyperkalemia that can be induced by succinylcholine
Quinidine	Digitalis (digoxin)	Can produce digitalis intoxication	Decreases digitalis clearance and increases concentration of digitalis
Propranolol	Heparin	Myocardial depression	Heparin increases free fatty acids, which displace propranolol from plasma protein binding sites leading to increased free propranolol
Quinidine	Myasthenia gravis plus skeletal muscle relaxants	Postoperative respiratory depression	Blockade of acetylcholine receptors at neuromuscular postsynaptic membrane
Digitalis	Thiazide diuretics	Increased potassium excretion by the kidneys	Combined effect of the two drugs on the kidneys promotes potassium excretion
Antibiotics			
Neomycin Streptomycin Dihydrostreptomycin Polymyxin A Polymyxin B Colistin Viomycin Paromomycin Kanamycin Lincomycin Gentamicin Tetracycline	Nondepolarizing skeletal muscle relaxants	Potentiates nondepolarizing muscle relaxants, respiratory depression	Neuromuscular blockade due to a reduction in the amplitude of the end-plate potential
Narcotics			
Morphine Meperidine Sublimaze Sufentanil	Inhalation anesthetics	Potentiation, respiratory and cardiovascular depression	Depressant effects of inhalation anesthetics and the narcotics are additive
Meperidine	Enovid Norinyl	Birth control pill potentiates meperidine	Excess female sex hormones with oral contraceptive therapy, which may slow the metabolism of meperidine
Sympathomimetic Amines			
Epinephrine	Halothane Enflurane	Cardiac arrhythmias	Anesthetic agents sensitize the myocardium to endogenous and exogenous catecholamines
Electrolytes			
Increased extracellular potassium	Skeletal muscle relaxants	Increased resistance to depolarization and greater sensitivity to nondepolarizing muscle relaxants	Acute increase in extracellular potassium increases end-plate transmembrane potential, causing hyperpolarization

Table continued on following page

Table 12–1. DRUG-DRUG OR DRUG-INDUCED INTERACTIONS IN THE PACU *Continued*

Drug(s)	Interact(s) with	Result	Mechanism
Decreased extracellular potassium	Skeletal muscle relaxants	Increased effects of depolarizing muscle relaxants and increased resistance to nondepolarizing muscle relaxants	Acute decrease in extracellular potassium lowers resting end-plate transmembrane potential
Increased calcium levels	Nondepolarizing skeletal muscle relaxants	Decreased response	Calcium increases the quantal release of acetylcholine and enhances the excitation-contraction coupling mechanism
Magnesium ions	Muscle relaxants	Potentiation	Magnesium ions cause a partial muscle relaxation by blocking the release of acetylcholine
Calcium chloride	Digitalis	Additive effect on the heart	High concentrations of calcium inhibit the positive inotropic actions of digitalis and potentiate digitalis toxicity
Miscellaneous Echothiopate iodide	Succinylcholine	Prolonged apnea	Echothiopate is a cholinesterase inhibitor, and succinylcholine is destroyed by pseudocholinesterase
Tolbutamide	Dicumarol	Intensification of the effects of tolbutamide leading to hypoglycemia	Dicumarol displaces tolbutamide from its binding site on plasma proteins and makes more tolbutamide available in the free form
Succinylcholine	*d*-Tubocurarine	Prolonged apnea	Both drugs act at the acetylcholine receptor, causing a synergistic effect on the myoneural junction
Procaine Nesacaine Pontocaine	Succinylcholine	Prolonged apnea	All these drugs are metabolized by the enzyme pseudocholinesterase. The concomitant use of these drugs may reduce the effective plasma concentration of the enzyme
Furosemide Thiazide Ethacrynic acid	Nondepolarizing skeletal muscle relaxants	Intensified neuromuscular block	Electrolyte imbalance (hypokalemia)
Aminophylline	*d*-Tubocurarine Pancuronium	Antagonized neuromuscular blockade	End-plate effect antagonized by the increase in neurotransmitter
Procaine Lidocaine	Nondepolarizing and depolarizing skeletal muscle relaxants	Enhanced neuromuscular blockade	Decreased end-plate potential
Lithium	Pancuronium Succinylcholine	Potentiated neuromuscular blockade	Lithium ions substituted for sodium ions at a presynaptic level
Chlorpromazine	Nondepolarizing skeletal muscle relaxants	Enhanced neuromuscular blockade	Potentiation of neuromuscular blockade
All inhalation anesthetics	Nondepolarizing skeletal muscle relaxants	Augment block in a dose-dependent manner in the following decreasing order of potency: isoflurane and enflurane, halothane, nitrous oxide	Central nervous system depression or presynaptic inhibition of acetylcholine
Insulin	Corticosteroids, oral contraceptives, loop and thiazide diuretics	Reduction in effects	Insulin antagonizes effects
Diethylstilbestrol (Stilphostrol)	Succinylcholine	Prolonged neuromuscular blockade	Decreased plasma cholinesterase
Hydrocortisone Dexamethasone Prednisolone	Phenobarbital	Decreased effects of the steroids	Increased metabolism

patient who also receives halothane, the anesthetic action may be prolonged considerably, lasting well into the PACU phase. This is caused by the prolonged retention of thiopental in the adipose tissue owing to the circulatory depressant action of halothane. Hence, at the end of the period of anesthesia, the redistribution and subsequent elimination of thiopental are delayed, resulting in a prolonged hypnotic effect.

Elimination

Biotransformation. When patients are administered enzyme-inducing agents, such as the barbiturates and the antibiotic rifampin, the activity of the enzyme systems of the liver will be increased. This results in a more rapid metabolism and excretion of drugs that are metabolized by a particular liver enzyme system. For example, if a barbiturate were administered to a patient who is on a stabilized dose of the anticoagulant warfarin, the warfarin blood level might be reduced, which would result in a lowered prothrombin time. If this situation were to occur (stabilization by an anticoagulant and administration of an enzyme-inducing agent) and the barbiturate were to be discontinued, the nurse would have to monitor the patient for the potentially more serious problem of excessive anticoagulation and hemorrhage.

The drug cimetidine (Tagamet) is sometimes administered preoperatively to reduce the amount of gastric secretion and increase the gastric pH. Cimetidine is a potent inhibitor of drug metabolism and can slow the elimination of antipyrine, warfarin, diazepam, and propranolol. This effect results in an increased drug concentration and enhanced pharmacologic effect of the latter drugs.

Excretion. The pharmacokinetic parameters of concern in excretion have to do with one drug either facilitating or hindering the excretion of another. An example of this occurs when probenecid is administered together with penicillin. The outcome of this interaction is that the pharmacologic actions of penicillin are prolonged because of the slower $T\frac{1}{2}_\beta$ produced by probenecid. Certainly, this can be considered a desirable drug-drug interaction.

Pharmacodynamic Interactions

Pharmacodynamic interactions occur when one drug alters the pharmacologic effects of another drug. For example, when a patient is being treated with an antibiotic such as an aminoglycoside or polymyxin and receives a skeletal muscle relaxant such as curare, a prolonged neuromuscular blockage may result. Another example is a patient receiving thiazide diuretic therapy who has resultant hypokalemia. If the patient is administered digitalis, digitalis toxicity may result. Also, if the patient on thiazide therapy is administered a nondepolarizing muscle relaxant, the neuromuscular blockade will be intensified.

DRUG-DRUG INTERACTIONS AND THE PACU

Antibiotics

Aminoglycoside and polymyxin antibiotics have been reported to interact with some anesthetic agents as well as skeletal muscle relaxants. Streptomycin and the other aminoglycoside antibiotics produce a partial neuromuscular blockade by inhibiting the release of acetylcholine from the presynaptic membrane and by stabilizing the postsynaptic membrane. The order of decreasing potency of aminoglycosides for causing a partial neuromuscular blockage is neomycin, kanamycin, amikacin, gentamicin, and tobramycin. When a nondepolarizing skeletal muscle relaxant, such as curare and pancuronium, is administered to a patient receiving an aminoglycoside antibiotic, the neuromuscular blockade will be intensified and difficult to reverse pharmacologically. Studies indicate that the aminoglycoside neuromuscular blockade can sometimes be partially reversed by calcium and neostigmine, whereas the neuromuscular blockade produced by polymyxin B is enhanced by neostigmine and not reversed by calcium. The antibiotics that prolong the actions of the nondepolarizing skeletal muscle relaxants are neomycin, streptomycin, dihydrostreptomycin, kanamycin, gentamicin, polymyxin A, polymyxin B, colistin, lincomycin, and tetracycline. The antibiotics that enhance the pharmacologic actions of the depolarizing skeletal relaxant succinylcholine include neomycin, streptomycin, kanamycin, polymyxin B, and colistin. These drugs must usually be given for at least 2 weeks before any clinically significant depression in the neuromuscular transmission occurs; such a depression may produce only slight muscular weakness in the patient. Antibiotics that have no skeletal muscle relaxant properties are penicillin, chloramphenicol, and the cephalosporins.

Sympathomimetic Amines

The volatile inhalation anesthetics, particularly halothane, can sensitize the heart to sympathomimetic amines, such as epinephrine, producing cardiac arrhythmias. Patients who are recovering from halothane anesthesia in the PACU still have a significant amount of halothane in their bodies. Consequently, epinephrine or other sympathomimetic amines should not be administered to them. If epinephrine must be used for hemostasis or for vasoconstriction in a local anesthetic, the epinephrine concentration should not be greater than 1:100,000 to 200,000 and the total adult dose should not be greater than 10 ml of 1:100,000 solution in 10 minutes, or the total dose should not exceed 30 ml of 1:100,000 solution in 1 hour.

Antihypertensives

It is estimated that 1 to 2 million hypertensive patients are anesthetized each year in the United States. Anesthetic agents have been reported to produce changes in cardiac output, peripheral resistance, and regional blood flow patterns in normotensive and hypertensive patients.

Hypertension is treated by lowering systemic vascular resistance or by reducing cardiac output, or both. Antihypertensive drugs alter the circulatory hemostasis, strongly influence the activity of pressor amines, and may alter the response to muscle relaxants and narcotic analgesics. Antihypertensive drugs can produce systemic conditions that may result in a hypotensive crisis during anesthesia and in the immediate postoperative period. Therefore, PACU patients who have been on long-term antihypertensive medication therapy and who have received a 100 percent potent inhalation anesthetic should be specifically monitored for cardiac dysrhythmias and hypotension. If a hypotensive crisis occurs in the PACU, the patient should have his or her legs elevated, and oxygen and, if necessary, vasopressors should be administered. The anesthesiologist and surgeon should be notified immediately so that specific treatment can be instituted.

Narcotics

Every PACU nurse has probably observed the drug-drug interaction between narcotics administered in the PACU and the inhalation anesthetic agents administered in the operating room. If the patient has not completely eliminated the anesthetic agent and is administered a narcotic, a synergistic effect between the two drugs will occur. The outcome of this interaction is usually respiratory depression, because both drugs are respiratory depressants.

If the two drugs have interacted in this way, a narcotic (opioid) antagonist, such as naloxone (Narcan), can be administered to reverse the respiratory depression produced by the narcotic. However, naloxone will not reverse respiratory depression produced by the inhalation anesthetic agents such as halothane (Fluothane), enflurane (Ethrane), or isoflurane (Forane).

Naloxone reverses respiratory depression and analgesia produced by an opioid. In the PACU, it is usually advantageous to reverse the respiratory depression and preserve some postoperative analgesia using nalbuphine (Nubain). The pharmacology of nalbuphine is discussed in detail in Chapter 15.

Steroids

Although exogenous steroids administered to a steroid-dependent patient is not actually an interaction of two drugs that alters one of the pharmacokinetic parameters, the problems resulting from this circumstance will be presented.

Patients experiencing adrenocortical insufficiency cannot withstand the stress of anesthesia and surgery. For example, if a patient with chronic obstructive pulmonary disease has been treated with long-term steroids, there will usually be some degree of adrenocortical insufficiency. Hence, because of the alteration in the receptor site, the patient may react to surgery and anesthesia with hypotension, respiratory depression, or delayed recovery. To prevent a hypotensive crisis during the perioperative period, these patients are usually maintained on corticosteroids until, through, and after the surgical procedure.

Should these symptoms appear in a PACU patient who did not receive this steroid coverage, the preferred treatment would be hydrocortisone (see Chapter 6).

References

1. Barash, P., Cullen, B. and Stoelting, R.: Clinical Anesthesia. 2nd ed. Philadelphia, J. B. Lippincott, 1992.
2. Gilman, A., Rall, T., Nies, A., et al.: Goodman and Gilman's The Pharmacological Basis of Therapeutics. 8th ed. New York, Pergamon Press, 1990.

3. Guyton, A.: Textbook of Medical Physiology. 8th ed. Philadelphia: W. B. Saunders, 1991.
4. Longnecker, D., and Murphy, F.: Dripps/Eckenhoff/ Vandam Introduction to Anesthesia. 8th ed. Philadelphia, W. B. Saunders, 1992.
5. Miller, R. (ed.): Anesthesia. 3rd ed. New York, Churchill Livingstone, 1990.
6. Stoelting, R.: Pharmacology and Physiology in Anesthetic Practice. 2nd ed. Philadelphia, J. B. Lippincott, 1991.
7. Stoelting, R. and Miller, R.: Basics of Anesthesia. 2nd ed. New York, Churchill Livingstone, 1989.
8. Waugaman, W., Foster, S., and Rigor, B.: Principles and Practice of Nurse Anesthesia. 2nd ed. Norwalk, CT, Appleton & Lange, 1992.
9. Wood, M., and Wood, A.: Drugs and Anesthesia: Pharmacology for the Anesthesiologist. 2nd ed. Baltimore, Williams & Wilkins, 1990.

CHAPTER 13

Inhalation Anesthesia

To anticipate how a patient will react when emerging from an inhalation anesthetic, the post anesthesia care unit (PACU) nurse should have a thorough understanding of the pharmacologic concepts of inhalation anesthesia. Although the complexity of these agents, coupled with drug interactions and the various levels of physical health, makes it difficult to predict the exact nature of each patient's emergence from inhalation anesthesia, an understanding of some general principles will prepare the PACU nurse for the most commonly expected outcomes.

BASIC CONCEPTS

Evolution of the Signs and Stages of Anesthesia

The five components of anesthesia are hypnosis, analgesia, muscle relaxation, sympatholysis, and amnesia. In the past, when diethyl ether was the primary general anesthetic administered, assessment of anesthetic depth using the signs and stages of anesthesia was quite simplistic—the patient could be monitored by assessment of the pupils, respiratory activity, muscle tone, and various reflexes. The ether signs and stages were devised to give some means of assessing the depth of anesthesia. The first three stages were described by Plomley in 1847, and a year later John Snow added a fourth stage, that of overdose. During World War I, Guedel more accurately defined and described the signs and stages of anesthesia. A graphic representation of these signs and stages is provided in Figure 13–1.

With the advent of modern anesthesia, which included the addition of fluorinated inhalation anesthetic agents, muscle relaxants, and various pharmacologic adjuncts, the usual predictable signs and stages as described by Guedel were abolished. However, in the PACU, many of these pharmacologic adjuncts have been reversed or the effects have dissipated in the patient recovering from anesthesia. The classic signs and stages do provide some help in the assessment and care of the postoperative patient. Consequently, a brief description to include the incorporation of some of the pharmacology of the modern anesthetics will be given.

Stage I begins with the initiation of anesthesia and ends with the loss of consciousness. It is commonly called the *stage of analgesia*. This stage has been described as the lightest level of anesthesia and represents sensory and mental depression. Stage I is the level of anesthesia used when nitrous oxide is employed. Patients are able to open their eyes on command, breathe normally, maintain protective reflexes, and tolerate mild painful stimuli.

Stage II starts with the loss of consciousness and ends with the onset of a regular pattern of breathing and the disappearance of the lid reflex. This is also called the *stage of delirium*. It is characterized by excitement, and, because of this, many untoward responses such as vomiting, laryngospasm, and even cardiac arrest may take place during this stage. With the use of anesthetic agents that act much more rapidly than ether, this stage is passed rather quickly. In addition, the induction of anesthesia is usually facilitated by short-acting barbiturates, which expedite a short duration of stage II.

Stage III is the *stage of surgical anesthesia*. Using ether anesthesia, it is defined as lasting from the onset of a regular pattern of breathing to the cessation of respiration. At this stage of anesthesia, there is an absence of response to surgical incision. The modern concept of minimum alveolar concentration (MAC) is predicated in part by the signs and stages of surgical anesthesia. MAC is exceeded by a factor of 1.3 in stage III because most patients do not respond to surgical incision at this level of anesthesia (see later discussion). Patients receiving 1.3 MAC anesthesia experience a depression in all elements of nervous system function, that is, sensory depression, loss of recall, reflex depression, and some skeletal muscle relaxation. From this point on, using the modern an-

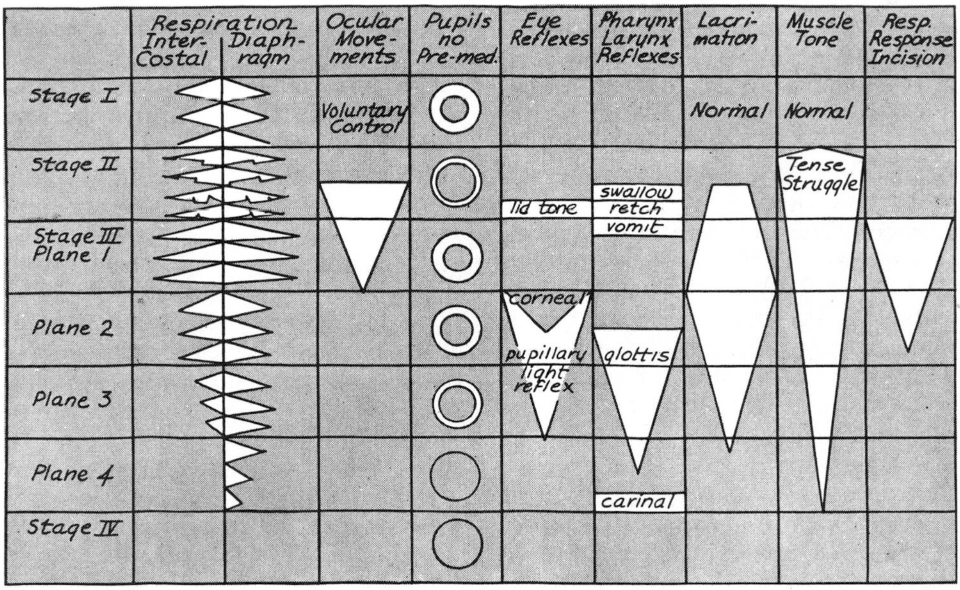

FIGURE 13–1. The signs and reflex reactions of the stages of anesthesia. (Adapted from Gillespie, N. A.: Signs of anesthesia. Anesth. Analg., 22:275, 1943.)

esthetics, increased MAC results in further respiratory, cardiovascular, and central nervous system depression. The difficulty is that each of the newer agents affects the clinical signs, such as blood pressure, differently. Consequently, monitoring the level of anesthesia depends on the particular properties of each agent.

Most surgical procedures in which ether anesthesia was used were performed at this stage of anesthesia, which is divided into four planes. *Plane 1* is entered when the lid reflex is abolished and respiration becomes regular. It is during this plane that the vomiting reflex is gradually abolished. It is important for the nurse working in the PACU to know that swallowing, retching, and vomiting reflexes tend to disappear in that order during induction and reappear in the same order during emergence from anesthesia.

Plane 2 lasts from the time the eyeballs cease to move and become concentrically fixed to the beginning of a decrease of activity of the intercostal muscles, or thoracic respiration. The reflex of laryngospasm disappears during this plane. *Plane 3* is entered when intercostal activity begins to decrease. Complete intercostal paralysis occurs in lower plane 3, and respiration is carried on solely by the diaphragm. *Plane 4* lasts from the time of paralysis of the intercostal muscles to the cessation of spontaneous respiration.

Tracheal tug often appears in association with deep anesthesia and intercostal paralysis. This represents an unopposed action of the diaphragm, displacing the hilum of the lung and thereby increasing traction on the trachea.

Stage IV lasts from the time of cessation of respiration to failure of the circulatory system. This level of anesthesia is considered the stage of overdose.

When ether is used as the sole inhalation agent, these signs and stages will be seen in reverse order on emergence from the anesthetic. No one clinical sign can be considered a reliable indicator of anesthetic depth by itself. All clinical signs must be viewed in the context of the patient's status along with the particular characteristics of the individual anesthetic agent used.

Some of the more reliable indicators of depth of anesthesia for the more modern inhalation anesthetics include changes in breathing pattern, eye movement, lacrimation, and muscle tone. Because the ventilation is under autonomic control, it is the most sensitive indicator of depth of anesthesia. In the PACU a patient who is using diaphragmatic ventilation without the use of the intercostal muscles should be considered to be in surgical anesthesia. As the ventilatory pattern returns to a more normal rate, rhythm, and pattern, the patient can be considered to be under light anesthesia and about to experience total emergence. Eye movement as opposed to pupillary size is a good indicator of anesthetic depth. Light anesthesia is present when there is eye movement. Deeper anesthesia is present when the eyes are close together in a cross-eyed position. Lacrimation does not occur during surgical anesthesia when a patient is receiving enflurane (Ethrane), isoflurane (Forane), or halothane (Fluothane). Conversely, if a patient received one of those drugs and is tearing, light anesthesia can be considered to be present. As the depth of anesthesia is increased, the amount of muscle tone decreases. Therefore, if a patient in the PACU lacks muscle tone, especially in the jaw and abdomen, the patient should be considered to be in a surgical depth of anesthesia. When making the assessment of the degree of muscle tone, it is important that the PACU nurse critically assess the degree of reversal of skeletal muscle relaxants (see Chapter 16) before making a determination of the depth of anesthesia using the criterion of muscle tone. Finally, because of the determinants of anesthesia depth have such a high degree of variability, all possible assessment tools should be incorporated into the care of the PACU patient. It goes without saying that the bottom line is constant vigilance of the patient's physiologic parameters during his or her emergence from anesthesia and the institution of appropriate nursing interventions based on an ongoing assessment.

Pharmacokinetics of Inhalation Anesthetics

The pharmacokinetics of inhalation anesthetics, as described by Stoelting, involves uptake, distribution, metabolism, and elimination. Basically, this involves a series of partial pressure gradients starting in the anesthesia machine, to the patient's brain for induction, and vice versa for emergence. The object of anesthesia is to achieve a constant and optimal partial pressure in the brain. The key to attaining anesthesia is having the alveolar partial pressure (PA) in equilibrium with the arterial (Pa) and brain partial pressure (Pbr) of the inhaled anesthetic. The partial pressure of an inhalation anesthetic in the brain determines the depth of anesthesia. The more potent the anesthetic, the lower the partial pressure of the agent required to produce a certain depth of anesthesia.

Movement of Inhalation Anesthetic from Anesthesia Machine to Alveoli. The determinants of the PA are the inspired partial pressure of the inhalation anesthetic, the characteristics of the anesthesia machine's delivery system, and the patient's alveolar ventilation. The inhaled partial pressure (PI) is the concentration of the inhalation anesthetic that is delivered

from the anesthesia machine. The impact of the PI on the rate of increase in the PA is called the *concentration effect*. The higher the inhaled concentration, the more rapidly the induction of anesthesia. The anesthesia machine's delivery system has an impact on the depth of anesthesia and the speed of induction and emergence. For example, the rate of uptake of an anesthetic agent administered by inhalation can be reduced by the diffusion of the anesthetic agent into the rubber tubing of the anesthesia machine; the small losses of anesthetic agent from the body by diffusion across skin and mucous membranes; and, to a lesser extent, the metabolism of the agents by the body.

Alveolar ventilation plays the primary role in delivery of the anesthetic gas. It is determined in large part by the minute ventilation ($\dot{V}_E$). If the $\dot{V}_E$ is high, the anesthetic concentration increases quickly in the alveoli, as does the concentration in the arterial blood. This is an important concept to understand because the reverse also is true. In the emergence phase of anesthesia, it is important to have a good $\dot{V}_E$ to ensure elimination of the anesthetic agent.

Movement of Inhalation Anesthetic from Alveoli to Arterial Blood. The movement of the inhalation anesthetic agent from the alveoli to the arterial blood depends on the blood-gas partition coefficient and the cardiac output. The rate at which the anesthetic is taken up by the blood and tissues is governed in part by the solubility of the agent in blood. This is expressed as the *blood-gas partition coefficient,* or the *Oswald solubility coefficient.* It is defined as the ratio of the concentration of an anesthetic in blood to that in a gas phase when the two are in equilibrium (Table 13–1). This is a difficult concept to understand because the more soluble the anesthetic agent is, the slower the agent is in producing anesthesia. This is because the blood serves as a reservoir, and a large volume of the agent must be introduced to attain an equilibrium between the blood partial pressure and the partial pressure in the lungs.

The blood conveys the anesthetic agent to the tissues. Consequently, a normal cardiac output is needed to facilitate the movement of the inhalation anesthetic through the tissues to the brain. The partial pressure increases most rapidly in the tissues with the highest rates of blood flow. Of interest is the great variation in blood perfusion of certain tissues in the body. The body tissue compartments can be divided into the following major groups:

Table 13–1. PROPERTIES OF INHALANT ANESTHETIC AGENTS

Agent	Partition Coefficient			Minimum Alveolar Concentration (% in oxygen)
	Blood-Gas	Oil-Gas	Blood-Brain	
Methoxyflurane (Penthrane)	12.0	970.0	1.4	0.16
Halothane (Fluothane)	2.37	224.0	2.0	0.75
Enflurane (Ethrane)	1.9	98.5	1.4	1.68
Isoflurane (Forane)	0.97	93.7	1.6	1.15
Desflurane (Suprane)	0.42	18.7	1.3	6.58
Sevoflurane	0.69	53.4	1.7	1.71
Nitrous oxide	0.47	1.4	1.1	104.0

1. The *vessel-rich group*, which consists of the heart, brain, kidneys, hepatoportal system, and endocrine glands.
2. The *intermediate group* of perfused tissues, which consists of muscle and skin.
3. The *fat group*, which includes marrow and adipose tissue.
4. The *vessel-poor group*, which has the poorest circulation per unit volume and is composed of tendons, ligaments, connective tissue, teeth, bone, and other avascular tissue.

The vessel-rich group of tissues receives 75 percent of the cardiac output; thus, the brain becomes saturated rapidly with an anesthetic agent administered by inhalation. On termination of the anesthetic, the reverse takes place, and there is rapid removal of the agent from the brain.

The tissue tensions of the inhaled anesthetic increase and approach the arterial blood tension and ultimately the PA. One of the tissue groups that has an impact on both the induction and emergence from anesthesia is the fat group. The oil-gas partition coefficient best exemplifies the process involved with the affinity of anesthesia agents to adipose tissue and, ultimately, the emergence from anesthesia. The *oil-gas partition coefficient* is defined as the ratio of the concentration of the anesthetic agent in oil (adipose tissue) to that in a gaseous phase when the two are in equilibrium (see Table 13–1). The oil-gas partition coefficients seem to parallel anesthetic requirements. In fact, one can calculate the MAC by knowing the oil-gas partition coefficient. Using the constant of 150, the calculated MAC for an anesthetic with an oil-gas partition coefficient of 100 would be 1.5 percent.

Because some anesthetic agents are highly fat soluble, they tend to be readily absorbed by the adipose tissue. This characteristic affects uptake of the anesthetic agent, but of more importance is the prolonged recovery phase that usu-

ally ensues with a high oil-gas partition coefficient, such as in the case of halothane. Because adipose tissue is poorly perfused by blood, at the termination of the anesthesia the adipose tissue releases the agent slowly to the blood. Redistribution then takes place: some of the agent is eliminated by the lungs, which are vessel rich, and some is distributed to the brain. The recovery period becomes significantly extended when the administration time of the anesthetic agent is prolonged to allow for complete saturation of the adipose tissue.

Halothane has an oil-gas partition coefficient that is about twice that of isoflurane or enflurane. Consequently, some authors question the use of halothane in the ambulatory surgical setting. However, clinical observation indicates that patients who receive halothane appear to emerge from anesthesia at about the same rate as they do from isoflurane. Therefore, even with its relatively high oil-gas partition coefficient, halothane remains a popular inhalation anesthetic for use in the ambulatory surgical setting.

Movement of Inhalation Anesthetic from Arterial Blood to the Brain. The transfer of the inhalation anesthetic from the arterial blood to the brain is dependent on the blood-brain partition coefficient of the agent and the cerebral blood flow. The blood-brain partition coefficient for most the inhalation anesthetics is between 1.3 and 2 (see Table 13–1). The concentration gradient during induction of anesthesia is

$$PA > Pa > Pbr$$

During maintenance of surgical anesthesia, the brain tissue becomes saturated with the anesthetic agent, and the brain tissue is in equilibrium with the alveolar and arterial concentration. Consequently,

$$PA = Pa = Pbr$$

Emergence of Inhalation Anesthesia

When the administration of the anesthetic is terminated, a reverse gradient takes place. In this instance, the PA is almost zero, because only oxygen is administered during the emergence phase. The gradient that develops is

$$PA < Pa < Pbr$$

This gradient favors the removal of the anesthetic agent from the brain tissue. Then the partial pressure in the tissues declines first, followed by that in the arterial blood. The agent returns to the lungs and is then eliminated into the atmosphere. The factors that affect the rate of elimination of the agent are the same ones that determine how rapidly an anesthetic agent takes a patient to surgical anesthesia. If a short procedure is performed (less than 1 hour), complete equilibrium among PA, Pa, and Pbr might not have occurred and the recovery from anesthesia will be more rapid. The reverse is true: during long procedures in which equilibrium occurs, a prolonged emergence may be anticipated.

Potency of Inhalation Anesthetic Agents

Potency is determined by factors such as absorption, distribution, metabolism, excretion, and affinity for a receptor. The *potency* of the anesthetic agent refers to its ability to take the patient through all the stages of anesthesia to respiratory and circulatory arrest without the occurrence of hypoxia or the use of preanesthetic medication. Certainly, circulatory and respiratory arrest are not desired outcomes of the use of anesthetic agents; this feature is used merely to describe the potency of anesthetic agents that are used clinically. For example, halothane is 100 percent potent as compared with nitrous oxide, which is 15 percent potent. Halothane, when administered with oxygen to meet the patient's metabolic needs, and when given without premedication, takes the patient to circulatory and respiratory arrest, whereas nitrous oxide administered with oxygen takes the patient only to the first portion of surgical anesthesia and no further. Therefore, clinically speaking, potency of a drug makes little difference as long as the drug that is to be administered has an effective dose for a particular patient. This is why the concept of effective dose (ED) was developed. The ED is the dose of a drug necessary to produce certain effects in a certain percentage of patients. For example, an ED_{50} means that a drug produces a particular effect in 50 percent of the patients.

Another way of determining potency is with the use of the MAC. The MAC is found by determining the alveolar concentration (at 1 atm) required to prevent gross muscular movement in response to painful stimuli in 50 percent of anesthetized patients. The lower the MAC value, the more anesthetic potency the inhalation anesthetic has. The MAC of halothane in oxygen required to prevent patient movement in response to surgical incision is 0.75 percent. A geriatric patient may be administered 0.38 percent halothane in oxygen, which is commonly referred to as *half-MAC. MAC hours* is the concentration in MAC units multiplied by the duration in hours of anesthetic administration. Consequently, the MAC hours for this patient is 0.76 (0.38 × 2). When 70 percent nitrous oxide is added to the halothane, the MAC decreases to 0.29 percent. Thus, when halothane (or any 100 percent potent agent) is combined with a premedication and nitrous oxide, the MAC will decrease (see Table 13–1). *MAC awake* is the anesthetic dose at which patients respond to commands. It is also the dose of anesthetic at which most patients lose consciousness and recall. MAC awake usually corresponds with stage I of anesthesia. Another term used with MAC is *MAC-BAR*. This is the MAC required to block the adrenergic and cardiovascular responses to incision, and it corresponds to stage III, plane III anesthesia. The MAC is reduced in patients who are hypothermic, elderly, or pregnant. Narcotics, clonidine, diazepam, nitrous oxide, reserpine, and methyldopa also decrease the MAC. On the other hand, amphetamines, which release catecholamines, increase the MAC.

TECHNIQUES OF ADMINISTRATION

The inhalation anesthetics are usually administered by means of an *anesthesia machine* (Fig. 13–2). The anesthesia machine is essentially a breathing circuit that conveys the agent and oxygen to the patient. It consists of a mask, corrugated tubing, an absorber to remove expired carbon dioxide, unidirectional valves, a reservoir bag, a pop-off valve, and vaporizers (Fig. 13–3).

Circle Systems

A variety of techniques can be used to deliver gaseous agents with the anesthesia ma-

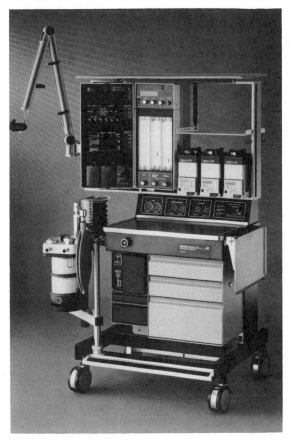

FIGURE 13–2. Anesthesia machine apparatus. (Permission granted by Ohmeda, A Division of BOC Health Care, Inc., Madison, WI.)

chine by adding or removing certain features. The most common technique used is the *semiclosed circle method*, in which some rebreathing of expired gases occurs by opening the pop-off valve to vent some of the gas to the atmosphere. The *closed circle method* is used when explosive gases are being administered or when low gas flows are desired for nonexplosive agents. In this technique, the pop-off valve is completely closed and complete rebreathing of expired gases occurs. A carbon dioxide absorber is used in both the semiclosed and the closed techniques.

Insufflation Technique

The *insufflation technique* involves the delivery of large volumes of fresh gases administered continuously to the mouth by means of a hook made of hard plastic or metal. This technique permits the least rebreathing of expired gases, and, although not often used now, has the advantages of posing little resistance to breathing and not requiring complex equipment.

Open Systems

The *open,* or *nonrebreathing, technique* ensures that the patient will inhale only the anesthetic mixture delivered by the anesthesia machine. Valves such as the Leigh, Fink, Rubin, or Stephen-Slater are used, and there is minimal rebreathing of the anesthetic gas.

Semiopen Systems

The *semiopen system* allows exhaled gases to pass into the surrounding atmosphere, and some of the exhaled gases are rebreathed. Essentially, the semiopen method works without carbon dioxide absorption. The types of semiopen systems used are the open drop method, the Ayre T-piece, the Magill attachment, and the Bain anesthesia circuit.

The *open drop method* was one of the first anesthesia methods ever used, and it requires the least equipment. A volatile anesthetic agent is dripped over a wire mask covered with gauze. Oxygen is usually administered by the insufflation technique to supply the metabolic needs of the patient. The open drop technique is not used in today's anesthesia practice because the anesthetic agents required in this technique are flammable and explosive.

The *Ayre T-piece* was devised to facilitate endotracheal anesthesia for infants and children (Fig. 13–4). One end of the T-piece is connected to the endotracheal tube, and the other end is open to the atmosphere. At the middle portion and at a right angle to the main limb a tube is attached, forming the T, through which the delivery of the anesthetic agent is accomplished. The modified Ayre T-piece consists of a rebreathing bag connected by corrugated tubing to the escape end of the T-piece. This arrangement gives the system more versatility and provides a means of positive pressure to support ventilation. This method is simple and is used for children 4 years of age and younger.

The *Magill attachment* is similar to the modified Ayre T-piece, except that an expiratory valve is inserted into the circuit close to the face mask and is separated from the reservoir bag by corrugated tubing (Fig. 13–5).

The *Bain anesthesia circuit,* introduced in 1972, consists of a tube within a tube. The inner noncorrugated tube, which provides fresh gases to

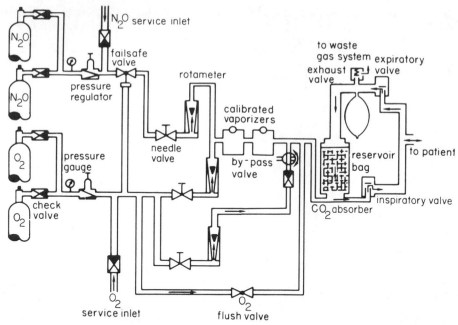

FIGURE 13–3. Anesthesia machine circuit. Oxygen and nitrous oxide enter the machine from cylinders or from the hospital service supply. Pressure regulators reduce cylinder pressure to about 3 kg per cm². Check valves prevent transfilling of cylinders or gas flow from cylinders to the service line. The fail-safe valve prevents the flow of nitrous oxide if the oxygen supply fails. Needle valves in the flowmeters control flows to rotameters. Calibrated vaporizers provide a preselected concentration of volatile anesthetics. Gases are delivered to the circle absorber, where unidirectional valves ensure flow from the patient through the carbon dioxide absorber. Excess gas is vented through the exhaust valve into a waste gas scavenger system. The reservoir bag compensates for variations in respiratory demand. (Adapted from Dripps, R. D., Eckenhoff, J. E., and Vandam, L. D.: Introduction to Anesthesia: The Principles of Safe Practice. 7th ed. Philadelphia, W. B. Saunders, 1988, p. 55.)

the patient, is surrounded by a wider corrugated tube that conveys exhaled gases away from the patient. The circuit attaches to a bag mount that is attached to the anesthesia machine. The bag mount incorporates an exhaust valve and a bag port for attachment of an anesthesia bag or ventilator tubing (Fig. 13–6). The major advantage of this circuit is its versatility: It may be used for both children and

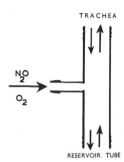

FIGURE 13–4. The Ayre T-piece. Nitrous oxide–oxygen supplemented with ether enters through the side tube. The tracheal end of the T-piece is connected to the endotracheal tube. The end marked "reservoir tube" is open to the air. (From Ayre, P.: The T-piece technique. Br. J. Anaesth., 28:520, 1956.)

adults; it has no directional valves; it is especially useful in surgical procedures involving the head and neck; and it does not require carbon dioxide absorption (no soda lime), yet patients may be maintained at a normal Pa_{CO_2} and pH.

THE INHALATION AGENTS

Inhalant anesthetic substances may be divided into two groups: *volatile* and *gaseous*. Volatile anesthetic agents are chemicals in the liquid state at room temperature that have a boiling point above 20°C. Ethyl chloride, which has a boiling point of 12°C, is also included in this class of anesthetic agents. The volatile inhalation anesthetic agents are divided into two major categories: the *halogenated hydrocarbons* and the *ethers*. Examples of the halogenated hydrocarbons are halothane, chloroform, and trichloroethylene. Enflurane, methoxyflurane, isoflurane, and diethyl ether are examples of the ethers. The gaseous anesthetic agents, such as nitrous oxide and cyclopropane, are those in the gaseous state at room temperature. The an-

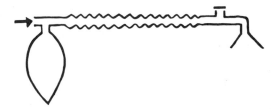

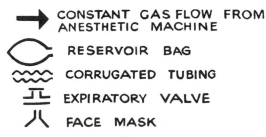

→ CONSTANT GAS FLOW FROM ANESTHETIC MACHINE

⟨⟩ RESERVOIR BAG

〰 CORRUGATED TUBING

⊥ EXPIRATORY VALVE

人 FACE MASK

FIGURE 13–5. The Magill attachment. (From Dripps, R. D., Eckenhoff, J. E., and Vandam. L. D.: Introduction to Anesthesia: The Principles of Safe Practice. 6th ed. Philadelphia, W. B. Saunders, 1982, p. 140.)

esthetic agents currently in use have evolved from the traditional inhalation anesthetics such as cyclopropane, chloroform, and diethyl ether. For that reason they will be described briefly before the current inhalation agents are presented in detail.

Traditional Inhalation Anesthetics

Chloroform (Trichlormethane)

Chloroform was the most potent anesthetic agent available until the 1970s. It offered many advantages, such as excellent muscle relaxation, no irritation of the respiratory tract, rapid

induction and emergence, and nonflammability. However, the disadvantages of chloroform are clinically significant. Because deep anesthesia can be achieved rapidly with small changes in concentration, it has a narrow margin of safety. The major problem with chloroform is that it is hepatotoxic and cardiotoxic and therefore is no longer administered to humans.

Because chloroform is a hydrocarbon, it has some excellent qualities that were preserved when researchers developed newer hydrocarbon inhalation anesthetic agents, such as halothane. In this way, chloroform served as a model for the modern inhalation anesthetics.

Cyclopropane

Cyclopropane was introduced into clinical anesthesia in 1934. It is a colorless gas with the characteristic odor of petroleum ether. It is stored in orange metal cylinders as a liquid under pressure. The most notable property of this drug is its speed of induction and emergence owing to its blood-gas partition coefficient of 0.42. In fact, anesthesia can be induced in five or six deep tidal breaths in a premedicated patient.

The simplest of the cyclic hydrocarbons, cyclopropane is flammable and explosive in air and in oxygen. Like other explosive inhalation anesthetic agents, cyclopropane is no longer used in anesthesia practice.

Diethyl Ether

Ether, one of the first inhalation anesthetics administered in the United States, is rarely used today; therefore, it is presented to the reader for its historical significance only. Ether

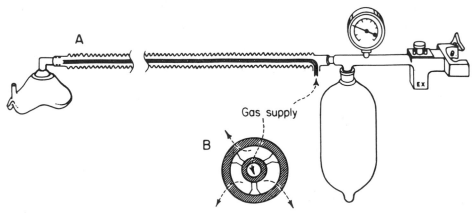

FIGURE 13–6. Bain system breathing circuit. *A*, tube-within-tube design. *B*, cross section of tubing. *Arrows* show air inflow and outflow. (*A* and *B* from Chu, Y. K., Rah, K. H., and Boyan, C. P.: Is the Bain breathing circuit the future anesthesia system? Anesth. Analg., *56*:84, 1977.)

has the relatively high blood-gas partition coefficient of 12.1. Consequently, when ether is administered alone, without any premedication, the induction time is long—usually 30 to 40 minutes. The same holds true for emergence. When the patient awakens, he or she usually has some degree of analgesia. Because of its rather high blood-gas partition coefficient, ether has a built-in safety factor that provides a wide margin of safety for the patient. This consists of the fact that it is difficult to deepen the anesthesia rapidly; thus, the anesthetist has a reasonable length of time to appraise the patient's status and make corrections before a deeper anesthetic plane is induced.

Ether has other advantages: It improves the blood pressure and causes excellent muscle relaxation; in addition, it can be used with all techniques and is inexpensive. The disadvantages of ether are that it is flammable and explosive and has been implicated in the occurrence of convulsions, nausea, and vomiting.

Ethylene

Ethylene, discovered in 1923, resembles nitrous oxide in its usage in anesthesia practice. The gas is about 25 percent potent and takes the patient to the lower border of stage III, plane 1 of anesthesia while supplying the metabolic oxygen requirement. A unique property of this agent is that it is lighter than air and will rise. Ethylene is a very rapid-acting agent because of its blood-gas partition coefficient of 0.14. This agent has been eliminated from use in anesthesia departments solely because of its flammability and explosive properties.

Fluroxene (Trifluoroethyl Vinyl Ether, Fluoromar)

Fluroxene was the first of the fluorine-containing hydrocarbons to be introduced into clinical practice. It is a mixed halogenated aliphatic ether that is flammable, although less so than the nonfluorinated ethers. Because fluroxene is a derivative of ether, post anesthetic nausea and vomiting are not uncommon with its use. Because it is explosive and has strong emetic properties, it is not used today.

Methoxyflurane (Penthrane)

Methoxyflurane is a fluorinated alkyl ether that was introduced into anesthesia practice in 1959. It is nonflammable and nonexplosive in air, oxygen, or nitrous oxide mixtures at normal room temperature. Methoxyflurane can produce any desired depth of anesthesia in the absence of hypoxia and therefore meets the requirements for a 100 percent potent agent. The drug has a high blood-gas partition coefficient of 13 and thus features excellent controllability and analgesia, with good muscle relaxation.

Methoxyflurane was originally thought to be exhaled unchanged, but it is now known to be partially metabolized into several substances that contribute to renal dysfunction. The most important metabolite is free inorganic fluoride, which is nephrotoxic. The renal syndrome caused by methoxyflurane is called *vasopressin-resistant high-output renal failure*. Because methoxyflurane is nephrotoxic, it is no longer used in anesthesia practice.

Trichloroethylene (Trilene)

Like chloroform and ether, trichloroethylene is not used today in anesthesia practice. The drug is related chemically to chloroform and ethylene. Because the drug decomposes to dichloroacetylene when it is exposed to soda lime, it was used only for its analgesic qualities in obstetrics, dentistry, and short surgical procedures. It was administered by techniques such as inhalers, insufflation, and blow-through vaporizers that did not have to incorporate soda lime in the circuit.

Modern Inhalation Anesthetics

Enflurane (Ethrane)

Enflurane is a halogenated ether that is enjoying significant popularity in the practice of anesthesia. It is nonflammable, 100 percent potent, and very rapid acting. Enflurane promotes a fair amount of muscle relaxation and strongly potentiates any nondepolarizing skeletal muscle relaxant, such as *d*-tubocurarine and pancuronium.

Enflurane, like halothane, causes cerebral vasodilatation, which results in an increase in cerebral blood flow if the patient is normotensive. When the patient is hypotensive, enflurane can reduce the cerebral blood flow. This agent may cause no change or small and inconsistent increases in intracranial pressure in neurosurgical patients who are hyperventilated. The hemodynamic effects of enflurane are similar to those of halothane; however, it depresses arterial blood pressure, stroke volume, and systemic vascular resistance. The cardiac depression that enflurane produces appears to be the result of direct negative inotropic effects on the heart, and it also produces a reduction in the peripheral vascular resistance. Enflurane tends to increase the heart rate, or it may keep it normal, and bradycardia does not usually occur. Enflurane sensitizes the myocardium to the effects of endogenous and exogenous catecholamines. However, a lower incidence of dysrhythmias has been associated with enflurane as compared with halothane. In comparison with halothane, enflurane is a more potent respiratory depressant and blunts a patient's response to hypercarbia.

Like methoxyflurane (another fluorinated ether), enflurane is metabolized to inorganic and organic fluoride. However, the maximum serum concentrations are not high enough to cause renal toxicity. However, a fluoride-induced nephrotoxicity is a potential hazard following the metabolism of enflurane. There is much debate in this area because the amount of fluoride produced by enflurane needed to produce any clinical signs of nephrotoxicity is rather low. There have been some reports suggesting that enflurane causes slight hepatic dysfunction. These reports describe a mild, self-limited postoperative hepatic dysfunction that is most likely caused by inadequate hepatocyte oxygenation during enflurane anesthesia. Hence, enflurane may not be the anesthetic of choice for a patient with compromised hepatic function.

The patient regains consciousness from enflurane quickly, partly because of its low blood-gas partition coefficient of 1.37. There usually is no residual analgesia; therefore, when the patient regains consciousness, it is important to assess his or her pain and administer a narcotic analgesic if indicated. Some anesthetists administer a short-acting narcotic, such as fentanyl, at the end of the surgical procedure to reduce the amount of postoperative pain experienced by the patient in the PACU. Therefore, the PACU nurse should note at admission whether the patient has received any pain-relieving drugs during the intraoperative period.

The incidence of nausea and vomiting has been minimal with enflurane. Some patients have exhibited shivering during emergence and recovery that is unrelated to body temperature. Because enflurane is a halogenated agent, it continues to be studied as a possible cause of liver problems; however, it has yet to be linked with any hepatic syndrome.

Advantages of enflurane include marked cardiovascular stability, good operative analgesia, pleasant induction and emergence, and good patient acceptance. Enflurane is contrain-dicated in seizure disorders; in diabetes mellitus; with administration of catecholamines; in obstetric usage, especially in the first trimester of pregnancy; and in patients receiving enzyme inducers, particularly phenobarbital and phenytoin (Dilantin).

Halothane (Fluothane)

Halothane is a saturated hydrocarbon. Unlike the traditional inhalation anesthetic agents, halothane was a product of planned research by chemists and pharmacologists whose aim was to synthesize a volatile compound that combined the properties of anesthetic potency with nontoxicity and nonflammability. Halothane is 100 percent potent and a very rapid-acting drug. It is also easily controlled, in that the depth of anesthesia can be changed quickly. Because it is such a potent agent, it is administered by finely calibrated vaporizers. Recovery to consciousness is rapid owing to the small amounts absorbed by the brain tissue and the low blood-gas partition coefficient of 2.37.

Halothane has demonstrated a low incidence of post anesthesia nausea and vomiting. It does, however, sensitize the heart to catecholamines. Therefore, epinephrine should be administered cautiously to a patient in the PACU who has received halothane intraoperatively, because serious dysrhythmias may result. For the patient who is emerging from halothane (within 30 minutes of the termination of the intraoperative anesthetic), the following guidelines for the administration of epinephrine in the PACU will reduce the incidence of dysrhythmias: The epinephrine concentration should be no greater than 1:100,000 to 1:200,000, with a total adult dose not exceeding 10 ml of 1:100,000 solution in 10 minutes, or a total dose of 30 ml of 1:100,000 solution in 1 hour.

When the position of a patient is being changed during emergence from halothane, the maneuver should be carried out slowly and gently because compensatory vasoconstrictor mechanisms are depressed. Bronchial dilatation, myocardial depression, peripheral vasodilatation, and nonirritation of respiratory tissues are other features of this agent.

The use of halothane anesthesia as a possible cause of hepatitis continues to be the subject of research studies. It is well known that postoperative jaundice and liver failure may be caused by factors other than the anesthetic agent. However, because of the possibility that halothane may cause hepatitis in certain sensitized patients, it is usually not the anesthetic of choice when the patient has had recent exposure to halothane or has had any type of liver disease.

Halothane is widely used for all types of surgical procedures in patients of all age groups. The importance of maintaining the blood volume within reasonably normal limits should be stressed because of the peripheral-vasodilating action of halothane. Diminution of the blood volume by preoperative fluid restriction, diuretic therapy, and hemorrhage augment the hypotensive effect of halothane and should be corrected by intravenous infusions of the appropriate solutions.

Because the recovery phase of halothane is generally short, the *postoperative analgesic phase is also short.* Evaluation of postoperative pain should be thorough before a narcotic analgesic is administered to the patient, because the synergistic effect of halothane and a narcotic may result in marked respiratory depression.

Isoflurane (Forane)

Isoflurane, an analogue of enflurane, is also a halogenated methyl ethyl ether. It produces a dose-related depression of the central nervous system. But, in contrast with enflurane, this anesthetic agent does not produce convulsive electroencephalographic abnormalities. Isoflurane reduces the systemic arterial blood pressure and total peripheral resistance. However, during isoflurane anesthesia, the heart rate is usually increased and the cardiac output usually remains within normal limits. This agent produces respiratory depression as well as skeletal muscular relaxation in a dose-related fashion, because isoflurane markedly potentiates the actions of the nondepolarizing muscle relaxants. Of interest to the PACU nurse is the fact that isoflurane does not sensitize the myocardium to catecholamines to the same extent as does halothane. Thus, the chance of dysrhythmias is reduced when the patient has received isoflurane anesthesia.

The recovery phase is rapid owing to isoflurane's low blood-gas partition coefficient of 0.97. The patient not only awakens promptly but is also quite lucid within 15 to 30 minutes after termination of the anesthetic. However, clinical observation indicates that if the anesthesia time using isoflurane is longer than 45 to 60 minutes, the patient will probably experience a slower emergence phase than would be expected given that the drug has such a low blood-gas partition coefficient.

The lung volumes and capacities, as measured by the Wright respirometer, return to normal in less than 30 minutes along with the ability to raise the head, protrude the tongue, cough on command, and converse clearly. The blood pressure and pulse remain stable. Shivering is seen in 2 percent of patients, and nausea and vomiting occurs only occasionally.

Isoflurane possesses some excellent qualities, that is, a lack of sensitization of the heart to catecholamines, cardiovascular stability, limited biodegradation, good neuromuscular relaxation, and no central nervous system excitatory effects. Since its introduction into anesthesia practice, isoflurane has enjoyed continuing success among both anesthesia practitioners and PACU nurses.

Sevoflurane

Sevoflurane is a 100 percent potent inhalation anesthetic agent that has a blood-gas solubility coefficient of 0.69, which is near nitrous oxide, making it an extremely rapid-acting agent. Consequently, patients emerge from sevoflurane anesthesia in a matter of minutes when they have received this drug as the sole agent. It must be remembered that a rapid recovery from an inhalation anesthetic usually mandates the need for analgesic drugs in the immediate postoperative period.

The drug is nonirritating to the respiratory tract, and the degree of patient acceptance is high. It can be used in place of halothane for the induction of anesthesia in children. Sevoflurane tends to decrease the blood pressure by decreasing the systemic vascular resistance. Like all other inhalation agents, this drug is a respiratory depressant and blunts the ventilatory response to an increased $PaCO_2$. This drug does undergo some metabolism at about the same degree as does enflurane. The metabolites of sevoflurane include fluoride and hexafluoroisopropanol, and from a number of studies, no evidence of toxicity has been demonstrated in regard to the biodegradation of this agent. This is probably due to sevoflurane's rapid ventilatory excretion, in which the metabolic by-products do not seem to be significantly detrimental to the patient.

Like the other ethers, sevoflurane does not sensitize the heart to catecholamines and hence does not predispose to arrhythmias. This inhalation agent does reduce cerebrovascular resistance and can increase intracranial pressure in a dose-related manner. In regard to its effect on skeletal muscle function, it does enhance the action of the skeletal muscle relaxants. However, because of its rapid elimination, this characteristic does not have a significant impact on the care of a patient in the PACU who has received sevoflurane intraoperatively.

Sevoflurane possesses many outstanding qualities, such as great precision and control over anesthetic depth, does not depress kidney or liver function, has little effect on heart rate, and most of all, is extremely rapid, which will speed up the emergence of the patient in the PACU.

Desflurane (Suprane)

Desflurane is a fluorinated ether that is similar to isoflurane. This drug has a blood-gas partition coefficient that is the same as cyclopropane (0.42) and even less than nitrous oxide, making it extremely rapid acting. As with sevoflurane, patient emergence is extremely rapid, and analgesia is needed in the immediate postoperative period. This drug produces a dose-related decrease in blood pressure and cardiac output that is slightly greater than the depression seen with equivalent doses of isoflurane. Because this drug is an ether-type inhalation agent, the incidence of cardiac dysrhythmias when epinephrine is administered is extremely low.

The pungency of desflurane irritates the respiratory tract and causes coughing, breathholding, and laryngospasm. Consequently, it is not recommended as an inhalation induction agent, especially in the pediatric age group. This drug depresses respiration in the same fashion as does sevoflurane and thus blunts the response to an increased Pa_{CO_2}. Because this drug decreases cerebrovascular resistance, it will produce in a dose-related fashion. Desflurane also enhances the neuromuscular blockade produced by skeletal muscle relaxants. However, like sevoflurane, this action is not of consequence for the patient in the PACU, owing to its extremely rapid ventilatory excretion during emergence. Finally, as opposed to sevoflurane, this drug resists biodegradation and is almost totally eliminated by the respiratory system and therefore does not have a negative effect on either the kidney or liver.

Desflurane represents a new era in inhalation anesthesia in regard to its impact on the care of the patient in the PACU. More specifically, because of its low solubility, rapid emergence will become quite common, and a more rapid release from the PACU and a shorter length of stay in the hospital may be possible.

Nitrous Oxide

Nitrous oxide is the only inorganic gas used as an anesthetic agent. It is marketed in blue steel cylinders as a colorless liquid under a pressure of 30 atm. As the pressure is released, nitrous oxide returns to the gaseous state. It is readily soluble in water and heavier than air. Nitrous oxide was probably the first anesthetic agent to be used extensively. The fact that it is still being used indicates that, when used properly, it is a valuable and safe anesthetic agent.

Nitrous oxide supports combustion; that is, if a burning match is put into a jar containing nitrous oxide, it will continue to burn. However, this agent is not explosive. Although the nitrous oxide molecule contains oxygen, that oxygen is unavailable for respiration because nitrous oxide does not decompose in the body.

Nitrous oxide is a 15 percent potent agent; therefore, the maximum depth of anesthesia that can be produced while supplying the patient's metabolic need for oxygen is the middle of plane 1 of stage III anesthesia. This agent has no side effects unless hypoxia is present. It is nontoxic and nonirritating; however, nitrous oxide can cause postoperative nausea and vomiting. This is particularly true in the ambulatory surgical setting when the procedure lasts 1, and quite probably 2 or more hours. Nitrous oxide is a rapid-acting agent owing, in part, to its blood-gas partition coefficient of 0.47. This agent does not combine with hemoglobin but is carried in physical solution in the blood. It is excreted mostly unchanged by the lungs, although a small fraction is excreted through the skin. It does not sensitize the heart to epinephrine, and it provides a fair amount of analgesia. Even in subanesthetic concentrations it has an analgesic effect in humans, and 20 percent concentrations of the gas have been claimed to be as effective as 15 mg of morphine sulfate. If this agent were more potent, it would probably be considered an almost perfect anesthetic.

In current anesthesia practice, nitrous oxide serves an important role, because it is administered alone and in combination with various agents. Recently, the balanced technique of anesthesia has been favored, owing to the number of negative factors associated with some of the more potent volatile inhalation anesthetics. The *balanced technique* consists of the administration of narcotics that may or may not be in combination with a tranquilizer, a muscle relaxant, nitrous oxide, oxygen, and barbiturates. All the elements of anesthesia or nervous system depression are met: sensory block (analgesia), motor block (muscle relaxation), reflex block, and mental block (narcosis). For short procedures, when only light anesthesia is desired, a *pent-nitrous technique* is sometimes used. This consists of nitrous oxide, oxygen, and sodium thiopental. This technique provides narcosis and limited analgesia for brief, simple procedures.

When nitrous oxide is administered with a potent volatile inhalation anesthetic such as halothane, it acts as a carrier and also provides an additional analgesic effect. The second gas effect occurs because of nitrous oxide's rapid uptake, after which the potent volatile agent takes the patient to the desired surgical plane. The reverse takes place at termination of the anesthetic.

The solubilities of nitrogen and nitrous oxide differ greatly. Nitrous oxide is 30 times more soluble than nitrogen. An enclosed gas-filled space in the body expands if gas within it is more soluble than the gas respired. For this reason, any enclosed gas-filled cavity in the body expands because of the slow exchange of nitrogen from the cavity for the rapid exchange of large volumes of nitrous oxide from the blood. This is why the use of nitrous oxide is not recommended in surgical procedures for intestinal obstruction or pneumothorax. Nitrous oxide has been shown to dislodge a tympanoplasty graft owing to the expansion of the air pocket in the middle ear. Consequently, in surgical procedures involving the middle ear, the administration of nitrous oxide is usually avoided. Of interest to the PACU nurse is the possible role nitrous oxide has in altering the pressures in the middle ear, as it has been suggested that nitrous oxide may cause nausea and vomiting due to the resulting increased pressure in that area.

Diffusion hypoxia following nitrous oxide anesthesia is another area of concern for the PACU nurse. This is sometimes referred to as the *Fink phenomenon*. It occurs when not enough nitrous oxide is removed from the lungs at the end of the surgical procedure. Normally, 100 percent oxygen is administered at the end of the procedure to remove the nitrous oxide. This is referred to as *nitrous oxide washout*. Diffusion hypoxia is directly related to the dilution of alveolar gas by the rapid diffusion of the nitrous oxide out of the blood. This outpouring of nitrous oxide into the alveoli occurs during the first 1 to 5 minutes after the nitrous oxide has been discontinued. Along with this, the rapid movement into the alveoli can cause a dilutional effect of the $Paco_2$ and ultimately, a reduction in the stimulus to breathe. It is therefore highly advisable to administer oxygen by mask to all patients who are admitted to the PACU. This maneuver forestalls the development of severe hypoxia, should some un-

predicted airway problem occur. Another measure for avoiding this complication is to provide adequate verbal and physical stimulation to the patient to promote good ventilatory effort. This approach should include encouraging the patient to sigh every 5 minutes to ensure adequate removal of the anesthetic gases.

ASSESSING THE EFFECTS OF INHALATION AGENTS IN THE PACU

When assessing the patient's degree of emergence from inhalation anesthesia, it is important for the nurse to understand the pharmacologic effects of each anesthetic agent and of the preoperative medications used. Along with this, the rate of recovery from inhalation anesthesia is predictable based on the solubility of the anesthetic agent, alveolar ventilation, and duration of the anesthetic. Each anesthetic agent is essentially a depressant drug. Certain volatile agents, such as halothane, enflurane, and isoflurane, possess a high degree of myocardial and respiratory depressant properties. One parameter for monitoring the emergence phase when these agents have been administered is the vital signs. Preanesthetic baseline vital sign readings are reliable indicators of the patient's cardiorespiratory status postoperatively and can be used to assess the patient's stage of recovery. When this assessment is being made, however, all other factors of the patient's condition must also be considered. Total assessment of the patient recovering from anesthesia is discussed in Chapter 20. Most inhalation anesthetics cause some degree of depression of the respiratory system. Consequently, there is an increase in the $Paco_2$ in a dose-related manner and an increase in frequency accompanied with a reduction in the tidal volume. Because of the respiratory depression that all patients have following anesthesia and surgery, it is important that the PACU nurse use the stir-up regimen that encourages the patient to perform the sustained maximal inspiration maneuver (see Chapter 20).

To understand the emergence phase of inhalation anesthesia, the nurse also needs a basic understanding of *blood-gas* and *oil-gas partition coefficients*. Anesthetic agents are usually administered in combinations, often with nitrous oxide as the carrier gas. The combination of agents usually consists of a 100 percent potent agent, a carrier agent, and oxygen to meet the metabolic needs of the patient. The agent with the highest blood-gas partition coefficient takes the longest time to be removed from the body. Therefore, if a halothane–nitrous oxide–oxygen combination were administered to a patient, the halothane, having the highest blood-gas partition coefficient, would be eliminated the most slowly.

Along with the factors attributed to the blood-gas partition coefficient, those attributed to the oil-gas partition coefficient should be considered in an evaluation of length of time of emergence from the anesthetic. When the intraoperative phase is of long duration, an agent that has a high oil-gas partition coefficient will redistribute into the adipose tissue. As mentioned previously, because the vascular supply to adipose tissue is sparse, the release of the agent to the blood is slow and the emergence is prolonged. Both coefficients must be kept in mind when predicting the length of the emergence phase from an inhalation anesthetic agent. Halothane, for example, has the low blood-gas partition coefficient of 2.37, and one would expect a rapid recovery from its administration. However, halothane has a high oil-gas partition coefficient of 224, so when it is administered for longer than 1 hour, the adipose tissue will be saturated and emergence from the anesthetic agent prolonged. Nitrous oxide, enflurane, and isoflurane have low blood-gas and oil-gas partition coefficients.

Inhalation agents, because of their depressant effect on the hypothalamus, cause a disruption in the regulation of body temperature that may be manifested by either a reduction or an elevation, depending on the environmental temperature. In the recovery phase, the emerging patient should be monitored for *hypothermia* or *hyperthermia.* Serious heat loss may occur in newborns, creating difficulties in the re-establishment of adequate ventilatory effort after surgery. Body temperature should be monitored in patients who were febrile before surgery and who received atropine before or during the operative procedure. Agents such as halothane, which have a direct vasodilatory effect on vascular smooth muscle, can cause a temperature drop of 1°C in esophageal temperature. Shivering and tremors have been reported during the postoperative period following the use of halothane anesthesia, although this phenomenon has mostly been associated with a generalized loss of muscle tone during surgery and anesthesia.

Water and electrolyte balance is affected by inhalation anesthesia. Pituitary and adrenocortical systems appear to be affected in such a way that there is water and sodium retention and potassium loss following anesthesia. This bal-

ance is also affected, in part, by the stress of surgical trauma. Decreased glomerular filtration, increased tubular reabsorption, and varying degrees of oliguria exist in the recovery phase because of renal vasoconstriction. If renal blood flow is not impaired, glomerular function quickly returns to normal after the operation. The increased tubular reabsorption of water usually persists for 36 to 48 hours but may continue for several days in the elderly.

References

1. Barash, P., Cullen, B., and Stoelting, R.: Clinical Anesthesia. 2nd ed. Philadelphia, J. B. Lippincott, 1992.
2. Benumof, J., and Saidman, L.: Anesthesia and Perioperative Complications. St. Louis, Mosby-Year Book, 1992.
3. Block, R., Ghonem, M., and Ping, S.: Efficacy of therapeutic suggestions for improved postoperative recovery presented during general anesthesia. Anesthesiology, 75:746–755, 1991.
4. Breslow, M., Miller, C., and Rogers, M.: Perioperative Management. St. Louis, C. V. Mosby, 1990.
5. Chu, Y., Rah, K., and Boyan, C.: Is the Bain breathing circuit the future anesthesia system? An evaluation. Anesth. Analg., 56:84–87, 1977.
6. Dorsch, J., and Dorsch, S.: Understanding Anesthesia Equipment. 2nd ed. Baltimore, Williams & Wilkins, 1989.
7. Drug Evaluations Annual 1991. Milwaukee, American Medical Association, 1991.
8. Eger, E.: Clinical pharmacology of nitrous oxide: An argument for its continued use. Anesth. Analg., 71:575–585, 1990.
9. Eger, E., Saidman, L., and Bradstater, B.: Minimum alveolar anesthetic concentration: A standard of anesthetic potency. Anesthesiology, 26:756, 1965.
10. Goodman, A., Rall, T., Nies, A., et al.: Goodman and Gilman's The Pharmacological Basis of Therapeutics. 8th ed. New York, Pergamon Press, 1990.
11. Jones, R.: Desflurane and sevoflurane: Inhalation anaesthetics for this decade? Br. J. Anaesth., 65:527–536, 1990.
12. Katoh, T., Suguro, Y., Nakajima, R., et al.: Blood concentration of sevoflurane and isoflurane on recovery from anaesthesia. Br. J. Anaesth., 69:259–262, 1992.
13. Kulli, J., and Koch, C.: Does anesthesia cause loss of consciousness? Trends Neurosci., 14(1):6–10, 1991.
14. Litwick, K.: Core Curriculum for Post Anesthesia Nursing Practice. 3rd ed. Philadelphia, W. B. Saunders, 1994.
15. Longnecker, D., and Murphy, F.: Dripps/Eckenhoff/Vandam Introduction to Anesthesia. 8th ed. Philadelphia, W. B. Saunders, 1992.
16. Mazze, R.: The safety of sevoflurane in humans. Anesthesiology, 77:1062–1063, 1992.
17. Miller, R. (ed.): Anesthesia. 3rd ed. New York, Churchill Livingstone, 1990.
18. Saidman, L.: The role of desflurane in the practice of anesthesia. Anesthesiology, 74:399–401, 1991.
19. Stancer-Smiley, B., and Paradise, N.: Does the duration of N$_2$O administration affect postoperative nausea and vomiting? Nurse Anesth., 2(1):13–18, 1991.
20. Stoelting, R.: Pharmacology and Physiology in Anesthetic Practice. 2nd ed. Philadelphia, J. B. Lippincott, 1991.

21. Stoelting, R., and Miller, R.: Basics of Anesthesia. 2nd ed. New York, Churchill Livingstone, 1989.
22. Tsai, S., Lee, C., Kwan, W., and Chen, B.: Recovery of cognitive functions after anaesthesia with desflurane or isoflurane and nitrous oxide. Br. J. Anaesth., *69*:255–258, 1992.
23. Waugaman, W., Foster, S., and Rigor, B. (eds.): Principles and Practice of Nurse Anesthesia. 2nd ed. Norwalk, CT, Appleton & Lange, 1992.
24. Wood, M., and Wood, A.: Drugs and Anesthesia: Pharmacology for Anesthesiologists. 2nd ed. Baltimore, Williams & Wilkins, 1990.

CHAPTER 14

Nonopioid Intravenous Anesthetics

The time-tested use of the inhalation anesthetic agents has proved that they possess some definite disadvantages. Because of the biotransformation hazards that have been reported with the halogenated inhalation anesthetics, other techniques have been sought to provide general anesthesia. Intravenous anesthetics are now enjoying a wide range of use in the perioperative period. In fact, in current anesthesia practice, the use of intravenous drugs is now commonplace. Intravenous anesthetics are now grouped by primary pharmacologic action into nonopioid and opioid intravenous agents. The nonopioid agents are further grouped into the barbiturates, nonbarbiturates, and tranquilizers. These drugs can be injected in a rapid intravenous fashion to induce anesthesia, or they can be used via continuous infusion pump to facilitate maintenance of anesthesia. These drugs have certainly found their place in the practice of anesthesia to enhance patient outcomes.

MECHANISM OF ACTION OF THE NONOPIOID INTRAVENOUS ANESTHETICS

The nonopioid drugs appear to interact with gamma-aminobutyric acid (GABA) in the brain. GABA is an inhibitory neurotransmitter, and activation of the GABA receptors by GABA on the postsynaptic membrane causes inhibition of the postsynaptic neuron. The barbiturates appear to bind to the GABA postsynaptic receptor, with the net result of hyperpolarization of the postsynaptic neuron and inhibition of neuronal activity and, ultimately, loss of consciousness. Conversely, etomidate (Amidate), which is a nonbarbiturate induction agent, probably antagonizes the muscarinic receptors in the central nervous system (CNS) and also acts as an agonist to the opioid receptors. The resultant action of these drugs is a loss of wakefulness.

Tranquilizers such as the benzodiazepines bind to specific receptors in the limbic system. These benzodiazepine receptors utilize GABA as part of the neurotransmitter system. After the benzodiazepines have bound to the receptor, the action of GABA is enhanced, leading to the hyperpolarized state and, ultimately, inhibition of neuronal activity. The drug flumazenil is a specific benzodiazepine receptor antagonist. Consequently, after the administration of a benzodiazepine agonist, flumazenil can be administered. The pharmacologic actions on the benzodiazepine receptor will be reversed, and neuronal activity will resume.

THE BARBITURATES

Intravenous anesthesia began with barbiturate anesthesia. The long-acting barbiturates were introduced clinically in 1927. It was not until 1934 that Tovell and Lundy began using thiopental in clinical anesthesia practice. Since then, barbiturate anesthesia has enjoyed great popularity and is still widely used in clinical anesthesia.

Thiopental (Sodium Pentothal)

Thiopental is most commonly injected intravenously to induce or sustain surgical anesthesia. It is usually used in conjunction with a potent inhalation anesthetic and nitrous oxide–oxygen combinations. The main reason for the use of other anesthetic agents with thiopental is that thiopental is a poor analgesic. For surgical procedures that are short and require minimal analgesia, thiopental and nitrous oxide–oxygen combinations can be used. This technique is commonly referred to as the *pent-nitrous technique.* Thiopental is also used (1) to maintain light sleep during regional analgesia, (2) to control convulsions, and (3) to quiet a patient rapidly who is too lightly anesthetized during a surgical procedure.

The mode of action of thiopental involves a

phenomenon of redistribution. Thiopental has the ability to penetrate all tissues of the body without delay. Because the brain, as part of the vessel-rich group, is highly perfused, it receives approximately 10 percent of the administered intravenous dose within 40 seconds after injection. The patient usually becomes unconscious at this time. The thiopental then redistributes to relatively poorly perfused areas of the body. In the brain, the level of thiopental decreases to half its peak in 5 minutes and to one tenth in 30 minutes. Recovery of consciousness usually occurs during this period. Recovery may be prolonged if the induction dose was excessive or if circulatory depression occurs that would slow the redistribution phenomenon. Thiopental is metabolized in the body at a rate of 10 to 15 percent per hour.

Thiopental is a respiratory depressant. The chief effect is on the medullary and pontine respiratory centers. This depressant effect is dependent on the amount of thiopental administered, the rate at which it is injected, and the amount and type of premedication given to the patient. The response to carbon dioxide is depressed at all levels of anesthesia and is abolished at deep levels of thiopental anesthesia. Therefore, apnea can be an adverse outcome of high-dose thiopental.

Myocardial contractility is depressed and vascular resistance is increased after injection of thiopental, with the result that blood pressure is hardly affected, although it may be transiently reduced when the drug is first administered (when the vessel-rich group is highly saturated).

In addition to its being nonexplosive, the advantages of thiopental are (1) rapid and pleasant induction, (2) reduction of post anesthetic excitement and vomiting, (3) quiet respiration, (4) absence of salivation, and (5) speedy recovery after small doses. The disadvantages of the drug are adverse respiratory actions, including apnea, coughing, laryngospasm, and bronchospasm. Extravenous injection may result in tissue necrosis because of its highly alkaline pH (10.5 to 11).

PACU Care. Because thiopental may have an antianalgesic effect at low concentrations, some patients who have pain may be irrational, hyperactive, and restless during the initial recovery phase. The patient may exhibit some shivering related to lowered body temperature, which may result from a cold operating suite. Of concern to the PACU nurse is the patient admitted with cold, clammy, cyanotic skin. This effect occasionally occurs with thiopental and is caused, in part, by the peripheral vasoconstrictive action of the drug.

If the anesthesia time exceeds 1 hour, or if the total dose of thiopental exceeds 1 g, patients may have a delayed awakening time owing to the redistribution of thiopental. This phenomenon is particularly common in obese patients, because the drug is highly fat soluble. At present, no antagonist exists for the barbiturates. Therefore, airway management and monitoring of cardiovascular status are important.

Methohexital (Brevital)

Methohexital is an ultra–short-acting barbiturate intravenous anesthetic agent. It is usually indicated for short procedures in which rapid, complete recovery of the patient is required. Methohexital is about three times as potent as thiopental, and the recovery time from anesthesia is extremely rapid (4 to 7 minutes) because the drug is redistributed from the CNS to the muscle and fat tissues and a significant portion of the drug is metabolized in the liver. Consequently, the clearance of methohexital is about four times faster than that of thiopental. Methohexital causes about the same degree of cardiovascular and respiratory depression as does thiopental. It should be mentioned, however, that this drug can cause coughing and hiccups, and that, after injection, excitatory phenomena such as tremor and involuntary muscle movements may appear.

THE NONBARBITURATES

Etomidate (Duranest)

Etomidate, which is a derivative of imidazole, is a short-acting intravenous hypnotic that was synthesized in the laboratories of Janssen Pharmaceutica in Beerse, Belgium. It is not related chemically to the commonly used hypnotic agents. This drug is a mere hypnotic and does not possess any analgesic actions. Etomidate is quite safe to administer to patients, because it has a high therapeutic index. Metabolism of this drug is accomplished by hydrolysis in the liver and by plasma esterases, with the final metabolite being pharmacologically inactive. The cardiovascular effects of etomidate are minimal; when the drug is injected in therapeutic doses, only a small blood pressure decrease and a slight heart rate increase may be observed. Studies have also shown that etomidate does cause a minimal reduction in the cardiac index and the peripheral resistance. This drug does not seem to produce arrhythmias. In regard to the respiratory system, etomidate causes a dose-related reduction in the tidal volume and respiratory frequency to include apnea. Laryngospasm, cough, and hiccups can occur during injection of this drug; however, the severity of these clinical phenomena can be reduced when the patient receives an opiate premedication.

Although this drug does cause some pain at the site of injection, it does not appear to effect a release of histamine. Spontaneous involuntary movements and tremor have been observed after the injection of etomidate. These involuntary movements can be reduced by an opiate premedication. Etomidate reduces both intracranial and intraocular pressure and therefore is considered safe to use in patients with intracranial pathologic conditions. This short-acting hypnotic is particularly well suited for the induction of neuroleptanalgesia and inhalation anesthesia. The induction dose ranges from 0.2 to 0.3 mg per kg, which produces sleep in 20 to 45 seconds after injection, with the patient awakening within 7 to 15 minutes after induction.

Research has demonstrated that etomidate inhibits steroid synthesis and that patients who receive etomidate by continuous infusion have marked adrenocortical suppression for as long as 4 days. Even when etomidate is administered as a single dose, adrenal function is suppressed for 5 to 8 hours. Consequently, after the administration of etomidate there is a decrease in cortisol, 17-alpha-hydroxyprogesterone, aldosterone, and corticosterone levels. Because of this, etomidate is administered only to selected patients and is no longer administered by continuous intravenous infusion.

Propofol (Diprivan)

Propofol is a rapid-acting nonbarbiturate induction agent. It is administered intravenously as a 1 percent solution. The dosage for induction is 2 to 2.5 mg per kg. The dosage should be reduced in elderly patients and in patients with cardiac disease or hypovolemia. Along with this, propofol in combination with midazolam (Versed) acts synergistically. In fact, the dosage of propofol can be reduced by 50 percent when it is administered in combination with midazolam. When propofol is used as the sole induction agent, it is usually administered over 15 seconds and produces unconsciousness within about 30 seconds. Emergence from this drug is more rapid than from thiopental or methohexital. This is because propofol has a half-life of 2 to 9 minutes. Hence, the duration of anesthesia after a single induction dose is about 3 to 8 minutes, depending on the dose of the propofol. A major advantage of this drug is its ability to allow the patient a rapid return to consciousness with minimal residual CNS effects. Along with this, what is of particular importance to PACU care is that this drug has a low incidence of nausea and vomiting. In fact, propofol may possess antiemetic properties.

Propofol decreases the cerebral perfusion pressure, cerebral blood flow, and intracranial pressure. It does produce a reduction in the blood pressure similar in magnitude to or greater than thiopental in comparable doses. The decrease in blood pressure is also accompanied by a reduction in cardiac output or systemic vascular resistance. This reduction in blood pressure is more pronounced in elderly patients and in patients with compromised left-ventricular function. As opposed to the reduction in blood pressure, the pulse usually remains unchanged after the administration of propofol owing to a sympatholytic or vagotonic effect of the drug. Therefore, in some patients, bradycardia may be assessed after injection of propofol, and in this instance, an anticholinergic drug such as atropine or glycopyrrolate (Robinul) can be administered to reverse the bradycardia.

In regard to ventilation, propofol has a profound depressant effect on both the rate and depth of ventilation. In fact, after the induction dose is administered, apnea normally occurs. In fact, the incidence of apnea is greater after propofol than thiopental and may approach 100 percent. Consequently, if propofol is administered in the post anesthesia care unit (PACU), the post anesthesia nurse should be prepared to support the patient's ventilation and, if necessary, intubate the patient (see Chapter 21).

Clinically, this drug is useful for intravenous induction of anesthesia, especially for outpatient surgery. It is also an excellent choice for procedures requiring a short period of unconsciousness, such as cardioversion and electroconvulsive therapy. Also, propofol can be used for sedation during local standby procedures. This drug does not interfere with or alter the effects of succinylcholine because it has such a rapid plasma clearance. Propofol can be used in a continuous intravenous infusion intraoperatively, and the patients will still emerge from anesthesia in a rapid fashion without any CNS depression.

PACU Care. When a patient has received

propofol for induction or even via continuous infusion, the PACU nursing care should be based mainly on the other drugs that were used intraoperatively. This is because propofol is so rapid and has no cumulative effects—its effects are normally dissipated within 8 to 10 minutes. Consequently, the patient usually arrives in the PACU awake and in pain. Therefore, analgesics should be titrated to effect. Titration is recommended in the immediate postoperative period because propofol and opioid analgesics can have a synergistic effect.

Propofol is an excellent addition to clinical anesthesia practice. It offers many advantages and few disadvantages. More specifically, propofol has one major advantage over all the other intravenous induction agents: early awakening. It can be used in the PACU if indicated. The major concern for the PACU care of the patient who has received this drug is the level of postoperative pain. The nursing assessment and appropriate interventions for pain are the most important aspects of care of the patient who has received this drug (see Chapter 22).

THE TRANQUILIZERS

The Benzodiazepines

The benzodiazepines, which are tranquilizers, have enhanced the anesthetic outcomes of the surgical patient. They exert their activity by depressing the limbic system without causing cortical depression. Opiates and barbiturates enhance the hypnotic action of the benzodiazepines.

Diazepam (Valium)

Diazepam is one of the more popular drugs used in anesthesia practice today. Because of its ability to allay apprehension, diazepam is indicated for use as a premedicant, as an adjunct to intravenous anesthesia, and as an induction agent. Recovery is usually not prolonged when diazepam is used for the induction of anesthesia. Diazepam can be used as the sole anesthetic agent for short diagnostic and surgical procedures and can also be used to provide sedation to make local anesthesia more acceptable to the patient.

Its principal action is to depress limbic system function. Important actions of diazepam are its ability to produce anterograde amnesia for as long as 48 hours postoperatively, to reduce anxiety, and to provide minimal cardiovascular depressant effects. Clinical doses of diazepam cause a slight degree of respiratory depression, although when combined with an opiate, the chance of respiratory depression, including apnea, is greatly increased.

Diazepam may possess some muscle-relaxant properties. It has been reported that diazepam is antagonistic to depolarizing neuromuscular blocking agents such as succinylcholine and that the action of the nondepolarizing neuromuscular blocking agents, such as d-tubocurarine, pancuronium, and gallamine, are potentiated. Diazepam has been used clinically for psychomotor and petit mal seizures because of its anticonvulsant actions.

Because many patients who undergo cardioversion are debilitated, diazepam may be used to provide sedation for this procedure. Increments of 2.5 to 5 mg can be given at 30-second intervals until the speech of the patient is slurred or light sleep occurs. At the time of electrical discharge, there may be a brief muscle contraction and slight arousal of the patient. When this technique is employed, a significant number of the patients have complete amnesia regarding the event. Diazepam can also be used to provide anesthesia in endoscopic and dental procedures and to control behavior on emergence from ketamine. Finally, this drug also has strong anticonvulsant activity and can stop generalized seizure activity.

Diazepam, when administered by the intramuscular route, can be quite painful to the patient. Along with this, the absorption is often poor. Also, when diazepam is administered by the intravenous route, thrombophlebitis frequently occurs. When diazepam is administered intravenously, it should be injected slowly, directly into a large vein. The drug should not be mixed with other drugs or diluted. The onset of action of diazepam administered intravenously is immediate, and the duration of action varies from 20 minutes to 1 hour. When administered intramuscularly, its onset of action is about 10 minutes and the duration of action may be as long as 4 hours. Adverse reactions to diazepam include hiccups, nausea, phlebitis at the site of injection, and occasional acute hyperexcited states.

Midazolam (Versed)

Midazolam has become a popular drug used in anesthesia practice and in the post anesthesia care of the surgical patient. Midazolam can be used for premedication, cardioversion, endoscopic procedures, and induction of anesthesia and as an intraoperative adjunct for inhalation anesthesia. It also is an excellent agent to provide sedation during regional anesthetic techniques. Midazolam's principal action is on the benzodiazepine receptors in the CNS, particularly on the limbic system, which results in a reduction in anxiety and profound anterograde amnesia. This drug also has excellent hypnotic, anticonvulsant, and muscle-relaxant properties.

This water-soluble benzodiazepine that may offer some advantages over diazepam. This drug causes depression of the CNS by inducing sedation, drowsiness, and, finally, sleep with increasing doses. Midazolam, when compared with diazepam, is about three times as potent, has a shorter duration of action, and produces less incidence of injection pain and postinjection phlebitis and thrombosis. More specifically, this drug has a rapid onset of action, a peak in action between 10 and 30 minutes, and a duration of action between 1 and 4 hours. Midazolam, administered at a dose of 0.2 mg per kg, produces a decrease in blood pressure, an increase in heart rate, and a reduction in systemic vascular resistance. Midazolam should be used with caution in patients with myocardial ischemia and those with chronic obstructive pulmonary disease. Postoperative patients who have a substantial amount of hypovolemia should not receive midazolam. Along with this, midazolam does not have an effect on intracranial pressure. Consequently, this drug can be used safely in neurosurgical patients in addition to patients with intracranial pathophysiology.

Because this drug can be administered in the PACU, it is of utmost importance to the post anesthesia nurse to monitor the patient for respiratory depression after injection. This is because midazolam causes a dose-dependent respiratory depression. Given that every patient in the PACU has received a plethora of depressant drugs intraoperatively, midazolam can be potentiated quite easily when administered in the PACU. Because of this potentiation factor, *any* dose of midazolam administered in the PACU should be considered effective enough to cause profound respiratory depression. Therefore, oxygen and resuscitative equipment must be immediately available, and a person skilled in maintaining a patent airway and supporting ventilation should be present. Along with this, extra care should be observed in patients with limited pulmonary reserve and in the elderly and debilitated by reducing the dosage of midazolam by 25 to 30 percent.

Lorazepam (Ativan)

Lorazepam, a long-acting benzodiazepine, is used mainly as a premedication in current clinical anesthesia practice. This drug has actions similar to those of diazepam but has a slow onset of action of 20 to 40 minutes; the pharmacologic activity may last as long as 24 hours. Lorazepam produces profound anterograde amnesia, tranquilization, and a reduction of anxiety, and the drug provides good cardiovascular and respiratory stability. Therapeutic plasma concentrations are achieved in about 3 hours when the drug is given orally. The drug is well absorbed via the intramuscular route; however, the patient experiences a significant amount of pain during the injection of the drug. Lorazepam can also be injected intravenously, and the patient may experience some burning on injection. Because of its slow onset and long duration, lorazepam is mainly used as a preanesthetic medication. If this drug has been administered in the preoperative period, the effects of lorazepam may last well into the postoperative period because of its prolonged action. If a narcotic is administered in the PACU to a patient who received lorazepam preoperatively, the nurse should monitor for increased narcotic sedation and respiratory depression because of the potentiation of the narcotic by lorazepam.

Flunitrazepam

Flunitrazepam is a new long-acting benzodiazepine that is similar to diazepam. It is approximately 10 times more potent than diazepam when given intravenously. It is characterized by a high patient variability in regard to its effects. However, it does produce pharmacologic actions similar to diazepam in regard to its cardiovascular, amnesic, and sedative-hypnotic properties. The major problems with this drugs are its slow onset of action and prolonged recovery time.

The Benzodiazepine Antagonists

Physostigmine (Antilirium)

Physostigmine is an anticholinesterase that crosses the blood-brain barrier. Its action is to inhibit the enzyme acetylcholinesterase, which will result in an increase in the availability of acetylcholine at the receptors that are affected by the benzodiazepines in the CNS. The preponderance of acetylcholine counteracts the negative effects of glycine and GABA. Consequently, this drug provides a nonspecific reversal of the CNS side effects of the benzodiazepines scopolamine and ketamine. The dosage is 0.5 to 1 mg, and it should be administered slowly to prevent untoward cholinergic side effects. Because this drug is a nonspecific agent, a number of vagally mediated cholinergic side effects can occur after its administration. These effects include nausea, vomiting, salivation, bradycardia, bronchospasm, and seizures. Hence, because of its nonspecific properties, physostigmine is rarely used for the reversal of the untoward effects of the benzodiazepines.

Flumazenil (Romazicon)

Flumazenil, a new benzodiazepine antagonist, has recently been introduced into clinical practice in the United States. When introduced, the trade name was Mazicon; however, because the name was similar to the trade name Mavacron (mivacurium chloride), a neuromuscular-blocking agent, the name was changed to Romazicon. This drug antagonizes or reverses the effects of benzodiazepine-induced sedation at the benzodiazepine receptors. Consequently, it reverses the CNS effects of benzodiazepines such as the sedation and amnesia that are produced by diazepam and midazolam, for example. This drug also reverses the other effects produced by benzodiazepines agonists, including their anxiolytic, muscle-relaxant, ataxic, and anticonvulsant actions. However, flumazenil may not be effective in the treatment for benzodizepine-induced hypoventilation or respiratory failure. This drug is specific for the benzodiazepines and, more specifically, their receptors. Consequently, this drug does not reverse the effects of barbiturates, opiates, and ethanol. Flumazenil should be used with great caution in patients who have a history of epilepsy or chronic benzodiazepine usage because reversal with flumazenil in these patients can result in seizures. The incidence of postoperative nausea and vomiting is increased after flumazenil has been administered.

The usual reversal dose for flumazenil is 0.4 mg administered intravenously in 0.1 increments. Flumazenil should be administered very slowly to avoid the adverse consequences of abrupt wakening. A maximum dose for this drug is 1 mg. The onset of action is usually within 5 minutes with a duration of action between 1 and 2 hours. Flumazenil has a shorter duration of action than most of the benzodiazepines and, consequently, the risk of resedation can occur after the initial reversal dose was administered. This is especially true when high doses of benzodiazepines were previously administered. Therefore, after the administration of flumazenil, the patient should be monitored

for resedation and other residual effects of benzodiazepines in the PACU and on the receiving unit. Should the patient develop signs of resedation, flumazenil should be given at 20-minute intervals as needed to reverse the sedation. In this situation, no more than 1 mg should be given at any one time and no more than 3 mg should be given within a 1-hour period. This drug should prove to be a valuable asset in the care of the patient who has received an excessive dose of a benzodiazepine such as midazolam and diazepam. Consequently, flumazenil will be useful intraoperatively, postoperatively, and in the intensive care unit.

The Butyrophenones

The butyrophenones are a class of tranquilizers that are characterized by producing a state of profound calm and immobility in which the patient appears to be pain free and dissociated from his or her surroundings. They are a potent inhibitor of the chemoreceptor trigger zone–mediated nausea and vomiting. These drugs have some profound side effects but do seem to be useful in anesthesia and post anesthesia care of the surgical patient. The two major butyrophenones used in clinical practice are haloperidol and droperidol.

Haloperidol (Haldol)

Haloperidol is a butyrophenone tranquilizer that has limited use in anesthesia practice because of its very long duration of action and its high incidence of extrapyramidal reactions. It is not approved for intravenous use and is usually administered intramuscularly at a dose ranging from 2 to 5 mg. It is used in the treatment of psychoses and as an antiemetic.

Droperidol (Inapsine)

Droperidol, which was originally investigated by Janssen Pharmaceutica, can be used alone or in combination with fentanyl (Sublimaze) as part of a neuroleptanalgesic technique. It produces a state of calm, disinclination to move, and disconnection from surroundings. It has an alpha-adrenergic blocking effect, which offers some protection against the vasoconstrictive components of shock; it leads to good peripheral perfusion; and it unmasks hypovolemia. More specifically, when a patient has compensated for a borderline hypovolemic state by activation of the alpha-vasoconstriction mechanisms, vital signs will be normal.

When a drug such as droperidol is administered to this patient, by virtue of droperidol's alpha-blocking properties, the signs of hypovolemia will appear. Hence, the patient's hypovolemia is "unmasked." Droperidol also protects against epinephrine-induced arrhythmias and has an antiemetic effect. In fact, because of its excellent antiemetic properties, droperidol is sometimes administered toward the end of the surgical procedure or in the PACU to reduce the risk of vomiting and aspiration in anxious patients. The antiemetic dose of droperidol is between 1 and 2.5 mg, which can be given intravenously. Also, by virtue of its alpha-blocking properties, this drug may be administered in the PACU on a short-term basis to reduce the afterload.

Droperidol is similar to chlorpromazine (Thorazine) in its CNS effects; however, its mechanism of action is different. Droperidol is more selective than chlorpromazine, because it provides more tranquillity with less sedation and has less effect on the autonomic nervous system. Droperidol has been classified as a neuroleptic and is the main tranquilizing component of Innovar (see following discussion in this section). Among its negative effects, droperidol may cause hypotension by virtue of its alpha-adrenergic blocking effect and peripheral vasodilatation. It may cause extrapyramidal excitation, such as twitchiness, oculogyric seizures, stiff neck muscles, trembling hands, restlessness, and, occasionally, psychologic disturbances such as hallucinations. These can be reversed with atropine or antiparkinsonian drugs such as benztropine mesylate (Cogentin) and trihexyphenidyl hydrochloride (Artane). Clinically, patients who have received droperidol have reported the dichotomy of appearing outwardly calm while feeling terrified inside and unable to express how they feel. Hence, the PACU nurse should provide emotional support to all patients who have received droperidol.

Droperidol is known to potentiate the action of barbiturates and narcotics. It has a high therapeutic margin of safety with a rapid onset of 10 minutes, and its activity is lessened in 2 to 4 hours, although some effects last as long as 10 to 12 hours.

Droperidol is the prototype neuroleptic drug. A *neuroleptic* drug is one that reduces motor activity, lessens anxiety, and produces a state of indifference in which the person can still respond appropriately to commands. *Neuroleptanalgesia* is a state of profound tranquilization with little or no depressant effect on the cortical centers. Therefore, neuroleptanalgesia

is achieved by the combination of a neuroleptic such as droperidol and a potent narcotic analgesic such as fentanyl. A fixed-dose mixture of droperidol and fentanyl is called *Innovar*. Each milliliter of Innovar contains 0.05 mg of fentanyl and 2.5 mg of droperidol. When the fixed-dose approach is not desired, fentanyl (0.004 mg per kg) and droperidol (0.2 mg per kg) can be administered in slow intravenous doses. Going a step further, *neuroleptanesthesia* is the combination of a neuroleptanalgesic (droperidol plus fentanyl), a skeletal muscle relaxant, and nitrous oxide and oxygen. The main objective in developing neuroleptanesthesia is to provide a technique for all types of operations that does not depress the metabolic, circulatory, or central nervous systems as severely as do the inhalation anesthetics when used alone.

PACU Care. In the immediate postoperative period, the awakening from neuroleptanesthesia is usually rapid, extremely smooth, and uneventful. A striking feature is the extension of analgesia well into the postoperative period. It is difficult to explain the mechanism of such a prolonged pain-relieving effect with a drug such as fentanyl, in which the onset is so rapid and the duration of action is so short.

Nursing personnel in the PACU should constantly assess the patient for signs of respiratory depression. Narcotics should be avoided in patients who have received droperidol, or they should be given in minimal amounts. It is recommended that the dosage of narcotic agonists be reduced to as little as one fourth to one third the usual dose owing to the additive potentiating effects of droperidol.

The patient should be encouraged to cough and perform the sustained maximal inspiration (SMI) maneuver in the PACU (see Chapter 20). Patients who have received droperidol or Innovar tend to drift back to sleep unless they are encouraged to move about. The PACU nurse will find the patient who has received neuroleptanesthesia more willing to cough and perform the SMI, because the analgesia extends into the postoperative period. Innovar depresses both the respiratory rate and the tidal volume. The PACU nurse should use verbal stimulation with these patients. This is because, if ordered, the patient will be able to take a deep breath, but otherwise respiration may remain slow and shallow or the patient may even become apneic. Consequently, the PACU nurse must remain with the patient, provide verbal stimulation, and actively monitor for any signs of respiratory depression.

The PACU nurse should monitor for extrapyramidal symptoms; although rare, they have been detected as long as 24 hours after a single administration of droperidol or Innovar. Most of the reported extrapyramidal reactions occurred in children younger than 12 years of age. Because of the length of action of droperidol, it is recommended that the PACU nurse provide information about the drug to the nursing personnel on the surgical units via hospital in-service education programs.

Because of droperidol's long duration of action and tremendous potentiating effects, all PACU personnel should be alerted when a patient has received this drug either intraoperatively or postoperatively. Hence, it is suggested that the patient's bed have a tag on it to indicate that the patient has received either droperidol or Innovar and serve as a visual reminder for the staff to reduce the dose of any narcotics or barbiturates given in the PACU.

THE DISSOCIATIVE ANESTHETICS

Ketamine

Traditionally, general anesthetic agents achieved control of pain by depression of the CNS. An anesthetic agent, ketamine, has been introduced that has a totally different mode of action. It selectively blocks pain conduction and perception, leaving those parts of the CNS that do not participate in pain transmission and perception free from the depressant effects of the drug. Ketamine is termed *dissociative* because patients who are totally analgesic usually do not appear to be asleep or anesthetized but rather disassociated from their surroundings. The drug is nonbarbiturate and non-narcotic. It is administered parenterally, and its effects are of a short duration. Early laboratory studies using ketamine suggested that most of the drug's activity is centered in the frontal lobe of the cerebral cortex.

The clinical characteristics of ketamine consist of a state of profound analgesia combined with a state of unconsciousness. The patient usually has marked horizontal and vertical nystagmus. The eyes are usually open and shortly become centered and appear in a fixed gaze. The pupils are moderately dilated and react to light. Respiratory function is usually unimpaired, except after rapid intravenous injection, when it may become depressed for a short time. Ketamine is sympathomimetic in action and is beneficial to asthmatic patients because of its bronchodilating effect. When patients receive ketamine, their pharyngeal and laryngeal reflexes remain intact. The tongue usually does not become relaxed, so the airway usually remains unobstructed. Ketamine accelerates the heart rate moderately and increases both the systolic and the diastolic pressure for several minutes, after which the pulse and blood pressure return to preinjection levels. Finally, ketamine increases cerebral blood flow and, consequently, intracranial pressure. Therefore, this drug is definitely contraindicated in patients who are at risk for increased intracranial pressure.

Ketamine can be administered intramuscularly or intravenously. The intramuscular dose is 4 to 6 mg per lb, and the anesthesia lasts from 20 to 40 minutes. The intravenous dose is usually 0.5 to 2 mg per lb with anesthesia lasting 6 to 10 minutes. Complete recovery from ketamine varies according to the duration of surgery and the amount of ketamine used throughout the procedure. When a single dose of intravenous ketamine is used, recovery time is usually rapid and does not exceed 30 minutes. When supplemental intravenous doses need to be administered, more particularly when supplemental intramuscular doses are required, recovery is often markedly prolonged, sometimes as long as 3 hours.

PACU Care. When patients are emerging from ketamine anesthesia, they may go through a phase of vivid dreaming, with or without psychomotor activity manifested by confusion, irrational behavior, and hallucinations. The PACU nurse should be aware that such psychic aberrations are usually transient and appear to be preventable by avoiding early verbal or tactile stimulation of the patient, which helps prevent fear and anxiety reactions. Short-acting barbiturates administered intravenously can effectively control the psychic responses sometimes seen after the administration of ketamine. Pediatric patients seem to be less prone to these psychic disturbances. Results of a study revealed that droperidol, the tranquilizer component of Innovar, may be effective in eliminating some of the adverse psychic emergence phenomena of ketamine. Other tranquilizers such as diazepam have also been found effective in suppressing these phenomena. Thus, the nurse should be aware of any tranquilizers the patient may have received when admitting him or her to the PACU.

Once the patient has arrived in the PACU, he or she should be secluded from auditory, visual, and tactile stimuli and be observed for any signs of respiratory depression. Mechanical airway obstruction, particularly when caused by marked salivation, accounts for most of the instances of respiratory insufficiency after ketamine anesthesia. When the patient does not have adequate respiratory exchange, oxygen should be administered by mask until it is restored. Other important signs to watch for are persistent blood pressure elevation, tachycardia, bradycardia, dreaming, delirium, hallucinations, euphoria, and increased muscle tone. It should be stressed to all PACU personnel that attempts to rouse patients while they are still unable to see, hear, and orient themselves may set off a chain of anxiety reactions that may ultimately lead to severe psychomotor responses and even more irrational behavior.

The widespread use of ketamine requires an entirely new approach to anesthesia and PACU nursing care. Certainly, the agent has many deficiencies, but one fact frequently overlooked is that it is one of the safest anesthetics used. Its safety justifies its important place in the drugs used by the anesthesiologist. Ketamine appears to be an excellent anesthetic for pediatric patients, as the sole agent for short procedures, for inducing anesthesia in extremely poor-risk patients, and for patients with burns that require surgical treatment. Certain adult orthopedic and diagnostic procedures have also been found suitable for the use of ketamine anesthesia.

Ketamine is the first of several drugs that will probably achieve clinical usage as dissociative agents. Its actions, therefore, should be well understood by the PACU staff to ensure effective, informed care of the patient.

OTHER AGENTS

Propanidid

Propanidid is a nonbarbiturate hypnotic-anesthetic agent. The drug may be used as an induction agent or to produce transient anesthesia. It exerts a biphasic effect on respiration. After injection intravenously, an initial period of hyperventilation ensues that is caused by stimulation of the carotid chemoreceptors. This is followed by a short period of hypoventilation, periodic breathing, or apnea. When propanidid is administered, some degree of hypotension, usually due to cardiac depression, will be observed. Other side effects of propanidid are rigidity, coughing, hiccups, phonation, and uncontrollable movements.

The action of this drug is terminated by its being rapidly metabolized enzymatically by plasma pseudocholinesterase, whereas the ultra-short-acting barbiturates have their anesthetic action terminated by redistribution. Recovery from propanidid is usually more complete, and accumulation does not occur with repeated administration in contrast with the barbiturates. Patients who receive propanidid usually have a smooth recovery with no "hangover" effect. During the emergence phase of this drug, headaches, nausea, and vomiting are more frequent than with thiopental. The patient may also complain of an unpleasant taste postoperatively. Propanidid has been in clinical use in Europe for many years; it is currently under investigation and therefore not available in the United States.

Steroid Anesthesia

Steroid anesthesia involves using steroids, administered intravenously, to produce an anesthetized state (loss of consciousness and immobility in response to stimuli). Currently, the major use of steroid anesthetics is as a substitute for the commonly used intravenous barbiturates.

Althesin

Althesin, which is currently enjoying wide popularity in Great Britain, is a combination of two steroids: alphaxalone and alphadolone acetate. At present, this drug is not available in the United States. Used mainly as an induction agent, althesin has a similar onset and about a 5- to 10-minute longer duration of action when compared with thiopental. This drug does not seem to alter the cardiac output and often causes a short period of hyperventilation, which is sometimes followed by apnea. The major disadvantage of althesin is in the realm of hypersensitivity reactions. These reactions, which may be caused by histamine release, range from severe circulatory collapse, bronchospasm, and edema to a generalized erythematous reaction.

References

1. Barash, P., Cullen, B. and Stoelting, R.: Clinical Anesthesia. 2nd ed. Philadelphia, J. B. Lippincott, 1992.
2. Brown, B. (ed.): New Pharmacologic Vistas in Anesthesia. Philadelphia, F. A. Davis, 1983.
3. Drain, C.: Innovar: A neuroleptic drug. Am. J. Nurs., 74:895–896, 1974.
4. Drain, C.: Recovery room care of the ketamine patient. RN, 36(11):OR1–2, 1973.
5. Gilman, A., Rall, T., Nies, A., et al.: Goodman and

Gilman's The Pharmacological Basis of Therapeutics. 8th ed. New York, Pergamon Press, 1990.

6. Gold, M., Sacks, D., Grosnoff, D., et al.: Comparison of propofol with thiopental and isoflurane for induction and maintenance of general anesthesia. J. Clin. Anesth., 1(4):272–276, 1989.

7. Katz, R. (ed.): Propofol: A critical assessment. Semin. Anesth., 6(1, Suppl):1–54, 1992.

8. Korttila, K., Ostman, P., Faure, E., et al.: Randomized comparison of recovery after propofol–nitrous oxide versus thiopentone-isoflurane–nitrous oxide anaesthesia in patients undergoing ambulatory surgery. Acta Anaesthesiol. Scand., 34:400–403, 1990.

9. Miller, R. (ed.): Anesthesia. 3rd ed. New York, Churchill Livingstone, 1990.

10. Reves, J., Fragen, R. J., Vinik, H. R., et al.: Midazolam: Pharmacology and uses. Anesthesiology, 62:310–324, 1985.

11. Sebel, P., and Larson, J.: Propofol: A new intravenous anesthetic. Anesthesiology, 71:260–277, 1989.

12. Short, T., and Chui, P.: Propofol and midazolam act synergistically in combination. Br. J. Anaesth., 67:539–545, 1991.

13. Short, T., and Galletly, D.: Acute tolerance from benzodiazepine night sedation. Anaesthesia, 46:929–931, 1991.

14. Spiess, B.: Two new pharmacological agents for the 1990s: Flumazenil and propofol. J. Post Anesth. Nurs., 5(3):186–189, 1990.

15. Stoelting, R.: Pharmacology and Physiology in Anesthetic Practice. 2nd ed. Philadelphia, J. B. Lippincott, 1991.

16. Waugaman, W., Foster, S., and Rigor, B.: Principles and Practice of Nurse Anesthesia. 2nd ed. Norwalk, CT, Appleton & Lange, 1992.

17. Wood, M., and Wood, A.: Drugs and Anesthesia: Pharmacology for the Anesthesiologist. 2nd ed. Baltimore, Williams & Wilkins, 1990.

CHAPTER 15

Opioid Intravenous Anesthetics

Modern anesthesia care is now using many new drugs and techniques in an effort to optimize patient outcomes. Opioid intravenous anesthetics constitute a major portion of the clinical anesthesia process. These drugs enhance the effectiveness of the inhalation anesthetics. More specifically, the opioids meet much of the analgesic portion of the anesthesia process. Also, by adding the opioids to the drugs used to provide general anesthesia, the concentration of the inhalation anesthetic can be reduced, and as a result, a safer anesthetic can be administered to the patient. Because opioids are used to manage acute and chronic pain and are administered for general inhalation anesthesia and sedation and pain relief during regional anesthesia, their implications for the post anesthesia nursing care of the surgical patient are profound. Consequently, it is imperative that the post anesthesia care unit (PACU) nurse be well informed in all aspects of the pharmacology of the opioid intravenous anesthetic agents.

THE CONCEPT OF OPIOIDS AND OPIOID RECEPTORS

Opioids are the substances, either natural or synthetic, that are administered into the body (exogenous) and bind to specific receptors, producing a morphinelike, or opioid agonist, effect. The endogenous opioids are the endorphins. The endorphins, which are produced in the body, attach to the opioid receptors in the central nervous system (CNS) to activate the body's pain modulating system. The term *opioid* was derived because of the multitude of synthetic drugs with morphinelike actions, and with the advent of receptor physiology, it has replaced the term *narcotic*. *Narcotic* is derived from the Greek word for stupor and usually refers to both the production of the morphinelike effects and the physical dependence.

The natural occurring alkaloids of opium are divided into two classes: phenanthrenes and benzylisoquinolines. The principal phenanthrene series of drugs includes morphine, codeine, and thebaine. Papaverine and noscapine, which lack opioid activity, are representatives of the benzylisoquinoline alkaloids of opium.

The synthetic opioids have been produced by the modification of the chemical structure of the phenanthrene class of drugs. Drugs such as fentanyl (Sublimaze) and meperidine (Demerol) are examples of synthetic opioids.

The identification of specific opioid receptors has enhanced the understanding of the agonist and antagonist actions of this category of drugs. The opioid receptors are located in the CNS, principally in the brain stem and spinal cord. These receptors have been determined by the pharmacologic effect they produce when stimulated by a specific agonist along with how the effect is blocked by a specific antagonist. The four major categories of opioid receptors are the mu, delta, kappa, and sigma receptors.

The *mu receptors* are mainly responsible for the production of supraspinal analgesia effects when stimulated. These receptors are further divided into mu-1 and mu-2 types. Activation of the mu-1 receptors results in analgesia, and when the mu-2 receptors are stimulated, hypoventilation, bradycardia, physical dependence, euphoria, and ileus can result. The mu receptors are activated by morphine, fentanyl, and meperidine. The drug that is specific to the mu-1 receptor is meptazinol. The *delta* opioid *receptors*, when stimulated, serve to modulate the activity of the mu receptors. Stimulation of the *kappa receptors* results in spinal analgesia, sedation, and miosis with little effect on ventilation. The drugs that possess both opioid agonist and antagonist activities, such as nalbuphine (Nubain), have their principal action on the kappa opioid receptors. The last category of opioid receptors is the *sigma receptors*, and activation of these receptors results in dysphoria, hallucinations, hypertonia, tachycardia, tachypnea, and mydriasis. The drug naloxone (Narcan) attaches to all the opioid receptors and thus serves as an antagonist to all the opioid agonists.

THE OPIOIDS

Narcotics, or opioids, are becoming quite popular in anesthesia practice. They are usually used in the *nitrous-narcotic (balanced) techniques*, which involve the use of a narcotic, nitrous oxide, and oxygen, with or without a muscle relaxant, and thiopental for induction.

The effects of narcotics generally last well into the PACU phase, and every PACU nurse should have a good knowledge of the pharmacologic actions of each narcotic that is administered to the patient in the perioperative phase of the surgical experience.

The administration of opioids in the perioperative period is not without the concern of overdosage. The major signs of overdosage of opioids are miosis, hypoventilation, and coma. If the patient becomes severely hypoxemic, mydriasis can occur. Airway obstruction is a strong possibility because the skeletal muscles become flaccid. Along with this, hypotension and seizures may occur. The treatment for an opioid overdosage is mechanical ventilation and the slow titration of naloxone. Consideration must always be given to the fact that some patients who become overdosed with an opioid may indeed be already physically dependent and the use of naloxone can precipitate an acute withdrawal syndrome.

Meperidine Hydrochloride (Demerol)

Meperidine was discovered in 1939 by Eisleb and Schauman. Because it is chemically similar to atropine, it was originally introduced as an antispasmodic agent and was not used as an opioid anesthetic agent until 1947. The main action of this drug is similar to morphine, and it stimulates the subcortical mu receptors, resulting in an analgesic effect. Meperidine is about one tenth as potent as morphine and has a duration of action of about 2 to 4 hours. The onset of analgesia is prompt (10 minutes) after subcutaneous or intramuscular administration. All pain, especially visceral, gastrointestinal, and urinary tract, is satisfactorily relieved. This drug causes less biliary tract spasm than morphine; however, when compared with codeine, meperidine causes greater biliary tract spasm. It produces some sleepiness but causes little euphoria or amnesia. Meperidine increases the sensitivity of the labyrinthine apparatus of the ear, which explains the dizziness, nausea, and vomiting that sometimes occur in ambulatory patients.

This narcotic may slow the rate of respiration, but the rate generally returns to normal within 15 minutes after intravenous injection. The tidal volume is not changed appreciably. In equivalent analgesic doses, meperidine depresses respiration to a greater extent than does morphine. Some authors have noted that meperidine may release histamine from the tissues. Occasionally, one may notice urticarial wheals that have formed over the veins where meperidine has been injected. The usual treatment is to discontinue the use of meperidine and, if the reaction is severe, to administer diphenhydramine (Benadryl). Diphenhydramine further sedates the patient, however, and should be administered only if truly warranted.

Meperidine does not, in therapeutic doses, cause any significant untoward effects on the cardiovascular system. When this drug is administered intravenously, it usually causes an increase in heart rate that is usually transient. When it is administered intramuscularly, no significant change in heart rate will be observed. One of the major concerns with this drug is that of orthostatic hypotension, probably owing to the fact that meperidine interferes with the compensatory sympathetic nervous system reflex. Hence, after a patient has received meperidine, he or she should be repositioned slowly, moving in a "staged" approach so as to avoid any possibility of hypotension.

Meperidine is generally metabolized in the liver; less than 5 percent is excreted unchanged by the kidneys.

Because of its spasmolytic effect, meperidine is the drug of choice for biliary duct, distal colon, and rectal surgery. It offers the advantages of little interference with the physiologic compensatory mechanisms, low toxicity, smooth and rapid recovery, prolonged postoperative analgesia, excellent cardiac stability in elderly and poor-risk patients, and ease of detoxification and excretion.

Morphine

Morphine, one of the oldest known drugs, has only recently been used as an opioid intravenous anesthetic agent. Alkaloid morphine is from the phenanthrene class of opium. The exact mechanism of action of morphine is unknown. In humans, it produces analgesia, drowsiness, changes in mood, and mental clouding. The analgesic effect can become profound before the other effects are severe and can persist after many of the side effects have almost disappeared. By direct effect on the respiratory center, morphine depresses respiratory rate, tidal volume, and minute volume. Maximal respiratory depression occurs within 7 minutes after intravenous injection of the drug and 30 minutes after intramuscular administration. Following therapeutic doses of morphine, the sensitivity of the respiratory center begins to return to normal in 2 or 3 hours, but the minute volume does not return to preinjection level until 4 or 5 hours have passed.

The greatest advantage of morphine is the remarkable cardiovascular stability that accompanies its use. It has no major effect on blood pressure, heart rate, or heart rhythm, even in toxic doses, when hypoxia is avoided. Morphine does, however, decrease the capacity of the cardiovascular system to adjust to gravitational shifts. This is important to remember because orthostatic hypotension and syncope may easily occur in a PACU patient whose care requires a position change. This phenomenon is primarily the result of the peripheral vasodilator effect of morphine. Therefore, a position change for a patient who has received morphine should be accomplished slowly, with constant monitoring of the patient's vital signs.

Morphine may cause nausea and vomiting, especially in ambulatory patients, by virtue of direct stimulation of the chemoreceptor trigger zone. The emetic effect of morphine can be counteracted by narcotic antagonists and phenothiazine derivatives such as chlorpromazine (Thorazine), prochlorperazine (Compazine), and benzoquinamide (Emete-con). Histamine release has been noted with morphine, and morphine also causes profound constriction of the pupils, stimulation of the visceral smooth muscles, and spasm of the sphincter of Oddi.

Morphine is detoxified by conjugation with glucuronic acid. Ninety percent is excreted by the kidneys, and 7 to 10 percent is excreted in the feces via the bile.

Morphine is used in the balanced, or nitrous-narcotic, technique with nitrous oxide, oxygen, and a muscle relaxant. This technique is useful for cardiovascular surgery, along with other types of surgery in which cardiovascular stability is required. The patient may arrive in the PACU still narcotized from morphine with an endotracheal tube in place. Mechanical ventilation for 24 to 48 hours is usually warranted. Morphine may or may not be supplemented during the time of ventilation. This type of recovery procedure facilitates a pain-free state and maximum ventilation of the patient during the critical phase of recovery. Morphine can

also be used to provide basal narcosis when regional anesthesia is employed.

In the PACU, morphine is an excellent drug to use in the control of postoperative pain. When given intravenously, this drug has a peak analgesic effect in about 20 minutes, with a duration of about 2 hours. When it is administered intramuscularly, the onset of action is about 15 minutes, with a peak effect attained in about 45 to 90 minutes and a duration of action of about 4 hours.

Fentanyl (Sublimaze)

Janssen and associates introduced a series of highly potent meperidine derivatives that were found to render the patient free of pain without affecting certain areas in the CNS. Fentanyl appeared to be of special interest. In regard to analgesic properties, fentanyl is approximately 80 to 125 times as potent as morphine, and it has a rapid onset of action of 5 to 6 minutes, a peak effect within 5 to 15 minutes, with the analgesia lasting 20 to 40 minutes when administered intravenously. Via the intramuscular route, the onset of action is 7 to 15 minutes, with analgesia usually lasting 1 to 2 hours. When fentanyl is administered as a single bolus, 75 percent of the drug will undergo "first-pass" pulmonary uptake. That is, the lungs serve as a large storage site, and this nonrespiratory function of the lung (see Chapter 6) limits the amount of fentanyl that actually reaches the systemic circulation. If the patient receives multiple doses of fentanyl by single injections or infusion, the first-pass pulmonary uptake mechanism will become saturated and the patient will have a prolonged emergence owing to increased duration of the drug. Consequently, during the admission of the patient to the PACU, the post anesthesia nurse must determine the frequency and amount of intraoperative fentanyl administration. Patients who have received a significant amount of fentanyl by infusion or by titration should be continuously monitored for persistent or recurrent respiratory depression. Along with this, fentanyl has been implicated in what is called a *delayed-onset respiratory depression*. In some patients, a secondary peak of the drug concentration in the plasma occurs about 45 minutes after the apparent recovery from the drug. This syndrome may occur owing to the fact that some of the fentanyl can become sequestered in the gastric fluid and then can become recycled into the plasma in about 45 minutes. Hence, in the PACU, all patients who have received fentanyl should be *continuously* monitored for respiratory depression for at least 1 hour from the time of admission to the unit.

Intraoperatively, fentanyl can be administered at three different dose ranges, depending on the type of surgery and the desired effect. For example, the low-dose range of 2 to 20 μg per kg attenuates moderately stressful stimuli. The moderate dose range is 20 to 50 μg per kg and strongly obtunds the stress response, and the megadose range of as much as 150 μg per kg blocks the stress response and is particularly valuable when protection of the myocardium is critical.

Fentanyl shares with most other narcotics a profound respiratory depressant effect, even to the point of apnea. Rapid intravenous injection can provoke bronchial constriction as well as resistance to ventilation caused by rigidity of the diaphragmatic and intercostal muscles. This is commonly referred to as the *fixed chest syndrome* and can occur when any potent narcotic analgesic is administered too rapidly by the intravenous route. Should this syndrome occur, intravenous succinylcholine (15 to 25 mg) will relieve the rigidity of the chest wall muscles. Once succinylcholine is administered for this purpose, the PACU nurse should be prepared to ventilate the patient until the skeletal muscle relaxant properties of succinylcholine subside.

Fentanyl, unlike most narcotics, has little or no hypotensive effects and usually does not cause nausea and vomiting. Because of its vagotonic effect, it may cause bradycardia, which can be relieved by atropine or glycopyrrolate. Fentanyl can be reversed by the narcotic antagonist naloxone, which also reverses analgesia. Should fentanyl be reversed by naloxone in the PACU, the PACU nurse should continue to monitor the patient for the possible return of respiratory depression, because the duration of the respiratory depression produced by the fentanyl may be longer than the duration of action of naloxone.

Fentanyl can be used alone in a nitrous-narcotic technique. It also is used in the PACU in the form of a low-dose intravenous drip for pain relief. Fentanyl is the narcotic portion of Innovar (see Chapter 14).

Sufentanil (Sufenta)

Sufentanil is an analogue of fentanyl and is approximately five to seven times as potent as fentanyl. Anesthesia with sufentanil can be in-

duced more rapidly, using basically the same technique as that used for fentanyl, without increasing the incidence of chest wall rigidity. However, sufentanil can produce chest wall rigidity, so if it is administered in the PACU, equipment for administering oxygen by positive pressure and the skeletal muscle relaxant succinylcholine should be on hand. The incidence of hypertension with sufentanil is lower than with comparable doses of fentanyl. Bradycardia is infrequently seen in patients who receive sufentanil, and when high-dose sufentanil is used in combination with nitrous oxide–oxygen, the mean arterial pressure and cardiac output may be decreased. The recovery time from sufentanil from the time of injection is about the same as with fentanyl. This is because sufentanil is very rapidly eliminated from tissue storage sites and, consequently, the duration of action of sufentanil is about the same as with fentanyl. Also, initial studies indicate that the incidence of postoperative hypertension, the need for vasoactive agents, and the requirements for postoperative analgesics are generally reduced in patients administered moderate or high doses of sufentanil as compared with patients given inhalation agents. Of particular interest to the PACU nurse is that sufentanil has an additive effect that is exhibited in patients receiving barbiturates, tranquilizers, other opioids, general anesthetics, or other CNS depressants. This is especially true of benzodiazepines, because they can potentiate a profound hypotensive action. Hence, when sufentanil is combined with any of these drugs, particular attention should be paid to any signs of decreased respiratory drive, increased airways resistance, and hypotension. Immediate countermeasures include maintaining a patent airway by proper positioning of the patient, by placement of an oral airway or endotracheal tube, and by the administration of oxygen. If indicated, naloxone should be employed as a specific antidote to manage the respiratory depression. The duration of respiratory depression following overdosage with sufentanil may be longer than the duration of action of the naloxone. Consequently, the patient should be constantly observed for the recurrence of respiratory depression, even after the initial successful treatment with naloxone. Hypotension can be treated with reversal with naloxone; however, fluids and vasopressors may be indicated (see Chapter 5).

Alfentanil (Alfenta)

Alfentanil is another analogue of fentanyl that is about one tenth as potent and has about one third the duration of action of fentanyl. The onset of action of this drug occurs in about 1 or 2 minutes, and the duration of action is 20 to 30 minutes. Alfentanil appears to have significant advantages over currently available opioid anesthetics. For example, it has no cumulative drug effects, and once the infusion of alfentanil is terminated, the emergence time is quite predictable. Alfentanil, like fentanyl, produces minimal hemodynamic effects and offers a high therapeutic index. In fact, the therapeutic index for alfentanil is higher than those of fentanyl and other opioids. A *therapeutic index* is the ratio of the lethal dose to the effective dose, and the higher the therapeutic index, the farther away the lethal dose is from the dose used to get the desired effect. More specifically, the therapeutic index of fentanyl is 270, which means that it is about four times safer than morphine. Alfentanil's therapeutic index is about 2.5 times more favorable than that of fentanyl.

Alfentanil, in addition to having a place in the operating room, may also have important uses in the PACU. Its rapid onset and very brief duration of action make it advantageous for the immediate pain relief needs of PACU patients. As previously stated, the drug has about one third the potency of fentanyl, but its onset of action is at least three times faster; its duration is one third that of fentanyl, and it has a high therapeutic index, making alfentanil well suited for pain relief in the immediate postoperative period. The drug produces few cardiovascular effects and thus should be of great value in the prevention of dangerous reflexes, such as tachycardia during intubation. Clinical observation indicates that the recovery time for this drug is extremely rapid. Hence, patients who receive this drug intraoperatively will most likely experience pain early in the *immediate* postoperative period, and the appropriate analgesic should be administered.

Pentazocine (Fortral; Talwin)

Pentazocine, an opioid agonist and antagonist analgesic, was first synthesized in 1959. The drug has significant activity and a low addiction potential. It is approximately one third as potent as morphine when given by the intramuscular route. It has an advantage over morphine in that it can be given by the oral route. It can be used preoperatively as well as postoperatively for the relief of pain from abdominal, cardiac, genitourinary, orthopedic, neurologic, and gynecologic surgery. The observed side effects of this drug include sedation, dizziness, nausea, and vomiting, but these occur infrequently.

Studies of the relative potency of this drug indicate that 30 mg of pentazocine is analgesically equivalent to 10 mg of morphine and 75 mg of meperidine. It has been established that pentazocine can relieve severe pain and is approximately two to four times less potent than morphine when administered parenterally.

Pentazocine can be used in the nitrous-narcotic technique. The respiratory depression produced by pentazocine is potentiated when general anesthetics are used concomitantly. Pentazocine produces an increase in systolic blood pressure and does not appear to have depressant effects on cardiac output. The drug should be used with caution in patients with renal or hepatic impairment. Pentazocine depresses the respiratory system in a manner comparable to morphine in equivalent analgesic doses. Tolerance to the analgesic effect of the drug does not appear to develop as it does with other narcotics. Because pentazocine is a narcotic antagonist at the mu receptors, administration of this drug to a patient who is dependent on opiates may induce abrupt withdrawal symptoms.

The onset of analgesic activity of pentazocine is approximately 2 or 3 minutes when it is given intravenously and 15 to 20 minutes when given intramuscularly. The duration of action is about 3 hours. When given orally, the drug is about one third as potent as when it is given intramuscularly.

Butorphanol (Stadol)

Butorphanol is a synthetic analgesic that is chemically related to the nalorphine-cyclazocine series with both narcotic and antagonist properties. More specifically, it serves as an agonist at the kappa and sigma opioid receptors. In regard to its analgesic potency, it is about 5 times more potent than morphine, 30 times more potent than meperidine, and 20 times more potent than pentazocine. Butorphanol can produce sedation, nausea, and respiratory depression. The respiratory depression is plateaulike in that 2 mg of butorphanol depresses respiration to a degree equal to 10 mg of morphine. The magnitude of respiratory depression with butorphanol is not appreciably increased at doses of 4 mg. The duration of the respiratory depression is dose related and is reversible by naloxone. Intravenous administration of butorphanol can produce increased pulmonary artery pressure, pulmonary wedge pressure, left-ventricular end-diastolic pressure, systemic arterial pressure, and pulmonary vascular resistance. Consequently, this drug increases the workload of the heart, especially in the pulmonary circuit. Because of its antagonist properties, butorphanol is not recommended for patients who are physically dependent on narcotics, because butorphanol can precipitate withdrawal symptoms in those patients. See Table 15–1 for an overview of the clinical pharmacology of butorphanol.

Nalbuphine (Nubain)

Nalbuphine is a potent analgesic with narcotic agonist and antagonist actions. It is chemically related to oxymorphone and naloxone. This drug is an antagonist at the mu receptors, a partial agonist at the kappa receptors, and an agonist at the sigma receptors. Nalbuphine is as potent as morphine and about three times as potent as pentazocine on a milligram basis. At a dose of 10 mg per kg, nalbuphine causes the same degree of respiratory depression as does 10 mg of morphine. At higher doses, nalbuphine exhibits the same plateau effect as butorphanol; that is, respiratory depression is not appreciably increased with higher doses. The respiratory depression that is produced by nalbuphine can be reversed by naloxone. Nalbu-

phine does not appear to increase the workload of the heart or to decrease cardiovascular stability. This drug has a lower abuse potential than does morphine, but if it is given to a patient who is physically dependent on narcotics, withdrawal symptoms may appear. Signs of withdrawal include abdominal cramps, nausea and vomiting, lacrimation, rhinorrhea, anxiety, restlessness, elevation of temperature, and piloerection. Should these symptoms appear after the injection of nalbuphine, the administration of small amounts of morphine can relieve the objective effects of the syndrome. See Table 15–1 for an overview of the clinical pharmacology of nalbuphine.

Dezocine (Dalgan)

Dezocine is a strong analgesic drug that has both agonist and antagonist activities. Its potency, onset, and duration of action are similar to those of morphine, and its analgesic effects appear to be at the mu opioid receptors. Dezocine produces a degree of respiratory depression similar to that of morphine when given in similar analgesic doses. Respiratory depression does not increase progressively in doses higher than 30 mg per kg. The depression of respiration produced by dezocine can be reversed by naloxone. The effects of dezocine on the cardiovascular system appear to be minimal.

Table 15–1. COMPARISON OF SEVEN ANALGESICS

	Morphine	Meperidine	Pentazocine	Butorphanol	Nalbuphine	Dezocine	Ketorolac
Indication	Moderate to severe pain	Moderate to severe pain	Moderate to severe pain	Moderate to severe pain	Moderate to severe pain	Moderate to severe pain	Moderate to severe pain
Recommended IM Dose	10 mg	25–50 mg	30 mg	2 mg	10 mg	5–15 mg	15–30 mg
Recommended IV Dose	4–10 mg	100 mg	30 mg	1 mg	10 mg	2.5–10 mg	Do not give IV
Time Required for Onset of Analgesia	Rapid IV 30 min IM	Rapid IV 30 min IM	Rapid IV 20 min IM	Rapid IV 30 min IM	Rapid IV 15 min IM	5–15 min IV 15–30 min IM	— 30–60 min IM
Duration of Analgesia	4 hr	2–4 hr	3–4 hr	3–4 hr	3–6 hr	2–3 hr	4–6 hr
Respiratory Depression	High	High	Occurs, but less than morphine	Occurs, but less than morphine	Occurs, but less than morphine	Occurs, but less than morphine	None
Cardiovascular Effect	Decreases cardiac workload	Decreases cardiac workload	Increases cardiac workload	Increases cardiac workload	Good cardiac stability	Good cardiac stability	Good cardiac stability
Abuse Potential	High	High	Occurs; induces withdrawal syndrome	Occurs; induces withdrawal syndrome	Occurs; induces withdrawal syndrome	Occurs; induces withdrawal syndrome	None

Adapted from Wood, M., and Wood, A.: Drugs and Anesthesia: Pharmacology for the Anesthesiologist. Baltimore, Williams & Wilkins, 1982.

Dezocine is available in three concentrations (5, 10, and 15 mg per ml) for either intravenous or intramuscular administration. For relief of postoperative pain, an intravenous dose of 2.5 to 10 mg can be used, and for the intramuscular route of administration, 5 to 15 mg is standard. The onset of analgesia is usually about 15 minutes for intravenous administration and 30 minutes for the intramuscular route. The peak analgesic effect and duration of action are about the same, regardless of the route of administration. Remedication with dezocine may be needed within 2 or 3 hours after its initial administration.

Dezocine should not be administered to patients who have developed a significant tolerance to opioid drugs from long-term use. This precaution is necessary because dezocine has some opioid antagonist properties, and if it is given to a patient who is physically dependent on narcotics, acute withdrawal symptoms can occur. Finally, because dezocine contains sodium metabisulfite, it should not be given to any patient who is allergic to this sulfite. In addition, asthmatics are more sensitive to sulfites than are nonasthmatics. Hence, an asthmatic patient with a strong allergy history probably should not receive this drug.

Buprenorphine (Buprenex)

Buprenorphine is a parenteral opiate analgesic with agonist-antagonist properties that is 30 times as potent as morphine sulfate. This drug is a derivative of the opium alkaloid thebaine and has a low abuse potential. It is proposed that the mechanism of action of buprenorphine involves the binding of the drug to the opiate receptors in the CNS. More specifically, this drug is a partial agonist at the mu opiate receptors. Buprenorphine at a dose of 0.3 mg has about the same respiratory depressant effect as 10 mg of morphine. This drug may cause a decrease or, rarely, an increase in pulse and blood pressure. Given by the intramuscular route of administration, the onset of analgesia is within 15 minutes, with a peak analgesic effect in 1 hour and a duration of 6 hours. When administered intravenously, the onset and peak times are shortened.

Of importance to the PACU nurse is the fact that the respiratory depressant effects of buprenorphine can be only partially reversed by naloxone. At present, there is no completely reliable specific antagonist available to reverse the respiratory depressant effects produced by buprenorphine. Consequently, patients who have been administered this drug should be assessed for respiratory depression for the next 6 hours. When a PACU patient is transferred, the nursing staff on the surgical units must be advised of the administration of and ramifications of the use of this drug.

Ketorolac (Toradol)

Ketorolac is an analgesic that is classified as a nonsteroidal anti-inflammatory drug (NSAID). Its mode of action is to inhibit the prostaglandin synthetase enzyme. Therefore, it has analgesic, anti-inflammatory, and antipyretic actions. On a dosage basis, 30 mg of this drug, given intramuscularly, is equal to about 12 mg of morphine or 100 mg of meperidine in degree of postoperative pain relief. This drug should *not* be administered intravenously and, hence, can be administered only by the intramuscular route. When it is used with supplemental opioids, ketorolac will afford excellent postoperative analgesia. For acute postoperative pain, an initial loading dose of 30 mg can be administered intramuscularly. Ketorolac can be administered every 6 hours thereafter at a dose of 15 mg. The duration of analgesia, but not the peak analgesic effect, is increased when the dose is increased beyond its recommended dosage range of 15 to 60 mg. Ketorolac should be given at a lower dose range for patients with renal disease, for the elderly (older than 70 years of age), and in patients weighing less than 50 kg. Because this drug is an NSAID and not an opioid, its lack of effect on psychomotor activities and on the respiratory system makes it an ideal analgesic for outpatient surgery.

Clinically, to take advantage of the peak effects of ketorolac, it is sometimes administered intramuscularly about 1 hour before the end of the surgical procedure. In this instance, the patient usually emerges from anesthesia in an analgesic state that lasts well into the immediate postoperative period. Hence, to effectively design an analgesic plan in the PACU, it is important for the post anesthesia nurse to determine if ketorolac was given intraoperatively so as to avoid analgesic overmedication.

The Narcotic Antagonists

Narcotic antagonists are used to reverse narcotic-induced respiratory depression. An opioid antagonist, such as naloxone, is a drug that completely antagonizes the effect of a narcotic. Drugs such as nalorphine (Nalline) and levallorphan (Lorfan) best typify the agonist-antagonists. These drugs partially reverse the effects of narcotics but also produce autonomic, endocrine, analgesic, and respiratory depressant effects similar to those of morphine.

Naloxone (Narcan)

Naloxone, a pure antagonist, reverses the depressant effects of narcotics. More specifically, this drug antagonizes the opioid effects at the mu, kappa, and sigma receptors. This drug also reverses the analgesic effect of the narcotic, which is important to remember when assessing the patient's respiratory effort. Naloxone should be titrated according to the patient's response. Usually, 0.1 to 0.2 mg given slowly intravenously should be adequate for reversal. The onset of action of naloxone is 1 or 2 minutes, and if after 3 to 5 minutes inadequate reversal has been achieved, naloxone administration may be repeated until reversal is complete. If the patient shows no sign of reversal, assessment of other pharmacologic agents administered is indicated. Drugs such as halothane, barbiturates, and muscle relaxants are not reversed by naloxone.

The duration of action of naloxone is 1 to 4 hours, depending on the route and amount of drug used. If long-acting narcotics were used, the patient must be monitored for respiratory embarrassment after the administration of naloxone, because the depressant activity of the narcotic may return. If this phenomenon occurs, supplemental doses of naloxone can be used. The intramuscular route of administration has been shown to produce a longer-lasting effect.

One adverse effect to watch for when an excessive dosage of naloxone is used is an increase in blood pressure that may be seen as a response to pain. Too-rapid reversal may induce nausea, vomiting, diaphoresis, or tachycardia. During the reversal procedure, the vital signs should be monitored, and naloxone should be used with caution in patients with cardiac irritability.

Naloxone does not produce respiratory depression as do other narcotic antagonists. It also does not produce any significant side effects or pupillary constriction. Naloxone reverses natural or synthetic narcotics, propoxyphene (Darvon), and the narcotic-antagonist analgesic pentazocine. Naloxone should be administered with great caution in patients who are physically dependent on opioids, because reversal may precipitate an acute withdrawal syndrome.

Naltrexone

Naltrexone is a pure mu receptor antagonist; therefore, its actions are similar to naloxone. This drug can be administered orally and can produce sustained opioid antagonist activity for as long as 24 hours.

Levallorphan (Lorfan)

Levallorphan is an agonist-antagonist of narcotic depression. It has essentially been replaced by naloxone. It acts as a narcotic antagonist in the presence of a strong narcotic effect. If used when no narcotic is present, respiratory depression may occur. It does not counteract mild respiratory depression and may in fact intensify it. Repeated doses decrease its effectiveness, and it eventually produces its own respiratory depression. Adverse reactions associated with levallorphan include dysphoria, miosis, drowsiness, nausea, and diaphoresis. It can also cause weird dreams, visual hallucinations, and disorientation.

SELECTED METHODS OF OPIOID ADMINISTRATION

Intrathecal and Epidural Routes of Administration

In an attempt to manage acute and chronic pain, the opioids can be administered via the subarachnoid or epidural space. The technique is called the *neuraxial* administration of opioids. This concept of pain relief is based on the fact that opioid receptors exist in the substantia gelatinosa on the dorsal horn of the spinal cord. More specifically, mu, kappa, and delta opioid receptors are located in the substantia gelatinosa. The pain relieved by the administration of neuraxial opioids is usually of the visceral as opposed to somatic type. When the opioid is administered via the epidural space, it crosses the epidural space to the opioid receptors in the spinal cord. Consequently, the dosage of the opioid, when administered into the epidural space, is usually 10 times the dosage of the opioid if it were to be administered via the subarachnoid space.

When 0.1 to 0.2 mg of preservative-free morphine (Duramorph) is administered into the subarachnoid space (intrathecal), the maximum concentration will be reached in about 5 to 10 minutes, with a duration of about 80 to 200 minutes. When morphine, 5 mg, is administered into the epidural space in the lumbar region, analgesia can last for as long as 24 hours. The patient should obtain pain relief in about 30 to 60 minutes after injection. If appropriate pain relief is not achieved, incremental doses of 1 to 2 mg can be administered. The maximum dose in a 24-hour period is 10 mg.

After spinal surgery, epidural morphine administered by the continuous epidural technique has both advantages and disadvantages. Its advantage is a profound degree of pain relief, especially for the first 12 to 18 hours postoperatively. However, disadvantages of this technique are related to displacement of the epidural catheter and the length of action of the epidural morphine. If the epidural catheter becomes displaced and the morphine has been injected, only partial pain relief ensues. Because of the possibility of profound respiratory depression, opioids must be administered cautiously. In fact, a nonopioid drug such as ketorolac may be especially useful in this circumstance. Depending on the anticipated amount and length of pain, a patient-controlled analgesia (PCA) device can be started on the patient and have an immediate result of pain resolution. Along with this, the post anesthesia nurse can have profound impact on reducing the pain threshold by repositioning and reassuring the patient. The new technology of apnea monitors can be quite useful to detect hypoventilation or apnea that can be created by the opioid in this technique. Hence, the use of the apnea monitor on patients receiving epidural morphine will certainly aid the post anesthesia nurse in monitoring for respiratory dysfunction.

Other opioids that can be administered epidurally are fentanyl and sufentanil. These drugs offer some advantages over morphine because they are more suited for continuous infusion techniques owing to their rapid onset and short duration of action. Also, because they have such a rapid clearance from the cere-

brospinal fluid, there is less chance for these drugs to spread toward the head (rostral spread). It has been demonstrated that rostral spread, which is associated more with morphine, produces side effects such as nausea, pruritus, and the previously discussed delayed respiratory depression syndrome. Naloxone reverses this side effect; however, the analgesic effect also is reversed. In this instance, nalbuphine administration should be considered to reverse the respiratory depression and preserve some of the analgesia.

Patient-Controlled Analgesia

To aid in the reduction of pain, the intramuscular injection of opioids and nonopioids has long been the standard route of administration used by nursing personnel. This method of administration has the advantage of simplicity and no requirement for specialized equipment. Its disadvantages include variable uptake, pain on injection, and patient dissatisfaction with the level of pain relief. Patient dissatisfaction is based on the cyclic effect of pain. If a level of analgesia were produced, the adverse effects of pain could be controlled. Intravenous administration offers some advantages over the intramuscular approach. The administration of an opioid via the intravenous route offers the patient an immediate reduction in pain. However, this reduction is only temporary because no appropriate blood level of the opioid has been established.

To achieve an appropriate level of analgesia, a "loading dose" followed by titration to effect, based on the pharmacokinetics of the opioid drug, is used intraoperatively. The maintenance of an appropriate blood level of the opioid to achieve and maintain a level of analgesia is the goal of this technique. The blood level of the drug is referred to as the *minimum*

Table 15–2. PROTOCOL FOR OPIOID ADMINISTRATION IN INTRAVENOUS PCA

Drug	Bolus Dose	Lockout (min)	Basal Rate/Hr*
Morphine	0.5–3 mg	6–10	0.5–2 mg
Meperidine (Demerol)	5–30 mg	6–10	5–20 mg
Hydromorphone (Dilaudid)	0.1–0.5 mg	6–10	0.1–0.3 mg
Fentanyl (Sublimaze)	15–75 µg	3–8	15–60 µg
Sufentanil (Sufenta)	2–10 µg	3–8	2–8 µg

*Basal rate is optional as the demand-only mode of PCA is often prescribed.
PCA = patient-controlled analgesia.
Adapted from Grass, J., and Harris, A.: Postcesarean section analgesia. Wellcome Trends Anesthesiol., 9(6):3–8, 1991.

Table 15–3. PROTOCOL FOR ADMINISTRATION OF FENTANYL* BY THE PCEA SYSTEM FOR POST-CESAREAN SECTION PATIENTS

	PACU	Surgical Unit	For Complaint of Pain
Bolus	100 µg	—	50–100 µg
Dose	40 µg	40 µg	50–60 µg
Lockout	10 min	10 min	10 min
Basal rate	60 µg/hr	60 µg/hr	60–80 µg/hr
Limit	260 µg/hr	260 µg/hr	310–380 µg/hr

*Mix fentanyl in 20 µg/ml solution.
PCEA = patient-controlled epidural analgesia.
Adapted from Grass, J., and Harris, A.: Postcesarean section analgesia. Wellcome Trends Anesthesiol., 9(6):3–8, 1991.

effective analgesic concentration (MEAC). Research has demonstrated that the MEAC is variable among individuals. Through the use of technology, the principles of this intraoperative technique have been continued into the immediate postoperative period. Intravenous PCA is the method of choice for those patients requiring continued analgesia. The peaks and valleys of analgesia can be avoided without the patient having to become totally dependent on the nurse's response for pain relief. PCA allows the patient more control of the situation by allowing him or her to "seek out" a particular level of analgesia—the MEAC.

In the PACU, the patient is administered a loading dose of the intravenous opioid to achieve the MEAC and then a PCA infusion pump is set up for the patient. The PCA pump is programmed for the administration of a particular opioid based on the patient's analgesic needs and the pharmacokinetics of the drug to be administered. The parameters to be programmed are the bolus dose, the lockout interval, and the low-dose continuous basal infusion rate. Consequently, by a "push of a

Table 15–4. PROTOCOL FOR ADMINISTRATION OF SUFENTANIL BY THE PCEA SYSTEM FOR POST-CESAREAN SECTION PATIENTS

	PACU	Surgical Unit	For Complaint of Pain
Bolus	30 µg	—	20 µg
Dose	8 µg	4 µg	8 µg
Lockout	10 min	10 min	10 min
Basal rate	6 µg/hr	6 µg/hr	6 µg/hr
Limit	46 µg/hr	26 µg/hr	26 µg/hr

PCEA = patient-controlled epidural analgesia.
Adapted from Grass, J., and Harris, A.: Postcesarean section analgesia. Wellcome Trends Anesthesiol., 9(6):3–8, 1991.

button" on the PCA pump, the patient can attain immediate analgesia and receive the benefits of controlled pain relief by low-dose continuous infusion of the opioid.

The amount of the *self-dose bolus* should be low so as to avoid an acute increase in blood levels of the drug above the MEAC because, along with the concern about overdosage, blood levels above the MEAC have no analgesic value. The *lockout interval*, or "delay," is the setting used to block the use of the self-dose bolus button for a period of time. During this time, the PCA pump does not deliver the drug, even when the patient pushes the button. The lockout interval is usually short, so the patient can self-administer small incremental doses to maintain his or her MEAC, yet the interval should be long enough to prevent overdosage. The *basal infusion rate* is usually set at a rate necessary to provide analgesia when the patient is resting. See Table 15–2 for a suggested protocol for drug administration in PCA.

Patient-Controlled Epidural Analgesia

The concept of PCA has been adapted to epidural analgesia. In this instance, the PCA infusion pump can be attached to the epidural catheter. The opioid drugs that can be used in this technique are fentanyl and sufentanil. They can be used with great success for analgesia after cesarean section. The basal infusion rate keeps the patient analgesic and comfortable. The patient can self-administer a bolus of the opioid if the analgesia provided by the basal infusion rate is not sufficient. Also, the bolus opioid facilitates additional analgesia needed for turning and early ambulation. A suggested protocol for both fentanyl and sufentanil is provided in Tables 15–3 and 15–4. Because of the possibility of rostral spread, it is suggested that an apnea monitor be used on patients who are receiving patient-controlled epidural analgesia.

References

1. Barash, P., Cullen, B., and Stoelting, R.: Clinical Anesthesia. 2nd ed. Philadelphia, J. B. Lippincott, 1992.
2. Butterworth, J.: Atlas of Procedures in Anesthesia and Critical Care. Philadelphia, W. B. Saunders, 1992.
3. Drug Evaluations, Annual 1991. Milwaukee, American Medical Association, 1991.
4. Estafanous, F.: Opioids in anesthesia: II. Symposia Reporter, 13(5):3–4, 1989.
5. Grass, J., and Harris, A.: Postcesarean section analgesia. Wellcome Trends Anesthesiol., 9(6):3–8, 1991.
6. Gilman, A., Rall, T., Nies, A., et al.: Goodman and

Gilman's The Pharmacological Basis of Therapeutics. 8th ed. New York, Pergamon Press, 1990.

7. Jacobsen, W.: Manual of Post Anesthesia Care. Philadelphia, W. B. Saunders, 1992.
8. Katzung, B. (ed.): Basic and Clinical Pharmacology. 2nd ed. Los Altos, Lange Medical Publications, 1984.
9. Miller, R. (ed.): Anesthesia. 3rd ed. New York, Churchill Livingstone, 1990.
10. Spindler, J., Mehlisch, D., and Brown, C.: Intramuscular ketorolac and morphine in the treatment of moderate to severe pain after major surgery. Pharmacotherapy, 10:51S–58S, 1990.
11. Stoelting, R.: Pharmacology and Physiology in Anesthetic Practice. 2nd ed. Philadelphia, J. B. Lippincott, 1991.
12. Vogelsang, J., and Hayes, S.: Butorphanol tartrate (Stadol): A review. J. Post Anesth. Nurs., 6(2):129–135, 1991.
13. Waugaman, W., Foster, S., and Rigor, B.: Principles and Practice of Nurse Anesthesia. 2nd ed. Norwalk, CT, Appleton & Lange, 1992.
14. White, P.: What's New in Intravenous Anesthesia. 1990 International Anesthesia Research Society Review Course Lectures. Cleveland, IARS, 105–114, 1990.
15. Wood, M., and Wood, A.: Drugs and Anesthesia: Pharmacology for the Anesthesiologist. 2nd ed. Baltimore, Williams & Wilkins, 1990.

CHAPTER 16

Muscle Relaxants

Neuromuscular blocking agents, or muscle relaxants, have been used in clinical anesthesia since the early 1940s. Significant advances have been made in understanding the physiology of neuromuscular transmission and the pharmacology of muscle relaxants, which have contributed greatly to clinical anesthesia as it is now practiced. Muscle relaxants are not used exclusively in the field of anesthesia; in post anesthesia (PACU) and intensive care units and in emergency department settings, these drugs may be required to enhance patient care.

Muscle relaxants are used (1) to facilitate endotracheal intubation; (2) for procedures requiring muscle relaxation, such as intraperitoneal and thoracic surgery; (3) in ophthalmic surgery to relax the extraocular muscles; (4) to terminate laryngospasm and eliminate chest wall rigidity, which may occur after rapid intravenous injection of a potent narcotic; and (5) to facilitate mechanical ventilation by producing total paralysis of the respiratory muscles.

PHYSIOLOGY OF NEUROMUSCULAR TRANSMISSION

Because of the frequent and routine intraoperative and postoperative use of drugs that alter the patient's neuromuscular function, it is important to review the anatomy and physiology of the neuromuscular system, with emphasis on the chemical changes that occur at the receptor sites.

Activation of skeletal muscle is both an electrical and a biochemical event. The term *conduction* refers to the passage of an impulse along an axon to a muscle fiber. *Transmission* applies to passage of a neurotransmitter substance across a synaptic cleft (neuromuscular junction). The combined electrical and chemical event is called *neurohumoral transmission*.

As the fine terminal branch of a motor neuron approaches the muscle fiber, it loses its myelin sheath and forms an expanded terminal that lies close to a specialized area of muscle membrane called the *end plate* (Fig. 16–1). Between the end of the muscle fiber and the end plate is the synaptic cleft or neuromuscular junction. This space between the nerve and muscle fibers is about 20 nm wide. *Acetylcholine* is the biochemical neurotransmitter involved in the initiation of muscle contraction. *Acetylcholine* or *cholinergic receptors* are classified as either nicotinic or muscarinic, respectively. The acetylcholine receptors are stimulated by acetylcholine. Anticholinesterase drugs such as neostigmine (Prostigmin), edrophonium chloride (Tensilon; Enlon), and pyridostigmine (Regonol) produce an increase in acetylcholine at the acetylcholine receptor. Therefore, the pharmacologic effects of the anticholinesterase drugs are on both the nicotinic and muscarinic receptors. The *nicotinic receptors* are further classified as either N_1 or N_2 receptors. The N_1 receptors are located at the autonomic ganglia, and the N_2 receptors are situated on the postsynaptic cleft in the neuromuscular junction. It is the nondepolarizing neuromuscular blocking agents such as pancuronium (Pavulon) that produce a block of the N_2 receptor—causing skeletal muscle paralysis. The *muscarinic receptors* are also subdivided into M_1 and M_2 receptors. M_1 receptors are located in the autonomic ganglia and the central nervous system, and the M_2 receptors are located in the heart and salivary glands. It should be noted that atropine and glycopyrrolate (Robinul) block both the M_1 and M_2 receptors.

Acetylcholine is formed in the body of the nerve cell and the cytoplasm of the nerve terminal and is stored in the small, membrane-enclosed *vesicles* for subsequent release. A *quantum* is the amount of acetylcholine stored in each vesicle and represents about 10,000 molecules of acetylcholine. The presynaptic membrane contains discrete areas of specialization that are thought to be sites of release of the transmitter. These presynaptic "active zones" lie directly opposite the N_2 cholinergic receptors, which are located on the postsynaptic membrane. This alignment ensures that the

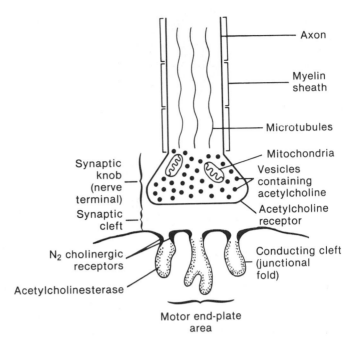

FIGURE 16–1. The myoneural junction at resting state.

Labels (clockwise from top right): Axon — Myelin sheath — Microtubules — Mitochondria — Vesicles containing acetylcholine — Acetylcholine receptor — Conducting cleft (junctional fold)

Labels (left side, top to bottom): Synaptic knob (nerve terminal) — Synaptic cleft — N_2 cholinergic receptors — Acetylcholinesterase

Motor end-plate area

acetylcholine diffuses directly to the N_2 receptors on the postsynaptic membrane quickly and in a high concentration. The N_2 receptor, which responds to the neurotransmitter acetylcholine, is a glycoprotein that is an integral part of the postsynaptic membrane of the neuromuscular junction (see Fig. 16–1). New evidence indicates that a positive feedback mechanism also exists at the neuromuscular junction. Acetylcholine has a presynaptic action and, hence, acetylcholine receptors are located on the presynaptic membrane. This positive feedback mechanism enhances the mobilization and release of acetylcholine. Finally, the enzyme that hydrolyzes acetylcholine is *acetylcholinesterase,* which is located in the neuromuscular junction.

The initiation of skeletal muscle contraction occurs as a result of application of a *threshold stimulus.* An action potential traveling down the axon causes *depolarization* of the presynaptic membrane. As a result of this depolarization, the membrane permeability for calcium ions is increased and the calcium enters, or influxes, into the presynaptic membrane. Calcium acts to unite the vesicle to the presynaptic membrane and causes the rupture of that coalesced membrane, releasing acetylcholine into the fluid of the synaptic cleft (Fig. 16–2).

The acetylcholine molecules released from the nerve terminal into the synaptic cleft are subject to two main processes: (1) attachment to N_2 cholinergic receptors located on the postsynaptic membrane, leading to an opening of calcium channels that results in the movement of sodium into the region, which generates an end-plate potential (EPP), and (2) attachment of acetylcholine to the presynaptic nicotinic receptor, which enhances the release of more acetylcholine. When enough EPPs are generated, an action potential will be propagated and will spread throughout the muscle and cause a change in the ionic permeability of the muscle sarcolemma. This process results in the release of calcium from the sarcoplasmic reticulum with a resultant increase in free calcium concentration in the muscle fiber. The process of *excitation-contraction (E-C) coupling* then takes place within that skeletal muscle cell. The physiologic outcome of E-C coupling is the contraction of the skeletal muscle. The increased concentration of calcium in the muscle fiber leads to an interaction between troponin-tropomyosin and actin. This interaction causes the active sites on actin to be exposed and interact with myosin and slide together, resulting in muscle contraction. This sliding of actin and myosin is sometimes referred to as the *ratchet effect.* The contraction of the muscle fibers is terminated when calcium is pumped back into the sarcoplasmic reticulum of the muscle fibers. The calcium is stored in the sarcoplasmic reticulum to be used when another action potential is generated.

Regulation and control of skeletal muscle contraction are also based on the enzymatic breakdown of acetylcholine. As previously discussed, the stimulus must be strong enough to

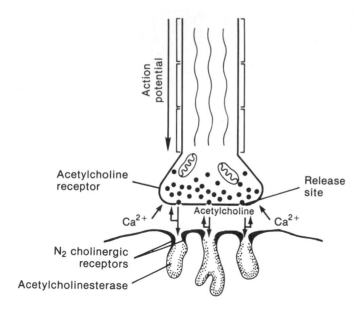

FIGURE 16–2. The myoneural junction when a threshold stimulus is applied.

release enough acetylcholine to bind to the postsynaptic N_2 cholinergic receptor. This process of competition between the postsynaptic N_2 receptor and acetylcholinesterase allows for some degree of regulation of the excitation process and for the recovery of the muscle cell membrane. The molecules of acetylcholine either diffuse in a random fashion to the N_2 receptor or are destroyed by acetylcholinesterase. As the concentration gradient begins to decrease owing to the destruction of acetylcholine by acetylcholinesterase, the N_2 receptor gives up its acetylcholine, which is then destroyed, and the skeletal muscle relaxes. A small portion of the acetylcholine can escape the acetylcholinesterase in the synaptic cleft and migrate into the extracellular fluid and from there into the plasma. Acetylcholine within the plasma is then destroyed by plasma acetylcholinesterase, or pseudocholinesterase, which is produced in the liver.

PHARMACOLOGIC OVERVIEW OF THE SKELETAL MUSCLE RELAXANTS

With the anatomy and physiology of neuromuscular transmission as a background, the principal pharmacologic actions of the nondepolarizing and depolarizing skeletal muscle relaxants will be discussed. Table 16–1 presents a pharmacologic overview of the commonly used skeletal muscle relaxants.

The prototypical nondepolarizing skeletal muscle relaxants are pancuronium and d-tubo-

curarine (curare). Pancuronium is an inhibitor of acetylcholine, is chemically viewed as two acetylcholine-like fragments, and has a bulky, inflexible nucleus. This drug attaches to the N_2 cholinergic receptors on the postsynaptic membrane and prevents depolarization. The skeletal muscle relaxant d-tubocurarine has the chemical structure of a monoquaternary compound. The principal pharmacologic action of this drug is to block the postsynaptic N_2 cholinergic receptor; in this way it stops acetylcholine from binding to the receptor, resulting in a competitive neuromuscular blockade. The nondepolarizing skeletal muscle relaxants also block the presynaptic cholinergic receptor, resulting in binding of the acetylcholine and thereby preventing activation of the positive feedback mechanism.

The pharmacologic actions of the nondepolarizing skeletal muscle relaxants can be reversed by anticholinesterase drugs such as neostigmine. In effect, these drugs increase the quantum of acetylcholine at the postsynaptic membrane by preventing destruction of the acetylcholine by acetylcholinesterase. This promotes a more effective competition by the released acetylcholine with the nondepolarizing skeletal muscle relaxant that is occupying the N_2 receptor. Because of the increased availability and mobilization of the acetylcholine, the concentration gradients favor acetylcholine and remove the nondepolarizing agents from the N_2 receptor, with the resultant return to normal contraction of the skeletal muscle.

The principal depolarizing skeletal muscle relaxant is succinylcholine (Anectine; Sucostrin). The molecular structure of this drug re-

Table 16-1. PHARMACOLOGIC OVERVIEW OF THE COMMONLY USED SKELETAL MUSCLE RELAXANTS

	Atracurium Besylate (Tracrium)	Pancuronium (Pavulon)	Vecuronium (Norcuron)	Doxacurium Chloride (Nuromax)	Pipecuronium Bromide (Arduan)	Mivacurium Chloride (Mivacron)	d-Tubocurarine	Metocurine (Metubine)	Succinylcholine (Anectine)
Nondepolarizing	Yes	Yes	Yes	Yes	Yes	Yes	Yes	Yes	No
Depolarizing	No	No	No	No	No	No	No	No	Yes
Intubation dose (IV mg/kg)	0.4–0.5	0.06–0.1	0.08–0.1	0.05–0.08	0.07–0.085	0.15	0.6	0.25–0.4	0.5–1.0
Intubation time (injection to relaxation in min)	2–2.5	4	2.5–3	4–5	2.5–3	2	6–8 (rarely used for intubation)	4	<1.0
Muscle relaxation dose (IV mg/kg)	0.2–0.5	0.04–0.08	0.05–0.06	0.025–0.08	0.05	0.15–2.0	0.3	0.2–0.3	0.1–0.2 mg/kg (IV drip)
Recovery time (min)	30–45	84–114		60–160	50–150	12–15	74–87	94–117	4–6
Reversible?	Yes	Yes	Yes	Yes	Yes	Yes	Yes	Yes	No
When? (in min after initial dose)	20–35	40–60	25–30 (for 0.1 mg/kg) 40–80 (for 0.2 mg/kg)	20–30	10–20	8–11	40–60	45–60	
Cumulative effects?	No	Yes	Slight	Yes	Yes	Slight	Yes	Yes	No
Fasciculations and muscle soreness	No	No	No	No	No	No	No	No	Yes
Risk of histamine release	Minimal	Slight to none	None	No	No	Yes	Significant	Moderate	Possible
Cardiovascular effects	Few	Slight ↑ in pulse and ↑ BP	None	None	None	Minimal	Hypotension	None	Slight ↓ in pulse

BP = blood pressure; IV = intravenous.

229

sembles two acetylcholine molecules back to back. Because of this structure, succinylcholine has the same effects as acetylcholine. Like acetylcholine, the succinylcholine molecule has a quaternary ammonium portion that is positively charged. This positively charged molecule is attracted by electrostatic action to the negatively charged N_2 receptor. Once the succinylcholine attaches to the receptor, a brief period of depolarization occurs that is manifested by transient muscular fasciculations. Succinylcholine also attaches to and activates the presynaptic acetylcholine receptor. This activation has an immediate effect of increased mobilization of acetylcholine in the motor nerve terminals. This explains why fasciculations are commonly observed after the administration of an intravenous bolus of succinylcholine. After the depolarization of the N_2 receptor takes place, succinylcholine promotes and maintains the receptor in a depolarized state and prevents repolarization. Succinylcholine has a brief duration of action because of its rapid hydrolysis of the succinylcholine by the enzyme pseudocholinesterase, contained in the liver and plasma. *The actions of succinylcholine cannot be pharmacologically reversed.*

NONDEPOLARIZING NEUROMUSCULAR BLOCKING AGENTS

Long-Acting Nondepolarizing Skeletal Muscle Relaxants

Tubocurarine Chloride (d-Tubocurarine Chloride; Curare)

d-Tubocurarine chloride was first known as an arrow poison used by South American Indians. *d*-Tubocurarine blocks access of acetylcholine to the N_2 receptor at the neuromuscular junction of skeletal muscle. The action is a combination of electrical and chemical transmission, with *d*-tubocurarine preventing depolarization by impeding leakage of the sodium ions necessary for depolarization.

The peak action of *d*-tubocurarine occurs 30 to 60 minutes after intravenous injection. Fifty to 70 percent of injected *d*-tubocurarine is excreted unchanged in the urine within 3 to 6 hours. In spite of this, the duration of action of *d*-tubocurarine is not unduly prolonged, even in the complete absence of renal function.

Side effects or variations in response to *d*-tubocurarine include histamine-like reaction, hypotension, increased airways resistance, and skin erythema. Consequently, asthmatic patients and those with a history of allergic reactions should receive a relaxant other than *d*-tubocurarine. *d*-Tubocurarine's ganglionic blocking action coupled with its histamine-like actions can cause hypotension in many patients.

Pancuronium Bromide (Pavulon)

Pancuronium bromide was introduced into clinical anesthesia in 1972. This drug has demonstrated value, particularly in terms of its safety, cardiovascular stability, and skeletal muscle relaxant properties, and is receiving widespread clinical usage.

Chemically, pancuronium bromide is a biquaternary aminosteroid and is related to the androgens; however, it has no hormonal activities. Pancuronium's action is similar to but five times more potent than the action of *d*-tubocurarine. Also, like *d*-tubocurarine, pancuronium is reversible by an anticholinesterase agent, such as neostigmine, that is administered in combination with an anticholinergic such as glycopyrrolate or atropine. It has been demonstrated clinically that this particular skeletal muscle relaxant is extremely difficult to reverse pharmacologically within the first 20 to 30 minutes after injection. In the PACU, if a skeletal muscle relaxant is required for a short duration, another reversible skeletal muscle relaxant, such as *d*-tubocurarine or atracurium, should be chosen. About 30 to 40 minutes after injection, pancuronium is easily reversed by the combination of an anticholinesterase and anticholinergic drug preparation. Pancuronium is best suited for surgical procedures lasting more than 1 hour. It is well suited for patients who require complete muscle relaxation when receiving continuous mechanical ventilation. The dosage for adults is approximately 0.08 to 0.1 mg per kg of body weight. Relaxation lasts 60 to 85 minutes. If relaxation is required past this initial period, subsequent doses should be decreased to 0.02 to 0.04 mg per kg of body weight.

Pancuronium bromide does not produce ganglionic blockade, but it does block the M_2 cholinergic receptors in the heart. Consequently, when pancuronium bromide is administered, a slight 10 to 15 percent increase in heart rate will be observed. Pancuronium activates the sympathetic nervous system by promoting the release of norepinephrine and blocking its uptake at the adrenergic nerve endings. Hence, after administration of this drug, a modest increase in mean arterial pressure and cardiac output will be produced. Although isolated cases of histamine release have been reported, pancuronium can probably be used in patients who have a marginal allergy history. Pancuronium bromide is compatible with anesthetic agents used clinically and is safe to use in most patients when a nondepolarizing skeletal muscle relaxant is indicated. However, pancuronium bromide is not indicated when a nondepolarizing muscle relaxant is to be used with caution. In addition, pancuronium should not be used in patients who are receiving chronic digitalis therapy because cardiac dysrhythmias have been reported. Finally, myocardial ischemia has been reported in patients with coronary artery disease when pancuronium is used. This ischemia is probably associated with the cardiac acceleration properties of the drug.

Pancuronium bromide should be avoided in patients with a history of myasthenia gravis. It is contraindicated in patients with true renal disease, because a major portion of the drug is excreted unchanged in the urine. This agent is contraindicated in patients known to be hypersensitive to it or to the bromide ion.

Gallamine (Flaxedil)

Gallamine, the first synthetic skeletal muscle relaxant, was introduced into clinical anesthesia practice 6 years after d-tubocurarine was initially used. This nondepolarizing skeletal muscle relaxant has been shown to be one fifth as potent as d-tubocurarine, with a 25 percent shorter duration of action. In clinical doses, gallamine blocks the M_2 cholinergic receptors (much like the muscarinic cholinergic blocking effects of atropine), which results in tachycardia. This property has been used to advantage when the drug is combined with halothane (Fluothane), which is normally a vagal stimulant. However, gallamine activates the sympathetic nervous system and also blocks the M_2 receptors. This leads to an imbalance in the autonomic nervous system in favor of the sympathetic nervous system. Ultimately, cardiac dysrhythmias can ensue following the administration of gallamine. Gallamine is excreted entirely unchanged by the kidneys, which explains reports of prolonged action of the drug in patients with poor renal function.

Metocurine Iodide (Metubine)

Metocurine, which was introduced into clinical anesthesia practice in 1948 as dimethyl-tubocurarine, is now regaining popularity.

Metocurine is a nondepolarizing neuromuscular blocking agent that is a trimethylated derivative of d-tubocurarine and, like d-tubocurarine, is quite reversible by the drug combination of an anticholinesterase and an anticholinergic. The dosage for surgical relaxation is 0.2 mg per kg, and to facilitate endotracheal intubation, a dosage of 0.3 to 0.4 mg per kg is required. It is about one or two times as potent as d-tubocurarine in neuromuscular blocking potency and yet is less potent than d-tubocurarine in its ability to inhibit autonomic responses and to release histamine. Consequently, the clinical cardiovascular and hemodynamic effects of metocurine seem to be much less than those of d-tubocurarine. Because metocurine produces minimal hemodynamic changes, it is useful in patients with hypertension and coronary artery disease.

Doxacurium (Nuromax)

Doxacurium is a long-acting nondepolarizing neuromuscular blocking agent. It is similar to pancuronium in its length of action and dependence on appropriate renal function for clearance, but it is twice as potent as pancuronium. It is similar to atracurium in chemical structure. It has no histamine-releasing properties, nor does it have any significant effect on the cardiovascular system; consequently, it offers excellent cardiovascular stability. The onset of action for the drug is about 4 to 9 minutes, with a duration of action of about 80 to 160 minutes that is potentiated by the inhalation anesthetics, particularly halothane. The dosage range for doxacurium is between 0.02 and 0.03 mg per kg for surgical relaxation and 0.05 to 0.08 mg per kg for facilitation of endotracheal intubation. Neostigmine 0.05 mg per kg as opposed to edrophonium should be used to reverse the neuromuscular blockade produced by doxacurium.

Doxacurium can be used in patients with liver failure with any change in onset and duration of action. In patients with renal failure, the time of onset is essentially the same; however, the duration is prolonged by about 30 minutes. Doxacurium can be used in the elderly patient, because the time of onset and duration of action is about the same as in the younger population. Finally, doxacurium does not appear to be a trigger agent for malignant hyperthermia, and for patients on mechanical ventilation in the PACU requiring a long-acting neuromuscular blocking agent, this drug would prove to be an excellent choice.

Pipecuronium Bromide (Arduan)

Pipecuronium is a long-acting nondepolarizing neuromuscular blocking agent with a chemical structure similar to pancuronium and vecuronium. The drug does not cause the release of histamine, nor does it have the circulatory side effects of tachycardia or hypotension. The dosage is 0.07 to 0.085 mg per kg. It has an onset of action of about 2 or 3 minutes, with a duration of action from 50 to 150 minutes. The neuromuscular blocking effects of the drug are prolonged more by isoflurane (Forane), followed by halothane, and lastly by nitrous-narcotic techniques. Pipecuronium can usually be reversed 10 minutes after it has been injected. For this particular drug, neostigmine is the preferred anticholinesterase-reversing drug. Because the kidney is its primary route of excretion, pipecuronium should not be used in patients with renal failure. This drug is more potent and shorter acting in infants than in children and adults.

Intermediate-Acting Nondepolarizing Skeletal Muscle Relaxants

Atracurium Besylate (Tracrium)

Atracurium is a nondepolarizing skeletal muscle relaxant that offers an advantage over other skeletal muscle relaxants in that it does not depend on renal or hepatic mechanisms for its elimination. In fact, this quaternary ammonium compound breaks down in the absence of plasma enzymes through what is called *Hofmann elimination* and, to a lesser extent, through ester hydrolysis. Hofmann elimination is a nonbiologic method of degradation that occurs at a physiologic temperature and pH.

Atracurium is less potent than pancuronium and has a rapid onset of 1 to 3 minutes and a duration of action of about 30 to 45 minutes. To facilitate endotracheal intubation in the PACU setting, 0.3 to 0.5 mg per kg of atracurium should provide adequate skeletal muscle relaxation for intubation in about 2.5 minutes. To maintain mechanical ventilation in the PACU setting, an infusion rate of 10 μg per kg per min of atracurium may be used. Once the infusion has been discontinued, spontaneous ventilation by the patient will occur in about 30 minutes. The effects can be reversed with a combination of anticholinesterase and antimuscarinic in about 12 to 15 minutes after the discontinuation of the atracurium infusion.

Atracurium has many distinct advantages, such as not having its neuromuscular blockade prolonged by renal failure or impaired hepatic function. Also, it has little or no cumulative effect and is not influenced significantly by the specific general inhalation anesthetic dosage or concentration. Finally, this drug has little or no cardiovascular effect and is easily antagonized by the combination of an anticholinesterase and an anticholinergic.

Vecuronium Bromide (Norcuron)

Vecuronium is a nondepolarizing skeletal muscle relaxant with a more rapid onset of action and shorter duration of action than pancuronium has. Actually, vecuronium is pancuronium without the quaternary methyl group in the steroid nucleus. Because of this structural difference, vecuronium has no effect on heart rate, arterial pressure, autonomic ganglia, or the alpha and beta adrenal receptors. The potency of vecuronium is equal to, or slightly greater than, that of pancuronium. Vecuronium has little or no cumulative effect. Although a portion of vecuronium is metabolized, most of the drug is excreted unchanged in the urine and bile. However, the neuromuscular blockade produced by vecuronium is not prolonged by renal failure. The duration of neuromuscular blockade produced by vecuronium is increased in patients with impaired hepatic function. It is of clinical interest that vecuronium, like atracurium, is less influenced by general inhalation anesthetics than are pancuronium and *d*-tubocurarine. The pharmacologic action of this drug is easily reversed by the combination of an anticholinesterase and an anticholinergic drug.

The onset of action of vecuronium is between 2.5 and 3 minutes, using the "normal" dosage of 0.08 mg per kg intravenously. Because of the rapid onset of action, vecuronium can be used for rapid-sequence intubation. In this instance, doubling the dosage of vecuronium to 0.2 mg per kg can achieve intubation conditions within 45 seconds to 2 minutes. Another method for using vecuronium for intubation is the "priming" technique. The object of this technique is to administer a small priming dose of vecuronium several minutes before the intubation dose is given to shorten the onset of neuromuscular blockade. The usual priming dose is 0.015 mg per kg, and after 3 minutes an intubation dose of 0.1 mg per kg is administered. The onset of neuromuscular blockade should be between 70 and 90 seconds. The main drawback of this technique is that some patients may develop symptoms of partial neuromuscular blockade. Sensations reported are heavy eyelids, blurred vision, and difficulty in swallowing. Therefore, if this technique is used in the PACU, the nurse should warn patients of the possible symptoms, and ventilatory support should always be available.

Because of concerns about the priming technique, the "timing" technique was developed. In the timing technique, which is used mainly in the operating room, the patient is given vecuronium before sodium pentothal. Consequently, the induction of anesthesia is specifically timed to the onset of clinical muscular weakness. In this technique, the patient is given 0.1 to 0.2 mg per kg of vecuronium, and at the onset of weakness, as determined by the peripheral nerve simulator, a 4 mg per kg bolus dose of sodium pentothal is given. Intubating conditions occur within 1 minute.

Short-Acting Nondepolarizing Skeletal Muscle Relaxants

Mivacurium Chloride (Mivacron)

Mivacurium is a skeletal muscle relaxant that was introduced into clinical practice in 1992. Research has demonstrated that this drug has a shorter duration of action than any other currently approved nondepolarizing agent. Thus, mivacurium may be suitable for providing skeletal muscle relaxation in surgical cases of short duration or for intubation when succinylcholine is not desirable. To facilitate good to excellent intubating conditions within 1.5 minutes, mivacurium can be given intravenously using the divided dose technique at a dose of 0.15 mg per kg; then, 30 seconds later, a second dose of 0.10 mg per kg should be given. Oxygen via bag-valve-mask system should be administered to the patient from the time of injection of mivacurium to the time of intubation. When mivacurium is administered in a bolus fashion, cutaneous flushing and arterial hypotension caused by systemic release of histamine have been reported. The average time of recovery from the drug is between 12 and 17 minutes after the last dose is given. Spontaneous recovery from mivacurium can occur without the use of reversal agents. However, if reversal agents are used, the recovery time is usually between 8 and 11 minutes.

Mivacurium is metabolized by pseudocholinesterase, which explains its short duration of action. Given in doses of 0.1 mg per kg or smaller, mivacurium does not cause facial flushing, hemodynamic changes, or histamine release. This skeletal muscle relaxant offers certain advantages over succinylcholine, such as its relative rapid rate of onset and short duration of action, its reversibility, and its approval for use in children and adolescents.

Alcuronium Chloride (Alloferin)

Alcuronium, which is chemically related to d-tubocurarine, is a new nondepolarizing skeletal muscle relaxant. It is about twice as potent as and much shorter in duration than d-tubocurarine. Administration of 0.2 mg per kg of alcuronium can produce muscular relaxation in 2 to 4 minutes that lasts about 20 minutes. Alcuronium is also reversible by combining an anticholinesterase and an anticholinergic drug. It produces about the same degree of hypotension as does d-tubocurarine and causes about the same amount of histamine release as does pancuronium. Because alcuronium is not metabolized and is excreted unchanged by the kidneys, it should be used with caution in patients with any type of renal dysfunction.

Rocuronium Bromide (Zemuron)

Rocuronium is a new nondepolarizing skeletal muscle relaxant with a chemical structure related to vecuronium. It has a rapid onset (1 to 1.5 minutes) and a short duration of action of 12 to 30 minutes. At a dose of 0.6 mg per kg, rocuronium provides excellent intubating conditions.

Rocuronium can be used in patients with renal failure and has a low potential for histamine release. Its actions are prolonged in patients with cirrhosis of the liver. Along with this, rocuronium's muscle relaxant actions are potentiated by the inhalation anesthetics.

Because rocuronium produces minimal cardiovascular effects and has such a fast onset and short duration of action, it is useful in intraoperative and postoperative periods.

Reversal of Nondepolarizing Neuromuscular Blocking Agents

To restore neuromuscular transmission, the antagonist must displace the competitive neuromuscular blocking agent from the nicotinic receptor sites and open the way for depolarization of the postjunctional membrane. The antagonist is an antiacetylcholinesterase that blocks the enzymatic action of acetylcholinesterase located in the postsynaptic clefts so that acetylcholine is not hydrolyzed. The result is a buildup of acetylcholine at the end plate at the N_2 cholinergic receptor. The accumulated acetylcholine displaces the competitive neuromuscular blocking agent, which diffuses back into the plasma, re-establishing neuromuscular transmission.

Neostigmine and pyridostigmine are usually the anticholinesterase drugs of choice because of their long duration of action and reliability as compared with edrophonium chloride. However, research has demonstrated that edrophonium chloride is an effective reversal agent of neuromuscular blockades produced by vecuronium and atracurium. Atropine or glycopyrrolate, both antimuscarinic (anticholinergic) drugs, can be administered immediately before, or in conjunction with, the anticholinesterase to minimize the muscarinic effects of the anticholinesterase drug. The muscarinic effects include bradycardia, salivation, miosis, and hyperperistalsis. These effects are produced at lower concentrations of the anticholinesterase-type drug when administered (acetylcholine nicotinic effects are at the autonomic ganglia and the neuromuscular junction). Consequently, when an anticholinesterase drug is administered to reverse the nondepolarizing neuromuscular blocking agent at the N_2 receptor, an antimuscarinic drug is also given to prevent the adverse muscarinic cholinergic effects associated with the high dosage of anticholinesterase. Generally, 2.5 mg of neostigmine is the maximum dose required for reversal; however, the suggested limit is 5 mg. The method is to give atropine, 0.4 mg, or glycopyrrolate, 0.2 mg intravenously, over a 1-minute period, to observe for an increase in pulse rate, and then to administer 0.5 mg neostigmine intravenously and monitor the reversal. This procedure can be repeated until reversal has been achieved or until the limit of neostigmine that can be given is reached. If edrophonium chloride is indicated for reversal, the dosage is 0.5 mg per kg with 0.007 mg per kg of atropine.

Neostigmine should be administered cautiously. Cardiac monitoring is essential, especially in elderly or debilitated patients and in patients with cardiac disease. Atrioventricular dissociation and other dysrhythmias can be initiated by the anticholinesterases.

Pyridostigmine is an analogue of neostigmine. It facilitates the transmission of impulses across the myoneural junction by inhibiting the destruction of acetylcholine by acetylcholinesterase. Clinical data indicate a lower incidence of muscarinic side effects with this drug than

with neostigmine. Like neostigmine, pyridostigmine should be administered with caution in patients with bronchial asthma or cardiac problems. Signs of overdosage are related to muscarinic and nicotinic receptor stimulation (Table 16–2). The muscarinic side effects are blocked with atropine or glycopyrrolate. Nicotinic responses can be blocked by drugs such as ganglionic or neuromuscular blocking agents. The recommended dosage for reversal is 0.15 mg per kg of intravenous pyridostigmine, in combination with 0.007 mg per kg of intravenous atropine. Full recovery occurs within 15 minutes in most patients; in others, it may require 30 minutes or more.

Another parasympatholytic agent, glycopyrrolate, has been substituted for atropine in the reversal technique. Its advantages over atropine are that it has a longer duration of action and a lower incidence of arrhythmias; it causes small, slow changes in the heart rate; and it does not cross the blood-brain barrier. The usual reversal dosage is 1 mg of neostigmine and 0.2 mg of glycopyrrolate in a 2-ml mixture. This dosage can be repeated if reversal is inadequate.

DEPOLARIZING NEUROMUSCULAR BLOCKING AGENTS

Succinylcholine (Anectine; Quelicin; Sucostrin)

Succinylcholine represents a valuable pharmacologic advance in modern anesthesia and in critical care, areas in which resuscitation of patients is required. This agent is usually included as one of the drugs available for emergencies, especially when endotracheal intubation is required. Outside the operating room,

Table 16–2. OBSERVABLE RESPONSES TO STIMULATION OF RECEPTORS

Nicotinic
Stimulation of autonomic ganglia—both sympathetic and parasympathetic
Stimulation of adrenal medulla, resulting in the release of both epinephrine and norepinephrine
Stimulation of skeletal muscles at the motor endplate

Muscarinic
Stimulation or inhibition of smooth muscle in various organs or tissues
Stimulation of exocrine glands (i.e., salivary and sweat glands)
Slowing of cardiac conduction
Decrease in myocardial contractile force

succinylcholine is used for electroshock therapy, to relieve profound laryngospasm, to control convulsions from tetanus, to manage ventilation of the flail chest, and during reduction of fractures or dislocations.

Although succinylcholine is widely used in the United States, it has side effects and complications that can be avoided through a basic understanding of the pharmacology of the drug.

Succinylcholine acts at the N_2 postsynaptic cholinergic receptor by causing a persistent depolarization of the end plate. It also acts on the presynaptic cholinergic receptor by causing an initial increase in acetylcholine at the motor end plate. This reaction is the reason that patients who receive succinylcholine have fasciculations when it is administered initially. It is a synthetic quaternary ammonium compound whose chemical structure closely resembles that of acetylcholine. The onset of action of succinylcholine is rapid on initial injection. Its length of action is approximately 3 to 5 minutes. The drug is hydrolyzed rapidly by plasma pseudocholinesterase, an enzyme produced by the liver, to succinylmonocholine and choline. Succinylmonocholine is further hydrolyzed by pseudocholinesterase and true cholinesterase, found in the erythrocyte, to succinic acid and choline (see equations at bottom of page).

Advantages and Uses. Succinylcholine has certain advantages that, in most instances, justify its clinical use. Its very rapid onset of action, coupled with its short duration of action, has made this drug valuable when (1) rapid intubation is required, (2) laryngospasm is irreversible with positive pressure; (3) the skeletal muscles are rigid and prevent good ventilatory excursion; (4) procedures require a short duration of skeletal muscle relaxation, such as reduction of dislocations and fractures; and (5) electroconvulsive therapy is used to decrease the negative effects of seizures. Continued use over a 30-year period has shown succinylcholine to produce complications that can, in most instances, be prevented if the basic pharmacodynamics of the drug are understood.

In emergencies, succinylcholine remains the major muscle relaxant to faciliate endotracheal intubation. When this drug is used for a rapid-sequence intubation, the succinylcholine-induced fasciculations and the associated increase in gastric pressure should be reduced or eliminated by an intravenous injection of a small amount (3 mg per 70 kg of body weight) of d-tubocurarine. This "defasciculating" dose of d-tubocurarine should be administered about 1 or 2 minutes before the intravenous bolus injection of succinylcholine of 1.5 mg per kg.

Untoward Reactions. Because hydrolysis of succinylcholine depends on enzymatic activity, it is important to understand the atypical responses that may occur. Pseudocholinesterase activity in the plasma may be increased or decreased. Cases with increased activity are congenital and occur rarely. Patients with atypical pseudocholinesterase are resistant to succinylcholine and do not relax well. The reductions in pseudocholinesterase activity may be acquired or congenital. Acquired deficiencies are more important to understand because they are more common. They occur with liver disease, severe anemia, malnutrition, prolonged pyrexia, pregnancy, and recent renal dialysis. Drugs such as quinidine and propranolol (Inderal) inhibit pseudocholinesterase, as do echothiophate iodide eye drops (Phospholine). Patients with low pseudocholinesterase activity exhibit a prolonged response to these drugs.

Atypical pseudocholinesterase occurs alone in about 1 in 2800 people; this atypical form is inherited. Patients with genetically induced deficiencies of pseudocholinesterase have remained apneic for as long as 48 hours after a usual dose of succinylcholine. These patients require mechanical ventilation and constant nursing care. Patients with documented pseudocholinesterase deficiency should be advised to wear a Medic Alert bracelet. If anesthesia is required, these patients should be administered nondepolarizing skeletal muscle relaxants, such as pancuronium, d-tubocurarine, and gallamine, because these drugs can usually be reversed.

Disadvantages and Side Effects. Succinylcholine can be administered by single injection or continuous infusion. The single-injection method is used when neuromuscular relaxation is required for a short time, such as to facilitate endotracheal intubation. The usual in-

---

Succinylcholine ————————————→ Succinylmonocholine and choline
　　　　　　Pseudocholinesterase

Succinylmonocholine ———————————————→ Succinic acid and choline
　　　　　True and pseudocholinesterase

tubation dosage of succinylcholine is 1 mg per kg intravenously. During the first intravenous injection, cardiovascular status usually remains normal. If the injection must be repeated, the patient may exhibit profound bradycardia and various arrhythmias. Therefore, it is important to monitor the patient's cardiovascular status when succinylcholine is administered, especially if the dose is repeated.

Because children and adolescent patients are more likely than adults to have undiagnosed myopathies, a nondepolarizing skeletal muscle relaxant such as mivacurium (Mivacron) should be used for routine procedures in the PACU. More specifically, *except when used for emergency tracheal intubation or in the instance where immediate securing of the airway is necessary, succinylcholine is contraindicated in children and adolescent patients.* This is because a patient with a myopathy in this age group who is administered succinylcholine can experience acute, fulminating destruction of skeletal muscle (rhabdomyolysis) resulting in hyperkalemia and cardiac arrest.

If succinylcholine must be administered to an adolescent or child, the patient must be monitored completely because he or she is especially prone to bradycardia, even on the initial injection of succinylcholine. This complication can be easily overcome by prior administration of glycopyrrolate (Robinul) or atropine sulfate, either alone or mixed with succinylcholine. This appears to be the safest way of administering intravenous succinylcholine in this age group.

A disadvantage of the single-injection method with succinylcholine is that it causes fasciculations of the muscles. These "mini" contractions are a result of the initial depolarization of the skeletal muscle due to the positive feedback mechanism of initial stimulation of the presynaptic acetylcholine receptor. These contractions frequently lead to muscle pain, which is usually noted by the patient the day after surgery. This is particularly true in patients who are ambulatory soon after surgery. In ambulatory patients, muscle pains occur in 60 to 70 percent of cases. The incidence decreases to 10 percent in those patients confined to bed. Complaints of these patients include pain when blinking their eyes, pain when smiling, and generalized pain when ambulatory. These objective symptoms are usually noticed first by the nurse in the PACU. The pain usually does not require analgesics and subsides in a day or two. The fasciculations can be prevented by administering 3 to 6 mg of *d*-tubocurarine 3 minutes before the injection of succinylcholine.

When succinylcholine is administered to patients in the presence of extensive burns, severe trauma, severe abdominal infections, tetanus, neuromuscular disease, or neurologic lesions such as paraplegia and quadriplegia, a release of potassium from the damaged muscle and nerve cells can result. The common denominator appears to be either massive tissue destruction or central nervous sytem injury with muscle wasting. This pathophysiologic process results when denervated muscle is stimulated by a nicotinic receptor agonist such as succinylcholine. After activation of the nicotinic receptor by succinyolcholine, there is an enhanced response in the ionic channels with a resultant increase in the release of potassium into the circulation. Elevation of the serum potassium level, which can be as high as 10 to 15 mEq per L, has been reported. The result of this potassium elevation is cardiac dysrhythmias and cardiac arrest. The peak time for this reaction is 7 to 10 days after the injury. However, the critical period for these reactions is between posttraumatic days 1 and 180. Consequently, *succinylcholine is contraindicated in patients who have injuries of major multiple trauma, extensive denervation of skeletal muscle, or upper motor neuron injury.*

Succinylcholine has been implicated as one of the trigger agents of *malignant hyperthermia* (MH). Chapter 43 contains a complete description of the pathophysiology and treatment of MH.

In pediatric and adult patients anesthetized with halothane, combined with succinylcholine as the muscle relaxant, there is an unusual incidence of plasma myoglobin. Myoglobin is an intracellular muscle protein and therefore should not be released into the plasma. If myoglobin is found in the plasma, it can only mean that the muscle membrane has been injured.

Succinylcholine can be administered in a drip infusion during a procedure that requires skeletal muscle relaxation for a longer period than a single injection can provide. It is usually administered in a 0.1 to 0.2 percent solution. If the infusion is administered for a prolonged period, the type of block can gradually change from a depolarizing block to a characteristic nondepolarizing block. The change is always from depolarization to nondepolarization, never in the reverse direction. This type of block is called a *dual* or *phase II block* (see later discussion). The exact time relationship and the mechanism of action are still uncertain. Treatment is by mechanical ventilation and by careful monitoring of the patient until the dual block disappears.

Succinylcholine increases intraocular pressure by about 7.5 mm Hg in both children and adults, owing, in part, to the contraction of the extraocular muscles. *d*-Tubocurarine, when administered before succinylcholine to prevent contraction of the extraocular muscles, does not completely extinguish the increase in intraocular pressure. Therefore, even if succinylcholine is used with *d*-tubocurarine, it is contraindicated in patients in whom an increase in intraocular pressure would be detrimental.

Hexafluorenium Bromide (Mylaxen)

Hexafluorenium bromide has both anticholinesterase and neuromuscular blocking effects. It is used clinically to potentiate the effects of succinylcholine and, consequently, to reduce the total amount of succinylcholine used during the surgical procedure. This approach averts the accumulation of breakdown products of succinylcholine and also reduces muscular fasciculations and twitching when succinylcholine is initially administered. Hexafluorenium bromide is not used much in clinical anesthesia practice because bronchospasm, tachycardia, hypotension, and cardiac dysrhythmias have been reported to occur frequently after its use.

Decamethonium Bromide (Syncurine)

Decamethonium was first used clinically in 1949. This drug's action is similar to that of acetylcholine in that it produces depolarization of the end plate of the neuromuscular junction. It liberates some histamine but only about half as much as is released by use of *d*-tubocurarine. Decamethonium has no action on the myocardium, but it does produce fasciculations like succinylcholine does. This drug is not metabolized in the body and is excreted largely unchanged by the kidneys. The intravenous route of administration is the only satisfactory one for this drug. The onset of action for decamethonium is about 30 to 40 seconds after injection; its duration of action is about 15 to 20 minutes. Because of the difficulty in reversal and the problems of histamine release and fasciculations, decamethonium is rarely used in clinical anesthesia practice.

FACTORS INFLUENCING THE NEUROMUSCULAR BLOCKING AGENTS

Fluid Balance

Patients who are dehydrated are reported to be extremely sensitive to skeletal muscle relaxants. This finding is probably true because (1) dehydration decreases neuromuscular excitability, (2) the contracted extracellular fluid compartment permits an increase in the plasma concentration of the relaxant and thus intensifies the relaxant action, and (3) renal function is slowed and the elimination time of the relaxant and its metabolites is prolonged.

Sodium

A deficit of sodium may prolong the neuromuscular block. Experimental evidence indicates that a sodium deficiency itself may result in a partial neuromuscular block.

Potassium

Potassium deficiency appears to increase the blocking action of *d*-tubocurarine and other nondepolarizing neuromuscular blocking agents. On the other hand, depolarizing neuromuscular blocking agents are required in larger amounts when potassium deficiency exists. Depolarization is prevented to some extent, because a potassium deficiency appears to stabilize the muscle end plate. Potassium depletion can occur from decreased intake or excessive loss, such as in chronic pyelonephritis, primary aldosteronism, chlorothiazide therapy, and chronic diarrhea.

Magnesium

An increase in magnesium concentration causes a flaccid paralysis clinically similar to that caused by a nondepolarizing neuromuscular blocking agent. The principal action of magnesium is that it can enter the nerve terminal and replace or decrease the amount of calcium that enters, which stabilizes the postsynaptic membrane. Ultimately, depression of the release of acetylcholine occurs and reduces the EPP, causing a partial neuromuscular block. Consequently, magnesium enhances a neuromuscular block produced by a nondepolarizing agent and, to a lesser extent, potentiates the block produced by succinylcholine.

Calcium

A deficiency in calcium prolongs the effects of nondepolarizing neuromuscular blocking agents by reducing the amount of acetylcholine released and by inhibiting neuromuscular transmission. The depolarizing neuromuscular blocking agents are also potentiated because a low calcium level aids depolarization. Conversely, the administration of calcium chloride solution in calcium deficiency states antagonizes the nondepolarizing effects of agents such as *d*-tubocurarine. Calcium chloride has a pronounced antagonism to the respiratory depressant effects of succinylcholine.

pH and Carbon Dioxide

The neuromuscular blocking effect of *d*-tubocurarine is intensified in acidosis and in states of elevated carbon dioxide tension. With drugs such as gallamine and succinylcholine, the neuromuscular blocking action is diminished. Alkalosis by itself decreases the effects of *d*-tubocurarine. Hyperventilation has been thought to augment the abdominal muscle relaxation produced by *d*-tubocurarine. One explanation of this phenomenon is that changes in pH or plasma concentrations of *d*-tubocurarine reflect a change in binding to the receptor substance.

Catecholamines

Epinephrine and ephedrine have an anticurare effect on skeletal muscle. Clinically, an antagonism to *d*-tubocurarine has been demonstrated. This effect is caused by an increase in acetylcholine release, the inhibition of acetylcholinesterase, a decreased excitability of muscle fibers, and the release of potassium when epinephrine and ephedrine are administered.

Mycins

Several antibiotics exhibit a nondepolarizing neuromuscular blocking property. This is because the aminoglycoside antibiotics potentiate the neuromuscular blockade by inhibiting the presynaptic release of acetylcholine. The resulting clinical difficulties are related to a combination of factors, including large doses of antibiotics, parenteral administration into body cavities that represent a large surface area for absorption, and concomitant use of a neuromuscular blocking agent. Neomycin and streptomycin have been most frequently implicated (Table 16–3).

Table 16–3. NEUROMUSCULAR BLOCKING PROPERTIES OF VARIOUS ANTIBIOTICS

Antibiotics that increase the action of the *nondepolarizing agents* include:

Neomycin	Polymyxin A
Streptomycin	Polymyxin B
Dihydrostreptomycin	Lincomycin
Kanamycin	Colistin
Gentamicin	Tetracycline

Antibiotics that increase the action of *succinylcholine* include:
Neomycin
Streptomycin
Kanamycin
Polymyxin B
Colistin

Antibiotics that do not exert any neuromuscular blocking activity include:
Penicillin
Chloramphenicol
Cephalosporins

Cardiac Antidysrhythmic Drugs

Lidocaine, when administered intravenously, potentiates a preexisting neuromuscular blockade. This occurs because lidocaine stabilizes the postsynaptic membrane and depresses the skeletal muscle fibers. Quinidine interferes with the presynaptic release of acetylcholine at the neuromuscular junction. Consequently, it intensifies the neuromuscular blockade of both depolarizing and nondepolarizing skeletal muscle blocking agents. Finally, calcium channel blocking agents inhibit the calcium entry with a resultant reduction in acetylcholine release followed by a reduction in neuromuscular function.

Temperature

Hypothermia antagonizes the action of *d*-tubocurarine and potentiates the action of succinylcholine or decamethonium. During the recovery phase of an anesthetic, when a neuromuscular blocking agent has been administered, young infants should be specifically monitored for return of skeletal muscle tone. This rule is especially in effect when a nondepolarizing relaxant is administered to infants, who are prone to have some hypothermia because of their immature heat-regulating system.

Inhalation Anesthetics

The inhalation anesthetics produce a dose-dependent enhancement of the neuromuscular blockade of the nondepolarizing neuromuscular blocking agents. More specifically, this blockade is most pronounced when a patient has received either enflurane (Ethrane) or isoflurane. Halothane has a moderate amount of potentiation qualities and the least with nitrous oxide. This potentiation of the neuromuscular blockade by the inhalation anesthetics is the result of depression of the central nervous system, and it ultimately reduces skeletal muscle tone. Consequently, patients in the PACU who have received nondepolarizing neuromuscular blocking agents intraoperatively and have not completely emerged from their inhalation anesthetic should be closely monitored for a reduction in skeletal muscle function by the use of a peripheral nerve stimulator. Also, an aggressive stir-up regimen should be instituted on these patients.

ASSESSMENT OF NEUROMUSCULAR BLOCKADE

Humans injected with d-tubocurarine at first have motor weakness, then their muscles become totally flaccid. The small, rapidly moving muscles, such as those of the fingers, toes, eyes, and ears, are involved before the long muscles of the limbs, neck, and trunk. The intercostal muscles, and finally the diaphragm, become paralyzed, and then respiration ceases.

The PACU nurse should know the order of the return of muscle function after a patient has received a nondepolarizing muscle relaxant such as d-tubocurarine. The recovery of skeletal muscle function is usually in reverse order to that of paralysis; therefore, the diaphragm is ordinarily first to regain function. The order of appearance of paralysis after injection with a nondepolarizing neuromuscular blocking agent can be assessed electromyographically as follows:

1. *Small-sized muscle groups:* oculomotor muscles, muscles of the eyelids; muscles of the mouth and face; small extensor muscles of the fingers, followed by the flexor muscles of the fingers.
2. *Medium-sized muscle groups:* muscles of the tongue and pharynx; muscles of mastication; extensor muscles of the limb, followed by flexor muscles of the limbs.
3. *Large-sized muscle groups:* neck muscles; shoulder muscles; abdominal muscles; dorsal muscle mass.
4. *Special muscle groups:* intercostal muscles; larynx; diaphragm.

The order of paralysis is essentially the same after injection with a depolarizing neuromuscular agent, except that the flexor muscles are paralyzed before the extensor muscles. Patients arriving in the PACU must be evaluated for residual effects from a neuromuscular blocking agent that was administered intraoperatively. In most instances, the action of the nondepolarizing neuromuscular blocking agent will be pharmacologically reversed at the end of the operation before the patient is admitted to the PACU; however, any patient who has received a neuromuscular blocking agent should be closely watched for signs of residual drug action. Table 16–4 describes the criteria for recovery from nondepolarizing neuromuscular blockade. The residual actions of the depolarizing muscle relaxants are similar to those of the nondepolarizing muscle relaxants, and the same nonrespiratory parameters and respiratory variables can be used to evaluate the neuromuscular blockade. The evoked (electrical stimulation) responses differ between the depolarizing and nondepolarizing neuromuscular blocking agents.

The PNS (Fig. 16–3A and B) can be used in the PACU to assess the type and degree of a neuromuscular blockade. This electrical device can be used to stimulate the ulnar nerve at the wrist or elbow, and, on stimulation of the ulnar nerve, the nurse can observe the contraction of

---

Table 16–4. CRITERIA FOR RECOVERY FROM NONDEPOLARIZING NEUROMUSCULAR BLOCKADE

Clinical Assessment of Neuromuscular Blockade
Nonrespiratory parameters
  Ability to open eyes wide
  Sustained protrusion of the tongue
  Sustained hand grip
  Sustained head lift for at least five seconds
  Ability to cough effectively
Respiratory variables
  Tidal volume of at least 5 ml/kg
  Vital capacity of at least 15–20 ml/kg
  Inspiratory force of 20–25 cm H_2O, negative pressure

Evoked Responses
Return of the single twitch to control height
Sustained tetanic response to high-frequency stimulation
Recovery of the train-of-four to a ratio above 75%

Adapted from Train-of-four technique facilitates assessment of NMB and correlation with recovery. Wellcome Trends in Anesthesiology/Symposium Perspectives, 3(6):8–10, 1985.

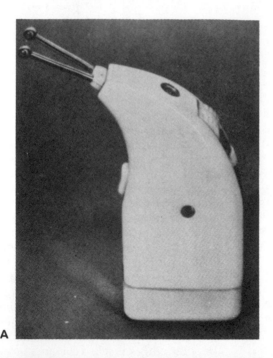

FIGURE 16–3. *A*, peripheral nerve stimulator. *B*, method of applying the peripheral nerve stimulator to the ulnar nerve at the wrist. (*A* and *B* from Wylie, W., and Churchill-Davidson, H. C. [eds.]: A Practice of Anesthesia. 4th ed. London, Lloyd-Luke Medical Books, 1978, p. 882.)

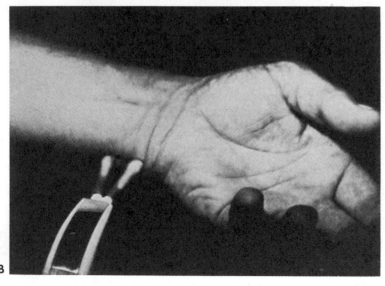

the fingers. The assessment of the depth of neuromuscular blockade using electrical stimulation is useful when more than 70 percent of the N_2 receptors are blocked by a skeletal muscle relaxant. However, in most instances, if the patient has a normal tidal volume, vital capacity, and maximal inspiratory force and can lift his or her head for 5 seconds, the use of the PNS is not warranted. If identification of the type of neuromuscular blockade used (depolarizing or nondepolarizing) is needed, or if some of the aforementioned parameters are marginal, the train-of-four or sustained tetanus using the PNS can be used to provide the objective data for assessment.

Although the mechanisms producing the nondepolarizing block differ from the depolarizing block, the diagnostic criteria using a PNS for assessing a nondepolarizing and phase II dual block are basically the same. Miller points out that the hallmark of a nondepolarizing neuromuscular blockade is an inability to sustain contraction in response to a tetanic stimulus and post-tetanic facilitation. A *tetanic stimulus* is the usual 50 Hz of current for 5 seconds (sustained tetanus) produced by a PNS. *Post-tetanic facilitation* is a twitch after the response to tetanic stimuli higher than the twitch immediately before tetanus. If a patient has a partial nondepolarizing neuromuscular block, an unsustained contraction called *fade* is seen after the initial tetanic stimulus (Fig. 16–4). Fade is caused by the decreased mobilization of acetylcholine in the nerve terminal because the presynaptic acetylcholine receptor is blocked by the nondepolarizing muscle relaxant. The responses to electrical stimulation are the result of the interaction of acetylcholine released and the number of N_2 cholinergic receptors occupied by the relaxant. In patients with a partial nondepolarizing neuromuscular block, the first three single electrical stimuli are of enough intensity to produce a twitch, but the twitch produced is not of the same magnitude as a twitch produced in a subject who has not received a nondepolarizing skeletal muscle relaxant (see Fig. 16–4). The three electrical stimuli cause the normal quantum of acetylcholine to be released at the synaptic cleft; however, in this instance, the reduction in twitch magnitude is the result of the number of acetylcholine receptors being occupied by the nondepolarizing relaxant. Consequently, if the patient has had a complete nondepolarizing neuromuscular block in which all the N_2 cholinergic receptors were occupied, no twitch would be elicited from the three electrical stimuli.

In a normal subject, when a tetanic stimulus is applied for 5 seconds, the quantum of acetylcholine that is released decreases during the stimulus period. Along with this, only a fraction of nicotinic cholinergic receptors are activated at any one time to trigger an action potential. The excess in nicotinic cholinergic receptors is the safety margin of neuromuscular transmission. Consequently, in the normal subject who receives a tetanic stimulus, the magnitude of the twitch response is maintained because of the large nicotinic cholinergic receptor pool; however, if 75 percent of the nicotinic receptors are occupied by a nondepolarizing neuromuscular relaxant, for example, the twitch response will not be maintained, and fade (unsustained contraction) will occur because the usual margin of safety of excess acetylcholine receptors has been abolished. Between the termination of a tetanic stimulus and the first single-twitch stimulus, a buildup of acetylcholine occurs in the presynaptic knob. Thus, after sustained tetanus, when the first electrical stimulus is administered, the height of the first twitch will be greater than the pretetanic twitches. These large post-tetanic twitches (post-tetanic facilitation) return to the pretetanic height as the acetylcholine mobilization also returns to the pretetanic level. Finally, more than 70 percent of the nicotinic cholinergic receptors must be occupied before this tetanic stimulation test will be sensitive enough to detect neuromuscular blockade.

The major drawback to the delivery of a 50-Hz tetanic stimulus to an awake patient in the PACU is pain and general discomfort. For the patient who is awake and reactive, it is better to use the *train-of-four stimulation* to assess the degree of neuromuscular blockade due to nondepolarizing skeletal muscle relaxants. In this test, the ulnar nerve is used, and four supra-

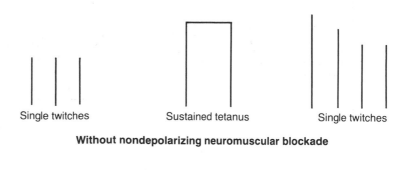

Without nondepolarizing neuromuscular blockade

Single twitches   Sustained tetanus   Single twitches

FIGURE 16–4. Magnitude of post-tetanic facilitation without and with nondepolarizing neuromuscular blockade. (Adapted from Donati, F.: Monitoring neuromuscular blockade. *In* Saidman, L., and Smith, N. T. [eds.]: Monitoring in Anesthesia. 3rd ed., p. 160. Woburn, MA, Butterworth, 1993. Copyright 1993, Butterworth-Heinemann.)

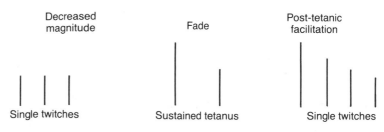

Decreased magnitude   Fade   Post-tetanic facilitation

Single twitches   Sustained tetanus   Single twitches

With nondepolarizing neuromuscular blockade

maximal electrical stimuli, 2 Hz 0.05 seconds apart, are administered by a PNS. This test, which produces minimal discomfort to the awake patient, is sensitive only when more than 70 percent of the nicotinic cholinergic receptors are occupied. The index of neuromuscular blockade in this test is the ratio of the fourth to the first twitch amplitude. More specifically, when the fourth response is abolished, a 75 percent block exists (Fig. 16–5). When the third and second responses to stimulation are abolished, the respective reductions in neuromuscular blockade are 80 and 90 percent. Finally, when all four twitch responses are absent, a 100 percent, or complete, block exists.

The depolarizing neuromuscular blockade is characterized by an absence of post-tetanic facilitation, a decreased response to a single impulse, a decreased amplitude (but sustained response to a tetanic stimulus), and, if present, a train-of-four ratio between the first and fourth stimulus that is greater than 70 percent.

SPECIAL PROBLEMS IN THE PACU

A prolonged response to succinylcholine sometimes occurs because a patient does not

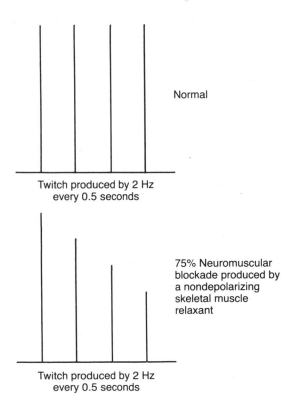

Normal

Twitch produced by 2 Hz
every 0.5 seconds

75% Neuromuscular blockade produced by a nondepolarizing skeletal muscle relaxant

Twitch produced by 2 Hz
every 0.5 seconds

FIGURE 16–5. Diagrammatic illustration of the train-of-four in normal response and 75 percent neuromuscular blockade produced by a nondepolarizing skeletal muscle relaxant.

possess the proper blood level of pseudocholinesterase. Other causes of a prolonged response include (1) overdosage, (2) temperature changes, (3) acid–base imbalance, (4) carcinoma, (5) antitumor agents, (6) antibiotics, (7) myasthenia gravis, and (8) liver disease.

If a patient who arrives in the PACU is apneic, controlled respiration must be initiated and maintained as long as necessary. Careful monitoring of vital signs and evaluation of renal function are important. The neuromuscular block can be identified with the PNS. If electrical stimulation results in vigorous contractions, it is unlikely that the apnea is the result of residual neuromuscular block. Consideration must then be given to other agents that may have caused the apneic state. The response of patients with neuromuscular disorders to muscle relaxants may include resistance, increased response, hyperkalemia, and even cardiac arrest. Table 16–5 is presented as a summary of the possible untoward responses in the clinical setting.

Phase II Block

Various terms are used to describe the different types of blocks that succinylcholine is able to produce. The phase I block is synonymous with the *depolarizing block* the drug ordinarily produces. It is characterized by a dose-dependent reduction in a single twitch without fade after a well-sustained tetanus and no post-tetanic facilitation when the PNS is used.

Phase II block is also known as a *dual block, desensitization,* or *open channel block.* This block is caused by a conformational change in the presynaptic and postsynaptic cholinergic receptors. This anatomic change results in a desensitization to the stimulation of acetylcholine. The characteristics of this block as demonstrated by the PNS are fade during the train-of-four and poorly sustained tetanus and post-tetanic facilitation. The same clinical features are seen when *d*-tubocurarine is used; however, this does not mean that the two blocks are the same, because there is good evidence that the *d*-tubocurarine and succinylcholine phase II blocks differ in several respects. Some clinicians believe that the phase II block produced by succinylcholine can be reversed with anticholinesterases such as edrophonium, which has a shorter duration of action than neostigmine. Edrophonium is used in this situation because it either reverses or potentiates the block. If potentiation occurs, it will be of a shorter duration than if neostigmine were

Table 16–5. SUMMARY OF THE RESPONSE OF PATIENTS WITH NEUROMUSCULAR DISORDERS TO MUSCLE RELAXANTS

Disorder	Pathophysiology	Response to Nondepolarizing Muscle Relaxant	Response to Depolarizing Muscle Relaxant
Hemiplegia	Sequelae of CVA; caused by an upper motor neuron in the cerebral motor cortex	Resistance	Hyperkalemia can occur as early as 1 wk and as late as 6 mo after stroke
Parkinson's disease	Extrapyramidal disorder	Normal	Hyperkalemia may occur
Multiple sclerosis	Demyelinating disorder of the CNS	Normal	Hyperkalemia may occur
Diffuse intracranial lesions	No focal neurologic deficits or muscular denervation or paralysis (i.e., ruptured cerebral aneurysm)	Normal?	Hyperkalemia and possible cardiac arrest
Tetanus	Acute infectious disease of the CNS caused by the endotoxin released by *Clostridium tetani*	Normal	Hyperkalemia and possible cardiac arrest
Paraplegia and quadriplegia	Traumatic or pathologic transection of the spinal cord and interruption of pyramidal tracts	Increased response	Hyperkalemia as early as 3 wks and as late as 85 d after spinal cord injury
Amyotrophic lateral sclerosis (ALS)	Degenerative disease of motor ganglia in the anterior horn of the spinal cord and of the spinal pyramidal tracts	Increased response	No reports of hyperkalemia in ALS; however, myotonia-like contracture may occur in ALS patients. Avoid succinylcholine in patients with significant muscular denervation
Muscular denervation	Result of traumatic peripheral nerve damage—muscles undergo atrophy	Normal response	Muscular contracture and hyperkalemia
Myasthenia gravis (MG)	Postsynaptic reduction in the number of ACh receptors caused by autoimmune disease	Increased response and prolongation of effects	Resistance and early appearance of phase II (dual) block
Myasthenic syndrome	Differs clinically and electromyographically from MG. Associated with small cell carcinoma of the lung resulting in presynaptic lesion at the neuromuscular junction	Exaggerated response	Exaggerated response
Myotonias	Lesion in the muscle fiber distal to the neuromuscular junction. Common symptom is delayed relaxation of skeletal muscles following voluntary contractions	Increased and prolonged. Some report normal response	Unpredictable. Many reports of increased rigidity
Muscular dystrophies (MD)	Disorder of the muscle fiber proper that may be secondary to a neurogenic disorder	Normal to prolonged response. Ocular MD has a very high sensitivity to *d*-tubocurarine	Unpredictable. Best to avoid use of succinlycholine

CVA = cerebrovascular accident; CNS = central nervous system; ACh = acetylcholine.

used. Most experts believe that routine reversal to antagonize the dual block is unwarranted. It is more advisable to ventilate the patient and wait for return of the normal neuromuscular transmission.

Recurarization

Recurarization is the reappearance postoperatively of the pharmacologic actions of a non-depolarizing skeletal muscle relaxant that was administered intraoperatively. The hazard of recurarization after the use of gallamine (Flaxedil) represents a significant problem that may be encountered in the PACU. This complication arises when renal insufficiency exists. The interesting facet of this complication is that even when the gallamine is reversed sufficiently at the end of the anesthetic, recurarization may still occur for as long as 8 hours. This reappearance may be partly caused by the fading of the effect of the neostigmine. Gallamine is normally excreted after 2 hours, but in renal insufficiency the excretion of the drug is poor and may take as long as 30 hours. Therefore, in patients with renal insufficiency in whom gallamine was used, signs of delayed excretion (weakness of the ocular muscles, difficulty in swallowing, or decrease in ventilation) should be sought. If symptoms appear, the required level of the reversal agent (neostigmine) must be maintained until that portion of the gallamine has been eliminated so that symptoms do not reappear. If recurarization occurs, the postoperative use of morphine and similar narcotics should be avoided, because these agents will enhance a residual neuromuscular block sufficiently to make it clinically significant.

Recurarization from *d*-tubocurarine does not usually occur because only 20 to 40 percent of the drug is excreted through the kidneys. In some reported cases, recurarization due to *d*-tubocurarine was caused by an increased sensitivity of the myoneural junction associated with a decrease in the plasma potassium concentration.

Bradycardia

Another problem occurring in the PACU is the appearance of bradycardia when a patient has received an atropine-neostigmine combination at the end of the anesthetic. The bradycardia is usually the result of the longer duration of action of neostigmine as compared with that of atropine. The treatment for this problem is glycopyrrolate. Glycopyrrolate should not be administered, however, until other causes of bradycardia are eliminated, such as pain, hypoventilation, and a full bladder.

References

1. Agoston, S., and Bowman, W.: Muscle Relaxants. 2nd ed. New York, Elsevier, 1990.
2. Azar, I.: The response of patients with neuromuscular disorders to muscle relaxants: A review. Anesthesiology, 61(2):173–187, 1984.
3. Basta, S., Savarese, K., Ali, H., et al.: Clinical pharmacology of doxacurium chloride: A new long-acting nondepolarizing muscle relaxant. Anesthesiology, 69:478–486, 1988.
4. Bradshaw, H., Drain, C., and Dutton, M.: A review of skeletal muscle contraction and neuromuscular function. AANA J., 48(4):334–343, 1980.
5. Brown, J., Foster, S., Anderson, C., et al.: The literature and perspectives on muscle relaxants for rapid-sequence induction. Nurse Anesth., 2(2):72–88, 1991.
6. Brown, M.: Antibiotics and anesthesia. Semin. Anesth., 9(3):153–161, 1990.
7. Emmott, R., Bracey, B., Goldhill, D., et al.: Cardiovascular effects of doxacurium, pancuronium, and vecuronium in anaesthetized patients presenting for coronary artery bypass surgery. Br. J. Anesth., 65:480–486, 1990.
8. Erkola, O., Karhunen, U., and Sandelin-Hellqvist, E.: Spontaneous recovery of residual neuromuscular blockade after atracurium or vecuronium during isoflurane anaesthesia. Acta Anaesthesiol. Scand., 33:290–294, 1991.
9. Gilman, A., Rall, T., Nies, A., et al.: Goodman and Gilman's The Pharmacological Basis of Therapeutics. 8th ed. New York, Pergamon Press, 1990.
10. Goldhill, D., Whitehead, J., Emmott, R., et al.: Neuromuscular and clinical effects of mivacurium chloride in healthy adult patients during nitrous oxide–enflurane anaesthesia. Br. J. Anaesth., 67(3):289–295, 1991.
11. Lambalk, L., De Wit, A., Wierda, J., et al.: Dose-response relationship and time course of action of Org 9426: A new muscle relaxant of intermediate duration evaluated under various anesthetic techniques. Anaesthesia, 46:907–911, 1991.
12. Larijani, G., Bartkowski, R. R., and Azad, S. S.: Clinical pharmacology of pipecuronium bromide. Anesth. Analg., 68:734–739, 1989.
13. Miller, R. (ed.): Anesthesia. 3rd ed. New York, Churchill Livingstone, 1990.
14. Miller, R., Rupp, S., Fisher, D., et al.: Clinical pharmacology of vecuronium and atracurium. Anesthesiology, 61(4):444–453, 1984.
15. Oduro, K.: Glycopyrrolate methobromide: Comparison with atropine sulfate in anaesthesia. Can. Anaesth. Soc. J., 22(4):466–473, 1975.
16. Ostheimer, G.: A comparison of glycopyrrolate and atropine during reversal of nondepolarizing neuromuscular block with neostigmine. Anesth. Analg., 56:182–186, 1977.
17. Pittet, J.: Neuromuscular effect of pipecuronium bromide in infants and children during nitrous oxide–alfentanil anesthesia. Anesthesiology, 73(2):432–436, 1991.
18. Reep, B.: Complications associated with the administration of succinylcholine. AANA J., 40(3):193–203, 1972.
19. Savarese, J., Hassan, H., and Antonio, R.: The clinical pharmacology of metocurine: Dimethyltubocurarine revisited. Anesthesiology, 47(3):277–284, 1977.
20. Schweinefus, R., and Schick, L.: Succinylcholine: "Good Guy, Bad Guy." J. Post Anesth. Nurs. 6(6):410–419, 1991.
21. Stoelting, R.: Pharmacology and Physiology in Anesthetic Practice. 2nd ed. Philadelphia, J. B. Lippincott, 1991.
22. Wicks, T.: Mivacurium chloride. Nurse Anesth., 3(4):173–182, 1992.
23. Wood, M., and Wood, A.: Drugs Used in Anesthesia: Pharmacology for the Anesthesiologist. 2nd ed. Baltimore: Williams & Wilkins, 1990.
24. Zarr, G.: Muscle relaxants. In Waugaman, W., Foster, S., and Rigor, B.: Principles and Practice of Nurse Anesthesia. 2nd ed., pp. 475–505. Norwalk, CT, Appleton & Lange, 1992.
25. Zuurmond, W., and van Leeuwen, L.: Atracurium versus vecuronium: A comparison of recovery in outpatient arthroscopy. Can. J. Anaesth., 35(2):139–142, 1988.

CHAPTER 17

Local Anesthetics

Local anesthetic agents are defined as pharmacologic agents capable of producing a loss of sensation in an area of the body. They were first used in 1884, when cocaine was employed as a topical anesthetic agent by Freud and Köller, and in 1885, when Halsted used cocaine to prevent nerve conduction in the lower extremities. The actual advent of the use of local anesthetics in anesthetic practice was not until 1943, when Lofgren synthesized procaine. Local anesthetics are used in all forms of regional anesthesia. The term *regional anesthesia* refers to the various anesthetic techniques that use local anesthetic agents to block nerve conduction in an extremity or a region of the body (see Chapter 18). Among the types of regional anesthesia are topical, infiltration, field block, and conduction. *Topical anesthesia* is produced when an anesthetic agent is applied to a surface, such as the skin, mucous membrane, urethra, nose, and pharynx. A new topical anesthetic that can be used on the skin to provide analgesia during venipuncture is called *EMLA*. This *eutectic mixture of local anesthetics* is composed of lidocaine and prilocaine. *Infiltration anesthesia* is produced by injecting a local anesthetic into the tissue to be cut. *Field block anesthesia* is produced by injecting a local anesthetic agent into the surrounding tissues of an area to be operated on. *Conduction anesthesia* is produced by injecting a local anesthetic agent into a nerve or nerves that supply a region of the body to eliminate sensation or motor control, or both. Epidural and subarachnoid blocks are *conduction blocks*.

The use of regional anesthesia has become popular in modern anesthesia practice because, when indicated, it offers many advantages over general inhalation anesthesia. To facilitate optimal recovery of the surgical patient from this type of anesthetic, the post anesthesia care unit (PACU) nurse must first have a complete knowledge of the physiology of nerve conduction as well as the pharmacology of local anesthetic agents, including their mechanism of action, effects, and toxicity.

PHYSIOLOGY OF NERVES, NERVE CONDUCTION, AND LOCAL ANESTHETICS

Nerves conduct impulses, or action potentials, that provide information to the central nervous system (CNS) about the type, degree, and magnitude of pain. As Wood and Wood describe, inside the nerve cell (including the axon) is cytoplasm containing potassium ions that are positively charged and proteins that are negatively charged. The potassium ions can freely move in and out of the cytoplasm, whereas the proteins are not freely difusible. The fluid outside the nerve cell and axon contains positively charged sodium ions and negatively charged chloride ions. These ions are freely diffusible into the cytoplasm. However, via a sodium pump, the sodium is quickly pushed out of the nerve cell. Outside the nerve cell, the concentration of the negatively charged ion chloride is large and the concentration of the positively charged potassium is low. Inside the nerve cell, this ratio is reversed—the concentration of potassium is high and the concentration of the negatively charged chloride ions is low. The freely difusible potassium ions are held inside the nerve cell by an excess of negatively charged ions. Because of the excess of negatively charged ions, an electrical potential exists of about -70 to -90 mV.

When the nerve impulse is conducted down the nerve fiber, the nerve membranes become permeable (owing to depolarization) to the positively charged sodium ions. These sodium ions are conducted through pores, or sodium channels, in which a "gate" regulates their passage to the inside of the nerve cell. As the sodium ions reach the inside of the nerve cell, the electrical potential changes to $+40$ mV. This change from negative to positive is about 110 mV and represents the movement of an action potential down a nerve fiber or, in neurophysiologic terms, propagation of an action potential. Once the sodium has reached a certain ionic concentration, the gate closes in the sodium channels. The membrane permeability to potassium increases, allowing potassium back into the cytoplasm, and sodium is pumped out of the nerve cell, which will slowly return the ionic potential to its resting level of -70 to -90 mV.

Local anesthetics are quite lipid soluble and, consequently, can diffuse through the cell membrane into the axoplasm. They ionize and occupy a receptor near the gate of the sodium channel. Thus, the local anesthetic prevents the opening of the gate, and sodium cannot enter the inside the nerve, which results in a slowing of the rate of depolarization. Consequently, a nerve action potential cannot be reached, and blockage of the nerve's electrical conduction system ensues.

The afferent nerve fibers that conduct impulses to the spinal cord are classified as A, B, and C, based on fiber diameter and conduction velocity. The A fibers are further divided into A-alpha, A-beta, A-gamma, and A-delta fibers. The large-diameter A fibers are myelinated and have the fastest conduction velocity. The A-alpha fibers have the largest diameter and the fastest conduction velocity. They provide innervation of motor function to the skeletal muscles. The moderately myelinated A-beta fibers are the next largest in diameter and speed, and they are responsible for touch and pressure. The sensation of proprioception and skeletal muscle tone are maintained by the A-gamma fibers, which are smaller in diameter and are slower than the preceding A-beta fibers. The A-delta fibers are lightly myelinated and are the smallest and slowest of the A fibers. They are responsible for conducting sensations of fast pain, touch, and temperature. The lightly myelinated B fibers are smaller than the A fibers and are the preganglionic autonomic fibers. The smallest fibers are the unmyelinated C fibers. They function as postganglionic sympathetic fibers and also conduct sensations such as slow pain and temperature.

Local anesthetics can penetrate and prevent nerve conduction in the smallest nerve fibers first and the large A-alpha fibers last. Consequently, during the emergence from conduction anesthesia, a particular order of return is seen that is based solely on the reduced concentration gradient of the local anesthetic and the fiber size (Table 17–1). For example, after epidural and peripheral nerve or plexus blocks, the large A-alpha fibers will return first and the patient will have a return of motor function. The next fibers to return are the A-beta and A-gamma, and the patient will have a return of

Table 17–1. EMERGENCE SEQUENCE OF A NERVE BLOCK

1. Motor paralysis
2. Proprioception (awareness of body or extremity position) lost
3. Pressure sense abolished
4. Tactile sense lost
5. Slow and fast pain
6. Temperature discrimination lost
7. Sensation of warmth by patient
8. Block of cold temperature fibers
9. Vasomotor block—dilatation of skin vessels and increased cutaneous blood flow

proprioception, touch, and pressure. Finally, a return of pain and a loss of a sensation of warmth occurs as a result of low concentration of local anesthetic in the A-delta, B, and C fibers.

Pain, which is called *nociception*, is a protective mechanism that occurs when tissues are damaged. There are two major types of pain: fast and slow. *Fast pain* is a well defined, stabbing sensation that is rather short in duration. Causes of fast pain include surgical incision and pin pricks. Fast pain is conducted via the small afferent, myelinated A-delta nerve fibers. *Slow pain* is not well defined and is characterized as a burning or aching sensation. In this type of pain, even after the pain stimulus is removed, the pain may continue. The efferent conducting nerves in this instance are the unmyelinated C fibers.

THE LOCAL ANESTHETICS

The ideal local anesthetic should have the following properties: selectivity of action, low toxicity, complete reversibility, nonirritation, short latency, good penetrance, sufficient duration, solubility in saline and water, stability, and compatibility with vasoconstrictors. Not all local anesthetic agents possess all these attributes. As new agents are discovered, they are measured against these criteria.

In regard to their analgesic activity, local anesthetic agents can be divided into three groups according to potency. Procaine and chloroprocaine are the least potent of the commonly employed agents, whereas lidocaine, cocaine, mepivacaine, and prilocaine are compounds of intermediate potency; that is, they are twice as potent as procaine. Tetracaine, bupivacaine, and etidocaine are drugs of high potency that are approximately six to eight times more active than procaine.

The local anesthetic agents are grouped pharmacologically into two categories: the amides and the esters (Table 17–2). The *amides* are metabolized in the liver, have no real history of documented allergic reactions, have good penetrance, and are stable. Drugs in this category are lidocaine, mepivacaine, prilocaine, etidocaine, and bupivacaine. The *esters*, except for cocaine, are hydrolyzed primarily in the plasma by plasma pseudocholinesterase and are metabolized more rapidly than the amides. Because the esters are metabolized to para-aminobenzoic acid, they are associated with an increased incidence of allergic reactions. In general, the esters have poor penetrance, rare allergic reactions, and fair to poor stability. Epinephrine is added to some local anesthetic agents because it is a vasoconstrictor and therefore prolongs the activity of the local agent and decreases its toxicity by slowing its uptake.

The Short-Duration Local Anesthetics

Procaine (Novocain)

Procaine is one of the first ester anesthetics, as it was first synthesized by Einhorn in 1905. Because it ionizes so fast, it has poor spreading and penetrating properties. Because it can produce vasodilatation, epinephrine is usually added to procaine to delay systemic absorption. The use of procaine is usually for infiltration anesthesia in a 1 or 2 percent solution or spinal anesthesia in a 5 percent solution. Allergic reactions have been reported after repeated doses of procaine.

Chloroprocaine (Nesacaine)

Chloroprocaine is an analogue of procaine with low toxicity, a rapid onset of 10 minutes, and a short duration of action of about 45 minutes. Because of its vasodilating effects, chloroprocaine is often used with a vasoconstrictor such as epinephrine. It can be used for most types of regional anesthesia. However, it is rarely administered epidurally (with preservatives) because of the risk of neurotoxicity due to accidental injection into the subarachnoid space. Along with this, chloroprocaine is not used for spinal anesthesia because of its potential of neurotoxicity. Preservative-free chloroprocaine can still be used for epidural anesthesia without risk of neurotoxicity. The multiple-dose vial containing chloroprocaine with preservatives (sodium bisulfite and methylparaben) should be used only for infiltration anesthesia. Rapid, inadvertent intrathecal injection of a low pH and bisulfite-containing solution can cause motor and sensory deficits.

The Intermediate-Duration Local Anesthetics

Cocaine

Cocaine has three distinctive actions: (1) it can block nerve conduction; (2) it can produce euphoria and sympathetic and CNS stimulation; and (3) it is highly addictive. Cocaine is used primarily for topical anesthesia and probably should not be administered parenterally. This is because it is addictive and has many toxic side effects when administered in any form other than topical. The major cardiovascular effect of cocaine is that it interferes with the re-uptake mechanism of catecholamines and, consequently, it can potentiate all vasopressors and cause cardiac dysrhythmias and seizures when administered in high doses.

Lidocaine (Xylocaine)

Lidocaine is one of the most widely used local anesthetics in the world. It can be used for topical, infiltration, field block, spinal, epidural, and caudal anesthesia. For topical anesthesia, a 4 percent solution is usually used, and in this form, its onset of action is about 5 minutes and its effects last for about 20 minutes. When lidocaine is administered for local infiltration in a 0.5 to 1 percent solution, the onset of anesthesia is from 2 to 5 minutes, with a duration of action of about 75 minutes. For brachial plexus (axillary) blocks, the drug has an onset of about 5 to 10 minutes and a duration of about 60 minutes without epinephrine and 120 minutes with epinephrine. A caudal block requires a 1 or 2 percent solution of lidocaine. The onset of anesthesia is between 5 and 15 minutes, with a duration of about 100 minutes with epinephrine and 60 minutes without epinephrine. A 5 percent solution of lidocaine in dextrose is used for spinal anesthesia. The onset is between 5 and 10 minutes, and the duration is about 60 minutes without epinephrine and 90 minutes with epinephrine.

Lidocaine can be used as a antidysrhythmic at an intravenous dose of 1 mg per kg. Infusion rates for this drug range from 20 to 50 µg per kg per min. Lidocaine can be used for postoperative analgesia when it is administered in a slow, continuous intravenous infusion. When

Table 17–2. LOCAL ANESTHETIC AGENTS: ESTERS AND AMIDES

Agent	Use	Discussion
Esters		
Cocaine	*Topical:* 4–20% for use in nose and throat procedures; duration, 10–55 min; maximum dose, 3 mg/kg	Topical use only; vasoconstrictor; CNS stimulant in abuse
Procaine (Novocain)	*Topical:* 10–20% required; *infiltration:* 0.25–0.5%; *nerve block:* 1–2%; duration, 20–30 min plain, 45 min with epinephrine; maximum dose, 10 mg/kg plain and 14 mg/kg with epinephrine	Low potency, rapid hydrolysis in plasma, mild acetylcholine inhibition, poor stability
Chloroprocaine (Nesacaine)	*Infiltration:* 10 mg/ml solution; *peripheral nerve block:* 10 and 20 mg/ml solution; *epidural block:* 20–30 mg/ml solution	Not topically active; more potent but shorter duration of action than procaine. The safest local anesthetic in regard to systemic toxicity. The onset of action is 6–12 min, and the duration of anesthesia is 30–60 min. Total dose should not exceed 1 g with epinephrine and 800 mg without epinephrine; 12 times more potent than procaine
Tetracaine (Pontocaine)	*Topical:* 0.5–1%, duration, 55 min; *infiltration:* 0.1–0.25%; *nerve block:* 0.25%, duration, 3–4 hr plain, 5–7 hr with epinephrine; maximum dose, 1.5–2 mg/kg plain and 2–3 mg/kg with epinephrine	
Amides		
Lidocaine (Xylocaine)	*Topical:* 2–4% onset, 2–4 min, maximum dose, 3 mg/kg; *nerve block:* 1–2%, maximum dose, 4–5 mg/kg plain or 7 mg/kg with epinephrine; duration, 1 hr plain, 2 hr with epinephrine; antiarrhythmic, 1 mg/kg bolus, then 1–2 mg/min intravenous drip	Rapid onset, intense analgesia, good penetration, stable. As antiarrhythmic, it depresses the automaticity of the Purkinje fibers and decreases their effective refractory period
Mepivacaine (Carbocaine)	*Infiltration:* 0.5–1%; *nerve block:* 1–2%, maximum dose, 5–6 mg/kg plain, and 7 mg/kg with epinephrine; duration, 1.5 hr plain, 2 hr with epinephrine	Derivative of lidocaine; less penetration, slower metabolism; ineffective topically
Bupivacaine (Marcaine)	*Infiltration:* 0.1–0.25%; *nerve block:* 0.25–0.5%; long-acting, up to 12 hr	Less penetration than other amides
Dibucaine (Nupercaine)	*Topical:* 2 mg/ml ointment, up to 15 ml; *spinal:* 2.5–5 mg/ml	Mainly used as topical anesthesia; rarely used for spinal anesthesia owing to high systemic toxicity
Etidocaine (Duranest)	*Infiltration:* 2.5–5 mg/ml solution; *peripheral nerve block:* 5 and 10 mg/ml solution; *epidural block:* 5 and 10 mg/ml solution	Greater potency and longer duration of action than lidocaine. Maximum dose of a single injection should not exceed 400 mg in the adult

using this technique, the plasma level of lidocaine should be between 1 and 2 μg per ml. Lidocaine can also reduce intracranial pressure when used in a slow, continuous intravenous infusion. Also, to prevent increases in intracranial pressure and hypertension associated with endotracheal intubation, a bolus dose of 1.5 mg per kg of lidocaine given intravenously is helpful. The upper limits of safe dosage for this drug are between 200 and 400 mg without epinephrine and 500 mg with epinephrine. Toxic symptoms develop when the blood level of lidocaine increases about 5 μg per ml. Seizures and respiratory and cardiac depression have been reported when the blood level of lidocaine is higher than 8 μg per ml.

Mepivacaine (Carbocaine)

Mepivacaine, an amide local anesthetic, is similar to lidocaine in its uses and onset of action; however, its duration of action is longer than lidocaine. Mepivacaine does not produce vasodilatation and, consequently, it is an attractive alternative to other local anesthetics that require epinephrine. Mepivacaine should not be used for topical anesthesia. The upper limits of safe dosage for the drug are 400 mg without epinephrine and 500 mg with epinephrine. At high doses, mepivacaine can depress both respiratory and cardiac functions.

Prilocaine (Citanest)

Prilocaine is quite similar to lidocaine in its uses and potency. However, it has a lower toxicity and shorter duration of action than lidocaine. The major reason why prilocaine is not as widely used as lidocaine is that it can cause significant complications. One complication associated with prilocaine is methemoglobinemia, especially when the dosage exceeds 500 mg. The treatment for this problem is usually methylene blue given over 5 minutes intravenously at a dosage of 1 to 2 mg per kg.

The Long-Duration Local Anesthetics

Bupivacaine (Marcaine; Sensorcaine)

Bupivacaine is an amide local anesthetic that is about four times as potent as lidocaine. Like lidocaine, it is widely used in clinical practice. For infiltration anesthesia, it can be used in a 0.125 to 0.25 solution without epinephrine. For this type of anesthesia, it has an onset of 5 to 15 minutes and a duration of about 200 minutes. The duration of action of bupivacaine can be doubled by the addition of epinephrine. For axillary block and other nerve block techniques, including epidural anesthesia, bupivacaine is administered in a 0.25 to 0.5 percent solution. In this instance, the onset of action is about 15 minutes and the duration is about 2 to 4 hours. For spinal anesthesia, 0.75 percent bupivacaine is in solution with dextrose. The dose range is between 5 and 20 mg, and the onset is between 8 and 15 minutes, with a duration of action between 2 and 4 hours. Bupivacaine is the drug of choice for lower extremity surgery when a tourniquet is used. Tourniquet pain is transmitted by the very small C fibers. Bupivacaine is able to better block the C fibers than is tetracaine.

A 0.75 percent, or 7.5 mg per ml, concentration of bupivacaine is not recommended for obstetric or intravenous regional anesthesia. The upper limits for safe dosage with this drug are 150 mg without epinephrine and 200 mg with epinephrine. In patients receiving diaze-

pam (Valium), bupivacaine can be potentiated because diazepam increases the bioavailability of bupivacaine. If bupivacaine is accidentally administered intravenously, acute cardiovascular collapse can ensue.

Etidocaine (Duranest)

Etidocaine resembles lidocaine in time of onset; however, its duration of action is considerably longer than lidocaine. It is effective in infiltration, spinal, epidural, and caudal anesthesia. It can cause a profound motor blockade and, consequently, should not be administered to obstetric patients. The safe dosage limit for etidocaine is 300 mg without epinephrine and 400 mg with epinephrine.

Tetracaine (Pontocaine)

Tetracaine is an ester local anesthetic that resembles procaine and chloroprocaine. It is metabolized by plasma pseudocholinesterase at a slower rate than other ester local anesthetics.

It is used predominately for spinal anesthesia in a 1 percent solution. The dosage range for spinal anesthesia is usually between 5 and 20 mg, with an onset of about 7 to 10 minutes and a duration of about 60 to 90 minutes. The addition of a vasoconstrictor increases the duration of the spinal block to about 120 to 180 minutes. Tetracaine can be potentiated by cimetidine (Tagamet). When the blood concentration of tetracaine exceeds 8 µg per ml, serious problems can occur, including seizures and severe depression of the respiratory and cardiovascular systems.

Ropivacaine

Ropivacaine is a new local anesthetic that resembles bupivacaine in potency and length of action. It may have certain advantages over bupivacaine when used in obstetrics. This is because it produces less motor blockage while it keeps the patient analgesic. Ropivacaine can be used for epidural anesthesia because it produces a rapid onset of sensory loss and has a duration of as long as 12 hours.

Complications of Use of Local Anesthetics

Allergic Reactions. Allergic reactions to local anesthetic drugs can be divided into four types: (1) contact dermatitis; (2) serum sickness, which

Table 17–3. SIGNS OF OVERDOSAGE OF LOCAL ANESTHETIC AGENTS

Central Nervous System
Stimulation of:
  Cortex: excitement, disorientation, euphoria, dizziness,
    hallucinations, muscle twitching, numbness of fingers
    or lips, and convulsions
  Medulla:
      Cardiovascular center: hypertension, tachycardia
      Respiratory center: increased respiratory rate and
        variations in rhythm
      Vomiting center: nausea and vomiting

Depression of:
  Cortex: unconsciousness
  Medulla:
      Vasomotor center: hypotension
      Respiratory center: apnea

Peripheral Nervous System
  Heart: bradycardia due to direct depression
  Blood vessels: vasodilatation from direct action

includes fever, lymphadenopathy, and urticaria 2 to 12 days after injection; (3) anaphylactic reaction, characterized by dyspnea, cyanosis, and death; and (4) atopic response, which includes bronchospasm, urticaria, and angioneurotic edema.

When the allergy is being evaluated, the first consideration is whether or not the reaction is caused by added epinephrine. Symptoms such as tachycardia, palpitations, restlessness, and anxiety indicate epinephrine as the causative agent.

Overdosage. Overdosage of local anesthetic agents can occur because of inadvertent intravenous injection of the local anesthetic, variation in patient response, or injection of the local anesthetic into a highly vascular area. Table 17–3 summarizes the signs of overdosage of the local anesthetic agents.

The treatment and nursing care of a patient who has had an overdosage of a local anesthetic agent begin with the administration of 100 percent oxygen. Oxygen should be administered to the patient at the first sign of local anesthetic toxicity. This should be followed by preparation for the management of convulsions, hypotension, and respiratory depression. Diazepam should be administered to suppress local anesthetic–induced seizures. Intubation and mechanical ventilation may be indicated. Vasopressors such as epinephrine may also be indicated.

References

1. Attia, R., Grogono, A., and Domer, F.: Practical Anesthetic Pharmacology. 2nd ed. Norwalk, CT, Appleton-Century-Crofts, 1987.
2. Barash, P., Cullen, B., and Stoelting, R.: Clinical Anesthesia. 2nd ed. Philadelphia, J. B. Lippincott, 1992.
3. Breslow, M., Miller, C., and Rogers, M.: Perioperative Management. St. Louis, C. V. Mosby, 1990.
4. Gilman, A., Rall, T., Nies, A., et al.: Goodman and Gilman's The Pharmacological Basis of Therapeutics. 8th ed. New York: Peragamon Press, 1990.
5. Guyton, A. Textbook of Medical Physiology. 8th ed. Philadelphia, W. B. Saunders, 1991.
6. Longnecker, D., and Murphy, F.: Dripps/Eckenhoff/Vandam Introduction to Anesthesia. 8th ed. Philadelphia: W. B. Saunders, 1992.
7. Miller, R. (ed.): Anesthesia. 3rd ed. New York, Churchill Livingstone, 1990.
8. Moore, D.: Regional Block. 4th ed. Springfield, IL, Charles C Thomas, 1976.
9. Saleh, K: Practical points in understanding local anesthetics. J. Post Anesth. Nurs., 7(1):45–47, 1992.
10. Stoelting, R.: Pharmacology and Physiology in Anesthesia Practice. 2nd ed. Philadelphia, J. B. Lippincott, 1991.
11. Waugaman, W., Foster, S., and Rigor, B.: Principles and Practice of Nurse Anesthesia. 2nd ed. Norwalk, CT, Appleton & Lange, 1992.
12. Wood, M., and Wood, A.: Drugs and Anesthesia: Pharmacology for the Anesthesiologist. 2nd ed. Baltimore, Williams & Wilkins, 1990.

CHAPTER 18

Regional Anesthesia

T he term *regional anesthesia* refers to the various anesthetic techniques that use local anesthetic agents to block nerve conduction in an extremity or a region of the body. The use of regional anesthesia has become popular in modern anesthesia practice because, when indicated, it offers many advantages over general inhalation anesthesia. To facilitate optimal recovery of the surgical patient from this type of anesthetic, the post anesthesia care unit (PACU) nurse should have a complete knowledge of all the particular regional anesthetic techniques employed.

SPINAL AND EPIDURAL ANESTHESIA

Anatomy of the Spine

The vertebral column comprises 33 vertebrae (7 cervical, 12 thoracic, 5 lumbar, 5 sacral, and 4 coccygeal). The ligaments of the vertebral column, which bind it together and protect the spinal cord, are the supraspinous ligament, intraspinous ligament, ligamentum flavum, posterior longitudinal ligament, and anterior longitudinal ligament (Fig. 18–1). When a midline spinal puncture is made, the needle will traverse the first three ligaments.

The spinal cord, which is a continuation of the medulla oblongata, occupies the upper two thirds of the vertebral canal. It is approximately 18 inches long, and it ends at the lower border of L1. The lower portion of the spinal cord then becomes the filum terminale, which connects to the bone of the coccyx vertebra and holds the spinal cord in place. The spinal cord is encased by three membranes: the dura mater, the arachnoid, and the pia mater. The outermost membrane is the dura mater, which consists of two layers (*periosteal* and *dural)* and ends at S2. Between the dura and the ligamentum flavum is the epidural space, which is a potential space filled with loose fatty tissue and blood vessels. It is in this space that local anesthetic solutions

are introduced when the epidural regional anesthetic technique is used. The arachnoid layer consists of a thin membranous sheath. The innermost layer is called the *pia mater*, and it is separated from the arachnoid layer by a subarachnoid space filled with cerebrospinal fluid (CSF). This space is where local anesthetic so-

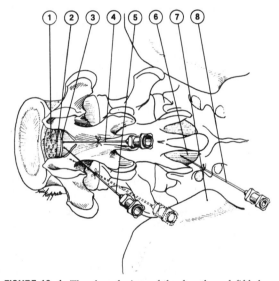

FIGURE 18–1. The dorsal view of the fourth and fifth lumbar vertebrae, their relationship to the sacrum and iliac bones, and the most frequently used approaches for needle puncture in subarachnoid and lumbar peridural techniques. Numerals represent the following: *(1)* the cauda equina; *(2)* the dura mater; *(3)* the ligamentum flavum at the L3–L4 interspace; *(4)* the midline approach for spinal and epidural techniques where the needle is introduced between the spines of L3 and L4 vertebrae, traversing the supraspinous and interspinous ligaments before piercing the ligamentum flavum; *(5)* the paramedian approach at this level where the needle puncture site is 1 to 2 cm lateral to the above midline approach; if the initial approach results in contacting the lamina of the vertebrae as shown in the dotted needle silhouette, then the needle is walked cephalad and medially until it slips off the lamina and contacts the ligamentum flavum as shown; *(6)* the large interspace between S5 and L1, which is situated 2 cm medial and cephalad from *(7)* the posterior superior iliac spine; *(8)* the needle can be introduced at this site in the Taylor approach for either subarachnoid or epidural puncture. (From Miller, R. [ed.]: Anesthesia. 2nd ed. New York, Churchill Livingstone, 1986.)

lutions are deposited when the spinal technique of producing regional anesthesia is used.

There are 31 pairs of spinal nerves that travel from the spinal column through the layers of the cord and exit at the intervertebral foramina. There are 8 cervical, 12 thoracic, 5 lumbar, 5 sacral, and 1 coccygeal pairs of spinal nerves. It is these nerves that are blocked by the local anesthetic drug to produce anesthesia.

Spinal Anesthetics

Techniques of Administration

Because a lumbar puncture may be performed in the PACU, a brief description of the procedure of lumbar puncture will be presented. Before the procedure is started, the PACU nurse should ensure that the spinal (or epidural) procedure is not contraindicated. The absolute contraindications are anatomic abnormalities, coagulation abnormalities, patient refusal, infection at the site of the needle insertion, and uncorrected hypovolemia. The relative contraindications are chronic back pain, bacteremia, neurologic disorders such as multiple sclerosis, and patients receiving minidose heparin.

Once it has been determined that the spinal procedure is not contraindicated, the PACU nurse should obtain the patient's baseline vital signs. These should include the blood pressure, pulse, respiratory rate, and oxygen saturation. The blood pressure cuff and pulse oximeter should remain in place throughout the procedure. Also, the nurse should describe the procedure to the patient and answer any questions he or she might have. Verbal contact with the patient throughout the procedure is important in reducing fear and anxiety.

Proper positioning of the patient is important in facilitating the success of this procedure. The lateral decubitus position is the best position to use in the PACU. The pregnant patient should always be placed in the left lateral decubitus position. Although it is technically easier to have the patient in the sitting position, this position should not be used because of the residual effects of anesthetics. To place the patient in the lateral decubitus position, the patient is turned on his or her side, the knees are then bent and drawn up near the patient's chin, and his or her back is arched out toward the person performing the lumbar puncture. A pillow may be placed under the patient's head to help align the spine and to add comfort during the procedure. The assistant should stand near

the patient's stomach, securing his knees and providing for his safety throughout the procedure. At this time the patient's back should be inspected for signs of any dermatologic infectious process that may be present. If an infectious process near the lumbar puncture site is found, the procedure should be canceled. Once the patient is properly positioned, the person performing the procedure should first wash his or her hands and then open the lumbar puncture tray so that the sterile components are available, and using sterile technique, don the sterile gloves. The drugs are then drawn into the syringes and the needles and equipment examined for any signs of damage. The back is then washed (prepped) with antiseptic solution, after which the sterile drapes are placed over the patient's back. Throughout the procedure, the PACU nurse should continue to explain each maneuver to the patient. An imaginary line, called *Tuffier's line*, is then drawn between the iliac crests. This line crosses the spine between the third or fourth lumbar interspace. Because the spinal cord terminates at the L2 interspace, from L3 and below are used when the lumbar puncture is performed. Once the interspace has been identified, a local anesthetic (usually procaine) is deposited subcutaneously and into the supraspinous ligament with a 25-gauge needle. A needle introducer is then placed through the skin, the supraspinous ligament, and interspinous ligaments. The spinal needle is inserted through the introducer and is passed through the ligamentum flavum and the dura and enters the subarachnoid space. The stylet is removed, and CSF can be seen at the hub of the needle. Blood-tinged CSF or lack of free flow is a contraindication to the injection of the anesthetic solution. If the blood-tinged CSF becomes clear, the anesthetic solution can be administered. Before the syringe is connected to the hub of the needle, the patient should be secured and told not to move or cough by the PACU nurse. The patient should also be told that his or her legs will feel warm after the anesthetic solution is injected. The syringe is then secured to the hub of the needle, and after aspiration to ensure that CSF is still present, the anesthetic solution is injected. After the solution is injected, the syringe is aspirated to verify the presence of CSF, confirming the introduction of the medications into the subarachnoid space. After confirmation, the syringe, needle, and introducer are removed simultaneously. Next, the patient is placed in the supine position by the PACU nurse and the person who performed the lumbar puncture. Before the patient is moved, he or she should be told not to try to move or cough because that would increase the spread of the anesthetics.

Once the patient is supine, his or her blood pressure, pulse, respiratory rate, and oxygen saturation should be assessed at 1-minute intervals for the first 5 to 10 minutes and then every 5 minutes during the next half hour. If the oxygen saturation drops below 94 percent or the blood pressure decreases by 20 percent of the baseline reading, the anesthesia practitioner should be notified immediately.

If a local anesthetic was administered into the subarachnoid space, the dermatome level (Fig. 18–2) should be closely monitored using a supersaturated alcohol sponge or a pin. With either method, patients should be informed

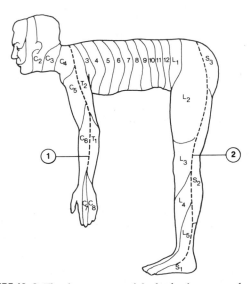

FIGURE 18–2. The dermatomes of the body show an orderly craniad to caudad sequence. By positioning the body as shown, the complex arrangement of dermatomes on the limbs is more readily understood. On the upper extremity, the limb dermatomes are distributed symmetrically about the axial line *(1)*. Note that dermatomes C5 and C6 are distributed on the preaxial border of the limb and the postaxial dermatomes, C8, T1, and T2, are distributed on the postaxial part of the limb. C7, which is the central dermatome of the limb, is distributed more distally, that is, over the middle finger. There is an orderly sequence on the trunk from T3 to L1. The dermatome distribution of the lower extremity is also arranged around the axial line *(2)*. Large areas of skin, that is, L2 and L3, have been borrowed from the trunk to supplement the true leg dermatomes of L4 through S3. Note that as in the upper extremity, the craniad dermatomes, L4 and L5, are distributed on the preaxial border of the limb and the caudad dermatomes, S2 and S3, are distributed on the postaxial border of the limb. The central dermatome S1 is distributed over the lateral aspect of the plantar surface and lateral border of the foot. (Adapted from Foerster O.: The dermatomes in man. Brain *56*:1, 1933; by permission of Oxford University Press.)

fully about the procedure to ascertain the dermatome level. In this procedure, the nurse touches the patient's shoulders with either the alcohol sponge or the pin. The patient is instructed to tell the nurse when he or she feels the same sensation. The nurse then touches the skin with the sponge or pin at about the sacral area and moves up slowly at intervals of about 1 inch, corresponding with the dermatomes. When the patient says the sensation is the same as the one felt on the shoulder, that dermatome is so noted (see Fig. 18–2) as the level of the anesthetic.

Mechanism of Action

After the local anesthetic drug is injected into the subarachnoid space, a level of anesthesia will be achieved that is dependent on the dosage of the agent used, the rate of injection, the specific gravity of the fluid injected, and the position of the patient following injection. The level of anesthesia is referred to as the *dermatome level* (see Fig. 18–2). A dermatome is that area of the skin that is supplied by a single spinal nerve. The face is supplied by the trigeminal nerve, and the remaining portions of the body's cutaneous areas are supplied in sequence by dermatomes C2 through S5. Some of the major topographic landmarks that can be depicted by a pinprick to detect sensory loss are L1 to T12, the inguinal ligament and iliac crest; T10, the umbilicus; T6, the xiphoid; T4, the nipples; T1, the clavicle; and C7, the middle finger. The order of blockage of the various nerve modalities is shown in Table 17–1 in Chapter 17.

During the recovery from a spinal anesthetic, the anesthesia works its way back from the extremities toward the site where the anesthetic was administered. Therefore, the areas near the site of injection are the last to recover.

Complications

The complications of spinal anesthesia are high spinal block, hypotension, nausea and vomiting, backache, palsies and paralysis, urinary retention, postspinal headache, and meningitis.

High Spinal Block. When the local anesthetic rises in the CSF, the major nerves exiting the spinal cord can be effectively blocked. The effects of the spread of the anesthetic into the cervical region are usually short lived, because dilution of the anesthetic produces a lower concentration of the drug. Some objective symptoms associated with a high spinal anesthetic are agitation, hypotension, nausea, diaphragmatic breathing (absence of intercostal muscle function), and an inability to speak in an audible fashion. The treatment of a high spinal block is initiated in the operating room and consists of efficient ventilation and oxygenation and the maintenance of the blood pressure by vasopressors. This block is a reversible complication; when the local anesthetic drug wears off, the patient will recover. PACU care consists of maintaining the treatment initiated in the operating room. The patient may be intubated and possibly placed on a ventilator. As the local anesthetic agent wears off, the patient may be unable to maintain tidal volume because of partial paralysis of the respiratory muscles. Ventilation of the patient should be assisted until an adequate tidal volume can be maintained. It is inadvisable to place the patient in a head-up position in an effort to limit the spread of the anesthetic—the anesthetic is already "fixed" at a level in the CSF, and raising the head can reduce cerebral blood flow, resulting in medullary ischemia.

The PACU nurse should establish verbal contact with the patient to decrease the anxiety and apprehension he or she may feel because of being partially sedated, having difficulty in breathing, and unable to move about.

To enhance the cardiac output, the patient's legs may be elevated to promote the return of venous blood from the lower extremities to the heart. If the vital signs still indicate neurogenic shock after this maneuver has been performed, vasopressor therapy will usually be instituted. Vasopressors used to treat this complication are usually of the alpha-adrenergic variety, because total spinal block produces a type of neurogenic shock. The alpha-adrenergic vasopressors produce peripheral vasoconstriction, which aids in returning the blood to the heart, thereby improving the cardiac output. Alpha-adrenergic vasopressors that may be used in this situation are phenylephrine (Neo-Synephrine) or norepinephrine (Levophed) and are discussed in Chapter 5.

Because of the height of the spinal block, the patient may also experience some bradycardia, which can be treated with atropine or glycopyrrolate (Robinul). Nausea and vomiting may also occur. Suction should be available, and antiemetics may have to be administered to the patient.

Hypotension. Postoperative hypotension due to a sympathetic blockade from a spinal anesthetic leads to venous dilation, resulting in a decreased venous return and a reduction in the cardiac output. This problem is most likely to occur during the first 30 minutes in the PACU, and, if the patient is hypotensive, it is important to assess for bleeding, which may be causing the hypotension. If bleeding is not the cause, treatment should be instituted and the anesthesiologist should be notified. If bleeding is the cause, the attending physician should be notified. The first line of treatment is to ensure that hydration is adequate. Often, the infusion of 500 ml of crystalloid along with the elevation of the legs corrects the postoperative spinal hypotension. If the hypotension continues, it can best be treated by vasopressors.

Nausea and Vomiting. Nausea and vomiting can be a result of hypotension, of hypertension due to the vasopressors, to motion during change in position, or to apprehension. If hypotension or hypertension is present, the anesthetist should be notified. It is important for the PACU nurse to assess the cause of the nausea and vomiting. Blood pressure should be taken and oxygen administered to the patient. Should vomiting occur, the patient should be placed in a Trendelenburg position with his or her head to the side, and a clear airway should be established and maintained. The anesthetist should be summoned if the patient experiences nausea or vomiting (see Chapter 9).

Palsies and Paralysis. Palsies and paralysis usually occur postoperatively in the peripheral nerves. Of the cranial nerves, the sixth cranial nerve is most often involved. In the PACU phase of the spinal anesthetic, the nurse should assess neurologic function of the extremities as the anesthetic wears off. If the patient has double vision or any other decrease in peripheral nerve function, the anesthetist and the surgeon should be notified.

Urinary Retention. Urinary retention is usually caused by trauma to the bladder during surgery or by a decrease in bladder tone due to the anesthesia. The patient complains of severe pain and may become hypertensive or bradycardic. If the condition is not diagnosed and corrected, the patient may become incoherent and thrash about in bed. The PACU nurse should assess the patient for a distended bladder or hypoxia, because the symptoms are almost identical. If urinary retention is the problem, the patient should be encouraged to void. If the patient cannot void, the surgeon should be notified and an order for catheterization of the bladder obtained.

Postspinal Headache. The true postspinal headache is caused by a persistent leak of CSF through the needle hole in the dura mater. Postspinal headache is usually transient but annoying to the patient. The pain usually becomes severe when the patient is upright and lessens when he or she is in a supine position. The location of the pain is usually occipital or frontal. The patient may also complain of tinnitus and diplopia.

As a prophylactic measure, most patients who have received a spinal anesthetic are encouraged to remain in the supine position for at least 6 to 8 hours following surgery. Some research indicates that the supine-bedrest prophylaxis is unnecessary and of no value in preventing postspinal headache. The advent of smaller-gauge needles has reduced the incidence of postspinal headache. Conservative treatment of the patient with this complication involves optimal hydration, analgesics, and reduction in environmental noise. However, if the postspinal headache becomes incapacitating or does not respond to conservative treatment within the first 2 days after the administration of the spinal anesthetic, an *epidural blood patch procedure* may be performed. This procedure involves administering 10 to 20 ml of the patient's own blood into the epidural space at the site of the previous lumbar puncture. This procedure seals the hole in the dura mater; prompt pain relief usually follows.

Epidural Anesthetics

Mechanism of Action

Epidural (peridural) block is produced by depositing an anesthetic agent in the epidural space. The location on the vertebral column or the segment where the epidural block is performed determines the type of epidural anesthesia the patient will receive. Thoracic epidural block, lumbar epidural block, and caudal epidural block or caudal anesthesia are the possible types of epidural anesthetic.

Techniques of Administration

Epidural block is usually performed in the same manner as the spinal block. The patient is placed into the lateral decubitus position, his or her back is prepped, and the needle is inserted into the epidural space. After it has been determined that the needle is in the epidural space, a test dose of the anesthetic solution is injected. Blood pressure, pulse, respiratory rate, and oxygen saturation are then determined. If vital signs are unchanged, the remainder of the anesthetic is administered. The needle may be removed, or a catheter may be placed through the needle into the epidural

space for the continuous (serial) epidural technique. Monitoring the patient after a epidural block is similar to monitoring after the spinal technique.

The morphine epidural technique is becoming popular as a way to reduce postoperative pain. Epidural morphine may be administered intraoperatively or in the immediate postoperative period. The pharmacology of epidural morphine is discussed in detail in Chapter 15. The major risk with epidural morphine is respiratory depression. Epidural morphine can depress respiration from 2.5 to 16.5 hours or longer. Consequently, monitoring for respiratory depression requires close surveillance of the patient's respiratory rate and oxygen saturation. To enhance the monitoring parameters, an apnea monitor should be used so as to have another alarm system to alert PACU personnel to the patient's respiratory depression. Fentanyl is also being used instead of morphine for epidural analgesia because it has a shorter duration of respiratory depression. This drug is discussed in Chapter 15.

The epidural block is the anesthetic technique of choice for cesarean section and is indicated in poor-risk patients and in those with cardiac, pulmonary, and metabolic diseases. It is also well suited for patients who have had thoracic or upper abdominal surgical procedures. In this instance, the epidural is usually placed intraoperatively and the patient receives both general and epidural anesthesia. This combination of two anesthesia techniques has been quite successful in reducing postoperative pulmonary complications and enhancing pain relief.

The epidural block is contraindicated in patients being given anticoagulants, when hemorrhage or shock is present, when the patient has had previous back surgery, and when local inflammation exists.

PACU Care After Spinal or Epidural Anesthesia

After the patient's arrival in the PACU, care must be exercised when moving him or her, as the block's residual effects, such as lack of motor and sensory function, are still present. Care should be taken in positioning the patient, because good body alignment is needed to reduce muscle soreness or injury. The patient's joints should not be hyperextended, and the bedclothes should not press on his or her toes.

If a patient has any residual spinal anesthesia while in the PACU, care should be taken to avoid rapid position change, which causes severe decreases in blood pressure. This is because the circulatory system cannot compensate adequately for rapid position change when anesthesia is present.

If intravenous sedation was given during the operation, respiratory function should be monitored closely by the use of a pulse oximeter. Oxygen should be administered to all block patients until their motor and sensory functions return adequately. The patient should be encouraged to cough and breathe deeply every 15 minutes to reduce the incidence of atelectasis.

The patient should be checked for any signs of bladder distention. Catheterization may be required, especially in patients who have had pelvic or perineal surgery.

AXILLARY OR BRACHIAL PLEXUS BLOCK

Nerve blocks are employed to produce anesthesia in specific areas of the body. They are usually used for orthopedic, obstetric, and vascular surgical procedures. They are relatively safe and usually have good patient acceptance.

The axillary or brachial plexus block is used to anesthetize the arm to facilitate surgery below the elbow. When this block is performed, either the axillary or the supraclavicular approach is used.

PACU Care After Axillary or Brachial Plexus Block

PACU care of the patient who has received an axillary block centers on patient education and observation for complications. The patient should be taught that motor function will be lost and that no attempts should be made to move his or her arm about. Injuries to the face and to the surgical site have been reported because the patient arm with reduced motor control managed to "flop" on his or her face or hit on the side rail.

If the supraclavicular approach was used, pneumothorax is a possible complication. The first sign is a complaint by the patient of pain in the chest that is accentuated by deep breathing. Other signs of pneumothorax are increased resonance to percussion, absence of or decreased breath sounds, lag in expansion on the affected side in comparison with the unaffected side, and difficulty in "getting breath."

PACU care involves administering oxygen and advising the anesthetist of the complication. Analgesics are usually administered and, after a chest radiograph is made, more definitive treatment may be instituted.

When the supraclavicular approach is used to perform the brachial plexus block, *Horner's syndrome* can result. This occurs when the anesthetic solution spreads so that it involves the stellate ganglion. Symptoms of this syndrome, which appear on the side where the block is performed, are flushing of the face, constricted pupils, ptosis, and stuffiness of the nose. Horner's syndrome clears as the block wears off.

Another complication caused by using the supraclavicular approach is *blockage of the phrenic nerve*. The incidence of this complication is related to the spread of anesthetic solution and is usually unilateral. Generally, there are no signs and symptoms, and the complication clears as the block dissipates itself.

Obliteration of the radial pulse is a possible complication of the axillary approach to the brachial plexus. It is caused by bleeding or the use of too large a volume of anesthetic solution. The radial pulse usually returns in 2 to 4 hours.

INTRAVENOUS REGIONAL ANESTHESIA

The intravenous regional, or Bier, block was named for August K. Bier, who originated it in 1908. It is useful for emergency procedures on the forearm and hand, especially for a procedure such as Colles' fracture reduction, and is simple to administer. The Bier block involves starting an intravenous infusion in the hand, exsanguinating the arm with an Esmarch latex bandage, inflating a double pneumatic tourniquet above the elbow, and then removing the Esmarch bandage and injecting the local anesthetic agent (bupivacaine or lidocaine) while the tourniquet remains inflated. At the end of the surgical procedure, the tourniquet is released and the analgesia will cease within 5 to 10 minutes. Usually, there are no sequelae from the anesthetic agent; by the time the venous blood from the limb has passed through the lungs and has mixed with the rest of the venous return, the systemic arterial blood levels are, because of the dilution effect, not clinically significant. Should the blood levels of the local anesthetic remain high, the patient will experience cardiovascular depression, which is usually manifested by bradycardia. This cardiovascular depression is usually quite transient. If this situation arises, vigilant monitoring, coupled with appropriate interventions such as oxygen and glycopyrrolate (Robinul) or atropine will usually correct the problem.

The intravenous regional technique can also be used for surgery on the lower leg and foot. Although it requires a larger tourniquet and more local anesthetic agent, it is an effective technique for this type of surgery.

PACU Care After Intravenous Regional Anesthesia

When the patient arrives in the PACU, all analgesia provided by the local anesthetic agent used in the intravenous regional anesthesia has usually dissipated. Medication for the relief of pain can be given soon after the patient's arrival. The PACU nurse should assess the patient's level of sedation, including the amount of premedication and sedation during the surgical procedure, before administering the pain medication.

References

1. Barash, P, Cullen, B., and Stoelting, R.: Clinical Anesthesia. 2nd ed. Philadelphia, J. B. Lippincott, 1992.
2. Cramer, C.: Morphine epidural anesthesia. J. Post Anesth. Nurs., 1(2):129–131, 1986.
3. Cramer, C.: Postanesthetic management of regional anesthesia. J. Post Anesth. Nurs., 1(4):236–243, 1986.
4. Gilman, A., Rall, T., Nies, A., et al.: Goodman and Gilman's The Pharmacological Basis of Therapeutics. 8th ed. New York, Pergamon Press, 1990.
5. Longnecker, D., and Murphy, F.: Dripps/Eckenhoff/Vandam Introduction to Anesthesia. 8th ed. Philadelphia, W. B. Saunders, 1992.
6. Miller, R. (ed.): Anesthesia. 3rd ed. New York, Churchill Livingstone, 1990.
7. Moore, D.: Regional Block. 4th ed. Springfield, IL, Charles C Thomas, 1976.
8. Wood, M., and Wood, A.: Drugs and Anesthesia: Pharmacology for the Anesthesiologist. 2nd ed. Baltimore, Williams & Wilkins, 1990.

Nursing Care
in the
PACU

Assessment and Monitoring of the Post Anesthesia Patient

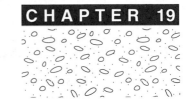

Patricia A. McGaffigan, M.S., R.N.,C.
Susan B. Christoph, D.N.Sc., R.N.

The primary purpose of the post anesthesia care unit (PACU) is the critical evaluation and stabilization of postoperative patients, with emphasis on anticipation and prevention of complications resulting from anesthesia or the operative procedure. It is, therefore, imperative that a knowledgeable, skillful nurse fully assess the condition of each patient not only at admission and at discharge but also at frequent intervals throughout the post anesthesia period. Assessment must be a continuous and complete process, leading to sound nursing judgments and the implementation of therapeutic care. Assessment includes gathering information from direct observation of the patient (the primary source), from the physician and other health care personnel, and from the medical record and the care plan.

Traditionally, PACU nurses have, with only limited information, performed the role of caring for the surgical patient in the vulnerable post anesthesia state. However, to assess the post anesthesia patient and plan and implement appropriate care, it is imperative that preoperative information be available as a basis for comparison with postoperative data. The PACU nurse has a professional obligation to consider the patient's history, clinical status, and psychosocial state. The necessary data may be gathered by chart review, personal preoperative visit, and consultation with other health care members providing care to the patient. The collection of such information should be a coordinated effort with all involved members of the health care team.

This chapter deals with the assessment of postoperative patients and their common needs. Specific assessments related to patient age, the type of surgical procedure, and problems resulting from complicated diagnoses are dealt with in the following chapters. The assessment and management of postoperative pain is presented in Chapter 22.

PREOPERATIVE ASSESSMENTS

Preoperative evaluation of both the physical and the emotional status of the surgical patient is extremely important, and nursing brings a unique perspective to this assessment. Nurses in a number of subspecialties, including PACU nurses, operative room nurses, and general unit nurses, have advocated making this assessment. Having each nurse who will care for the patient make a preoperative visit seems redundant and may be overwhelming for the patient. More appropriately, nurses should treat each other as colleagues, communicating needs for specific information, coordinating the collection of such information, and documenting data to be used for planning care. Multidisciplinary care conferences can be instrumental in educating all those who will care for the surgical patient and in developing communication patterns.

Because many PACU departments now include preoperative holding areas, it may be necessary for the PACU nurse to participate in the patient's preoperative interview and assessment. A complete preoperative nursing assessment should include relevant preoperative physical and psychosocial status, past medical history (including anesthesia history), length of fasting, understanding of the surgery and postoperative course, and the need for follow-up services. The preoperative physical assessment should include documentation of temperature, pulse, blood pressure, respirations, oxygen saturation, height, and weight and a review of systems. Nursing diagnoses are established based on analysis of data collected during the assessment phase, and an appropriate plan of care is generated.

ADMISSION OBSERVATIONS

Physical assessment of the post anesthesia patient must begin immediately on admission to the PACU. The patient is accompanied from the operating room to the PACU by the anesthesiologist (or anesthetist), who reports to the receiving nurse on the patient's general condition, the operation performed, and the type of anesthesia used for the surgery. In addition, the nurse should be informed of any problems or complications encountered during the surgery and anesthesia.

Because all anesthetics are depressants, postoperative assessment and care generally are the same, regardless of the specific agent used. For special precautions required for certain agents, review the chapters on anesthesia (see Chapters 12 through 18).

Rapid assessment of the life-sustaining cardiorespiratory system is of initial concern. Ensure that the airway is patent and that respirations are free and easy. Check and record the patient's blood pressure, pulse, rate of respiration, and oxygen saturation level. Quickly inspect all dressings and drains for gross bleeding. These baseline observations, made immediately on admission, should be reported to the anesthesiologist in attendance and recorded in the admission note.

Once these initial observations are made, it is essential to systematically assess the patient's total condition. This assessment may be made from head to toe or by systems, whichever the individual nurse prefers—the observations are essentially identical. Because our own preference is for a systems approach, the following outline of post anesthesia assessment is presented. It should be noted that each system of the body has an integral function, and therefore all observations are interrelated.

RESPIRATORY FUNCTION

Because the post anesthesia patient has experienced some interference with his or her respiratory system, maintenance of adequate gas exchange is a crucial aspect of care in the PACU. Any change in respiratory function must be detected early so that appropriate measures can be taken to ensure adequate oxygenation and ventilation. The most significant respiratory problems encountered in the immediate postoperative period include hypoventilation, airway obstruction, aspiration, and atelectasis.

Respiratory assessment is coupled with the related responses of the cardiovascular and neurologic systems to provide for total evaluation of the adequacy of gas exchange and ventilatory efficiency. Respiratory function is evaluated by clinical assessment. Additionally, pulse oximetry is used to assess arterial oxygenation, and capnography is used to evaluate the adequacy of ventilation. Arterial blood gas measurements may also be a part of the respiratory assessment (see Chapters 6 and 21).

Clinical Assessment

Inspection

The resting respiratory rate of a normal adult is approximately 16 to 20 breaths per min. Infants and children have a higher respiratory rate and a lower tidal volume than adults (see Chapter 39). Respirations should be quiet and easy, with a regular rate and rhythm. The chest should move freely as a unit, and expansion should be equal bilaterally. Alterations in symmetry may be due to many factors, including pain that may cause splinting at the incision site, consolidation, and pneumothorax. Note the character of the respirations: intercostal retractions, bulging, nasal flaring, or use of the accessory respiratory muscles are signs of respiratory distress. The depth of respiration is as important as the rate. Shallow respiration is the cardinal sign of continuing depression from anesthesia or preoperative medications, but it may be caused by many other factors, including incisional pain, obesity, tight binders, and dressings that restrict movements of the thoracic cage or abdomen. Shallow respirations and use of the neck and diaphragmatic muscles may also indicate recurarization from the use of skeletal muscle relaxants such as succinylcholine, atracurium, pancuronium, and vercuronium. The presence of chest movements alone, however, does not provide evidence that adequate gas exchange is occurring.

Airway obstruction may be present when the normal duration of inspiration versus exhalation is altered. Restlessness, confusion or anxiety, and apprehension are the earliest signs of hypoxemia and carbon dioxide (CO_2) retention and should receive immediate attention to determine their cause. The patient's color should also be regularly evaluated. Although this assessment is difficult, it provides important information about the respiratory function. However, it is crucial to remember that cyanosis is a late sign of severe tissue hypoxia; when it appears, immediate and vigorous efforts must be instituted to determine and correct the cause of hypoxia. The noninvasive monitors that are increasingly used in the PACU provide an effective means of continuously and objectively assessing gas exchange; pulse oximeters monitor hemoglobin oxygen saturation, and capnographs evaluate the adequacy of ventilation. These monitors will be discussed later in this chapter.

Note the presence of an artificial airway; airways are used primarily to maintain a patent air passage so that respiratory exchange is not hampered. Four types of airways commonly used are (1) the balloon-cuffed endotracheal tube (extends from the mouth through the glottis to a point above the bifurcation of the trachea); (2) the balloon-cuffed nasotracheal tube (extends from the nose to the trachea); (3) the oropharyngeal airway (extends from the mouth to the pharynx and prevents the tongue from falling back and obstructing the trachea); and (4) the nasopharyngeal airway (extends from the nose to the pharynx). The airway must be kept clear of secretions for adequate gas exchange to occur, and it may need to be suctioned if gurgling develops. The airway should not be removed until the laryngeal and pharyngeal reflexes return; these reflexes enable the patient to control the tongue, to cough, and to swallow. If the patient "reacts on the airway" (makes attempts to eject it), gagging may occur that progresses to retching and vomiting. The airway should be removed as soon as clinically possible in this instance to avoid aspiration.

An endotracheal tube can be removed as soon as the patient is adequately reversed and able to maintain the airway without it and when the danger of aspiration is over. This point may be difficult to determine; it is usually much easier to determine when a patient needs an airway than to decide when such an adjunct is not needed. Therefore, if PACU policy permits removal of an airway, it should definitely include insertion of an airway. Both procedures should, of course, be accompanied by appropriate education and skill training for the nurses who will perform them.

Palpation

Palpation and inspection of the chest may be carried out simultaneously to validate obser-

vations such as symmetry of expansion. In addition, crepitation may be heard or fremitus may be felt. The temperature, the level of moisture and general turgor of the skin, and the presence of any edema should be noted.

Percussion

The normal sound over the lungs is resonance. Dullness heard where there should normally be resonance indicates consolidation or filling of the alveolar or pleural spaces by fluid.

Listening and Auscultation

First, listen to the patient's respirations unaided. Normal respiration should be quiet; noisy breathing indicates a problem. Extraneous sounds always indicate some kind of obstruction; however, quiet breathing does not always indicate the absence of problems. An accumulation of mucus or other secretions evidenced by gurgling in any of the respiratory passages may cause airway obstruction and should be removed immediately. Purposeful coughing with good expiratory airflow is the most effective way of clearing secretions. If the patient is not yet reactive enough to do this alone, the secretions must be suctioned out orally and nasally. Nasotracheal suctioning may be useful to clear secretions and to stimulate cough, but the catheter is ineffective for reaching secretions distal to the carina. Obstruction may also occur from poor oropharyngeal muscle tone, resulting from the muscle-relaxant effect of general anesthesia plus the rolling back of the tongue. To relieve this obstruction, provide anterior pressure support on the angle of the jaw to open the air passages.

Crowing may indicate laryngospasm—a sudden, violent contraction of the vocal cords that may result in complete or partial closure of the trachea. If spasms continue, the airway must be maintained by the insertion of an endotracheal tube. Total blockage of the airway caused by laryngospasm produces no sound because of the absence of moving air. Equipment and medications for emergency tracheostomy should be readily available in the PACU.

Wheezing may indicate bronchospasm caused by a reflex reaction to an irritating mechanism. Bronchospasm occurs most often in patients with pre-existing pulmonary disease such as severe emphysema, reactive airway disease, pulmonary fibrosis, and radiation pneumonitis. Laryngeal edema following endotracheal intubation is not uncommon and can contribute significantly to airway obstruction. Acute changes in the patient's skin condition, cardio-vascular status, and bronchospasm after regional anesthesia must alert the nurse to a possible allergic reaction, but this event is rare.

Listen to the patient's chest with a stethoscope for quality and intensity of breath sounds. Locate and identify any abnormality, and describe it in the patient's medical record. Total absence of breath sounds on one side may signal the presence of pneumothorax (collapsed lung), obstruction, or fluid or blood within the pleural space. Auscultation of breath sounds in the PACU is often difficult, because the patient frequently cannot sit up or respond to commands to breathe deeply with the mouth open. Positioning the patient on alternating sides during the stir-up regimen provides an opportunity to examine the posterior lung field.

Monitoring Oxygenation by Pulse Oximetry

A pulse oximeter noninvasively measures the arterial oxygen saturation (SaO_2) in the blood (referred to as SpO_2 when measured by pulse oximetry). Therefore, it is a valuable adjunct to the clinical assessment of oxygenation. Many clinical indicators, such as the patient's color and the characteristics of the respirations, are subjective, and the physical signs of cyanosis are not evident until hypoxia is severe. Pulse oximetry monitoring is objective and continuous, and it provides an early warning of developing hypoxemia, allowing intervention before signs of hypoxia appear. Consequently, pulse oximetry has been widely adopted in the PACU as a tool for both safety monitoring and patient management. As a confirmation of its importance, the American Society of Post Anesthesia Nurses (ASPAN) *Standards of Post Anesthesia Nursing Practice* (1991) requires evaluation of all PACU patients with pulse oximetry at admission and discharge, and ASPAN recommends a pulse oximeter for every patient care unit in a Phase I PACU.

A pulse oximeter consists of a microprocessor-based monitor and a sensor (Fig. 19–1). In addition to an SpO_2 display, most oximeters display the pulse rate and have an adjustable alarm system that sounds when values register outside a designated range. A variety of sensors is available, each intended for application to specific sites and for use on patients of various sizes (the manufacturer's instructions describe these requirements). The sensor is applied to a site with a good arterial supply. The most common application site is a finger or toe (hand or foot in neonates); other sites include the nose, the forehead, or the temple. Both reusable sensors and disposable adhesive sensors are available, with disposable sensors allowing for patient-dedicated monitoring when infection control concerns are present.

Technology overview

A pulse oximeter uses plethysmography to detect the arterial pulse and spectrophotometry to determine SpO_2. The pulse oximetry sensor incorporates a red and an infrared light-emitting diode (also known as an *LED*) as light sources and a photodiode as a light detector. In the most common type of sensor—a transmission sensor—the light sources and detector are positioned on opposite sides of an arterial bed, such as around the finger. In a reflectance oximetry sensor, they are positioned on the same surface, such as on the forehead.

With both transmission and reflectance sensors, red and infrared light passes into the tissue, and the detector measures the amount of light absorbed. Because oxyhemoglobin and deoxyhemoglobin differ in their absorption of red and infrared light, the detector can determine the percentage of oxyhemoglobin in the arterial pulse.

Applications. Pulse oximetry is used in many clinical settings for safety monitoring and as a patient management tool. As a safety monitor, a pulse oximeter detects hypoxemia caused by unanticipated events such as severe atelectasis, bronchospasm, airway displace-

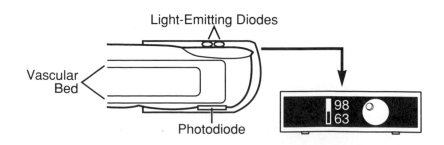

FIGURE 19–1. A pulse oximeter uses two light-emitting diodes and a photodiode to determine the arterial hemoglobin saturation.

ment, disconnections or kinks in the breathing circuit, and cardiac arrest. As a patient management tool, it is valuable in titrating oxygen therapy, weaning a patient from mechanical ventilation, and evaluating response to medications or other interventions that are intended to improve oxygenation.

In addition to these broad applications, certain uses of pulse oximetry are of particular value in the PACU. For example, postoperative patients can become significantly hypoxemic during transport to or from the PACU. Pulse oximetry during transport can diagnose undetected hypoxemia and identify a need for supplemental oxygen. Also, as indicated by the ASPAN standards, it is a valuable adjunct to clinical assessments in determining readiness for PACU discharge. When evaluated by pulse oximetry, some patients judged to be stable and ready for transfer based on clinical evaluation alone have been found to be hypoxemic.

Interpretation of SpO$_2$ Measurements. To adequately interpret SpO$_2$, it is essential to consider the mechanisms of oxygen transport. Approximately 98 percent of the oxygen in blood is bound to hemoglobin; SaO$_2$ and SpO$_2$ reflect this blood oxygen. The remaining blood oxygen is dissolved in plasma; blood gas analysis measures the partial pressure exerted by this oxygen dissolved in plasma (PaO$_2$). It is the dissolved oxygen that is used to meet immediate metabolic needs. The oxygen bound to hemoglobin serves as the reservoir that replenishes the pool of dissolved oxygen (see Chapter 6).

The rate at which oxygen binds to hemoglobin is primarily controlled by two factors: the PaO$_2$ and the affinity of hemoglobin for oxygen. This relationship between SaO$_2$ and PaO$_2$ is represented by the oxyhemoglobin dissociation curve. The curve is sigmoid in shape, and its position is affected by a number of physiologic variables that change the affinity of hemoglobin for oxygen (Fig. 19–2).

Many factors that shift the oxyhemoglobin dissociation curve are commonly seen in PACU patients. For example, a hypothermic patient may have a left-shifted curve. In such a patient, a given SpO$_2$ as measured by pulse oximetry may correspond to a lower than normal PaO$_2$. Although oxygen saturation may be adequate, hemoglobin will have a greater affinity for oxygen and be less willing to release oxygen to meet tissue needs. Warming the patient to a normothermic range facilitates oxygen unloading from the hemoglobin molecule and helps maintain adequate tissue oxygenation.

Clinical Issues. As with any technology, there are important clinical issues that must be considered to use pulse oximetry appropriately. As just discussed, shifts in the oxyhemoglobin dissociation curve that are caused by abnormal values of pH, temperature, PCO$_2$, and 2,3-diphosphoglycerate must be considered. It is also important to consider the patient's hemoglobin level because a pulse oximeter cannot detect a depletion in the total amount of hemoglobin. When using pulse oximetry on a postoperative patient with a low hemoglobin level, a high SpO$_2$ value may not be reflective of adequate oxygenation. The amount of hemoglobin, although well saturated with oxy-

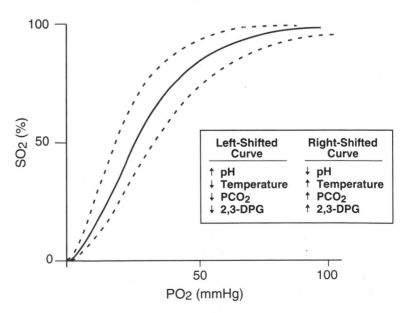

FIGURE 19–2. The normal oxyhemoglobin dissociation curve is indicated by the *solid line.* This curve may shift (indicated by the *broken lines*) whenever pH, temperature, PCO$_2$, or 2,3-DPG values are increased or decreased. So$_2$ = oxygen saturation; PO$_2$ = partial pressure of oxygen; PCO$_2$ = partial pressure of carbon dioxide; 2,3-DPG = 2,3-diphosphoglycerate.

Left-Shifted Curve	Right-Shifted Curve
↑ pH	↓ pH
↓ Temperature	↑ Temperature
↓ PCO$_2$	↑ PCO$_2$
↓ 2,3-DPG	↑ 2,3-DPG

gen, may be inadequate to meet tissue needs because there are fewer carriers available to transport oxygen.

Adequate oxygenation is a factor of not only adequate oxygen saturation and hemoglobin values but adequate oxygen delivery (which necessitates appropriate cardiac output) and the ability of the tissues to effectively utilize oxygen. When oxygen demand exceeds oxygen supply, tissue hypoxia results. Pulse oximetry readings, therefore, should be assessed in conjunction with all other indices of oxygenation.

Dysfunctional hemoglobins, variants of the hemoglobin molecule that are unable to transport oxygen, present a similar problem. Despite the high SpO$_2$ level, there may be insufficient hemoglobin available to carry oxygen. Carboxyhemoglobin is hemoglobin that is bound with carbon monoxide and therefore unavailable for carrying oxygen. Its effect must be considered in patients with burns or carbon monoxide poisoning and those who smoke. In methemoglobinemia, the iron molecule on the hemoglobin is oxidized from the ferrous to the ferric state. This form of iron is unable to transport oxygen. Methemoglobinemia, although rare, may occur in patients receiving nitrate-based and other drugs, as well as those exposed to a variety of toxins. When dysfunctional hemoglobins are suspected, assessment of oxygenation by pulse oximetry must be supplemented with arterial blood gas saturations measured by a laboratory co-oximeter to determine whether dyshemoglobins are present and oxygenation is adequate.

Perfusion at the sensor application site must be sufficient for the pulse oximeter to detect pulsatile flow. This is an important consideration for some PACU patients, such as those treated with vasoconstrictors, those who are markedly hypothermic, and those who have significantly reduced cardiac output. When applying the sensor, select a well-perfused site. If in doubt, check the pulse and adjacent capillary refill. If the monitor is unable to track the pulse, first evaluate the patient for adverse physiologic changes. Next, ensure that blood flow is not being restricted, such as by a flexed extremity, a blood pressure cuff, an arterial line, any restraints, or a sensor that is applied too tightly. Local perfusion to the sensor site can be improved by covering the site with a warm towel or by use of a convective warming device such as the Bair Hugger. Certain sensors, such as a nasal sensor, are designed for application to areas where perfusion is preserved even when peripheral perfusion is relatively poor. Finally, some pulse oximeters use an electro-cardiogram (ECG) signal as an aid in identifying the pulse, thus enhancing the instrument's ability to detect a weak pulse.

The patient movement seen in the PACU can produce false signals that interfere with the pulse oximeter's ability to identify the true pulse, leading to unreliable SpO$_2$ and pulse rate readings. When movement presents a problem, check whether the sensor is properly and securely applied; a sensor that is loosely attached or incorrectly positioned can magnify the effect of motion. If the problem persists, consider moving the sensor to a less active site. Also, pulse oximeters that use the ECG signal as an aid in identifying the pulse can have an enhanced ability to distinguish between the true pulse and artifacts produced by motion. The result is more reliable SpO$_2$ readings.

Normally, venous blood is nonpulsatile and is not detected by a pulse oximeter. In the presence of venous pulsations, the SpO$_2$ value provided by the pulse oximeter may be a composite of both arterial and venous saturations. Venous pulsations may occur in patients with severe right-sided heart failure or other pathophysiologic states that create venous congestion and in patients receiving high levels of positive end-expiratory pressure. They may also occur when the sensor is placed distal to a blood pressure cuff or occlusive dressing and when additional tape is wrapped tightly around the sensor. When venous pulsations are present, the PACU nurse should take care in interpreting the SpO$_2$ readings and, if possible, attempt to eliminate their cause.

Because pulse oximeters are optical measuring devices, the PACU nurse must be aware of additional factors that can influence the reliability of SpO$_2$ readings. To ensure good light reception, the sensor's light sources and detector must always be positioned according to the manufacturer's specifications. In the presence of bright lights, such as infrared warming devices, fluorescent lights, direct sunlight, and surgical lights, the sensor must be covered with an opaque material, or else incorrect SpO$_2$ readings may result. Also, agents that significantly change the optical-absorbing properties of blood, such as recently administered intravascular dyes, can interfere with reliable SpO$_2$ measurements. The use of pulse oximetry with certain nail polishes, especially those that are blue, green, and reddish-brown in color, may result in inaccurate readings. If nail polish in these shades cannot be removed, the sensor should be applied to an alternate unpolished site.

Monitoring Ventilation by Capnography

Monitoring CO_2 in respiratory gases provides an early warning of physiologic and mechanical events that interfere with normal ventilation. Capnography, which measures CO_2 at the patient's airway, is increasingly used in the PACU. It allows continuous assessment of the adequacy of alveolar ventilation, the function of the cardiopulmonary system, ventilator function, and the integrity of the airway and the breathing circuit. Consequently, it enables early detection of many potentially catastrophic events, including the onset of malignant hyperthermia, esophageal intubation, hypoventilation, partial or complete airway obstruction, breathing circuit leaks or disconnects, a large pulmonary embolus, and cardiac arrest.

Two variants of the instrument are available. A *capnometer* provides numeric measurement of exhaled CO_2 levels. A *capnograph* provides the same numeric information, and it also displays a CO_2 waveform. Both types of instruments usually incorporate an adjustable alarm system and often have trending and printing capabilities. The following discussion focuses on the use of capnographs, because they allow more complete and effective patient assessment than do capnometers. As discussed later, changes in the shape of the CO_2 waveform can provide crucial diagnostic information about ventilation, similar to the way in which the waveform provided by an ECG can provide crucial diagnostic information about the heart.

Technology overview

To measure exhaled CO_2, the most common type of capnograph passes infrared light at a wavelength that is absorbed by CO_2 through a sample of the patient's respiratory gas. The amount of light that is absorbed by the patient's gas is reflective of the amount of CO_2 in the sample.

Capnographs differ in the manner in which they obtain respiratory gas samples for analysis. *Sidestream* (or diverting) capnographs transport the sample through a narrow-gauge tubing to a measuring chamber. *Mainstream* (or nondiverting) capnographs position a flow-through measurement chamber directly on the patient's airway. Special adapters are available to allow sidestream capnographs to be used on nonintubated patients. The sample adapter should be placed as close to the patient's endotracheal tube or airway as possible.

Sidestream capnographs incorporate moisture-control features that are designed to minimize clogging of the sample tube, protect the measurement chamber from moisture-induced damage, and minimize the risk of cross-contamination. The design of these moisture-control systems significantly impacts a monitor's ease of use. Most rely on water traps, which must be emptied routinely. A new technology uses a special system of filters and tubing to dehumidify the sample, eliminating the need for water traps.

Capnographs also differ in their calibration requirements. Many require removal of the patient from the respiratory circuit and adjustment of the instrument with special mixtures of calibration gases. Advanced capnographic technology includes automatic calibration and does not require any user calibration skills or time.

The Normal Capnogram. To effectively use capnography, it is important to understand the components of the normal CO_2 waveform (capnogram), which are illustrated in Figure 19–3. Early in exhalation, air from the anatomic dead space, which is virtually CO_2 free, is measured by the instrument. As exhalation continues, alveolar gas reaches the sampling site and the CO_2 level increases rapidly. The CO_2 concentration continues to increase throughout exhalation, reaching the alveolar plateau, because alveolar gas dominates the sample. At the end of exhalation, the peak (end-tidal) CO_2 (ETCO$_2$) occurs, which in the normal lung is the best approximation of alveolar CO_2 levels. The CO_2 concentration then drops rapidly as the next inhalation of CO_2-free gas begins.

End-Tidal Versus Arterial CO_2. Under normal conditions, when ventilation and perfusion are well matched, ETCO$_2$ closely approximates arterial CO_2 (PaCO$_2$). The difference between the PaCO$_2$ and the ETCO$_2$ levels is referred to as the *alveolar-arterial CO_2 difference* (a − ADCO$_2$). ETCO$_2$ is usually as much as 5 mm Hg lower than PaCO$_2$. When the two measurements differ significantly, there is usually an anomaly in the patient's physiology, the breathing circuit, or the capnograph. Significant divergence between ETCO$_2$ and PaCO$_2$ is often attributable to increased alveolar dead space: CO_2-free gas from nonperfused alveoli mixes with gas from perfused regions, decreasing the ETCO$_2$ measurement. Clinical conditions that cause increased dead space, such as pulmonary hypoperfusion, cardiac arrest, and pulmonary embolus, can increase the a − ADCO$_2$. Changes in the a − ADCO$_2$ can be used to assess the efficacy of the treatment: as the patient's dead space im-

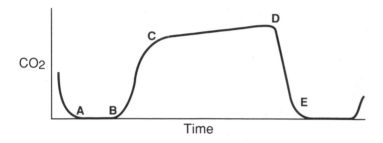

FIGURE 19–3. The normal capnogram. AB = beginning exhalation, dead space. BC = initial alveolar emptying. CD = end-alveolar emptying. D = end-tidal CO_2. E = inspiration (CO_2-free gas).

proves, the PaO_2 − PaO_2 narrows. Alternatively, a significant PaO_2 − PaO_2 can indicate incomplete alveolar emptying (such as with reactive airway disease), a leak in the gas-sampling system that allows loss of respiratory gas, and contamination of respiratory gas with fresh gas.

Interpretation of Changes in the Capnogram. An abnormal capnogram provides an initial warning of many events that warrant immediate intervention. Abnormalities may be seen on a breath-by-breath basis or when the CO_2 trend is examined. For this reason, it is preferable to visualize both the real-time waveform and the CO_2 trend on the monitor display. This discussion will provide a few examples of changes produced by significant events that commonly occur in the PACU.

A sudden decrease in $ETCO_2$ to a near-zero level indicates that the monitor is no longer detecting CO_2 in exhaled gases (Fig. 19–4). Immediate action is crucial to detect and correct the cause of this loss of ventilation. Possible causes include a completely blocked endotracheal tube, esophageal intubation, a disconnection in the breathing circuit, and inadvertent extubation. The latter three possibilities are

particularly likely if the decrease in $ETCO_2$ coincides with movement of the patient's head. Only after eliminating possible clinical causes for this decrease in $ETCO_2$, investigate whether a clogged sampling tube or instrument malfunction may be causing the problem.

An exponential decrease in $ETCO_2$ over a small number of breaths usually signals a life-threatening cardiopulmonary event that has dramatically increased dead space ventilation (Fig. 19–5). Sudden hypotension, pulmonary embolism, and circulatory arrest with continued ventilation must be considered.

A gradual increase in the $ETCO_2$ level while the capnogram retains its normal shape usually indicates that ventilation is inadequate to eliminate the CO_2 that is being produced (Fig. 19–6). This situation can be the result of a small ventilator leak or a partial airway obstruction that reduces minute ventilation. It can also reflect increased CO_2 production associated with increased body temperature, the onset of sepsis, or shivering. Of particular importance, a large increase in $ETCO_2$ can be one of the earliest signs of malignant hyperthermia, which may not begin until after emergence from anesthesia.

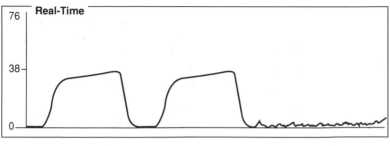
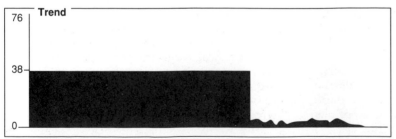

FIGURE 19–4. Sudden decrease in end-tidal CO_2 to near-zero level.

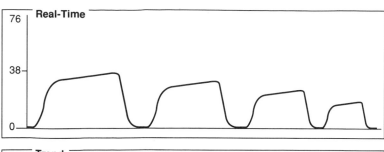

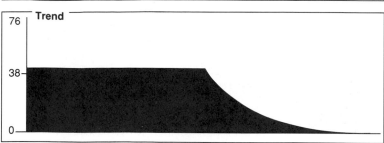

FIGURE 19–5. Exponential decrease in end-tidal CO_2.

A gradual decrease in the $ETCO_2$ level commonly occurs in the patient who is anesthetized, narcotized, hyperventilated, or hypothermic (Fig. 19–7).

Assessment of the capnogram can reveal information about the quality of alveolar emptying. For example, the patient with bronchospasm is unable to completely empty his or her alveoli, and the resulting capnogram will not have an alveolar plateau (Fig. 19–8). The $ETCO_2$ reported by the capnograph in this instance is not a good estimate of alveolar CO_2. Effective administration of bronchodilator therapy commonly improves alveolar emptying and results in a more normal capnogram.

Clinical Issues. In addition to the diagnostic usefulness of changes in the capnogram, there are specific applications of capnography that are particularly valuable in the PACU. Of primary importance is its ability to provide early warning of hypoventilation that, in the PACU, may be secondary to anesthesia, sedation, analgesia, or pain. A falling $ETCO_2$ may indicate pulmonary hypoperfusion due to blood loss or hypotension. During rewarming, $ETCO_2$ values are likely to increase as metabolic activity increases. Capnography can signal when shivering is producing an unacceptable increase in oxygen consumption and metabolic rate. During ventilator weaning, capnography is valuable in assessing the adequacy of ventilation.

Recent studies have demonstrated the value of capnography in monitoring the course and efficacy of cardiopulmonary resuscitation

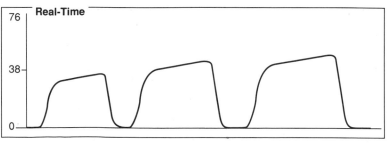

FIGURE 19–6. Gradual increase in end-tidal CO_2.

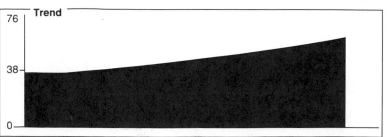

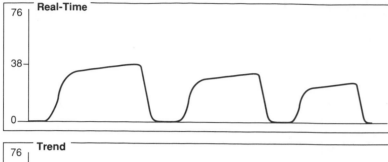

FIGURE 19–7. Gradual decrease in end-tidal CO_2.

(CPR). $ETCO_2$ measurements, which decrease during cardiac arrest, typically reach about 50 percent of normal levels during effective CPR. When spontaneous circulation is restored, $ETCO_2$ values increase dramatically.

The presence and persistence of normal $ETCO_2$ values are also useful determinants in confirming tracheal intubation, because CO_2 is not normally found in the esophagus. However, capnography cannot be substituted for chest auscultation and radiograph in eliminating the possibility of bronchial intubation.

CARDIOVASCULAR FUNCTION AND PERFUSION

The three basic components of the circulatory system that must be evaluated are (1) the heart as a pump, (2) the blood, and (3) the arteriovenous system. The maintenance of good tissue perfusion depends on a satisfactory cardiac output. Therefore, most assessment is aimed at evaluating cardiac output.

Clinical Assessment

Observe the overall condition of the patient, especially skin color and turgor. Peripheral cyanosis, edema, dilatation of the neck veins, shortness of breath, and many other findings may be indicative of cardiovascular problems. In addition to checking all operative sites for blood loss, note the amount of blood lost during surgery and the patient's most recent hemoglobin level.

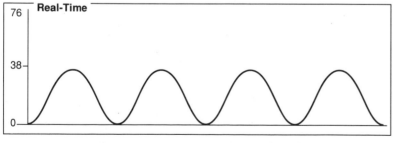

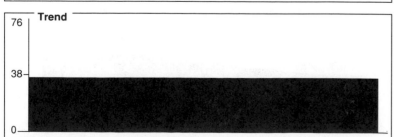

FIGURE 19–8. Incomplete alveolar emptying.

Blood Pressure Monitoring

Arterial blood pressure must be assessed in the preoperative physical assessment, on admission to and discharge from the PACU, and at frequent, regular intervals during the PACU stay. Arterial blood pressure is currently measured either noninvasively (indirectly) or invasively (directly). *Noninvasive* methods include manual cuff measurement with either an aneroid or mercury sphygmomanometer and automatic measurements with an electronic blood pressure monitor. *Invasive* measurement may be accomplished via a transduced arterial line. A clear understanding of proper technique is essential to ensure accurate and reliable readings with all the blood pressure measurement methods.

Noninvasive Measurement

Manual Method. An aneroid or mercury-type sphygmomanometer with inflatable cuff and stethoscope is required for the standard auscultatory blood pressure measurement technique. It is essential to use the correct cuff size. The width of the inflatable bladder that is encased inside the cuff should be 40 to 50 percent of upper arm circumference. A bladder that is too wide underestimates blood pressure, whereas a bladder that is too narrow overestimates blood pressure. The length of the bladder should be at least 80 percent of the arm circumference.

The cuff is placed on the extremity, with the inflatable bladder positioned directly over the artery at the level of the heart. The brachial artery is the site most commonly used for blood pressure measurement. If the upper extremities are unavailable for cuff placement owing to operative issues or other problems, the lower extremities may be used. The bladder of the cuff should be centered over the posterior surface of the lower third of the thigh, and pressure may be auscultated over the popliteal artery or at the ankle over the posterior tibial artery (just posterior to the medial malleolus). Systolic pressure in the legs is usually 20 to 30 mm Hg higher than in the brachial artery.

The cuff is inflated, and when cuff pressure exceeds the arterial pressure, arterial blood flow will cease and the pulse will no longer be palpated. As pressure is released by turning the valve of the inflation bulb, blood flow will resume and audible (Korotkoff) sounds will be noted with the stethoscope. These sounds change in quality and intensity throughout further cuff deflation and generally disappear.

The American Heart Association recommends that the systolic pressure be noted as the first audible sound in the cuff-deflating process. The diastolic pressure is marked by the disappearance of sounds in the adult patient and the muffling of sounds in the pediatric patient.

A common cause of error in blood pressure measurement is an auscultatory gap that may be present, especially in hypertensive patients. This gap is a silent interval between the systolic and diastolic pressures. During this gap, the pulse is palpable. Therefore, to avoid mistakenly low systolic readings, the cuff should be inflated until the pulse is obliterated. Blood pressure readings should be recorded completely, including the systolic pressure, the point at which the sounds become muffled and when they cease, and, if present, the range of the auscultatory gap.

Auscultatory blood pressure measurements may be completed quickly and easily under many circumstances. The accuracy and reliability of the readings may be affected by low flow states (including decreased cardiac output and vasoconstriction) or decreased sound transmission due to factors related to the patient (edema and obesity) or the environment (noise). Cuff size and placement, user error, and improperly calibrated manometers may also contribute to unreliable readings. Because measurements are intermittent and must be initiated by the user, blood pressure changes may go unnoticed in the postoperative patient with labile hemodynamics or sudden blood loss. The use of automatic blood pressure monitors that can be set to measure blood pressure at regular, frequent intervals can minimize some of this risk.

Automatic Method. Automatic blood pressure monitoring with electronic devices has become increasingly prevalent in the PACU. The devices are commonly used to provide frequent blood pressure measurements over relatively brief periods, when the need for arterial sampling is minimal to absent, and when the risks of arterial lines cannot be justified.

One of the most commonly used automatic noninvasive blood pressure methods is based on oscillometric technology. The cuff is chosen and applied according to conventional technique. Oscillations of the arterial wall are occluded as the cuff is inflated and are detected during cuff deflation. Systolic pressure is indicated at the onset of oscillations. As cuff pressure decreases, oscillations increase in amplitude and peak at the mean arterial pressure. The point at which oscillations disappear is the diastolic pressure (Fig. 19–9). All three pres-

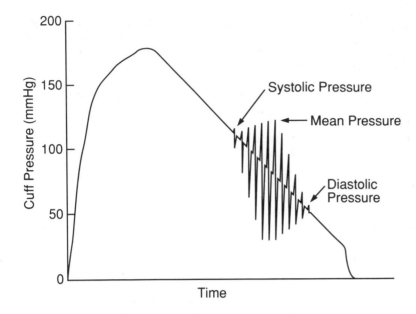

FIGURE 19–9. Oscillometric blood pressure measurement. Systolic pressure is indicated at the onset of oscillations. Mean arterial pressure occurs when oscillations peak in amplitude. The point at which oscillations disappear is the diastolic pressure.

sures are normally reported on oscillometric monitoring devices.

Automatic noninvasive blood pressure monitors may be set to cycle at various measurement periods. The instruments alarm when systolic and diastolic pressures register outside of a preset range. Equipment should be calibrated on a regular basis, and preventive maintenance should include assessment for leaks. The use of automatic devices may be limited in patients with low-flow states or high peripheral vascular resistance and in those who are severely obese or edematous. These devices provide only intermittent measurements and are less desirable for assessment of the labile patient.

Newer advances in noninvasive blood pressure technology, currently available for intraoperative monitoring of the anesthetized patient, include continuous monitoring capabilities that ensure detection in sudden blood pressure variations. The only other method of continuous blood pressure monitoring currently available is invasive arterial blood pressure technology.

Invasive Measurement

Invasive arterial pressure measurements are most commonly obtained via cannulation of the radial artery but may be obtained at other arterial sites as well. A continuous flush solution is connected to the intra-arterial catheter and is slowly infused into the arterial vessel under pressure. The pressure within the artery is transmitted through the column of fluid to the transducer. The transducer then converts this pressure to an electrical signal that can be converted to millimeters of mercury and displayed on the monitor. A corresponding arterial waveform, or pressure pulse, is also displayed on the monitor.

Arterial blood pressure measurements are continuous and are indicated for hemodynamically high-risk patients. Changes in patients' pressures can be observed on an ongoing basis. This technology may also be chosen in patients for whom indirect measurements fail, because of diminished or absent Korotkoff sounds (as in obese or edematous patients), and with high peripheral vascular resistance. The direct arterial access is also beneficial if the patient requires frequent blood samples for laboratory analysis.

To ensure more reliable arterial blood pressure readings, the clinician should balance and calibrate the system according to the manufacturer's specifications. The transducer must always be balanced and positioned at the fourth intercostal level at the midaxillary line. Aseptic technique must always be used during placement and maintenance of the arterial line and transducer.

Damping of the arterial waveform with subsequent unreliable readings may occur for a variety of reasons, including clotting and kinking of the arterial catheter, positioning of the catheter against the arterial wall, and the presence of air bubbles within the arterial line system. Loose connections, calibration error, and equipment failure may also contribute to unreliable readings.

An Allen test should be performed prior to radial artery cannulation to minimize the risk of hand ischemia (see Chapter 5). If arterial lines are discontinued in the PACU, constant pressure should be applied to the site for 10 to 15 minutes or until bleeding has ceased. A pressure dressing should be applied, and the site should be checked frequently for any bleeding.

Complications and risks of invasive arterial blood pressure monitoring include infection, thrombosis, emboli, tissue ischemia, hemorrhage, and vessel perforation. Arterial blood pressure monitoring is generally contraindicated in patients with septicemia, coagulopathies, irradiated arterial sites, anatomic anomalies, inadequate collateral blood flow, or thrombosis.

Clinical Issues. To assess their significance, blood pressure readings in the postoperative period must be compared with preoperative baseline measurements. A low postoperative blood pressure may be the result of a number of factors, including the effects of muscle relaxants, spinal anesthesia, preoperative medication, changes in the patient's position, blood loss, poor lung ventilation, and peripheral pooling of blood. The administration of oxygen to help eliminate anesthetic gases and to assist the patient in awakening causes an increase in blood pressure. Deep breathing, leg exercises, verbal stimulation, and conversation can be instituted to raise the blood pressure. A low fluid volume may be augmented by increasing the rate of intravenous fluids, which helps maintain the arterial pressure. Any method designed to raise the pressure must be instituted with consideration for the patient's overall condition.

An increase in blood pressure postoperatively is not uncommon because of the effects of anesthesia, respiratory insufficiency, or decreased respiratory rate and depth causing CO_2 retention. The surgical procedure, with its accompanying discomfort, also causes increased blood pressure. Emergence delirium, with its excitement, struggling, and pain, may also be a causative factor in a transient increase in blood pressure. Obviously, it is important to determine the cause before treatment is instituted. In patients with uncontrolled hypertension, continuous intravenous antihypertensive medications may be required. However, it is extremely important to diagnose the cause of the hypertension so that effective therapy may be employed rapidly.

Pulse Pressure Monitoring

Pulse pressure is an important determinant in the evaluation of perfusion. Because of the pulsatile nature of the heart, blood enters the arteries intermittently, causing pressure increases and decreases. The difference between the systolic and diastolic pressures equals the pulse pressure. The pulse pressure is affected by two major factors: the stroke volume output of the heart and the compliance (total distensibility) of the arterial tree. The pulse pressure is determined approximately by the ratio of stroke output to compliance. Therefore, any condition that affects either of these factors also affects the pulse pressure.

To evaluate the patient's cardiovascular status accurately, all signs and symptoms must be evaluated individually as well as within the body system as a whole. For example, cool extremities, decreased urine output, and narrowed pulse pressure may be indicative of decreased cardiac output, even in the presence of normal blood pressure.

Pulses

The rate and character of all pulses should be assessed bilaterally. Examine the pulses simultaneously to determine their equality and time of arrival. Peripheral arterial occlusion is not uncommon; if it is suspected, a Doppler instrument can be of great value in detecting the presence or absence of blood flow. Occlusion is an emergency and must be reported to the surgeon at once.

Irregularities in pulse are most frequently caused by premature beats, generally premature ventricular contractions (PVCs) or premature atrial contractions (PACs). These irregular rhythms should be thoroughly investigated before therapy is initiated.

ELECTROCARDIOGRAPHIC MONITORING

The PACU nurse must have a basic understanding of cardiac monitoring and should be able to interpret the basic cardiac rhythms and dysrhythmias and correlate them with expected cardiac output and its effects on the patient's condition. According to the most recent ASPAN standards, ECG monitoring should be available for each patient in a Phase I PACU and should be readily available for patients in Phase II units. Arrhythmias of any type may occur at any time and in any patient during the

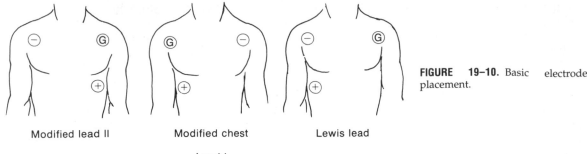

Modified lead II

Modified chest

Lewis lead

Lead I

FIGURE 19–10. Basic electrode placement.

postoperative period. Therefore, accurate ECG monitoring and interpretation are mandatory skills for the PACU nurse (see Chapter 5). This section is designed to provide an introduction to specific problems of cardiac monitoring in the PACU.

Any type of cardiac arrhythmia may be seen in the PACU. The causes of specific arrhythmias must be carefully differentiated before any treatment is instituted. Some commonly encountered problems are reviewed here, but the list is by no means complete.

All abnormal rhythms should be documented with a rhythm strip and recorded in the patient's progress record. Any questionable rhythms should be documented by a complete 12-lead ECG.

Electrical monitoring of the patient's heart is only one assessment parameter and must be interpreted in conjunction with other salient parameters before therapy is initiated. Cardiac monitors generally depict only a single lead. They do not detect all rhythm disturbances and alterations, and a 12-lead ECG is essential to define a conduction problem accurately.

Lead Placement

The skin where the electrode will be placed should be clean, dry, and smooth. Excessive hair should be removed; moisture or skin oils should be removed with alcohol or acetone and the skin mildly abraded to obtain good adherence of the electrode.

Site selection on the chest is based on a triangular arrangement of positive, negative, and ground electrodes. Avoid placing electrodes directly over the diaphragm, areas of auscultation, heavy bones, or large muscles. Allow adequate space for application of defibrillator paddles in the event that defibrillation should become necessary. Figure 19–10 depicts the most commonly used electrode leads. The modified lead II is the most commonly used

because it is the most versatile; it is useful in assessing P waves, PR intervals, and atrial arrhythmias. The modified chest lead I is useful for assessing bundle branch block and differentiating between ventricular arrhythmias and aberrations. This lead is useful when the patient is known to have pre-existing cardiac disease. The Lewis lead is useful when P waves are difficult to distinguish using other leads.

Sinus Arrhythmias

Sinus Bradycardia

Figure 19–11 shows a slow heart rate—less than 60 beats per min. Its rhythm may be irregular owing to accompanying sinus arrhythmias. All other complex features are normal.

Sinus bradycardia is commonly encountered in the PACU, owing to the depressant effects of anesthesia. Young, healthy adults, especially those who are normally physically active, often have bradycardia. Usually no treatment is necessary except to continue the stir-up regimen. Excessive parasympathetic stimulation from pain may cause bradycardia, in which case appropriate analgesics should be administered and other pain-relieving measures initiated. If the patient shows symptoms of low cardiac output, the physician should be notified and treatment instituted using atropine to block vagal effects or isoproterenol to stimulate the cardiac pacemaker. If temporary pacing wires are available, either atrial or ventricular pacing can be attempted.

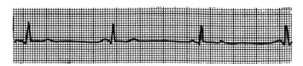

FIGURE 19–11. Sinus bradycardia (lead III). (From Guyton, A. C.: Textbook of Medical Physiology. 6th ed. Philadelphia, W. B. Saunders, 1981, p. 197).

Sinus Tachycardia

Figure 19–12 shows a fast heart rate—more than 100 beats per min. The rhythm may be slightly irregular, and all other complex features are normal.

Sinus tachycardia results from any stress and may be encountered in the PACU owing to numerous causes, including the stress of surgery, anoxia, fever, overhydration, hypovolemia, pain, anxiety, or apprehension, or any combination of these factors. Tachycardia is an important postoperative sign and should be fully evaluated before treatment is instituted. Increasing tachycardia is an early sign of shock and must be thoroughly investigated. Treatment must be specific and based on removal of the underlying cause (see Chapter 44). The patient should be assessed carefully for his or her ability to tolerate the rapid rate. The deleterious effects of tachycardias are generally related to diminished stroke volume and cardiac output. In general, the patient with previously normal cardiac function can tolerate tachycardias as high as 160 beats per min without manifesting symptoms. Poor tolerance with a resultant decrease in cardiac output occurs when the diastolic interval, and thus the ventricular filling time, is significantly impinged on.

Sinus Arrest (Atrial Standstill)

Sinus arrest is failure of the sinoatrial (SA) node to discharge, with resulting loss of atrial contraction. The rate remains within normal ranges. The rhythm is regular except when the SA node fails to discharge. P waves and QRS complexes are normal when the SA node is firing and absent when it fails to discharge.

Common causes of sinus arrest in the PACU are the depressant effects of anesthesia or analgesics and electrolyte disturbances. Treatment is aimed at eliminating depressant drugs from the body and correcting electrolyte imbalances. This arrhythmia must be brought to the attention of the physician immediately, because persistent sinus arrest constitutes an emergency, and CPR must be initiated.

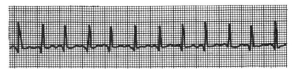

FIGURE 19–12. Sinus tachycardia (lead I). (From Guyton, A. C.: Textbook of Medical Physiology. 6th ed. Philadelphia, W. B. Saunders, 1981, p. 197).

Premature beat

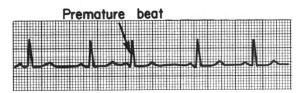

FIGURE 19–13. Atrial premature beat (lead I). (From Guyton, A. C.: Textbook of Medical Physiology. 6th ed. Philadelphia, W. B. Saunders, 1981, p. 200).

Supraventricular Arrhythmias

Supraventricular arrhythmias consist of supraventricular extrasystole (PAC), atrial tachycardia, atrial flutter, and atrial fibrillation. Supraventricular arrhythmias occur in about 10 to 40 percent of patients after coronary artery bypass graft surgery. These rhythms should be documented with a 12-lead ECG. Their cause has been related to a number of possible factors, such as an inflammatory reaction to surgical trauma, insufficient "protection" of the atria during surgery, atrioventricular (AV) node ischemia, and sudden withdrawal of beta blockers. There is a correlation between persistent atrial activity during cardioplegic arrest and postoperative supraventricular arrhythmias.

Premature Atrial Contraction

PAC, or atrial premature beat, occurs earlier than expected, resulting from an irritable focus in the atrium (Fig. 19–13). Cardiac rate and rhythm are normal except for their prematurity. The P wave configuration of the premature beat usually differs from that of the normal beat. The PAC is followed by a pause that is not fully compensatory.

This arrhythmia results from anxiety and is commonly encountered in the PACU. No treatment is necessary unless the PACs become frequent or the patient becomes symptomatic. If pharmacologic therapy becomes necessary, agents such as propranolol and verapamil can be administered.

Atrial Tachycardia

Atrial tachycardia is a rhythm disturbance that is a rapid, regular supraventricular heart rate, resulting from an irritable focus of five or more PACs in succession (Fig. 19–14). The rate is 150 to 200 beats per min, with a regular rhythm.

This rhythm should be documented with a full 12-lead ECG. The physician should be

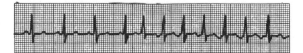

FIGURE 19–14. Atrial paroxysmal tachycardia—onset in middle of record (lead I). (From Guyton, A. C.: Textbook of Medical Physiology. 6th ed. Philadelphia, W. B. Saunders, 1981, p. 201).

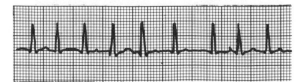

FIGURE 19–16. Atrial fibrillation (lead I). (From Guyton, A. C.: Textbook of Medical Physiology. 6th ed. Philadelphia, W. B. Saunders, 1981, p. 202).

notified to institute therapy. Maneuvers that enhance vagal tone, such as the Valsalva maneuver and carotid sinus massage, may be successful in terminating this arrhythmia. Antiarrhythmic agents such as digitalis, quinidine, and verapamil may cause the patient to revert to normal sinus rhythm. If these measures are unsuccessful, cardioversion with countershock will be necessary.

Atrial Flutter

Atrial flutter consists of rapid supraventricular contractions resulting from an ectopic focus with varying degrees of ventricular blocking (Fig. 19–15). Its cause is the same as that of PACs and atrial tachycardia. The rhythm is usually regular; the atrial rate is 250 to 350 beats per min. Treatment is the same as for atrial tachycardia.

Atrial Fibrillation

In atrial fibrillation, one or more irritable atrial foci discharge at an extremely rapid rate that lacks coordinated activity (Fig. 19–16).

Atrial fibrillation occurs commonly in patients with atrial enlargement from mitral valve disease or from long-standing coronary artery disease and is often preceded by PACs, tachycardia, or flutter. Clinically, the patient has an irregular heart beat, pulse rate, and, usually, a noticeable pulse deficit. Cardiac output decreases in varying degrees. Normally atrial filling and contraction account for 30 percent of ventricular filling. Without this atrial filling, or "atrial kick," of volume into the ventricle, stroke volumes and, thus, cardiac outputs are diminished. Treatment involves digitalis, quin-

idine, verapamil, atrial pacing, or cardioversion.

Ventricular Arrhythmias

Myocardial ischemia and perioperative myocardial infarction remain the two major causes of ventricular arrhythmias, although bradycardia, hypokalemia, hypoxemia, acidosis, and hypothermia are also potential causes.

Premature Ventricular Contraction

PVC is a rhythm disturbance involving an earlier-than-expected ventricular contraction from an irritable focus in the ventricle (Fig. 19–17). The rhythm is regular except for the premature beat, and the rate is normal.

The P wave is absent from the premature beat. A wide, bizarre, notched QRS complex that may be of a greater-than-normal ampli-

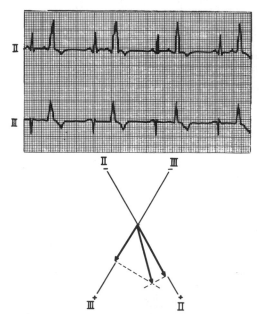

FIGURE 19–17. Premature ventricular contractions (leads II and III). (From Guyton, A. C.: Textbook of Medical Physiology. 6th ed. Philadelphia, W. B. Saunders, 1981, p. 200).

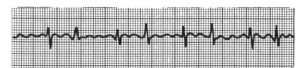

FIGURE 19–15. Atrial flutter—2:1 and 3:1 rhythm (lead I). (From Guyton, A. C.: Textbook of Medical Physiology. 6th ed. Philadelphia, W. B. Saunders, 1981, p. 202).

tude is present. A widened T wave of greater-than-normal amplitude is present after the premature beat and is of opposite deflection to that of the QRS complex.

The PVC is followed by a pause that is fully compensatory; that is, the time of the PVC plus the pause time equals the time of two normal beats.

PVCs are commonly encountered in the PACU and can occur in any patient. Occasional PVCs occur normally and need no treatment. Multiple PVCs may indicate inadequate oxygenation, and when they occur, the patient's respiratory status should be thoroughly assessed. Other causative factors of PVCs include electrolyte disturbances, acid–base imbalance, drug toxicity, and hypoxemia of the myocardium.

Treatment of PVCs is based on the underlying cause and obliteration of the irritable focus. Occasional, isolated PVCs need not be treated. If PVCs occur more frequently than five per minute, if a successive run of two or more occurs, if they are multifocal or occur during the vulnerable period on the ECG complex, they must be treated, because they are the precursors of the more lethal ventricular arrhythmias.

Ventricular arrhythmias present in the setting of bradycardia should be treated with atropine or with overdrive pacing to eliminate ventricular escape rhythms. Otherwise, lidocaine should be the first drug of choice to treat ventricular arrhythmias.

Ventricular Tachycardia

Three or more consecutive PVCs constitute ventricular tachycardia (Fig. 19–18). The rhythm is fairly regular, and P waves are not seen. Occasionally, patients may have ventricular tachycardia and be asymptomatic, but usually they experience anxiety, palpitations, fluttering, pounding in the chest, dizziness, faintness, and precordial pain. If ventricular tachycardia is prolonged, cyanosis, mental confusion, convulsions, and unconsciousness develop as a result of decreased blood and oxygen supply to the brain.

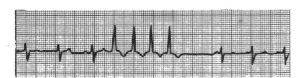

FIGURE 19–18. Ventricular paroxysmal tachycardia (lead III). (From Guyton, A. C.: Textbook of Medical Physiology. 6th ed. Philadelphia, W. B. Saunders, 1981, p. 202).

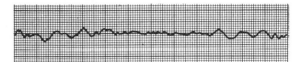

FIGURE 19–19. Ventricular fibrillation (lead II). (From Guyton, A. C.: Textbook of Medical Physiology. 6th ed. Philadelphia, W. B. Saunders, 1981, p. 203).

The causative factors of ventricular tachycardia are essentially the same as those for PVCs. Most commonly, ventricular tachycardia in the PACU is the result of hypoxia, drug toxicity, or underlying heart disease.

Ventricular tachycardia must be treated immediately. If the patient initially tolerates the arrhythmia, treatment should be instituted with lidocaine. If the patient has cardiac decompensation and circulatory insufficiency, cardioversion with direct-current (DC) electrical countershock should be immediately instituted. Immediate notification of the physician is essential.

Ventricular Fibrillation

A rapid, irregular quivering of the ventricles that is uncoordinated and incapable of pumping blood characterizes ventricular fibrillation (Fig. 19–19). This rhythm disturbance is the major death-producing cardiac arrhythmia. The immediate initial treatment is external DC countershock (Fig. 19–20). Ventricular fibrillation may occur spontaneously without any forewarning, or it may be preceded by evidence of ventricular irritability. Patients likely

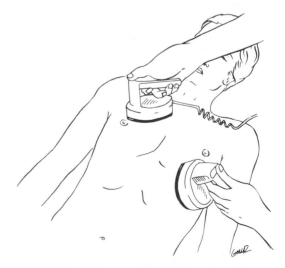

FIGURE 19–20. The emergency administration of external direct-current countershock. (From Sanderson R. C. [ed.]: The Cardiac Patient. Philadelphia, W. B. Saunders, 1972).

to develop ventricular fibrillation include those with underlying heart disease, those who evidenced ventricular irritability in the operating room during surgery, and those with symptoms of shock. All of these patients should be monitored continuously throughout their recovery period.

If ventricular fibrillation is not immediately terminated with countershock, CPR is instituted without delay. The anesthesiologist should be summoned immediately (see Chapter 45).

HEMODYNAMIC MONITORING

Although more prominent in cardiac surgery, additional hemodynamic monitoring is commonly used with higher acuity patients not cared for in many PACUs. Hemodynamic monitoring can be accomplished via the following invasive lines: a flow-directed pulmonary artery catheter, a central venous pressure catheter, a left-atrial or right-atrial catheter, a pulmonary artery thermistor catheter, or a peripheral arterial catheter (A line). The parameters obtained from these various lines, the catheter insertion sites, and the placement and monitoring methods are presented in Table 19–1 and depicted in Figure 19–21. Problems associated with maintaining these lines are summarized in Table 19–2.

Right-Atrial Pressure

The normal right-atrial pressure ranges from 0 to 7 mm Hg. Pressures exceeding that level can be the result of fluid overload, right-ventricular failure, tricuspid valve abnormalities, pulmonary hypertension, constrictive pericarditis, or cardiac tamponade. Values in the lower range are usually indicative of hypovolemia.

Pulmonary Artery Pressure

Pulmonary artery systolic pressures normally range from 15 to 25 mm Hg, whereas a normal pulmonary artery diastolic pressure is 8 to 15 mm Hg. Hypovolemia contributes to low pressure readings. Increased volume loads that can develop with an atrial or ventricular septal defect or left-ventricular failure can create elevations in pressure. Additionally, obstructions to forward flow that can be caused by mitral stenosis or pulmonary hypertension can lead to an elevation in pulmonary artery pressures.

Pulmonary Capillary Wedge Pressure

Normal pulmonary capillary wedge pressure (PCWP) recordings are between 6 and 15 mm Hg. Values in this range can be caused by an increased volume load, as is seen in left-ventricular failure, or created by an obstruction to forward flow. Such obstructions may be caused by mitral stenosis or regurgitation or by a pulmonary embolism. Lower values may be a result of hypovolemia or indicative of an obstruction to left-ventricular filling, which could occur with a pulmonary embolism, pulmonary stenosis, or right-ventricular failure.

Left-Atrial Pressure

Normal left-atrial pressures range from 4 to 12 mm Hg. As is seen with the PCWP, elevations in left-atrial pressure are associated with volume overloads or obstructions to forward flow, the latter of which may consist of left-ventricular failure states, mitral or aortic valve dysfunctions, or constrictive pericarditis. Lower recordings are generally a consequence of hypovolemia from inadequate volume or related to an obstruction to forward flow. Such an obstruction may be a pulmonary embolism or pulmonic valve stenosis, or it may result from right-ventricular failure.

Mean Arterial Pressure

Normal mean arterial pressures generally range between 80 and 120 mm Hg. In a postoperative cardiac surgical patient, pressures lower than 60 mm Hg are generally avoided, because coronary artery filling may be limited or impeded when parameters reach this level and may contribute to an ischemic or infarction state. Conversely, pressures higher than 120 mm Hg are avoided, because they place too much stress on newly created suture lines that could readily rupture under sustained pressures.

Cardiac Output and Cardiac Index

Cardiac output is the amount of blood ejected by the ventricle in 1 minute. Normal

Table 19–1. METHODS FOR INVASIVE MONITORING OF HEMODYNAMIC PARAMETERS

Parameters	Catheter Placement	Insertion Sites	Monitoring Method	Special Considerations
RAP	Proximal port of FDPAC lies in the right atrium	Brachial Jugular Subclavian	Water manometer	Intermittent readings at lowest fluctuation*
	Distal end of RAC or CVP lies in the right atrium	Direct insertion through RA wall†	Transducer‡	Intermittent or continuous readings on mean§
PAP	Distal end of FDPAC lies in right or left branch of pulmonary artery	Brachial Jugular Subclavian	Transducer	Readings on systole and diastole
	Distal end of PATC lies in main pulmonary artery	Direct insertion through PA wall†		
PCWP	Inflation of balloon on tip of FDPAC allows it to float into a wedged position in a smaller branch of the pulmonary artery	—	Transducer	Intermittent readings on mean§
LAP	Distal end of the LAC lies in left atrium	Direct insertion through LA wall†	Water manometer	Intermittent reading recorded at lowest fluctuation*
MAP	Distal end of catheter lies in a peripheral artery	Radial Brachial Femoral	Anaeroid manometer	Midpoint of needle fluctuation
			Transducer	Continuous readings on mean§

*Fluctuation indicates a patent catheter and good position in the thorax.
†Direct insertion is achieved during an open chest procedure via a median sternotomy incision. The exit site is via a stab wound at the distal portion of the median sternotomy. The catheter is attached to skin with suture. Removal is achieved by removing the suture and applying gentle traction to the catheter to free it from the chamber wall. The catheter is sutured to chamber wall with absorbable suture so that it releases easily. Chest tubes remain in place until such lines are removed, owing to the possibility of bleeding.
‡To convert mm Hg to cm H$_2$O, multiply mm Hg reading times 1.36.
§Biphasic waves are measured on mean.
Adapted from Whitman, G. R.: Bedside hemodynamic monitoring. In Horvath, P. T. (ed.): Care of the Adult Cardiac Surgery Patient. New York, John Wiley & Sons, Inc., 1984. Used with permission.
RAP = right-atrial pressure; PAP = pulmonary artery pressure; PCWP = pulmonary capillary wedge pressure; LAP = left-atrial pressure; MAP = mean arterial pressure; FDPAC = flow-directed pulmonary artery catheter; RAC = right-atrial catheter; LAC = left-atrial catheter; CVP = central venous pressure; PATC = pulmonary artery thermistor catheter.

cardiac output is 5 to 6 L per min; it is calculated by the formula:

$$SV \times HR = CO$$

where SV = stroke volume, HR = heart rate, and CO = cardiac output.

Cardiac index is calculated by the following formula:

$$\frac{CO}{BSA} = CI$$

where BSA = body surface area in m^2 and CI = cardiac index. Normal CI ranges from 2.5 to 3.5 L per min per m^2. Because CI takes body size into consideration, it is a better indicator of the patient's perfusion status.

Systemic Vascular Resistance

Systemic vascular resistance (SVR) is the resistance the left ventricle must work against to eject its volume of blood. Normal SVR is 900 to 1300 dynes per sec per cm^{-5}. An elevated SVR can create enough resistance to left-ventricular

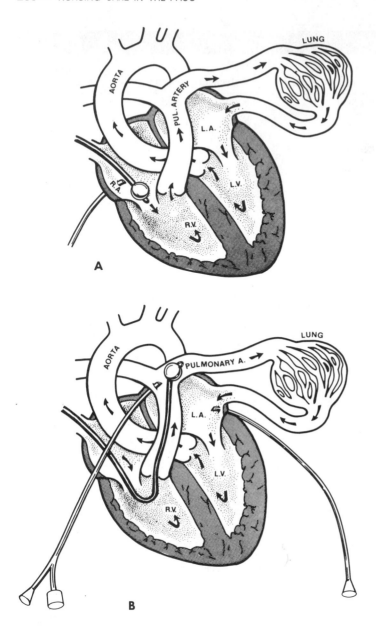

FIGURE 19-21. Placement of hemodynamic lines. *A,* distal tip of a flow-directed pulmonary artery catheter (FDPAC) lying in the right atrium as it floats toward the pulmonary artery, and the distal tip of a right atrial catheter directly inserted through the right atrial wall lying in the right atrium. *B,* distal tip of an FDPAC advancing into a wedged position. Also illustrated is the distal tip of a pulmonary artery thermistor catheter lying in the pulmonary artery after direct insertion through the pulmonary artery wall and the distal tip of a left atrial catheter lying in the left atrium after direct insertion through the left atrial wall near or in a pulmonary vein. Pul. = pulmonary; R.A. = right atrium; L.A. = left atrium; R.V. = right ventricle; L.V. = left ventricle; A. = artery. (*A* and *B* from Whitman, G. R.: Bedside cardiovascular monitoring. *In* Horvath, P. T. [ed.]: Care of the Adult Cardiac Surgery Patient. New York, John Wiley & Sons, 1984, pp. 31 and 33.)

ejection that cardiac output and cardiac index will decrease, which will lead to a state of hypoperfusion or shock. Infusion of vasodilators and afterload-reducing agents can counteract this elevation. SVR is calculated using the following formula:

$$SVR = \frac{(MAP - CVP) \times 80}{CO}$$

where MAP = mean arterial pressure and CVP = central venous pressure.

Pulmonary Vascular Resistance

Pulmonary vascular resistance (PVR) is the resistance the right ventricle must work against to eject blood into the pulmonary bed. Normal PVR is 80 to 240 dynes per sec per cm^{-5}. An elevated PVR can create enough resistance to right-ventricular ejection that right-sided failure or infarction can develop. Infusion of vasodilators or pulmonary artery dilators such as aminophylline can counteract these elevations.

Table 19–2. POTENTIAL PROBLEMS ASSOCIATED WITH INVASIVE HEMODYNAMIC MONITORING

Potential Problems	Etiology	Precautions/Treatment
Alterations in Pressure Wave Configurations		
Dampened tracings	Technical	
	Air in system	Check system for bubbles; flush bubbles out of system.
	Disconnection in system	Inspect and tighten all connections.
	Blood on transducer head	Flush until transducer dome clears of blood; change dome if necessary.
	Kinked catheter	Remove dressing to ascertain if catheter is kinked externally.
	Catheter tip against wall	Turn patient's head or reposition extremity that catheter is inserted into, watching for improvement in tracing. Gently aspirate catheter from various angles to determine at which angle the best flow is achieved; tape and redress the catheter at the angle at which the best flow is achieved. Gently flush catheter in an attempt to push tip away from vessel wall. NEVER flush a catheter in which a clot is suspected.
	Physiologic	
	Clot on catheter tip	Attempt to aspirate blood from catheter. If possible, keep aspirating until clot is retrieved or blood no longer seems thickened. Flush system until the line is cleared and a readable tracing reappears. If blood cannot be aspirated, notify the physician.
	With an FDPAC this may also indicate the catheter has advanced forward and is in a wedged position*	Make sure balloon is deflated. Recheck system and line. If no improvement, obtain a chest radiograph and notify physician.
Abrupt exaggeration of pressure tracings	Technical	Recalibrate and relevel transducer.
	Loss of calibration of level of transducer	
	Physiologic	
	Slippage of catheter out of chamber or vessel	Avoid traction on intravascular lines; tape catheter to skin or secure with suture.
	FDPAC slipping from pulmonary artery to right ventricle. This is characterized by a systolic pressure that remains the same while the diastolic pressure falls into the range of the right-ventricular end-diastolic pressure	Inflate balloon in attempt to let catheter float back into pulmonary artery. If catheter does not migrate back into pulmonary artery, obtain a chest radiograph and notify a physician.
	RAC, PAC, or PATC has slipped out of vessel wall into thoracic cavity	Attempt to aspirate to see if catheter is still in the vessel. If blood returns, flush system and attempt to obtain readable pressure tracings. If no blood return is achieved, notify physician and remove catheter, per protocol.
Alterations in vascular integrity		
Venous and arterial spasms	Irritation to vessels during prolonged insertion attempts	Apply local anesthetic to catheter surface or administer anesthetic by intravenous route. Use a guidewire to facilitate insertion. Cool catheter to make it less flexible and easier to insert.
Thrombophlebitis	Irritation to vessels from prolonged insertion attempts or from constant motion of catheter against vessel	*See "venous and arterial spasms" above.* Secure catheter in place with either tape or suture. Avoid prolonged infusions of chemically irritating medications. Maintain adequate dilutions. Observe for signs and symptoms of phlebitis, and notify physician for possible withdrawal of catheter. Distal placement of stopcocks, connecting catheters, and tubing permits atraumatic blood sampling and flushing.
Embolization	Clot embolization from thrombophlebitis or from clot on catheter tip	Always aspirate catheter first if clot is suspected. NEVER FLUSH.
	Pulmonary embolism with infarct from FDPAC	Observe for changes in chest radiograph that indicate pulmonary embolization.
	Cerebral embolization from LAC catheter	Observe for neurologic changes that may indicate embolization from LAC.
	Peripheral embolization with extremity ischemia from peripheral arterial lines	Observe for ischemic changes of the extremity in which the catheter is located.

Table continued on following page

Table 19–2. POTENTIAL PROBLEMS ASSOCIATED WITH INVASIVE HEMODYNAMIC MONITORING *Continued*

Potential Problems	Etiology	Precautions/Treatment
Air embolization	Loose connections	Secure and tighten all connections. Vigilantly observe LAC catheter, because even minute amounts of air in this system can lead to serious neurologic complications.
	Rupture of balloon on FDPAC due to overinflation or following normal use, because the latex layer on the balloon absorbs lipoproteins from the blood and slowly loses elasticity, thus increasing its incidence of rupture	Inflate balloon slowly, and do not overinflate. Limit inflations. Allow balloon to empty air passively back into syringe. Avoid aspirating air back, because this weakens integrity of balloon. Aspirate only if air fails to return passively. If air does not return and rupture is questioned, sterile saline can be injected into balloon and attempts made to aspirate it back. Failure to aspirate fluid back indicates a leak and the physician should be notified.
Vessel erosion or hemorrhage	Inadequate hemostasis following insertion	Apply firm pressure for 15–20 min.
Bleeding from insertion site: Rupture of a branch of the pulmonary artery	Overinflation of the balloon in a normal-sized vessel	Do not attempt to inflate the balloon if tracing already appears wedged. Inject only prescribed amount of air into balloon.
	Normal inflation of balloon in a too-small vessel	Inject air slowly, and stop injecting if resistance is felt. Inject only amount of air required to obtain a wedge tracing.
	Repeated normal inflations in a brittle or susceptible vessel	Limit wedge intervals in high-risk patients, such as patients with pulmonary hypertension or long-standing mitral valve disease.
Atrial dysrhythmias	Irritation of RA from RAC or during insertion of FDPAC	Withdraw CVP catheter to level of superior vena cava, and obtain readings from that area. Continue with insertion of FDPAC, because dysrhythmias are usually self-limiting and stop once catheter tip exits the right atrium.
Ventricular dysrhythmias	Irritation of right ventricle from tip of FDPAC during insertion procedure or from catheter tip slipping out of the pulmonary artery and back into the right ventricle	Continue with insertion of FDPAC, because dysrhythmias are usually self-limiting and stop once the catheter passes into the pulmonary artery. If catheter tip falls back into the right ventricle from the pulmonary artery, inflate the balloon, because this will cushion the tip of the catheter and may alleviate the dysrhythmias. Administer lidocaine if ventricular dysrhythmias continue. Notify physician, obtain a chest radiograph, and manipulate catheter, per hospital policy.
Infections		
Local infection	Faulty aseptic techniques during insertion or during subsequent dressing changes	Maintain sterility during insertion. Change dressings with sterile technique and tubings, per hospital policy.
Systemic infection	Faulty aseptic technique during insertion	Avoid spasms during insertion. Avoid development of thrombophlebitis along vessel. Change indwelling catheters and insertion sites every 48–72 hr. This may be impossible in patients with difficult vascular access sites. In these situations, rethreading a new catheter over a guidewire at the previous insertion site can be done every 48–72 hr. However, once the site is questionable or the patient develops symptoms of sepsis, such as elevated temperatures and white blood cell count, a new line at a new site is required.
Endocarditis	Extension of a local insertion site. Infection along the catheter and into the circulation	Culture, per hospital policy. Observe for the development of new murmurs.

*Note: Wedging of the catheter in a postoperative patient may be a common occurrence for two reasons: (1) the catheter may have advanced forward during operative procedure when the chest was open and the lungs were not fully inflated, because there was less resistance to forward advancement; and (2) as hypothermia is reversed and the patient and catheter rewarm, its increased flexibility may allow it to float forward.

See Table 19–1 for abbreviations.

Adapted from Whitman, G. R.: Bedside Hemodynamic Monitoring. *In* Horvath P. T.: Care of the Adult Cardiac Surgery Patient. New York, John Wiley and Sons, Inc., 1984.

PVR is calculated using the following formula:

$$PVR = \frac{[PAM - (PCWP\ or\ LAP)] \times 80}{CO}$$

where PAM = pulmonary artery mean pressure and LAP = left-atrial pressure.

CENTRAL NERVOUS SYSTEM FUNCTION

All anesthetics affect the central nervous system (CNS), and it can be assumed for the present, even though we do not know exactly how narcosis occurs, that anesthetics are general, nonselective depressants. The complexity of the CNS, coupled with our incomplete knowledge of how it functions, makes it a most difficult system to evaluate.

Assessment of the CNS in the PACU generally involves only gross evaluation of behavior, level of consciousness, intellectual performance, and emotional status. A more detailed assessment of CNS function is necessary for patients who have undergone CNS surgery, and that discussion occurs in Chapters 4 and 29.

Emergence from Anesthesia

Patients arrive in the PACU at all levels of consciousness, from fully awake to completely anesthetized. With modern anesthesia techniques, however, most patients respond appropriately by the time they are established in the PACU and become oriented quickly when the stir-up regimen is begun (see Chapter 20). With the use of fluorinated and narcotic anesthetics, emergence is generally quiet and uneventful. Occasionally, a patient will become agitated and thrash about; this seems to occur more often in adolescents and young adults than in patients of other age groups. Emergence delirium also tends to occur more frequently in patients who have undergone intra-abdominal and intrathoracic procedures (see Emergence Excitement in Chapter 20). Additional information on emergence can be obtained by reviewing the chapters on specific anesthetic agents (see Chapters 12 through 18).

The PACU nurse can facilitate patient orientation by telling the patient where he or she is, that the surgery is over, and what time it is as a part of the stir-up regimen. Reorientation occurs in reverse order from anesthesia: the patient first becomes oriented to person, then

place, then time. This order, of course, may not hold true for the patient who was somewhat confused or disoriented prior to surgery, which emphasizes the importance of recording accurate information about the mental status of the patient before anesthesia.

Alterations in cerebral function are often the first signs of impaired oxygen delivery to the tissues. Therefore, an orderly and periodic assessment of mental function is necessary to detect early evidence of abnormal cerebral function. Restlessness, agitation, and disorientation occurring in the PACU may be ascribed to a number of other causes and are often difficult to evaluate. The use of continuous pulse oximetry can assist the PACU nurse in determining whether symptoms may be related to hypoxemia.

THERMAL BALANCE

The measurement of the patient's body temperature in the PACU is particularly important. The most recent ASPAN standards state that, at minimum, the preoperative assessment, initial postoperative physical assessment, and discharge evaluation of the patient in Phases I and II PACUs should include documentation of temperature. Normal body temperature may vary from 35.9° to 38°C. In the normal healthy adult, body temperature remains fairly constant, owing to the balance between heat production and heat loss. Alterations in body temperature occur frequently in the postoperative patient. Factors that affect the body temperature in the PACU patient are listed in Table 19–3.

Premedications, anesthesia, and the stress of surgery all interact in a complex fashion to disrupt normal thermoregulation. Both hypothermia (temperature below 36°C) and hyperthermia (temperature above 39°C) are associated

---

Table 19–3. FACTORS INFLUENCING BODY TEMPERATURE OF THE PACU PATIENT

Anesthesia
Preoperative medications
Age of patient
Site and temperature of intravenous fluids
Vasoconstriction (secondary to blood loss or anesthetic agent)
Vasodilation (secondary to regional anesthesia or use of halothane)
Body surface exposure
Temperature of irrigations
Temperature of ambient air

Table 19-4. PHYSIOLOGIC ALTERATIONS ASSOCIATED WITH HYPOTHERMIA AND HYPERTHERMIA

Hypothermia	Hyperthermia
Bluish tint to skin (cyanosis)	Pale skin (mottled)
Increased metabolic rate with shivering, then decreased metabolic rate	Increased metabolic rate
Decreased oxygen consumption	Increased oxygen consumption
Decreased muscle tone	Decreased muscle tone
Decreased heart rate	Increased heart rate (rapid and bounding)
Dysrhythmias	Dysrhythmias
Decreased level of consciousness	Alterations in CNS (patient may be agitated)

with physiologic alterations that may interfere with recovery (Table 19-4).

Patients at the age extremes and those who are extremely debilitated are at even greater risk for the development of temperature abnormalities postoperatively.

The accuracy of axillary, rectal, or oral measurement is frequently debated. Core temperature (approximate value of temperature of blood perfusing the major metabolically active organs) is only estimated by oral and rectal temperature readings. Invasive techniques that use the thermistor on a pulmonary artery catheter, the tympanic membrane, or the bladder as a site for monitoring temperature are more accurate. Unless required during surgery or because of a specific problem, these temperature monitoring modalities are seldom used in the PACU.

Shell (skin) temperature may be measured at the axilla or forehead with conventional thermometers or liquid crystal temperature strips. Shell temperature does not accurately reflect core temperature, although it may at least indicate gross trends.

Infrared tympanic membrane thermometry is increasingly used in the PACU. It is noninvasive and nontraumatic and may be used with patients of all sizes. When placed over the outer third of the auditory canal, the sensor on this otoscope-like thermometer gathers emitted infrared energy from the ear and translates this energy into a temperature reading within seconds. The infrared tympanic thermometer has been found to accurately track core temperature as measured by the thermistor tip of a pulmonary artery catheter.

Management of the hypothermic patient is directed toward the restoration of normothermia and the avoidance of shivering. Warm blankets may be placed over the patient as specific hospital protocol allows. Convective warming devices, such as the Bair Hugger, provide a safe and effective means of gradually rewarming the patient. Hypothermia and hyperthermia are discussed in greater detail in Chapter 20.

FLUID AND ELECTROLYTE BALANCE

Evaluation of a patient's fluid and electrolyte status involves total body assessment. Imbalances readily occur in the postoperative patient owing to a number of factors, including the restriction of food and fluids preoperatively, fluid loss during surgery, and stress (Table 19-5). The normal body response to stress of surgery is renal retention of water and sodium. In addition, patients often have abnormal avenues of fluid loss postoperatively.

Fluid Intake

Each patient must be evaluated to determine his or her baseline requirements and the fluid needed to replace abnormal losses. The normal adult, deprived of oral intake, requires 2000 to 2200 ml of water per day to make up for urinary output and insensible loss.

Intravenous Fluids. Most patients admitted to the PACU from the operating room will be

Table 19-5. COMMON CLINICAL STATES AFFECTING FLUID AND ELECTROLYTE BALANCE IN THE PACU

Clinical State	Effect on Fluid and Electrolyte Balance
Pain Anesthesia Fear Trauma	Heightened response to stress Water and sodium retention
Acute renal failure	Impaired acid–base regulatory mechanism
Blood loss Immobilization	Impaired fluid circulation
"-ostomies" Nasogastric suction Bleeding Vomiting	Excessive loss of fluid by abnormal routes Potassium and sodium deficit
Thyroidectomy Treatment of acidosis Excessive administration of citrated blood	Calcium deficit

receiving intravenous fluids. The anesthetist must have an open intravenous line for the administration of necessary medications and replacement fluids intraoperatively, and an open line is needed postoperatively to supply necessary fluids, electrolytes, and medications. Because all efforts to substitute for normal oral intake of electrolytes and adequate volumes of fluid are, at best, temporary and inadequate, the first objective is to return the patient to adequate oral intake as soon as possible. Until this objective can be attained, an intravenous line must be maintained. The nurse should be aware of the type and amount of any fluid being administered and any medications that may have been added to it.

The intravenous site should be checked to ensure that the needle or cannula is still in the vein and that no extravasation has occurred. Watch for kinks or disconnected tubing, and ensure that the rate of infusion is accurate. The intravenous site should be positioned comfortably; a board may be helpful to maintain the intravenous site if the patient should become restless.

Pediatric patients may require a protective device over the site or soft restraints to prevent dislodging of the needle or cannula. A simple paper cup device can be helpful in preventing dislodgment of the intravenous from the scalp veins of small infants. Snip the bottom out of the cup, thread the cup over the tubing, place the large opening over the intravenous site, and secure the cup to the baby's head with tape crisscrossed over the entire cup. In addition to providing protection for the intravenous site, this method allows the nurse to check the insertion site frequently.

After ensuring that the intravenous fluids are infusing correctly, check to see what fluids, if any, are to follow or if the infusion is to be discontinued.

If the patient is receiving total parenteral nutrition and intralipids, only feeding solutions should go through this line—another intravenous pathway must be secured for other uses. Multilumen catheters allow for the administration of multiple fluids and medications and can be transduced to provide continuous hemodynamic monitoring, if indicated.

The flow of intravenous fluids in the patient receiving hyperalimentation, the patient who is fluid restricted, the infant and small child, and the patient receiving intravenous analgesia or vasopressors should always be regulated by electronic fluid administration devices.

Oral Fluids

Oral intake must be prohibited after anesthesia until the laryngeal and pharyngeal reflexes are fully regained, as evidenced by the patient's ability to gag and swallow effectively. If the patient is permitted oral intake, it is best to start with small amounts of ice chips, because these are less likely to cause nausea and vomiting. Some PACUs use isotonic ice chips that are made from a balanced electrolyte solution, such as Lytren. If ice chips are well tolerated, the patient can progressively increase oral intake to include water and other clear liquids. Kool-Aid and fruit-flavored popsicles are well tolerated and accepted by both children and adults. In addition, carbonated beverages may be soothing to a patient who feels slightly nauseated. The management of postoperative nausea and vomiting is discussed in Chapters 9 and 20.

Fluid Output

Normal output in the average adult results from obligatory urinary output and insensible avenues of loss, including evaporation of water from the skin and exhalation during respiration. The amount of urine necessary for the normal renal system to excrete waste products of a day's metabolism is approximately 600 ml. Optimally, 30 ml per hr or more of urine should be obtained from a catheterized adult to ensure proper hydration and kidney function. Urinary output should be closely monitored in the recovery phase; measurement of urinary output and urine specific gravity yields important clues to the overall status of the patient and may alert the nurse to overhydration or dehydration or the development of shock.

A lower than normal urinary output can be expected in the postoperative patient as a result of the body's normal reaction to stress; however, an unduly small volume of urine (less than 500 ml in 24 hours) may indicate the presence of renal insufficiency, and the physician should be notified.

If a Foley catheter is in place, a more accurate observation of hourly output is available. If urine volume is low and specific gravity remains fixed at a low level, renal insufficiency is indicated. A small urine volume plus a high specific gravity indicates dehydration. In addition to the volume and specific gravity of urinary output being noted, the urine should be examined for the presence of pus, blood, or casts.

The PACU nurse must evaluate abnormal as well as normal avenues of output. Abnormal ways include external losses from vomiting, nasogastric tubes, T-tubes, and fistula or wound drainage and temporary functional losses from fluid shifting within the body, such as hemorrhage into soft tissues and the edema of surgical wounds.

The surgical site should be noted on admission to the PACU, and the dressing should be checked for drainage. The PACU nurse must be aware of the presence of any drains and the expected amount of drainage. Drainage tubes should be checked to ensure patency, and the amount, color, and odor of any drainage should be observed and documented. All tubes should be secure and either clamped shut or connected to drainage apparatus as ordered by the physician. A summary of imbalances that may occur with abnormal avenues of output is presented in Table 19–6. Any deviations from the normally expected drainage in a specific route should be reported promptly to the surgeon.

Obviously, the accurate measurement and recording of all intake and output is vital to the assessment of each patient's fluid and electrolyte status. Keeping a running total on the postoperative flow sheet is essential for quick assessment of fluid status.

In addition to observing and assessing avenues of intake and output, the PACU nurse should be alert to symptoms of fluid and electrolyte imbalance, which are summarized in Table 19–7.

PSYCHOSOCIAL ASSESSMENT

Assessment of the patient's psychological and emotional well-being is an important component of PACU nursing. As with any other assessment, this must be made in the context of the whole patient. Illness, hospitalization, surgery, and pain all take on a variety of values, depending on the person experiencing them. The meaning of the surgery to the person must be explored preoperatively and will probably have been obtained by other health care providers; this information should be communicated to the PACU nurse who will care for the patient. Likewise, the PACU nurse must ensure that additional assessment information and psychosocial care in the PACU are shared with those who will care for the patient after his or her discharge from the unit.

Table 19–6. IMBALANCES THAT MAY OCCUR WITH ABNORMAL AVENUES OF OUTPUT

Fluid	pH	Content (mEq/L)		Likely Imbalances with Significant Losses
Gastric juice (fasting) (nasogastric suction)	1–3	Na^+	60	Metabolic alkalosis
		K^+	10	Potassium deficit
		Cl^-	85	Sodium deficit
		HCO^-_3	0–15	Fluid volume deficit
Small intestine (suction)				
Jejunum	7–8	Na^+	111	
		K^+	4.6	Metabolic acidosis
		Cl^-	104	Potassium deficit
		HCO^-_3	31	Sodium deficit
Ileum		Na^+	117	Fluid volume deficit
		K^+	5.0	
		Cl^-	105	
New ileostomy		Na^+	129	Potassium deficit
		K^+	11	Sodium deficit
		Cl^-	116	Fluid volume deficit
				Metabolic acidosis
Biliary tract fistula	7.8	Na^+	148	Metabolic acidosis
		K^+	5.0	Sodium deficit
		Cl^-	101	Fluid volume deficit
		HCO^-_3	40	
Pancreatic fistula	8.0–8.3	Na^+	141	Metabolic acidosis
		K^+	4.6	Sodium deficit
		Cl^-	76	Fluid volume deficit
		HCO^-_3	121	

Adapted from Bland, J.: Clinical Metabolism of Body Water and Electrolytes. Philadelphia, W. B. Saunders, 1963; and Guyton, A. C.: Textbook of Medical Physiology. 7th ed. Philadelphia, W. B. Saunders, 1986.

Table 19–7. SIGNS AND SYMPTOMS OF ACUTE FLUID AND ELECTROLYTE IMBALANCE

Imbalance	Symptoms and Findings
Hyperosmolarity Water excess Sodium deficit	Polyuria (if kidneys are healthy), twitching, hyperirritability, disorientation, nausea, vomiting, weakness, serum Na^+ ↑ 120 mEq/L
Isotonic disturbances Dehydration Circulatory collapse Volume excess	Weakness, nausea, vomiting, oliguria, postural drop in systolic blood pressure, elevated hematocrit, normal serum Na^+ → SHOCK Dyspnea, cough, sweating, edema
Hydrogen ion imbalances Metabolic acidosis	Apathy, disorientation, increased rate and depth of respiration → Kussmaul's respiration, symptoms of K^+ excess, ABG pH ↓ 7.35, HCO^-_3 ↓ 25, acid urine with pH ↓ 6.0
Metabolic alkalosis	Increased irritability, disorientation, shallow, slow respirations, periods of apnea, irregular pulse, muscle twitch, ABG pH ↑ 7.45, HCO^-_3 ↑ 29, alkaline urine with pH ↑ 7.0
Respiratory acidosis (CO_2 retention)	Increased rate and depth of breathing, tachycardia and other arrhythmias, drowsiness, ABG pH ↓ 7.4, Pco_2 ↑ 40, HCO^-_3 25–35
Potassium imbalances Deficit (hypokalemia)	Weakness, mental confusion, shallow respirations, hypotension, arrhythmias, serum K^+ ↓ 3.5 (this is a measurement of extracellular K^+ and only gives a vague reflection of intracellular balance)
Excess (hyperkalemia)	Intestinal colic, oliguria, bradycardia, cardiac arrest, serum K^+ ↑ 5 mEq/L
Calcium imbalances Deficit (hypocalcemia)	Tingling of the fingers, laryngospasm, facial spasms, painful muscle spasms, positive Trousseau's sign, positive Chvostek's sign, convulsions, palpitations, cardiac arrhythmias, serum Ca^{2+} ↓ 4.5 mEq/L
Excess (hypercalcemia)	Not usually seen in the PACU. Usually due to pathology involving the parathyroid glands

ABG = arterial blood gas.

Almost all surgical patients experience a degree of anxiety about anesthesia and the surgical procedure and a fear of postoperative pain. The physical signs and symptoms of anxiety are the same as those produced by any stressor. Reactions are mediated by the sympathetic nervous system and are listed in Table 19–8.

Symptoms of anxiety must be carefully differentiated from those of other causes. Differentiation is particularly difficult while the effects of anesthesia are still present.

A quiet, calm environment is important to the post anesthesia recovery of the surgical patient. A calm, confident nurse can do much to allay anxiety for the postoperative patient through both verbal reassurance and touch. Hearing is the first sense to return after anesthesia. It is not necessary to yell at patients—they may not respond even if they hear you. In fact, yelling at patients may increase their anxiety early in the PACU period, because they may believe they are not recovering as quickly as they should.

Attention to comfort, including minimal environmental noise and stimuli, and the reassuring presence of the nurse are calming. Once the patients have fully regained consciousness, simply talking to them may help allay anxiety. Simple, factual statements repeated often are best. At this point, the nurse may be able to explore the cause of the distress with the patients.

For the patient in acute distress due to anxiety, a mild tranquilizer, such as diazepam (Valium), midazolam (Versed), and lorazepam (Ativan), may be indicated; however, these benzodiazepines should be used judiciously. One advantage of their use is that they potentiate narcotics, often allowing a reduction of the narcotic analgesia dosage necessary to control pain. Because apnea is a common side effect when benzodiazepines are given to patients receiving narcotics, continuous respiratory monitoring with pulse oximetry and capnography is indicated.

Table 19–8. SIGNS AND SYMPTOMS OF ANXIETY

Tachycardia	Hyperventilation
Increased blood pressure	Increased muscle tone
Pale cool skin	Restlessness/agitation
Increased respiratory rate	Dilated pupils

Attention to the psychosocial ramifications of specific surgical interventions is provided in each of the following chapters on post anesthesia care. These comments are incorporated into the overall text whenever deemed appropriate. For further discussion of the relationship between pain and anxiety, see Chapter 22.

SUMMARY

Obviously, the PACU nurse must be an expert in assessment. The PACU nurse must not only understand the normal physiologic functioning of the human body but also be able to differentiate and evaluate the variety of pathologic symptoms that may arise in the post anesthesia patient. The PACU nurse must be aware of the interrelationships between mind and body and must be sensitive to the psychosocial factors influencing the patient's reactions. Knowledgeable assessment of the post anesthesia patient is essential for the provision of safe and effective medical treatment and nursing care.

References

1. Altsberger, D., and Shrewsbury, P.: Postoperative pain management: The PACU nurse's challenge. J. Post Anesth. Nurs., 3(6):399–403, 1988.
2. American Society of Post Anesthesia Nurses: Standards of Post Anesthesia Nursing Practice. Richmond, AS-PAN, 1991.
3. Cook, K. G.: Assessment and management of anxiety in recovery room patients. Curr. Rev. Recov. Room Nurses, 7(5):51–55, 1983.
4. Durbin, N.: The application of Doppler techniques in critical care. Focus Crit. Care, 10(3):44–46, 1984.
5. Fraulini, K. E.: Coping mechanisms and recovery from surgery. Assoc. Operating Room Nurses J., 37(6):1198–1208, 1983.
6. Henneman, E. A., and Henneman, P. L.: Intricacies of blood pressure measurement: Reexamining the rituals. Heart Lung, 18(3):263–273, 1989.
7. Holtzclaw, B. J.: Shivering: A clinical nursing problem. Nurs. Clin. North Am., 25(4):977–986, 1990.
8. Kataria, B. K., Harnik, E. V., Mitchard R., et al.: Postoperative arterial oxygen saturation in the pediatric population during transportation. Anesth. Analg., 67:280–282, 1988.
9. Kruse, D. H.: Postoperative hypothermia. Focus Crit. Care, 10(2):48–50, 1983.
10. McCarthy, E. J.: Ventilation-perfusion relationships. AANA J., 55(5):437–440, 1987.
11. Miller, K. M., and Taylor, B. T.: Standard care plans for the post anesthesia care unit. J. Post Anesth. Nurs., 6(1):26–32, 1991.
12. New, W.: Pulse oximetry. J. Clin. Monit., 1(2):126–129, 1985.
13. Pesci, B.: Neuromuscular blockage and reversal agents: A primer for post anesthesia nurses. J. Post Anesth. Nurs., 1(1):42–47, 1986.
14. Sanders, A.: End-tidal carbon dioxide monitoring during cardiopulmonary resuscitation: A prognostic indicator for survival. JAMA, 262(10):1347–1351, 1989.
15. Shields, J. R.: A comparison of physostigmine and meperidine in treating emergence excitement. MCN, 5:(3)170–175, 1980.
16. Shinozaki, T., Deane, R., and Perkins, F. M.: Infrared tympanic thermometer: Evaluation of a new clinical thermometer. Crit. Care Med., 16(2):148–150, 1988.
17. Skoog, R. E.: Capnography in the post anesthesia care unit. J. Post Anesth. Nurs., 4(3):147–155, 1989.
18. Swedlow, D. B.: Capnometry and capnography: The anesthesia disaster early warning system. Semin. Anesth., 5(3):194–205, 1986.
19. Toledo, L. W.: Pulse oximetry: Clinical implications in the PACU. J. Post Anesth. Nurs., 2(1):12–17, 1987.
20. Vaughn, M. S.: Shivering in the recovery room. Curr. Rev. Recov. Room Nurses, 6(1):3–7, 1984.

CHAPTER 20

Care of the Post Anesthesia Patient

Denise O'Brien, B.S.N., R.N., C.P.A.N.

Nursing care of post anesthesia patients emerging from anesthesia is reviewed in this chapter. Post anesthesia care includes the stir-up regimen, intravenous and transfusion therapy, maintenance of respiratory function, infection control, and general comfort measures. Emergence excitement and delayed emergence, which may alter the post anesthesia patient's recovery, are also reviewed.

STIR-UP REGIMEN

The stir-up regimen is probably the most important aspect of post anesthesia nursing care. Like most other post anesthesia care unit (PACU) activities, the basics of the stir-up regimen are aimed at prevention of complications, primarily atelectasis and venous stasis. Five major activities—deep-breathing exercises, coughing, positioning, mobilization, and pain management—constitute the stir-up regimen.

Deep-Breathing Exercises

The primary factor contributing to postoperative pulmonary complications is decreased lung volumes. The major factor contributing to low lung volumes in the PACU patient is a shallow, monotonous, sighless breathing pattern caused by general anesthesia, pain, and narcotics. Full inflation of the lungs prevents small areas of patchy atelectasis from developing and assists in the elimination of inhalation anesthetics, thus hastening the awakening process. Intravenous anesthesia differs from inhalation anesthesia in that, once injected, little can be done to expedite removal of the drug; however, the prevention of atelectasis by deep breathing remains just as important.

The patient must be stimulated to take three or four deep breaths every 5 to 10 minutes. Full expansion is important. This may be impeded by a number of factors discussed in the previous chapter. Every effort must be made to enhance the patient's ability to expand the lungs. Many devices and maneuvers have been proposed to improve postoperative lung expansion, but they have had limited success. One of the problems for the PACU patient is the inability to achieve a tight fit on the mouthpiece of the mechanical devices. Additionally, patients emerging from anesthesia may have difficulty participating in the activity owing to their reduced levels of consciousness and awareness.

The sustained maximal inspiration (SMI) maneuver is a method to enhance the lung volumes of postoperative patients. The SMI maneuver consists of the patient inhaling as close to total lung capacity as possible and, at the peak of inspiration, holding that volume of air in the lungs for 3 to 5 seconds before exhaling it. The SMI maneuver produces maximal alveolar inflating pressure, time, and volume. In controlled studies, the SMI maneuver has been more effective than simple deep breathing in preventing reduced lung volumes in the immediate post anesthesia period.

Ideally, the patient will have received instruction and coaching in the use of this maneuver preoperatively. During the immediate postoperative period, the patient must be coached with verbal and tactile (hands on the chest) cues to perform the SMI maneuver.

If the patient's vital capacity is inadequate or respiratory depression due to anesthesia is prolonged, deep breathing and the SMI maneuver may be augmented with a self-inflating bag connected to any oxygen source or with an intermittent positive-pressure breathing apparatus.

Incentive spirometry has become increasingly popular and is used to prevent or assist with reversing atelectasis, promote normal lung expansion, and improve oxygenation. The incentive spirometry devices allow patients visual feedback and observation of inspiratory volume. Instruction and practice before surgery provide patients the opportunity to master the device and establish a baseline for themselves before anesthetic and surgical interventions. Devices currently available include disposable flow-oriented and volume-oriented incentive spirometers that are inexpensive and can be used by the patient at home. Incentive spirometry may have greater use after the immediate post anesthesia period because patients are more awake and capable of manipulating the devices than they are in the PACU.

Coughing

The patient must be instructed to cough along with performing SMIs. The best way to clear the air passages of obstructive secretions is a purposeful cough. Cough effectiveness depends on the inspired tidal volume and the velocity of expired airflow. For the patient recovering from anesthesia, the cascade cough is the most effective cough maneuver. The patient should be taught to take a rapid, deep inspiration to increase the volume of air in the lungs, which will in turn dilate the airways, allowing air to pass beyond the retained secretions. On exhalation, the patient should perform multiple coughs at succeedingly lower lung volumes. With each cough during exhalation, the length of the airways undergoing dynamic compression will increase, enhancing cough effectiveness.

Coughing is most effective with the patient sitting up. Splinting of incisions and adequate analgesia facilitate a good cough. If the patient is unable to sit upright, positioning the patient in a side-lying position with hips and knees flexed or in a semi-Fowler's position with head and arms supported with pillows and knees flexed will decrease abdominal tension and allow maximal movement of the diaphragm, thereby improving the effectiveness of the cough.

Between cascade cough maneuvers, the patient should be encouraged to inhale and close the glottis. This dilates the airways and, by increasing the pleural pressure, further compresses the airways so as to "milk" the secretions toward the larger airways, where they can be removed in succeeding cough maneuvers.

If an effective cough cannot be produced, secretions from the respiratory passages must be suctioned manually. If the patient cannot or will not cough effectively, it may be necessary to stimulate cough by means of tracheal suctioning or manual pressure to the trachea. A cough is stimulated by finger pressure against the trachea just above the manubrial notch; the maneuver is also known as *tracheal tickle*. Because this maneuver may also produce retching and vomiting, it should be used cautiously.

Preoperative teaching of postoperative breathing exercises and cough and their importance is effective and should be included in the preoperative regimen whenever possible. Patients scheduled for surgery may attend formal teaching sessions before surgery or may receive instructions for coughing, deep breathing, and incentive spirometry through educational booklets, video programs, and one-on-one visits to preoperative testing departments.

Positioning

When possible, patients in the PACU should be maintained in a semiprone, side-lying position. The semiprone position promotes maintenance of a patent airway, prevents aspiration of vomitus into the trachea, and permits optimal ventilation of the lower lung lobes. Frequent repositioning of patients (at least every hour) is essential for the prevention of atelectasis and peripheral stasis. The patient's position should be changed from side to side. Care must be taken to ensure that all drainage tubes and intravenous catheters remain in place and patent and that no tension on any of these lines is created. As soon as they are able, patients should be encouraged to turn and change positions alone.

Mobilization

To prevent venous stasis, patients must be encouraged to move their legs and arms rhythmically. Have patients flex and extend their extremities. Mobilization and flexion of the muscles aid venous return, automatically cause deep breathing, and improve cardiac function.

Pain Management

Achievement of the stir-up regimen's first four activities is difficult if adequate pain relief is not provided. Narcotics depress the cough reflex and ciliary activity and may lower alveolar ventilation by direct depression of the respiratory center; they must not be used indiscriminately. If breathing is painful and splinting occurs, however, or if the patient refuses to cough or move because of pain, nothing is gained. Pain relief is discussed in detail in Chapter 22.

Modifications of the Stir-Up Regimen

Modifications of the stir-up regimen may be needed depending on the type of anesthesia used and the operative procedure performed. When ketamine is the anesthetic used, the stir-up regimen is eliminated from routine PACU care and verbal and tactile stimulation of the patient are avoided as much as possible. Cough must be eliminated after eye surgery and other delicate plastic procedures. Stimulation of the patient with increased or potentially increased intracranial pressure must be undertaken carefully to avoid dangerous and potentially life-threatening pressure changes.

Positioning is probably the activity most often modified in the stir-up regimen. Positioning of the patient and modifications of the stir-up regimen after specific surgical procedures and anesthetics are discussed in related chapters.

EMERGENCE EXCITEMENT

Most patients emerge from general anesthesia in a calm, tranquil manner. Some patients, however, emerge in a state of "excitement," a condition characterized by restlessness, disorientation, crying, moaning, or irrational talking. In the extreme form of excitement, which is referred to as *emergence delirium*, the patient screams, shouts, and thrashes about wildly.

The incidence of emergence excitement is high among children and is most common in healthy patients. As age increases, the incidence decreases. Premedication with barbiturates and anticholinergics, especially scopolamine, seems to increase its occurrence. Factors such as fear of disfigurement, fear of cancer, and a feeling of suffocation also increase the likelihood of emergence excitement.

The PACU nurse should assess the patient's status if emergence excitement is encountered. Check the patient's respiratory function and airway patency first because restlessness is a well-known manifestation of hypoxia. Other causes include a full bladder, cramped or sore muscles and joints from prolonged abnormal positioning on the operating table, the presence of pain, incomplete reversal of neuromuscular

blocking agents, withdrawal from alcohol and other drugs, acid-base disturbances, and electrolyte abnormalities.

The restless patient requires constant, careful observation. Gentle physical restraint may be required to prevent injury. Several nurses or attendants may be needed. If hypoxia, pain, and full bladder are ruled out, a change in position may have a quieting effect. Physostigmine may be used to reverse anticholinergic drug effects. Opioids and anxiolytics, such as midazolam, either alone or in combination, usually calm the patient. If narcotic or sedative treatment is instituted, the patient should be monitored for hypotension and respiratory depression.

DELAYED EMERGENCE

Occasionally patients awaken from anesthesia more slowly than expected. Causes include prolonged action of anesthetic and other drugs; metabolic problems such as hypoglycemia, hypocalcemia, hyponatremia, and hypermagnesemia; hypovolemia; hypothermia; and neurologic injury. Respiratory inadequacy with resultant hypercarbia and hypoxemia may be the result of narcotics, sedatives, other anesthetic agents and adjuncts, or neurologic causes.

Treatment consists of thorough assessment and identification of the cause or causes of the delayed arousal. Oxygenation and ventilation along with adequate cardiac output must be maintained. Residual anesthetic agents may be treated with maintenance of ventilation. Residual narcotics, sedatives, and anticholinergics may be reversed with the appropriate antagonists. Metabolic disturbances should be corrected. If hypothermia is the suspected cause, warming measures are instituted with appropriate temperature monitoring. Neurologic evaluation may be needed if other causes of delayed arousal have been excluded.

INTRAVENOUS THERAPY

Postoperative parenteral fluid requirements vary with the patient's preoperative status and with the surgical procedure. For a discussion of fluid and electrolyte balance, see Chapter 7.

TRANSFUSION THERAPY

The administration of whole blood or blood components (serum, plasma, red blood cells, platelets) is less common, although it is often a lifesaving treatment modality for the postoperative patient. However, the inherent dangers are numerous, and PACU nurses must be well aware of the principles of safe administration of blood and blood components.

Whole Blood

The only indication for whole blood transfusion in the PACU is hypovolemic shock to restore and maintain circulating blood volume that has been depleted from hemorrhage or trauma. The nurse may anticipate this need in patients who have required emergency surgery and in patients who have been subjected to extensive dissection. The only other indications for whole blood transfusions are exchange transfusions to remove toxic substances from the blood or to prime the oxygenating pump for cardiac surgery. These are rare occurrences in the PACU. Most other clinical situations requiring replacement therapy can be handled with blood components, plasma volume expanders, and crystalloids.

Patients anticipating blood loss requiring replacement during elective operative procedures may donate autologous blood before the scheduled procedure. As many as four units or more may be obtained through collections as frequently as every 96 hours. This preoperative autologous donation, acute normovolemic hemodilution (in which blood is removed immediately before the procedure and the patient infused with intravenous fluids; at the end of the procedure, the stored blood is reinfused), and autotransfusion of blood scavenged either intraoperatively or postoperatively are commonly used for replacement instead of homologous blood transfusions. Patients may also name designated donors to give blood for their operations, although the blood of these donors may be no safer than the blood of volunteer donors.

Every possible safeguard must be exercised to prevent the administration of incompatible blood to the patient needing replacement. Before any blood or blood component is administered, including autologous donor units, typing and crossmatching of the donor and the recipient blood must be done. Whether it is known in advance that the patient will need blood replacement for major surgery or only that the patient might need blood replacement based on possible planned operative procedures, this typing and crossmatching should be carried out before the start of surgery, and

compatible blood should be available for administration.

Great care must be taken in the identification of the recipients and the unit of blood prepared for them. An information form listing the donor's and recipient's types, crossmatches done and identification number, the recipient's name, and the date prepared must be crosschecked with the label on the unit of blood to be administered and with the patient's identification bracelet. At least two persons should be involved in the identification of the recipient, preferably two nurses or a physician and a nurse. Because PACU patients are often not well known by the nurse and are frequently only partially conscious owing to anesthesia, scrupulous attention must be directed toward positive identification of the recipient. If any discrepancy exists, do not give the blood until clarification is obtained. Once positive identification of the recipient and the unit of blood to be transfused is established, the blood must be inspected for hemolysis and abnormal cloudiness or color. Red blood cells settle to the bottom of whole blood, and plasma rises to the top. Before the transfusion is begun and from time to time during the transfusion, whole blood should be gently and thoroughly mixed by tilting the bag back and forth.

Blood and blood components should be administered via large-bore intravenous needles or by plastic cannulas in a large vein of the forearm or through a central venous catheter. Only blood administration sets designed for use with any plug-in type of blood, plasma, or serum container should be used for transfusion. The drip chamber must be filled enough to just cover the filter before the infusion is started. If the filter becomes clogged during the infusion, it may be cleared by squeezing the flexible drip chamber above the filter after the clamp has been completely closed. The level is then reset by squeezing the chamber. Squeezing the plastic drip chamber above the filter ensures that particulate matter will not be forced into the filter and that the filter will not be bent. Multiple transfusions and some blood components require special filters or administration sets, or both.

The recommended solution to infuse with blood and blood components is 0.9 percent sodium chloride, injection (USP). It is completely compatible with blood. Small clumps or globules of red blood cells may form when blood is administered with dextrose in water, and many of the balanced solutions (e.g., Ringer's injection, USP; lactated Ringer's injection, USP) contain calcium, which may cause citrated blood to clot. Solutions containing calcium or a potent drug (e.g., any anesthetic or neuromuscular blocking agent) should never be used in the primary infusion line when blood is administered by secondary or piggyback hookup.

Before beginning the blood administration, obtain baseline vital signs, including temperature, and note the status of the infusion site. Untoward reactions to blood generally occur with the first 50 ml of the transfusion; start the transfusion slowly (20 to 40 drops per min) for the first 15 minutes. If no symptoms of reaction develop, the rate of administration may be increased to 80 to 100 drops per min or the rate ordered by the physician.

A unit of blood is usually administered over a period of 1 to 2 hours; however, in emergency situations, such as shock or hemorrhage, a unit of blood can be infused within 10 minutes under pressure. A pressure cuff similar to a blood pressure cuff is slipped over the collapsible plastic blood container and pumped to compress the bag and literally push the blood into the patient's veins. When pressure transfusion equipment is used, every precaution must be exercised to prevent air from entering the system and causing air embolization. All tubing and the blood container itself must be checked for leaks. The infusion site must be monitored carefully for signs of infiltration to prevent the infusion of blood into subcutaneous tissue.

Blood may need to be warmed, especially in emergency situations and large volumes are infused or when the patient is hypothermic or has cold agglutinin disease. Rapid infusion of refrigerated blood can cause cardiac arrhythmias, especially when given through a central venous catheter, and hypothermia. Warming devices available include dry-heating and water-bath types.

Once the blood infusion is started, the flow rate should be checked frequently. Changing the height of the intravenous stand or the bed may alter the rate of the infusion, as will repositioning of the patient, changes in location of the catheter or needle in the vein, or alterations in the tone of the vein.

Transfusion Reactions

The exact incidence of transfusion reactions is unknown. Reports of their incidence vary from 0.2 to 10 percent, and some reactions are undoubtedly unrecognized and unreported.

Nurses in the PACU must be especially adept at assessing the patient receiving blood, because many of the signs and symptoms of an adverse reaction to blood may be difficult to separate from those caused by other variables such as the patient's illness, surgery, or medications (including anesthesia). In addition, the patient who is not fully conscious may not complain of symptoms. Blood transfusion reactions may be either immediate or delayed. Immediate reactions include hemolytic, febrile, bacterial contamination, and allergic reactions.

Hemolytic Reactions. Fifty to 75 ml of ABO-incompatible blood can precipitate a hemolytic reaction resulting in agglutination, or clumping, of red blood cells, which blocks the patient's capillaries, obstructing the flow of blood and oxygen to vital organs. In time, hemolysis of the red blood cells occurs, releasing free hemoglobin into the plasma. Free hemoglobin may plug the renal tubules and disrupt the work of the nephrons, resulting in renal failure. Improper storage, overheating, or freezing of blood may also cause hemolysis of the cells and release of free hemoglobin.

The clinical signs of the hemolytic reaction occur quickly and include sudden hypotension; tachycardia; substernal chest pain; abdominal, leg, and back pain; dyspnea; and sensorium changes, most often anxiety. Headache may be one of the awake patient's first complaints. Pain may occur along the vein path. Fever and chills develop later, along with hemoglobinuria, which leads to oliguria. Many of these symptoms may be significantly masked under the influence of anesthesia. Bleeding from the wound is strongly suggestive that the patient has received incompatible blood; it is also a poor prognostic sign.

Febrile Reactions. Febrile reactions are most often due to sensitivity to leukocytes and platelets and are seen most frequently in patients who have received multiple transfusions. A febrile reaction may also be attributed to bacterial contamination. In febrile or bacterial contamination reactions the patient may complain of headache and chills, followed by a rapid rise in temperature. Backache, nausea, vomiting, diarrhea, and abdominal pain follow. Hypotension and tachycardia develop quickly. Pyrogenic reactions caused by the polysaccharide products of bacterial metabolism are manifested by the same symptoms, except that blood pressure does not drop, and the temperature usually returns to normal within 12 hours.

Allergic Reactions. Allergic reactions occur in about 1 percent of all transfusions and are most often seen in patients who have a history of allergy. Symptoms include mild edema and hives, sometimes accompanied by itching, occasionally by fever and chills, and bronchial wheezing. More severe reactions include symptoms of asthma, bronchospasm, severe dyspnea, laryngeal edema, and finally, anaphylactic shock.

Treatment of Immediate Reactions. At the first sign of a reaction, the transfusion must be stopped and the physician notified. The donor blood unit and administration set, along with a sample of the recipient's blood, should be sent to the blood bank for transfusion reaction investigation. The first voided specimen should be sent to the laboratory and tested for hemoglobin and urobilinogen. Urine output must be monitored carefully. Ideally, a Foley catheter should be inserted and hourly output recorded. Vital signs must be monitored and the patient treated according to his or her symptoms. The intravenous line should be kept open with normal saline. Blood transfusion with properly matched blood may be needed to correct blood volume deficits and control shock. Vasoconstricting drugs may be required to control blood pressure but must be used with caution because they may contribute to renal damage, especially if blood volume has not been restored. Oxygen and epinephrine may be used to treat dyspnea and wheezing. Steroids and broad-spectrum antibiotics may be necessary to treat reactions caused by bacterial contamination. Antihistamines and antipyretics are given to the patient experiencing an allergic reaction. Diuretic therapy (e.g., furosemide) and the infusion of 0.9 percent sodium chloride or 5 percent dextrose in 0.45 percent sodium chloride may be prescribed to maintain hydration and urine flow of more than 100 ml per hr.

Delayed Reactions

Delayed reactions include the transmission of disease (hepatitis, cytomegalovirus, malaria, human immunodeficiency virus [HIV]-1), transfusion siderosis, graft-versus-host disease, circulatory overload, citrate intoxication, cardiac dysrhythmias, and bleeding due to depleted coagulation factors.

Circulatory overload results when fluid is infused into the circulatory system either too rapidly or in too great a quantity. Elderly patients and those with minimal cardiac reserve are particularly susceptible. The use of packed red blood cells in these patients should be considered carefully. Symptoms of circulatory overload include cough, dyspnea, edema, tachycardia, hemoptysis, and frothy, pink-tinged

sputum. If patients are conscious, they may complain of a pounding headache, a feeling of constriction around the chest, back pain, and chills. If these symptoms develop, the transfusion should be stopped and the physician notified.

When large amounts of banked blood are transfused, *citrate intoxication* may occur. If the blood is infused rapidly, the liver cannot metabolize the citrate ions, which combine with the calcium in the blood, causing calcium deficit symptoms, such as tingling of the fingers, muscular cramps, and nervousness. If the calcium deficit is not corrected, cardiac dysrhythmias, including ventricular fibrillation, may occur. Treatment consists of slow intravenous administration of calcium gluconate, 1 g for every 1000 ml of blood the patient received. If calcium gluconate is unavailable, calcium chloride may be used, but this is more irritating to the veins.

The rapid infusion of cold blood may result in *cardiac dysrhythmias.* Blood should be warmed to room temperature or passed through a warming coil, taking care not to overheat it, which would cause hemolysis of the red blood cells.

In cases of massive blood replacement, *bleeding from dilution of coagulation factors and platelets* can occur. If massive transfusions are required, it is suggested that several fresh blood infusions (<4 hours old) be used along with banked blood.

Blood must be properly stored and refrigerated at 5°C. In most instances, blood should be stored in the blood bank until required. If blood is to be kept in the PACU, proper storage requirements must be met. When units of blood prepared for a given recipient are not used, they should be promptly returned to the blood bank.

Blood Component Transfusions

Packed Red Blood Cells. The use of packed red blood cells can eliminate many of the problems associated with whole blood transfusion. Packed cells are prepared by drawing off about two thirds of the plasma, either through the natural settling-out process or by centrifugation. Patients who require red blood cells to improve the oxygen-carrying capacity of the blood should be treated with packed cells to minimize volume increase and the risks of circulatory overload or cardiovascular failure. In addition, a better balance of sodium, potassium, and ammonium ions is maintained, and citrate intoxication is prevented. When plasma is removed, the antibody content of blood is markedly reduced and hence minimizes reactions to plasma factors.

Platelets and Plasma Proteins. Other blood components that may be used in the PACU include platelets and the plasma proteins. Transfusion of platelets is the treatment of choice when bleeding occurs and the platelet count is less than 10,000 per μl. Platelets may be administered through a standard blood administration set or a special component administration set.

Plasma proteins may be used to treat specific deficits. *Albumin* is used to treat shock due to hemorrhage, trauma, or infection. It is prepared in concentrations of 5 percent in buffered saline and of 25 percent in salt-poor diluent. It is administered with a large-bore needle and may be infused through standard intravenous tubing.

Plasma protein fraction (PPF) is heat treated like albumin, destroying antibodies and thereby eliminating compatibility problems. Hepatitis and HIV cannot be transmitted by PPF or albumin because the pasteurization process destroys the viruses. PPF consists of 83 percent albumin and 17 percent globulins extracted from plasma. It is less pure than albumin and can cause hypotension due to vasoactive contaminants.

Fresh-frozen plasma thawed slowly forms a precipitate that is separated and refrozen. This *cryoprecipitate* consists of factor VIII and fibrinogen and is used to control bleeding due to factor VIII deficiency. It is also indicated for the treatment of von Willebrand's disease and for fibrinogen or factor XIII replacement.

Non-Blood Volume Substitutes

Dextran is a synthetic plasma substitute that may be used in acute hemorrhage until more specific blood components can be given. It is inexpensive, readily available, and carries no risk of disease transmission. Dextran may interfere, to some extent, with platelet function and may be associated with a transient prolongation of bleeding time. Hypersensitivity reactions can occur—patients should be closely monitored during the first 30 minutes of infusion. Certain blood typing and crossmatching methods are affected by dextran. Dextran is administered through standard intravenous tubing.

Hetastarch is an artificial colloid. It is a synthetic starch molecule derived from corn that closely resembles human glycogen. Available in a 6 percent hetastarch in 0.9 percent sodium chloride solution, hetastarch is claimed to be less likely to produce allergic reactions and to have minimal effects on coagulation when infused in moderate amounts (<1500 ml total volume). It is also used for volume replacement and expansion following acute blood loss from trauma, burns, and surgery.

MAINTENANCE OF RESPIRATORY FUNCTION

Oxygen Therapy

The optimal use of the oxygen-carrying capacity of arterial blood is the goal of oxygen therapy. All anesthetized patients have experienced some interference with their respiratory processes, and it is for this reason that most experts suggest routine oxygen administration to all post anesthesia patients in the PACU. However, oxygen is a drug and should be treated as such, with full prescription information provided by the anesthesia care provider. This information may be contained in standard orders that are individualized for each patient. Low-flow oxygen administration assists the patient in maintaining adequate oxygenation of all tissues. Optimal arterial oxygen tension should be between 70 and 100 mm Hg. Patients with chronic lung disease may be maintained with low-flow oxygen administration, which keeps the oxygen tension in the range of 50 to 70 mm Hg. Pulmonary processes should be monitored carefully in the PACU. Pulse oximetry monitoring of all patients who have received an anesthetic is recommended in the initial post anesthesia period.

Pulse oximetry, a noninvasive technique, measures arterial oxygen saturation of functional hemoglobin. In the post anesthesia setting, continuous monitoring of a patient's oxygen saturation assists in manipulating the fraction of inspired oxygen (FIO_2) levels and in identifying episodes of desaturation and hypoxia. Normal pulse oximetry values are 97 to 99 percent. Oxygen saturation as measured by pulse oximetry (SpO_2) values of 95 percent or greater are acceptable. Preanesthetic baseline SpO_2 values should be noted; patients may normally fall below the normal range on room air. Attempting to maintain higher oxygen saturation levels than the patient's baseline level may result in prolonged oxygen therapy and PACU stays.

Sensor site selection and application, ambient light, motion, electrical interference, and impaired blood flow (low perfusion states, excessive edema) may influence SpO_2 levels. Accurate measurement is affected by temperature, pH, $PaCO_2$, hemodynamic status, and anemia. These factors alter the oxyhemoglobin dissociation curve and oxygen delivery. Additionally, dysfunctional hemoglobins (carboxyhemoglobin, a by-product of smoking and smoke; methemoglobin, formed from drugs such as lidocaine and nitroglycerine) may result in false elevation of oximetry values.

Nurses should never be reluctant to draw arterial blood gases to aid in the assessment of a patient's status. For discussion of arterial blood gases and the method for obtaining their measurement, see Chapter 6.

Complications of oxygen therapy do occur, and nurses should be aware of them. Oxygen-induced hypoventilation, atelectasis, substernal chest pain, and toxicity may occur when high concentrations are administered over prolonged periods (FIO_2 >0.5 for >24 hours). For more detailed discussions of these complications, the reader is referred to the respiratory references at the end of this chapter.

Methods of Administration

Routine oxygen administration in the PACU can be accomplished with nasal cannula (prongs) or face masks. Table 20–1 lists frequently used oxygen delivery methods. Nasal cannulas are advantageous for routine short-term oxygen administration in the PACU. The cannula is made of plastic tubing with two soft plastic tips that insert into the nostrils for about 1.5 cm. The prongs deliver an oxygen concentration of 30 to 40 percent when a 4 to 6 l per min flow is used. The prongs are easily inserted, comfortable, inexpensive, and disposable. Simple, clear plastic disposable face masks may be used for oxygen administration in the PACU. They are also easy to apply and comfortable. The oxygen concentration delivered depends on the mask fit and the patient's inspiratory flow rate; however, an oxygen flow rate of 5 to 8 l per min yields an FIO_2 of approximately 40 to 60 percent. Face masks in the PACU must be clear to provide adequate observation of the patient's nose and mouth. The mask should be removed intermittently to dry the face.

Humidity

Surgery and anesthesia often interrupt the normal functioning of the nose in heating and humidification of inspired air. When oxygen is administered by nasal cannula at flow rates of less than 4 l per min or by Venturi mask, humidification is generally unnecessary because adequate amounts of humidified room air are inspired. At higher flow rates, humidification or nebulization may be needed in the PACU.

Humidifiers convert water from the liquid to the gaseous state, whereas nebulizers produce tiny water particles. Humidifiers are used to add water vapor to the airway, whereas a nebulizer can provide both water vapor and particulate water or medication or saline aerosols to the airway. Aerosol therapy can be used to administer antibiotics, bronchodilators, and corticosteroids.

Mechanical Ventilation

Rarely, some patients recovering from anesthesia may require some form of mechanical ventilation in the PACU. Various techniques such as positive end-expiratory pressure (PEEP), continuous positive airway pressure (CPAP), and intermittent mandatory ventilation (IMV) are used to improve the respiratory status of the patient. Table 20–2 gives the terminology of the common ventilatory modes.

Positive End-Expiratory Pressure. PEEP is a technique that can be used to help prevent collapse of the alveoli during the expiratory phase of ventilation, to increase the lung's functional residual capacity (FRC), and to reduce the amount of physiologic shunting. PEEP also increases the PaO_2, which will usually enable the FIO_2 to be reduced, thus lessening the chances of oxygen toxicity. In patients with pre-existing obstructive lung disease, PEEP should probably be used cautiously, because it may overexpand relatively normal alveoli. When it is used under such circumstances, the dead space increases and occasionally causes a decrease in the PaO_2 and an increase in the $PaCO_2$.

When a patient is placed on PEEP, hemodynamic status should be monitored because this ventilatory technique retards venous return and may cause a decrease in cardiac output, especially in the hypovolemic patient. In some instances, the reduced cardiac output can cause a decrease in systolic blood pressure. Other parameters to be monitored are vital signs, skin perfusion, and urine output.

Continuous Positive Airway Pressure. CPAP helps keep the lungs expanded. The patient breathes out against increased pressure as high as 10 to 20 cm H_2O, but the mechanics of ventilation do not change. The lung performs

Table 20–1. METHODS OF OXYGEN ADMINISTRATION

Method	FiO₂	Flow (l/min)	Comments
Low-Flow Methods			
Nasal cannula (prongs)	0.24–0.40	5–6	Comfortable to wear, patient can breathe orally or nasally and still raise F_{IO_2}; humidification unnecessary
Simple face mask	0.40–0.60	5–8	Adjustable to fit face; may be hot and uncomfortable for patients. Poorly tolerated, potential for skin irritation from tight fit and oxygen contact
Face tent	0.30–0.55	4–10	Less confining, useful when extra humidity needed
Partial rebreathing mask	0.35–0.60	6–10	Mask with attached reservoir bag; no valves on mask (exhalation ports open)
High-Flow Methods			
Non-rebreathing mask	0.40–1.00	6–15	Mask with reservoir bag; one-way valves on exhalation side ports of mask, one-way valve between mask and bag for inhalation
"Venturi" mask	0.24–0.55	2–14	Believed accurate delivery of desired F_{IO_2}; may be less if patient is hyperpneic or unable to keep mask in position on face
T-piece or Brigg's	0.21–1.00	2–10	Used with endotracheal or tracheostomy tube; provides accurate delivery of desired F_{IO_2} and humidification; most often used when weaning patients from ventilator assistance before endotracheal tube removed
Mechanical ventilator	0.21–1.00	Direct from supply	Pressure, volume, flow, and oxygen percentage all adjustable

F_{IO_2} = Fraction of inspired oxygen concentration.

at a larger, more inflated volume, thereby increasing the FRC and decreasing the tendency to atelectasis. CPAP is a technique that can be used for weaning a patient from a ventilator. When CPAP is being used, the patient should be monitored for tachypnea, tachycardia, increase in blood pressure, arrhythmias, or generalized distress, which should be reported to the physician, if detected.

Intermittent Mandatory Ventilation. IMV was originally devised to facilitate the weaning process from mechanical ventilation. It is currently used when a patient is first given mechanical ventilation. This technique allows patients to breathe on their own as often and as deeply as they would like; it also ensures that every minute a set tidal volume is delivered at a predetermined back-up rate. IMV allows gradual progression from complete ventilatory support by the ventilator to spontaneous provision of ventilation by the patient.

Nursing Responsibilities. All PACU nurses must be familiar with the specific types and modes of operation of ventilators used in their area (Figs. 20–1 and 20–2; see Table 20–2). There are, however, nursing responsibilities that remain the same regardless of the type of mechanical ventilator used.

1. Ascertain that the patient is being ventilated by frequently observing the chest for bilateral synchronous and equal expansion and by listening for bilaterally present and equal breath sounds.
2. Check the airway frequently for complete patency. See that the patient ventilator system is free of significant leaks by listening for air gurgling in the upper airway during ventilation and by comparing the exhaled volume with the tidal volume set on the ventilator.
3. Ensure that the cuff is *never* overinflated. Inflate the cuff until there is no leak on tidal ventilation and a small, barely audible leak on sigh volume.
4. Empty the ventilatory hoses frequently of excess water from condensation.
5. Be sure that proper humidification is being delivered to the patient by noting the presence of water droplets in the ventilator hoses.
6. The humidifier should be checked and

Table 20–2. TERMINOLOGY: COMMON VENTILATORY MODES

Abbreviation	Term
Mechanical Ventilation with Positive Airway Pressure	
PPV	Positive-pressure ventilation
MV	Mechanical ventilation
CV	Controlled ventilation
A-CV	Assist-control ventilation
AMV	Assisted mechanical ventilation
CMV	Controlled mechanical ventilation
IMV	Intermittent mandatory ventilation
SIMV	Synchronized intermittent mandatory ventilation
IAV	Intermittent assisted ventilation
IDV	Intermittent demand ventilation
PSV	Pressure support ventilation
IPPB	Intermittent positive-pressure breathing
IPPV	Intermittent positive-pressure ventilation
CPPB	Continuous positive-pressure breathing
CPPV	Continuous positive-pressure ventilation
PEEP	Positive end-expiratory pressure
HFJV	High-frequency jet ventilation
HFPPV	High-frequency positive-pressure ventilation
HFO	High-frequency oscillation
ILV	Independent lung ventilation
APRV	Airway pressure-release ventilation
Spontaneous Breathing (SB) with Positive Airway Pressure	
CPAP	Continuous positive airway pressure
EPAP	Expiratory positive airway pressure
IPAP	Inspiratory positive airway pressure

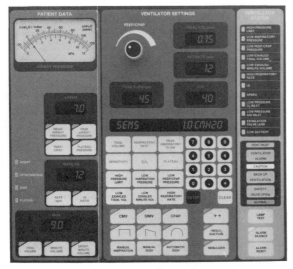

FIGURE 20–1. Top panel of 7200 Series system ventilator. The left side of the panel includes patient data indicators: airway pressure, mode, pressure in cm H₂O, rate with inspiratory, expiratory ratio. The middle of the panel indicates ventilator settings: tidal volume, rate, O₂%, peak flow, and a keyboard for entering parameters. Note the keys for manual inspiration and sigh. The right side of the panel has a light-emitting diode (LED) display to indicate alarm status and ventilator status. (Courtesy of Puritan-Bennett Corporation, Overland Park, KS.)

filled frequently to ensure proper humidification.

7. The temperature gauge should be between 90° and 98°F (32.2° and 36.6°C), and the ventilator hoses and the humidifier should be warm to the touch, never cold or hot.
8. There must *never* be any pull on the patient's endotracheal or tracheostomy tube.
9. Tracheostomy wound care should be performed as needed during the post anesthesia phase.
10. Ascertain frequently that all alarms on the ventilator are *on* and *functioning properly.*

The observations and checks of mechanical devices often seem simple and routine but are an important part of nursing the mechanically ventilated patient. Ideally, all these checks, along with measured parameters of the patient's respiratory status, should be recorded on a flow sheet attached to the patient's bed or to the ventilator. Such a flow sheet is vital for clinical evaluation of the patient's response to therapy. A sample flow sheet is shown in Figure 20–3.

Suctioning

When large amounts of secretions accumulate that cannot be handled effectively by coughing, suctioning must be instituted to assist the patient in clearing air passages.

Oral and Nasal Suctioning

Suctioning the nose and mouth is simple and safe. This procedure is commonly used to assist patients in eliminating secretions before they have regained full consciousness and cannot spit out secretions. The catheter used should be soft and pliable. The technique should be clean but need not be strictly sterile. A Yankauer or tonsil suction tip may be used to remove oral secretions from the mouth and over the tongue.

Tracheal Suctioning

Tracheal suctioning may be performed through the mouth or nose, via endotracheal tube, or through a tracheostomy tube (Fig. 20–4). Tracheal suctioning must be accomplished atraumatically using aseptic technique. A selection of sterile suctioning catheters in a variety of sizes should be kept at the bedside of every patient in the PACU along with sterile gloves and sterile water or normal saline. The catheter chosen for suctioning should not have an exter-

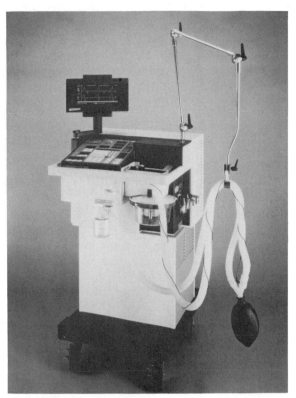

FIGURE 20–2. A volume ventilator used either to assist or to control a patient's respirations. (Courtesy of Puritan-Bennett Corporation, Overland Park, KS.)

nal diameter that exceeds by one third the internal diameter of the tube to be suctioned. Most commonly, a 14 or 16 French size is used for adult patients. The catheter must not completely occlude the trachea or endotracheal tube.

The procedure should be explained to the patients even if they are apparently totally unconscious. Explaining the procedure alleviates fear and also helps gain cooperation from the patients to the extent that they are able.

Before suctioning the patient, ensure proper ventilation. In most patients, suctioning lowers the arterial pressure of oxygen 30 to 35 mm Hg. Because suctioning removes oxygen, which may in turn initiate cardiac dysrhythmias, the nurse should assess the total physiologic condition of the patient before beginning the procedure. Are they restless, agitated, or disoriented? Although these conditions can be caused by other factors, they often indicate inadequate oxygenation. Conscious patients can be asked to take four or five deep breaths. The patient who cannot cooperate must be preoxygenated with an air-mask-bag unit (Ambu) or anesthesia bag. Ambus deliver variable oxygen

concentrations (FIO_2 between 30 to 95 percent) and volumes. Flow rates should be at least 10 to 15 l/min to achieve higher FIO_2. Higher volumes can be obtained by using two hands to compress the bag. If the patient has an endotracheal airway in place and is on a ventilator, several sigh volumes can be delivered at FIO_2 before suctioning.

To suction patients with no airway adjunct, have them stick out their tongues. Grasp the tongue with a gauze pad, and apply gentle traction to make the glottis open and move in line with the trachea. Lubricate the catheter tip with a small amount of water-soluble jelly. Gently insert the catheter into the nostril. A slight curvature in the tubing may facilitate intubation of the larynx. Advance the catheter until intubation of the trachea is accomplished. Listen through the catheter, or feel for air movement against your cheek through the proximal end of the catheter. An increasing intensity of breath sounds or more air against the cheek indicates nearness to the larynx. If the breath sounds decrease or the patient begins to gag, the catheter is in the hypopharynx. Draw back and advance again. A sudden cough indicates the presence of the catheter in the larynx; advance quickly with the next breath.

Once the catheter is positioned in the trachea, apply intermittent suction by alternately occluding and opening the vent of the Y-connector with the thumb and withdraw the catheter in a spiral motion. If an airway adjunct is present, suctioning may be accomplished through it.

Never apply suction until the catheter is in the trachea, and never apply suction longer than 15 seconds. One useful trick is to hold your breath while suctioning the patient to remind yourself of the time limits. Monitor the patient carefully during all suctioning procedures. Any form of suctioning can lead to dysrhythmias, and prolonged suctioning may produce hypoxia, asphyxia, and cardiac arrest. Remember that suctioning removes oxygen as well as secretions, so oxygenate the patient after the procedure as well as before.

Suctioning is not without risk of complication, nor should it be done routinely. Appropriate indications for suctioning are the presence of bronchial secretions, identified visually, by auscultation or, in the mechanically ventilated patient, by rising airway pressures from retained secretions. Hypoxemia is the most common complication that can lead to atelectasis and dysrhythmias. Other complications include mucosal trauma, infection, paroxysmal coughing, and increased systemic and intracranial pressures.

RESPIRATORY CARE PATIENT RECORD
UNIVERSITY HOSPITALS, UNIVERSITY OF MICHIGAN

DATE:	
V_t MECH/SPONT	
RR MECH/SPONT	
F_iO_2	
PRESS PEAK/PLAT	
ST COMP ml/cm H_2O	
FLOW LPM	
SIGH VOL/FREQ	
PRESS LIMIT V_t/SIGH	
PEEP cm H_2O	
SENSITIVITY	
O_2 ALARM HI LO	
AIRWAY TEMP	
LOW EEP PRESS	
LOW EXH V_t/TIME	
LOW EXH $\dot{V}_E$	
LOW INSP PRESS/TIME	
V_t	
Vc	
NIF - cm H_2O	
RR	
$\dot{V}_E$	
HR/BP	
%SAT a/v	
PO_2 a/v	
PCO_2 a/v	
pH a/v	
CUFF PRESS/ PLACEMENT	
THERAPIST-INITIAL	

NAME:	
REG. NO.:	
VENTILATOR:	
START DATE:	TIME:
FLOOR:	BED:
DC DATE:	TIME:
PHYSICIAN:	
SERVICE:	
DIAGNOSIS:	

TIME	ORDERS
	VENTILATOR:
	TREATMENTS:
	CARDIAC OUTPUTS:
	MISCELLANEOUS:

FIGURE 20–3. Sample respiratory care patient record. *Date and Time*: It is critical to know when certain measurements were made and under what clinical settings. *Ventilator settings:* V_T = tidal volume; RR = respiratory rate; FIO_2 = fraction of inspired oxygen concentration; Press = peak and plateau airway pressure; St Comp = static compliance; Flow = peak flow; Sigh = volume and frequency of sigh; Press limit = limits on tidal volume and sigh pressure; PEEP = positive end-expiratory pressure expressed in cm H_2O; Sensitivity = negative pressure required to generate a breath. *Alarm settings—the patient's measured respiratory parameters*: V_T = tidal volume; V_C = vital capacity; NIF-cm H_2O = negative inspiratory force; RR = respiratory rate; V_E = minute ventilation. *Vital signs and arterial blood gases*: HR/BP = heart rate and blood pressure; %SAT = percentage of hemoglobin saturated with oxygen; PO_2 = partial pressure of oxygen in the arterial blood as measured by the arterial blood gases; PCO_2 = partial pressure of carbon dioxide in the arterial blood; pH = hydrogen ion concentration. *Cuff pressure/placement*: pressure in cuff, location. (Courtesy of the University of Michigan Hospitals, Ann Arbor, MI.)

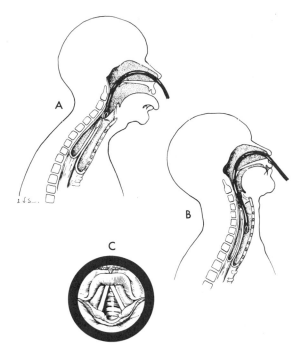

FIGURE 20–4. Technique of nasotracheal suctioning. *A*, optimal position of head to direct the catheter tip anteriorly into the trachea. The neck is flexed and the head is extended. The tongue is protruded (and held there by a 4 × 4 gauze). *B*, after the catheter has been advanced into the trachea, the tongue is released and the patient's head may be more comfortably positioned. *C*, view of the vocal cords from above. The cords are most widely separated during inspiration. (From Sanderson, R. G. [ed]: The Cardiac Patient. Philadelphia, W. B. Saunders, 1972, p. 304.)

Tracheostomy care is discussed in Chapter 23.

INFECTION CONTROL

Infection control in the PACU is always a problem. All postoperative patients are exceedingly vulnerable to infection because their body defenses are depressed. Prevention of the spread of infection involves blocking infectious agents from the three major avenues of transmission in the PACU: air, human carriers, and inanimate objects used in the care of patients, particularly instruments.

When a patient is received in the PACU for whom air may reasonably be expected to act as a vector, that patient should be isolated in a single room and the hospital's standard isolation techniques carried out. Ideally, a separate isolation room with glass partitions should be planned for the PACU to allow for separation of contaminated cases. Ease of observation of a

patient placed in the isolation room is essential. If patients in isolation cannot be fully observed, they should be attended until complete recovery from anesthesia. The Centers for Disease Control and Prevention's recommendations for isolation precautions and the institution's own system for isolation precautions should be reviewed regularly.

The Occupational Safety and Health Administration (OSHA) mandates that universal precautions (the treating of blood and certain body fluids as if infectious), engineering controls, work practice controls, personal protective equipment, and housekeeping protocols be complied with in the health care environment. Pertinent references can be found in the list at the end of the chapter.

Primary to infection control and prevention of disease transmission is handwashing. All personnel should wash their hands thoroughly after caring for each patient, and there should be no deviation from this practice. Handwashing facilities must be easily accessible to the observation area. In an emergency or if handwashing facilities are not readily available, antiseptic hand cleaners must be provided.

Disposable patient care items such as drinking glasses, catheter sets, and irrigation sets have contributed immensely to infection control programs. Many of these products are used in the PACU; they must be used as specified and then discarded and must not be resterilized for reuse. All items that are not disposable should be cleaned and sterilized appropriately after use before contact with a new patient. OSHA standards address the disposal of regulated waste and cleaning of reusable items.

Personnel must be scrupulous in their personal hygiene. Personnel should never work in the PACU if they know or suspect that they have any infectious disease, especially an upper respiratory infection. Open cuts or sores should disqualify a person from working with postoperative patients.

The wearing of scrub attire in the PACU has been questioned. Although recommendations for its use continue, no definitive studies exist to indicate that scrub suits should be mandatory. The proximity and access to the operating suite may determine the dress code for staff and visitors.

Every hospital has its own physical limitations, and modifications in isolation techniques must be made to fit the circumstances. Good practice dictates using scientific principles and knowledge when making plans to prevent the spread of infection.

GENERAL COMFORT AND SAFETY MEASURES

General comfort and safety measures are important parts of post anesthesia care. For safety, there should always be at least two nurses (one of whom is a registered nurse) present whenever patients are recovering. An unconscious patient should never be left alone, and side rails should be raised on the bed whenever direct patient care is not being provided. The wheels of the bed should be locked to prevent sliding when care is being rendered.

General physical measures such as cleanliness should not be overlooked in the PACU. Comfort measures, important to the total well-being of the patient, are often forgotten in the hustle of caring for post anesthesia patients. As soon as the patient is settled into the unit and assessment has been accomplished, all excess skin preparations and electrodes should be removed; in addition to providing comfort, washing off excess skin preparations gives the nurse an excellent opportunity to further assess the patient's general condition. A backrub at this time may prevent later complaints of discomfort from positioning for long periods in the operating room. This is also a good time to change the patient's position, assist with range of motion exercises, and encourage deep breathing. Frequent position changes help prevent atelectasis, promote circulation, and prevent pressure from developing on the skin surfaces.

Mouth care with lemon-glycerin swabs may be comforting to the patient who has not only had nothing by mouth but who has been medicated with an anticholinergic or glycopyrrolate to reduce secretions. When patients are fully conscious and their laryngeal reflexes have returned, they can rinse their mouths with mouthwash and water. Ice chips and small sips of water or juice may be offered to the patient who can tolerate fluids. A petrolatum-based ointment should be applied to the lips after mouth care to prevent drying and consequent cracking.

Patients often complain of being cold when returning from the operating suite. This is due in part to the effects of anesthesia and premedications and in part to the cool atmosphere of the operating suite and the PACU. This must be explained to the patient. Warming measures should be instituted on arrival to the PACU if the patient is hypothermic. Warmed cotton blankets, thermal foil drapes, radiant lamps, and convective warming devices are available.

The normothermic patient may shiver or complain of feeling cold; warm blankets may provide psychological comfort, and pharmacologic and active warming interventions may be needed to reduce or eliminate shaking. Blankets of any type should not, however, obscure the intravenous lines, arterial lines, or other monitoring apparatuses from the direct view of the attending nurse. The patient's temperature must be monitored closely to avoid overheating.

In addition to physical comfort measures, remember to provide psychological comfort. Reorientation, especially to time and place, is important to the post anesthesia patient, as is constant reassurance that the surgery is completed and that all went well. The nurse's presence at the bedside or gentle touch may also be comforting to the patient.

TRANSFER OF THE PATIENT FROM THE PACU

When the patient has recovered from the effects of anesthesia, vital signs will have stabilized; if no surgical complications have arisen, the patient is ready for transfer to the nursing unit or discharge area. The patient's post anesthesia recovery score, if this system is used, should be 10, unless criteria for exception are noted. The patient should have regained a satisfactory level of consciousness to the point of being oriented and able to call for assistance, if necessary, and should be clean, dry, and dressed in appropriate hospital garb. All dressings should be dry and intact, and all drainage receptacles should be emptied.

No patient should be discharged immediately after receiving an initial dose of a narcotic medication. Discharge should be delayed to assess the patient for pain relief and adverse side effects of the medication.

A summarizing PACU discharge note should be written on the patient's progress record indicating condition and time of transfer. The nurse should alert the receiving unit that the patient is being transferred and request the preparation of any specialized equipment for care and the assignment of a receiving nurse.

Patients may be transferred on a stretcher or bed as required by their condition and the operative procedure. Ensure that the patient is adequately covered with bed linens, including a warmed blanket if hallways are kept cool. Lock the side rails of the stretcher in place, and secure the safety straps comfortably around the patient. Ideally, two persons should be used to wheel the stretcher to the receiving unit: the person in back pushes, the person in front steers, both moving at a reasonable speed. Transport personnel vary by institution, and who transports may vary based on the patient's condition, staffing, and unit needs.

A receiving nurse should meet the patient on arrival to the unit and direct the transfer to the patient's room. The patient is transferred to the bed along with all apparatuses. Safety precautions must be strictly followed. Always use at least two people to transfer the patient. A third person may be necessary to assist with the patient transfer if extra equipment or multiple drainage tubes are present. Stabilize both the bed and the stretcher by locking the wheels when transferring the patient from one to the other. Ensure that all drainage tubes and catheters are safely transferred, that no kinking occurs, and that they do not become tangled underneath the patient. All drainage receptacles should remain below the level of the patient. Intravenous tubing and solution must be carefully transferred from the portable stand attached to the stretcher to the bedside stand or holder. Drainage tubes should be connected to suction or gravity drainage as indicated, and their proper functioning checked. Ensure that the patient's call light is positioned within the patient's reach along with any other items that may be needed. Check the intravenous infusion rate, and adjust as necessary. Side rails on the bed should be raised.

The report may be written, telephoned, or given in person to the receiving nurse. The PACU nurse should give a complete report to the receiving nurse, including pertinent facts about the following:

1. The operative procedure performed.
2. The anesthesia used and any reversal agents given.
3. The patient's general condition and post anesthesia course.
4. The incision, any drains placed, and the dressing.
5. Any drainage tubes or catheters.
6. Intake and output, including intravenous fluids (colloid and crystalloid) given, estimated blood loss, and time of void or catheterization. The flow sheet should be reviewed.
7. Any medications given in the PACU, especially analgesics, and the patient's response and level of comfort.

References

1. American Society of Anesthesiologists: Questions and Answers About Transfusion Practices. 2nd ed. Park Ridge, IL, American Society of Anesthesiologists, 1992.
2. American Society of Post Anesthesia Nurses: Standards of Post Anesthesia Nursing Practice 1992. Richmond, VA, American Society of Post Anesthesia Nurses, 1992.
3. Association of Blood Banks, American Red Cross, and Council of Community Blood Centers: Circular of Information for the Use of Human Blood and Blood Components. ARC no. 1751, December 1, 1991, revised. American Red Cross, Washington, DC.
4. Black, J. M., and Matassarin-Jacobs, E.: Luckmann and Sorensen's Medical-Surgical Nursing: A Psychophysiologic Approach. 4th ed. Philadelphia, W. B. Saunders, 1993.
5. Boggs, R. L., and Wooldridge-King, M.: AACN Procedure Manual for Critical Care. 3rd ed. Philadelphia, W. B. Saunders, 1993.
6. Bruning, L. M.: The bloodborne pathogens final rule. AORN J., 57(2):439–461, 1993.
7. Campbell, A., and Johnston, C. A.: OR-PACU reports: What they should tell you about your postoperative patient. Nursing 91, 21(10):49–51, 1991.
8. Centers for Disease Control: CDC Guidelines for Isolation Precautions in Hospitals (HHS publication No. CDC 83-8314). Atlanta, Centers for Disease Control, 1983.
9. Centers for Disease Control: Update: Universal precautions for prevention of transmission of human immunodeficiency virus, hepatitis B virus, and other bloodborne pathogens in the health care setting. Morbidity and Mortality Weekly Report, 37(3):377–388, 1988.
10. Dettenmeier, P. A.: Pulmonary Nursing Care. St. Louis, Mosby-Year Book, 1992.
11. Guiffre, M., Finnie, J., Lynam D. A., et al: Rewarming postoperative patients: Lights, blankets, or forced warm air. J. Post Anesth. Nurs., 6:387–393, 1991.
12. Longnecker, D. E., and Murphy, F. L.: Dripps/Eckenhoff/VanDam Introduction to Anesthesia. 8th ed. Philadelphia, W. B. Saunders, 1992.
13. Luce, J. M., Pierson, D. J., and Tyler, M. L.: Intensive Respiratory Care. 2nd ed. Philadelphia, W. B. Saunders, 1993.
14. McConnell, E. A.: Preventing postop complications: Minimizing respiratory problems. Nursing 91, 21(11): 35–39, 1991.
15. Occupational Exposure to Bloodborne Pathogens: Final Rule. Federal Register 56 (235) (December 6), 64,175–64,182 (FR Doc 91-28886), 1991.
16. Shannon, M. T., and Wilson, B. A.: Govoni & Hayes Drugs and Nursing Implications. 7th ed. Norwalk, CT, Appleton & Lange, 1992.
17. Summers, S., Dudgeon, N., Byram, K., et al: The effects of two warming methods on core and surface temperatures, hemoglobin oxygen saturation, blood pressure, and perceived comfort of hypothermic post anesthesia patients. J. Post Anesth. Nurs., 5:354–364, 1990.
18. Thompson, J. M., McFarland, G. K., Hirsch, J. E., et al: Mosby's Clinical Nursing. 3rd ed. St. Louis, Mosby-Year Book, 1993.
19. Vender, J. S., and Speiss, B. D.: Post Anesthesia Care. Philadelphia, W. B. Saunders, 1992.
20. Yount, S., and Schoessler, M.: Description of patient and nurse perceptions of preoperative teaching. J. Post Anesth. Nurs., 6:17–25, 1991.

Assessment and Management of the Airway

Airway assessment and management are principal skills required of all personnel in the post anesthesia care unit (PACU). Intubation of the trachea is a skill that should be reserved for nursing personnel who are specifically trained to perform this maneuver. The PACU nurse should be familiar with the intubation technique and capable of performing it quickly and efficiently. Airway management skills, including endotracheal intubation, can be developed in the operating room setting under the mentorship of a nurse anesthetist or an anesthesiologist. Using the same mentor, the PACU nurse should continue to practice the intubation skills on a monthly basis in the operating room.

ORAL AIRWAY MANAGEMENT

Patients may arrive in the PACU still experiencing the depressant effects of the anesthetic, and because they are obtunded, airway obstruction can occur. Some of the indications of airway obstruction include increased respiratory effort, retraction of the various muscles of respiration, a rocking chest motion, abnormal breath sounds, and evidence of hypoxemia and hypercarbia. In some instances, the obtunded patient's tongue and epiglottis may fall back on the posterior pharyngeal wall, occluding the airway. When this happens, the nurse should place the patient in a supine position, with the head tilted backward and the neck hyperextended. The nurse should then lift the angle of the lower jaw upward using moderate pressure (Fig. 21–1). Often, this maneuver is all that is required for spontaneous respirations to return. If spontaneous respirations do not return, the oral cavity should be inspected for foreign material and the oral pharynx suctioned if necessary. If large particles are present, the nurse should turn the patient's head to the side and remove the particles manually.

If spontaneous ventilation does not occur, positive-pressure breathing must be instituted.

If possible, a bag-valve-mask unit, connected to an oxygen source, should be used. (The requirements for a bag-valve-mask unit are addressed in Table 21-1.) The PACU nurse should be positioned behind the patient's head, not at his or her side. The mask should be fitted over the patient's mouth and nose with his or her neck hyperextended. The lower jaw should be lifted at its angle with the other fingers of the hand holding the mask. The thumb of that hand should be placed at the top of the mask, pushing down to provide compression over the bridge of the nose so as to reduce air leaks (Fig. 21–2).

After the mask is properly applied, the patient should be ventilated. While the PACU nurse is ventilating the patient, an assistant should assess the adequacy of the positive-pressure breathing by auscultating the chest. If an assistant is not present, the PACU nurse should check to see if the chest rises and falls or if air escapes during expiration. These are rough estimates of ventilation, and they may not be completely accurate about adequacy of ventilation. If breath sounds are not heard during auscultation or if the rough estimates are inconclusive, an oropharyngeal airway should be inserted (Fig. 21–3). This airway can be extremely stimulating to patients in the PACU who are awake or lightly anesthetized. The results of stimulation of reflexes include bradycardia, retching, vomiting, and laryngospasm.

The oropharyngeal airway may relieve the airway obstruction by providing a mechanical conduit for air to pass between the base of the tongue and the posterior oropharynx. To place an oropharyngeal airway, the PACU nurse should first open the patient's mouth with the right hand and, using the left hand, place a tongue blade toward the posterior aspect of the tongue. Slight pressure should then be applied to draw the tongue forward. Holding the oropharyngeal airway in the right hand, the nurse should slip it in over the tongue blade into the oropharynx. The airway should not be twisted or forced into place, and the airway insertion procedure should be accomplished quickly and

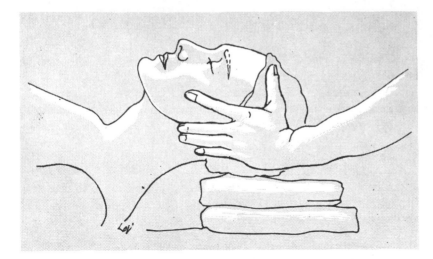

FIGURE 21-1. Technique of lifting the jaw by placing the fingers behind the mandible to overcome soft-tissue obstruction of the upper airway. (From Dripps, R., Eckenhoff, J., and Vandam, L.: Introduction to Anesthesia: The Principles of Safe Practice. 6th ed. Philadelphia, W. B. Saunders, 1982, p. 111.)

carefully so as to avoid trauma to the soft tissue and teeth.

Compared with the oropharyngeal airway, the nasopharyngeal airway is less stimulating to the irritant receptors in the upper airway, especially in awake or lightly anesthetized patients. The nasopharyngeal airway should be lubricated with a local anesthetic water-soluble lubricant, such as 1 percent lidocaine, and gently passed with the right hand through the nares along the curvature of the nasopharynx to the oropharynx. The nasopharyngeal airway should not be forced. If resistance is encountered, the other naris should be used. When positioned properly, the nasopharyngeal airway should rest between the base of the tongue and the posterior pharyngeal wall. This airway should not be used in a patient with a nasal septal deformity, a leakage of cerebrospinal fluid from the nose, or a coagulation disorder.

Once the oropharyngeal or the nasopharyngeal airway has been placed properly, ventilation should be continued. Then, assessment of adequacy of ventilation should be repeated. With insertion of the oropharyngeal airway, the patient will often resume ventilation. In this instance, the patient should be given a breath via the bag-valve-mask unit to assist his or her breathing effort and to help remove excess carbon dioxide. If the patient continues to be apneic, positive-pressure breathing should be continued by using large tidal volumes (10 to 12 ml per kg) at a rate of 14 to 16 breaths per min.

Table 21-1. REQUIREMENTS FOR BAG-VALVE-MASK UNIT

Self-refilling, but without sponge rubber inside (because of the difficulty in cleaning and disinfecting, and in eliminating ethylene oxide, and because of fragmentation)
Nonjam valve system at 15 L/min oxygen inlet flow
Transparent, plastic face mask with an air-filled or contoured, resilient cuff
Standard 15 mm/22 mm fittings
No popoff valve, except in pediatric models
System for delivery of high concentrations of oxygen through an ancillary oxygen outlet at the back of the bag or by an oxygen reservoir
True nonrebreathing valve
Oropharyngeal airway
Satisfactory practice on mannequins
Available in adult and pediatric sizes

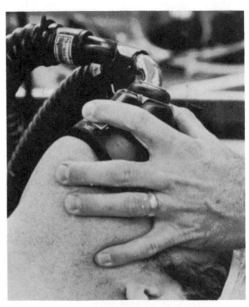

FIGURE 21-2. Holding the mask with one hand. (From Dorsch, J., and Dorsch, S.: Understanding Anesthesia Equipment. Baltimore, Williams & Wilkins, 1975, p. 225.)

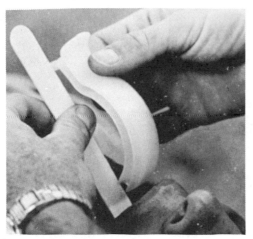

FIGURE 21–3. Insertion of an oral airway. The airway is inserted with the use of a tongue blade to displace the tongue forward. (From Dorsch, J., and Dorsch, S.: Understanding Anesthesia Equipment. Baltimore, Williams & Wilkins, 1975, p. 228.)

INTUBATION OF THE TRACHEA

If the PACU nurse cannot ventilate the patient, even after placement of an oropharyngeal or nasopharyngeal airway, endotracheal intubation should be performed. *Endotracheal intubation* and *intratracheal intubation* are synonymous terms indicating the placement of a tube directly into the trachea. When the endotracheal tube is placed through the mouth, the method is referred to as *orotracheal intubation.* Other indications for endotracheal intubation in the PACU are inability of the patient to protect his or her airway, prolonged mechanical ventilation, cardiac arrest, and respiratory arrest.

The PACU nurse should be familiar with the technique of tracheal intubation and be capable of performing it quickly and efficiently, knowing that the conditions under which intubation is performed in the PACU are less than ideal. The patient's position in the bed, excess upper airway secretions, and intact reflexes all increase the difficulty in performing this maneuver in the PACU.

Equipment for Tracheal Intubation

Adult and pediatric intubation equipment should be kept in the PACU at all times. This equipment should be inspected daily and after each use. For a list of the suggested items to be kept in the PACU, see Table 21–2. Table 21–3

Table 21–2. SUGGESTED EQUIPMENT FOR PACU PEDIATRIC AND ADULT ENDOTRACHEAL TRAYS
Pediatric Endotracheal Equipment
Small laryngoscope handle
No. 2 Macintosh curved blade
No. 1 Miller straight blade
Pediatric oral airways
Assorted pediatric masks
Child's anatomic masks
Randell-Baker-Soucek masks
Assorted tracheal tubes
Reverse-angle endotracheal tubes
Cole tubes
Reinforced latex tube with stylet
Plastic thin-walled tube
Adult Endotracheal Equipment
Laryngoscope handle
Laryngoscope blades
No. 2 and 4 Miller
No. 3 Macintosh
Stylet
Sterile gauze with topical water-soluble anesthetic lubricant
Sizes 6- through 9-mm cuffed tracheal tubes
10 ml syringe to inflate the cuff
Small hemostat
Tongue blades for airway insertion
Assorted-sized oropharyngeal airways

shows the recommended sizes for endotracheal tubes. Because of their importance, the laryngoscope and tracheal tubes will be discussed in detail.

Laryngoscope. The *laryngoscope* is used to visualize the larynx and the anatomic structures in close proximity to the larynx (Fig. 21–4). The laryngoscope has two main parts: the handle and the blade. The *handle* holds the laryngoscope and houses batteries that provide

Table 21–3. RECOMMENDED SIZES FOR ENDOTRACHEAL TUBES*	
Age	Endotracheal Tube (internal diameter in mm)
Newborn	3.0
6 months	3.5
18 months	4.0
3 years	4.5
5 years	5.0
6 years	5.5
8 years	6.0
12 years	6.5
16 years	7.0
Adult (female)	8.0–8.5
Adult (male)	8.5–9.0

*One size larger and one size smaller should be allowed for individual variations.

Reprinted with permission © American Heart Association.

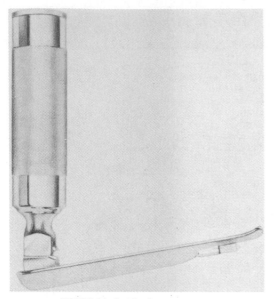

FIGURE 21–4. The laryngoscope.

electricity for the light on the side of the blade. The *blade* consists of three sections: the spatula, the flange, and the tip. The *spatula* can be straight or curved; it is the long main shaft of the blade. It serves to compress and move the soft tissue of the lower jaw to facilitate direct vision of the larynx. The *flange*, which is on the side of the spatula, deflects tissue that may obstruct the direct vision of the larynx. The *tip*, at the distal end of the spatula, is either curved or straight and serves to elevate the epiglottis, either directly or indirectly. The blade is attached to the handle at a connection called the *hook-on fitting*. The PACU nurse is strongly encouraged to practice connecting the blade to the handle before using the laryngoscope in an emergency.

The Macintosh and Miller blades are the most popular types in clinical use. The Macintosh is a curved blade with the flange on the left side to aid in moving the tongue so as to enhance visual exposure of the larynx. The Macintosh blade (Fig. 21–5) comes in four sizes: no. 1 for the infant, no. 2 for the child, no. 3 for the medium adult, and no. 4 for the large adult. For most adults, the no. 3 medium adult is the blade of choice. The Miller blade (see Fig. 21–5) is a straight spatula with a curved tip. This blade has five sizes: no. 0 for the premature infant, no. 1 for the infant, no. 2 for the child, no. 3 for the medium adult, and no. 4 for the large adult. The Miller nos. 0 and 1 are the blades of choice for premature and full-term infants, whose anatomic structures are more receptive to the use of a straight blade. Many anesthesia practitioners use the no. 2 Miller to intubate adults. The PACU nurse is encouraged to use both the straight and the curved blades and then to decide on the blade of preference. In most instances, the curved blade is easier to use than the straight blade; however, the exposure of the vocal cords is not as good as with the straight blade.

Tracheal Tube. The *tracheal tube* is also called the *endotracheal tube*, *intratracheal tube*, or *catheter* (Fig. 21–6). It is usually made from natural or synthetic rubber or plastic. The *proximal*, or *machine end*, protrudes from the patient's mouth and receives the adaptor. The *distal*, or *patient end*, has a slanted portion called the *bevel*. An uncuffed tracheal tube should be used on patients who are 8 years of age or younger. Endotracheal tubes are numbered according to their internal diameter in millimeters. Near the distal end of the tracheal tube is a *cuff*. Also leading away from the cuff is an inflating tube with a *pilot balloon* at its proximal end to indicate whether the cuff is inflated. Above the pilot balloon is a plug or *one-way valve* to which the inflation syringe is attached.

The cuff is an inflatable sleeve that provides a leak-resistant fit between the tube and the trachea when inflated. It also prevents aspiration and allows positive-pressure ventilation of the lungs. The cuff is permanently attached to the tracheal tube at the distal end. Concerning inflation volume, there are high- or low-residual-volume cuffs, referring to the amount of air that can be withdrawn from the cuff after it has

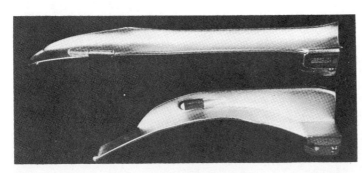

FIGURE 21–5. The most frequently used laryngoscope blades: Miller *(top)* and Macintosh *(bottom)*. (From Miller, R. [ed.]: Anesthesia. New York, Churchill Livingstone, 1981, p. 237.)

been inflated and allowed to deflate spontaneously with the tube patent and open to the air. The high-residual-volume cuff is also referred to as a *low-pressure cuff*. The low-residual-volume cuff is also called a *high-pressure cuff*. The arterial pressure in the tracheal wall is about 30 torr and the venous pressure in that area is about 20 torr. Most clinicians agree that a low-pressure (high-residual-volume), thin-walled cuff should be inflated to a pressure of about 17 to 23 torr. Local tracheal complications are associated with the cuff, especially after longer periods of intubation. Excessive cuff pressure is the primary factor causing ulceration, necrosis, and tracheal stenosis. These complications occur because high cuff pressure reduces the blood supply in the tracheal mucosa. For long-term ventilation, the cuffs should be long, with a large residual volume.

In an emergency, the PACU nurse should choose an endotracheal tube that is one size smaller than the size normally recommended for the patient. When making this choice, many clinicians look at the little finger of the patient, because a small-sized little finger indicates that the patient has an opening at the vocal cords that is smaller than normal. Also, a stylet made of malleable metal or plastic should be inserted inside the endotracheal tube to improve its cur-

vature and maintain its shape. Before the stylet is placed inside the tracheal tube, it *must* be covered with a water-soluble lubricant to ease its withdrawal from the tube after placement. The end of the stylet should be about 3 cm from the distal end of the tracheal tube and *should not protrude beyond the bevel* because damage to the vocal cords can occur.

Oral Endotracheal Intubation

Before oral endotracheal intubation is attempted, additional equipment should be immediately available and ready for use. Such equipment includes a tonsil suction connected to a working suction device, McGill forceps, 1-inch tape, a 10-ml empty syringe, and an anesthesia bag system or bag-valve unit. Also, throughout the procedure, the patient's oxygen saturation should be monitored continuously with a pulse oximeter.

The essential steps in the technique of oral endotracheal intubation are positioning the patient, positioning his or her head, inserting the blade of the laryngoscope, raising the epiglottis, visualizing the vocal cords, placing the tracheal tube, and assessing the patient. The

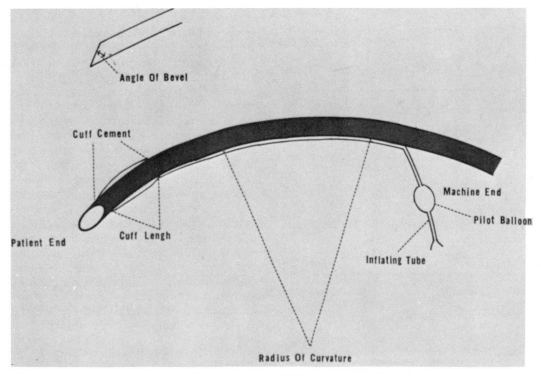

FIGURE 21–6. The curved tracheal tube. (From Dorsch, J. and Dorsch, S.: Understanding Anesthesia Equipment. Baltimore, Williams & Wilkins, 1975, p. 249.)

methods for accomplishing these steps are as follows.

Positioning the Patient. Move the patient up so that his or her head is at the top of the bed. Raise the head of the bed (or the entire bed, if possible) so that the patient's face is approximately at the level of the standing PACU nurse's xiphoid process.

Positioning the Head. Place a firm 4-inch pillow or ring under the head. Flex the patient's head at the neck. This position is called the *sniffing position* (Fig. 21–7), because of the

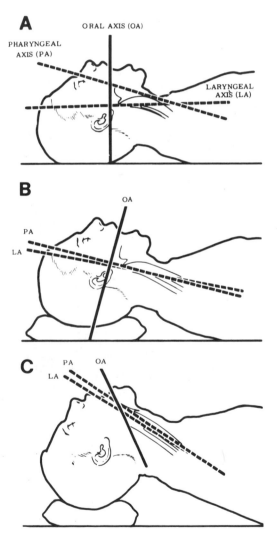

FIGURE 21–7. Positioning for endotracheal intubation. *A,* the patient is in the supine position—with alignment of the oral, pharyngeal, and laryngeal axes. *B,* placement of pad or ring under the patient's occiput (sniffing position) aligns the pharyngeal and laryngeal axes. *C,* extending the patient's head at the atlanto-occipital joint now aligns all three axes, which provides the shortest distance and most nearly straight line from the mouth to the larynx. (From Miller, R. [ed.]: Anesthesia. New York, Churchill Livingstone, 1981, p. 234.)

flexion of the head at the neck and extension of the head. Place your right hand on the patient's forehead to extend the head.

Inserting the Blade. With the fingers of the right hand, open the jaw wide, making sure that the lips are spread away from the teeth. With the laryngoscope in the left hand, insert the moistened or lubricated blade between the teeth at the right side of the patient's mouth. Advance the blade slowly inward, past the tonsillar pillars and toward the midline of the oral cavity, sweeping the tongue toward the left side of the mouth. A major key to a successful intubation is moving the tongue to the left, out of the visual path to the vocal cords. At this point, the right hand can be placed under the patient's occiput to extend the head. The epiglottis should now be visualized; it is a red, leaf-shaped structure that will appear behind the tip of the blade as the laryngoscope is advanced down the oral cavity.

Raising the Epiglottis and Visualizing the Vocal Cords. With the epiglottis under direct vision, slip the straight blade just beneath the tip of the epiglottis and gently lift the blade forward and upward at a 45-degree angle, holding the wrist rigid (Fig. 21–8). If a curved blade is used, such as the Macintosh, slip the tip of the blade between the epiglottis and the base of the tongue (see Fig. 21–8). With the left hand, lift forward and upward on the handle at a 45-degree angle. The epiglottis will fold onto the blade, and the vocal cords should then be visible.

Whether using a curved or straight blade, do not use the handle as a lever with the upper teeth acting as a fulcrum, because the tip of the blade will push the larynx up and out of sight and the teeth can become chipped or broken.

At this point, if the vocal cords cannot be visualized, have an assistant apply gentle external downward pressure on the larynx (the Sellick maneuver)—the vocal cords should come into view. If the blade is passed too far, it will enter the esophagus. If this happens, withdraw the blade, ventilate the patient with 100 percent oxygen, and perform the procedure again. While ventilating the patient, think about what went wrong, and design an alternative strategy to facilitate a successful intubation of the trachea.

Placing the Tracheal Tube. When the vocal cords are visualized, an assistant should place the tracheal tube—with a stylet properly inserted to maintain a curve and the cuff deflated—in the right hand. Pass the tracheal tube with the right hand to the right of the tongue and blade through the vocal cords until

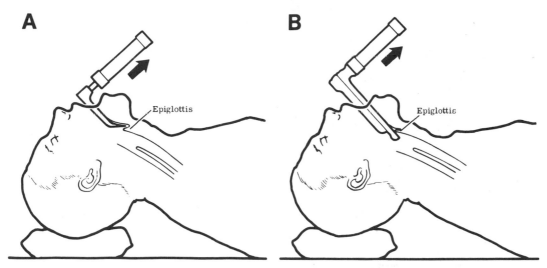

FIGURE 21–8. Proper positioning of the laryngoscope blade to facilitate endotracheal intubation. *A,* using a curved blade (i.e., Macintosh), the tip is placed into the space between the base of the tongue and the pharyngeal surface of the epiglottis, which is called the *vallecula. B,* using a straight blade (i.e., Miller), the tip is placed on the laryngeal surface of the epiglottis. Regardless of the type of blade used, once the blade is in position, the forward and upward movements on the handle (as denoted by the *arrows*) exert pressure on the long axis of the blade, which serves to elevate the epiglottis and expose the vocal cords. (From Miller, R., [ed.]: Anesthesia. New York, Churchill Livingstone, 1981, p. 238.)

the cuff disappears behind the vocal cords or until the tip of the tracheal tube protrudes 2 or 3 cm into the trachea.

Assessing the Patient. Once the tracheal tube is in place, while holding on to the tube with the right hand, remove the blade with the left hand. Place the laryngoscope on the patient's bed or on a table, and slowly remove the stylet without dislodging the tracheal tube. The patient end to the tracheal tube should then be connected to a bag-valve unit or an anesthesia bag system and ventilated while an assistant auscultates the chest for breath sounds. The breath sounds should be assessed in all four quadrants, and the stomach also should be auscultated. If no breath sounds are heard or if a "gurgling" sound is heard over the stomach, deflate the cuff, remove the tracheal tube, and ventilate the patient with a mask using 100 percent oxygen. While ventilating the patient, think about why the attempt was unsuccessful, review the procedure, and reintubate the patient. If breath sounds are heard on only one side of the chest (usually the right side, not the left), withdraw the tube at 1-cm intervals until the breath sounds are bilateral. Using a 10-ml syringe full of air, inject a volume of air (about 4 to 6 ml) into the pilot balloon until there is minimal or no air leakage around the cuff. The cuff leak is assessed by placing the bell of the stethoscope over the larynx. Once tube placement and cuff pressure are correct, insert an oral airway and secure the tube with adhesive tape.

Documentation of the procedure should include the number of attempts, the degree of visualization of the vocal cords, whether the intubation was traumatic or atraumatic, the quality of breath sounds, the amount of air injected into the cuff, the cuff pressure, and the tracheal tube size, and the laryngoscope blade type and size.

Ventilating the Patient. The adult patient should be ventilated approximately 14 to 18 times per min at a tidal volume of 8 to 10 ml per kg. Infants should be ventilated at approximately 26 to 30 times per min at a volume large enough to raise their chest on inspiration. However, when time permits, a tidal volume of 7 ml per kg should be used. Children should be ventilated at a rate of 18 to 24 breaths per min. The tidal volume to be delivered can be determined in the same manner for infants.

Nasotracheal Intubation

When the tube is inserted through the nose, the method is referred to as *nasotracheal intubation*. When nasotracheal intubation is done without the use of a laryngoscope, the method is referred to as a *blind nasotracheal intubation*. *Direct-vision intubation* is the insertion of an endotracheal tube with the aid of a laryngoscope. When using the direct-vision method to perform a nasotracheal intubation, the PACU nurse may use Magill forceps (Fig. 21–9). A

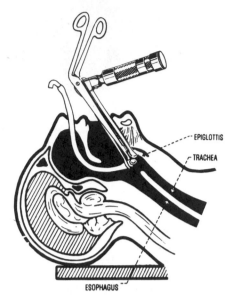

EPIGLOTTIS

TRACHEA

ESOPHAGUS

FIGURE 21-9. Use of Magill forceps for nasal intubation. (From Collins, V. J.: Principles of Anesthesiology. 2nd ed. Philadelphia, Lea & Febiger, 1976, p. 334.)

description of the nasal intubation technique can be found in many anesthesia textbooks.

Intubation has many advantages. It provides a route for mechanical ventilation, reduces the amount of anatomic dead space, and protects the patient from aspiration of blood, mucus, or foreign material into the tracheobronchial tree. It also relieves upper airway obstruction and provides an access route for removing excess secretions in the airways.

The disadvantage of intubation is that it may produce trauma to the teeth, lips, soft palate, epiglottis, vocal cords, and other tissues in that region.

PACU Care of the Intubated Patient

Nursing care of the intubated patient involves (1) frequent auscultation of the chest for bilateral breath sounds to ensure correct placement of the endotracheal tube; (2) frequent suctioning of the oral cavity and, if clinically required, suctioning down inside the endotracheal tube to remove secretions; and (3) maintenance of verbal communication with the intubated patient to reduce anxiety. The PACU nurse must reassure the patient that the attendants are constantly observing him or her. In addition, the nurse should provide the patient with a means of communication. *Warning:* When suctioning down an endotracheal tube, *always* administer at least five maximal venti-

lations of 100 percent oxygen before performing the suctioning procedure.

Extubation of the Intubated Patient

When it is determined that the patient can be extubated, the PACU nurse should first ensure that all intubation, suction, and ventilation equipment is at the patient's bedside and is operational. Then, the entire procedure should be explained to the patient. Depending on the amount and location of secretions, the trachea, the nasopharynx, or both, should be suctioned. All secretions must be aspirated from the upper airway to reduce the incidence of coughing and laryngospasm. Next, the patient should be ventilated with 100 percent oxygen for about 2 minutes. A syringe is then placed into the side valve, and the tracheal tube cuff is deflated. The patient should be asked to take a deep breath, and at the end of the inspiration, the tube should be gently removed. If the patient is completely awake and responding, the oral airway should also be removed. Then, 100 percent oxygen should be administered by mask and the patient assessed for dyspnea, stridor, and airway obstruction. Oxygenation should be assessed continually by the pulse oximeter.

Adverse Sequelae After Tracheal Intubation

Hoarseness and Sore Throat. On emergence from anesthesia, some patients who have been intubated intraoperatively will complain of a very sore throat. Although the incidence of a sore throat after intubation is low, it is a significant discomfort to the patient. The incidence of sore throat increases dramatically when the patient's head is turned frequently or is placed in an abnormal position intraoperatively.

Assessment of the patient complaining of sore throat should include visual assessment of the oropharynx and auscultation of the chest. Abnormal findings should be reported to the anesthesiologist. Counseling the patient is probably the most important nursing intervention. The nurse should review the anesthesia record to determine if the patient was intubated and if the procedure was traumatic (such as multiple attempts and difficult intubation). Sore throats usually result from traumatic intubations.

Interventions consist of telling the patient that he or she had a tube in the throat during surgery to help with breathing and that throat discomfort may occur for 1 to 3 days. Often when the patient understands the reason for the discomfort and learns that it is not life threatening, the discomfort will become less severe. If treatment is required, dexamethasone (Decadron) may be given to reduce the inflammation; also, an ice bag or chips of ice may be given to the patient to relieve the symptoms.

Laryngospasm. Partial or complete closure of the vocal cords can occur owing to increased secretions or as a reflex caused by stimulation of the irritant receptors. Assessment reveals reduced or no breath sounds. If partial laryngospasm is present, the patient will make crowing sounds, especially on inspiration. Interventions include the administration of 100 percent oxygen under positive pressure with a bag-valve-mask unit and, if the patient cannot be ventilated, administration of succinylcholine intravenously and reintubation are mandated (see Chapter 5).

Aspiration of Gastrointestinal Contents. Aspiration of gastrointestinal contents is a complication that may be seen in weak and debilitated patients and those with neurologic disease or intestinal obstruction. See Chapter 9 for a complete discussion of this syndrome.

References

1. Austin, R.: Respiratory problems in emergence from anesthesia. Int. Anesthesiol. Clin., 29(2):25–36, 1991.
2. Barash, P., Cullen, B., and Stoelting, R.: Clinical Anesthesia. 2nd ed. Philadelphia, J. B. Lippincott, 1992.
3. Class, P.: Nursing considerations for airway management in the PACU. Curr. Rev. Post Anesth. Care Nurses, 14(1):3–7, 1992.
4. King, T., and Adams, A.: Failed tracheal intubation. Br. J. Anaesth., 65:400–414, 1990.
5. Longnecker, D., and Murphy, F.: Dripps/Eckenhoff/Vandam Introduction to Anesthesia. 8th ed. Philadelphia, W. B. Saunders, 1992.
6. Miller, R.: Anesthesia. 3rd ed. New York, Churchill Livingstone, 1990.
7. Motoyama, E., and Davis, P.: Smith's Anesthesia for Infants and Children. 5th ed. St. Louis, C. V. Mosby, 1990.
8. Pesola, G., and Kvetan, V.: Ventilatory and pulmonary problem management. Anesthesiol. Clin. North Am., 8(2):287–309, 1990.
9. Waugaman, W., Foster, S., and Rigor, B.: Principles and Practice of Nurse Anesthesia. 2nd ed. Norwalk, CT, Appleton & Lange, 1992.
10. Whitten, C.: Anyone Can Intubate. 2nd ed. San Diego, Medical Arts Publications, 1990.

CHAPTER 22

Assessment and Management of Postoperative Pain

Susan B. Christoph, D.N.Sc., R.N.

Although pain is often considered a protective mechanism, postoperative pain serves no useful purpose and can be deleterious. Despite this knowledge and the increased sophistication of available pain relief modalities, postoperative pain continues to be undertreated and patients continue to suffer from it.

The postoperative pain experience is so common that it is an expected consequence of surgical intervention. Pain can be a frightening experience; in fact, the fear of postoperative pain ranks second only to the fear of death in surgical patients.

Physiologic Impact of Pain

Post anesthesia care unit (PACU) nurses are familiar with the decreased lung volume, increased oxygen consumption, immobility, and depletion of energy that occur when a patient must cope with pain. Pain disrupts rest and sleep, thereby further depleting the body's natural reserve for healing.

Post anesthesia patients experience altered respiratory function; therefore, attention must be directed specifically to maintaining adequate gas exchange. The "stir-up" regimen is aimed at preventing complications, primarily atelectasis and venous stasis, that may occur as a consequence of inadequate gas exchange and immobility. The stir-up regimen must therefore include adequate relief of pain so that the other required activities, such as deep-breathing exercises, coughing, repositioning, and mobilization, can be accomplished.

Psychological Impact of Pain

It is clear that pain is more than just a physiologic experience—it is a psychological one as well. Just as emotional and sociocultural factors influence the pain experience, the pain experience may influence the patient's general psychological responses. In the surgical patient, a variety of factors may influence the level of anxiety, including fear of surgery, fear of pain, or fear of the unknown. The multiplicity of uncontrollable intervening variables has made it difficult for researchers to demonstrate the exact relationship between anxiety and pain. It is generally accepted that a positive relationship exists between the two at moderate levels (Fig. 22–1).

Feelings of helplessness or lack of control may also contribute to anxiety and fear and, hence, influence the perception of pain (Fig. 22–2). These feelings may be enhanced by the constraints of postoperative care, such as a flat-lying position in bed and the presence of casts, dressings, and other apparatus needed for care.

It is hoped that most patients will emerge from general anesthesia in a calm, tranquilized manner. Some patients, however, emerge in a state of excitement, a condition characterized by restlessness, disorientation, crying, moaning, or irrational talking. In the extreme form of excitement, referred to as *emergence delirium*, the patient screams, shouts, and thrashes about wildly. Postoperative pain or discomfort from prolonged maintenance of an abnormal position on the operating table, as well as fears of disfigurement or cancer and a feeling of suffocation, all contribute to the likelihood of emergence excitement.

The patient depends on the health care team, specifically the nurse, to manage and control postoperative pain. How well the patient's pain is managed can greatly influence the sense of trust that is central to the therapeutic nurse-patient relationship.

ASSESSMENT OF POSTOPERATIVE PAIN

Pain is an extremely complex phenomenon and may well be the most difficult symptom to

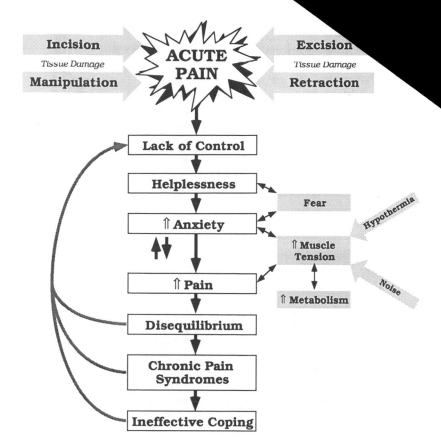

FIGURE 22–1. Christoph's conceptual model of postoperative pain relationships.

assess. Postoperative pain is stimulated by tissue damage and is modified by myriad other factors, including the anesthetic technique and agents used. Age, personality, culture, and emotional state modify the patient's responses to pain. The effectiveness of the post anesthesia pain treatment plan depends on the accuracy of the pain assessment. Assessment of the post anesthesia patient's pain experience is often difficult because of the residual effects of anesthesia, which alters consciousness; communication may be difficult owing to the patient's clouded sensorium or constraints from mechanical devices such as nasogastric tubes and artificial airways.

Influence of Anesthetic Agents and Technique

The anesthetic technique and the anesthetic agents used influence the postoperative pain experience. The inhalation agents, including enflurane (Ethrane), isoflurane (Forane), and halothane (Fluothane), are commonly used, short-acting ones that provide little or no residual analgesia postoperatively. The intravenous

agent sodium pentothal (Thiopental) is a poor analgesic and may even have an antianalgesic effect. Therefore, post anesthesia patients with pain may become irrational, restless, and hyperactive.

A balanced anesthetic technique that includes the administration of narcotics, such as meperidine (Demerol), morphine, sublimaze (Fentanyl), sufentanil (Sufenta), and alfentanil, is commonly used. When the patient has received meperidine, morphine, sublimaze, or sufentanil, some residual analgesia may be expected. These drugs may exacerbate respiratory depression, so the patient should be monitored carefully. Alfentanil has an extremely short recovery time, and patients who receive this drug as the narcotic portion of a balanced-

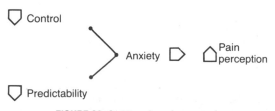

FIGURE 22–2. Visual analogue scale.

...likely experi-
...ostoperative pe-
...algesia.

...with a narcotic
...rgery. The PACU
...any antagonist ad-
...igns and symptoms
...ure and pain. The
...o symptoms of with-
drawal in ... have a history of narcotic drug use. With...wal symptoms may include anxiety, jittery behavior, rhinorrhea,
hypotension, muscle twitching, sweating, pupillary dilation, gooseflesh, and nausea and
vomiting. Treatment for withdrawal should include the administration of narcotic analgesia.

The patient who receives regional anesthesia
(local, spinal, and epidural blocks) may have
residual analgesia during the postoperative recovery period; however, the analgesia may be
short lived. The nurse should assess the patient's level of sedation, including the amount
of premedication and sedation used during the
surgical procedure, before administering pain
medication.

The nature of pain makes it a most difficult
symptom to assess. The patient is the only expert on what he or she is feeling. There are no
reliable invariable signs or symptoms of pain;
however, there are indications that a person is
suffering.

The assessment of pain is based on a variety
of observable behavior and physiologic manifestations. The physiologic and psychological
reactions to pain are as individualistic as the
person who experiences it. It is the grouping of
associated symptoms or constellation of pain
indicators that is most helpful in assessing pain
in the post anesthesia patient.

Pain Indicators

Verbalizations

The patient's own verbalizations are one of
the most reliable indicators of pain. As the patient emerges from the second stage of anesthesia, there may be a period of excitement and
overreaction to all stimuli, including pain. As
the patient emerges from the first stage of anesthesia (analgesia), there may be enough pain-
relieving effect left from the anesthetic so that
he or she awakens, complains of pain, and then
falls asleep again.

The post anesthesia patient may experience
pain yet be unable to verbalize it accurately.
Children, especially those who are preverbal,
may not be able to communicate their discomfort in words. Groaning, grunting, screaming,
sobbing, and crying are probable indicators
that pain is present. Despite difficulties with
communication in the PACU, the nurse must
collaborate with the patient to identify the location, intensity, and quality of pain being experienced before implementing a plan for pain
control.

The patient's description of pain can greatly
assist the nurse with assessment of pain and
the development of a plan for management.
The nurse may have to aid the patient with
directive questioning to get the descriptions of
the most important characteristics of the pain:
location, intensity, quality, onset, duration, and
variations. Listening carefully to the words
chosen by the patient to describe these characteristics will provide important clues to the nature of the pain being experienced.

Location

Where is the pain being felt? It may not always be easy for patients to localize the pain.
It may be felt in more than one place, or it may
cover an extensive area. Patients may be asked
to point to the location of the pain on their own
bodies or on a drawing or doll.

Postoperative pain, although certainly influenced by many factors, is largely governed by
the site and the nature of the operation. Patients who have undergone abdominal and intrathoracic operations generally experience the
most pain, and this may be the reason that post
anesthesia delirium and excitement most commonly occur after these procedures. Posterolateral incisions tend to be more painful than anterolateral ones. The incisions for major
vascular surgery are long and painful. Surgery
on the joints, back, and anorectal area is also
generally quite painful. Pain is uncommon
after eye surgery. The fear and anxiety of having one's eyes operated on, however, may
evoke responses of pain.

Complaints of pain or discomfort by the
postoperative patient may not be brought on
by incision pain, as might be assumed, but
rather by headache or sore throat as a result of
anesthesia technique, by discomfort at the site
of intravenous infusion, or by irritation from
other associated apparatuses, such as nasogastric tubes. Each cause would require a different
intervention.

Pain may arise from other causes, such as
angina pectoris, and this type of pain must be
differentiated from surgical pain. A common
source of postoperative pain and restlessness is

a distended bladder, and this possibility must not be overlooked. Other common sources of pain or discomfort in the PACU that may be easily corrected by removing their source are open safety pins on dressings, improper positioning so that stress is placed on a suture line, and dressings and casts that are too tight and are restricting circulation or creating friction.

Intensity

The intensity of pain may range from mild discomfort or irritation to severe, completely debilitating pain. There is no direct correlation between stimulus and pain perception. The patient's report of intensity is influenced by the patient's threshold and tolerance for pain. *Threshold* refers to the point at which pain is first perceived and has been thought to be fairly constant from person to person. Evidence now indicates that threshold varies from person to person and may vary within the person from situation to situation. *Tolerance* refers to the point at which a person reports that he or she cannot or will not withstand the noxious stimulus. Because threshold and tolerance vary so greatly from person to person and within the same person from one time to another, intensity may be extremely difficult for the nurse to judge.

Several tools have been developed to assist in the assessment of pain intensity. Although not in common use in the PACU, the verbal rating scale and the visual analogue scale (VAS) are simple to use, easily explained—even to the patient in the post anesthesia state—and can greatly improve the consistency of pain assessment. These tools depend on anchors at either end of a scale on which the patient rates his or her pain. The anchors are arbitrary. The verbal rating scale asks the patient to rate pain on a scale ranging from 0 to 10 or 100. The pain score is the patient's chosen number, and it can be recorded for comparison with later complaints of pain or to evaluate the effectiveness of relief measures.

The VAS is a 10-cm line with anchors of "no pain" at the left end and "severe pain" or "pain as bad as it can be" at the right end. The distance in centimeters from the left end of the line to the point marked by the patient on the line constitutes the measurement (Fig. 22–3). With the VAS, there is an infinite number of points between the extremes, which allows sensitivity for many grades of pain as experienced by the patient without forcing the patient to translate a feeling into words.

For children, various assessment tools have

Please make a mark on the line (_____|_____) that best describes the pain you are experiencing right now.

NO PAIN _____ SEVERE PAIN

FIGURE 22–3. Wire diagram of direct relationships between control, predictability, anxiety, and pain perception.

been developed that use colors or faces that the child can choose to communicate pain and discomfort.

Quality

The quality of pain may be the most difficult characteristic for the patient to describe. The language of pain is varied, and many patients lack the vocabulary to relate what they are feeling. Superficial pain is often described as *pricking* or *burning*. Deep pain is more likely to be described as *aching*, *throbbing*, or *radiating*. Intensity may be described as *gnawing* or *tiring*.

Variations

It is important to determine whether or not the pain is associated with any other discernible factors such as movement, swallowing, and changes in posture. Time associations may be particularly diagnostic. Unfortunately, the patient often cannot or will not admit that pain is present while in the PACU.

Increased blood pressure, increased pulse and respiratory rates, pallor, dilated pupils, increased muscle tension, cold perspiration, and nausea are physical indicators of pain. Restlessness is a common manifestation of pain and, when present, must be carefully evaluated to differentiate it from restlessness due to hypoxemia. The patient's vocalizations, including groaning, grunting, and crying, as well as statements about having pain, must be carefully evaluated.

Physiologic Changes

The physiologic indicators of pain result primarily from autonomic stimulation. Pain elicits sympathetic responses that include pallor, increased respirations, increased heart rate, increased blood pressure, dilated pupils, and increased muscle tension. The colon, rectum, and bladder, however, are innervated through the sacral parasympathetic nerves; therefore, trauma involving these viscera may elicit parasympathetic pain responses, including nausea and vomiting, decreased heart rate, and decreased blood pressure.

Behavioral Cues

Excitement, irritability, anger, hostility, depression, unusual quietness, or withdrawal may indicate that the patient is experiencing pain. The patient in pain may hold the body or the painful part rigid and immobile in an attempt to limit pain. On the other hand, activity may increase. The patient may rock, rub a painful body part, become restless, or exhibit purposeless activity. Facial expressions such as clenched teeth, tightly shut lips, or widely opened eyes may indicate pain. These signs may be especially useful in the assessment of children's pain.

Influence of Nurses' Attitudes and Perceptions

Nurses are the primary assessors of pain in the PACU. An accurate assessment of the patient's pain forms the basis for the selection of an appropriate intervention. A number of authors have described the influence that the nurse's perceptions, attitudes, and personal biases may have on the assessment of the patient's pain.

Nurses respond more readily to physiologic indicators of pain than to the patient's verbal reports. Investigators have also found that the nurse's perception of the patient's pain is influenced by the nurse's personal experience with pain. In general, nurses who have experienced intense pain are more sympathetic to a patient's suffering. The assessment of pain is also influenced by the nurse's learned behavioral responses from a given culture or subculture. It is important, therefore, that PACU nurses be aware of how their own biases may influence their assessment.

MANAGEMENT OF POSTOPERATIVE PAIN

Prevention

The prevention of pain and the promotion of comfort should be major goals in the care of the post anesthesia patient. Recent evidence demonstrates that opiate premedication and the use of local anesthetic blocks reduce postoperative pain. It is suggested that anesthetic blocks and small narcotic dosages prevent the barrage of surgically created stimuli on the central nervous system and thereby prevent the development of a hyperexcitable state. This ev-

idence also provides a sound rationale for the prompt treatment of postoperative pain with appropriate analgesia before the development of severe pain. Once severe pain exists, much larger dosages of narcotic analgesics are necessary to suppress the hyperexcitable state and to bring the pain response under control.

Once surgery is over, the prevention of pain requires attention to detail to reduce noxious stimuli. Positioning to avoid stress on incisions and to promote adequate ventilation is especially important in the PACU. Injured tissue must be handled carefully and further trauma avoided whenever possible. Careful attention to positioning body parts that may still be paralyzed by regional anesthesia is important in the prevention of discomfort later in the postoperative period. Good body alignment and frequent changing of position help prevent muscle contractions and spasms. Injured parts should be supported to prevent muscular strain and fatigue. Often, the patient is the best judge of how to avoid stimulating pain. Incisions or operative sites should not be placed under tension or pressure. Sometimes, something as slight as the minimal pressure of a bedsheet may produce noxious stimuli.

Postoperative patients should have been taught preoperatively how to splint abdominal and thoracic incisions externally to minimize noxious stimuli during ventilatory exercises, but they will probably need assistance during the post anesthesia period. Emergency surgical patients may not have been prepared at all for surgery and will need primary teaching and intensive coaching to manage respiratory maneuvers in the post anesthesia period. A semirigid splinting device, such as a folded blanket or a firm pillow, is useful for splinting incisions.

Attention to comfort details can reduce sensory stimulation and support pain tolerance. A clean, dry, wrinkle-free bed in a quiet environment improves comfort. A dry mouth, which is frequently a problem after anesthesia, can be relieved with ice chips, moistened gauze, and petrolatum ointment applied to the lips. All drainage tubes should be checked frequently for patency to avoid distention of the drainage site. A common source of postoperative pain and restlessness is a distended bladder, and this possibility must not be overlooked. Any apparatus attached to the patient should be checked frequently to ensure that it is secure and will not cause irritation of the tissue from movement or create tension from pulling. The nurse must ensure that the dressings and casts are not too tight and do not restrict circulation or create irritating friction.

Sensory stimulation, including noise and bright lights, should be reduced as much as possible, because sensory overload reduces pain tolerance. Reassurance that the surgery is over and the patient is doing well, as well as explanations of what is going on and what sensations will be experienced, do much to allay anxiety.

Pharmacologic Management

Analgesics

A large number of pharmacologic agents have been incorporated into the list of medications used for pain relief in the PACU. The more commonly used analgesics are listed in Table 22–1. The analgesics are categorized as non-narcotic and narcotic. The non-narcotic analgesics are generally administered orally and are fairly weak. They have few side effects, however, and may be useful in conjunction with other modalities to provide relief of mild to moderate pain states for the patient who can tolerate oral medications and fluids.

Concern for the side effects of narcotic analgesia (Table 22–2) has drastically limited treatment with narcotics that could be effective if used properly. Although it is true that the narcotics eventually cause addiction, this has never been a significant problem when they are used to treat acute pain. Respiratory depression occurs with the use of narcotics, and the patient should be monitored carefully for adequacy of ventilation as part of the standard

Table 22–1. COMMON ANALGESICS USED IN THE PACU	
Generic Name	Trade Name
Non-Narcotics	
Aspirin	Various
Acetaminophen	Tylenol, Tempra, Datril, Panadol
Ibuprofen	Motrin, Nuprin
Fenoprofen	Nalfon
Phenacetin	Various
Narcotics	
Codeine	Codeine
Oxycodone	Percocet
Pentazocine	Talwin
Meperidine, Pethidine	Demerol
Morphine	Morphine
Hydromorphone	Dilaudid
Methadone	Dolophine
Levorphanol	Levo-Dromoran, Levorphan
Fentanyl	Sublimaze

Table 22–2. SIDE EFFECTS OF NARCOTIC ANALGESIA	
Respiratory depression	Vomiting
Cardiovascular depression	Clouding of sensorium
Nausea	Drowsiness

practice within the controlled environment of the PACU. The possibility of respiratory depression should not preclude the use of narcotic analgesia when it is needed. In fact, narcotics can be titrated to produce appropriate analgesia by observing for normalcy of respiratory pattern, such as the presence of expiratory pause versus the shortening or absence of expiratory pause in the respirations of a patient in pain.

Assessment of analgesic requirements

Just as there are no objective indicators of pain, there are no reliable indicators of analgesic requirements. Drugs are often prescribed based on body weight, but weight does not seem to be a reliable predictor of the amount of analgesic needed. The best pain measures and indicators have limitations, and there is little or no relationship between analgesic medication used or requested and reported pain. The frequency or amount of narcotic analgesics used is not a good measure of pain experienced when the administration of analgesics is sporadic and related to both patient and nurse characteristics.

Age Considerations. The elderly patient is often undermedicated for severe, acute pain because it is assumed that the elderly have a higher pain threshold or tolerate pain better. This assumption is not necessarily accurate. The elderly patient should be assessed for concomitant physical problems, such as decreased circulation and decreased kidney and liver function, which affect both uptake and clearance of analgesic drugs and therefore prolong the duration of action of these drugs. This effect does not change the amount of drug per administration needed to control pain for these patients. Narcotics must be used judiciously in the patient with chronic obstructive lung disease. A history of myasthenia gravis should alert the nurse to the potential need for a reduced reliance on narcotic pain relief. The anticholinesterases potentiate morphine and other narcotics; therefore, dosages should be reduced initially and increased only if required. The nurse should also be alert to the increased likelihood of drug interactions if other medications are being administered for other associated disease processes.

Children are also undermedicated for post-operative pain, mainly owing to misinformation about pain and how it is manifested in children. Children do experience pain but have quite different ways of expressing it. The small child may be able to express pain only by crying. Comfort and reassurance may be provided for infants and small children by holding and rocking them. Codeine is the narcotic of choice for severe pain in infants and children because of its wide margin of safety due to limited respiratory or cardiovascular depression. Dosages must be adjusted for the individual child.

Previous Narcotic Use. The patient should be evaluated for previous narcotic use, because this influences the dosages of narcotics necessary to control pain. Patients who are physically dependent on narcotics, including those persons who have been in drug rehabilitation programs and are on a methadone maintenance schedule, require larger doses of narcotics to prevent the symptoms of withdrawal during this vulnerable time.

Analgesic administration

Intravenous Analgesia. The plethora of new analgesics is not an indication that good analgesics have not been found but rather that we are still not using appropriate methods of drug delivery. For the post anesthesia patient, the intramuscular route of administration is clearly inferior to the intravenous route. The peak levels of serum drug concentration are variable, partly because of the variable absorption rates from muscle. Administration of postoperative analgesia should be via the intravenous route because of the inability of most post anesthesia patients to tolerate anything orally. An added advantage to the intravenous route is the assurance of accurate dosage and absorption and more prompt action and, thus, relief from pain. Administering small amounts of a narcotic frequently via the intravenous route to maintain serum drug concentrations controls pain more effectively than by the oral or intramuscular routes of administration.

Patient-Controlled Analgesia. The patient-controlled analgesia (PCA) device (Fig. 22–4) is an electronically controlled infusion device that includes a timer and a mechanism for presetting dosages of analgesics. This device allows the patient to self-administer analgesia as necessary. A lockout mechanism can be set to preclude inadvertent overdosages, but initial evidence indicates that patients do a much better job of assessing the dosage of analgesics needed to relieve pain without deleterious side effects than do either nurses or physicians. Blood serum concentrations are maintained at a more stable level, preventing the development of severe pain that is more difficult to abate without producing drowsiness (Fig. 22–5). The beneficial aspects of this device are obvious: it combines individualized analgesic therapy, based on each patient's subjective appreciation of pain, with the reassurance and sense of control that patients derive from knowing that pain relief is at hand.

Data from clinical trials of this device indicate that patients need far more analgesia in the immediate postoperative period to relieve pain than was previously supposed but that patients taper off their narcotic usage more quickly when they regulate the administration themselves. Use of this device in the PACU is gaining in popularity.

Intrathecal and Epidural Analgesia. Intraspinal administration of narcotics has become increasingly popular for the management of postoperative pain owing to the relatively high-quality, long-lasting pain relief achievable with small quantities of medication. These techniques are particularly useful in managing the pain after thoracotomy and orthopedic, abdominal, and extensive vascular surgical procedures.

Intrathecal opioids are placed directly into the cerebrospinal fluid and attach readily to spinal cord receptor sites, preventing the transmission of pain impulses. The use of intrathecal techniques is fairly limited, and side effects seem to be more common. Intrathecal analgesia is usually administered in a single dose intraoperatively, and the epidural catheter is removed before the patient's admission to the PACU.

Epidural opioid analgesia is accomplished via a catheter placed in the epidural space, a potential space between the dura mater and the vertebral canal that extends from the cranium to the sacrum. Pain relief results from drug levels in the spinal cord, not the plasma. The narcotic diffuses into the cerebrospinal fluid in the subarachnoid space, where it binds the opiate receptors in the dorsal horn. This is thought to block substance P and, thus, transmission of pain impulses to the cerebral cortex.

Many narcotics have been used for intraspinal analgesia, including meperidine, hydromorphone (Dilaudid), sufentanil, alfentanil, clonidine (Catapres), and ketamine (Ketaject;

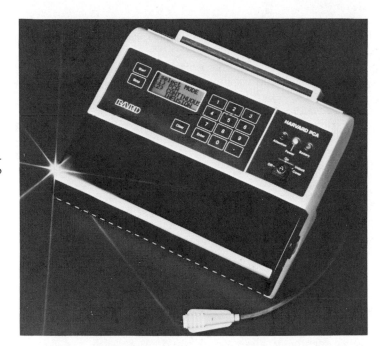

FIGURE 22–4. The patient-controlled analgesia device (PCA). (Courtesy of Bard Electro Medical Systems, Inc., Englewood, CO.).

Ketalar). Most commonly, preservative-free morphine sulfate or fentanyl citrate is used. Analgesia administered in this manner is advantageous in that patients are comfortable and cooperative with postoperative activities, especially deep breathing, coughing, and early ambulation.

A standard protocol for care of these patients should be written and available on the unit. The site of the intrathecal catheter should be inspected for leakage or skin excoriation. If an epidural catheter is in place, it should be secured with a transparent dressing and be free of any kinks or entanglements with other catheters. The epidural catheter should be clearly labeled to avoid any confusion. Strict aseptic technique should be adhered to in the care of this catheter.

Pain assessment should be accomplished at least every hour and should include an objective measure that can be documented. No additional parenteral narcotics should be administered while epidural analgesia is being used. Additional dosages of epidural opioids are not generally required in the PACU; however, should the PACU nurse need to administer additional narcotic, the catheter site should be inspected carefully. The catheter should be gently aspirated prior to injection of an additional narcotic dose. No clear fluid (cerebrospinal fluid) or blood should appear. The aspiration of fluid indicates that the catheter may have migrated or entered a blood vessel, and the physician should be notified immediately. The narcotic dose should be very slowly injected so as to avoid pain on injection.

The side effects of intraspinal analgesia are listed in Table 22–2. All patients should be evaluated carefully for respiratory adequacy by assessment of the rate and depth of respirations and monitoring of oxygen saturation via pulse oximetry. Although respiratory depression seems to be the greatest concern, it occurs relatively infrequently (i.e., less than 1 percent

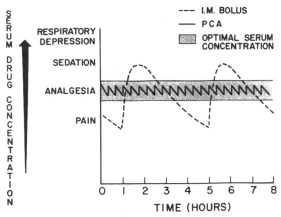

FIGURE 22–5. Narcotic analgesics exhibit a hierarchy of response to increasing serum drug concentrations. Typically, there is an optimal concentration in which the patient is both analgesic and unsedated. Intermittent intramuscular injections of narcotics produce much wider swings in serum drug concentrations than do smaller, more frequently administered intravenous boluses. (From Bennett, R. L., and Griffen, W. O.: Patient-controlled analgesia. Contemp. Surg., 23:186–191, 1983.)

of cases). Respiratory depression is more common in patients who have never received narcotics and in patients with concomitant respiratory disease. Should respiratory depression occur, 0.1 to 0.4 mg of naloxone should be administered intravenously in repeated doses until respirations are adequate.

A dural headache may occur. Treatment for this headache includes keeping the patient in a supine position and ensuring adequate fluid intake.

Pruritus is common and is most often associated with the use of morphine sulfate. The pruritus from epidural analgesia must be differentiated from that which may occur during a transfusion reaction if blood products have been or are being administered. Usually, this pruritus is not too bothersome for the patient, but if it is, it can be controlled with small doses of naloxone and cool compresses.

Urinary retention is fairly common in post anesthesia patients and may be caused by epidural anesthesia alone or in conjunction with the patient's position in bed and immobility. Urinary retention due to epidural analgesia responds to naloxone, or it may be relieved with catheterization.

Nausea and vomiting may occur as a side effect of epidural administration of narcotic therapy. The cause of these symptoms must be determined prior to treatment, because other causes may include gastric distention or a nonfunctioning nasogastric tube. Nausea and vomiting from the use of epidural analgesia can be controlled with antiemetics such as promethazine hydrochloride (Phenergan) and droperidol (Inapsine).

Analgesic Adjuncts

Analgesic adjuncts include drugs developed to alter a component of disease or injury that may contribute to the pain phenomenon or to relieve associated symptoms of pain. Retching and vomiting aggravate the effects of noxious stimuli, and alleviation of these symptoms may significantly reduce the pain experience. Often, an antiemetic such as promethazine or chlorpromazine (Compazine) may be ordered to be given concurrently with an analgesic. Droperidol has been used successfully in the PACU as an antiemetic. Anxiety may be alleviated by the administration of a mild tranquilizer, such as diazepam (Valium). Drugs administered to promote sleep, to relax muscles, or to reduce inflammatory processes also are useful in augmenting pain relief from the narcotics. An advantage of the concurrent administration of these drugs is the potentiation of the narcotic. The nurse must be alert, however, for an exaggeration of respiratory depression when these adjuncts are administered in the post anesthesia period.

Noninvasive Interventions

Transcutaneous Electrical Nerve Stimulation

Transcutaneous electrical nerve stimulation (TENS) involves external stimulation of nerves through electrodes placed over the skin. The stimulation is produced by electrical current activated by a battery-powered device (Fig. 22–6). The electrical current produces a mild tingling or vibrating sensation over the area of application.

Controlled studies have demonstrated TENS to be particularly effective for the alleviation of acute incision pain. It is not satisfactory as the sole modality but can significantly reduce the dosages of narcotic analgesia needed to provide comfort. It seems to work better when the patient is drug naïve. Patients report that it potentiates relief from analgesics and gives them a sense of control over pain.

A number of different units are on the market; most are simple to use. Generally, elec-

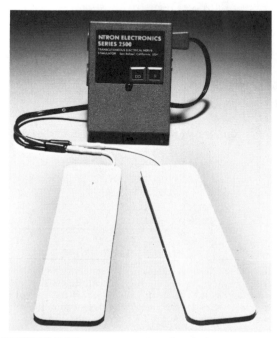

FIGURE 22–6. The transcutaneous electrical nerve stimulation device (TENS). (Courtesy of NTRON International Sales Co., San Rafael, CA.)

trodes, similar to those used for cardiac monitoring, are applied to the area to be stimulated, and the current flow is adjusted until the patient reports discomfort. The current flow is then reduced until stimulation is felt but is a comfortable sensation. Each patient must make this determination.

In the event a patient does not identify the stimulation as uncomfortable but a muscle response becomes apparent, the current flow should be reduced until the muscle response is obliterated. On many models, pulse rate and pulse width may be adjusted in a similar manner.

Because there are no deleterious side effects associated with TENS, it is an excellent adjunct for pain relief in the PACU. It has been particularly effective in relieving the incision pain associated with large thoracic and abdominal incisions. It may also be effective for relieving pain associated with chest tubes and sternal pain following open heart surgery. Initially, the use of TENS for patients scheduled for cardiac surgery or who had either internal or external pacemakers was contraindicated. Evidence now indicates that it is safe for these patients to use TENS, although it should be used with caution and the patient observed closely for any adverse effects. TENS may interfere with electrical monitoring equipment, and this should be observed for. Caution should also be exercised when TENS is used for patients who are taking anticoagulant medications, for those who are pregnant, and for those with myasthenia gravis.

Relaxation

Relaxation has been studied repeatedly as a pain relief adjunct with demonstrated effectiveness for increasing tolerance to pain and reducing narcotic analgesia necessary to control pain. Relaxation reduces anxiety and muscle tension and theoretically depresses the autonomic responses, thereby reducing pain. Learning the techniques and practicing take time, which is seen by some as a disadvantage. However, there are major advantages in that relaxation is fairly simple to learn, is noninvasive, and is not associated with known deleterious effects. Furthermore, the patient can easily transfer the technique from one situation to another.

The effective use of cognitive relaxation techniques appears to depend on coaching, and this may be another means by which the patient's family can contribute to care.

Relaxation is usually not effective when used as the sole pain relief modality but can be useful to augment analgesics and increase tolerance by providing a sense of control over pain, which reduces anxiety.

Not to be overlooked are alternative methods for inducing relaxation, including back rubs or massage, light stroking, application of heat, and the reassurance of personal attention. Pain management is often neglected in the PACU, and the patient is relegated to the surgical unit before pain assessment and comfort measures are instituted. For humanitarian reasons as well as for promotion of physical well-being, pain management should be a priority for the patient in the PACU, because pain is known to decrease lung volumes, increase oxygen consumption, and deplete patient energy. Pain involved with specific procedures and its management is also discussed in each of the individual chapters in this section.

References

1. al Absi, M. A., and Rokke, P. D.: Can anxiety help us tolerate pain? Pain, 46:43–51, 1991.
2. Austin, K. L., Stapleton, J. V., and Mather, L. E.: Multiple intramuscular injections: A major source of variability in analgesic response to meperidine. Pain, 8:47–62, 1980.
3. Bieri, D., Reeve, R. A., Champion, G. D., et al.: The faces pain scale for the self-assessment of the severity of pain experienced by children: Development, initial validation, and preliminary investigation for ratio scales properties. Pain, 41:139–150, 1990.
4. Borokas, L.: Factors affecting nurses' decision to medicate pediatric patients after surgery. Heart Lung, 14:373–379, 1985.
5. Bragg, C. L.: Practical aspects of epidural and intrathecal narcotic analgesia in the intensive care setting. Heart Lung, 18(6):599–608, 1989.
6. Caplan, R. A., Ready, L. B., Olsson, G. L., et al.: Transdermal delivery of fentanyl for postoperative pain control [Abstract]. Anesthesiology, 65:A210, 1986.
7. Christoph, S. B.: A comparison of patient-controlled transcutaneous electrical nerve stimulation with traditional analgesics for relief of postoperative pain [Dissertation]. Washington, D. C., Catholic University, University Microfilms, 1985.
8. Christoph, S. B.: Pain. In Kinney, M. R., Packa, D. R., and Dunbar, S. B. (eds.): AACN's Clinical Reference for Critical Care Nurses. 2nd ed. New York, McGraw-Hill, 1988, pp. 372–398.
9. Christoph, S. B.: Pain assessment. Crit. Care Nurs. Clin. North Am., 3(1):11–16, 1991.
10. Christoph, S. B.: Pain in the postoperative patient. In Puntillo, K. A. (ed.): Pain in the Critically Ill. Gaithersburg, MD, Aspen, 1991, pp. 211–221.
11. Donovan, M., Dillon, P., and McGuire, L.: Incidence and characteristics of pain in a sample of medical-surgical inpatients. Pain, 30:69–78, 1987.
12. Eland, J. M., and Coy, J. A.: Assessing pain in the critically ill child. Focus Crit. Care, 17(6):469–475, 1990.
13. Gilbert, H. C.: Pain relief methods in the post anesthesia care unit. J. Post Anesth. Nurs., 5(1):6–15, 1990.
14. Gourlay, G. K., Kowalski, S. R., Plummer, J. L., et al.:

The transdermal administration of fentanyl in the treatment of postoperative pain: Pharmacokinetics and pharmacodynamic effects. Pain, 37:193–202, 1989.

15. Holland, M. S., Gammill, B. G., and Mackey, D. C.: New techniques in anesthesia: Update for nurse anesthetists—alternatives for postoperative pain management. AANA J., 58(3):201–210, 1990.

16. Holm, K., Cohen, F., Dudas S., et al.: Effect of personal pain experience on pain assessment. Image, 21(2):72–75, 1989.

17. Ketovuori, H.: Nurses' and patients' conceptions of wound pain and the administration of analgesics. Pain, 38:213–218, 1987.

18. Litwack, K., and Lubenon, T.: Practical points in the management of continuous epidural infusions. J. Post Anesth. Nurs., 4(5):327–330, 1989.

19. Moltner, A., Holzl, R., and Strian, F.: Heart rate changes as an autonomic component of the pain response. Pain, 43:81–89, 1990.

20. Musgrave, C. F.: Postoperative pain: A treatable symptom. Curr. Rev. Post Anesth. Care Nurses, 13(8):59–63, 1991.

21. Olsson, G. L., Leddo, C. C., and Wild, L.: Nursing management of patients receiving epidural narcotics. Heart Lung, 18(2):130–137, 1989.

22. Thomas, B. L.: Pain management for the elderly: Alternative interventions. AORN J., 52(1):126–132, 1991.

23. Van Poznak, A.: Role of respiratory patterns in the treatment of pain and anxiety. In Luczun, M. E. (ed.): Post Anesthesia Nursing. Rockville, MD, Aspen, 1984.

24. Wall, P. D.: The prevention of postoperative pain [Editorial]. Pain, 33:289–290, 1988.

25. White, P. F.: Use of parenteral narcotics in the postoperative period. Curr. Rev. Recov. Room Nurses, 15(7):118–123, 1985.

26. Yeager, M. P., Glass, D. G., Neff, R. K., et al.: Epidural anesthesia and analgesia in high-risk surgical patients. Anesthesiology, 66:729–736, 1987.

Post Anesthesia Care of the Ear, Nose, Throat, Neck, and Maxillofacial Surgical Patient

CHAPTER 23

Lynda Marks, R.N.
Anita Gurwin, B.S.N., R.N.
Sharon Farrar, B.S.N., R.N.

SURGERY ON THE EAR

Otologic surgery has been revolutionized by antibiotics, the operating microscope, new and more delicate instruments, and an increased understanding of the anatomic structures involved (Figs. 23–1 and 23–2). New methods have been devised to treat hearing loss surgically by correcting conduction apparatus abnormalities, and selected patients can now be surgically relieved of the disabling symptoms of sensorineural hearing loss.

Definitions

Cochlear implant: a prosthesis with internal electrode is surgically implanted into the cochlea so that an external microphone can be applied later to stimulate the eighth cranial nerve and provide sound for a deaf person.
Fenestration: reconstruction of the outer and middle parts of the ear by means of a new drum or skin flap; creation of a new window into the internal ear mechanism with a newly established drum or skin flap.
Labyrinthectomy: opening of the labyrinth to destroy the inner ear in an attempt to relieve medically uncontrollable symptoms of unilateral Meniere's syndrome.
Mastoidectomy: removal of mastoid air cells and of the tympanic membrane. Radical mastoidectomy also involves removing the malleus, incus, chorda tympani, and mucoperiosteal lining.

Myringotomy: incision of the tympanic membrane under direct vision and insertion of tubes to facilitate drainage.
Ossiculoplasty: reconstruction of the ossicular chain.
Stapedectomy: removal of the stapes (Fig. 23–3A), followed by the placement of a prosthesis (Fig. 23–3B).
Tympanoplasty (myringoplasty): reconstruction of the tympanic membrane.

Most otologic procedures are now performed in the day surgery arena. The immediate post anesthesia care for patients who have undergone surgery on the ear is generally the same, no matter what the procedure. Immediate postoperative complications are rare. Occasionally, excessive bleeding may occur, especially if a large blood vessel has been entered during the operation. If bleeding has occurred, it should be reported to the post anesthesia care unit (PACU) nurse who will provide care for the patient on admission to the PACU. Immediate post anesthesia assessment should follow the same format as for any patient undergoing general anesthesia. In addition, post anesthesia assessment should include testing for function of the facial nerve. Have the patient frown, smile, wrinkle the forehead, close the eyes, bare the teeth, and pucker the lips. Inability to perform these actions indicates injury to the facial nerve and should be appropriately indicated in the patient's medical record and reported to the surgeon.

If surgery has been performed near the brain (inner ear), check for clear fluid in the ear or on the dressings that may indicate cerebrospinal

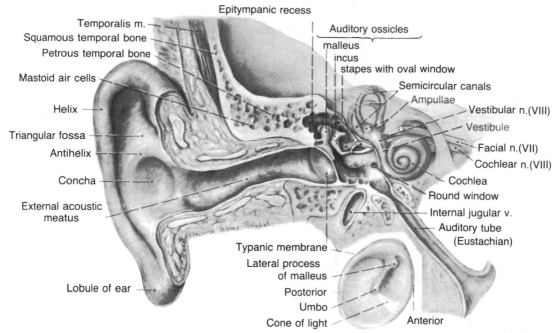

FIGURE 23–1. Frontal section through the outer, middle, and internal ear. (From Jacob, S. W., and Francone, C. A.: Elements of Anatomy and Physiology. 2nd ed. Philadelphia, W. B. Saunders, 1989, p. 134.)

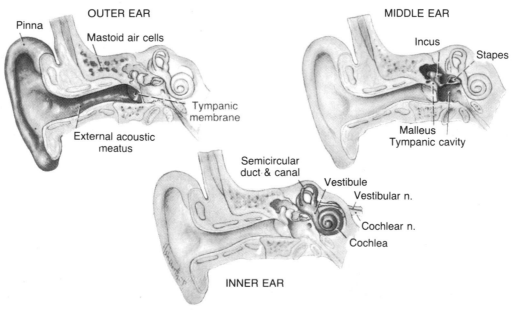

FIGURE 23–2. Three divisions of the ear. (From Jacob, S. W., and Francone, C. A.: Elements of Anatomy and Physiology. 2nd ed. Philadelphia, W. B. Saunders, 1989, p. 134.)

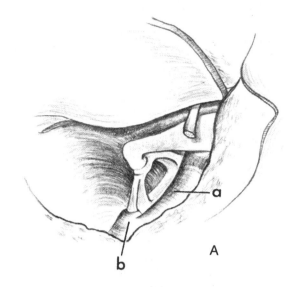

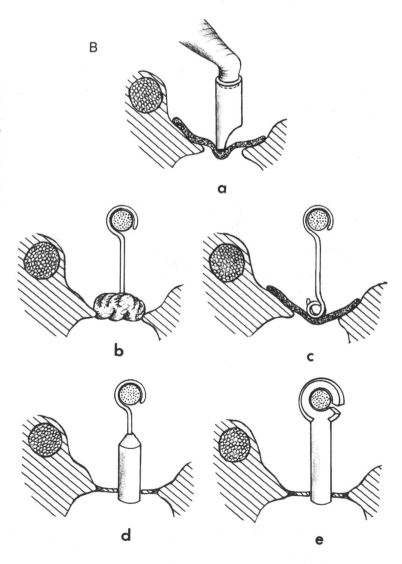

FIGURE 23–3. *A,* stapedectomy. Adequate footplate exposure is achieved when the facial canal (a) and the pyramidal process (b) are seen. *B,* stapedectomy prostheses: (a) vein/polyethylene strut (Shea); (b) wire/fat (Schuknecht); (c) wire on compressed Gelfoam (House); (d) wire/Teflon piston; (e) Teflon piston (Shea). (*A* and *B* from Paparella, M. M., and Shumrick, D. A.: Otolaryngology. Vol. 2. Philadelphia, W. B. Saunders, 1973, p. 304.)

fluid leakage. Aseptic technique for all dressings and protection from infection are especially important elements in the care of the patient who has undergone surgery on the ears, because infection can easily be transmitted to the meninges and the brain. The outer ear is highly vascular and susceptible to circulatory damage and excoriation. The outer ear may even become necrotic if circulation is impaired by excessive pressure from or malpositioning of a dressing. Assessment of the dressing should therefore include proper positioning.

Post anesthesia positioning of the patient who has undergone ear surgery should be indicated by the surgeon. If position is unimportant, the patient should be allowed to assume a position of comfort, usually with the head of the bed elevated to facilitate drainage. This position also decreases the need to move the head to see. Generally, lying on the unoperated side is the most comfortable position for the patient.

Nausea, vertigo, and nystagmus commonly occur in patients following ear surgery. The patient may minimize discomfort by remaining in the position ordered, moving slowly, and avoiding quick, jerky movements. Advise the patient to take slow, deep breaths through the mouth to minimize nausea. Antiemetic drugs and sedatives such as dimenhydrinate (Dramamine), diazepam (Valium), droperidol (Inapsine), and chlorpromazine (Thorazine) may be ordered to prevent or treat nausea and vertigo. Avoid jarring the bed. When approaching the patient, place your hand on top of the patient's head as a reminder not to turn toward you suddenly when you speak. Avoid sudden turns and move slowly while transporting this patient. Particular attention must be paid to maintaining the integrity of the airway should nausea and vomiting occur.

Special Considerations

Myringotomy. This is the most common procedure performed on infants and small children. Special pediatric considerations must be given in the immediate post anesthesia phase to airway management, safety, parental involvement, and outpatient teaching. Position the patient so as to promote drainage from the ear. A small piece of sterile cotton may be placed loosely in the external ear to absorb the drainage that commonly occurs. The cotton should be changed frequently to avoid contamination.

Mastoidectomy. A firm, bulky dressing is placed over the ear and held in place with a circular head bandage after mastoidectomy. This dressing may be reinforced, if necessary, but should be changed only by the physician. Minimal serosanguineous drainage may be expected, but bright bloody drainage should be reported to the surgeon.

The patient should be placed in a position of comfort, usually on the unoperated side. Grafts are often taken from the arm or leg for radical mastoidectomy and the donor sites should be assessed for drainage and treated according to local policy. Dizziness and vertigo are common following mastoidectomy and may be treated with the previously mentioned measures.

Tympanoplasty. Patients are usually positioned on the unoperated side after tympanoplasty. Care must be taken to keep bandages and grafts in place. Patients should be instructed not to blow their noses or cough and to avoid sneezing to prevent disruption of the grafts.

Fenestration. Fenestration is not commonly performed; however, it may occasionally be the procedure of choice for patients who have lost effective hearing in both ears. It is a major surgical procedure and is usually performed under general anesthesia. Nausea, vertigo, and pain on moving the jaws can be expected following fenestration. The patient is usually placed on the operated side to keep drainage from the operative site from entering the ear. The patient may be allowed to change position from the operated side to the back for nursing care and comfort.

Stapedectomy. Patients who have undergone stapedectomy are usually admitted to the PACU with ear packing in place, and this packing should not be disturbed. Occasionally, patients complain of vertigo postoperatively. Patients should be advised not to blow their noses or cough and to avoid sneezing.

Cochlear Implant. Patients who have undergone a cochlear implant require the same post anesthesia care as any other ear surgery patient. It is important to verify the integrity of the facial nerve. These patients do not have hearing immediately postoperatively and require emotional support and a means of communication.

SURGERY ON THE NOSE AND SINUSES

Nasal and sinus surgery may be accomplished under local or general anesthesia. The disposition of the patient is determined by the nature and type of surgery and anesthesia as well as the post anesthesia course related to complications and sedation required in the PACU. It may be necessary to observe the patients in an inpatient setting overnight before their discharge from the hospital.

The anatomy of the nasal cavity is shown in Figure 23–4.

Definitions

Endoscopy: nasal surgery performed using direct vision with endoscopic equipment.
Ethmoidectomy: removal of ethmoid bone.
Intranasal antrostomy (antral window): creation of an opening in the lateral wall of the nose under the middle turbinate and the removal of the anterior end of the inferior turbinate.
Radical antrostomy (Caldwell-Luc operation): use of an incision into the canine fossa of the upper jaw and exposure of the antrum for removal of bony, diseased portions of the antral wall and contents of the sinus; establishment of drainage by means of a counteropening into the nose through the inferior meatus to establish a large opening in the nasoantral wall of the inferior meatus, which will ensure adequate gravity drainage and aeration and

will permit removal of all diseased tissue in the sinus under direct vision.
Submucosal resection: removal of either cartilaginous or osseous portions of the septum that lie between the flaps of the mucous membrane and the perichondrium to establish an adequate partition between the left and right nasal cavities, thereby providing a clear airway for both the internal and external cavities and the parts of the nose.

Nasal Surgery

Conscious patients admitted to the PACU after nasal surgery should be placed in a semi-Fowler position to promote drainage, reduce local edema, minimize discomfort, and facilitate respiration. Some postoperative serosanguineous drainage is expected; however, the nurse should observe closely for gross bleeding. The patient is usually admitted with one or both nostrils packed and a "mustache dressing" in place to catch any drainage from the packing. The position of the nasal packs and the amount of drainage should be checked frequently. The mustache dressing may be changed as necessary; it is not unusual for it to be changed two or three times within a 4-hour period. Another method commonly used to facilitate postoperative drainage is the insertion of nasal stents. This approach affords more comfort and permits nasal breathing.

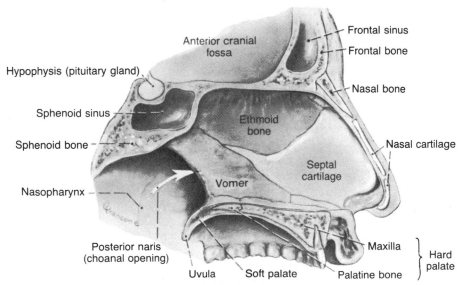

FIGURE 23–4. Sagittal section through the nose showing components of the nasal septum. (From Jacob, S. W., and Francone, C. A.: Elements of Anatomy and Physiology. 2nd ed. Philadelphia, W. B. Saunders, 1989, p. 226.)

The back of the patient's throat should be checked frequently for blood. Frequent belching (from the accumulation of blood in the stomach) and frequent swallowing as well as the classic signs of hemorrhage, such as tachycardia, are additional signs of unusual bleeding. The patient should be instructed not to blow his or her nose and not to swallow secretions but rather to spit them into a basin. An ample supply of disposable tissues along with an emesis basin should be placed within easy reach of the patient.

Airway obstruction or laryngeal spasm may occur if a postnasal pack accidentally slips out of place. A flashlight, scissors, and a hemostat for emergency removal of nasal packing and emergency airway equipment must be kept readily available at the patient's bedside.

Fluids are withheld until bleeding is controlled, vomiting and nausea have subsided, and independent airway management has been established. Occasionally, an antiemetic may be ordered to alleviate nausea and vomiting.

Mouth breathing, bleeding, and postnasal drainage create a dryness and an offensive taste and odor in the patient's mouth, so once the gag reflex has returned, oral hygiene is a priority. Lemon-glycerine swabs or mouthwash may be used for mouth care and to make the patient more comfortable. A petrolatum-based ointment may be applied to the lips to prevent drying and cracking.

Ice packs across the nose may be ordered to minimize pain, edema, discoloration, and bleeding. These ice packs should be small and lightweight.

Oxygen should be delivered via cool mist mask through a face tent because dry mucous membranes often produce coughing, dyspnea, and decreased respiratory exchange. Ice chips may be a comfort measure if intake is warranted.

Sinus Surgery

Following surgery on the sinuses, the patient is usually admitted to the PACU with packing in place. It is not unusual for the patient to report feelings of numbness in the upper lip and teeth. Following general anesthesia, the patient should be positioned well on one side to prevent aspiration of drainage. The conscious patient should be placed in a semi-Fowler position, with the head elevated 45 degrees to promote drainage and minimize edema. The same general care, including oral hygiene and instructions to the patient not to blow his or

her nose, should be followed as for the patient with nasal surgery.

SURGERY ON THE TONGUE

Definitions

Ankyloglossia ("tongue tied"): a short lingual frenulum that may cause difficult suckling in the infant and subsequent speech impairment. It is treated surgically by clipping of the frenulum.
Glossectomy: removal of the tongue.

The tongue occupies a large portion of the floor of the mouth. Surgery on the tongue generally involves excision of benign or malignant lesions, correction of congenital anomalies, or repair of traumatic lacerations. Lesions may be excised without associated neck dissection; however, when the lesion is malignant, surgical treatment usually involves a combined operation that may include radical neck dissection and resection of both the mandible and the tongue.

Local anesthesia is used for minor surgical procedures such as incision and longitudinal closure of the frenulum in ankyloglossia. Local infiltration is also used when repairing lacerations due to trauma. More extensive surgical procedures on the tongue require endotracheal anesthesia.

Postoperatively, the patient must be placed in a side-lying position with the head slightly dependent to allow for the drainage of secretions out of the mouth. When protective reflexes have returned, the patient should be placed in a sitting position to promote venous and lymphatic drainage.

Maintenance of the airway is the most crucial nursing concern. Suctioning equipment with soft-tipped catheters must be immediately available at the bedside. The patient should be instructed to allow saliva to run out of the mouth. A wick of gauze may be placed in the patient's mouth to assist in the elimination of secretions. Swelling of the tongue may occur, causing obstruction of the airway. Therefore, an intubation tray should be readily available.

Because of the vascular nature of the tongue and oral cavity, postoperative bleeding may be a problem. If excessive bleeding occurs, local pressure should be applied until the surgeon can be notified and repair effected in the operating room.

THROAT SURGERY

Definitions

Laryngectomy: removal of the larynx; *total laryngectomy* is the complete removal of the cartilaginous larynx, the hyoid bone, and the strap muscles connected to the larynx and possible removal of the pre-epiglottic space along with the lesion (Fig. 23–5 and Table 23–1).

Laryngofissure: opening of the larynx for exploratory, excisional, or reconstructive procedures.

Laryngoscopy: direct examination of the interior of the larynx with a laryngoscope.

Paletouvuloplasty: the reconstruction of the posterior section of the palate and the uvula.

Tonsillectomy and adenoidectomy (T&A): surgical removal of the tonsils and adenoids (Fig. 23–6).

Tracheostomy: opening of the trachea and insertion of a cannula through a midline incision in the neck below the cricoid cartilage (Fig. 23–7).

Surgery on the throat and neck is generally accomplished under general anesthesia. Aside from routine care and assessment, specific post anesthesia care for the patient who has undergone surgery on the throat involves (1) close observation for bleeding from the surgical site, (2) maintenance of a patent airway, (3) prevention of aspiration of secretions, and (4) awareness of possible cerebral neurologic complications that may develop.

The most common procedures are tonsillectomy, either alone or in combination with adenoidectomy, and tracheostomy.

Tonsillectomy and Adenoidectomy

Most patients undergoing tonsillectomy and adenoidectomy (T&A) are children and young adults. Patients who have undergone T&A with local anesthesia or are admitted to the PACU fully conscious may be positioned on their backs with their heads elevated 45 degrees. Patients who return following general anesthesia and who are unconscious or semiconscious must be placed in the tonsillar posi-

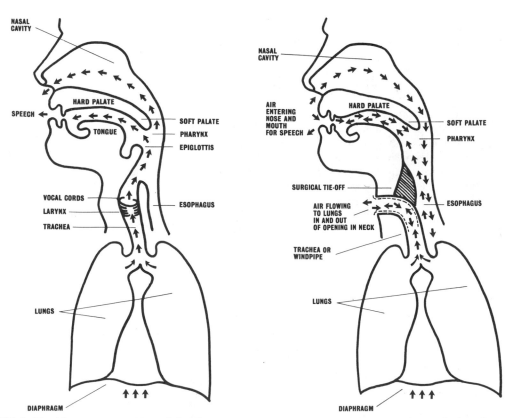

FIGURE 23–5. Total laryngectomy. (From Rehabilitating Laryngectomies. © 1960, American Cancer Society, Inc., 4R–50M–2/69–No. 4506-PS. *In* Luckmann, J., and Sorensen, K. C.: Medical-Surgical Nursing. 2nd ed. Philadelphia, W. B. Saunders, 1980, p. 2099.)

Table 23–1. LARYNGECTOMY

Structures Removed	Structures Remaining	Postoperative Conditions
Total Laryngectomy		
Hyoid bone	Tongue	Loses voice; breathes through tracheostomy; no problem swallowing
Entire larynx (epiglottis, false cords, true cords)	Pharyngeal walls	
Cricoid cartilage	Lower trachea	
Two or three rings of trachea		
Supraglottic or Horizontal Laryngectomy		
Hyoid bone	True vocal cords	Normal voice; may aspirate occasionally, especially liquids; normal airway
Epiglottis	Cricoid cartilage	
False vocal cords	Trachea	
Vertical (or Hemi-) Laryngectomy		
One true vocal cord	Epiglottis	Hoarse but serviceable voice; normal airway; no problem swallowing
False cord	One false cord	
Arytenoid	One true vocal cord	
One half thyroid cartilage	Cricoid	
Laryngofissure and Partial Laryngectomy		
One vocal cord	All other structures	Hoarse but serviceable voice; occasionally almost normal voice; no airway problem; no swallowing problem
Endoscopic Removal of Early Carcinoma		
Part of one vocal cord	All other structures	May have a normal voice; no other problems

tion—well over on the side with the face partially down. The Trendelenburg position may be used to facilitate drainage. The patient's airway and chest expansion must be in full view of the nurse to ensure maximum respiratory integrity at all times. In this position, secretions are easily drained from the mouth. An oral airway should be left in place until the swallowing reflex has returned and the patient can handle secretions. The patient should be advised to spit out secretions as much as possible and to try not to cough, clear the throat, blow the nose, or talk excessively. An ice collar may be applied to minimize pain and postoperative bleeding. The administration of cool, humidified air to the T&A patient provides comfort, helps minimize swelling, and supplies oxygen.

The most common complication of T&A is postoperative bleeding. Frequent swallowing, clearing of the throat, and vomiting of dark blood are indications of possible bleeding. The nurse should frequently check the back of the throat with a flashlight for trickling blood. If any of the cardinal symptoms of hemorrhage occur, such as decreased blood pressure, tachycardia, pallor, and restlessness, the surgeon should be notified. Because the surgeon may wish to treat a bleeding episode in the PACU, a tonsil tray should be available (Table 23–2). An electrocautery unit and appropriate illumination with a headlight should be available, along with suction equipment. Postoperative bleeding after T&A can often be controlled by the application of vasoconstrictors via nasal

packing with pressure. If significant bleeding occurs, however, the patient may have to return to the operating room for suturing or cauterizing of blood vessels.

With the advent of laser dissection of tonsils and adenoids, swelling of the tissue in the hypopharyngeal area is increased. Close observation as well as measures to alleviate swelling are crucial. The advantage of laser dissection is that the potential for bleeding is significantly decreased.

Once the patient is conscious and the reflexes have returned, ice chips and fluids may be offered. Large swallows of lukewarm fluids seem to cause the least discomfort to these patients.

Table 23–2. CONTENTS OF TONSIL TRAY

Tongue depressors
1 Hurd retractor
2 Mouth gags
1 Allis clamp
2 Tonsil hemostats
1 Short sponge forceps
1 Pair scissors
Sterile towels
Epinephrine hydrochloride (adrenalin) 1:1000
1 Set tonsil suture needles
1 Needle holder
1 Glass medicine cup
1 Sterile basin
Cotton balls
Tonsil tampons
1 Soft rubber catheter
Petrolatum

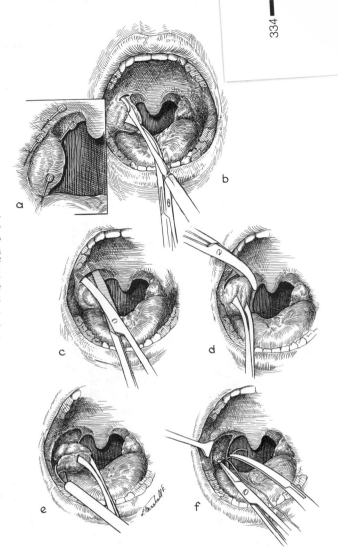

FIGURE 23–6. A method of dissection tonsillectomy. *a*, points of infiltration for local anesthesia. *b*, start of incision with tonsil knife at attachment of anterior pillar to the tonsil superiorly. *c*, separation by scissor dissection of the superior pole of the tonsil. *d*, continuation of dissection of tonsil from its attachment to pillars and bed of tonsillar fossa. *e*, separation of the tonsil by snare at the lower pole, including the plica triangularis. *f*, hemostasis. (*a* through *f* from Boies, L. R., Hilger, J. A., and Priest, R. E.: Fundamentals of Otolaryngology: A Textbook of Ear, Nose, and Throat Diseases. 4th ed. Philadelphia, W. B. Saunders, 1964, p. 415.)

Sucking may precipitate bleeding, so a straw should not be offered to the patient. Oral hygiene, including alkaline mouthwash, may provide comfort. Apply petrolatum ointment to the lips to prevent drying and cracking.

Patients who have undergone T&A are especially prone to laryngospasms and must be observed closely for patency of the airway. Airway obstruction may be created by swelling of the palate or nasopharynx, swelling in the retropharyngeal space, or swelling of the tongue and nose. If laryngospasm does occur, positive pressure via Ambu bag and 100 percent fraction of inspired oxygen (FIO_2) is administered. If this is not effective in breaking the spasm, it may be necessary to reintubate the patient, with the administration of succinylcholine and narcotics as prescribed.

Laryngoscopy

Laryngoscopy may be accomplished with local or general anesthesia. If the patient's gag and cough reflexes have been obliterated, the patient should not be given anything orally until these reflexes have fully returned. The conscious patient may be placed in a semi-Fowler position, lying on either side. If unconscious, the patient should be placed in the side-lying position to avoid aspiration. Cool mist, sips of water, and intravenous narcotics may help relieve coughing that often occurs.

These patients are especially susceptible to the development of laryngospasm, and the most important observations in the postlaryngoscopy patient are aimed at ascertaining the patency of the airway. Laryngeal stridor, dysp-

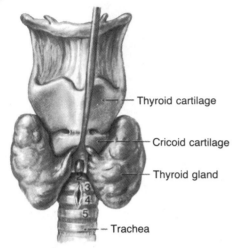

Thyroid cartilage

Cricoid cartilage

Thyroid gland

Trachea

FIGURE 23–7. Incision for a tracheostomy. (From Jacob, S. W., and Francone, C. A.: Elements of Anatomy and Physiology. 2nd ed. Philadelphia, W. B. Saunders, 1989, p. 229.)

Table 23–3. CONTENTS OF TRACHEOSTOMY TRAY

1 Adson or Poole suction (without guard)
No. 3 knife handle with No. 15 blade
No. 11 Blade
1 Metzenbaum scissors
1 One-point sharp scissors
1 Curved tenotomy scissors
1 Collier needle holder
1 6-inch needle holder
2 Adson forceps
1 Tissue forceps
1 Dressing forceps
4 Curved mosquito forceps
2 Straight mosquito forceps
2 Allis clamps
4 Small towel clips
1 Sponge stick (or forceps)
1 Probe
1 Grooved director
1 Goiter right-angle retractor
1 Tracheostomy hook
2 Vein retractors
2 Army-Navy retractors
1 Tonsil suction with tip screwed on
1 10-ml, 3-ring syringe
1 25-gauge × ⅝-inch needle
1 Prep cup
1 Medicine glass
Tracheostomy tubes, 1 each, sizes 00–8
4 Hand towels
1 Trousseau tracheal dilator

nea, decreased oxygen saturation, or shortness of breath should alert the nurse to respiratory impairment, and the anesthesiologist should be notified. Equipment for endotracheal intubation and emergency tracheostomy should be immediately available at the bedside should laryngeal edema or laryngospasm develop (Table 23–3).

A certain amount of throat discomfort can be expected and may be relieved by the use of an ice collar. The administration of high-humidity oxygen by face tent or mask decreases throat irritation. After the cough and gag reflexes have returned, the patient may be allowed sips of warm normal saline, which is soothing to irritated tissues. If severe pain occurs in either the throat or the chest, the physician should be notified. Watch for signs of hemorrhage, including coughing or regurgitation of blood, apprehension, and the classic signs of tachycardia and lowered blood pressure.

In patients who have had a laryngoscopy (with biopsy) or removal of polyps, vocal rest is important. Coughing should be avoided if possible, and paper and pencil or a "Magic Slate" should be made available so the patient can communicate without talking. If intractable coughing does occur, it may be necessary to consult the anesthesiologist for further measures of control, including pharmacotherapeutics such as codeine and lidocaine to suppress the cough reflex.

Tracheostomy

A tracheostomy—the making of an incision into the trachea and the insertion of a can-

nula—may be done as either an emergency or an elective procedure. Ideally, a tracheostomy is performed in the operating suite under controlled conditions. Tracheostomies are done to improve the airway and to provide access for suctioning of secretions from the trachea and bronchi. The PACU nurse should know what condition necessitated the tracheostomy.

PACU personnel should anticipate the arrival of a tracheostomized patient and have the necessary items at the bedside, as listed in Table 23–4.

A variety of tracheostomy tubes are available, and the nurse should be familiar with those used in the particular institution. Several common types are shown in Figure 23–8.

Immediate post anesthesia care of the newly tracheostomized patient includes a complete assessment of the patient's general condition as well as detailed attention to respiratory status and tracheostomy wound care. Because of the many nursing needs and the necessity of intensive, ongoing respiratory assessment, the newly tracheostomized patient requires constant attendance.

Assessment of respiratory function should include all parameters mentioned in previous chapters. The nurse should auscultate the pa-

Table 23–4. BEDSIDE EQUIPMENT NEEDED FOR A PATIENT WITH TRACHEOSTOMY

Suction equipment
Respirator
Ambu or anesthesia bag
Extra sterile tracheostomy tray, including tracheostomy
 tubes of proper size, sterile forceps, tracheal hook, and
 Trousseau tracheal dilator (see Table 23–3)
Sterile gauze squares
Sterile scissors
Tracheostomy ties
Cleaning solutions for the tracheostomy tube and the
 incision
Syringe
Hemostat (for inflating the tracheostomy tube cuff)

tient's chest frequently for normal bilateral breath sounds and report any adventitious sounds or indications of pulmonary congestion. Pulse oximetry should be used to assist in assessment.

Suctioning and Tracheostomy Care. Patency of the newly created airway is vital, and frequent suctioning is necessary owing to increased secretions from the tracheobronchial tree as a result of trauma. Suctioning the tracheostomy must be sterile and atraumatic—a sterile disposable catheter and glove should be used for each procedure. A suction catheter in a plastic sleeve provides a means of suctioning without the use of gloves and is most convenient for use in the PACU. Catheters should be smooth and small enough to pass easily into the lumen of the tracheostomy tube without obstructing it.

As with any suctioning technique, the patient should be hyperventilated with increased FIO_2 both before and after the procedure. To suction, insert the catheter 6 to 8 inches into the tracheostomy tube. Do not apply suction during insertion. Apply suction intermittently by occluding the air valve with the thumb, at the same time slowly withdrawing the catheter in a twisting motion. Suctioning should not continue for longer than 5 seconds. Time should be allotted between each suctioning for adequate oxygenation of the patient. Suctioning often stimulates forceful coughing, which is effective in bringing up secretions, so the nurse should be prepared to wipe expelled secretions away from the tracheostomy tube orifice with plain gauze squares. To determine the effectiveness of the suctioning, the chest should be auscultated immediately afterward.

If deep suctioning is indicated, a coudé-tip catheter should be used. Insert the catheter with the tip pointing in the direction of the

main stem bronchus to be suctioned. Recent evidence indicates that positioning the patient's head to the left or the right has little effect, if any, on which bronchus will be entered.

If the patient's secretions are exceptionally thick, the physician may order instillation of 3 to 5 ml of sterile normal saline into the tracheostomy tube to help loosen secretions and promote coughing. Although this is a common procedure, it is questionable whether or not it is actually effective, and if the normal saline is not immediately removed by suctioning, it may produce the effects of any inhaled fluid as well as acting as a contaminant. More effective measures to ensure liquefaction of secretions include providing inspired air that is well humidified and making sure that the patient is well hydrated.

Immediate post anesthesia care of the newly tracheostomized patient also includes care and cleaning of the tracheostomy tube, which may be necessary as often as every hour. A variety of methods may be used to clean the inner cannula of the tracheostomy tube, including normal saline and hydrogen peroxide or 2 percent sodium bicarbonate solution. A small test tube brush or pipe cleaners may be used to scrub off sticky crusts of mucus. Whatever the method used, it must be a sterile procedure, and no supplies should be used that may leave on the cannula any lint or other debris that may be inhaled by the patient.

Wound drainage from the tracheostomy is generally minimal; however, soiling of the tracheostomy dressing occurs from secretions and sweating. The dressings should be changed as often as necessary, and the skin should be kept clean and dry to prevent maceration and infection. The skin around the stoma should be cleansed with hydrogen peroxide and normal saline and dried with sterile gauze pads, and an antibiotic ointment such as bacitracin should be applied. The tracheostomy dressing should be plain gauze with the edges bound and should have no cotton filling or loose strings. Special tracheostomy "pants" that fit over the tracheostomy tube and have all edges sewn make the best dressing. Sterile gauze may be cut halfway to the center and fitted over the tube (Fig. 23–9); however, this approach has the disadvantage of cut edges that may fray and allow bits of gauze to enter the wound or the trachea.

Fabric tapes or ties or Velcro devices are used to secure the tracheostomy tube in place. These should be checked frequently to ensure the proper tension. If they are too tight, they

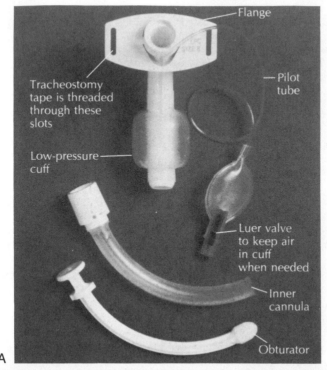

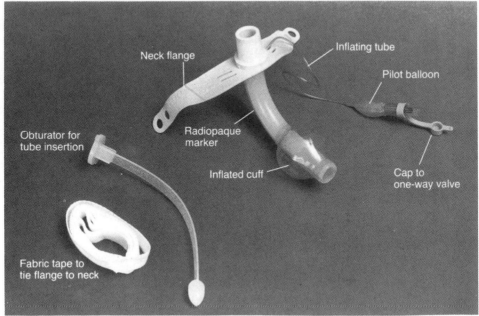

FIGURE 23–8. *A,* polyvinylchloride tracheostomy tube and obturator. (*A* courtesy of Shiley, Inc., Irvine, CA.) *B,* single-lumen tracheostomy tube (Portex). (*B* from Kersten. L. D.: Comprehensive Respiratory Nursing: A Decision-Making Approach. Philadelphia, W. B. Saunders, 1989.)

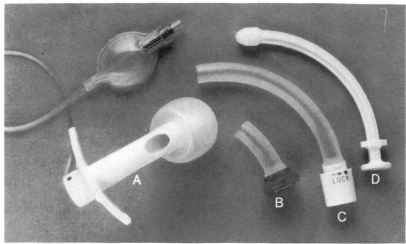

C

FIGURE 23–8 *Continued C,* Shiley fenestrated low-pressure cuffed tracheostomy tube, showing (A) the outer cannula with a fenestration above the cuff; (B) decannulation cannula used to plug the tracheostomy tube; (C) inner cannula; and (D) obturator. (C courtesy of Shiley, Inc., Irvine, CA.)

will be uncomfortable for the patient and may compress the external jugular veins. If they are too loose, the cannula will slide up and down in the trachea or even be expelled. When the tapes are tied so that one finger can easily slip underneath, the tension is right.

Complications. Complications of a tracheostomy do occur, and PACU nurses should be especially astute in observing for signs of danger. The most common complication is respiratory obstruction due to external pressure, foreign bodies, tracheal edema, or excessive secretions. If suctioning does not relieve airway obstruction, the tracheostomy tube may be removed immediately, the tracheal stoma held open with a tracheal dilator and hook or for-

ceps (Fig. 23–10), and the surgeon or anesthesiologist summoned.

Occasionally, a tube is coughed out either because the ties are not sufficiently tight or because the tube is too short. If a tube is accidentally expelled, it must be reinserted by persons qualified to do so. In some institutions, nurses practice changing tracheostomy tubes under the supervision of physicians so that if accidental expulsion should occur in the PACU, the nurse will be skilled in replacement. If the tube cannot be inserted easily, the stoma should be held open and the surgeon called. Misplacement or displacement of the tube is a common complication and must be corrected immediately (Fig. 23–11).

Obstruction below the tracheostomy tube may create respiratory insufficiency. Respiratory adventitious sounds, unequal lung expansion, and marked respiratory efforts, including

FIGURE 23–9. Gauze square cut to use as tracheostomy dressing. (From Sutton, A. L.: Bedside Nursing Techniques in Medicine and Surgery. 2nd ed. Philadelphia, W. B. Saunders, 1969, p. 357.)

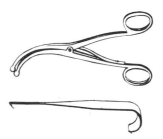

FIGURE 23–10. Tracheal dilator and hook. (Adapted from Sutton, A. L.: Bedside Nursing Techniques in Medicine and Surgery. 2nd ed. Philadelphia, W. B. Saunders, 1969, p. 353.)

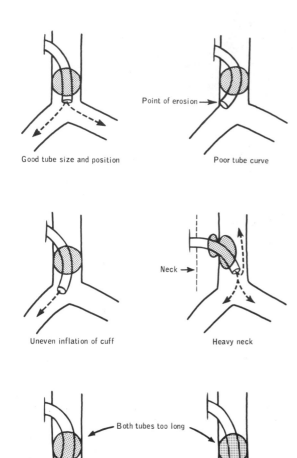

Good tube size and position

Point of erosion →

Poor tube curve

Uneven inflation of cuff

Neck →

Heavy neck

← Both tubes too long →

Carina

FIGURE 23–11. Tracheostomy tube positions and factors affecting them. (From Murphy, E. R.: Intensive nursing care in a respiratory unit. Nurs. Clin. North Am., 3:433, 1968.)

supraclavicular, intercostal, and substernal retractions, should alert the nurse to this problem, and the physician should be notified.

Some bloody secretions from the tracheal stoma may be expected in the immediate postoperative period, but frank bleeding is abnormal and the surgeon should be notified. Sometimes, there is bleeding from a thyroid vein or other neck vessel next to the tube, and blood, which runs down into the trachea, is sprayed about with every cough. This is usually not serious and can often be controlled with local packing with petrolatum gauze. Occasionally, however, serious bleeding does occur, and the patient must be taken back to the operating room, where the wound is reopened and the bleeding vessel ligated.

Subcutaneous emphysema may occur as a complication of tracheostomy if the wound is su-

tured too tightly about the tracheostomy tube, allowing air to enter the subcutaneous tissues, or it may be the result of an overly large incision or a partially obstructed tube. Although subcutaneous emphysema is annoying, it is usually not serious and generally clears after several days. If the nurse notices a crackling sensation under the skin of the neck, chest, or face of the patient, it should be reported to the surgeon, because removal of a suture or two may readily correct this problem.

The complications of tracheostomy in infants and children are almost always more serious, because the relative size of the airway is smaller and there is little tolerance for any obstruction.

Emotional support of the patient with a new tracheostomy is important and begins immediately upon the patient regaining consciousness. Even though the patient may have been well prepared with regard to the loss of ability to speak, awakening in that state is still a traumatic event. A pad and pencil should be readily available to allow the patient to communicate.

Laryngectomy

Partial laryngectomy (see Table 23–1) is the surgical treatment of choice for patients with a limited malignant process of the vocal cords. It is commonly performed through a laryngofissure, and tracheostomy is usually performed concomitantly to ensure a good airway during the immediate postoperative period. Post anesthesia nursing care is essentially the same as that for a posttracheostomy patient.

Subcutaneous emphysema is not uncommon postoperatively and should be reported to the surgeon. Laryngectomy patients have trouble swallowing and need frequent suctioning and reassurance.

Supraglottic laryngectomy is performed for carcinoma of the epiglottis and adjacent structures above the level of the true vocal cords. A tracheostomy is mandatory for these patients; they also have a great deal of difficulty swallowing and require close observation and assistance with elimination of saliva and other secretions.

Total laryngectomy is reserved for patients with advanced carcinoma of the true cords. Tracheostomy is always performed. Some means of communication should be established preoperatively for postoperative use.

The primary nursing concern after laryngectomy is maintenance of an adequate airway.

Tracheostomy care, as previously discussed, should be deftly carried out and the air well humidified. In the immediate post anesthesia period, the patients need frequent suctioning not only of the tracheostomy but also of the nose and mouth, because they cannot blow their noses and may have difficulty spitting. Frequent mouth care provides additional comfort, and a petrolatum ointment should be applied to the lips to prevent drying and cracking.

Postoperatively, the patient should be positioned on the side until full consciousness is regained. When conscious, the patient may be positioned in a low semi-Fowler position with the head elevated about 30 degrees. This position promotes drainage, minimizes edema, prevents uncomfortable pressure on suture lines, and facilitates respirations.

Dressings should be checked frequently for excessive drainage and reinforced or changed as necessary. Sometimes, drainage catheters are placed under the wound flaps to remove fluid from the potential dead space left after removal of the larynx and related structures. Drainage catheters must be connected to a constant vacuum source at 40 to 60 mm Hg, and free drainage must be maintained within the system. This may be accomplished by use of a Hemovac drainage device (Fig. 23–12). Excessive bloody drainage should be reported to the surgeon. The most common site of hemorrhage is the base of the tongue.

Laryngectomy patients are frequently very apprehensive upon awakening and should have someone in close attendance at all times. Although patients may be prepared for their loss of voice preoperatively, their first experiences of being voiceless and unable to call for help are always extremely frightening. A bell to ring or other noisemaker is more reassuring in this instance than the routine pencil-and-paper communication system.

RADICAL NECK SURGERY

The radical neck procedure itself is a relatively simple one involving removal of all the subcutaneous fat, lymphatic channels, and some of the superficial muscles within a prescribed area of the neck (Fig. 23–13). Generally, the procedure involves the removal of the sternocleidomastoid muscle, omohyoid muscle, internal and external jugular veins, and all lymphatic tissue on one side of the neck. It is the purposeful resection of the 11th cranial (spinal accessory) nerve that causes atrophy of the large trapezius muscle. In the modified neck dissection, the accessory nerve and the internal jugular vein are spared.

Post anesthesia nursing care of the patient after radical neck surgery is somewhat less demanding than that after laryngectomy, because these patients do not have a tracheostomy and can talk and eat normally. The patient should be placed in a low semi-Fowler position with the head elevated 30 to 45 degrees to improve venous return. Pillows must be used cautiously when patients are positioned to avoid restricting venous return or compressing the bases of pedicle flaps. Venous congestion, when present, gives the patient's face a purplish hue. This hue can be differentiated from cyanosis due to inadequate ventilation by observing the color of the extremities to confirm good circulation and close monitoring of oxygen saturation. Postoperative pain is usually minimal after radical neck dissection and can be managed with the usual analgesics.

Dressings are minimal. Skin flaps are secured over drainage tubes, which should be connected to constant suction at 40 to 60 mm Hg. The suction catheters constantly working under the skin flaps suck them firmly against the neck. Approximately 70 to 120 ml of serosanguineous drainage can be expected the day of operation. This amount drastically decreases the second day and becomes minimal (less than 30 ml) the third day. If the dressing soaks through with blood, the surgeon should be notified immediately.

Edema of the recurrent laryngeal nerve and of the nerves to the pharynx may cause difficulty in swallowing and in expectorating secretions; therefore, frequent, gentle suctioning of oral secretions may be needed. Extreme care must be taken to avoid any trauma to the internal suture lines. A gauze wick placed in the corner of the patient's mouth can alleviate the annoyance of constant dribbling of mucus and saliva. Mouth care is important for the comfort of this patient and can be accomplished by any of the conventional methods.

Complications. Edema of the lower part of the face on the same side as the surgery is to be expected. Lower facial paralysis may occur, owing to injury of the facial nerve during dissection. The most common complication following radical neck dissection is hemorrhage, which is most often the result of inadequate hemostasis in the immediate postoperative period. The most serious complication is rupture of the carotid artery ("carotid blowout"). This is an uncommon event and occurs almost exclusively when radical neck dissection is com-

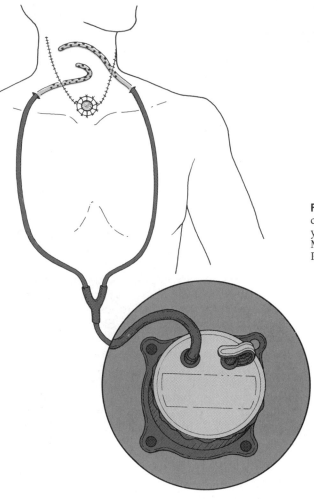

FIGURE 23–12. Use of Hemovac drainage device as a closed suction apparatus and blood receptacle after laryngectomy. (From Ignatavicius, D. D., and Bayne, M. V.: Medical-Surgical Nursing: A Nursing Process Approach. Philadelphia, W. B. Saunders, 1991, p. 1969.)

bined with total laryngectomy. It is more likely to occur in a patient who has had a course of radiation therapy preoperatively or who has a fistula that bathes the carotid artery in secretions. If the danger of a blowout of the carotid artery is present, all personnel should be aware of it and know what to do if it occurs.

If a carotid blowout occurs, digital pressure with gauze pads, bath towels, or anything available should be applied immediately and help summoned. Intravenous fluids must be started immediately if they are not already infusing. Fluids should be administered at an increased rate to replace loss and combat shock. Inflate the cuff on the tracheostomy tube, and perform tracheal suctioning to prevent aspiration of blood. Most important, maintain a patent airway and administer oxygen. Patients on "carotid precautions," that is, those who may experience this complication, should be typed and cross-matched for whole blood, and appropriate emergency equipment, including gauze

pads, vascular clips, and suture ties, should be immediately available at the bedside.

Reconstruction Surgery in Head and Neck Cancer

Any of a large variety of reconstructive procedures may be employed to re-establish both contour and function after the removal of large areas of the head and neck for malignant disease. Skin grafts have largely been replaced with skin flaps or muscle-skin combined flaps that can cover extensive areas both inside and outside the neck. These flaps provide a lining of the throat or mouth and can also replace excised skin on the external surfaces. The commonly used flaps are the pectoralis major muscle–skin unit and the deltopectoral flap, both from the anterior chest area. In rare instances, a free flap may be used. This flap is usually a muscle-skin flap that is moved a long distance

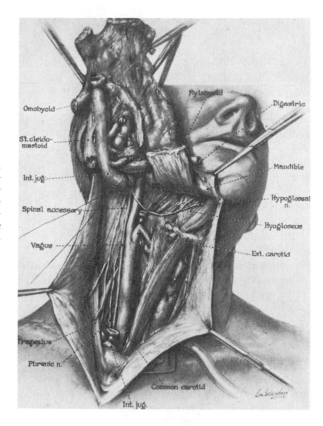

FIGURE 23–13. Drawing showing the extent of the usual radical neck dissection. The specimen is retracted superiorly. As is shown, resection of the posterior belly of the digastric muscle permits high ligation of the internal jugular vein and also facilitates dissection around the hypoglossal nerve. (From Converse, J. M. [ed.]: Reconstructive Plastic Surgery. Vol. 3. Philadelphia, W. B. Saunders, 1964.)

from one area of the body to another. To be successful, this type of flap requires the microsurgical repair of its tiny artery and vein with an artery and vein in its new location. In general, these reconstructive flaps must be free of any pressure or dressings. A light coat of antibacterial ointment is usually applied along the suture lines, and the area is frequently observed for color, warmth, and bleeding. Because these flaps depend on a single small artery and vein, any kinking or external pressure may result in the death of the flap.

MAXILLOFACIAL SURGERY

The care of patients with extensive maxillofacial surgery follows the principles outlined earlier for tracheostomy care and care after laryngectomy or radical neck dissection. The care of these patients is extremely demanding, and attention to detail is the basis for the prevention of complications.

Maxillofacial surgery may be required to correct trauma and fractures or to correct congenital skeletal deformities. Following this type of surgery, the patient will be in intermaxillary fixation (IMF) with his or her jaws wired shut. Care revolves around protection of the airway.

Some additional emergency equipment is required at the bedside of patients who are admitted with IMF, including wire cutters, a suture set, additional nasal airways, small suction catheters, and gauze pads. On admission of the patient, the surgeon should review placement of the IMF wires with the nurse. A line drawing of these wires indicating which ones to cut in case of extreme emergency (e.g., cardiac or respiratory arrest) should be posted at the head of the bed.

Preoperative preparation of the patient undergoing IMF is particularly important and should include instructions on how to clear secretions or remove vomitus while remaining in IMF. The patient should also be taught how to use the suction catheter. These instructions will have to be repeated frequently in the PACU as the patient recovers. Having the jaws wired closed is a frightening experience for any patient, no matter how well prepared that patient is. Blood, emesis, lingual and pharyngeal edema, hematoma formation, or laryngospasm may further compromise the oral airway, which is already obstructed as much as 90 percent by fixation of the jaws. Reassurance is provided by maintaining proximity to the patient, ensuring a means to attract attention, and explaining fully all treatments and procedures.

The patient will arrive in the PACU with a nasotracheal tube in place. Extubation should not be considered until the patient is fully awake and reflexes have returned sufficiently to allow handling of secretions. A soft nasal airway may be inserted following extubation to assist in maintaining a patent airway.

Observe closely for bleeding. Some oozing of blood is normal, but excessive amounts should be reported to the surgeon. Frequent, gentle suctioning with a small catheter assists in keeping the airway clear by removing blood and saliva. The patient may be more comfortable doing this independently when able. It is reassuring to these patients to have a suction catheter in hand for use as necessary.

Vomiting, and subsequent aspiration, is a significant risk for this patient. A nasogastric tube is frequently used to reduce the likelihood of nausea and vomiting. Ensure that it is correctly positioned and patent. Antiemetics should be administered as necessary, and pain should be treated promptly to prevent the development of nausea and vomiting.

Despite all efforts to prevent it, vomiting may occur. If still drowsy, the patient should be turned immediately to the lateral or semi-prone position and the emesis suctioned out via the nose or mouth. If the patient is awake, assist him or her to sit up, lean over, and allow emesis to flow out of the mouth and nose. Retract the cheeks by holding them out with the fingers. Most important, repeat instructions and reassurances quietly but confidently to keep the patient calm. It is rarely necessary to cut the wires.

The patient should be positioned with the head of the bed elevated 30 degrees to assist in maintaining the airway by controlling edema. Ice packs are usually ordered postoperatively to assist in controlling edema and promote comfort. A surgical glove partially filled with cracked ice can be used, or ice collars can be molded to the jaws, chin, or nose. Iced saline gauze pads may be applied to the eyes.

Petrolatum ointment or other emollient cream should be applied to the lips and corners of the mouth to relieve tenderness and prevent drying and cracking. Dental wax can be molded and applied to protruding wires, which are quite irritating to the oral mucosa.

When the patient is fully awake and protective reflexes have sufficiently returned, rinsing the mouth with warm saline will provide additional comfort. The patient may then also have small sips of liquids.

References

1. Arnet, G., and Basehore, L. M.: Dentofacial reconstruction. Am. J. Nurs., 84(12):1488–1490, 1984.
2. Balkany, T. J.: The Cochlear Implant. Otolaryngol. Clin. North Am., 19:217–449, 1986.
3. Ball, K. A.: Lasers: The Perioperative Challenge. St. Louis, C. V. Mosby, 1990.
4. Darvich-Kodjouri, C.: Nursing care of the patient with a new tracheostomy. Curr. Rev. Recov. Room Nurses, 3(7):18–23, 1985.
5. Frost, C. M., and Frost, D. E.: Nursing care of patients in intermaxillary fixation. Heart Lung, 12(5):524–528, 1983.
6. Gotta, A.: Airway management for maxillofacial trauma. Curr. Rev. Post Anesth. Nurses, 10(5):34–39, 1988.
7. Litwack, K., and Zeplin, K.: Practical points in the management of laryngospasm. J. Post Anesth. Nurs., 4(1):36–39, 1989.
8. Lyons, R. J., and Coren, D. A.: The head and neck patient. AORN J., 40(5):751–760, 1984.
9. Mapp, C.: Trach care: Are you aware of all the dangers? Nursing 88, 18(7):34–43, 1988.
10. Patton, C.: The critical airway. Curr. Rev. Post Anesth. Nurses, 13(5):35–39, 1991.
11. Rook, J. L., and Rook, M.: Head and neck cancer. J. Post Anesth. Nurs., 4(6):263–277, 1989.
12. Saunders, W. H., Havener, W. H., Keith, C. F., et al.: Nursing Care in Eye, Ear, Nose, and Throat Disorders. St. Louis, C. V. Mosby, 1979.
13. Smalley, P. J.: Lasers in otolaryngology. Nurs. Clin. North Am., 25(3):645–655, 1990.

Post Anesthesia Care of the Ophthalmic Surgical Patient

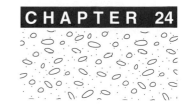

CHAPTER 24

Carolyn Zehren, R.N., C.P.A.N.

The assessment and care of patients who have had surgery on their eyes are always a challenge for the post anesthesia care unit (PACU) nurse. As with all other types of patients, the PACU nurse must consider not only the elements of surgery performed but the whole patient. Eye surgery is performed on patients of all ages. The special precautions that apply to specific age groups must therefore be taken into account. For the elderly patient, it is wise to keep in mind that those who need an operation on the eyes may also have hypertension, cancer, diabetes, emphysema, or congestive heart failure. In addition, the PACU nurse's assessment and care of the ophthalmic patient are greatly influenced by the type of anesthesia used intraoperatively.

Many eye surgical procedures are performed under local anesthesia and are increasingly being performed as day surgery. Cataract surgery, after which few restrictions are necessary, is often performed on an outpatient basis. Postoperative care instructions should be discussed with the patient and a significant other both preoperatively and postoperatively. Instructions should also be written so that they may be reviewed as necessary after discharge. Special care of the patient undergoing day surgery is outlined in Chapter 37.

The anatomy of the normal eye is shown in Figure 24–1.

Definitions

Blepharoplasty: surgical removal of a segment of skin from the eyelid.

Cataract: an opacity of the lens. Surgical treatment consists of removal of the lens.

Chalazion: a chronic granulomatous inflammation of one or more of the meibomian glands in the tarsal plate of the eyelid. Surgical treatment consists of incision and curettage.

Dacryocystitis: infection of the lacrimal sac.

Dacryocystorhinostomy: creation of a new pathway from the lacrimal sac to the nasal cavity.

Dermatochalasis: relaxation of the skin of the eyelid due to atrophy. Surgical treatment is blepharoplasty.

Ectropion: eversion of the margin of the eyelid. Surgical treatment is to shorten the lower lid in a horizontal direction.

Entropion: inversion of the margin of the eyelid; usually affects the lower lid but may affect the upper lid. Surgical treatment involves either removing a base triangle of skin, muscle, and tarsus and suturing the edges together to evert the lid margin or exposing the orbicular muscle, dividing it, and suturing it to the lower border of the tarsus.

Enucleation: removal of the entire eyeball after the eye muscles and optic nerve have been severed.

Epiphora: excess tearing; may be caused by blocked lacrimal drainage system. Surgical treatment for epiphora and dacryocystitis caused by blockage is probing of the lacrimal duct.

Evisceration of the eye: removal of the contents of the eye, leaving the sclera intact and the muscles attached to the sclera.

Exenteration of the eye: removal of all orbital contents.

Glaucoma: a disease of the eye characterized by increased intraocular pressure. Surgical treatment is aimed at establishing an evacuation route for outflow of aqueous fluid.

Goniotomy: surgery for congenital glaucoma wherein the trabecular meshwork is incised.

Intraocular lens (IOL) implant: synthetic lens used to replace the crystalline lens after cataract surgery (Fig. 24–2).

Iridectomy: removal of a section of iris tissue (Fig. 24–3).

Keratoplasty: corneal transplant (Fig. 24–4).

Plaque: a localized patch that is tailored to the size and extent of the tumor, onto which io-

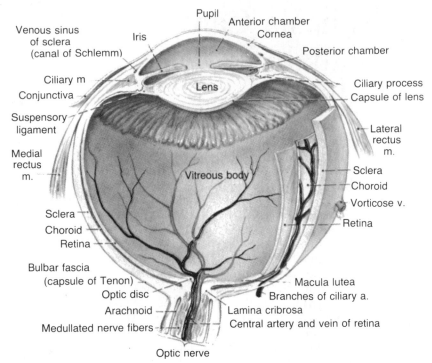

FIGURE 24–1. Anatomy of the normal eye. A midsagittal section through the eyeball shows the layers of the retina and the blood supply. (From Jacob, S. W., Francone, C. A., and Lossow, W. J.: Structure and Function in Man. 5th ed. Philadelphia, W. B. Saunders, 1982, p. 331.)

dine seeds are attached; it is then surgically applied to the sclera over the tumor.

Pterygium: a fleshy triangular encroachment on the cornea. Surgical treatment is by excision.

Ptosis: drooping of the upper eyelid. Surgical treatment involves either elevating the lid with a sling or shortening the levator muscle of the lid (levator resection).

Retinopexy: surgical correction of retinal detachment (Fig. 24–5) by sealing the hole. Sealing is accomplished by causing scar formation with heat, electrical current, or cold.

Scleral buckle: surgical correction of a retinal detachment by compression of the sclera to rejoin the underlying retinal pigment epithelium to the detached sensory retina; used in conjunction with retinopexy.

Strabismus: condition in which the eyes are not simultaneously directed toward the same object. *Esotropia* is inward deviation of the eyes, and *exotropia* is outward deviation. Surgical treatment involves changing the relative strength of individual muscles either by resection (the shortening of a muscle by removal of part of the tendon) or by recession (the surgical transfer of a muscle insertion backward from the original attachment on the eye).

Trabeculectomy: creation of a drainage channel from the anterior chamber to the subconjunctival space; used to treat intractable glaucoma.

Vitrectomy: surgical removal of vitreous from the eye, usually to clear opacified vitreous for better visualization or to sever vitreous traction bands (Fig. 24–6).

ANESTHESIA

Ophthalmic procedures are often performed under local anesthesia, and many patients are treated in the day care or ambulatory surgical center. For cooperative adult patients, local anesthesia is generally preferred to avert the restlessness and nausea or vomiting that may occur after general anesthesia. Infants, children, uncooperative or particularly anxious patients, and psychotic persons usually require general anesthesia. General anesthesia is also indicated when a local anesthetic might accentuate an eye problem; when surgery is to be performed on a lacerated cornea, ruptured globe, or optic nerve decompression; or when the surgery planned is extensive, as in enucleation or evisceration. The ophthalmic patient who has undergone general anesthesia must be assessed and cared for as previously described for pa-

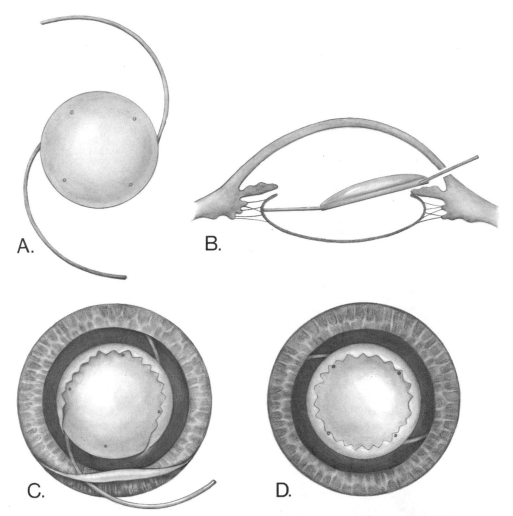

FIGURE 24–2. Simcoe C-loop posterior chamber lens (intraocular lens) *(A)* with "in-the-bag" insertion technique *(B through D)*. (From Spaeth, G. L.: Ophthalmic Surgery: Principles and Practice. 2nd ed. Philadelphia, W. B. Saunders, 1990, p. 166.)

tients undergoing general anesthesia. The special precaution for these patients is that modifications in care must be made to prevent stress on the eyes and surrounding musculature (see Fig. 24–1).

PACU CARE

Positioning

The patient usually arrives in the PACU awake, and the nurse should begin to orient the patient as soon as he or she enters the PACU. It is particularly important to warn the patient when he or she is about to be moved and to prepare the patient for being touched to avoid any startle reflexes. Every caution should be observed when the patient is transferred from stretcher to bed to avoid bumping and

jarring. Movement should be kept to a minimum and should be slow and smooth. To prevent pressure on the operated eye, the patient should be positioned on his or her back or on the unaffected side. The patient who has had vitreoretinal surgery may require special positioning of the head to allow proper approximation and healing of the retina. The surgeon should provide explicit positioning instructions for all special cases. The patient assumes this position when fully recovered from the anesthetic.

If the patient has had only one eye operated on or has only one eye bandaged, it is important to determine just how much sight exists in the unaffected eye before a plan of care is formulated. It is not safe to assume that the patient can see with the unoperated eye. One may choose to patch the unaffected eye to remind the nursing personnel that this is a sightless

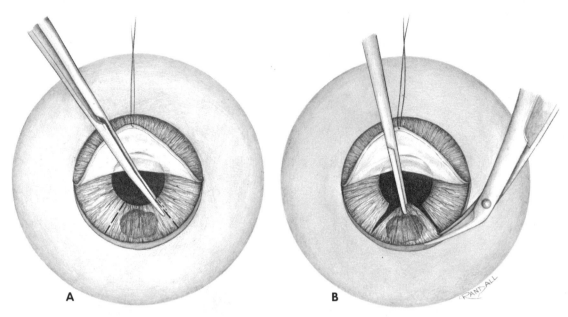

FIGURE 24–3. Technique of sector iridectomy for iris tumor. *A*, a limbal incision has been made for 180 degrees, and two radial cuts are made from the pupillary margin to the iris root *(dotted lines)*. *B*, after the radial incisions are done, the iris is cut at its base to free it from the anterior portion of the ciliary body. (*A* and *B* from Spaeth, G. L.: Ophthalmic Surgery: Principles and Practice. 2nd ed. Philadelphia, W. B. Saunders, 1990, p. 714.)

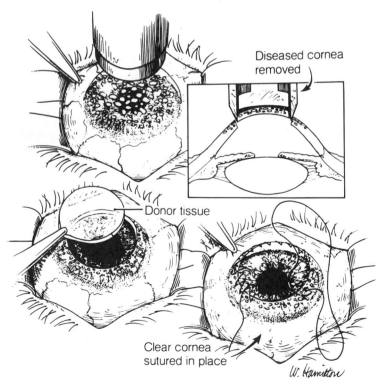

Diseased cornea removed

Donor tissue

Clear cornea sutured in place

FIGURE 24–4. Corneal transplant surgery. *Upper,* the diseased cornea is removed. *Lower,* the donor corneal tissue is placed in the opening and is sewn in place using a very fine suture. (Courtesy of the Department of Medical Illustration and Audio Visual Education, Baylor College of Medicine, Houston, TX.)

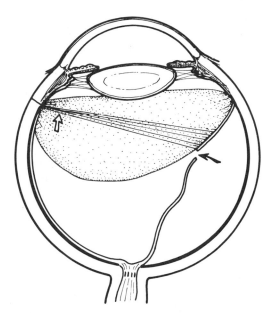

FIGURE 24–5. Retinal detachment following penetrating injury. The break *(thin arrow)* is caused by contraction of fibrovascular tissue that has proliferated from the entry wound *(open arrow).* (From Spaeth, G. L.: Ophthalmic Surgery: Principles and Practice. 2nd ed. Philadelphia, W. B. Saunders, 1990, p. 413.)

patient who requires additional care. The nurse should tell the patient exactly what to expect and what is expected of him or her.

Cardiorespiratory Assessment and Care

Assessment of the cardiorespiratory system should proceed as described in other chapters.

Vital signs should be assessed, and the stir-up regimen should be started. The challenge is in keeping the patient's lungs clear without increasing intraocular pressure. Deep rhythmic breaths at frequent intervals assist in the prevention of atelectasis. The nurse should spend more time than usual coaching this type of patient in deep inspirations because coughing must be avoided. If the patient feels the urge to cough, help him or her concentrate on breathing, which may help dispel that feeling. Sucking on ice chips, throat lozenges, or hard candy may soothe the throat and prevent coughing. In some instances, codeine, meperidine (Demerol), or an antitussive suspension may be administered to control coughs. If coughing does occur and cannot be controlled, the surgeon must be notified.

Vomiting, sneezing, straining, or any exertion on the part of the patient may increase intraocular pressure, which may be damaging to the affected eye. These reactions must therefore be avoided, if at all possible. As a precaution against the development of nausea and vomiting after general anesthesia, oral fluids and diet are routinely delayed for a brief period. Ophthalmologists routinely order an antiemetic drug as needed for the first 24 hours after surgery. The patient should be instructed to alert the nurse immediately if he or she begins to feel nauseated so that an antiemetic such as prochlorperazine (Compazine), trimethobenzamide (Tigan), or dimenhydrinate (Dramamine) can be administered without delay. In addition, deep breathing and sucking on ice chips or hard candy may help alleviate nausea. If vomiting occurs in spite of these interventions, the surgeon should be notified. Pain

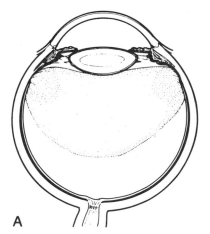
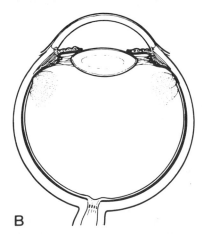

FIGURE 24–6. A, simple vitreous hemorrhage with complete posterior vitreous detachment. B, central vitreous removed by vitrectomy. (A and B from Spaeth, G. L.: Ophthalmic Surgery: Principles and Practice. 2nd ed. Philadelphia, W. B. Saunders, 1990, p. 405.)

accompanied by nausea and vomiting may indicate intraocular hemorrhage, which requires immediate intervention by the ophthalmologist.

The exertion of hard crying, often a problem with children and infants, must be prevented. Some children respond well to being held by the nurse. All infants and children should be assessed for pain and medicated depending on their age, surgical procedure performed, and severity of pain.

No patient should be restrained, because exertion against the restraints increases intraocular pressure. In some instances, in both children and adults, tranquilizers may be required to ensure patient cooperation and a smooth recovery course.

Pain Management

Pain is uncommon after most eye surgery. The eye is usually quite comfortable, owing to the intraoperative use of topical steroids and cholinergic blockers, such as atropine, which paralyze the ciliary muscle. In addition, medications in ointment form are often applied to the eye prior to patching. These ointments soothe the eye and promote comfort.

Complaints of itching, scratchy or grating feelings, or a "pins and needles" sensation should be interpreted as pain and treated as such. Eye discomfort that may occur with more common ophthalmic procedures can usually be controlled with acetaminophen (Tylenol), propoxyphene hydrochloride (Darvon), and similar analgesics.

Patients undergoing vitreoretinal procedures may experience significant pain. The administration of narcotic analgesia as well as the application of ice packs to the operative site should control the pain. If meperidine, codeine phosphate, or other opiates are necessary for pain relief, they should be used in conjunction with an antiemetic, because they frequently cause nausea and subsequent vomiting when used alone. Significant pain that is not relieved with the prescribed analgesics is so unusual that investigation by the surgeon is warranted.

Dressings

Dressings are often not required, especially after relatively minor procedures or plastic ophthalmic surgery. Hemorrhage or excessive discharge is uncommon. A slight, blood-tinged, watery discharge from the eyes is not unusual and may be gently wiped from the face, taking care not to apply pressure to the eye. Although an infrequent occurrence, hemorrhage may be a problem after enucleation, exenteration, or orbital surgery. If bleeding occurs in the PACU, the surgeon may be able to control it with pressure, but in some instances, the patient may have to return to the operating room.

Frequently, one or both of the eyes are bandaged. If bandages are present, these should not be disturbed. The patient must be prevented from disturbing the bandage or inadvertently rubbing the eyes.

Following enucleation, a firm pressure dressing is applied for 24 hours. An alternative to enucleation for treatment of ocular tumors is the use of iodine plaque irradiation. The iodine plaque is sutured over the base of the tumor under local anesthesia. The plaque remains in place for a calculated amount of time, depending on the strength of the iodine plaque and the size of the tumor. A lead shield is placed over the operative eye to protect the health care personnel and visitors from radiation exposure (Fig. 24–7). Whenever both eyes are bandaged,

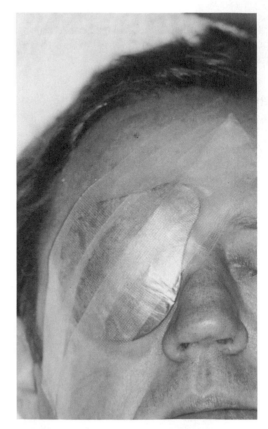

FIGURE 24–7. Patient with a lead shield after surgical application of iodine plaque. (Courtesy of Wills Eye Hospital, Philadelphia, PA.)

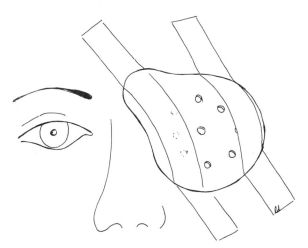

FIGURE 24–8. Plastic eye shield. (Courtesy of Wills Eye Hospital, Philadelphia, PA.)

extra care must be taken to orient the patient and to provide reassurance. Frequently, plastic eye shields are placed over the dressing as an additional protection for the eye (Fig. 24–8). Dressings should not be changed unless ordered by the surgeon, and if accidentally dislodged, they should be replaced and the physician notified. The tape used to hold eye patches or shields in place should not extend to the maxilla, because movement of the jaw may cause disruption of the dressing.

Psychological Aspects of Care

Caring for the patient who has undergone ophthalmic surgery requires not only physical assessment skills but also a great deal of sensitivity to the meaning of sight and a creative approach to promoting comfort and preventing complications.

The post anesthesia care of the patient who has undergone eye surgery involves a great deal of empathy and reassurance. Our eyes and the sense of sight are precious—when sight is threatened by disease or surgery, we are understandably anxious and apprehensive. Injuries, particularly those produced by imbedded foreign bodies, may provoke even greater anxiety for the patient who often goes to surgery with the prognosis for visual acuity completely unknown. It is important that the PACU nurse be armed with factual information from the surgeon about expectations for the patient so that reassurances offered are realistic. In addition, the PACU nurse must be prepared to provide significant support through both verbal communication and touch.

References

1. Boyd-Monk, H., and Steinmetz, C. G. III: Nursing Care of the Eye. East Norwalk, CT, Appleton & Lange, 1987.
2. Clanton, C., and Means, M. E.: Quality and appropriateness of care. J. Ophthal. Nurs. Technol., 7(4):130–133, 1988.
3. Duane, T. D.: Ophthalmic Surgery, vol. 5. In Clinical Ophthalmology. Hagerstown, MD, Harper & Row, 1980.
4. Hill, B. J.: Sensory information, behavioral instructions, and coping with sensory alteration surgery. Nurs. Res., 31(1):17–21, 1982.
5. Hirschman, H.: Intraocular lens implantation: Faster, more complete rehabilitation of the cataract patient. J. Am. Geriatr. Soc., 25(1):35–38, 1977.
6. Kornzweig, A. L.: New ideas for old eyes. J. Am. Geriatr. Soc., 28(4):145–152, 1980.
7. Marta, M.: A guide to the posterior vitrectomy. Today's OR Nurse, 5(1):26–29, 69, 1983.
8. Moore, C. R.: Scleral buckling for retinal detachment. AORN J., 36(3):495–506, 1982.
9. Murphy, S. B., and Donderi, D. C.: Predicting the success of cataract surgery. J. Behav. Med., 3(1):1–14, 1980.
10. Saunders, W. H., Havener, W. H., Keith, C. F., et al.: Nursing Care in Eye, Ear, Nose, and Throat Disorders. 4th ed. St. Louis, C. V. Mosby, 1979.
11. Shields, J. A., and Shields, C. L: Intraocular Tumors: A Text and Atlas. Philadelphia, W. B. Saunders, 1992.
12. Shipley, S. B.: Patient teaching and day care anesthesia. Focus, 9(4):14–16, 1982.
13. Smith, J. F., and Nachazel, D. P.: Ophthalmic Nursing. Boston, Little, Brown, 1980.
14. Whitton, S.: Penetrating keratoplasty: The gift of sight. Today's OR Nurse, 5(1):20–24, 72, 1983.
15. Zack, P. L., and Smirnow, I. H.: IOL implantation. Today's OR Nurse, 5(1):12–18, 68, 1983.

Post Anesthesia Care of the Thoracic Surgical Patient

Thoracic surgery involves procedures on the structures contained within the chest cavity, including the lungs, heart, great vessels, and esophagus. In this chapter, discussion primarily centers on surgical procedures performed on the lungs. Detailed instructions are given on the care of the patient following the insertion of chest tubes, because any time the thoracic cavity is entered, chest tubes are required to re-expand the lungs and allow healing of the chest wall to occur. Specific post anesthesia care following cardiac surgery is discussed in Chapter 26; care following surgery of the great vessels is discussed in Chapter 27; and care following surgery of the esophagus is discussed in Chapter 31.

Surgical procedures on the lungs involve diagnostic procedures as well as the removal of tumors, or diseased parts, or all of the lung. In addition, thoracic surgery may be performed to correct congenital or acquired chest wall injuries and to repair traumatic damage to the lung.

Definitions

Atelectasis: collapse of the alveoli, caused primarily by obstruction of the lower airways. Obstruction is most commonly caused by the accumulation of respiratory secretions, although it may be caused by tumors, bronchospasm, foreign bodies, or any other form of obstruction.

Bronchoscopy: visualization of the tracheobronchial tree by use of a lighted scope (Figs. 25–1 to 25–3).

Chylothorax: collection of lymph in the pleural space. Although a rare occurrence, this condition can develop following chest trauma or surgical procedures performed through the pleural space on mediastinal structures.

Decortication (of the lung): removal of fibrinous deposits or restrictive membranes on the pleural lining that interfere with ventilatory action.

Hemothorax: a collection of blood or serosanguineous fluid, or both, within the pleural cavity (Fig. 25–4).

Lobectomy: removal of one or more lobes of the lung.

Mediastinoscopy: visualization of lymph nodes or tumors at the tracheobronchial junction, subcarina, or upper lobe bronchi via a lighted scope. This is done by passing the mediastinoscope through a small incision at the suprasternal area and then down along the anterior course of the trachea.

Pectus excavatum: (trichterbrust or chonechondrosternon): a structural defect, usually congenital, of the anterior thoracic wall, characterized by a posterior depression of the sternum; also called a *funnel chest*.

Pneumonectomy: removal of the lung.

Pneumothorax: collection of air or gas within the pleural cavity (see Fig. 25–4).

Segmental resection of the lung: excision of individual bronchovascular segments of the lobe of the lung with ligation of segmental branches of the pulmonary artery and vein and division of the segmental bronchus.

Sternotomy: incision through the sternum.

Thoracentesis: insertion of a needle through the chest wall into the pleural space to remove either fluid or air.

Thoracoplasty: removal of ribs or portions of the ribs to reduce the size of the thoracic space and to collapse a diseased lung.

Thoracotomy: incision into the chest cavity. Closed thoracotomy (intercostal drainage) is the insertion of a drain (i.e., catheter, chest tube, or thoracotomy tube) through the intercostal space to establish drainage of accumulated air or fluid from the pleural cavity and to restore the normal negative pressure of the pleural space.

Wedge resection: the excision of a small, wedge-shaped section from the peripheral portion of a lobe of the lung.

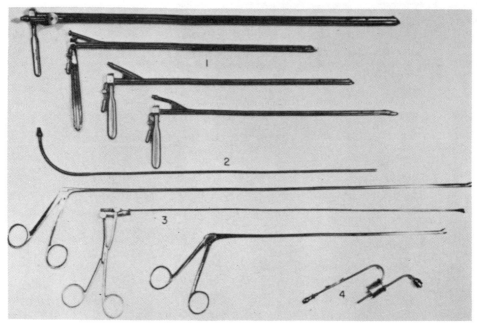

FIGURE 25–1. Rigid bronchoscope. (From DeWeese, D. D., and Saunders, W. H.: Textbook of Otolaryngology. St. Louis, C. V. Mosby, 1968.)

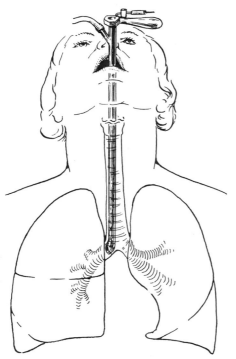

FIGURE 25–2. Diagram of a bronchoscope in place. Note that during bronchoscopy the patient's hair and eyes would be covered. (From DeWeese, D. D., and Saunders, W. H.: Textbook of Otolaryngology. St. Louis, C. V. Mosby, 1968.)

INVASIVE DIAGNOSTIC PROCEDURES

Invasive diagnostic procedures involving the thoracic cavity include bronchoscopy, mediastinoscopy, thoracentesis, and needle biopsy. In addition to being diagnostic, these procedures may be therapeutic. They may be performed at the bedside, in a special procedures room, or in the operating suite, depending on the urgency of the procedure, the reason it is being performed, and the condition of the patient.

Bronchoscopy

Bronchoscopy is performed to visualize the structures of the tracheobronchial tree; to remove secretions, washings, mucus plugs, or foreign bodies; to perform a tissue biopsy; or to apply medication. Bronchoscopy may also be performed to accomplish bronchography, which involves the instillation of a radiopaque medium into the tracheobronchial tree, making it visible on radiograph. Laser therapy is also used with bronchoscopy. Ablation of tracheal and bronchial obstructions can be accomplished by using a laser beam in conjunction

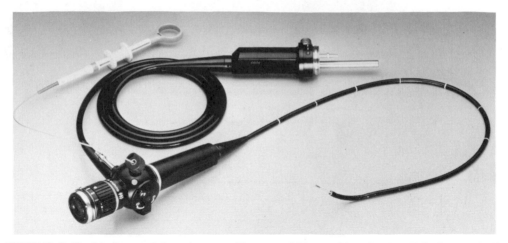

FIGURE 25-3. Flexible fiber-optic bronchoscope. (Courtesy of Olympus America, Inc., Lake Success, NY.)

with a bronchoscope. Carbon dioxide and neodymium-YAG lasers are the laser sources most frequently used in these techniques.

Bronchoscopy can be performed with either topical or general anesthesia. The choice is determined by the patient's condition and the anesthetist's preference. Prior to the procedure, the patient is required to abstain from liquids for at least 6 hours. Premedication generally consists of midazolam. Preprocedure patient education and instructions should include these routines, as well as a brief description of and rationale for the procedure itself.

If a topical anesthesia is used, 4 percent lidocaine hydrochloride (Xylocaine) solution is sprayed or instilled into the pharyngeal and laryngeal areas. Other agents that can be used include tetracaine hydrochloride (Pontocaine) and hexylcaine hydrochloride (Cyclaine). Toxic reactions can occur with any of these agents, and emergency equipment should be available. If general anesthesia is used, propofol (Diprivan) for induction followed by the administration of narcotics and a muscle relaxant is the preferred technique.

On return to the post anesthesia care unit (PACU), the patient is placed flat in the side-lying position or on his or her side with the head of the bed raised 20 to 30 degrees. Nursing observations and care are directed toward maintenance of a patent airway. The patient must be carefully observed for the development of laryngeal edema or laryngospasm, either of which requires prompt action to restore an open airway. Intubation equipment, along with an emergency tracheostomy tray, must be immediately available. The application of a light crushed-ice collar and the administration of warmed, humidified oxygen help prevent the development of edema and promote comfort.

The patient must be given nothing by mouth until the pharyngeal and laryngeal reflexes have returned (after 2 to 8 hours). Once the gag reflex has fully returned, the patient may gargle with warmed saline or suck on anesthetic throat lozenges to relieve the sore throat that is inevitable following bronchoscopy. Patients should be advised to rest their voices and to avoid coughing or clearing their throats. After

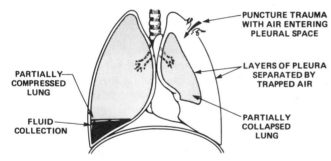

FIGURE 25-4. Schematic representation of a hemothorax versus a pneumothorax.

the gag reflex has returned, fluids and soft foods are allowed as desired and tolerated.

If a needle biopsy was also performed, the patient must be observed for bleeding. Sputum that is pink tinged or streaked with blood can be expected following this procedure; however, grossly bloody sputum or coughing up of frank blood should be reported. Subcutaneous emphysema or dyspnea indicates perforation of the trachea or bronchus. Pain experienced in this area may be mistaken by the patient for heartburn. If any of these symptoms is present, the patient must be given nothing by mouth and the physician notified immediately.

Mediastinoscopy

Care following mediastinoscopy is similar to that after bronchoscopy, although general anesthesia is almost always used for this procedure. A small dressing is placed over the stab wound and should be inspected for any drainage.

Thoracentesis

Thoracentesis is performed to remove air or fluid from the pleural space to relieve lung compression or for diagnostic purposes. Fluid removed is evaluated for chemical, bacteriologic, and cellular composition. Thoracentesis is almost always performed at the bedside with only local anesthesia.

Post-thoracentesis care includes positioning the patient in the side-lying position on the unoperated side and observing for complications, which are rare. The thoracentesis site is sealed with a small piece of petrolatum-impregnated gauze, and a sterile dressing is applied. The site should be checked for drainage.

A decreasing blood pressure along with an increasing pulse rate may indicate the development of shock due to hemorrhage from a damaged blood vessel and should be reported. This is most likely to occur when large amounts of fluid are removed; the patient must also be observed for symptoms indicating mediastinal shift, including pallor or cyanosis, dyspnea, increased respiratory and pulse rates, and a deviation of the larynx and trachea from their normal midline position in the neck. Mediastinal shift is a serious complication and must be reported at once. Compression of the great vessels and decreased blood return to the heart compromise the cardiorespiratory system

quickly, so mediastinal shift must be corrected without delay.

Hemoptysis, vertigo, syncope, decreased blood pressure, increased pulse rate, uncontrollable or persistent cough, dyspnea, cyanosis, tightness in the chest, and subcutaneous emphysema alone or in combination are danger signs and indicate damage to the lung that could result in pneumothorax, tension pneumothorax, or the reaccumulation of fluid in the intrapleural space. If any of these distress symptoms develops, the physician should be notified immediately and preparations made for the insertion of thoracotomy tubes and the institution of closed chest drainage.

Needle Biopsy

Needle biopsy may be performed to remove tissue specimens from the pleura or lungs for diagnostic purposes. Needle biopsy is generally performed with only local anesthesia, and care is essentially the same as that following thoracentesis. Complications are infrequent, but the patient should be observed closely over several hours for signs and symptoms of damage to the lungs.

CHEST TUBES AND CLOSED CHEST DRAINAGE

Surgery on the structures of the chest involves entrance into the thoracic cavity and the creation of a pneumothorax (atmospheric air admitted into the pleural cavity and collapse of the lung) under controlled conditions. General endotracheal anesthesia is required. Endotracheal anesthesia allows the anesthetist to control fully both inspiration and expiration as the lung is ventilated on the unoperated side.

The surgical approach to the chest cavity may be made through a median incision in the sternum (sternotomy) or through variously placed lateral thoracic incisions through a rib or between two ribs (Fig. 25–5). Resective surgery on the lung is approached by way of a posterolateral parascapular incision through the fourth, fifth, sixth, or seventh intercostal space or an anterior incision through the third, fourth, or fifth intercostal space. Generally, less pain and disability result from the anterior approach.

Indications and Method of Insertion

Following thoracotomy (except after pneumonectomy), the surgeon strategically places

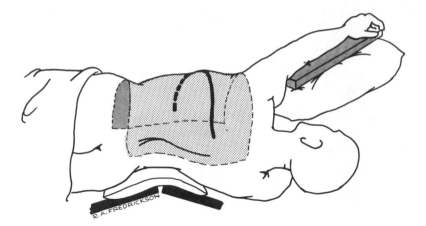

FIGURE 25–5. Position for a left thoracotomy, a standard thoracotomy incision, and extent of the prep. (From LeMaitie, G. D., and Finnegan, J. A.: The Patient in Surgery. 3rd ed. Philadelphia, W. B. Saunders, 1975, p. 406.)

large chest tubes in the intrapleural space to remove air and blood or other accumulated fluid, to restore the normal negative pressure, and to allow re-expansion of the lung on the operative side. Contrary to popular belief, care of the patient with chest tubes is logical and follows simple principles. The reader is advised to review the principles of normal ventilatory mechanics as discussed in Chapter 6 if necessary.

Chest tubes are placed after thoracic surgery to remove both air and fluid. Because blood or other fluids are heavier than air, they tend to accumulate in the lower portion of the pleural space, with air tending to accumulate in the upper portion. Therefore, usually two chest tubes are placed through the chest wall by way of stab wounds or the incision: one for fluid and one for air. An upper or anterior chest tube

is placed anteriorly in the second intercostal space to allow for air removal. A lower or posterior chest tube is positioned in the sixth to eighth intercostal space just anterior to the postaxillary line to allow for drainage of fluid from the pleural space (Fig. 25–6). Occasionally, two lower or posterior chest tubes are used to drain fluid. The two posterior chest tubes are positioned in the same intercostal space approximately 4 cm apart. This decreases postoperative pain for the patient and minimizes intercostal damage.

As the surgeon places the chest tubes and closes the chest, the anesthetist mechanically expands the lung of the operated side as fully as possible. The chest tubes are sutured to the patient's skin and also securely taped with regular cloth adhesive to prevent accidental removal (Fig. 25–7). Because regular cloth adhesive can cause skin breakdown, it is advisable to place Stomahesive on the skin around the chest tube site and then to place the tape over the Stomahesive. Because the chest tube is inserted between two ribs, any back-and-forth movement of the tube against the insertion site can be painful. Making sure that the tube is anchored with an appropriate dressing is therefore essential to minimize the patient's discomfort. Each chest tube is then connected to its appropriate drainage system. These systems are sterile and must remain so until the tubes are removed.

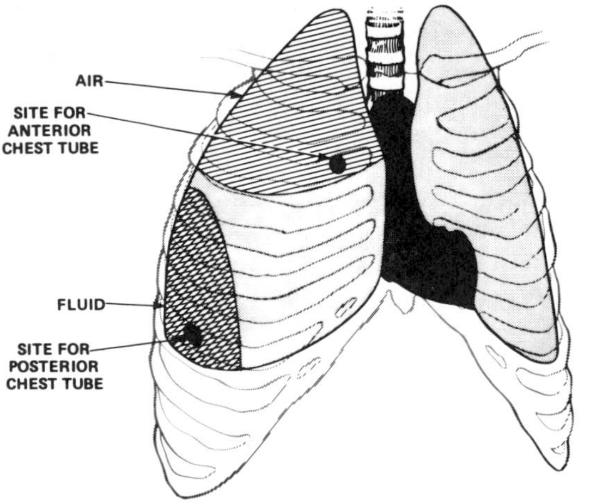

FIGURE 25–6. Because air rises to the top of the cavity, chest tube placement for treatment of a pneumothorax is at the second intercostal space, close to the sternum. Chest tube placement for fluid removal is generally at the level of the 6–8 lateral intercostal space, because this is where fluid will collect.

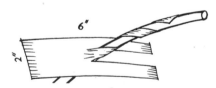

FIGURE 25–7. Taping the chest tube. (From Sutton, A. L.: Bedside Nursing Techniques in Medicine and Surgery. 2nd ed. Philadelphia, W. B. Saunders, 1969, p. 226.)

Types of Drainage Systems

The purpose of chest tube drainage systems is to provide a means by which air and fluid can be removed from the intrapleural space. Once air and fluid are removed, the visceral and parietal pleurae are brought back together and the pressure in the intrapleural space becomes negative once again. Evacuation of air and fluid is facilitated by three forces: positive pressure, gravity, and suction. The trapped air itself in the intrapleural space creates the positive pressure. As long as it is present, it facilitates the functioning of the chest tube system by helping draw air into the system. Gravity assists primarily in fluid evacuation; suction, when applied, assists in removing both air and fluid. All systems use these three forces to varying degrees to assist in re-expanding the lung.

One-way drainage systems primarily depend on the forces of positive pressure and gravity. Figure 25–8 illustrates a one-bottle water-seal drainage system. Air and fluid pushed from the patient's chest by positive pressure facilitated by gravity drainage enters the water-sealed tube. The tube is generally immersed in 1 to 2 cm of water. The force of the patient's exhalation pushes air out through the bottom of the tube. The air then bubbles to the surface and can escape into the atmosphere via the other outlet. During inhalation, air is prevented from entering the tube by the water sealing it. During inhalation, water rises in the water-sealed tube, owing to the suction that inhala-

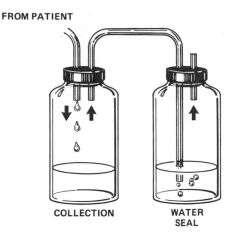

FROM PATIENT

COLLECTION   WATER SEAL

FIGURE 25–9. A two-bottle water-seal drainage system in which one bottle collects fluid and the other serves as a water seal.

tion produces. How deeply the tube is submerged plays a role in how difficult it is for the patient to push air through the water seal—the more deeply the tube is submerged, the more difficult it is. This, then, is perhaps not the best system to use if the patient has significant fluid accumulation, because this will increase the level of submersion of the tube. If this occurs, the bottle needs to be emptied at frequent intervals, or a second bottle can be attached (Fig. 25–9). With this setup, the water-sealed tube is in the second bottle. This system is particularly useful for fluid collection. Again, both of these systems work owing to the forces of positive pressure and gravity. Another one-way system is the Heimlich valve (Fig. 25–10). This is a sterile plastic disposable device that employs a rubber diaphragm to act as a one-way valve. This device is not commonly used in the PACU but rather replaces the water-seal system 2 or 3 days postoperatively, when patient activity is

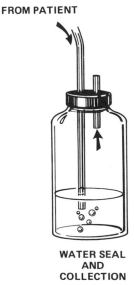

FROM PATIENT

WATER SEAL
AND
COLLECTION

FIGURE 25–8. A one-bottle water-seal drainage system.

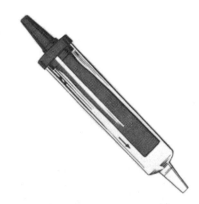

FIGURE 25–10. B. P. Heimlich chest drainage valve. (Courtesy of Becton, Dickinson and Co., Rutherford, NJ.)

increased and mobility is hampered by the cumbersome water-seal system. The valve is not gravity dependent and functions in any position.

Suction

Suction is the third force that can facilitate fluid and air removal and can be added to both the one- and the two-bottle systems. The purpose of the suction is to lower the pressure over the surface of the fluid in the water-seal system. By doing this, the pressure of the water that the patient must displace to force air out through the water seal is decreased. Suction requires adding another bottle to the current system for suction control (Fig. 25–11). The suction control bottle is attached to the water-seal bottle via the air vents. The suction control bottle also has one outlet that is attached to the suction source and another inlet for air, called the *manometer tube*. When the suction is applied, bubbles are created at the bottom of the manometer tube. When the manometer tube is pushed up close to the surface of the fluid, the suction exerted against the patient's pleural space decreases, because most of the suction

can pull in atmospheric air through the tube. In this instance, it is harder for the patient to exhale. As the manometer tube is submerged to a greater depth, the suction exerted on the patient's pleural space increases and exhalation is easier. Orders usually request that 20 cm of negative pressure be applied to the system. In this instance the manometer tube should be submerged 20 cm below the water level in the control bottle. The suction machine or wall vacuum outlet is, of course, also set to produce 20 cm of negative pressure. If a wall vacuum outlet is used, a valve and meter must be connected between the outlet and the water-seal bottle to control the suction.

Immediate PACU Care

As soon as the patient is returned to the PACU, the chest tubes are attached to water-seal drainage if this has not already been accomplished in the operating room. All connections are inspected to ensure that they are secure and airtight. (All connections must be airtight so that the system will work properly.) The connections should be wrapped with adhesive tape as double protection against air

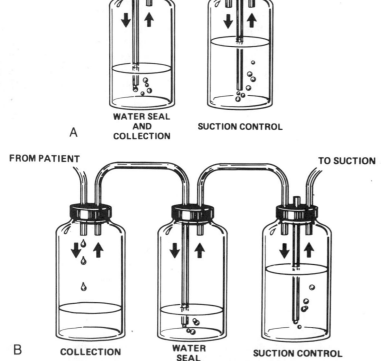

A FROM PATIENT — TO SUCTION
WATER SEAL AND COLLECTION — SUCTION CONTROL

B FROM PATIENT — TO SUCTION
COLLECTION — WATER SEAL — SUCTION CONTROL

FIGURE 25–11. Two methods to establish suction control. *A,* this system is primarily designed for controlling the amount of suction and removing air from the chest cavity. *B,* this system facilitates fluid collection, maintains the water seal, and allows for the application of suction.

leaks and accidental disconnections. All tubing and receptacles must be kept below the level of the patient's chest to maintain gravitational flow. If they are raised above the patient's chest, fluid and air may return to the pleural space.

The bottles of the apparatus should be securely fastened at the patient's bedside in a special rack designed for this purpose, or they should be placed on a large-rimmed, wheeled cart at the bedside.

Monitoring Volume of Drainage

The drainage water-seal bottles (these are the same in the one-bottle system) are marked with a strip of adhesive tape if they are not already marked by the manufacturer, and the level of water in the water-seal bottle is indicated. Usually 100 ml of sterile water or saline is used initially. As drainage collects, the time and volume are marked on the tape at the fluid level. In the two- or three-bottle system, a separate drainage bottle is provided, and the water-seal fluid and drainage do not mix. The advantage of this system is that the volume and character of the chest drainage can be assessed more accurately. Marking the bottle at 2- to 4-hour intervals, depending on how fast the drainage is accumulating, allows personnel to evaluate the volume of chest drainage and its rate of accumulation. If a one-bottle system is used, the water-seal tube must be elevated as drainage accumulates so that it remains only 1 to 2 cm below the fluid level.

If the drainage bottle becomes more than two-thirds full, it should be replaced. Under no circumstances should the drainage be allowed to accumulate to the point that openings to the air vent or tubing to the control bottle or suction machine are occluded. A full drainage bottle will not allow the system to function properly and may, in fact, be dangerous to the patient. If replacement of the drainage bottle becomes necessary, a person who is thoroughly familiar with the apparatus should perform this procedure. All necessary equipment must be gathered and arranged prior to making the replacement. Remember that the entire system must remain sterile. The chest tube of the system that needs to be replaced (usually only the lower or posterior tube) is clamped at the end close to the patient's chest wall to prevent air from entering the pleural cavity, and the full bottle is replaced with the new setup and the clamps removed. This should be accomplished swiftly and deftly so that the chest tube is clamped only momentarily. Prolonged clamp-

ing of the chest tube may produce tension in the cavity, allowing air or fluid, or both, to accumulate within the pleural space.

Most institutions currently use prefabricated disposable chest drainage units such as the Pleur-Evac (Fig. 25–12) and the Argyle double-seal system (Fig. 25–13). The principles of positive pressure, gravity, and suction apply equally to these systems. The Pleur-Evac system consists of a collection chamber, a water-seal chamber, and a suction control chamber. The Argyle double-seal system is a four-chambered system with a collection and suction control chamber and two water-seal chambers. The second water-seal chamber serves as a safety vent for the patient.

Ensuring Patency of Tubing

The flexible drainage tubing that connects the chest catheters to the drainage apparatus must be long enough to allow the patient to turn fully and to sit up in bed but not so long that dependent loops of tubing are formed. The tubing must be draped and secured in such a way that it forms a straight line to the recepta-

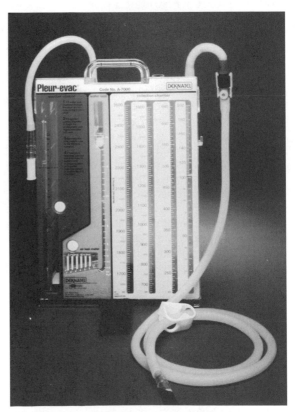

FIGURE 25–12. Disposable Pleur-Evac A-7000 unit. (Courtesy of Krale Laboratories, a Division of Deknatel, Inc., Fall River, MA.)

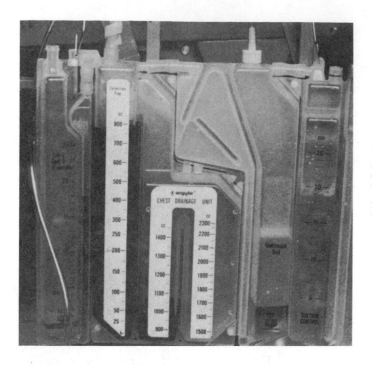

FIGURE 25-13. Disposable plastic pleural drainage system. The fluid collection chamber is in the center, the suction control is on the right, and the water-seal chamber is on the left. (Courtesy of Argyle, Division of Sherwood Medical, St. Louis, MO.)

cles to allow unobstructed gravitational flow. The tubing can be secured to the bed linen by wrapping a rubber band or a piece of adhesive tape around it and then pinning the tape or rubber band to the sheet. Excess tubing should be coiled flat on the bed. If more than two loops of tubing are present, a length of tubing should be removed to make the connection shorter. Excess tubing gets in the way of patient care, obstructs the smooth flow of drainage, is likely to fall off the bed into dependent loops, and is more likely to become kinked, tangled, or constricted.

Patency of the system and proper functioning should be checked frequently. In the first 2 or 3 hours postoperatively, this should be checked every 30 minutes or so along with the vital signs. If straight gravitational closed chest drainage is used, proper functioning is evidenced by fluctuation of the fluid in the water-seal tubing in response to the patient's respiration. If mechanical suction is being used with a two- or three-bottle system, the apparatus must be changed to the setup of the simple water-seal system to check the patency of the system. This is accomplished by disconnecting the tubing from the suction machine or outlet and leaving it open to atmospheric air to provide an air vent.

The fluid moves up the tubing approximately 2 to 6 cm as the patient inhales, owing to decreased intrapleural pressure, and then moves back down the tubing as the patient exhales, owing to increased intrapleural pressure. If fluctuation does not occur, check the tubing for obstruction due to kinking, compression, or the presence of blood clots. Ensure that the tubing has not become obstructed by the patient lying on it.

During positive-pressure ventilation, the opposite occurs: with positive-pressure inspiration, intrapleural pressure approaches or exceeds atmospheric pressure, and therefore the drainage tube fluid is forced downward.

"Milking," or "stripping," the chest tubing may dislodge clots of blood blocking the tubing (Fig. 25-14). Start close to the chest wall and

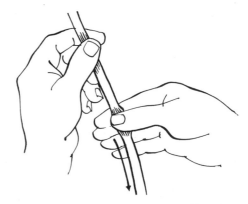

FIGURE 25-14. Technique for milking the chest tube. (From Sutton, A. L.: Bedside Nursing Techniques in Medicine and Surgery. 2nd ed. Philadelphia, W. B. Saunders, 1969, p. 226.)

work toward the drainage bottle. Never work toward the patient, because fluid or clots may be forced into the pleural space. Gently compress the tubing inch by inch down its entire length. This may be done by holding an alcohol swab in the hand stripping the tube, while the other hand holds the tube firmly in place and prevents traction on the insertion site. The hand-over-hand method may also be used: Gently squeeze the tubing with one hand and then the other, working in this fashion down its entire length. Some chest tubes are provided with chest tube strippers (Fig. 25–15). Whenever chest tubes are stripped, the procedure should be carried out gently, because it changes intrapleural pressure in the patient's chest cavity and may produce pain. Some studies have indicated that stripping chest tubes can create negative pressures considerably higher than the normally prescribed suction pressures of 15 to 20 cm H_2O. Therefore, each clinical situation should be evaluated individually before routine stripping is initiated. If large amounts of clotted blood appear in the chest tube, it seems reasonable to attempt to strip the tube. A chest tube draining only air does not require routine stripping.

Having the patient turn, cascade cough, and perform the sustained maximal inspiration (SMI) may improve patency of the chest tube. If fluctuation does not occur after these measures, the surgeon should be notified, and a radiograph will probably be ordered. The cessation of fluctuation may indicate full re-expansion of the lung, but this is a most unusual occurrence in the relatively short period the patient resides in the PACU. Most commonly, the system is blocked somewhere. If the tubing appears patent and milking has not improved the system's functioning, the physician may try irrigating the chest tube with a small amount of sterile saline.

Maintaining Proper Functioning

Intermittent bubbling in the water-seal bottle as the patient exhales or coughs indicates that the system is working properly and that air is being removed from the pleural space. Continuous bubbling in the water-seal bottle, however, indicates an air leak in the system that should be remedied immediately. Check all connections to ensure that they are snug. Check the entire length of the tubing for small leaks that can be corrected by taping. Check the dressing and the catheter at the insertion site on the patient's chest: If the catheter appears loose at the insertion site, gather skin around it and apply sterile petrolatum gauze around the skin and catheter to form an airtight seal. Cover with gauze and tape firmly. If no leak can be found and corrected and bubbling continues, the physician must be notified, because this may indicate an incision or tear in lung tissue that is allowing a large amount of air leakage from the lung.

In the closed chest drainage apparatus attached to suction, continuous bubbling should occur and indicates proper functioning. Proper functioning can be determined by examining the suction control tube. This tube should be emptied periodically of fluid and then refilled. If continuous bubbling does not occur, check all the connections and the suction machine. Check for air leaks as described earlier.

Do not clamp chest tubes unless specifically ordered. Clamping chest tubes, which may allow the development of a tension pneumothorax, is considerably more dangerous than allowing an open pneumothorax to occur. If something disrupts the system, correct the problem. If the water-seal bottle is tipped and the seal is disrupted, return the bottle to the upright position to re-establish the seal. If the water-seal bottle is inadvertently raised above the level of the patient's chest, lower the bottle at once to re-establish drainage. If the water-seal bottle is broken, or if the tubing becomes disconnected, sterilize the end of the tubing with antiseptic solution and reconnect it, or connect another sterile water-seal bottle. Make

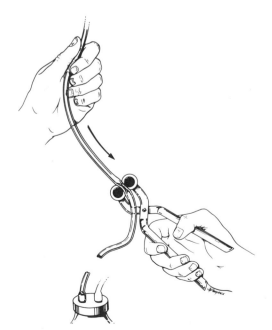

FIGURE 25–15. Technique for stripping the chest tube using a chest tube stripper.

sure to retape all connections after they are fit snugly together.

Once the problem is remedied, have the patient breathe deeply and cough to assist in forcing out any air or fluid that may have entered or accumulated within the pleural space during disruption of the system. If a large pneumothorax was precipitated by the event, as evidenced by asymmetric chest expansion, chest pain, and difficult breathing, a chest radiograph should be ordered and the physician notified.

GENERAL CARE FOLLOWING THORACIC SURGERY

Thoracic surgical patients recovering from general inhalation anesthesia are in the highest risk group for developing postoperative respiratory insufficiency. Nerve blocks along with continuous epidural anesthesia help reduce the amount of postoperative pain that the patient will be enduring. However, because of the size of the dressings, chest tubes, nasogastric tubes, and immobility, the patient is still at significant risk. Consequently, a rigorous modified stir-up regimen must be instituted on these patients.

Positioning

Positioning following chest surgery varies— check the surgeon's orders. Generally, the patient is kept in the supine position until reflexes begin to return. The supine position reduces the threat of hypoventilation by preventing restriction of thoracic expansion, and the abdominal organs do not impinge on the diaphragm or cause pressure on the mediastinal structures. The Trendelenburg position is contraindicated after chest surgery, even in the presence of shock, because it causes the abdominal organs to press against the diaphragm, thus restricting movement and creating pressure on the mediastinal contents, which decreases venous return and cardiac output. If hypotension develops owing to venous pooling of blood in the legs, apply elastic stockings or raise the legs.

Once the patient's reflexes have started to return and vital signs are stabilized, the head of the bed is raised 30 to 45 degrees to allow the diaphragm to drop to normal position, thus enhancing lung expansion and facilitating chest tube drainage. The specific surgical procedure will determine what changes in position can be made during the first 24 to 48 hours postoperatively. Surgeons differ in the theory of positioning, but several guidelines may be generally followed. After pulmonary resection (such as lobectomy, segmentectomy, and wedge resection), the patient may be turned to a full lateral position on either side to allow full expansion of lung tissue on both the operated and the unoperated sides. Occasionally, a surgeon does not want the patient turned onto the operated side to enhance full expansion of remaining lung parenchyma on that side; however, this ignores the necessity for full ventilation on the unoperated side, the lack of which may be just as detrimental. After median sternotomy the patient may be positioned on the back, which is the most comfortable position, or on either side. The patient with a pneumonectomy may be positioned on the back or turned on the operative side. Extreme lateral positioning on the nonoperative side is contraindicated after pneumonectomy, because the mediastinum is no longer confined by lung tissue and may move freely and cause compression of the remaining lung or create traction or torsion phenomena on the vena cava. Additionally, if the bronchial stump is ruptured while in this position, the unaffected lung would be drowned with secretions from the pneumonectomy site.

Position changes are an important part of the stir-up regimen. During the first 4 to 6 hours, the patient should be turned every half hour, then every hour until ambulatory. Ambulation is started as soon as possible after recovery from anesthesia and stabilization of vital signs. Mobilization, through position change, exercise, and ambulation, is important to promote drainage of secretions and chest tube drainage of fluid and air, to prevent venous stasis, and to promote comfort. When turning the patient or helping him or her to sit or slide up in the bed, support the back of the head and assist from the unoperated side. The patient can help in turning by grasping the side rail and pulling. A draw sheet may be kept under the patient for the first 4 to 6 hours to assist in turning the patient comfortably. When changing the patient's position, ensure that chest tubes remain free, that they remain patent (i.e., without kinking or compression), and that no dependent loops are formed. Active and passive arm exercises are initiated within the first postoperative day. Simple exercises, such as arm circles and lifting the arm out to the side on the affected side, are encouraged.

Chest Tubes

Thoracotomy tubes are connected to a sterile, closed chest drainage system with or without suction, as the surgeon specifies, if this has not already been accomplished in the operating room. Chest drains are not usually placed after pneumonectomy because serous fluid accumulation, which eventually consolidates and fills the empty thoracic space left by removal of the lung, is desirable to prevent mediastinal movement of the heart and remaining lung. Occasionally, a clamped chest tube is placed as a monitoring device to check bleeding and for measuring and regulating pressure in the thoracic space. The chest tubes are cared for as previously described.

Chest tube drainage must be checked frequently for character, volume, and rate of formation. The drainage is usually grossly bloody for the first 3 to 4 postoperative hours, after which it becomes more serous and only pink tinged. Approximately 100 to 300 ml of drainage can be expected in the first 2 hours, after which it should slow to 50 to 100 ml per hour. Total drainage in the first 24 hours postoperatively will be 500 to 1000 ml. If drainage of more than 50 ml of grossly bloody fluid per hour persists 3 hours after surgery, hemorrhage should be suspected and the surgeon notified. These quantities must be interpreted in light of patient activity, because a sudden gush of 50 ml of drainage at one time would not be unusual after turning the patient to the operated side or having him or her cough and breathe deeply. Check the patient's vital signs and urine output for interrelated features of developing shock.

Vital Signs

All vital signs are measured and recorded every 15 minutes for the first 2 hours and then every 30 minutes until stable. A central venous pressure line, Swan-Ganz catheter, or arterial line may be present to assist in monitoring the patient. They must be correctly connected to monitoring devices and maintained with flushing solution. All flushing solutions must be included in the parenteral intake computations.

Nursing assessment and intervention are aimed at maintaining adequate respiratory and circulatory function and at preventing complications from hypoxia, hypoxemia, and circulatory insufficiency.

SPECIFIC ASPECTS OF POSTOPERATIVE CARE

Respiratory Functions

Maintenance of a Patent Airway

Maintaining a patent airway depends primarily on assessment and initiation of the modified stir-up regimen as outlined in Chapter 20. Assess air movement—stridor, wheezing, gurgling, decreased chest expansion, and decreased breath sounds on auscultation may indicate airway obstruction. If obstruction is not relieved by repositioning of the head and jaw or suctioning the airway, notify the anesthesiologist. Emergency equipment, including laryngoscope, endotracheal tubes, Ambu or anesthesia bag, and tracheostomy sets, must be immediately available.

Assessment of Respiratory Function

Vital signs are taken every 15 minutes for the first 2 hours (at least until reflexes are returning), then every 30 minutes to an hour until stable. The frequency of vital sign measurement will be determined by the discrepancies among preoperative, intraoperative, and postoperative levels. Observe respiratory rate, rhythm, and depth, and auscultate for adventitious or diminished breath sounds. Observe the quality of respirations—labored breathing, dyspnea, stridor, retraction, nasal flaring, and asymmetry of chest expansion may indicate obstruction. Intrapleural air or fluid (blood), or both, may compress lung tissue and decrease ventilation markedly.

Paradoxical respiration, or flail chest (Fig. 25–16), which may occur after thoracoplasty, is extremely deleterious. Paradoxical respiration results not only in hypoventilation but also in obstruction owing to accumulation of secretions that the patient cannot effectively remove by coughing. Tight dressings, binders, or abdominal distention may also restrict chest excursion. Restlessness, irritability, disorientation, inappropriate behavior, and other cerebral symptoms offer significant evidence of hypoxia. Although these symptoms may be difficult to assess and may be attributable to pain and other causes, inadequate oxygenation should be the first possibility that comes to mind.

Measurements, including arterial blood gases and spirometry (the measurement of tidal volume, minute volume, and vital capacity), are also used to assess respiratory function. An ar-

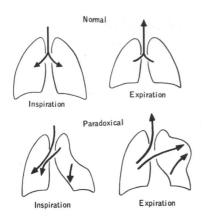

FIGURE 25–16. Paradoxical motion of the flail chest. (From Sutton, A. L.: Bedside Nursing Techniques in Medicine and Surgery. 2nd ed. Philadelphia, W. B. Saunders, 1969, p. 217.)

terial line should be present so that frequent arterial samples may be obtained easily. Blood gas measurements are extremely important in guiding oxygen therapy. (For information on analysis of blood gases, see Chapter 6). Along with this, oxygen saturation measurements have proved to be an excellent parameter in the evaluation of respiratory function. When the percent oxygen saturation is determined, the PACU nurse can use an oxygen dissociation curve to determine the patient's partial pressure of oxygen. For example, an oxygen saturation of 90 percent has a partial pressure of 57.8 mm Hg under standard conditions of pH and temperature. The reader is encouraged to review the oxygen dissociation curve as discussed in Chapter 6.

Institution of Oxygen Therapy

All patients should receive supplemental humidified oxygen in the PACU. Some degree of hypoxemia while breathing room air is usually present for 5 to 7 days following thoracic surgery. This because the pressure-volume curve on these patients as described in Chapter 6 will remain shifted to the right for as long as 7 days postoperatively. Therefore, the patient should use the SMI in the PACU and the incentive spirometer for 7 days postoperatively. The SMI maneuver is designed to help shift the pressure-volume curve back to the left and facilitate normal matching of ventilation to perfusion. As stated previously, oxygen should be viewed and treated as a drug, and the physician should individualize dosage and administration route for each patient. Preferably, oxygen is administered via catheter or cannula, because the pa-

tient needs to cough up secretions at frequent intervals. Oxygen administration, humidification, and airway adjuncts are discussed in more detail in Chapter 20.

Initiation of the Modified Stir-Up Regimen

The modified stir-up regimen, including positioning, mobilization, SMI, cascade coughing, and pain relief, is especially important for this patient. Positioning and mobilization have already been discussed. The SMI and cascade coughing exercises are the easiest ways to maintain a patent airway after the patient is reactive to verbal commands. Preoperative teaching is extremely important; the patient who has been well educated and knows what is expected of him or her postoperatively can cooperate by taking a deep breath, holding it for 3 seconds and then exhaling (the SMI), and then taking a deep breath and coughing throughout exhalation (the cascade cough). Effective preoperative teaching will enhance the effectiveness of the modified stir-up regimen even if the patient is not fully reactive.

Once the patient is fully conscious, rigorous SMIs and cascade coughing are continued every hour. This regimen is most effective with the patient sitting up to allow full lung expansion. If the patient cannot sit up, raise the head of the bed and have him or her bend the knees to relax the abdominal muscles. The patient is instructed to take a deep inspiration and hold it for 3 seconds to expand the lungs and relax the abdominal muscles so that the belly pouches out. Four to five SMIs are taken, and then the patient is instructed to perform the cascade cough to clear the tracheobronchial tree of accumulated secretions. After the patient performs about three cascade coughs, a "forceful" cough will then usually be produced spontaneously, thus clearing the airways of secretions. Endotracheal secretions are usually excessive after thoracic surgery, owing to trauma to the tracheobronchial tree during the operation and intubation, to decreased lung ventilation, and to a decreased cough reflex. Pain or fear, or both, may interfere with the patient's ability to perform the SMI and cascade cough.

Pain Relief

The thoracic surgical patient should be told preoperatively to expect a fair amount of incisional pain postoperatively but that breathing deeply and coughing are essential. The patient should be ensured that the nurses will assist in this and that medications will be provided to alleviate pain.

Postoperatively, the nurse must provide adequate analgesia to allow the patient to cooperate effectively with the stir-up regimen. Postthoracic surgical patients generally experience a great deal of incisional pain and pain caused by the chest tubes. Posterolateral incisions tend to be more painful than anterolateral ones. Narcotic analgesics such as morphine sulfate and meperidine hydrochloride (Demerol) are usually the agents of choice for pain control. Naloxone hydrochloride (Narcan), a narcotic antagonist, is usually kept readily available to reverse the effects of the analgesics if they begin to depress respiratory functioning; because both morphine and meperidine depress respiration and the cough reflex, they must be administered judiciously. Meperidine may be preferred to morphine, because it seems to be somewhat less of a depressant and acts as a bronchodilator. The opiates, such as codeine, are generally contraindicated, because they severely depress the cough reflex, stimulate bronchospasm, and produce thickened secretions. Frequently, a potentiating drug such as hydroxyzine (Atarax, Vistaril) or promethazine hydrochloride (Phenergan) is added to the narcotic so that the dosage of the narcotic can be reduced, yet pain is adequately relieved.

The smallest dose of narcotic that will give adequate pain relief should be administered. Small doses given frequently decrease their tendency to depress respiratory centers. An order such as meperidine 15 to 25 mg intravenously every 1 to 2 hours as necessary for pain is advantageous, because the nurse can use discretion and give the minimal dose necessary to provide adequate analgesia.

The patient should be observed closely after the administration of narcotics for indications of depression. The administration of analgesics 15 to 30 minutes before the performance of the SMI, cascade coughing, and mobilization assists the patient in cooperative efforts and decreases physiologic splinting and restriction of chest movement.

Pain can also be reduced and fear lessened by providing proper manual support for the incision during cascade coughing (Fig. 25–17). Patients often fear that they may tear the incision or that a lung may protrude through the incision if they breathe too deeply or cough too rigorously. They should be reassured verbally that this will not occur, and the nurse can support the incision with the hands to reassure the patient physically and prevent pain. Manual

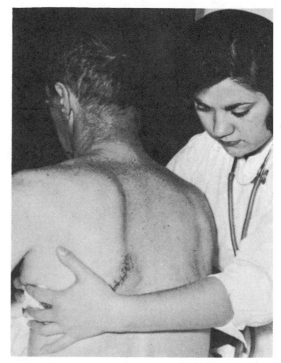

FIGURE 25–17. Correct position for "splinting" a patient's chest. (From MacVicar, J., and Mendelsohn, H. J.: In Meltzer, L. E., Abdellah, T., and Kitchell, J. R. [eds.]: Concepts and Practices of Intensive Care for Nurse Specialists. Philadelphia, Charles Press, 1969.)

support decreases stretching of the incision, thereby decreasing pain, and assists in depressing the thoracic cage during expiration.

To splint the incision correctly, stand to the side of the patient with your face posterior to the patient's head for protection from the cascade cough and to be able to listen to the chest. Apply firm, even pressure with your open palms placed anteriorly and posteriorly over the incision. Do not squeeze across the chest, depress the sternum, or restrict movement of the lower rib cage. The diaphragm contributes more than 50 percent to the ventilatory process and must not be restricted. The thoracic incision may also be splinted by applying firm pressure upward underneath the incision and exerting pressure on the shoulder of the patient's affected side with the other hand.

Auscultate the patient's chest after the performance of the SMI and cascade coughing. If the lungs are not clear, allow the patient to rest for a brief period and repeat the SMI and cascade coughing. If the chest does not clear, other methods of mobilizing and removing secretions and fully inflating the lungs may have to be instituted. Syncope may occur while the patient is performing SMI and cascade coughing, but recovery is usually quick, because syncope is self-limiting. Syncope during these exercises is probably caused by (1) impeded venous return from the increase in intrathoracic pressure with subsequent reduced cardiac output and cerebral ischemia, and (2) the sudden reduction of carbon dioxide in the blood owing to hyperventilation, which, if not reversed, can result in loss of consciousness.

The best way to clear the tracheobronchial tree of secretions is by an effective cascade cough. If the patient cannot clear the airway of secretions effectively with the SMI and cascade coughing, other methods must be instituted; for example, respiratory therapy adjuncts may be ordered to assist the patient.

Other pain control methods that can be used include single-dose intercostal nerve blocks, continuous intercostal nerve blocks via indwelling intercostal analgesic catheters, or the use of transcutaneous electrical stimulation. In this last method, stimulation of large myelinated fibers is accomplished by the placement of small electrodes on either side of the thoracotomy incision. Stimulation via these electrodes inhibits the pain response of the small unmyelinated fibers.

Tracheal Suctioning

Tracheal suctioning of the post-thoracic surgical patient may be necessary to assist in removing accumulated secretions. Suctioning technique has been described in Chapter 20.

The patient should be in the sitting position. The catheter is introduced into the nares, and the pharynx is suctioned. This removes secretions and also stimulates a good cough, which may be all that is necessary to mobilize secretions from the lower airway. Tracheal suctioning must be accomplished carefully, especially after pneumonectomy, when a suture line may be interrupted by introduction of the catheter. If the catheter is difficult to pass, pull the tongue forward. Do not force the catheter. There is no evidence that turning the patient's head or neck will help pass the catheter to the left main stem bronchus, although this is a frequently advocated procedure. If the airway does not clear after suctioning, the physician may have to perform a bronchoscopy to remove secretions. Remember that suctioning removes oxygen as well as secretions, and the patient must be hyperventilated before and after suctioning.

Humidification

Reservoir nebulizers and humidifiers with aerosol masks, face tents, continuous positive airway pressure masks, and T-tubes can provide both supplemental oxygen and dense water vapor or medicated mist, all of which are effective methods of thinning tracheobronchial secretions, thus permitting the ciliary mechanism and coughing to clear the airway.

The most effective therapy device is the ultrasonic nebulizer, which generates a fine mist of saline droplets, 2 to 4 μ in diameter, which are carried down to the smallest and most distal bronchioles. This mist should be used only intermittently. Mist treatments may be administered via mask (tracheostomy mask, if tracheostomy is present) or in a mist tent. The mask is definitely preferable in the PACU to allow close, direct observation of the patient.

Fluid Balance

Maintenance of Optimal Hydration

Optimal hydration of the post-thoracic surgical patient is exceptionally important to prevent increased viscosity of mucus to facilitate the removal of secretions. Oral fluids may be started as soon as the patient recovers from anesthesia and the danger of nausea and vomiting has passed.

Accurate intake and output measurement is especially important to ensure that optimal hydration is maintained without letting vascular overload develop. Removal of large segments or of the total lung significantly reduces the size of the pulmonary circulation, predisposing the patient to development of pulmonary edema if fluids are administered too rapidly or in too large a volume. Increased permeability of the capillaries that results from hypoxia increases the risk of pulmonary edema developing in this patient. Unless the surgeon specifically directs otherwise, the intravenous fluid rate should not exceed 200 ml in an hour.

Circulatory Functions

Maintenance of Adequate Circulation

Accurate assessment of the patient's cardiovascular status is important to ensure adequate circulation and thus oxygen delivery to the tissues. Vital signs, including blood pressure, pulse, and respirations, are monitored frequently to detect trends that may indicate level of circulatory efficiency. The incision and the dressings should be checked frequently for drainage, and accurate intake and output records, including chest tube drainage, should be kept and evaluated.

Urine output volume is measured as an indicator of hypovolemia. Should the urinary output decline precipitously (i.e., less than 0.5 ml·kg^{-1}·hr^{-1}, the surgeon should be notified immediately. Level of consciousness and sensory changes are evaluated, and heart rhythm may be electrically monitored, especially if the patient is known to have underlying cardiac disease. Central venous pressure should be maintained between 6 and 12 mm Hg because determinations in that pressure range suggests that the patient has an adequate blood volume.

Maintenance of Optimal Blood Volume

In addition to measuring degree of hydration, blood loss must be estimated. Blood loss during thoracic surgery is usually great, because the incision is quite long and capillary oozing is significant, thoracic adhesions and tissue planes are usually extensive and quite vascular, and the thoracic arteries are large. Re-expansion of blood volume with intravenous infusions, blood, or plasma expanders is indi-

cated if blood loss is significant and the patient shows signs of hypovolemia.

Prevention and Detection of Complications

Hypoxemia and Atelectasis

Hypoxemia and atelectasis have already been discussed in this chapter and in Chapter 6. The PACU nurse must make astute observations to quickly identify the symptoms of developing hypoxemia and institute treatment to correct the cause (Fig. 25–18).

Airway obstruction leads rapidly to the development of postoperative atelectasis, which may in turn lead to pneumonitis. The presence of decreased breath sounds and increased temperature should alert the PACU nurse to the need for greater efforts at maintaining a clear airway, because this is the essence of treatment. The modified stir-up regimen should be accomplished more frequently; more SMIs, cascade coughing, and suctioning are necessary. Bronchoscopy may be necessary to remove obstructive secretions or mucoid plugs. Respiratory

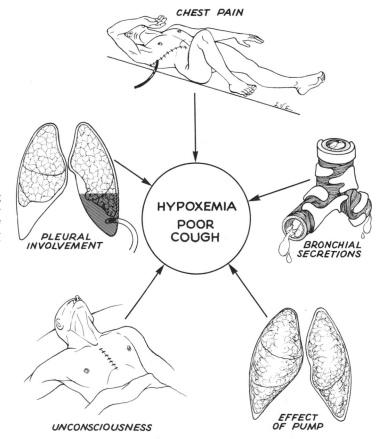

FIGURE 25–18. Postoperative factors leading to hypoxemia. (From Thomas, A. N.: Respiratory care. In Sanderson, R. G. [ed.]: The Cardiac Patient. Philadelphia, W. B. Saunders, 1972, p. 233.)

therapy adjuncts, including percussion and postural drainage, mist inhalation, and intermittent positive-pressure breathing, with or without the addition of detergent aerosols, may be used to increase ventilatory efforts and remove secretions. The surgeon may elect to start the patient on antibiotic therapy to prevent the development of infection.

Infection

Pulmonary infection following thoracic surgery is rare when preventive measures are followed. The use of sterile suctioning technique, the maintenance of sterility of the chest drainage system and of a patent airway (see earlier), and nose, mouth, and skin care to promote cleanliness are safeguards against the development of pulmonary infection. Definitive symptoms of infection rarely appear within the relatively short period the patient spends in the PACU. Nurses on the receiving unit must be alert to symptoms of hypoxia, increasing temperature, increased production of secretions, or change in the color of secretions from clear or pale yellow to yellow or green. These symptoms may indicate the presence of pulmonary infection. If infection develops, culture and sensitivity studies are done to identify the causative organism and the antibiotics that will be effective.

Ventilatory Mechanical Complications

Pneumothorax, tension pneumothorax, and mediastinal shift have been discussed previously. Maintenance of the patency of chest tubes and correct positioning of the postoperative patient are preventive measures. If symptoms of these complications develop, rapid intervention to correct intrapleural pressure, including the placement of thoracotomy tubes, is necessary, because these are life-threatening conditions.

Subcutaneous emphysema, or the accumulation of air in the subcutaneous tissue of the neck and chest, especially around the site of chest tube insertion, is common after thoracic surgery and does not usually cause serious problems. The PACU nurse should note its presence, however, and mark the boundaries of accumulation with a skin-marking pencil so that its rate of formation can be evaluated. Subcutaneous emphysema of the neck may be evaluated by measuring neck circumference. Small areas of subcutaneous emphysema are tender and may be uncomfortable for the adult but do not require specific treatment; however,

compression of the vena cava or trachea by distended tissues may occur in the infant, so air must be removed. A progressive increase in subcutaneous emphysema in any patient should alert the nurse to the possibility that chest drainage tubes are not properly functioning or that a bronchopleural fistula is present, or, in the patient with pneumonectomy, that air is leaking through the bronchial stump. Treatment in these patients is aimed at correcting the underlying cause, ensuring patency of chest drains, replacing the chest tube, adding or increasing suction to the drainage system, aspirating the mediastinum, or repairing the bronchial stump to make it airtight.

Gastric dilatation may occur in the postoperative period as a result of depression of gastric motility, air swallowing, or insufflation of anesthetic gases. Gastric distention is more common after surgery involving the left chest and occurs in the immediate postoperative period. Treatment involves decompression of the stomach with the use of a nasogastric tube.

Bleeding, Hypovolemia, and Shock

Blood loss or fluid depletion that results in hypovolemia is the most common cause of circulatory inadequacy in postoperative patients. Any signs and symptoms of blood loss, including increased pulse rate, decreased blood pressure, progressive oliguria, and changes in the sensorium, as well as external bleeding, should alert the nurse to possible hypovolemia, which could result in shock if the cause is not corrected. The surgeon should be notified if any of these signs and symptoms occur. Preoperative and postoperative hematocrit values may assist in determining the presence of hypovolemia and the types and amounts of replacement fluids necessary to correct the problem. Vasopressors may be used to support blood pressure while waiting for fluid replacement to take effect. A return to the operating room may be necessary to correct continued bleeding.

If bleeding occurs into the intrapleural space and it cannot escape through the chest tubes, a hemothorax will result. All chest tubes should be checked frequently to ensure that they are functioning correctly. If the patient becomes dyspneic, if pulse and respiratory rates increase, and if blood pressure decreases, the surgeon should be notified. Chest tubes may have to be inserted or replaced to remove blood from the intrapleural space, or surgical evacuation of the blood and direct control of bleeding may have to be accomplished in the operating room.

Cardiac Arrhythmias

Underlying cardiac disease should be carefully evaluated and documented before surgery. Any patient with pre-existing cardiac dysfunction should be electrically monitored on a continuous basis in the PACU, because these patients commonly develop cardiac dysrhythmias in the anesthesia recovery period. Sinus tachycardia and atrial fibrillation are the most commonly encountered dysrhythmias in the early recovery phases, but any disturbance in cardiac rate, rhythm, or electrical conduction may be cause for alarm.

Neurogenic Hypotension

Neurogenic reflexes due to pain or chest trauma may cause hypotension via vasodilatation in the postoperative period. This hypotension must be carefully evaluated to rule out other possible causes, including blood loss, volume depletion, or cardiac disease. Neurogenic hypotension may be treated by providing adequate analgesia to remove the pain stimulus. The patient must be observed carefully after administration of analgesia for depression of respiratory or cardiac function. The return of a preoperative blood pressure level should be sought.

References

1. Allan, D.: Chest tube patient. Nurs. Times, *81*(5):24–25, 1985.
2. Barash, P., Cullen, B., and Stoelting, R.: Clinical Anesthesia. 2nd ed. Philadelphia, J. B. Lippincott, 1992.
3. Drain, C.: Postoperative care of the surgical patient. *In* Waugaman, W., Foster, S., and Rigor, B. (eds.): Principles and Practice of Nurse Anesthesia. 2nd ed. Norwalk, CT, Appleton & Lange, 1992, pp. 813–822.
4. Kaplan, J. (ed.): Thoracic Anesthesia. 2nd ed. New York, Churchill Livingstone, 1991.
5. Katz, J., Benumof, J., and Kadis, L.: Anesthesia and Uncommon Diseases. 3rd ed. Philadelphia, W. B. Saunders, 1990.
6. Miller, R. (ed.): Anesthesia. 3rd ed. New York, Churchill Livingstone, 1990.
7. Vender, J., and Spiess, B.: Post Anesthesia Care. Philadelphia, W. B. Saunders, 1992.

Post Anesthesia Care of the Cardiac Surgical Patient

CHAPTER 26

Karen D. Keeler, R.N., B.S.N., C.C.R.N., C.E.N.

The concept of cardiac surgery as a viable option for patients with heart disease or trauma did not develop until the late 1800s, largely because of the emotional as well as technical difficulties inherent in the concepts of the heart itself. The perceived seat of the soul and a vital hemodynamic structure, the heart was viewed as untouchable on both fronts. The first surgical manipulation occurred in 1896, when Rehn successfully closed a stab wound in the ventricle of an unconscious man. Since then, success in the treatment of cardiac trauma has continued, and major developments have occurred in many aspects of treatment. In the 1950s, the development of the cardiopulmonary bypass machine and techniques made open heart surgery a viable option. Today, procedures ranging from valve and myocardial structure repair and replacement and direct manipulation of the coronary arteries to transplantation, implantation of assist devices, and total mechanical replacement of the heart are common.

In many institutions, patients are transferred directly from surgery to a special cardiac surgical intensive care unit (ICU), where they remain for 1 to 3 days before transfer to a regular nursing unit. During this period these patients require intensive hemodynamic monitoring and rapid intervention to prevent many of their normal postoperative states (e.g., hypothermia and hypertension) from progressing to postoperative complications (e.g., myocardial infarction and hemorrhage). Discharge from the hospital usually occurs within 7 to 10 days after the surgical intervention.

The length of the preoperative period and thus patient preparation time can vary greatly. The post anesthesia care unit (PACU) nurse should be aware of the level of knowledge, understanding demonstrated, and anxieties that both the patient and the family are experiencing. It is helpful, although not always practical, for the PACU nurse to provide the preoperative instruction for the patient and family or to make an introductory visit to them before surgery.

This chapter is designed to familiarize the PACU nurse with postoperative care for the cardiac patient. Additional study is a necessity, and the reader is directed to the reference list at the end of this chapter for sources that deal with the continuum of care needed by the patient hospitalized for cardiac surgery.

Definitions

Annuloplasty: a surgical technique in which the annulus of the valve is manipulated to decrease the size of the valvular orifice and thus limit valvular regurgitation; this can be accomplished by suturing portions of the valvular annulus. More recently, this has been done by using a plication ring, which is a cloth-covered flexible metal ring that is placed over the valve orifice, with the annulus of the valve attached to the ring (Fig. 26–1). This procedure is most frequently performed on tricuspid and mitral valves.

Aortic regurgitation: a condition that occurs when the aortic valve does not totally close because the cusps do not completely approximate with each other during diastole. This can occur as a result of congenital or rheumatic heart disease, infective endocarditis, trauma, aortic dissection, or Marfan's syndrome. This lesion is also known as *aortic insufficiency.*

Aortic stenosis: a narrowing of the orifice of the aortic valve itself or of the areas adjacent to the aortic valve. These narrowings create an obstruction to left-ventricular outflow and can be generally classified as three different types: valvular, subvalvular, and supravalvular. In the most common type, the valvular, there is a fusion of the commissures of

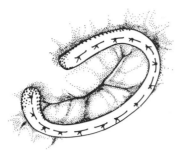

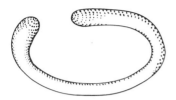

FIGURE 26–1. Plication ring.

the valve leaflets that leaves only a small opening. This lesion can occur as a congenital process, as in the bicuspid valve, or as an acquired disease process, such as in rheumatic heart disease. The second most common type is a subvalvular aortic stenosis. This lesion is usually caused by a fibrinous diaphragm located a few millimeters below the valvular leaflets. Another type of subvalvular stenosis occurs when the intraventricular septum becomes hypertrophied and creates an obstruction to left-ventricular outflow. This lesion is known as *idiopathic hypertrophic subaortic stenosis* or *hypertrophic obstructive cardiomyopathy*. The most infrequently seen form of aortic stenosis is the supravalvular type in which the aorta is constricted just above the ostia of the coronary arteries. This lesion may be considered a coarctation of the ascending aorta. Figure 26–2 illustrates the different types of left-ventricular outflow tract obstructions.

Aortic valve disease: a disease that is usually caused by rheumatic involvement of the aortic valve in which the valve cusps become thick and fibrotic or that is the result of a congenital bicuspid valve. Aortic valve disease places increased amounts of work on the left ventricles, resulting in increased afterload, left-ventricular hypertrophy, and decreased compliance. The left-ventricular cavity becomes reduced, and the atrial contribution to cardiac output becomes important to maintain adequate preload and forward flow of blood and to contribute to a more forceful ventricular contraction. Loss of

this atrial contribution, or "kick," through the development of atrial arrhythmias can result in a marked decrease in cardiac output with resultant pulmonary edema.

Aortocoronary bypass grafts: see *Myocardial revascularization*.

Atrial septal defect (ASD): a hole through the atrial septum. An *ostium secundum defect* is a defect high in the atrial septum for which no etiologic factors are known. Some secundum defects are associated with anomalous pulmonary veins returning oxygenated blood into the superior vena cava or into the right atrium. An ostium primum lesion is a defect low in the atrial septum and may involve the tricuspid and mitral valves and the upper portion of the intraventricular septum. Ostium primum defects develop following arrested embryonic development of the endocardial cushions that normally meet with the ventricular and atrial septa to form the four chambers of the heart. *Atrioventricularis communis* is a severe lesion caused by extensive nondevelopment of the endocardial cushions. In this lesion there is an ostium primum defect, portions of the mitral and tricuspid leaflets form a common valve, and a ventricular septal defect exists. Both ostium primum defects and atrioventricularis communis are also known as *endocardial cushion defects* or *atrioventricular canal defects,* owing to their similar embryonic origins. Closure of septal defects is accomplished by suturing or patching the defect with a graft of pericardium or prosthetic material. Appropriate manipulation and reconstruction of the involved valves are also performed if necessary. Anomalous pulmonary veins are diverted to the left atrium. Figure 26–3 illustrates the areas affected by these lesions.

Automatic implantable cardioverter-defibrillator (AICD): a device, first introduced in 1980, that converts the electrocardiogram (ECG) to a probability density function (PDF) of the ventricular activity and delivers a shock within 15 seconds. The PDF determines the amount of time the ECG signal spends on and away from the baseline. The PDF differentiates between lethal ventricular arrhythmias and supraventricular tachycardia, sinus tachycardia, and atrial fibrillation. The rate-detecting lead allows for detection of ventricular tachycardia (VT), the precursor to ventricular fibrillation (VF), and a greater chance for successful cardioversion.

Patients with documented sustained VT or VF are considered candidates for the AICD if prior drug therapies have failed. The device

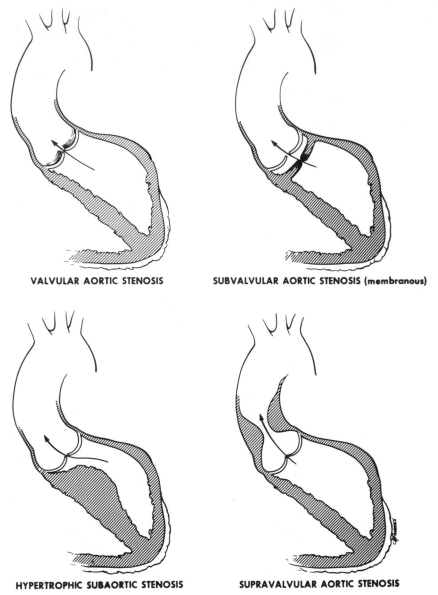

VALVULAR AORTIC STENOSIS

SUBVALVULAR AORTIC STENOSIS (membranous)

HYPERTROPHIC SUBAORTIC STENOSIS

SUPRAVALVULAR AORTIC STENOSIS

FIGURE 26–2. Schematic representation of various types of left-ventricular outflow tract obstructions.

is not considered appropriate if the patient has frequent episodes of sustained VT or self-terminating, nonsustained VT for longer than 5 seconds. In these circumstances, the AICD discharges frequently in the former and discharges when the VT has terminated in the latter example. The procedure is done under general anesthesia. The system may consist of two patches (either intrapericardial or extrapericardial) or a superior vena cava spring-coil electrode and an apical patch.

When the two-patch technique is used, the patches are placed over the diaphragmatic surface and over the posterobasal portion of the left ventricle via anterior thoracotomy. The objective is to cover the largest amount of myocardial mass between the two patches. Testing of the sensing and cardioversion thresholds is performed in the operating room by inducing VT and VF. If sufficient, the generator is turned on and tested for adequate sensing and cardioversion-defibrillation. If defibrillation is adequate, the generator is turned off and placed in a square pocket in the left upper quadrant of the patient's abdomen.

The AICD is activated when the patient is transferred out of the PACU or ICU. Compli-

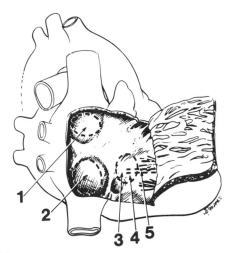

FIGURE 26-3. Schematic representation of areas involved with various atrial septal defects: 1. anomalous pulmonary vein; 2. ostium secundum defects; 3. ostium primum defects; 4. ventricular septal defect; and 5. leaflet of mitral valve.

cations are rare, and studies have shown 98 percent freedom from sudden death at 1 year and 94 percent at 5 years.

Cardiac catheterization: a technique in which a radiopaque plastic catheter is inserted into the right or left heart via a percutaneous puncture or a cutdown into the femoral or brachial artery or vein to obtain pressure, volume, and oxygen saturation determinations from the intracardiac chambers and the great blood vessels (i.e., superior and inferior vena cava, pulmonary artery, and aorta). In addition, injection of a contrast medium can be used to assist in identifying intracardiac and intracoronary artery structural alterations, as well as in obtaining cardiac output and ejection fraction values and wall motion studies. Generally, a "right-heart" catheterization yields data concerning the inferior and superior vena cava, the right atrium and ventricle, and the pulmonary artery. A "left-heart" catheterization yields information concerning the left atrium and ventricle, the aorta, and the coronary arteries, if a selective coronary arteriography study is performed.

Cardioplegia: a paralysis of the heart or cardiac arrest. Although there are different methods that can be used to induce this arrest, the term *cardioplegia* is most commonly used to refer to hyperkalemic solutions that produce this arrest effect. Infused into the aortic root, these solutions enter the ostia of the coronary arteries and perfuse the myocardium. In addition to potassium, these solutions can have numerous additives, such as other electro-

lytes, blood, and antiarrhythmic agents. The purpose of these other agents is to provide a physiologically balanced environment, to provide energy substrates, and to decrease ventricular irritability.

Cardiopulmonary bypass (CPB): a temporary substitution for the heart and lungs by an oxygenator pump. With CPB, direct visualization and manipulation of a noncontracting heart are achieved. At the same time, blood is oxygenated, carbon dioxide is removed, and systemic blood flow is sustained. Venous access is achieved by placing cannulas in the venae cavae and the right atrium. Blood is then circulated through the CPB circuit where it becomes oxygenated. It is then returned to the patient via arterial cannulas that are located in the aorta or femoral or iliac arteries. Commonly used types of oxygenators are the rotating disk, the bubble, and the membrane (Fig. 26-4).

Coarctation of the aorta: a narrowing of the aorta that can occur anywhere between the aortic arch and the femoral bifurcation. There are generally two types of coarctations: preductal and postductal (Fig. 26-5). In the *preductal type*, the pulmonary artery communicates with the distal aorta through a ductus. In this situation, blood flow from the right ventricle and the pulmonary artery supplies the lower half of the body, whereas flow from the left ventricle and the aorta supplies the upper torso. With this anomaly there are usually other concurrent intracardiac defects, such as ventricular septal defects and transposition of the great arteries. In the *postductal type*, there is a localized constriction, usually just distal to the left subclavian artery. This narrowing is usually followed by poststenotic dilatation. Correction is accomplished by excising the coarctation and then performing an end-to-end anastomosis, with or without a graft, to establish continuity. In the preductal type, appropriate correction of the associated intracardiac defects is also performed.

Commissurotomy: the opening or separation of fused valvular commissures. Either closed or open commissurotomy may be performed. In mitral stenosis, closed commissurotomy with a transventricular dilator can be performed, in which a dilator is inserted through the left-atrial appendage and then through the mitral valve. The valve is then dilated to the appropriate degree. If the patient is suspected of having a left-atrial thrombus that could be easily embolized, an open procedure is performed, in which both a dilator and digital pressure are used.

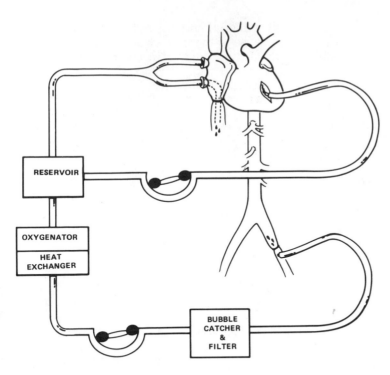

FIGURE 26–4. Schematic representation of a standard cardiopulmonary bypass circuit.

Hypothermia: the elective cooling of the patient during cardiac surgery. Two general methods are used: systemic and local. *Systemic cooling* is accomplished by lowering the patient's temperature to 25° to 30°C with the use of the CPB circuit. *Local cooling* refers to cooling the myocardium to levels of 0 to 10°C. This can be accomplished by placing an ice slush solution in the pericardial area as well as by administering a cold cardioplegic solution. The purpose of both the local and the systemic use of hypothermia is to diminish cellular demands and limit ischemic injury.

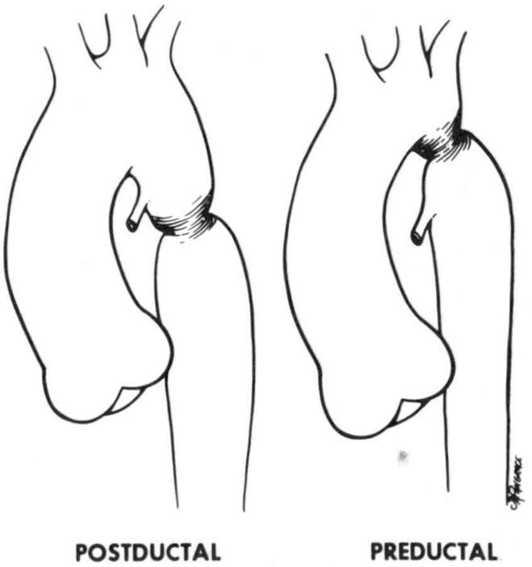

Mechanical assist devices: these devices can be divided into two general types: *temporary assist* and *permanent assist.* The purpose of temporary assist devices is to provide the failing heart with support over a short period, such as hours or days. Examples of temporary assist devices include the intra-aortic balloon pump (IABP) and the external left-ventricular and right-ventricular assist devices (LVAD; RVAD).

The intra-aortic balloon is a sausage-shaped balloon mounted on a catheter that is inserted most often through the femoral artery and is then placed distal to the left subclavian artery in the descending thoracic aorta. The action of the balloon is to inflate and deflate during diastole. Inflation allows the blood to be pushed cephalad into the aortic root, which increases coronary artery blood supply. Deflation of the balloon, just prior to systolic ejection, creates a negative intra-aortic pressure and therefore decreases afterload. Afterload is the impedance against which the ventricle must work to open the aortic valve. By increasing coronary blood flow and decreasing afterload, the total work of the heart is reduced, thereby providing an environment that supports the recovery of a failing myocardium.

Another variety of temporary cardiac assist de-

POSTDUCTAL   **PREDUCTAL**

FIGURE 26–5. Postductal and preductal types of coarctation of the aorta.

vices, the external ventricular assist device, is indicated for use in patients with markedly impaired ventricular function who, following cardiac surgery, develop ventricular failure unresponsive to pharmacologic and IABP support. Although these devices vary in their specific design, their technique generally consists of removing blood via cannulas from the left atrium or ventricle and reinfusing it into the aortic root. This technique bypasses the ventricle and therefore requires no ventricular contraction. Blood flow in these systems can be either pulsatile or nonpulsatile and can be propelled by roller, centrifugal, or pneumatically powered drive systems. In these temporary systems, the cannulas and pumps are most often situated outside the chest cavity.

Research on a permanently implantable mechanical heart assist device is advancing in two directions. The totally artificial heart, developed by Jarvik at the University of Utah, has arrived at the stage of clinical usage. This system consists of two pneumatically driven, elliptic, artificial ventricular chambers. Blood flows through these chambers in a manner similar to that in the natural heart, going from the right side through the lungs and then into the left chamber. At this point the blood is ejected into the systemic circulation. The pumping action in the chambers is supplied by a pusher-plate system that is controlled by a console external to the patient. The chambers are attached to the console via drive lines that exit from the patient in the abdominal region. This system requires complete excision of the natural myocardium. The other thrust in the development of a permanent artificial device is toward a permanently implantable LVAD in which the natural heart would remain in place, while cannulas and a pump system divert blood flow from the left atrium or ventricle into the aorta. Implanted in the chest cavity, this device would also require external drive lines and a drive system. The advantage to this system is that if there were a catastrophic failure of the artificial pump, the natural pump—the heart—could maintain the patient until arrival at a medical facility. This device currently has numerous successes in animal models. For both of these systems, technology to eliminate the cumbersome drive systems is less than half a decade away.

Mitral regurgitation: a condition that occurs when the mitral valve does not totally close because the leaflets do not completely approxi-

mate with each other during diastole. This lesion can occur as a result of a rheumatic process in which there is a progressive shortening of the leaflets and the chordae tendineae. The ischemia or infarction that is associated with coronary artery disease can cause a rupture or elongation of the papillary muscles or the chordae tendineae and also create a regurgitant state. In addition, connective tissue disorders, syphilis, Marfan's syndrome, and systemic lupus erythematosus can produce this state by their effect on the papillary muscles and on the chordae.

Mitral stenosis: a narrowing of the normal aperture of the mitral valve due to one or a combination of the following: a growth of rheumatic nodules on the valve where the leaflets meet, a thickening of the valves, a fusion of the commissures, or a shortening and thickening of the chordae tendineae. It is most frequently seen as a consequence of rheumatic heart disease.

Myocardial protection techniques: techniques or procedures designed to expedite the surgical procedure and to limit the amount of ischemic tissue injury that can occur. These techniques and procedures consist of the following: (1) electrical arrest of the myocardium with alternating current during diastole. This allows a quiet operative field, which expedites surgical repair and, hence, limits ischemic time; (2) anoxic arrest, produced by crossclamping the aorta. The effect of this technique is similar to (1); (3) hypothermia, both local and systemic, which serves to decrease cellular metabolism and thus limits ischemic damage (see *Hypothermia*); and (4) chemical cardioplegia, the infusion into the aortic root of electrolyte, pharmacologic, or blood solutions that assist in chemically arresting the myocardium. This also limits the amount of cellular damage (see *Cardioplegia*). In addition to these techniques, care is taken to prevent VF, because this arrhythmia increases wall tension and oxygen consumption.

Myocardial revascularization: surgical intervention in which blood flow is diverted past significant obstructions in the coronary arteries to inadequately perfused myocardium distal to the obstruction. This allows adequate oxygenation of these ischemic sections. Most often, portions of the saphenous vein harvested from the patient's leg are used as the conduits for blood flow. One portion of the vein is anastomosed in an end-to-side fashion to the aorta, and the other end is similarly anastomosed to the coronary artery distal to the obstruction (Fig. 26–6). In addition to using the saphenous vein, the right and left internal mammary arteries are well suited for myocardial revascularization. Arising from the aorta, these vessels extend along the inside of the chest wall. For revascularization purposes, they are distally dissected off the chest wall and are left attached proximally to the aorta. Their distal ends are then attached to vessels on their respective sides. Other conduit vessels that are attached in the same manner as the saphenous vein include portions of the cephalic vein and of a specially processed human umbilical vein. Bypass grafts are usually performed on the major coronary arteries, such as the right coronary artery, the two major branches of the left coronary artery, the left anterior descending artery, or the circumflex artery. However, grafts can be attached to any vessel that has a 1-mm diameter. Because of this, other vessels, such as the diagonal artery, or other branches of the major arteries, such as the posterior descending artery of the right coronary artery, also can be revascularized. Myocardial revascularization is also known as *coronary artery bypass* (CABG) or *aortocoronary grafting.*

Patent ductus arteriosus (PDA): a duct between the pulmonary artery and the aorta. This structure, which is normally present in fetal life, usually closes within 1 or 2 weeks after birth. Failure to close can predispose the patient to the development of pulmonary hypertension or cardiac failure. Closure can be surgically achieved by ligation of the ductus or by division of the ductus followed by oversewing of the ends.

Percutaneous transluminal coronary angioplasty (PTCA): a widely accepted nonsurgical treatment modality for acute or chronically obstructed coronary arteries. The exact mechanism in which angioplasty improves vessel patency is still debatable, but it appears to restore patency by compression and rupture of the atherosclerotic plaque creating a crack or fracture down to the internal elastic membrane. These "cracks" extending from the lumen appear to improve vessel patency by creating new channels for coronary blood flow. Healing at the angioplasty site may, in itself, mimic the original atherosclerotic plaque, causing a restenosis of the vessel. Restenosis occurs in 25 to 35 percent of patients and usually recurs within 3 to 6 months after the angioplasty procedure.

PTCA is performed in a cardiac catheterization laboratory using fluoroscopy to guide catheter placement. Local anesthetics and mild sedation are employed to help relax the patient and reduce discomfort. The patient needs to be awake, alert, and able to verbalize the occurrence of chest discomfort, shortness of breath, or other adverse reactions. The patient is monitored for arrhythmias and the presence of ischemia and injury. The guide

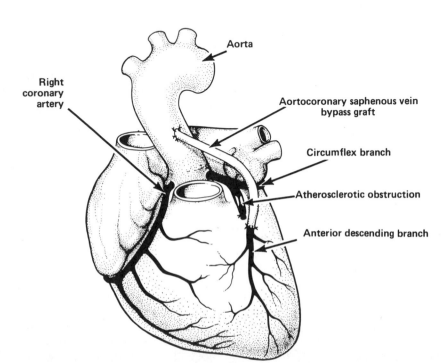

FIGURE 26–6. Saphenous vein bypass graft attached proximally to the aorta and distally to the anterior descending coronary artery past the atherosclerotic obstruction.

catheter is inserted through a cutdown over the right femoral artery. The balloon is inflated in a stepwise manner; the amount of pressure applied to inflate the balloon and the duration of the inflation are determined by the physician based on the patient's symptoms, the presence of ischemia, and the percentage of dilatation achieved with each inflation. Complications from the PTCA procedure include prolonged chest pain or myocardial infarction or coronary artery dissection or spasm often necessitating an emergency CABG. Other techniques have been developed using rotoblation and the transluminal extraction catheter (TEC) device when the catheter "drills" through the lesion, with the former pulverizing the lesion into minuscule particles to be absorbed by the body and the latter pulverizing the lesion with the TEC device "sucking out" the particles into an attached vacuum bottle. Laser angioplasty is also being used as well as the insertion of stents to maintain vessel patency. Care of the patient after PTCA includes monitoring of vital signs and cardiac rhythm to detect early signs of ischemia and impending infarction, assessing for bleeding at the site of the right femoral artery, and palpating pulses in the extremities for possible arterial thrombosis. Sheaths may be left in place overnight, and once removed, direct pressure, most often by the use of 5-lb sandbags, is applied to the site for approximately 6 hours. The patient is maintained on bedrest for about 8 hours after the procedure to prevent any potential bleeding from the cannulation site. Patients generally are discharged home the following day.

Pericardiectomy: the partial excision of an adhered, thickened, fibrotic pericardium to relieve constriction of a compressed heart and great blood vessels. In patients with chronic cardiac effusions, the creation of a pericardial window between the pericardial sac and the pleural space can also be accomplished. The opening to the pleural space allows chronically accumulating fluid to be reabsorbed.

Pulmonary artery banding: a procedure in which the pulmonary artery is constricted with tape to reduce its diameter and to decrease the pulmonary blood flow. This is usually performed as one of several stages prior to a complete surgical correction. The goal of this technique is to prevent the development of pulmonary hypertension.

Pulmonary stenosis: fusion of the valve cusps at the commissures, which creates an obstruction to the right-ventricular outflow tract. In infundibular stenosis, fibromuscular obstruction occurs proximal to the valve. Most frequently, repair is accomplished via an open procedure under direct visualization. The stenotic valve is opened wide, and the fused commissures are sharply excised back to the annulus. Correction can also be performed by a closed procedure in which, via a right ventriculotomy, a valvulotome is inserted and the stenotic leaflets are separated when it is withdrawn.

Tetralogy of Fallot: a congenital entity with four distinctive features (Fig. 26–7): (1) a high ventricular septal defect, (2) pulmonary stenosis, (3) overriding of the ventricular septal defect by the aorta, and (4) hypertrophy of the right ventricle. The current trend is to proceed with an elective procedure for correction, generally when the patient is 3 to 5 years old. If the child is severely symptomatic prior to this age, either a corrective or a palliative procedure is performed, according to the surgeon's preference. Currently, the most frequently performed palliative procedure is the Blalock-Taussig or systemic-pulmonary anastomosed technique. In this procedure, the subclavian artery is anastomosed to the pulmonary artery, thereby producing an increase in blood flow to the lungs. In a corrective procedure, a complete resection of the infundibular or pulmonary valve stenosis and closure of the ventricular

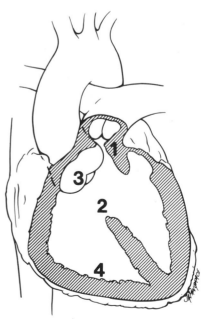

FIGURE 26–7. Four features of tetralogy of Fallot: 1. pulmonary stenosis; 2. ventricular septal defect; 3. overriding aorta; and 4. right-ventricular hypertrophy.

septal defect are performed. If previously constructed palliative shunts are present, they are closed prior to the initiation of the corrective procedure.

Transplantation: With the improvement in pharmacologic management and infection prophylaxis, cardiac transplantation 1-year survival rates are approaching 90 percent. Potential candidates are patients who are considered to be in the New York Heart Association's functional class IV and who have less than a 10 percent chance of surviving for 6 months. Contraindications for transplantation include significant pulmonary hypertension, the presence of systemic disease, a recent pulmonary infarction, or active systemic infection. Heart donors are persons with irreversible, catastrophic brain injury who are younger than 30 years of age and do not have atherosclerotic heart disease. Removal of the donor heart is accomplished by transection of the vena cava, the pulmonary artery and veins, and the aorta. The donor heart is then transported to the recipient's institution in an iced saline bath with ischemic times of less than 4 hours. The recipient's heart is surgically removed once the donor heart has arrived in the operating room. The posterior and lateral atrial walls, the vena caval inflow tracts, the pulmonary vein orifices, and the atrial septum remain intact while the remainder of the heart is excised. The donor heart is then attached at the atria, the pulmonary artery, and the aorta. Except for the addition of infection and rejection monitoring, these patients receive the same postoperative care given other general cardiac surgery patients. If no complications ensue, they are generally discharged from the hospital in 3 weeks.

Transposition of the great arteries (TGA): a congenital anomaly in which the pulmonary artery arises from the left ventricle and carries oxygenated blood back to the lungs, and the aorta arises from the right ventricle and carries unoxygenated blood into the systemic circulation. An uncommon anomaly, this condition is incompatible with life unless a concomitant anomalous shunt, such as a septal defect or PDA between the systemic and pulmonary circulations, is also present. These lesions allow adequate mixing of the blood between the two circulations. To maintain the patency of the atrial septal defect, a balloon atrial septostomy is usually performed. In addition, prostaglandin E is administered to maintain the patency of the PDA. A variety of corrective procedures can be used to achieve a repair, with the selection of the procedure being dictated by the patient's anatomic structure and the surgeon's preference. Arterial, ventricular, and intra-atrial repairs can be performed. The two intra-arterial repairs are the Senning and the Mustard procedures. In both of these types, the atrial chambers are reconstructed so that pulmonary venous blood returns to the right atrium and systemic venous blood returns to the left atrium. Surgical correction of this anomaly is undertaken as early as possible.

Tricuspid regurgitation: a condition that occurs when the tricuspid valve does not totally close because the leaflets do not completely approximate in diastole. This lesion is more common than tricuspid stenosis and can develop because of rheumatic changes, following a right-ventricular infarction, or, transiently, from annular dilatation resulting from right-ventricular failure.

Tricuspid stenosis: a narrowing of the orifice of the tricuspid valve. Although this condition occurs infrequently, it can be associated with rheumatic heart disease or bacterial endocarditis.

Valve replacement: a surgical procedure in which the natural valve is replaced with an artificial valve. Whatever the cause, repair consists of excising the natural valve and its attached apparatus, such as the chordae tendineae of the mitral valve, and inserting a prosthetic valve. Prosthetic valves can be classified into two groups: mechanical and biologic. Types of mechanical valves currently used are the caged-ball, the tilting-disk, and the bileaflet valves (Fig. 26–8). The caged-ball valve consists of a metallic cage attached to a sewing ring. In the center of the cage is a hollow metal or plastic ball that moves forward in the cage, allowing blood to flow through the valve. When the ball rests on the sewing ring, it impedes flow. An example of the caged-ball type is the Starr-Edwards valve.

The tilting-disk valve consists of a free-floating, thin, lens-shaped disk occluder made of pyrolytic carbon mounted on a semicircular sewing ring. The disk tilts or pivots upward when the valve is open, allowing blood flow, and when the valve is closed, the disk lies on the sewing ring. Examples of the tilting disk valve are the Björk-Shiley and the Lillehei-Kaster valves. More recently, a bileaflet valve, the St. Jude Medical prosthesis, has been developed. The St. Jude valve consists of a sewing ring in which reside two semicircular leaflets that open centrally. This valve is well suited for use in children and adults

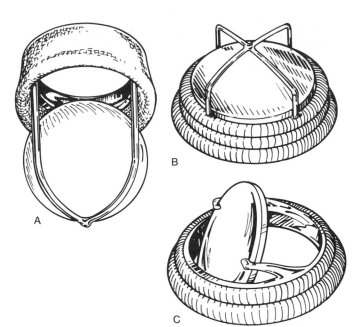

FIGURE 26–8. Schematic representation of various types of mechanical valves: *A*, cage and ball; *B*, cage and disk; and *C*, tilting disk.

with small aortic roots because of its size and design.

Mechanical valves are extremely durable and withstand wear over a long period. One disadvantage associated with their use is the high incidence of thromboembolic events. For this reason, patients with these valves need lifelong anticoagulation therapy. This is usually initiated 3 to 5 days after surgery, when all their intracardiac lines and chest tubes are discontinued and immediate postoperative hemorrhage is no longer a concern. Oral coumarin therapy is then started and titrated appropriately to achieve prothrombin times two and a half times normal.

Biologic valves can be classified as *xenograft* (from animal cadaver tissues) or *homograft* (from human cadaver donor tissue). Xenografts can be made from porcine aorta or bovine pericardium. The Hancock and Carpentier-Edwards valves are porcine valves. The Ionescu-Shiley valve is an example of a bovine pericardial valve. The advantage of biologic valves resides largely in the decreased incidence of thromboembolic events associated with their use. Despite this, some physicians maintain their patients on prophylactic anticoagulation drugs for 6 months after biologic valve replacement, particularly if the patient has had a history of a mural thrombus, atrial fibrillation, or an enlarged left atrium. Disadvantages of biologic valves are that they are not as durable as mechanical valves; they are prone to tissue degeneration and calcification of their leaflets and

may therefore require reoperation and replacement earlier than mechanical valves.

An occasional postoperative problem after valve replacement for aortic stenosis is the *hyperdynamic left-ventricle syndrome*, which may also occur in patients with long-standing hypertension. This syndrome is characterized by extreme hypertension that occurs in the immediate postoperative period that is not responsive to increasingly larger dosages of vasodilators. Widening pulse pressure secondary to a diastolic decrease in blood pressure from effects of the vasodilators is seen with a consequential decrease in myocardial oxygen supply. Simultaneously, oxygen demand increases as a result of systemic hypertension and tachycardia. If left untreated, left-ventricular failure occurs with decreased cardiac output, increased pulmonary artery wedge pressure (PAWP) with eventual hypotension, and cardiac arrest. Medical management includes lowering the rate of vasodilators, adding a director peripheral vasodilator to treat hypertension, and using beta blockers if tachycardia coexists.

Conversely, patients with aortic insufficiency (AI) have a volume-overloaded ventricle with increased compliance. Irreversible left-ventricular dysfunction may result from chronic volume overload in patients with AI. Some of these patients may not benefit from having the aortic valve replaced. Massive AI with dilated chambers and large changes in volume are associated with minimal changes in pressure. This factor limits the usefulness of postoperative left-atrial or PAWP pressures. After valve replacement for acute or chronic AI, a state of peripheral vasodilation with low diastolic pressure sometimes occurs. If ventricular performance is hampered and there are no contraindications, an alpha-adrenergic agonist may be used. This approach is often used in septic patients with acute AI from infectious endocarditis.

Patients undergoing mitral valve replacement need to be observed for both right-ventricular and left-ventricular failure. Right-ventricular failure may occur intraoperatively at the time CPB is discontinued or in the early post anesthesia period. Low cardiac output despite adequate preload, increased central venous pressure, normal or low PAWP, and right-ventricular distention should alert the nurse to the onset of right-ventricular failure.

Patients with chronic mitral insufficiency have an enlarged left ventricle that is accustomed to low-pressure "pop-off" of the incompetent valve. Implantation of a prosthesis or repair of a dysfunctional valve results in a competent mechanism that creates a postoperative afterload mismatch. Sodium nitroprusside (Nipride) is often used preoperatively to decrease the afterload caused by the new competent valve.

Acute mitral insufficiency is better tolerated than acute AI. The most frequent causes of acute mitral insufficiency are papillary muscle rupture or dysfunction secondary to ischemia or injury and ruptured chordae tendineae. The left-atrial pressure increases because it cannot accommodate the regurgitant volume. This high left-atrial pressure is transmitted to the pulmonary veins. Large "V" waves can be seen on PAWP tracings. Forward output decreases, resulting in pulmonary edema. Management of these patients includes digoxin, diuretics, inotropic support with dopamine or dobutamine, and afterload reduction with sodium nitroprusside or nitroglycerine.

Ventricular aneurysm repair: a surgical technique used to correct a ventricular aneurysm. Ventricular aneurysms most often result from a large myocardial infarction or numerous smaller adjacent infarctions in which a portion of the myocardial wall becomes necrotic, thin, and weak. This portion then does not contract during systole but instead bulges outward, which decreases the patient's cardiac output. Additionally, the endothelial layers of the aneurysm become roughened, which promotes the development of large mural thrombi, leaving the patient at high

risk for an embolic event. Also, the perimeter around the necrotic area, because it consists largely of varying amounts of fibrous tissue, can alter conduction pathways and create re-entrant ventricular arrhythmias. The surgical technique consists of excising the aneurysm at its perimeter and carefully removing the thrombus inside to avoid embolization. Then, the edges of the ventricle are joined with sutures. If the patient has been experiencing recurrent VT, an endomyocardial mapping might also be performed. With this technique, the aneurysm is first removed; next, a small electrode probe is attached to the surgeon's fingers and passed over the edges of the endothelial portion of the remaining ventricle; and finally, activation potentials are observed. This procedure assists in differentiating fibrous tissue from viable tissue. The endothelium is then peeled back, removing all the fibrous tissue. This eliminates tissues that are a source of re-entrant rhythms. The edges of the ventricle are then closed as previously described (Fig. 26–9).

Ventricular septal defect: a defect consisting of a hole through the ventricular septum. This defect is usually located in the upper portion of the septum just anterior to the membranous septum. A ventricular septal defect can be congenital or acquired; those of congenital origin sometimes close spontaneously. In an adult, these are most commonly acquired from myocardial ischemia following an infarction of the septal wall (Fig. 26–10). In both types, closure of the defect can be accomplished either with the use of a synthetic patch or by oversewing the edges, depending on the size of the defect.

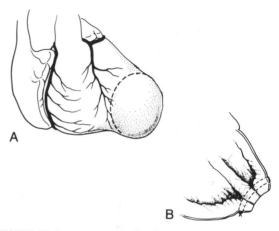

FIGURE 26–9. *A,* a ventricular aneurysm is illustrated. *B,* repair consists of excision of the aneurysm and approximation of the edges of the left ventricle.

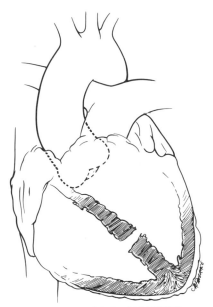

VENTRICULAR SEPTAL DEFECT

FIGURE 26–10. Schematic representation of a ventricular septal defect. The size and location of the defect vary from patient to patient.

INTRAOPERATIVE CONSIDERATIONS

The most commonly used approach in cardiac surgery is the median sternotomy. However, anterolateral or posterolateral thoracotomy incisions or a transverse sternotomy with a bilateral thoracotomy can also be used. The median sternotomy approach allows exposure of the anterior mediastinum without entry into the pleural cavities. With this approach, the sternum is split with a saw. At the conclusion of the procedure, the sternum is closed with stainless steel wires, and the skin is approximated subcutaneously with suture. The pericardium that was incised during the surgery is left open at the end of the procedure. Pericardial chest tubes are placed anteriorly and posteriorly in the pericardium to facilitate drainage. They exit via stab wounds at the distal portion of the mediastinal incision. If either of the pleurae was opened during the procedure, then pleural chest tubes are also inserted.

Once the sternum is opened, the patient is placed on CPB, and hypothermia and cardioplegic infusions are initiated. Although CPB is an essential component of cardiac surgery, it is not without potential problems. With prolonged use of an oxygenator pump (usually 4 hours or longer), various coagulation, volume, respiratory, and neurologic dysfunctions may develop.

Physiologic Changes Associated with Cardiopulmonary Bypass

Patients who undergo surgery requiring CPB are subject to several physiologic changes. Personnel involved with the care of these patients should be familiar with the physiologic changes that occur during the initial post anesthesia period. There is a marked elevation of epinephrine and norepinephrine levels during CPB. Hyperglycemia and impaired insulin responses are present, resulting in the utilization of fat stores for energy until carbohydrate metabolism returns to normal levels. There is also an increased secretion of antidiuretic hormone and aldosterone that is stimulated by different mechanisms associated with the physiologic components of stress. Serum complement that is activated, in combination with the crystalloid solutions employed to prime the CPB pump, causes a marked increase in total body water and interstitial edema.

With an understanding of these mechanisms, one can expect to see excess fluid in the interstitial spaces. Postoperative fluid requirements should be minimal, especially when rewarming has been instituted. Rewarming itself also causes fluid shifts. This excess fluid usually redistributes itself by the second or third day postoperatively and will be excreted spontaneously or from the use of diuretic therapy. CPB and hypothermia also alter coagulation factors and platelet formation. When exposed to the foreign surfaces of the CPB pump, platelets clump together. A decrease in the remaining number of platelets occurs along with a decrease in the aggregative and adhesive functions of remaining platelets. Release of vasoactive substances occurs as platelets are destroyed. In addition, exposure to the CPB pump causes a breakdown of plasma proteins, including gamma globulin, which in turn may cause fat microemboli release, microcoagulation, and clotting factor consumption and increased vascular permeability. The stresses of CPB also cause destruction of erythrocytes and leukocytes.

Also of importance is hypothermia-related hypocarbia. The body temperature usually remains lower than normal during the early postoperative hours. Slowly, the body temperature returns to normal, and occasionally rebound hyperthermia occurs. The problem that arises is that as rewarming takes place, so does the production of carbon dioxide; consequently, the potential exists for the development of hypercarbia, and ventilator settings should be adjusted to produce a minute volume necessary to facilitate normocarbia. In addition, if rebound hyperthermia occurs or if rewarming devices are not regulated and monitored appropriately, a hyperthermic overshoot will occur. Again, this reaction is undesirable, because hyperthermia increases myocardial oxygen demand and consumption.

Anesthesia

Anesthesia for cardiac surgery varies from hospital to hospital and also can vary depending on the type of cardiac repair undertaken. For example, in the repair of a mitral valve when there is evidence of significant pulmonary involvement, agents that increase pulmonary vascular resistance should be avoided. Commonly employed inhalation agents include halothane, enflurane, methoxyflurane, and nitrous oxide. Barbiturates, such as thiopental and methohexital, are used to accomplish the rapid sequence of induction and intubation. Other induction agents, such as etomidate and ketamine, can be used depending on the physiologic status of the patient. Morphine sulfate, sufentanil, or fentanyl are the narcotic analgesics that are most frequently used. Morphine can assist in increasing the cardiac index, because it decreases systemic vascular resistance. Also, because fentanyl has a negligible myocardial effect, it is also a commonly used analgesic. Antianxiety agents such as diazepam and midazolam, in addition to narcotic analgesics, are employed in the early postoperative period.

PACU CARE

Following cardiac surgery, most patients require monitoring of their heart rate, arterial blood pressure, and oxygen saturation during transport from the surgical suite to the PACU or cardiac ICU. This is because these patients can develop acute circulatory instability owing either to their normally recovering physiologic state or to inadvertent movement or displacement of the numerous invasive lines and tubes they require. On admission to the PACU, the nurse should assess these parameters immediately. If either of these parameters indicates circulatory or ventilatory dysfunction, immediate resuscitative measures should be instituted.

If, at a quick glance, circulatory and ventilatory status appear adequate, then admission routines should be begun. The respiratory therapist or anesthesiologist usually attaches the

patient to the ventilator, establishes the initial ventilator settings, and sets the alarms. Once the patient is attached to the ventilator, the nurse auscultates both lung fields and repeats that assessment frequently until the patient's discharge from the PACU. Arterial blood gas values are determined on admission and as needed thereafter. Patients remain intubated until the effects of anesthesia subside and hemodynamic stability is achieved and maintained. Controlled ventilation is used initially. As patients begin to generate their own respirations, they are switched to intermittent mandatory ventilation modes, in which they gradually increase their spontaneous respirations to maintain adequate minute ventilations. Once patients are maintaining an adequate respiratory rate, they are switched to continuous positive airway pressure (CPAP) systems. With CPAP, the patient determines the respiratory rate, and the ventilator provides the positive pressure to the airway that the glottis normally provides when the patient is not intubated. The use of CPAP prevents microatelectasis and increases the functional residual capacity of the lung. Once the patient maintains adequate arterial blood gas levels on CPAP, extubation usually follows quickly. After extubation, face masks or nasal cannulas are used to deliver supplemental oxygen.

A continuous ECG recording is established, alarm limits are set, and a strip recording is obtained. A 12-lead ECG is obtained as soon as possible and is repeated daily for the first 3 days. Recorded rhythm strips are then obtained every 2 hours and documented. Lead selection varies, but MCL_1, in which the left-atrial and right-atrial leads are in their respective places and the third lead is placed on the fourth right intercostal space, is commonly used. Electrode placement with this lead does not interfere with defibrillation procedures or with mediastinal or chest tube dressing placement. The apical pulse is auscultated and validated with the ECG recording. If the patient has a temporary external pacer in place, the nurse should check and record the type of pacing, the mode, the rate, and the milliamperage and determine if the pacer is functioning adequately. If the patient is not being paced, then the nurse needs to ensure that the unused pacemaker wires are covered with gauze, placed in a plastic covering (a finger cot), and securely dressed and attached to the chest to protect the patient from electrical hazard. Usually, two ventricular and two atrial pacing wires are attached to the epicardium with absorbable suture prior the chest being closed. These wires then exit the chest via stab wounds on either side of the sternal incision. The atrial wires are usually on the right and the ventricular wires on the left. They are most often left in place for a few days after surgery and may be used to assist in cardiac rhythm control. Before the patient is discharged from the hospital, the wires are totally removed by gentle traction or they are clipped off at the skin level, leaving a portion of them attached to the epicardium and residing in the subcutaneous tissues.

All intravascular lines are attached to transducers or manometers. Their patency is ascertained and their values or wave tracings or both are continuously displayed and recorded. Commonly measured intravascular parameters include the following pressures: mean arterial, right atrial, mean pulmonary artery, pulmonary artery systolic, pulmonary artery diastolic, pulmonary capillary wedge, and left atrial. In addition to providing these directly measured parameters, these values assist in calculating indirect or derived hemodynamic parameters, such as cardiac output and cardiac index, systemic vascular resistance, and pulmonary vascular resistance. All of these parameters assist in assessing both left-ventricular and right-ventricular status and are invaluable in determining pharmacologic, fluid, and mechanical therapies for the postoperative cardiac surgery patient. Once these intravascular lines are appropriately monitored, the nurse reviews and assesses with the anesthesiologist all intravascular lines and solutions with regard to type, drugs being infused, flow rates, patency, and expiration times, if applicable. Intake and output recordings with running totals are made and documented hourly. Volume administration and replacement treatments are largely determined by the individual patient's hemodynamic parameters, and responses can vary greatly from hour to hour.

The patient's neurologic status is assessed on admission and every 30 to 60 minutes thereafter until arousal from anesthesia. Once the patient has been aroused, neurologic assessments are decreased to every 2 hours. The Glasgow coma scale can be used for these checks (see Chapter 29).

Chest tube drainage systems are established. Water-seal drainage or autotransfusion systems with 15 to 20 cm of negative suction are most frequently used. The amount and type of chest tube drainage are frequently assessed and recorded on an hourly basis. Drainage exceeding 100 ml per hr should be brought to the attention of the physician. Chest tubes are usually removed on the first or second postoperative day, providing intracardiac lines have been removed, there is no evidence of fluid accumulation on the chest radiograph, and there has been less than 200 ml of drainage in the last 6 hours. Most patients will have one or two mediastinal chest tubes that facilitate pericardial drainage after surgery. If the pleural spaces were opened during the procedure or the internal mammary arteries were dissected off the chest wall, or both, then pleural chest tubes will also be present to facilitate drainage and to prevent a pneumothorax.

An admission temperature is obtained, and rewarming therapies are instituted, if necessary. During rewarming, temperatures are recorded hourly, and rewarming devices are discontinued just before the patient reaches normothermia. This slightly premature discontinuation is performed to avoid a hyperthermic overshoot, which is common. In this situation, temperatures may overshoot the 37°C (98.6°F) level and elevate to levels of 38° to 40°C (100.4° to 104°F).

An abdominal assessment is performed on admission and every 2 hours thereafter until bowel sounds return. A nasogastric tube is in place to relieve gastric distention and facilitate removal of gastric contents. It is usually attached to low intermittent suction or gravity drainage and removed at the time of extubation. Analysis of pH and tests for the presence of occult blood may be performed on gastric secretions if they begin to resemble coffee grounds. Once the nasogastric tube is removed, the patient is given ice chips and resumes a clear liquid diet within the first 24 hours.

A retention catheter is in place, and urinary outputs are recorded on admission to the PACU and then hourly. The appearance of the urine is also monitored closely. During the first few hours after surgery, massive diuresis of 2 to 3 L of pale, dilute urine is usually common. This is a result of use of diuretics that are generally administered during the discontinuation of CPB pumping to facilitate the removal of fluid that has sequestered during surgery in the interstitial space. Once this initial diuresis resolves, urine color and consistency return to normal. At that time, it is desirable to keep urinary output at levels higher than 0.5 ml per kg per hr.

Peripheral pulses as well as skin color and temperature are assessed and recorded hourly. All incisions and intravascular and tube insertion sites are observed. The patient is placed in a semi-Fowler position with his or her legs supported at the knees and calves slightly elevated. This facilitates venous return from the legs and limits swelling, particularly in patients with saphenous vein incisions. Legs are wrapped from toes to hips with elastic leg wraps or antiembolism stockings.

Following these admission routines, a written assessment is performed. The frequency of assessing and documenting the hemodynamic parameters discussed earlier and routines is dictated by the patient's response to and recovery from surgery. Recovery time varies from patient to patient but generally occurs within 12 to 48 hours. During that time, owing largely to the techniques of CPB, hypothermia, anesthesia, and surgical manipulation of the myocardium, numerous normal postoperative physiologic alterations occur. With correct interventions, these normal physiologic responses are short-lived and reversible. However, two problems do exist. First, although these alterations are reversible, if they are not identified early and quickly reversed, they can lead to complications. Such is the case with uncontrolled hypertension that can develop into hemorrhage if fresh suture lines are disrupted. Second, these normal alterations frequently resemble complications and thus may be missed in their early stages. For example, the initial absence of a pedal pulse may be attributed to hypothermia and vasoconstriction only to be traced later to a vascular embolism. For these reasons, it is incumbent on the PACU nurse to be knowledgeable about the causes, assessment factors, and interventions for both normal physiologic alterations and complications that can occur after cardiac surgery. In the following section, these alterations and potential complications will be briefly reviewed.

COMPLICATIONS

Cardiovascular System

A number of predisposing factors are known to increase the incidence of postoperative complications and early mortality. These include preoperative cardiac conditions such as myocardial dysfunction, recent myocardial infarction, and previous CABG surgery or systemic conditions such as advanced age, obesity, diabetes mellitus, and chronic obstructive pulmonary disease.

The surgical risks of CABG can be assessed quite accurately preoperatively, and complications can be anticipated by taking preoperative risk factors into consideration.

Complications related to CABG and valvular surgery can generally be classified as either cardiac or noncardiac. *Cardiac complications* include myocardial infarction, congestive heart failure, tamponade, decreased cardiac output, arrhythmias, and postoperative hypertension. *Noncardiac complications* include hemorrhage, wound dehiscence and infection, and neurologic, renal, pulmonary, and gastrointestinal problems. Each complication will be addressed individually.

Cardiac Complications of CABG and Valvular Surgery

Myocardial Infarction. Despite better myocardial protection with hypothermia, cardioplegic arrest, and topical hypothermia during surgery, myocardial infarction still remains the most common and serious postoperative complication and the main cause of early death after surgery. Suboptimal myocardial protection may result secondary to uneven distribution of cardioplegic solutions in the coronary arteries. Subendocardial ischemia may occur secondary to a distended left ventricle and incomplete revascularization. All serve as frequent causes of new infarction.

Hemorrhagic infarction may occur 1 to 4 hours postoperatively as a result of reperfusion injury. It is often manifested as a malignant reperfusion arrhythmia such as VT that is unresponsive to antiarrhythmic therapy, and cardiogenic shock develops quickly. Sudden reperfusion of an ischemic area is thought to cause hemorrhagic necrosis owing to a rapid influx of calcium ions into the ischemic myocardial cells. The appearance of new Q waves postoperatively has been shown to adversely affect early and late survival. A number of other predictors of perioperative myocardial infarction include left main stenosis, multivessel disease, absence of collateral circulation, the number of grafts, and the duration of CPB.

Ischemic changes sometimes occur within the first 48 hours after surgery as a result of spasm of bypassed or unbypassed coronary arteries. Treatment with intravenous nitroglycerine or calcium channel blockers is usually effective in relieving the spasm.

Congestive Heart Failure (alterations in myocardial contractility). Although relatively uncommon after CABG surgery, congestive heart failure remains a serious complication and is the second most common cause of early mortality.

Alteration in myocardial contractility with resultant low cardiac outputs and shocklike states can also develop postoperatively. The causes include a perioperative myocardial infarction or an ischemic state, faulty surgical repair, myocardial edema from surgical manipulation, metabolic disturbances, and depression from hypothermia and anesthesia. The patient clinically demonstrates a decrease in cardiac output and cardiac index, hypotension, elevated systemic vascular resistance, elevated filling pressures, acidosis, tachycardia, and decreased urine output. If the condition is the result of faulty surgical repair, the patient should immediately be returned to the surgical suite for correction.

The treatment includes a balance of pharmacologic and mechanical circulatory support throughout the period of recuperation, which may last from 1 to 5 days. Depending on the hemodynamic status of the patient, different combinations of inotropic and vasopressor agents are used as initial therapy, with the addition of mechanical support if cardiac output remains low despite inotropic stimulation and optimal filling pressures, as indicated by a pulmonary capillary wedge pressure higher than 22 to 25 mm Hg.

In most instances, decreased cardiac output occurs as a result of terminating CPB, and immediate attention is required. Temporary support by resuming CPB for about 30 minutes may be enough to relieve myocardial ischemia and improve ventricular contractility to a level that will allow smooth weaning with low dosages of inotropic support.

Cardiac Tamponade. Cardiac tamponade develops when there is an accumulation of blood or fluid in the pericardial cavity sufficient to compress the heart. This compression of the heart results in ineffective filling and ejection. Signs therefore consist of low cardiac output and cardiac index, hypotension, tachycardia, equalization of the right-atrial and left-atrial pressures, development of pulsus paradoxus, narrowed pulse pressure, muffled heart sounds, widening of the mediastinum on chest radiograph, and alteration in neurologic status. Observation of the quality of chest tube drainage is critical in this situation. Normally, chest tube drainage in cardiac surgical patients is thin, red, and nonclotted. This is because blood resides in the chest cavity for a brief period before it exits via the chest tubes. Because of this residence time, it is exposed to the mechanical effects of the contracting heart and the motion of the lungs. This allows the blood that normally begins to clot once it leaves its vessel to lyse the clot it forms and thus become thin, nonclotted drainage by the time it exits the chest tube. If clots begin to appear in the chest tubes, this indicates that relatively fresh bleeding is occurring, because blood has no residence time in the chest cavity. In this situation, the incidence of tamponade is higher, because the chest tubes become clotted off easily. Therefore, sudden cessation of previously heavily clotted drainage is a primary indicator for the nurse at the bedside that a tamponade may be developing. Tamponade most frequently occurs in the first 6 hours after surgery. The specific cause can be either rapid, active bleeding from a suture line or continuous, slow oozing from a coagulopathy that exceeds the ability of the chest tube to drain it. A tamponade may also develop after the removal of intracardiac lines, as a result of which bleeding occurred. Treatment consists of reoperation. If the patient becomes acutely unstable, the chest will be reopened in the PACU. Opening of the chest cavity frequently relieves the compression enough that relatively stable vital signs immediately ensue. The patient can then be taken to the surgical suite for complete repair on a less emergent basis. A reoperation to relieve a tamponade does not usually delay the patient's recovery or prolong hospitalization.

Dysrhythmias. Rhythm disturbance can occur postoperatively in as many as 30 percent of patients undergoing cardiac surgery. Caused by ischemic, pharmacologic, metabolic, or iatrogenic effects, these disturbances can range from atrial to ventricular in nature. Ischemia due to infarction, hypoxemia, or hypotension may serve as the precipitant drive for dysrhythmia. Inotropic drugs, with their contractile and chronotropic effects, or acid–base imbalances and electrolyte abnormalities may also be the causative factors. Iatrogenically, mechanical irritation from some intracardiac lines and from the patient's endogenous catecholamine release may create irregularities. The high incidence of dysrhythmias demands that continuous monitoring be performed for the first 48 hours on these patients, even if they are discharged to a regular nursing unit in that period. Aggressive treatment of electrolyte imbalances and correction of hypoxic states are the first priorities. The massive diuresis some patients experience frequently precipitates hypokalemia and thus numerous arrhythmias. Therefore potassium replacement is aggressive, and efforts are made to maintain serum potassium concentrations at levels higher than 4 mEq per L. If correction of these imbalances fails to eliminate the dysrhythmia, pacing may be undertaken via the temporary external pacing wires inserted during the surgical procedure.

Peripheral Vasoconstriction (postoperative

hypertension). Factors that contribute to the development of peripheral vasoconstriction include the patient's own sympathetic drive triggered by anxiety and the surgical manipulation of the heart and the great vessels with their attached pressor receptors. Additionally, CPB, systemic hypothermia, and vasoactive drugs contribute to this vasoconstriction. The patient physically presents with pale, cold extremities; temperature lower than 37°C (98.6°F); increased systemic vascular resistance; absent pulses; tachycardia; and varying degrees of hypertension. If left unattended, the hypertension can disrupt new surgical anastomoses, and the increased systemic vascular resistance can assist in creating a state of myocardial depression owing to the high afterload effect it creates. Treatment approaches consist of immediate rewarming and administration of vasodilating agents, including intravenous sodium nitroprusside, nitroglycerine, and phentolamine. These agents have relatively immediate effects and can be easily reversed once their use is discontinued. The PACU nurse usually titrates the dosage of these agents to maintain the mean arterial blood pressure at 60 to 120 mm Hg and to bring systemic vascular resistance back to normal levels.

Noncardiac Complications of CABG and Valvular Surgery

Hemorrhage. Coagulation difficulties and hemorrhage pose a potential threat to the post anesthesia CABG surgical patient. Coagulation dysfunction often occurs as a result of using the oxygenator pump 4 hours or longer. Bleeding difficulties may occur as a result of direct trauma to the blood components from solid synthetic surfaces and systemic heparinization associated with CPB.

Preoperative evaluation should detect most coagulation disturbances and dictate treatment for correction prior to surgery. Prior health problems should also be taken into account as possible causes of coagulation disturbances, such as in patients with uremic and hepatic diseases.

The main causes of postoperative mediastinal bleeding include inadequate surgical hemostasis and coagulation disorders. Surgical hemostasis at the end of CPB is the best prophylactic measure against postoperative bleeding. Particular attention to the internal mammary artery sites is required because of the extensive dissection from the chest wall. Risk of bleeding often is the result of pericardial adhesions that have formed. Adequate heparin

reversal with confirmation by an whole-blood activated coagulation time (ACT) or activated partial thromboplastin time (APTT) should be performed (see Chapter 5). Even if the results of these studies are normal, heparin may still be released from body stores, causing a heparin rebound phenomenon. Therefore, an initially normal ACT or APTT result does not guarantee that subsequent bleeding is unrelated to the effects of heparin. Another prophylactic measure to reduce intraoperative and postoperative bleeding is the use of the drug aprotinin. This anti-inflammatory agent has been used traditionally to manage pancreatitis. Aprotinin may be indicated for patients undergoing repeat or complicated CABG procedures and for patients who have taken aspirin in the perioperative period who have had a CABG procedure performed.

Mediastinal exploration is indicated when signs of cardiac tamponade develop with bleeding of more than 500 ml per hr or less or more than 300 ml per hr for 6 hours or longer. The decision to reoperate should be made before the patient becomes hemodynamically unstable. On re-exploration for bleeding, oozing from the mediastinal wound is more commonly found as opposed to active bleeding. After evacuation of clots and hematomas, bleeding can usually be controlled.

Sternal Wound Dehiscence and Infection. Three to four percent of the postoperative CABG patients have difficulty with sternal wound healing. Although sterile dehiscence of the sternal bone is possible, superficial wound infection, sternal osteitis, and mediastinitis are more common. Predisposing factors include advanced age, obesity, diabetes mellitus, and chronic obstructive pulmonary disease. Postoperative bleeding necessitating re-exploration significantly contributes to sternal wound infection. Infection may occur at any time, but it is usually diagnosed 6 to 12 days postoperatively. Treatment consists of intravenous antibiotics, opening of the wound, débridement, and removal of all foreign objects, including sutures. Once the sternal wound is clean, reconstruction can take place about 1 or 2 weeks after débridement. Intravenous antibiotics are continued for at least 1 week after wound closure.

Inadequate Volume Status. Inadequate volume status can easily develop in postoperative patients. Hypovolemia can be induced by inadequate volume management in conjunction with or following rewarming in which there is rapid vasodilatation. Hypovolemia can also be associated with diuretic and vasodilator therapies; hemorrhage from active or slow-oozing bleeders in the chest or from coagulopathies associated with CPB; or inadequate reversal of the effects of the heparin used during CPB. Hypervolemia develops as interstitial fluid moves back into the intravascular space or if overaggressive volume replacement occurs. Assessment of these states requires extensive hemodynamic monitoring and understanding of the numerous processes involved. Signs and symptoms specific to hypovolemia or hypervolemia should be sought. Interventions for hypovolemia consist first of replacement with crystalloid agents. If the patient is suspected of having a moderate capillary leak syndrome due to prolonged bypass times, or if the patient had significant peripheral edema, then colloidal solutions are more appropriate. If persistent hemorrhage from coagulopathies exists, transfusion with replacement factors such as fresh-frozen plasma, platelet concentrates, and other factors may be indicated. If hemorrhage is related to technical factors, reoperation is required, and replacement solutions in the interim can be autotranfused blood, whole blood, or packed cells.

Respiratory System

The effects of anesthesia, sedation, and CPB commonly create moderate episodes of impaired gas exchange with concurrent moderate alterations in the arterial blood gas values. These episodes, largely atelectatic in nature, are usually self-limiting or easily resolved with the sustained maximal inspiration (see Chapter 19), chest physiotherapy, and the administration of supplemental oxygen. A hemothorax or a pneumothorax may develop. In these situations, more negative pressure may be added to the drainage systems, or placement of additional chest tubes may be required. A volume overload from overaggressive replacement or mobilization of fluid from the third spaces may exist that can hamper gas exchange. In this situation, diuretic therapy would be instituted. In rare instances, a noncardiac permeability pulmonary edema can develop. Because this entity is associated with a high mortality rate, mechanical ventilatory assistance and pharmacologic and fluid therapies are quite intensive.

Nervous System

Temporary and permanent sensory, motor, perceptual, and cognitive deficits can occur during the perioperative period.

Permanent deficits can usually be attributed to a low cerebral perfusion state from inadequate cardiac output or to an embolic phenomenon from intracardiac thrombi, calcified valve fragments, plaque embolization from the aortic crossclamp, or air embolization from intracardiac lines. The magnitude of the deficit is determined by the degree of neurologic involvement. These are usually identified early in the postoperative period when the effects of anesthesia have resolved. Some of these deficits may not be identified until after extubation. Transient deficits that can last from hours to days can occur in as many as one fourth of patients undergoing cardiac surgery. These transient deficits can range from a slowness to arouse to confusion and delirium.

Renal System

Prerenal and acute renal failure states can develop after cardiac surgery. Inadequate cardiac output from myocardial depression or inadequate volume replacement can lead to prerenal oliguria. In this situation, blood urea nitrogen and serum sodium levels increase and serum creatinine levels remain the same. There is a low sodium content in the urine as the body attempts to save sodium and thus increase its intravascular volume; the urine plasma osmolality ratio remains 1:1.5. If these states continue for prolonged periods, acute renal failure can ensue. Treatment focuses on maintaining an adequate volume replacement and on increasing cardiac output, perhaps with an inotropic agent. In addition, renal emboli from intracardiac thrombi or hemolysis from blood transfusions can also lead to the development of acute renal failure. In the event of acute renal failure, serum creatinine and urea levels elevate and remain in a 10:1 ratio, urine sodium levels increase, and the plasma urine osmolality ratio falls to a 1:1 ratio.

Transient hematuria can occur following discontinuation of CPB or after autotransfusion of shed mediastinal blood. These events are usually short-lived and either clear up themselves or resolve following infusion of an osmotic diuretic such as mannitol.

Gastrointestinal System

Gastric complications that can develop include mesenteric or splenic ischemia or infarction from intracardiac thrombi or air emboli. Immediate surgical intervention may be necessary in these situations. Gastric distention can occur if the patient swallows air. This distention can cause cardiac problems as well as pulmonary complications. Stress ulceration can also develop; however, in recent years its incidence has decreased with the more frequent use of cimetidine, ranitidine, or famotidine.

Peripheral Vascular System

Vascular complications can include both venous and arterial thrombus formation and embolism development. Venous thrombus can develop, owing to stasis from immobilization and inactivity in the immediate postoperative period. Arterial complications are largely associated with various intravascular devices such as intra-arterial lines and intra-aortic balloon catheters. Assessment of pulses should be ongoing, but particular attention should be given to the performance of the Allen test following radial artery line removal. The Allen test assesses for the patency of the radial and ulnar arteries. In addition, the status of lower extremity pulses, skin color and temperature, and motor activity should be monitored closely in the presence of an intra-aortic balloon catheter, particularly during insertion and removal. Passive and active range-of-motion exercises and early ambulation are advocated and encouraged in these patients to prevent some of the foregoing complications. In the recovery areas, the patient is instructed and assisted in performing active dorsiflexion and extension of the feet and ankles. These maneuvers facilitate venous return and decrease stasis.

References

1. Barash, P., Cullen, B., and Stoelting, R.: Clinical Anesthesia. 2nd ed. Philadelphia, J. B. Lippincott, 1992.
2. Baue, A.: Glennis Thoracic and Cardiovascular Surgery. 5th ed. Norwalk, CT, Appleton & Lange, 1991.
3. Benumof, J., and Saidman, L.: Anesthesia and Perioperative Complications. St. Louis, Mosby-Year Book, 1992.
4. Dervan, J., and Goldberg, S.: Acute aortic regurgitation: Pathophysiology and management. Cardiovasc. Clin. North Am., 16(2):1281–1288, 1986.
5. Gerson, M.: Cardiac Nuclear Medicine. 2nd ed. New York, McGraw-Hill, 1991.
6. Goldberger, E.: Treatment of Cardiac Emergencies. 5th ed. St. Louis, Mosby-Year Book, 1990.
7. Grossman, W., and Baem, D.: Cardiac Catheterization, Angiography, and Intervention. 4th ed. Philadelphia, Lea and Febiger, 1991.
8. Kaplan, J.: Thoracic Anesthesia. 2nd ed. New York, Churchill Livingstone, 1991.
9. Kapur, P.: Anesthesia and the beta-blocked patient. Semin. Anesth., 10(2):87–96, 1991.
10. Kayser, S.: Pharmacology and hematology: Antithrombin III, heparin, and warfarin. Anesth. Today, 2(2):15–17, 1990.
11. Kirklin, J., and Baratt-Boyes, B.: Cardiac Surgery. New York, John Wiley and Sons, 1986.
12. Miller, R.: Anesthesia. 3rd ed. New York, Churchill Livingstone, 1990.
13. Moreno-Cabral, C., Mitchell, R., and Miller, D.: Manual of Postoperative Management in Adult Cardiac Surgery. Baltimore, Williams & Wilkins, 1988.
14. Pelletier, L., and Carrier, M.: The immediate postoperative period. In Care of the Patient with Previous Coronary Bypass Surgery. Philadelphia, F. A. Davis, 1991, pp. 96–120.
15. Rosow, C., and Eckhardt, W.: The pharmacology of cardiopulmonary bypass. Semin. Anesth., 10(2):122–128, 1991.
16. Smith, P.: Postoperative care in cardiac surgery. In Sabiston, D., and Spencer, F.: Surgery of the Chest. 5th ed. Philadelphia, W. B. Saunders, 1990, pp. 202–251.
17. Stinson, E., and Swerdlow, C.: Recurrent ventricular tachycardia, ventricular fibrillation: The AICD. In Austen, W., and Vlahake, G. (eds.): Current Therapy in Cardiothoracic Surgery. Philadelphia, B. C. Decker, 1990.
18. Topol, E.: Textbook of Interventional Cardiology. Philadelphia, W. B. Saunders, 1990.
19. Underhill, S. L., Woods, S. L., Sivarajan, E. S., et al.: Cardiac Nursing. 2nd ed. Philadelphia, J. B. Lippincott, 1989.
20. Waller, B.: Pathology of coronary balloon angioplasty and related topics. In Topol, E. (ed.): Textbook of Interventional Cardiology. Philadelphia, W. B. Saunders, 1990, pp. 395–451.

Post Anesthesia Care of the Vascular Surgical Patient

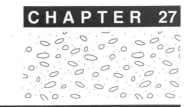

CHAPTER 27

Kathleen A. Daly, M.S., R.N., C.C.R.N.

Integrity and patency of the vascular system, including the arteries, veins, and lymphatic vessels, are essential to the life of human tissues. Before 1950, the patient with impaired vascular patency was treated only medically. Loss of limb or life resulting from impaired blood flow was common, and surgery on the vascular system was only in the experimental stage. The advancement of vascular surgery from the experimental laboratory to accepted procedure in the clinical setting resulted from the successful development of diagnostic tools, such as arteriography, improvements in antibiotics and anticoagulants, and refinements in vascular surgical instruments and techniques.

In the past decade there has been an explosion in the field of vascular surgery. This explosion has resulted in the development of new methods of noninvasive diagnosis and the treatment of disease. Although arteriography continues to be the mainstay in invasive diagnosis, noninvasive procedures include the use of ultrasonography, computed tomographic scanning, magnetic resonance imaging, and subdigital arteriography complement the picture. The nonsurgical treatment options include percutaneous transluminal angioplasty with and without laser and fibrinolytic therapy. Despite the fact that these options are nonsurgical in nature, these patients require close observation in the post anesthesia care unit (PACU). Therefore, it is imperative that PACU nurses are aware of these new procedures so that adequate care can be delivered.

Definitions

Aneurysm: a localized, abnormal dilatation, distention, or sac in an artery.

Angiography (arteriography): the injection of radiopaque dye into the arteries followed by rapid-sequential radiographs of the vascular tree to determine abnormalities.

Angioscopy: a procedure using a specialized scope in the operating room to visualize the pathway within blood vessels and to assess graft patency after revascularization procedures.

Bypass: a rerouting of the vascular system by construction of another arterial route by use of a vein graft or a synthetic (Dacron or Teflon) artery, and re-establishment of functional integrity.

Embolectomy: the surgical removal of an embolus from a blood vessel.

Embolus: a bit of free-floating foreign matter (may be clotted blood, air, tumor, or other tissue cells; amniotic fluid; fat; or other foreign bodies) carried by the blood stream.

Endarterectomy: opening of the artery over an obstruction and removal of the obstruction, or excision of atheromatous material creating the blockage.

Fibrinolytic therapy: the injection of streptokinase or urokinase (plasminogen activators) through a catheter to dissolve a clot.

Ischemia: a lack of adequate blood supply to meet the tissue needs.

Ligation: tying or binding of a blood vessel; in vascular surgery, a technique used to prevent embolism (Fig. 27–1).

Percutaneous transluminal angioplasty (PTA): the use of a special catheter with a balloon at the distal tip that is passed percutaneously to the area of stenosis. The balloon is inflated and deflated to compress the area of stenosis and widen the vessel lumen.

Plication: the creation of folds in the wall of a vessel or other methods of reducing intraluminal size (see Fig. 27–1).

Subdigital arteriography: a procedure used in conjunction with arteriography to localize regions of peripheral arterial disease. The dye is injected through the catheter, and the computer subtracts all background layers (i.e.,

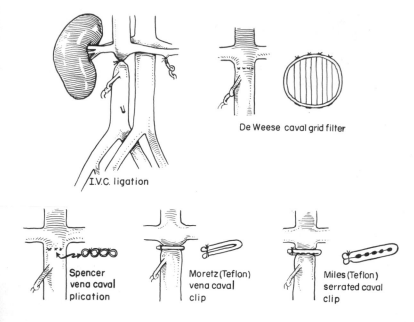

De Weese caval grid filter

I.V.C. ligation

Spencer vena caval plication

Moretz (Teflon) vena caval clip

Miles (Teflon) serrated caval clip

FIGURE 27–1. Various surgical techniques available for preventing embolism from pelvic and lower extremity veins. IVC = inferior vena cava. (Adapted from Fairbairn, J. F. II, Juergens, J. L., and Spittel, J. A., Jr.: Allen-Barker-Hines Peripheral Vascular Diseases. 4th ed. Philadelphia, W. B. Saunders, 1972, p. 579.)

bone), leaving only the image of dye-filled vessels.

Sympathectomy: the resection of selected portions of the sympathetic nervous system to denervate the vascular system, producing vasodilatation.

Thrombectomy: the surgical excision of a thrombus from within a blood vessel.

Thrombus: a stationary blood clot or atheromatous plaque that partially or totally occludes a blood vessel.

NONINVASIVE TREATMENT OF VASCULAR DISEASE

The three major noninvasive treatments for peripheral vascular disease include percutaneous transluminal angioplasty (PTA), PTA with laser (light amplification by the stimulated emission of radiation), and fibrinolytic therapy. These procedures are performed in the radiology department by the radiologist in conjunction with the surgeon. Although the aforementioned procedures are performed with local anesthesia, the patients require postprocedural nursing care in the PACU. The nursing care for this patient population is similar to that of patients undergoing other revascularization procedures. The catheter site has to be watched for bleeding and hematoma formation. Pulses, color, movement, sensation, and vital signs must be assessed frequently.

PTA has been performed on superficial femoral, iliac, popliteal, and tibial occlusions. Ma-

jor complications arising after PTA include bleeding, hematoma, and acute restenosis of the vessel. PTA is often used in conjunction with surgery and laser treatment.

Laser-assisted PTA is still considered an experimental procedure. The procedure is essentially the same as PTA, except that the laser is used first. The reason it is coupled with angioplasty is that it does not widen the vessel enough to significantly improve flow. A channel is created by the laser, and PTA follows to increase the diameter of the vessel. The major complication is vessel rupture. Owing to the high incidence of vessel rupture, nurses must monitor the patient's cardiovascular status more closely, including hemoglobin and hematocrit levels and perfusion to the extremity. Research continues to improve both the equipment and the techniques in this area so that laser-assisted PTA can be applied to a broader patient population.

Fibrinolytic therapy is also considered experimental. The specialized catheter is placed in the area of stenosis, and the infusion of urokinase or streptokinase is initiated. Urokinase is presently the drug of choice. This therapy is started in the radiology department; the patient is then transferred to the PACU for close observation while the drug is being infused. Reperfusion is evident when the patient complains of a burning-type pain and the extremity is warm. Arteriograms are done at regular intervals to evaluate clot lysis. A successful outcome is complete lysis. Therapy is discontinued by the physician when (1) the clot is lysed, (2) there is increased symptomatology, (3) bleeding that requires transfusion occurs, or (4) there is a lack of response. The major complication of therapy is bleeding. Nursing care revolves around monitoring for this complication. Because the agents used are plasminogen activators, prothrombin and partial thromboplastin times and hematocrit and hemoglobin levels must be monitored on admission and at least every 4 hours.

GENERAL CONSIDERATIONS

Vascular surgery is now commonly practiced in most institutions, and the PACU nurse must be prepared to care for these patients postoperatively and to evaluate their vascular status. Vascular occlusive disease is most often treated with surgical revascularization procedures. Other forms of adjunct treatments, namely PTA, laser, and fibrinolytic therapies, are achieving increasing success. These noninvasive therapies are generally reserved for patients (1) who are poor surgical candidates because of their general health status, (2) whose surgical reconstructions are limited or prohibited, and (3) who sustain graft thrombosis after one or more revascularization procedures. These forms of therapy were briefly discussed in the previous section.

Many vascular impairments are amenable to surgery, especially when localized. Vascular surgery generally involves eliminating an obstruction by excision and removal of thrombi and emboli, the bypassing of atherosclerotic narrowing, and the resection of aneurysms. Occasionally, sympathectomy is performed to treat vasospastic disease, but its success is limited to patients whose vascular systems are still elastic enough to dilate. Veins may be ligated or plicated to prevent emboli from passing up the vena cava into the heart and lungs. Research in vascular disease continues, and new techniques and surgical devices are introduced for trial almost daily. The nurse should be familiar with all of the procedures being performed in the local setting and with any specific care involved postoperatively. Only the more common procedures will be discussed here.

Vascular problems may be acute and constitute a life-threatening or limb-threatening emergency; they may be chronic conditions for which surgery is performed only as a last resort after medical treatment has failed. In either instance, the PACU nurse must be sensitive to the feelings of these patients and be prepared

for the questions about limb viability that will invariably arise when the patient awakes.

Post anesthesia care of vascular surgical patients is determined by the surgical site, the extent of surgical revision, and the anesthesia used.

Method of Anesthesia

Anesthesia may be local, spinal, or general, depending on the surgical site and the patient's condition. Peripheral embolectomy may be accomplished with only local anesthesia and appropriate sedation, whereas an aortoiliac bypass graft requires prolonged general anesthesia. Anesthetic management of bypass graft patients is exceptionally important, because they are often elderly and in poor physical condition and present with many risk factors. Patients who undergo thoracic or abdominal aortic surgery are considerably more labile than patients who undergo peripheral vascular surgery, and they are frequently transferred directly from the operating suite to the intensive care unit for monitoring and special care. The goals of treatment in vascular surgical patients are to support the vascular system, to remove the cause of the problem, and to prevent further episodes of ischemia.

DIAGNOSTIC PROCEDURES

Arteriography is commonly performed prior to any vascular surgery to determine the exact location of the problem. It is usually accomplished within the radiology department. The patient may be returned to the PACU for a brief period of observation, depending on the policies of the hospital and the patient's post anesthesia recovery (PAR) score (see Table 3–3). Arteriography is generally accomplished with the use of only local anesthesia at the catheter insertion site.

Postarteriography care includes observation of the catheter site for bleeding. Usually, a pressure dressing is applied to the site for several hours. The injection site may become irritated or thrombosed, and, occasionally, the patient may have an allergic reaction to the radiopaque dye. Postarteriography care includes the following:

1. Observing the catheter site for bleeding and hematoma.
2. Palpating pulses distal to the catheter site

(i.e., pedal pulses if the femoral artery is used).
3. Maintaining bedrest for 6 to 8 hours with the extremity kept straight.
4. Hydrating with intravenous fluids to clear the radiopaque dye.

The cardiovascular status of the patient should be carefully monitored if pulmonary arteriography is performed, because passage of the catheter may create myocardial irritability.

The patient is often apprehensive following arteriography and anxious to know the results. The nurse should be familiar with the information given to the patient by the physician and be able to reinforce or reinterpret it for the patient if necessary.

PERIPHERAL VASCULAR SURGICAL PROCEDURES

Treatment for peripheral vascular disease may be performed directly on the involved vessels or sympathectomy may be done, depending on the nature of the problem and the age and general condition of the patient.

Peripheral procedures include embolectomy, thrombectomy, endarterectomy, and ligation and stripping of veins (see Fig. 27–1). Some specific procedures are the femoral-popliteal bypass graft (Fig. 27–2), peripheral artery embolectomy, carotid endarterectomy or bypass, and venous ligation and stripping of the lower extremities.

The method of anesthesia used may be local, as for embolectomy; spinal, as for surgery on the lower extremities; or general, as for more extensive procedures or when the patient cannot tolerate local or spinal anesthesia.

PACU Care

Positioning

On return to the PACU, the patient is placed in the supine position, with head of the bed maintained in a semi-Fowler position and the head and neck turned to the side. Some controversy exists over the positioning of the patient after vein stripping. In the author's experience, surgeons have preferred to elevate the patient's legs slightly (20 to 30 degrees) to aid venous return. The surgeon's preference should be fol-

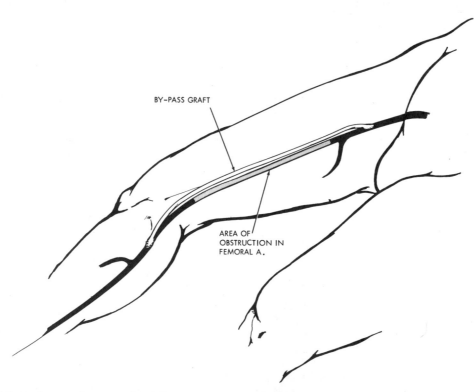

BY-PASS GRAFT

AREA OF OBSTRUCTION IN FEMORAL A.

FIGURE 27–2. Saphenous femoropopliteal bypass graft in place, going around the femoral artery obstruction. (From LeMaitre, G. D., and Finnegan, J. A.: The Patient in Surgery: A Guide for Nurses. 4th ed. Philadelphia, W. B. Saunders, 1980, p. 310.)

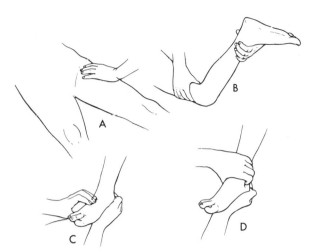

FIGURE 27–3. Method of palpation for pulsations in the peripheral arteries. *A*, femoral artery, *B*, popliteal artery. *C*, dorsalis pedis artery. *D*, posterior tibial artery. (Adapted from Fairbairn, J. F. II, Juergens, J. L., and Spittell, J. A., Jr.: Allen-Barker-Hines Peripheral Vascular Diseases. 4th ed. Philadelphia, W. B. Saunders, 1972, p. 34.)

lowed; if that preference is not specified, the nurse should ask for clarification.

Circulatory Status

Checking the circulation to the operated extremity is one of the most important nursing functions. Careful, explicit recording of observations is important for determining any changes. The circulatory status of the patient and the pulses present should be reported to the nurse by the surgeon. It is helpful to PACU

personnel for the surgeon to mark on the skin those places where the pulses can be evaluated best.

All pulses on the affected extremity are evaluated frequently and compared with pulses on the unaffected side (Fig. 27–3). The pulses should be checked not only for their presence but also for pulse volume and occlusion pressure. A reduction in pulse volume or occlusion pressure is more likely to be detected if the same nurse cares for the patient during the entire stay in the PACU. If assignments need to be changed—for instance, if a shift change occurs—a direct report, with direct inspection, palpation, and evaluation of the pulses, should be made from nurse to nurse so that the relieving nurse has accurate baseline observations for future assessments.

The PACU should have an ultrasonic Doppler device to assist with evaluating pulses (Fig. 27–4). The Doppler can indicate the presence of adequate blood flow even when pulses are not palpable. The affected part should remain warm, dry, and normal in color. Capillary refill should be checked by the examiner applying pressure on the skin surface and nail bed with his or her fingers, which should produce blanching. Normal pink color should return quickly when pressure is released (normal capillary refill is less than 3 seconds). Coolness, pallor, numbness, and tingling may be danger signs that vascular problems have developed. If pulses previously present become more difficult to palpate or are absent, the surgeon should be notified immediately.

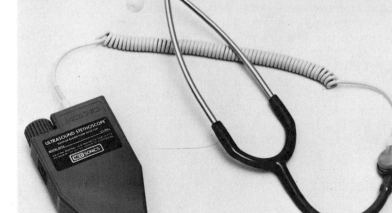

FIGURE 27–4. Doppler instrument for the detection of blood flow. (Courtesy of Medasonics, Inc., Fremont, CA.)

Dressings

All dressings should be checked for drainage. Dressings following bypass grafting and embolectomy are usually light, and they should remain dry and intact. If frank bleeding occurs, the surgeon should be notified, because this may indicate an interrupted arteriotomy or graft anastomosis site. A tourniquet or a blood pressure cuff should be kept at the bedside for immediate use if rupture on an arterial operative site should occur. If a cuff is used, it should be applied proximal to the incision site and inflated carefully and slowly until bleeding just stops. The pressure necessary to stop bleeding is normally just below the systemic systolic blood pressure.

After venous ligation and stripping, the legs are wrapped with Kerlix or similar elastic gauze dressings, and compression is applied with Ace wraps or antiembolism stockings from toes to groin. Some seepage of blood may occur, but the dressings should not soak through. Excessive bleeding should be reported to the surgeon.

Pain Relief

Pain following any of these procedures should be mild and easily controlled with moderate doses of the narcotic analgesics. Severe, unrelieved pain should be reported to the surgeon because it may indicate ischemia or graft occlusion.

Intake and Output

The PACU course for these patients is usually smooth and uneventful. Fluids may be instituted orally as soon as the patient recovers the pharyngeal reflexes, and solids can then be given progressively as tolerated.

The patient may experience urinary retention, which is especially likely to occur after spinal anesthesia. Check for abdominal distention. Some surgeons allow male patients to stand for voiding. If measures to enhance the ability to void are not effective, a catheterization order must be obtained.

Sympathectomy

Some carefully selected patients with vasospastic disease are amenable to sympathectomy, which results in vasodilatation of the vessels in the extremity by removing the vasoconstrictive effects of the sympathetic nervous system.

Cervicodorsal Sympathectomy

Cervicodorsal sympathectomy is performed to denervate the upper extremity and improve circulation. The most common approach used is the transaxillary-transpleural incision. Resection of the thoracic ganglia, T2 through T6, and half of the stellate ganglia, C8 through T1, is accomplished.

Anesthesia is general. On return to the PACU, the patient is placed in the supine position until sufficiently recovered from anesthesia to be able to tolerate the head of the bed being elevated 30 to 45 degrees. A chest tube is present because a thoracic incision has been made, and it should be cared for as outlined in Chapter 25. Because the chest tube is inserted primarily to remove air to correct the surgically created pneumothorax, bleeding should be negligible. Accumulation of more than 200 ml of blood in the collection receptacle in 8 hours or less is excessive and should be reported to the surgeon.

Bilateral breath sounds should be evaluated. Circulation to the hand and arm must be assessed by evaluating pulses, temperature, and color. As soon as pharyngeal reflexes have returned, the patient may be started on oral fluids and the diet progressed as tolerated. The dressings should remain dry and intact. The patient's cardiovascular status should be assessed and any downward trends reported, because these may indicate hemorrhage from the intercostal vessels, thoracic aorta, or subclavian artery. Damage to these vessels causes excessive bleeding, and hypovolemic shock can develop quickly.

Lumbar Sympathectomy

Lumbar sympathectomy is performed to denervate the lower extremity and improve circulation. A flank incision is used to approach the lumbar ganglia (L1 through L4), and the ganglia are resected. This particular procedure is not commonly performed. Lumbar sympathectomy is accomplished under general anesthesia. The patient may be placed in the supine or side-lying position when returned to the PACU. The light flank dressing on the operative side should remain dry and intact. If bleeding occurs, the surgeon should be notified, because this may indicate damage to one of the lumbar veins. Drainage from the incision site must be carefully assessed. The presence of urine in the drainage suggests that damage to the ureter may have occurred during surgery.

Postoperative pain should be minimal and easily controlled with small dosages of narcotic analgesics. If the patient complains of severe flank pain not associated with the incision, the surgeon should be informed, because this may indicate inadvertent ligation of the ureter. Ligation of the ureter leads to dilatation of the renal pelvis with urine. If the patient is unable to void normally within 8 to 10 hours, catheterization will probably be required.

The patient may develop an ileus and should be given nothing by mouth for the first 24 hours postoperatively. Bowel sounds should be monitored for return. Fluid intake is provided intravenously. Occasionally, a nasogastric tube is required to decompress the stomach, and this should be cared for as outlined in Chapter 31. Circulation to the lower extremities should be assessed by evaluating the pulse, temperature, and color.

After sympathectomy, especially the lumbar type, the patient has an increased sensitivity to changes in body position, so turning and sitting up should be accomplished slowly. This patient is also more sensitive to changes in room temperature and should be provided with warmed blankets or a Bear Hugger (hypothermia unit) in the PACU to conserve body heat.

Carotid Endarterectomy

Special mention must be given to the post anesthesia nursing care for the patient following carotid endarterectomy.

Positioning

After surgery on the carotid arteries, the patient is placed in the supine position, with the head of the bed elevated 25 to 30 degrees to minimize venous oozing in the neck. Sudden changes in head position should be avoided during the immediate postoperative period. Raising the head suddenly or more than 30 degrees can precipitate hypotension, and lowering the head can precipitate hypertension, owing to a temporary inability of the great vessels to compensate for changes in head position.

Circulatory Status

After carotid endarterectomy or bypass, circulation to the head and neck is checked by

assessing the patient's level of consciousness. If local anesthesia has been used, the patient's degree of orientation is a useful sign. If general anesthesia has been employed, consciousness is more difficult to evaluate; however, the pharyngeal reflexes, the lid (or blink) reflexes, and the patient's response to pain stimuli are helpful indicators of the level of consciousness. As the patient emerges from anesthesia, specific levels of response should be noted along with the time of response, so that any relapse will be detected. Check pupillary response and motion of the extremities to further assess neurologic status.

As with all surgical procedures, the dressing should be checked for excessive drainage, which should be reported to the physician. A Penrose drain may be placed to facilitate drainage. Hematoma formation is a major complication. The nurse must assess neck size, comparing the operative side with the nonoperative side to determine if a hematoma is forming. Hematoma can compromise the airway, and the surgeon should be notified immediately. The patient may require reoperation for evacuation of the hematoma.

Neurologic Function

All patients recovering from general anesthesia require close monitoring for the return of neurologic function. This aspect of care is vital with this group of patients because the carotid artery is the main blood supply for the brain. During surgery, plaque or microemboli from the surgical bed can become dislodged and travel to the brain. Assessing neurologic status includes level of consciousness, mentation, movement of extremities, and cranial nerve function (Table 27–1).

Meticulous blood pressure monitoring must be performed for these patients, owing to the risk of hypotension or hypertension during the immediate postoperative period. Postoperative carotid endarterectomy patients may exhibit a labile blood pressure owing to manipulation of the carotid sinus. As a result of surgical trauma, the baroreceptor located in the carotid sinus may not function properly in the immediate postoperative period. Postoperative orders should include parameters indicating when to notify the physician.

Operations on the Large Vessels

Operations on the large vessels include embolectomy and thrombectomy; bypass proce-

Table 27–1. CRANIAL NERVE ASSESSMENT FOR THE CAROTID ENDARTERECTOMY PATIENT

Cranial Nerve	Function	Assessment
VII (facial)	Muscles of facial expression, saliva secretion	Smile, frown
IX (glossopharyngeal)	Swallowing, pharyngeal muscle	Pharyngeal reflexes, swallowing
X (vagus)	Pharyngeal and laryngeal muscles	Speech
XII (hypoglossopharyngeal)*	Muscles of tongue	Stick tongue out, move side to side

*This nerve traverses the internal carotid artery.

dures on the aorta, iliac arteries, and renal arteries; and ligation and plication of the vena cava (Figs. 27–5 through 27–7).

Surgery on the great vessels still is associated with rather high rates of morbidity and mortality. Patients are usually in a precarious physical state before surgery, owing to the cardiovascular problem. These patients are often elderly, and, in addition to the specific problem for which surgery is being performed, they often have diffuse cardiovascular and respiratory diseases affecting all of the vital organs. Vascular surgery on the large vessels, especially abdominal and thoracic aortic surgery, is often prolonged and is quite shocking to the system.

As with postoperative cardiac patients, these patients should be cared for in the immediate recovery period by at least two professional nurses. All physiologic functions must be assessed accurately and continually. In some institutions, a special unit is set aside for the postoperative care of cardiac and vascular patients. If these patients are sent to the general PACU, adequate numbers of well-trained personnel must be available to manage their care. After recovery, these patients must be transferred to the surgical intensive care unit, where close monitoring and special care can be provided until they are fully stable and until the time has passed during which the most common complications occur.

Anesthesia for these procedures is general and may be prolonged. Surgery may take as long as 10 hours in some instances. The procedure may involve extensive blood loss, and the

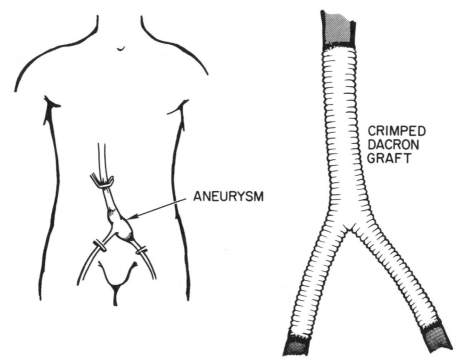

ANEURYSM

CRIMPED DACRON GRAFT

FIGURE 27–5. Aneurysm of the distal aorta. *Right,* the crimped Dacron graft has been inserted. (From LeMaitre, G. D., and Finnegan, J. A.: The Patient in Surgery: A Guide for Nurses. 4th ed. Philadelphia, W. B. Saunders, 1980, p. 321.)

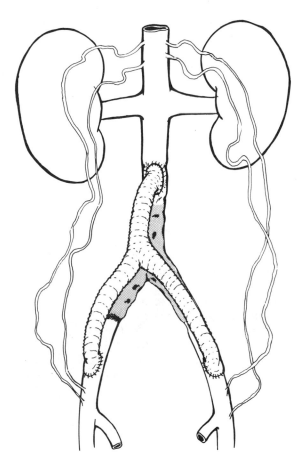

FIGURE 27–6. An aortoiliac Dacron bypass graft in place. (From LeMaitre, G. D., and Finnegan, J. A.: The Patient in Surgery: A Guide for Nurses. 4th ed. Philadelphia, W. B. Saunders, 1980, p. 314.)

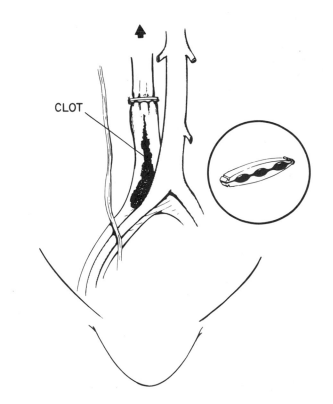

CLOT

FIGURE 27–7. A partially occluding Teflon clip on the vena cava, preventing a caval embolism (visible below clip) from reaching lungs. (From LeMaitre, G. D., and Finnegan, J. A.: The Patient in Surgery: A Guide for Nurses. 4th ed. Philadelphia, W. B. Saunders, 1980, p. 339.)

incisions used are commonly long, involving both thoracic and abdominal entrances. For a review of care of the patient and management of chest tubes following thoracic incisions, see Chapter 25.

Positioning and Initial Care

On return to the PACU, the patient is placed in the supine position with head and neck turned to the side. As soon as the patient can tolerate it, the head of the bed is elevated 30 to 45 degrees to promote respiratory function. After vena cava plication, the patient is kept supine, or the bed may be placed in the Trendelenburg position, as directed by the surgeon.

The surgeon and anesthesiologist should give the receiving nurse a detailed report on the anesthesia, the procedure accomplished, blood loss and replacement, other fluid replacement, the patient's overall condition, and any special instructions. At the same time, all necessary monitors and support systems should be hooked up, all drainage tubes and catheters cared for appropriately, and baseline measurements of all physiologic functioning determined and documented.

Cardiopulmonary Status

Most commonly, owing to systemic shock from the procedure, the extent of anesthesia, and the general condition of the patient, respiratory support with a volume-controlled ventilator is provided for at least 8 to 24 hours postoperatively. A 24-hour period of assisted or controlled respiration gives the patient a rest and assists in stabilizing his or her condition more rapidly. The reader should review Chapter 21 for information on the care of the patient with an endotracheal airway and management of the respirator.

Because of the age of the average patient undergoing this type of surgery, respiratory care is especially important. The patient should be suctioned frequently, following the guidelines in Chapter 21, and the patient's position should be changed at least every hour. Because thoracic and abdominal incisions are long and painful, adequate analgesia must be maintained to promote respiratory function as well as comfort. An order for morphine sulfate, typically 2 to 4 mg intravenously every 1 to 2 hours, gives the nurse flexibility in medicating the patient appropriately for both of these purposes while controlled ventilation is still being used.

The patient's cardiac status should be monitored electronically. Any arrhythmias not previously present must be investigated and an explanation for their presence sought. The nurse must, of course, be prepared to treat immediately any lethal arrhythmias that develop. Frequently, the cause of premature ventricular contractions is inadequate oxygenation. Arterial samples for blood gas analysis are frequently necessary to evaluate the patient's cardiorespiratory status. It is, therefore, highly advantageous to have an arterial line present from which to draw specimens. The arterial line is also helpful in monitoring the patient's systolic blood pressure continuously. Systolic blood pressure should be recorded every 10 to 15 minutes during the first 2 postoperative hours and every 30 minutes thereafter. Because these procedures involve a moderate to extensive blood loss and are shocking to the system, a systolic blood pressure of 100 mm Hg is generally acceptable if the patient was not hypertensive preoperatively.

Hypertension control is also essential when surgery has been performed on the great vessels. Extreme elevations in blood pressure can stress the suture line, precipitating oozing and rupture of the operative site. In some institutions, standard orders, according to physician preference, allow pharmacologic treatment of systolic blood pressure higher than 150 mm Hg.

A pulse rate of 80 to 100 beats per min is generally acceptable. Moderate tachycardia is expected as a result of the stress of surgery. Central venous pressure or Swan-Ganz monitoring may also be instituted to assist in the evaluation of the patient's cardiovascular function and fluid balance.

Circulatory Status

Circulation to the extremities must be checked every hour and results recorded along with the vital signs. All peripheral pulses should be present. The surgeon should indicate the parameters within which he or she would like the patient's vital signs to remain. Trends in these measurements are more important indicators of the patient's status than any one number. Any indication of hypotension or impending shock should be reported to the surgeon. Hemorrhage and shock are the most common complications of vascular surgery and may result from the primary surgery or from associated injury to the aorta, the vena cava, or the nearby vessels, including the iliac or renal arteries and veins or the lumbar veins. Massive bleeding is particularly likely if anticoagulant therapy was instituted preoperatively.

Temperature

The temperature should be taken hourly for several hours postoperatively. An electronic axillary or rectal temperature or the core temperature from the pulmonary artery catheter is most accurate. Many PACUs use FirstTemp, a product that provides a highly accurate measure of core temperature. The presence of a nasogastric tube, an endotracheal tube, or a connected respirator makes oral temperature readings impossible, and the paraphernalia present make rectal readings difficult. A temperature elevation to 38.36° or 38.86°C (101.6° or 102.6°F) is common after these extensive procedures and is not indicative of infection. A temperature of 39.46°C (103.6°F), however, is significant and may indicate respiratory problems such as pulmonary atelectasis. In this instance, efforts at pulmonary toilet must be increased, and the surgeon may institute an antibiotic regimen if it has not already been ordered.

Intake and Output

Adequate fluid intake is provided by intravenous infusions maintained throughout the postoperative period. The quantity and content of the fluids needed are determined by the surgeon, based on the patient's cardiovascular status and urine output. Blood replacement may be necessary. Hematocrit and hemoglobin determinations are usually performed 4 and 8 hours postoperatively. At least four units of blood, typed and crossmatched for this patient, should be kept available in the blood bank until it is released by the surgeon.

A Foley catheter should be connected to straight gravitational drainage with a calibrated measuring device. Urine output is measured and recorded hourly. At least 0.5 ml per kg per hr (approximately 30 ml per hr) of urine output should be expected, and the surgeon should be notified if any downward trend occurs. Decreased or inadequate urine output may indicate hypotension due to hypovolemia or impending shock with renal shutdown. The urine should be examined for the presence of blood or for cloudiness. Blood in the urine may indicate injury to a ureter or kidney, reaction to blood transfusion, or massive hemorrhage. Descending thoracic aneurysms may require cardiopulmonary bypass, which can cause hematuria secondary to red blood cell damage.

A nasogastric or long intestinal tube will be present and is cared for as described in Chapter 31. It should be connected to low intermittent suction. The drainage and all stools should be given a guaiac test for occult blood, and its presence should be reported to the surgeon immediately, the presence of blood may be indicative of impending infarction of the colon, which must be treated immediately. Occasionally, a gastrostomy must be performed in this situation; it is cared for in the routine manner.

All intake and output measurements must be done accurately and then recorded. The intake and output record assists in the evaluation of hypotensive states, pulmonary congestion, edema, and renal shutdown, all of which are common problems encountered after major vascular surgery.

Pain Relief

The incisions for major vascular surgery are long and painful, and significant dosages of narcotic analgesics are often required to keep the patient comfortable and promote respiratory effort. All vital signs must be monitored continuously following administration of medication, because the narcotics commonly alter the patient's cardiorespiratory status. Transcutaneous electrical nerve stimulation (TENS) has been effective in controlling incision pain in these patients. Although not satisfactory as the sole pain relief modality, TENS, in conjunction with narcotic analgesia, may significantly reduce the dosage of narcotics necessary to control pain. This is advantageous, because it allows the patient to breathe and ambulate more easily.

Dressings

Abdominal incisions are not usually drained, so all dressings should remain dry and intact. If dressings become soaked with serosanguineous drainage, the surgeon should be notified. The surgeon should change the dressing and inspect the incision.

Neurologic Status

The state of consciousness, facial function, movement, and strength of all extremities, as well as pupillary size and reaction and carotid pulses, must be evaluated frequently as parameters of cerebral function. Cerebrovascular accidents are not uncommon postoperatively, owing to the dislodgment of emboli during surgery.

References

1. Bilodeau, M., and Capasso, V.: Peripheral arterial thrombolytic therapy. Crit. Care Nurs. Clin. North Am., 2(4):673–680, 1990.
2. Blank, C. A., and Irwin, G. H.: Peripheral vascular disorders. Nurs. Clin. North Am., 25(4):777–793, 1990.
3. Bondy, B.: An overview of arterial disease. J. Cardiovasc. Nurs., 1(2):1–11, 1987.
4. Borgini, L., and Almgren, C.: Peripheral vascular angioscopy. AORN J., 52(3):543–550, 1990.
5. Dixon, M. B., and Nunnelee, J.: Arterial reconstruction for atherosclerotic occlusive disease. J. Cardiovasc. Nurs., 1(12):36–49, 1987.
6. Durbin, N.: The application of Doppler techniques in critical care. Focus Crit. Care, 10(3):44–46, 1983.
7. Ernst, C., and Stanley, J.: Current Therapy in Vascular Surgery. Toronto, B. C. Decker, 1987.
8. Fahey, V.: Vascular Nursing. Philadelphia, W. B. Saunders, 1988.
9. Fahey, V., and Riegel, B.: Advances in diagnostic testing for vascular disease. Cardiovasc. Nurs., 25(3):13–18, 1989.
10. Fode, N.: Carotid endarterectomy: Nursing care and controversies. J. Neurosci. Nurs., 22(1):25–31, 1990.
11. Moore, W.: Vascular Surgery: A Comprehensive Review. Philadelphia, W. B. Saunders, 1991.
12. Sakalaris, B.: Laser therapy for cardiovascular disease. Heart Lung, 16(5):465–471, 1987.
13. Seabrook, G., Mewissen, M., Schmitt, D., et al.: Percutaneous intra-arterial thrombolysis in the treatment of thrombosis of lower extremity arterial reconstructions. J. Vasc. Surg., 13:646–651, 1991.

CHAPTER 28

Post Anesthesia Care of the Orthopedic Surgical Patient

Sandra S. Barnes, M.S., R.N., C.P.A.N.

Orthopedic nursing in the post anesthesia care unit (PACU) is challenging and rigorous. In this highly technologic age, the care demanded by the orthopedic patient requires both vigilant general post anesthesia care and a sound knowledge of orthopedic surgical procedures. The PACU nurse must possess astute nursing observation and inspection skills to ensure a low incidence of morbidity in this patient population. The psychosocial challenges are generally more evident within this group because, more frequently, the goal of the surgery is focused on restoring mobility and relieving pain and disability. The nurse must be sensitive to heightened anxieties and be empathetic to individual needs.

Definitions

Anesthesia: local or systemic loss of sensation caused by trauma or injury.

Arthrodesis: surgical fixation or fusion of a joint.

Arthroplasty: reconstruction of joints to restore motion and stability.

Arthroscopy: surgical examination of the interior of a joint by the insertion of an optic device (arthroscope) capable of providing an external view of an internal joint area.

Arthrotomy: surgical exploration of a joint.

Articulation: the connection of bones at the joint.

Cineplastic (kineplastic) amputation: an amputation that includes a skin flap built into a muscle; a portion of the prosthetic mechanism is activated by the muscle.

Disarticulation: amputation at a joint.

Diskectomy (discectomy): removal of herniated or extruded fragments of an intervertebral disk.

External fixators: equipment used to manage open fractures with soft-tissue damage (provides stabilization for the fracture while it permits treatment of soft-tissue damage).

Fasciotomy: surgical separation of the fascia (a fibrous membrane that covers, supports, or separates the muscles) to relieve muscle constriction or reduce fascia contracture.

Harrington rods: equipment used in spinal fixation for scoliosis and for some spinal fractures.

Hemiarthroplasty: replacement of the femoral head with a prosthesis.

Internal fixation: the stabilization of a reduced fracture by the use of metal screws, plates, nails, and pins.

Joint replacement: the substitution of joint surfaces with metal or plastic materials.

Laminectomy: removal of the lamina to expose the neural elements in the spinal canal or to relieve constriction.

Lordosis: abnormal anterior convexity of the lower part of the back.

Luque rods: spinal fixation, applying transverse force, for scoliosis.

Meniscectomy: surgical removal of the damaged knee joint fibrocartilage.

Open reduction: the reduction and alignment of a fracture through surgical dissection and exposure of the fracture.

Osteoporosis: diminished amount of calcium in the bone.

Osteotomy: surgical cutting of the bone.

Paresthesia: describes numbness and a tingling sensation.

Scoliosis: lateral curvature of the spine.

Sequestrectomy: surgical removal of necrotic bone.

Spinal fusion: a fusion of the cervical, thoracic, or lumbar region of the spine using an iliac or other bone graft, primarily fusing the laminae and sometimes the joints, most often through the posterior approach.

Syme amputation: modified ankle disarticulation (below-the-ankle) amputation of the foot.

Volkmann contracture: the final state of unrelieved forearm compartment syndrome; contractures of tendons to wrist and hand.

GENERAL POST ANESTHESIA CARE

Specific nursing care related to the orthopedic patient that begins in the PACU includes positioning, neurovascular assessment, care of immobilization devices, wound care, range-of-motion exercises, and observation for complications.

Positioning

After the initial assessment of the orthopedic patient is made, attention is turned to positioning. Proper body alignment is important for all these patients and requires a sound knowledge of operative procedure and body mechanics. Each surgeon generally has specific directives for positioning, but general guidelines apply to all patients. The goal is to provide optimum comfort and safety for the operated limb. The upper extremities should be held close to the body; elevation should be achieved without undue pressure on the elbow or shoulder. The lower extremities are in a neutral position, with support provided for their entire length, and heels are off the bed.

Elevation of operative limbs is usually indicated to increase venous return, reduce swelling, and promote comfort. When elevating a hand or an arm, the hand must be higher than the heart, and there should be no pressure on the elbow. This position can be achieved by the use of a stockinette device for suspension on an intravenous (IV) pole. Measure the stockinette from elbow to approximately 12 inches beyond the finger tips. Cut a piece double this length. Fold it in half, and rest the elbow in the fold. Using safety pins, close the sides around the limb to form a tube, making sure the fingers are exposed (to assess neurovascular status). With the excess material, tie a knot and suspend the end from the IV pole. Be careful to properly support the elbow. If using a pillow for elevation, remember to allow the arm slight flexion for maximum comfort, and provide additional support for the elbow and shoulder.

Lower extremity elevation is most effective if the toes are above the heart. The limb, if not in an immobilization device, is kept in a position of extension. This position is achieved by elevating the foot of the bed rather than the use of pillows. If pillows are used, be sure to support the entire length of the limb and keep the heels off the bed.

Shoulder immobilization can be accomplished with a sling or shoulder immobilizer.

An airplane splint may be applied for rotator cuff repairs. If a sling is used, the patient is instructed to keep his or her arm close to the chest with the wrist and elbow supported. The shoulder immobilizer requires special care to pad areas where skin is in contact with skin.

The patient with a hip pinning is positioned with proper body alignment, and the legs are in a proper neutral position. Care is given to avoid stress to the operative area with exaggerated flexion or rotation. A pillow is placed between the knees when turning to prevent adduction and rotation. For the patient with a total hip replacement, proper body alignment is achieved by the use of an abduction pillow placed between the knees at all times. Most important with these patients is to avoid flexion and adduction of the newly placed joint. If the abduction pillow straps are not in use, it is necessary to support the lateral aspect of the leg to avoid external rotation. This can be accomplished by the use of rolled towels or sheets.

The PACU nurse should also be familiar with various types of orthopedic equipment that may be used and that can affect positioning. Often, the patient with a total knee replacement and those with more extensive knee arthrotomy are placed in a continuous passive motion (CPM) machine. The purpose of CPM is to enhance the healing process by providing CPM to the joint, increasing circulation and movement. Traction may also be used with various patients to immobilize and align a specific area. The PACU nurse is not usually involved in setting up the traction but should be aware of some basic principles for maintenance: (1) the traction must be continuous; (2) the patient is centered in bed in good alignment to maintain the line of pull in line with the long bone; (3) weights should hang freely, not resting on the floor or bed; and (4) the pulley ropes should be in alignment and free of knots. One type of traction is depicted in Figure 28–1.

Neurovascular Assessment

Critical to the care of the orthopedic patient is assessment of the neurovascular status of the operative limb. Any alteration in blood flow to the extremity or nerve compression requires immediate intervention. Assessment is recommended every 30 minutes because problems can occur as soon as 2 to 4 hours. Baseline neurovascular indicators should be noted in the admission nursing assessment. These can

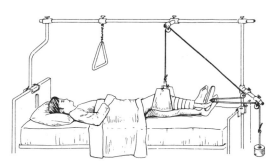

FIGURE 28–1. Russell's skin traction (single) with overhead frame and trapeze. (From Rambo, B. J., and Wood, L. A.: Nursing Skills for Clinical Practice. Philadelphia, W. B. Saunders, 1982, p. 359.)

be used to establish whether or not there have been any deleterious effects from the surgery and to avoid the masking of potential complications. Both the affected and unaffected limbs are assessed.

The hallmarks of neurovascular changes due to constriction and circulatory embarrassment are pain, discoloration (skin that is pale or bluish), decreased mobility, coldness, diminished or absent pulses, altered capillary refilling, and swelling. Pain is common with orthopedic patients, and the approach to treatment must be individualized. Pain unrelieved by conventional methods, such as elevation and repositioning and the administration of narcotics, must be further assessed. Color indicates circulatory compromise. Cyanosis suggests venous obstruction; pallor suggests arterial obstruction. Mobility is assessed by determining the range of motion of the fingers or toes and is a strong indicator of neural compromise. Fingers are flexed, extended, spread, and wiggled. Toes should be dorsiflexed, plantarflexed, and wiggled. Inability to move the fingers or toes, pain on extension of the hand or foot, or coldness of the extremity is indicative of ischemia. Sensation is described as *normal, hypesthetic* (dulled), *paresthetic,* or *anesthetic.* Alteration in sensation suggests nerve compression or circulatory compromise. Limb perfusion is further assessed by the presence of peripheral pulses and capillary refilling. Capillary refilling is assessed by compression of the nail bed, which causes it to blanch; when the compression is released, color briskly returns. Compromise delays the filling time. With the development of pulse oximetry, a more reliable method of perfusion assessment is available. With placement of the oximeter sensor on a finger or toe of the affected limb, the pulsation will be sensed and oxygen saturation displayed. This method is more reflective of perfusion than capillary refilling and is valuable when pulses cannot be assessed owing to the presence of a cast or dressing.

Care of Immobilization Devices (Cast Care)

Immediate assessment of the orthopedic patient in PACU should include the type of immobilization device applied. The soft knee immobilizer should be checked for proper placement and closure and the surgical dressing checked for drainage. For care involving traction, refer to the section on positioning earlier in this chapter.

The cast is a rigid immobilization device molded to the contours of the part to which it is applied. The cast has a dual purpose: to immobilize in a specific position and to provide uniform pressure on the encased soft tissue. The cast should be inspected for visibility of fingers and toes for neurovascular assessment. If the cast is bivalved, the edges should be inspected for roughness to avoid discomfort and potential skin breakdown. When the patient arrives in PACU, the cast will probably still be wet, and special care must be taken to prevent indentations. A wet cast must be handled carefully using the palms of the hand to avoid pressure caused by fingertips. Support the cast on a pillow, avoiding hard, flat surfaces. Improper handling and flat surfaces can cause indentations that may lead to the development of pressure sores. More frequently, a fiberglass cast is applied with quicker drying properties, but the same general principles still apply. Any drainage noted on the cast should be circled, and the time should be noted. This documentation can provide a guide for postoperative blood and fluid loss and can alert the nurse if the drainage appears to be excessive. Note that orthopedic wounds tend to ooze and bleed more than other surgical wounds.

Wound Care

All surgical dressings should be checked for drainage and closure. Orthopedic patients are highly susceptible to infection; therefore, strict asepsis when changing dressings or handling drains is required. Drains may be placed in the wound to minimize blood accumulation and the possibility of infection. Care must be taken to attend these drains to maintain suction.

It is not uncommon for a patient with total joint replacement to have a large amount of blood loss in the immediate postoperative period. This loss can be as great as 250 to 300 ml in the first hour. The retrieval of this blood for reinfusion (autotransfusion), when coupled with preoperative autologous blood donation, has substantially reduced the need for homologous transfusions. Autotransfusion is accomplished by the use of self-contained disposable systems (e.g., Solcotrans® Plus Orthopaedic Autotransfusion System, as shown in Fig. 28–2) that are designed for easy setup and safe use.

Range-of-Motion Exercises

Range-of-motion exercises can be initiated in the PACU as soon as the patient is alert and cooperative. Flexion, extension, and rotation of joints distal to the operative area assist in stimulating circulation and strengthening muscles. Prevention of venous stasis decreases the incidence of thromboembolism, and early movement of joints promotes healing and stabilization.

Observation for Complications

Postoperative complications for the orthopedic patient include deep vein thrombosis, pulmonary embolism, fat embolism syndrome, compartment syndrome, shock, and urinary retention.

Deep Vein Thrombosis. Thrombosis is the formation of a blood clot associated with three conditions outlined by Virchow in 1846: venous stasis, altered clotting mechanism, and altered vessel wall integrity. Immobilization and the insult of the surgical procedure place the orthopedic patient at high risk. Immobilization impairs the leg muscle action needed to move the blood sufficiently, and the surgical procedure causes injury to vessel walls that activates altered clotting mechanisms. An inflammation process begins within the vessel wall, leading to deep vein thrombosis. The patient usually complains of pain and tenderness. Signs include swelling and sometimes localized redness. Palpation of the calf reveals firmness or tension of the muscle. A positive Homan's sign may be exhibited.

Venous complications can usually be prevented by early initiation of exercise, but if they occur, exercise should cease; anticoagulant therapy is usually initiated. Anticoagulant therapy is routinely begun postoperatively on the higher risk patients, such as those with total joint replacements. Antiembolism stockings or pneumatic hose should be used on all patients who will not be ambulatory, who have hip or lower extremity injury, who are elderly, or who have a previous history of thrombophlebitis. These stockings provide compression that enhances venous flow rates. The pneumatic stockings (alternating–pressure-gradient stockings) provide automatically a consistent compression-decompression system. These stockings are growing in popularity and should be considered for the higher risk total hip replacement and spinal surgical patients.

Pulmonary Embolism. The most serious sequela of deep vein thrombosis is pulmonary embolism. If the patient has been inactive and movement has been restricted prior to surgery, the risk of clot formation is greatly enhanced. Embolization of this clot leads to pulmonary embolism. The severity of symptoms depends on the size and number of clots. Symptoms range from none if the clot is small to a myriad that may include—with increasing severity—anxiety, dyspnea, tachypnea, hemoptysis, substernal pain, stabbing "pleuritic" pain, tachycardia, cough, signs and symptoms of cerebral ischemia, fever, elevated sedimentation rate, shock, and sudden death. Immediate nursing care involves administration of oxygen and relief of pain.

Fat Embolism Syndrome. Fat embolism syndrome is a condition that leads to respiratory insufficiency and is related to multiple fractures, especially of the long bones. It is caused by fat droplets released into the circulation

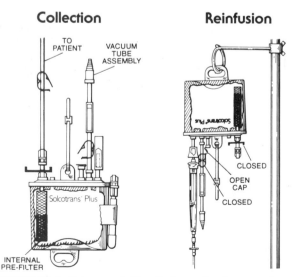

Collection   **Reinfusion**

TO PATIENT
VACUUM TUBE ASSEMBLY
Solcotrans Plus
INTERNAL PRE-FILTER
CLOSED
OPEN CAP
CLOSED

FIGURE 28–2. Solcotrans® Plus Orthopaedic Autotransfusion System. (Courtesy of Davol, Inc., Cranston, RI, Subsidiary of C. R. Bard, Inc.)

from the bone marrow and local tissue trauma. Similar to pulmonary embolism, these fat globules migrate to the lungs, causing occlusions. The fat globules break down into acids, irritating vascular walls and causing extrusion of fluids into the alveoli. The lung involvement alters ventilation and leads to hypoxemia. Fat embolism syndrome may lead to adult respiratory distress syndrome. The symptoms related to lung involvement include tachypnea, tachycardia, anxiety, petechiae over the chest, Po_2 less than 60 mm Hg, fever, pallor, and confusion. Brain involvement is evidenced by agitation, confusion, delirium, and coma. Immediate nursing care of this sometimes fatal complication includes administering oxygen, keeping the patient quiet, and preventing motion at the fracture site.

Compartment Syndrome. Compartment syndrome is a condition in which increased pressure within a muscle compartment causes circulatory compromise, leading to diminished function of the limb. Left undetected, the compression may cause permanent damage to the extremity. The compartment is described as a fascial sheath enclosing bone, muscle, nerves, blood vessels, and soft tissue. The two main causes of increased pressure to this space are (1) constriction from the outside, such as a cast or bandage that decreases the size of the compartment, or (2) increased pressure within the compartment, such as swelling. The hallmark symptoms of compartment syndrome include intense pain unrelieved by conventional methods, paresthesia, and sharp pain on passive stretching of the middle finger of the affected arm or the large toe of the affected leg. Progressive symptoms include decreased strength, decreased sensation (numbness and tingling), and decreased capillary refilling; peripheral pulses are not generally compromised. Immediate intervention includes elevation of the extremity, application of ice, and release of restrictive dressings. Fasciotomy may be required if conservative measures are unsuccessful.

Shock. Because of the highly vascular composition of bone and secondary injury to the soft tissue, hemorrhage is always a potential risk in the trauma and postoperative orthopedic patients. Vigilant observation of the operative area and blood pressure and pulse will alert the PACU nurse to any impending danger. Immediate nursing measures include keeping the patient warm and flat in bed, monitoring vital signs, and replacing fluid volume. The surgeon is notified immediately, and more definitive treatment is initiated (see Chapter 44).

Urinary Retention. *Urinary retention* refers to the inability to void despite the urge or desire. This condition may occur in adult patients on whom hip or back surgery has been performed. The retention may be the result of spinal anesthesia or, possibly, inability to void in the supine position. These patients should be monitored for bladder distention and complaints of pain in the lower abdomen. The surgeon should be notified if distention occurs or if the patient is unable to void within 8 hours after the surgery is completed.

POST ANESTHESIA CARE AFTER HAND SURGERY

The hand surgical patient usually is admitted to the PACU with a large bulky dressing in place on the hand and forearm. An elastic bandage to apply pressure may also be in place outside the dressing. The hand should be elevated above the level of the heart at all times to prevent edema and hemorrhage. The hand may be placed on pillows on the chest of the patient or suspended from the bed frame or IV pole by stockinette. The elbow should be supported by a pillow. Support under the shoulder and wrist aids in decreasing pressure to the elbow. If a drain is present, it should be checked to ensure that it is activated, or it may be connected to a vacuum blood tube. The drain is placed to minimize the bleeding into the wound and to reduce the possibility of infections. Drains should be checked every 1 or 2 hours to maintain a proper vacuum and the output recorded on the intake and output records. The tips of the fingers should be visible, and the neurovascular status should be assessed every 30 minutes for signs of change. It should be remembered that hand surgery is often done with the use of an axillary block and that sensation and movement may not fully return for several hours after surgery. Baseline neurovascular indicators should be noted in the admission nursing assessment. These can be used to establish whether or not there have been any deleterious effects from the surgery.

POST ANESTHESIA CARE AFTER ARM AND FOREARM SURGERY

Post anesthesia care of the patient recovering from arm and forearm surgery centers on elevating the extremity, observing for excessive bleeding, and monitoring for neurovascular changes. The radial pulse should be taken every 30 minutes and compared with that of the unaffected limb. If pulses cannot be assessed because of a dressing or cast, the pulse oximeter sensor should be placed on a finger of the affected arm—the pulsation will reflect perfusion to the limb. Any decrease in intensity of the pulse or in bilateral strength of the hand, any excessive bleeding, and any changes in neurovascular status should be reported to the surgeon. Symptoms of excessive pain, weakness, or decreased sensation, especially on passive extension of the fingers, are usually indicative of compartment syndrome, which constitutes an orthopedic emergency. Patients should be encouraged to perform active range-of-motion exercises with their wrist and hand.

POST ANESTHESIA CARE AFTER SHOULDER SURGERY

Shoulder surgery may include arthroscopy, arthrotomy, or total shoulder joint replacement. The patient is admitted to the PACU with a bulky pressure dressing in place along with a sling-style shoulder immobilizer. Make sure that the immobilizer does not interfere with chest expansion because this would inhibit adequate respiratory exchange. The surgical dressing should be inspected for bleeding because the shoulder is a vascular area in which hemorrhage is difficult to manage.

Inspection should include checking to see if any skin surface is in contact with another. If this is the case, a protective pad should be inserted between the two skin surfaces. The radial pulse should be monitored because flexion of the arm in the immobilizer can reduce blood flow to the hand. The immobilizer should be checked for areas that might be causing pressure to the shoulder and arm. Remember to support the elbow and wrist to prevent any undue pressure to the ulnar and radial nerves. Again, neurovascular observations are a critical part of the post anesthesia assessment of these patients. The patient should be encouraged to perform active range-of-motion exercises with that hand.

POST ANESTHESIA CARE AFTER HIP OR FEMORAL SURGERY

When the patient who has had hip or femoral surgery is admitted to the PACU, nursing assessment should include pulmonary and neurovascular function, body alignment, and the amount and type of bleeding from the surgical incision. Owing to advancing age and long bone trauma, these patients represent the highest risk group for post orthopedic complications.

Pre-existing medical conditions and the effects of anesthetic agents compromise respiratory function. Coughing and deep breathing, sustained maximal inspirations, and position changes, when possible, are of utmost importance. The incentive spirometer can be used to facilitate good lung expansion. Any change in the pulmonary dynamics should be reported to the anesthetist.

Because swelling at the operative site can reduce blood flow to the feet, neurologic signs along with pulses of the affected foot should be monitored and compared with those of the unaffected foot. The dorsalis pedis pulse can be palpated on the dorsum of the foot and lateral to the extensor tendon of the great toe. The posterior tibial pulse can be palpated just behind and slightly below the medial malleolus of the ankle. The extremity is elevated where indicated.

The body should be aligned as normally as possible. The legs and feet are maintained in a neutral position, elevated as indicated, and supported to avoid rotations of and pressure on the heels. Traction may be applied and has been discussed earlier in this chapter. Observe for peroneal nerve compression in any patient with lower limbs wrapped in elastic bandages or strapped as in an abductor pillow. Compression may occur where the peroneal nerve crosses the knee at the head of the fibula. Decreased sensation over the dorsum of the foot, tingling, extremity weakness, and an inability to bring the foot up are signs indicative of this injury, which is a common cause of foot-drop. The patient should be encouraged to perform active range-of-motion exercises of the ankle to enhance venous return.

The patient with total hip replacement has an abduction pillow placed between the knees at all times. This position must be maintained to avoid adduction and internal rotation of the newly placed joint. The patient should not be allowed to flex the hips at a greater than 30- to 40-degree angle or to adduct the leg of the affected side. The muscle groups are weakened, and dislocation of the joint is a potential risk. If turning is required, the patient may be turned to the unoperated side no more than 45 degrees with hip abduction maintained and total leg support provided. The head of the bed may be elevated no more than 45 degrees.

An autotransfusion system or Hemovac

drain is usually inserted at the operative site to facilitate the removal of blood; the color and amount should be inspected frequently. If the color is bright red or the drainage is more than 300 ml in an 8-hour period, the surgeon should be notified. The patient with total hip replacement may experience a large blood loss, which becomes a problem if the loss is sustained or if it increases.

POST ANESTHESIA CARE AFTER KNEE SURGERY

Post anesthesia care of the patient who has had surgery of the knee involves observation for complications and proper knee positioning. The surgical procedure may involve repair of ligaments and tendons or removal of all or of a portion of the meniscal cartilage. Patients may undergo a total knee replacement when degenerative processes have caused the knee joint to become nonfunctional.

The knee joint is formed by the articulation of rounded condyles of the femur with shallow depressions in the tibia, also called *condyles*. At the periphery of the articulation between the femoral and tibial condyles are the wedge-shaped meniscal cartilages that function primarily in joint lubrication and in cushioning. Located within the joint capsules, the medial and lateral cruciate ligaments are primarily responsible for lateral stability, and the anterior and posterior cruciate ligaments within the intercondylar notch are primarily responsible for anteroposterior stability. Externally, the joint is strengthened by tendons of the quadriceps muscle stabilized by the patella.

After knee surgery, the patient arrives in the PACU with a bulky compression dressing in place. Ice over the surgical site may be ordered to provide comfort and minimize swelling. The leg should be elevated and positioned in full extension. This can be facilitated by elevation at the ankle so that maximum extension of the leg can be accomplished. Remember to avoid pressure to the heel. An effective means of providing compression and cold is the use of the CryoCuff (Fig. 28–3). The CryoCuff is a large vinyl bladder that fits over the knee. The cuff, anchored by Velcro straps to the leg, is then filled with ice water via a portable canister. When filled, safe cooling and compression are provided to the operative area.

Assessments of neurovascular status should be performed every 30 minutes. Any decrease in sensation over the dorsum of the foot should be noted, because this can represent compres-

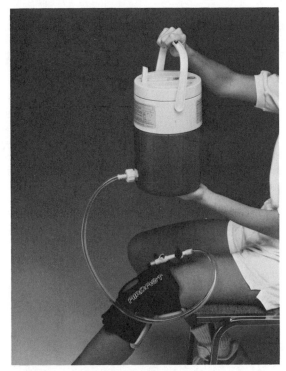

FIGURE 28–3. CryoCuff system. (Courtesy of Aircast, Summit, NJ.)

sion of the peroneal nerve where it crosses the fibula at the knee. The surgeon should be notified if any neurologic or circulatory change is found, because early detection and correction prevent permanent nerve deficit or ischemic muscular injury. If the patient received a spinal anesthetic, it will be necessary to wait for the motor function to return before initiating neurologic assessment.

These patients should be encouraged to flex, extend, and rotate their ankles as soon as possible to improve circulation. Knee-strengthening exercises may also be started in the PACU. Isometric exercises and quad sets aid in healing the muscle and providing stability to the joint. Isometrics involve a 6-second contraction of the entire leg followed by relaxation. The quad sets require contraction of the quadriceps muscle while pressing the knee to the bed for 5 to 10 seconds and then relaxation.

Arthroscopic examination of the knee is done to facilitate minor repairs and the diagnosis of more extensive damage to the knee; in general, there are fewer postoperative complications because this is a less invasive procedure. However, neurovascular assessment remains an important part of the post anesthesia care of these patients.

The patient with total knee replacement and

those patients who have undergone extensive arthrotomy knee repairs are sometimes placed in a continuous passive motion (CPM) machine (Fig. 28–4). This device provides a safe method of elevation, comfort, and continuous range-of-motion to the operative knee. The CPM promotes healing by increasing circulation and movement of the knee joint. The machine should be inspected to ensure proper positioning of the limb. The flexion and extension settings of the machine should be determined by the physician and are generally 0 to 30 degrees at slow speed initially.

Extensive knee procedures generally have large amounts of drainage. An autotransfusion device or Hemovac drain is present to facilitate removal of drainage from the wound. The Hemovac drain is emptied and reactivated as necessary. Autotransfusion is discussed in Chapter 20. Drainage amounts of 250 to 300 ml in 1 to 2 hours are not uncommon.

POST ANESTHESIA CARE AFTER FOOT SURGERY

The patient who has had a surgical procedure performed on the foot has either a cast or a bandage over the operative site. The amount and color of bleeding should be noted. Neurovascular signs should be monitored every 30 minutes. The extremity should be elevated above the level of the heart, with pillows supporting the entire length of the leg.

POST ANESTHESIA CARE AFTER SPINAL SURGERY

There are several types of spinal procedures. The important features of the postoperative assessment relate mostly to the surgical area of the spine. Patients who have had a cervical procedure should be monitored for neurologic signs of the upper extremities. Symptoms such as weakness and radiating pain should be reported to the surgeon. Patients in halo traction should be monitored for any deficiency in the sixth cranial (abducent) nerve. Any decrease in the lateral movement of the eye is indicative of injury to the abducent nerve.

If the surgical procedure involves C3, C4, or C5, respiratory movements should be monitored, because the diaphragm muscle is innervated by the spinal outflow from these vertebrae. The patient with this nerve deficit exhibits lack of diaphragmatic excursion, as well as shortness of breath and the use of intercostal and accessory muscles in breathing. If these symptoms appear, oxygen should be administered, and assistance in ventilation may be necessary.

Patients who have had midthoracic or lower spinal surgery may develop an ileus. This complication is signaled by abdominal distention, diminished or absent bowel sounds, and tympany on percussion of the abdomen. The usual treatment is to withhold oral food and fluids and to decompress the stomach with a nasogastric tube.

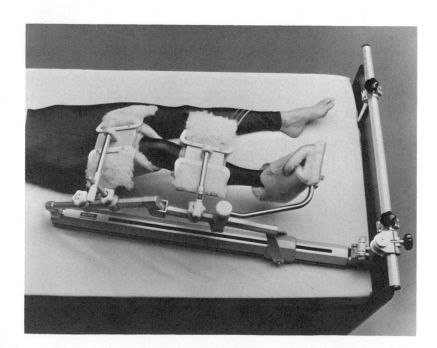

FIGURE 28–4. LiteLift continuous passive motion machine. (Courtesy of Sutter Corporation, San Diego, CA.)

Patients who have had lumbar or sacral spinal surgery should be observed for loss of strength in the lower extremities and bladder distention. Bladder distention may be indicated by diaphoresis, hypertension, tachycardia, tachypnea, and a feeling of distress. If the patient has a catheter in place, it should be irrigated to remove any obstruction. If there is no urinary catheter and the patient cannot urinate, the surgeon should be notified.

Patients with progressive curvature of the spine (scoliosis) may undergo a Harrington or Luque rod insertion for correction or stabilization of the spine. The procedure entails a spinal fusion followed by rod placement. The post anesthesia assessment entails those features included in the assessment of the thoracic and the lumbosacral spine surgical patient.

Patients who have surgery on the spine should also be observed for bleeding from the site of the operation. The patient should be turned from side to side to help reduce stasis of fluids in the lungs. The technique for turning the spinal patient is called *logrolling*. All parts of the patient's body should move in unison. To facilitate this, a pillow may be placed between the patient's knees and the knee opposite the side the patient will be turned to should be flexed. Using a draw sheet can also help to facilitate turning in one smooth motion. Pillows should be placed to support the length of the back and buttocks along with the pillow between the patient's knees. This method of turning the patient puts the least amount of pressure on the spine. With the advent of microdisk surgery, there is minimal disturbance to the stability of the spine, and these patients are generally allowed activity as desired.

All spinal patients with restricted movement should have antiembolism or pneumatic stockings on, and ankle pumping and rotation should be encouraged to decrease the stasis of blood in the lower extremities. The patient should be encouraged to use the incentive spirometer every hour to reduce the stasis of fluids in the lungs. Neurovascular evaluation is performed every 30 minutes to assess any improvements or deficiencies. Pain is a relative experience for the spinal surgical patient. In many instances, the relief from nerve compression pain is so dramatic that the operative site pain is minimized. In other instances, the pain from spinal fusion is often difficult to manage. As discussed earlier in this chapter, the pain experience must be individualized and treated appropriately. The nurses's goal is to help the patient perceive the pain as something that can be controlled rather than a fearful, unrelenting burden.

POST ANESTHESIA CARE AFTER LIMB AMPUTATION

Patients who have had an amputation of the leg are admitted to the PACU with a dressing or a cast applied to the extremity. A cast is used to provide uniform pressure to the soft tissue, to control swelling, and to position the limb to avoid contracture. See cast care discussed earlier in this chapter in the section on immobilization devices. To prevent hip contracture, elevation of the lower extremity with a soft compression dressing should be achieved by elevating the foot of the bed rather than using a pillow. The patient with an amputation of the arm usually has a bulky compression dressing in place. The dressing should be assessed for drainage. The extremity should be elevated, and ice may be applied to reduce postoperative edema and discomfort.

References

1. Allard, J. L., and Dibble, S. L.: Scoliosis surgery: A look at Luque rods. Am. J. Nurs., *84*(5):609–611, 1984.
2. Callahan, J.: Compartment syndrome. Orthop. Nurs., *4*(4):11–14, 1985.
3. Farrell, J.: Orthopedic pain: What does it mean? Am. J. Nurs., *84*(4):466–469, 1984.
4. Farrell, J.: Positioning postoperative orthopedic patients. Today's OR Nurse, *6*(10): 12–16, 1984.
5. Genge, M.: Orthopedic trauma: Pelvic fractures. Orthop. Nurs., *5*(1):11–18, 1986.
6. Gregory, B., and Van Valkenburgh, J.: The athlete's knee. J. Post Anesth. Nurs., *5*(6):414–417, 1990.
7. Herron, D., and Nance, J.: Emergency department nursing management of patients with orthopedic fractures resulting from motor vehicle accidents. Nurs. Clin. North Am., *25*(1):71–83, 1990.
8. Johnson, J.: Respiratory complications of orthopedic injuries. Orthop. Nurs., *5*(1):24–28, 1986.
9. Maier, P.: Take the work out of range-of-motion exercises. RN, *49*(9):46–49, 1986.
10. Miller, B. K., and Gregory, M.: Carpal tunnel syndrome. AORN J., *38*(3):525–537, 1983.
11. Mims, B.: Back surgery: Helping your patient get through it. RN, *48*(5):26–32, 1985.
12. Rodts, M.: Orthopedic nursing and sports nursing. Nurs. Clin. North Am., *26*(1):1–240, 1991.
13. Shenkman, B., and Stechmiller, J.: Fat embolism syndrome: Pathophysiology and current treatment. Focus Crit. Care, *11*(6):26–35, 1984.
14. Thompson, M. B.: An overview of arthroscopy. Today's OR Nurse, *4*(11):9–13, 1983.
15. Turner, P.: Caring for emotional needs of orthopedic trauma patients. AORN J., *36*(4):566–570, 1982.
16. Urbanski, P. A.: The orthopedic patient: Identifying neurovascular injury. AORN J., *40*(5):707–711, 1984.
17. Voluz, J. M.: Surgical implants: Orthopedic devices. AORN J., *37*(7):1341–1352, 1983.
18. Willert, D., and Barden, R.: Deep vein thrombosis, pulmonary embolism, and prophylaxis in the orthopedic patient. Orthop. Nurs., *4*(4):27–32, 1985.
19. Wise, L.: A comparison of orthopedic casts: Breaking the mold. MCN, *11*(3):174–176, 1986.

Post Anesthesia Care of the Neurosurgical Patient

John K. Hawkins, M.H.S., R.N., C.R.N.A.
Virginia C. Hawkins, M.S.N., R.N., C.C.R.N.

Many health care facilities have specialized neurologic care units that receive neurologic surgical patients directly from the operating room, but most facilities require that these patients first be recovered from anesthesia in the post anesthesia care unit (PACU) before returning to the routine care units. Neurosurgical patients, or those with underlying neurologic conditions, present a challenge to the post anesthesia nurse. In addition to being familiar with routine post anesthesia care, the nurse must have a basic understanding of the nervous system and of the types of pathologic conditions or injuries that may affect this system, and he or she must be able to translate this knowledge into the skills necessary to assess, provide care for, and evaluate the neurosurgical patient.

This chapter is divided into two sections: cranial surgery and spinal surgery. The division is made solely for this discussion, because there are aspects of care related to each topic that are common to both areas. In addition, disease or injury in any portion of the nervous system may also affect other organs and systems of the body. In caring for the neurosurgical patient, the nurse must consider each structure of the nervous system (see Chapter 4) as it relates to the individual as a whole.

Definitions

Baroreceptor: a sensory nerve cell aggregate present in the wall of a blood vessel that is stimulated by changes in blood pressure.
Compliance: the ability of the brain to yield when a pressure or force is applied.
Crepitus: a crackling sound produced by the rubbing together of fractured bone fragments or by the presence of subcutaneous emphysema.
Decompensation: the inability of the heart to maintain adequate circulation due to an impairment in brain integrity.
Diabetes insipidus: a metabolic disorder caused by injury or disease of the posterior lobe of the pituitary gland (the hypophysis).
Focal deficit: any sign or symptom that indicates a specific or localized area of pathologic alteration.
Gibbus: a hump or convexity.
Laminectomy: excision of the posterior arch of a vertebra to allow excision of a herniated nucleus pulposus.
Phrenic nucleus: a group of nerve cells located in the spinal cord between the levels of C3 and C5. Damage to this area abolishes or alters the function of the phrenic nerve.
Pyramidal signs: symptoms of dysfunction of the pyramidal tract, including spastic paralysis, Babinski sign, and increased deep tendon reflexes.
Rhizotomy: surgical interruption of the roots of the spinal nerves within the spinal canal.
Spinal shock: a state that occurs immediately after complete transection of the spinal cord. It may sometimes occur after only partial transections. All sensory, motor, and autonomic activities are lost below the level of the transection, and reflexes are absent. Paralysis is of a flaccid nature and includes the urinary bladder. Autonomic activity gradually resumes as spinal shock subsides. Once autonomic activity has returned, bladder and bowel training programs may be begun. Flaccid paralysis may develop into varying degrees of spastic paralysis, as evidenced by spasms of flexor or extensor muscle groups. The presence of autonomic activity also allows for episodes of autonomic hyperreflexia.

Subarachnoid block: the injection of a local anesthetic into the subarachnoid space around the spinal cord.

Subluxation: partial or incomplete dislocation.

Tonoclonic movements: tense muscular contractions alternating rapidly with muscular relaxation.

Valsalva maneuver: contraction of the thorax in forced expiration against the closed glottis; results in increases in intrathoracic and intraabdominal pressures.

CRANIAL SURGERY

Diagnostic Tools

Some of the techniques used to ascertain the presence and extent of cranial injury or disease are invasive. In many hospitals, patients on whom these procedures are performed spend some time in the PACU. In most instances, anesthesia care is not necessary for these procedures; however, anesthesia support may be needed when these procedures are performed on pediatric, elderly, combative, or medically compromised patients. A brief discussion of invasive as well as noninvasive diagnostic procedures is included here to familiarize the PACU nurse with the techniques and the special considerations necessary in the care of these patients.

Invasive Techniques

Pneumoencephalography. This procedure can usually be performed with the use of local anesthesia and mild sedation. However, because of the incidence of severe headache, nausea and vomiting, shock, and impaired consciousness, general anesthesia may be used.

A lumbar puncture is performed, and the cerebrospinal fluid (CSF) removed is replaced with air or gas. The patient is usually placed in a chair designed for easy movement and positioning while radiographs are being made. Even when this procedure is performed under general anesthesia, the patient often experiences a severe headache for some time after the procedure. Therefore, it is considerate to place the patient in an area where extraneous noise and activity are minimal but where frequent observations are possible. Analgesics and antiemetics can be given to provide comfort for the patient who experiences headache, nausea, and vomiting.

Pneumoencephalography is rarely used because of the availability of modern, more effective diagnostic tools such as computed tomographic (CT) scanning and magnetic resonance imaging (MRI).

Ventriculography. Ventriculography is usually performed under local anesthesia with the patient in the same type of chair as that used in pneumonencephalography. Performing a ventriculographic examination involves puncture of the ventricle through burr holes made in the cranium. CSF is removed and replaced with gas or air. Radiographs are made; the size, shape, and position of the ventricular, cisternal, and subarachnoid spaces are visualized; and the presence of space-occupying lesions may be noted.

As with the pneumoencephalogram patient, the postventriculogram patient may experience nausea, retching, and headache, although not usually as severely. Both types of patient require frequent observation of vital signs, neurologic status, and level of consciousness (LOC). Intravenous fluids are usually continued for 24 hours or until the danger of shock reaction and vomiting has ended. This period is variable and depends on the patient's general condition and tolerance of the procedure. Headaches may persist for 2 to 4 days, and mild analgesics may be prescribed.

As with pneumoencephalography, ventriculography has now become obsolete and is rarely used.

Arteriography. Arteriography, or angiography, is employed to visualize the pattern and patency of the cerebral vasculature. A cannula is introduced into the femoral or axillary artery and threaded to the level of the common carotid artery. Radiopaque dye is then injected, and radiographs record its path through the cerebral vasculature. Arteriovenous malformations (AVMs), aneurysms, thromboses, occlusions, space-occupying lesions, and abscesses may be detected by this method (Fig. 29–1). During and after arteriography, the patient may experience an allergic reaction to the dye used that may range from mild urticaria to anaphylaxis. Resuscitative equipment must be immediately available until the danger of allergic reaction has passed.

Irritation brought on by use of the dye may manifest itself by altered states of consciousness, hemiparesis, or speech difficulties that are usually transient in nature. It is imperative that the site of injection be examined closely at frequent intervals for the presence of bleeding that, when present, occurs beneath the skin and defies casual detection. The effects of the local anesthetic agent often last for several hours and prevent the patient from detecting and re-

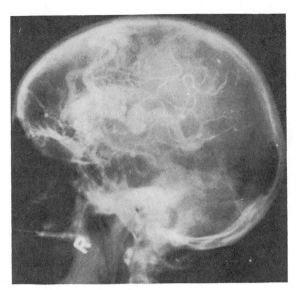

FIGURE 29–1. Arteriographic demonstration of an intracranial arteriovenous malformation. (From Sabiston, D. C., Jr. [ed.]: Davis-Christopher Textbook of Surgery: The Biological Basis of Modern Surgical Practice. 14th ed. Philadelphia, W. B. Saunders, 1991, p. 1250.)

porting the pain caused by hemorrhage. The site is often swollen, becoming painful after the anesthetic effect has worn off. This pain and edema can be minimized by the prompt placement of a pressure dressing and an ice pack over the area. A weighted device, such as a small sand bag or a liter bag of fluids, can be placed over the dressing for additional pressure to help control hemorrhage. Intravenous fluids are maintained until the danger of untoward reaction has passed and the patient is no longer experiencing the transient nausea that occasionally occurs.

Brain Scanning. A radioactive compound is injected intravenously and is taken up by brain tissue. The pattern of this uptake is detected by a scintillation scanner, and a visual record is made. Uptake may be altered at the site of a disorder and may reflect the presence of cerebral neoplasms, hematomas, abscesses, and AVMs.

CT Scanning. CT scanning (sometimes called *computerizd transverse axial* or *electromagnetic interference scanning*) creates a cross-sectional picture that separates various densities in the brain by means of an external radiation beam. A computer-based apparatus allows the assessment of brain-emitted radiation after the intravenous injection of a radioactive isotope. The computer performs thousands of simultaneous equations on the radiation input and output data stored on its tapes and delivers an

accurate, detailed picture of the brain and of any abnormalities (Fig. 29–2).

CT scanning has the advantages of accuracy and rapidity; both are essential in emergency situations. Unfortunately, the procedure requires the patient's maximum cooperation for sustained periods and is therefore difficult, if not impossible, to use in an agitated, confused, or restless patient.

Magnetic Resonance Imaging. Also known as *nuclear magnetic resonance*, MRI is a technique for obtaining cross-sectional pictures of the human body without exposure of the patient to ionizing radiation. MRI yields anatomic information comparable in many ways to the information supplied by a CT scan but is often able to discriminate more sensitively between healthy and diseased tissues. In fact, many studies have demonstrated that MRI is superior and will eventually make CT scanning obsolete as it becomes more available.

MRI is able to visualize soft organs by differentiating the number of hydrogen molecules present in the water content of the tissues. The water content for each type of tissue, including abnormal tissue, varies and, when assessed by a skilled radiologist, serves almost as its signature.

The patient to be scanned is placed within a cylindrical high-powered magnet. Body tissues are then subjected to a magnetic field, causing some of the hydrogen ions to align themselves with the field. A burst of low-energy radio waves is then applied that knocks atomic protons within the tissues out of alignment. When

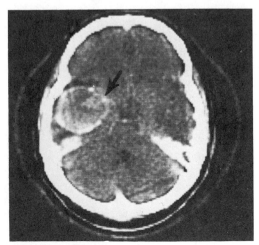

FIGURE 29–2. CT scan of large congenital aneurysm *(arrow)* of middle cerebral artery in left middle fossa. (From Sabiston, D. C., Jr. [ed.]: Davis-Christopher Textbook of Surgery: The Biological Basis of Modern Surgical Practice. 11th ed. Philadelphia, W. B. Saunders, 1977, p. 1472.)

the radio waves are discontinued, these protons release tiny amounts of energy that are "read" by a computer. Then the MRI generates an image based on this information, yielding a detailed picture of the structural content and contours of the internal organs.

Positron Emission Tomography. Currently, positron emission tomographic (PET) scanning is used mainly in research settings and has limited, although promising, clinical application because of difficulties in interpreting its images. In this type of study, the state of the functioning of the tissues or organs is assessed. The patient is injected with a glucose analogue that is tagged with a radionuclide. As the radionuclide decays in the tissue, the protons emitted are recorded by detectors, and a computerized picture is generated. Now used mostly in assessing brain function, PET scans have been helpful in identifying schizophrenia, Alzheimer's disease, and other brain disorders.

Noninvasive Techniques

Conventional Radiography. Skull films show bony fragments and fractures and any shift in the calcified pineal gland from the midline. Epidural hematoma almost always shows an accompanying linear fracture across the temporal fossa. Except in nondisplaced linear skull fracture, positive skull radiographs are almost always followed up with other diagnostic tests (Fig. 29–3).

Electroencephalography. An electroencephalogram (EEG) is the tracing and recording of the electrical activity at the surface of the brain. Aberrations in the rate and amplitude signal the presence of tumors, abscesses, scars, hematomas, or infection and may aid in the localization of such lesions.

Echoencephalography (ultrasonography). This technique is used to detect shifts in the midline structures of the brain. The pineal gland, septum pellucidum, and wall of the third ventricle are used as the target structures of the ultrasound waves. These waves are then echoed back to the instrument, revealing the exact location of the midline structure. When the midline structures are off center, a space-occupying lesion is assumed to have altered their position. In this manner, hematomas, massive cerebral infarcts, and neoplasms are detected. Echoencephalography has the advantages of being rapid and noninvasive, but its use is sometimes limited by imprecise or inconclusive results.

Injuries and Pathologic Conditions of the Brain

Types of Injuries

When a head injury occurs, the most crucial concern is the extent of injury to the brain itself. Linear skull fractures in and of themselves are of little significance, but when the fracture involves depression of fragments into the brain, penetration of a foreign object, leakage of CSF, expanding hematomas, or signs and symptoms of herniation, surgery is required to relieve the increased intracranial pressure (ICP) that results.

Concussion, a jostling of the brain without contusion, is caused by a violent jar or shock to the skull. The patient may be dazed, "see stars," or experience a period of impaired consciousness. On regaining consciousness, these patients often experience post-traumatic amnesia, remembering nothing of the injury itself or, frequently, nothing of the events immediately preceding the injury.

More serious than concussion is *contusion,* a multiple bruising of the brain or hemorrhage on its surface. Consciousness may be lost for a considerable period. Death may occur within a few hours, or if the contusion is less severe, stupor and confusion may persist for days or weeks. These patients characteristically resent attempts to arouse them and may be disoriented, agitated, or violent.

Contusion of the brain is usually incurred through one of two types of *blow-counterblow injury.* In a *coup-contrecoup injury,* the brain is injured directly beneath the site of the striking force. As the blow thrusts the brain against bony prominences of the inner surface of the opposite side of the skull, further injury results. The vasculature of the brain may be lacerated, and considerable hemorrhage may result. The second type of blow-counterblow injury is the *acceleration-deceleration injury.* In a trauma involving abrupt impact, such as a motor vehicle accident, the internal soft-tissue structures, including the brain, continue to travel for a fraction of a second longer than the external body and receive further injury as they are pressed against the rigid structures of the body. The brain is slapped *by* the surrounding skull and then is slapped *against* it. Rebound occurs, and further damage is done as it strikes the unyielding bony ridges of the inside of the skull. Severe bruising or laceration may occur.

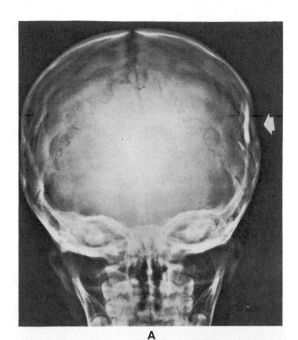

A

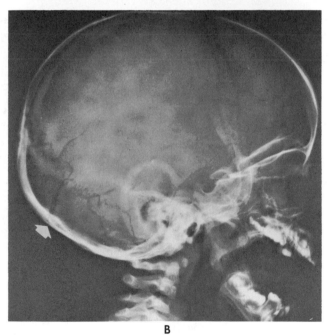

B

FIGURE 29-3. *A*, depressed skull fracture of the left parietal bone and adjoining portion of temporal bone *(arrow)*. *B*, lateral view of the skull demonstrating a linear fracture of the occipital bone with no detectable depression of the fragments *(arrow)*. (*A* and *B* from Meschan, I.: Synopsis of Analysis of Roentgen Signs in General Radiology. Philadelphia, W. B. Saunders, 1976, p. 191.)

Consequences of Injury

Concussion or contusion, as well as intrinsic medical conditions, may produce different kinds of injury to the brain, including subdural, epidural, and intracerebral hematomas and supratentorial herniation (Fig. 29-4), all requiring surgical intervention. The signs and symptoms of brain ischemia and increased ICP vary with the speed at which the functions of vital centers are altered. A small clot that accumulates rapidly may be fatal. On the other hand, the patient may survive a slowly developing, much larger hematoma through effective compensatory mechanisms.

An *epidural hematoma* accumulates in the epidural space (between the skull and the dura mater) and is arterial in nature. Frequently, the

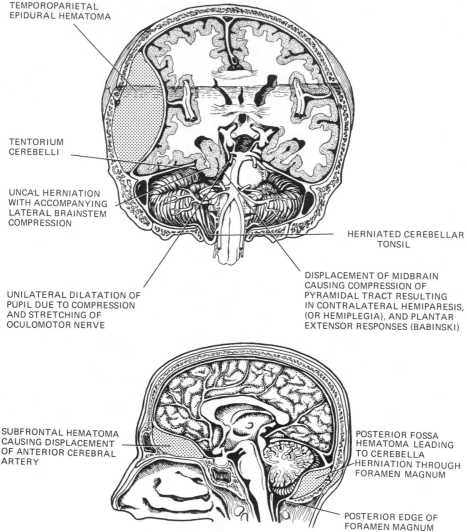

FIGURE 29–4. Pathophysiology of head injuries. (From Kintzel, K. C.: Advanced Concepts in Clinical Nursing. 2nd ed. Philadelphia, J. B. Lippincott, 1977, p. 679.)

cause is the rupture or laceration of the middle meningeal artery, which runs between the dura and the skull in the temporal region. Bleeding along a fracture line is another possible cause. Epidural hematomas most frequently occur in the temporal area but may appear elsewhere, depending on the area of trauma or arterial rupture. Epidural hematoma requires rapid emergency surgery. Owing to its arterial nature, the hemorrhage may be massive, and neurologic deficit and death may occur imminently. Treatment consists of evacuation of the clot through burr holes made in the skull.

Subdural hematoma may result from trauma. Venous blood usually accumulates beneath the dura and spreads over the surface of the brain. A subdural hematoma may be acute, subacute, or chronic, depending on the size of the vessel involved and the amount of blood present. Acute subdural hematomas exhibit a rapid progression of signs and symptoms, and the patient is critically ill.

Subacute subdural hematomas fail to show acute signs and symptoms at their onset. Brain swelling is not great, but the hematoma may become large enough to produce symptoms. Progressive hemiparesis, obtundation, and aphasia often appear 3 to 10 days after injury. The degree of ultimate recovery depends on the extent of damage produced at the time of injury.

Chronic subdural hematomas are most frequently seen in infants and adults older than middle age. A history of head injury may be lacking, because the causative injury is often minimal and long forgotten or deemed insignificant by the patient. The history is usually one of progressive mental or personality changes with or without focal symptoms. Papilledema may be present. As blood slowly accumulates, it compresses the brain. The blood itself becomes thicker and darker within 2 to 4 days and within a few weeks resembles motor oil in character and color. Subdural hematoma may mimic any disease affecting the brain or its coverings and is often incorrectly diagnosed initially as a stroke, neurosis, or psychosis. Treatment consists of evacuation of the defibrinated blood through multiple burr holes or craniotomy incision.

Intracerebral hematomas are more frequently found in the elderly, often following a fall, but are also seen as a result of spontaneous rupture of a weakened blood vessel. Hemorrhaging may be scattered or isolated. Surgical evacuation of an isolated or well-defined clot may be attempted, but the mortality rate remains high.

Supratentorial herniation is regarded as an emergency more severe than that occurring with epidural hematoma. The tentorium is an extension of the dura mater, which forms a transverse partition or shelf dividing the cerebral hemispheres from the cerebellum and brain stem. The superior portion of the brain stem passes upward through an aperture in the tentorium known as the *tentorial hiatus*. No space-occupying mass or lesion expanding within the cerebral hemispheres can escape upward or outward because of the unyielding confinement of the skull. Consequently, expansion within and compression of the hemispheres cause herniation of its contents (usually a portion of the temporal lobe known as the *uncus*) through the tentorial hiatus.

Uncal herniation is accompanied by compression of the lateral brain stem on the same side, shutting off its blood supply and suppressing certain basic functions. The third cranial nerve (oculomotor) is in close proximity to the herniated uncus, and the pupil on the injured side becomes fixed and dilated. The reticular-activating system located in the brain stem that is responsible for waking and alertness becomes affected, and the patient rapidly becomes less and less responsive. Displacement of the midbrain causes compression of the pyramidal tract, resulting in contralateral hemiparesis or hemiplegia and plantar extensor responses (Babinski sign). The respiratory center in the medulla may be affected, which will result in changes in the respiratory pattern or cessation of respiration altogether.

In addition to these changes, the cerebellum itself may be so compressed that the cerebellar tonsil herniates inferiorly through the foramen magnum (see Fig. 29–4). This usually results in immediate death, as the centers vital to life are compressed or sheared. The best treatment for supratentorial herniation is prevention through early detection and treatment of increased ICP and its causes.

If efforts to minimize edema and increased ICP fail, surgical intervention is required as a life-saving measure.

Types of Pathologic Conditions

Cerebral aneurysms are round dilatations of the arterial wall that develop as a result of weakness of the wall due to defects in the medial layer of the artery. Most cerebral aneurysms occur at bifurcations close to the circle of Willis, usually involving the anterior portion. Common bifurcations include those with the internal carotid, the middle cerebral, and the basilar arteries and in relation to the anterior and posterior communicating arteries. The exact cause or precipitating factor is not well defined but may be related to congenital abnormality, arteriosclerosis, embolus, or trauma. Aneurysms are usually asymptomatic and present no clinically detected problem to the patient unless rupture occurs, resulting in neurologic deficits. Ruptured cerebral aneurysm is the major cause of subarachnoid hemorrhage. Intracerebral hemorrhage may occur alone or with the subarachnoid bleed. Morbidity and mortality rates are high owing to rebleeding of the aneurysm and cerebral vasospasm of adjacent arteries. Surgical intervention involves identification and clipping of the aneurysm through a craniotomy.

AVM is a vascular network appearing as a tangled mass of dilated vessels that create an abnormal communication between the arterial and venous systems. The communication may be singular or multiple and resembles an arteriovenous fistula in that there is no connecting capillary system between the arteries and the veins. AVMs most frequently occur in the supratentorial structures and usually involve the vessels of the middle cerebral arteries. AVMs are usually present at birth as a result of congenital abnormalities but may exhibit a delayed age of onset, with symptoms most commonly occurring between the ages of 10 and 20 years. Symptoms may include headache, seizures, altered LOC, and intracranial hemorrhage with resultant increased ICP. The treatment of choice is complete surgical excision by dissection or obliteration by ligation of feeder vessels. Radiation is used to treat AVMs that are surgically inaccessible.

Intracranial tumors are space-occupying lesions that destroy brain tissue and nerve structures by invasion, infiltration, and compression and produce increased ICP.

Intracranial tumors can be primary or metastatic. Primary tumors are classified as primary intracerebral (intra-axial) tumors, which originate from glia cells, or primary extracerebral (extra-axial) tumors, which originate from supporting structures of the nervous system. Metastatic tumors most commonly arise from breast malignancies in women and lung malignancies in men. Clinical manifestations can be both localized and generalized in nature. Local pathophysiologic changes, such as focal neurologic deficits, seizures, visual disturbances, cranial nerve dysfunction, and hormonal changes, result from the tumor itself destroying tissue at a particular site in the brain. Generalized pathophysiologic changes result from the effects of increased ICP. The treatment for cerebral tumors is surgical excision or surgical decompression if total excision is not possible. Surgery is often performed before or after radiation treatment and chemotherapy.

Hydrocephalus, in and of itself, is not a disease entity but rather a clinical syndrome characterized by excess fluid within the cerebral ventricular system, the subarachnoid space, or both. Hydrocephalus occurs because of abnormalities in overproduction, circulation, or reabsorption of CSF. Hydrocephalus can be classified into two categories: noncommunicating (obstructive) or communicating (nonobstructive). *Noncommunicating hydrocephalus* is the result of an obstruction in the ventricular system or the subarachnoid space that prevents the flow of CSF to the location of the arachnoid villi, where reabsorption occurs. The obstruction may be owing to congenital abnormalities or space-occupying lesions. *Communicating hydrocephalus* occurs when the flow of CSF is normal but there is impaired absorption of the fluid at the arachnoid villi. Common causes of communicating hydrocephalus include inflammation of the meninges, subarachnoid hemorrhage, congenital malformation, and space-occupying lesions.

Intracranial Pressure Dynamics

ICP is pressure that is exerted against the skull by its contents: solid brain matter and intracellular water, CSF, and blood. These contents are essentially noncompressible, and a volume change in any compartment requires a reciprocal change to occur in one or both of the other compartments if the ICP is to remain constant (Monro-Kellie hypothesis). Owing to the communications between their intracranial and extracranial compartments, CSF and blood can be translocated extracranially in partial compensation for increased ICP. These compensation capabilities are limited because of the small amount of CSF that the spinal subarachnoid space can hold, and total displacement of cerebral blood results in cerebral ischemia. Normal ICP is 0 to 15 torr. Intracranial hypertension occurs when there is a sustained increased ICP at the level of the head exceeding 15 torr.

Volume may be added to any of the cerebral compartments and results in increased ICP when the compensatory capacity is exceeded. Brain volume can be increased by a tumor, a hematoma, or edema. Blood volume can be increased through dilatation of the vascular bed. CSF volume can be increased through obstruction in the ventricles, resistance to reabsorption, or, in rare instances, increased production of the CSF. Large brain tumors increase pressure by their mass or by blocking the rate of CSF reabsorption, or both. If the tumor is near the surface of the brain, it can cause inflamed meninges that may exude large quantities of fluid and protein into the CSF, increasing ICP. Hemorrhage or infection also causes increases in ICP. Large numbers of cells suddenly appear in the CSF and can almost totally block CSF absorption through the arachnoid villi. Regardless of the mechanism, when the volume added exceeds the volume that can be displaced, intracranial compliance is greatly reduced and ICP begins to increase.

Figure 29–5 illustrates the relationship between intracranial volume and pressure. Phase I demonstrates the success of compensatory mechanisms in maintaining a constant ICP despite early increases in volume. In phase II, the limited capability of compensatory mechanisms has been exceeded, and ICP begins to rise. In phase III, even a slight increase in volume causes a dramatic rise in ICP, resulting in complete decompensation and death. The shape of the curve may be altered by the rate at which the volume increases. Slowly developing increases in volume broaden the curve, whereas rapid increases narrow it.

Post anesthesia care for the patients with the potential for increased ICP requires an understanding of cerebral blood flow (CBF) and the factors affecting it, because it is these factors

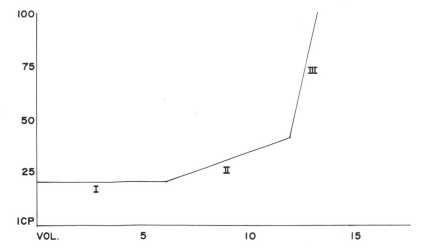

FIGURE 29-5. Pressure-volume curve.

that become defective during increased ICP and are manipulated to reduce ICP. CBF is directly proportional to cerebral perfusion pressure (CPP) and inversely proportional to cerebrovascular resistance. CPP is the difference between the mean arterial pressure (MAP) and the right atrial pressure. When ICP is greater than right atrial pressure, the CPP is determined by the difference between the MAP and ICP.

$$CPP = MAP - ICP$$

and

$$CBF = (MAP - ICP) \, CVR$$

where CPP = cerebral perfusion pressure, MAP = mean arterial pressure, ICP = intracranial pressure, CBF = cerebral blood flow, and CVR = cerebrovascular resistance.

Consequently, any increase in ICP or reduction in MAP reduces CPP and resultant CBF. Normal CBF is 45 to 60 ml per 100 g per min. The CBF below which cerebral ischemia occurs has been termed the *critical CBF*, which is at flow rate of 16 or 17 ml per 100 g per min. Normal CPP is 80 to 100 torr. CBF begins to fail at a CPP of 30 to 40 torr. Irreversible hypoxia occurs at a CPP below 30 torr. When ICP equals MAP, CPP equals zero and CBF ceases.

Factors that influence CBF regulation are PaO_2 and $PaCO_2$ (metabolic regulation), arterial blood pressure and autoregulation, and venous blood pressure. Metabolic regulation works in two ways. The first is by regulation of blood flow based on the tissue needs for metabolic substrates—oxygen and glucose. As the activity of neuronal and glial cells in the brain increases, the demand for oxygen and glucose increases. The increased demand causes vaso-

dilatation of arterioles, which increases CBF. Likewise, if the metabolic demand decreases, vasoconstriction occurs and CBF decreases.

The second, and most significant, way metabolic regulation affects CBF is by the presence of metabolic by-products, specifically carbon dioxide. Carbon dioxide is the most potent vasodilator of cerebral blood vessels. Normal cerebral vessels respond to changes in carbon dioxide by dilating when carbon dioxide increases and constricting when carbon dioxide decreases. The relationship between CBF and carbon dioxide is linear, and changes in CBF are in direct proportion to changes in carbon dioxide. There is a decrease of 1 ml per 100 g per min in CBF for every 1 torr decrease in carbon dioxide. When treating elevated ICP, carbon dioxide levels of 25 to 30 torr are used to lower CBF.

Autoregulation is the ability of the cerebral vasculature in normal brain tissue to alter its resistance so that CBF remains relatively constant over a wide range of CPP. This mechanism causes vasoconstriction when perfusion pressure increases and vasodilatation when perfusion pressure decreases. The limits of autoregulation are at a CPP of approximately 60 torr at the lower end and 160 torr at the upper end. Beyond the limits of autoregulation, CBF becomes passively dependent on CPP. When CPP increases above the upper limit of autoregulation, it exceeds the ability of the vasculature to constrict; CBF becomes directly related to and possibly dependent on CPP.

The lower limit of CBF autoregulation is the blood pressure below which vasodilatation becomes inadequate and CBF decreases. When CPP decreases below 60 torr owing to increases in ICP, it is at this point that autoregulation ceases to be beneficial or effective in regulating

CBF. Defective autoregulation aggravates pressure increases and creates critical or irreversible levels of ICP by increasing the blood volume within the cranium in an effort to maintain CBF. Defective autoregulation generally occurs when ICP exceeds 30 to 35 torr. Eventually, autoregulation ceases altogether, and blood flow fluctuates passively with changes in arterial pressure, regardless of metabolic activity or regulation.

When ICP is increased, CPP and CBF are reduced, rendering the tissues ischemic. Ischemic cerebral tissue releases acid metabolites that cause a relatively fixed reduction in cerebrovascular tone. Autoregulation ceases, and any increase in MAP causes further increase in cerebral blood volume, eliciting a further increase in ICP. CPP is reduced, causing ischemic areas (such as those surrounding an expanding intracranial mass) to enlarge. As can be seen in Figure 29–6, a pathologic cycle ensues in which the outcome is that ICP and MAP eventually equilibrate, the CPP drops to zero, CBF stops, and death occurs.

Anesthetic Agents and Intracranial Pressure

Anesthetic agents alter ICP by their ability to increase or decrease CBF and cerebral metabolic rate. In addition to their effects on ICP, some of these agents may also reduce systemic blood pressure and cause cerebral ischemia due to inadequate CPP.

Inhalation Anesthetics. The inhalation anesthetic agents generally decrease blood pressure and may increase ICP in the cranial surgical patient. They produce a clinically significant degree of cerebrovascular vasodilatation and metabolic depression and can modify autoregulation. In fact, high dosages of volatile anesthetic agents can cause a total loss of autoregulation. The resulting increase in CBF will ultimately lead to increased ICP. In patients with decreased intracranial compliance secondary to neurologic disease, anesthetic agents that increase CBF may produce marked changes in ICP.

Halothane (Fluothane) produces dose-related elevations in CBF. Low concentrations produce minimal changes in CBF and ICP, whereas higher concentrations can increase CBF nearly threefold. Introduction of halothane simultaneously with the initiation of mechanical hyperventilation sufficient to lower $Paco_2$ to 25 torr does not reliably prevent drug-induced elevations in CBF and ICP. Conversely, establishment of hypocarbia before adding halothane prevents increases in ICP; however, this also may not be totally reliable. Presumably, prior hypocarbia attenuates or blocks the cerebral-vasodilating effects of halothane that lead to increased CBF.

Enflurane (Ethrane), like halothane, can cause abrupt increases in ICP. As with halothane, hypocarbia produced simultaneously with the administration of enflurane does not always protect against an increase in ICP. In addition to increased CBF, the increased ICP may reflect the ability of enflurane to increase

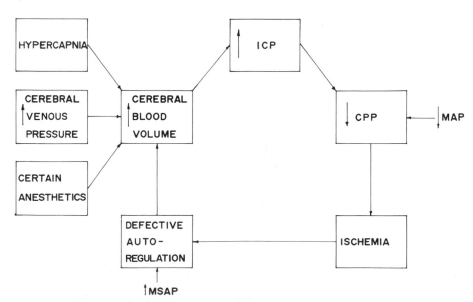

FIGURE 29–6. Intracranial pressure dynamics with failed compensatory mechanisms.

both the rate of production and resistance to reabsorption of CSF. Enflurane also has the ability to produce central nervous system seizure activity that can occur in pathologic or nonpathologic conditions. The likelihood of enflurane-evoked seizure activity is increased when high concentrations are used or when hyperventilation of the lungs lowers $PaCO_2$ below 30 torr. These characteristics make enflurane unsuitable for patients undergoing neurosurgical procedures.

Isoflurane (Forane), at normocarbia, has been shown to increase ICP. Unlike halothane, the initiation of hyperventilation simultaneously with the introduction of isoflurane prevents the increase in ICP that occurs at normocarbia. Unlike enflurane, isoflurane does not alter production of CSF and actually decreases resistance to absorption. Isoflurane does not cause excitation of the central nervous system as enflurane does. Isoflurane produces reductions in cerebral metabolic rate that exceed those produced by an equivalent-dose concentration of halothane, and there is less impairment of autoregulation as compared with halothane. The greater decrease in cerebral metabolic rate may explain why CBF increases are minimal at low concentrations.

Nitrous oxide, in contrast to the volatile agents (halothane, enflurane, and isoflurane), has less effect on CBF and is unlikely to increase ICP in patients maintained at normocarbia. Any increases in CBF or ICP that may occur can be attenuated by hyperventilation under most conditions. To a small extent, nitrous oxide is a cerebral vasodilator and does not interfere with autoregulation of the CBF.

Intravenous Anesthetics. Intravenous anesthetic agents (with the exception of ketamine) are usually the anesthetics of choice in cranial surgery.

Barbiturates such as thiopental (Pentothal) are potent cerebral vasoconstrictors capable of reducing CBF with subsequent reduction in elevated ICP. Cerebral vasoconstriction produced by barbiturates and the impact on CBF and ICP are dose related. The reduction in CBF produced by barbiturates is even greater if hypocarbia is also present and maintained at a constant level. Deep thiopental anesthesia during normocarbia results in about a 50 percent reduction in both cerebral metabolic rate and CBF.

Benzodiazepines, such as diazepam (Valium) and midazolam (Versed), produce sedation and amnesia by stimulating specific receptors in the brain. The benzodiazepines produce dose-related reductions in cerebral metabolic rate and CBF. When central benzodiazepine receptors are pharmacologically saturated, these drugs may decrease cerebral metabolic rate as much as 40 percent.

Narcotics, such as fentanyl, morphine, and meperidine, are typically classified as cerebral vasoconstrictors, with resultant reductions in CBF. This effect is readily abolished by vasodilatation that can accompany narcotic-induced ventilatory depression and the resultant increase in $PaCO_2$. In humans maintained at normocarbia, fentanyl does not alter CBF. During normocarbia, the combination of nitrous oxide and morphine does not significantly alter CBF or autoregulation. Fentanyl, and the combination of fentanyl and droperidol (Innovar), causes a reduction in CBF and ICP in patients with normal CSF pathways. Alfentanil and sufentanil may in fact cause an increase in ICP in patients with compromised cerebral compliance.

Etomidate (Amidate) produces a maximal 45 percent decrease in cerebral metabolic rate and CBF; like the barbiturates, it is capable of producing complete EEG suppression and appears to be comparable in lowering ICP. Unlike the barbiturates, etomidate has less effect on MAP and offers greater stability in hemodynamically compromised patients.

Propofol (Diprivan), in a dose-dependent manner, reduces cerebral metabolic rate, CBF, and ICP and increases cerebrovascular resistance. The use of propofol in patients with elevated ICP may not be appropriate owing to the substantial decrease in MAP and resultant decrease in CPP.

Ketamine (Ketalar; Ketaject) can rapidly increase ICP and frequently reduce CPP, despite mild increases in blood pressure. Ketamine is generally contraindicated for use in neurosurgical patients unless the fontanelles are open, CSF aspiration is instituted, or ventilatory control is maintained.

The use of controlled ventilation to produce $PaCO_2$ levels in the range of 25 to 30 torr and the administration of nitrous oxide and oxygen and possibly low concentrations of isoflurane, together with narcotics and muscle relaxants, is a generally accepted anesthetic technique for the neurosurgical patient.

Adjunctive Drugs Used to Reduce Intracranial Pressure

Diuretics. Mannitol and furosemide (Lasix) are diuretics frequently used to control increased ICP. Mannitol, an osmotic diuretic, is the agent of choice for ICP reduction. It has replaced urea because it is less irritating to veins and its larger molecular size tends to better impede its penetration across the blood-brain barrier. Mannitol is administered intravenously in doses of 0.25 to 1 g per kg in a 20 percent solution over 30 to 60 minutes, with the maximum effects occurring in 1 or 2 hours. Urine output can reach 1 or 2 L within 1 hour. Appropriate infusion of crystalloid and colloid solutions is often necessary to prevent adverse changes in plasma concentrations of electrolytes and intravascular fluid volume owing to the rapidity of diuresis.

Potential complications of the use of mannitol include hyperosmolarity, electrolyte loss, changes in blood viscosity and coagulation, transient intravascular hypervolemia, and rebound or secondary elevation of ICP.

Furosemide is a loop diuretic that, when administered intravenously at a dose of 1 mg per kg to patients with normal ICP undergoing craniotomy, is more effective in reducing ICP than is mannitol. Furosemide may be the intracranial decompressive agent of choice in patients with congestive heart failure.

Furosemide, when combined with mannitol, has been shown to potentiate the ICP-reducing effects of mannitol at the cost of rapid loss of intravascular volume and electrolytes. The ICP effects of these drugs are lost after 1 or 2 hours.

Corticosteroids. The drugs most frequently used are dexamethasone and methylprednisolone. Steroids are effective in lowering increased ICP due to localized vasogenic cerebral edema associated with mass-type lesions, such as neoplasm, abscess, and intracerebral hematoma. The mechanism for the beneficial effect of corticosteroids is not known but may in-

volve stabilization of capillary membranes, reduction in the production of CSF, blood-brain barrier repair, prevention of lysosomal activity, enhanced cerebral electrolyte transport, improved brain metabolism, and promotion of water and electrolyte excretion.

Intracranial Pressure Monitoring

The most precise indicator of the pressure state within the cranium is the CSF pressure. Measurement of this pressure may be obtained from the lateral ventricle, lumbar subarachnoid space, cisterna magna, or epidural or subdural spaces. Values from these areas are meaningful as indicators of ICP only if pressure is freely transmitted between these compartments. Because injury and disease of the brain often create obstruction in CSF flow, the most accurate values are those obtained from the ventricle.

Lumbar puncture values reflect only a relative index of the actual ICP. These values depend on the state of the spinal canal and all the factors that affect it. On the other hand, measurement of the ventricular fluid pressure gives a direct and absolute value of the ICP, regardless of the influence or condition of the spinal canal. Lumbar puncture has other limitations. Its use is limited to those patients without suspected intracranial mass or to those whose ICP is not elevated or is elevated only slightly. In patients with these conditions, there is risk of herniation of the brain tissue with the removal of CSF. ICP monitoring does not present this risk and can be used in a variety of conditions.

ICP monitoring requires a sensor, a transducer, and a display and recording instrument (Fig. 29–7). The sensor is usually implanted in

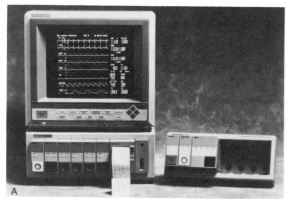
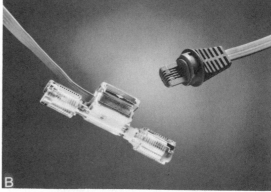

FIGURE 29–7. *A,* bedside pressure display and recording monitor, showing cardiac rhythm, blood pressure, central venous pressure, and pulmonary artery waveforms. It is also used to display intracranial pressure waveforms. (*A* courtesy of Hewlett Packard Company, Andover, MA.). *B,* external pressure transducer capable of converting mechanical impulses transmitted from the cerebrospinal fluid into electrical impulses, which are then displayed on the bedside monitor. (COBE CDX III Disposable Transducer. *B* courtesy of COBE Cardiovascular, Inc., Arvada, CO.)

the nondominant hemisphere in the ventricle or the subarachnoid or epidural space. The transducer itself may be implanted intracranially, or it may be placed outside the cranium. Intracranial transducers decrease the risk of infection but are often heat sensitive and may produce false ICP readings, because they cannot be recalibrated once implanted. The greater the distance from the sensor to the transducer, the greater the incidence of artifact and imprecise waveforms. Other complications possible with any of these devices include CSF leakage, producing inaccurately low ICP readings, and contamination resulting in ventriculitis or meningitis.

The methods of continuous monitoring of the ICP include the subarachnoid screw, the subdural bolt, the intraventricular catheter (IVC), and the intracranially implanted ICP transducers. The *subarachnoid screw* was developed in 1973 and requires only a twist-drill hole in the skull and a nick in the dura for insertion. As the name implies, the sensor lies in the subarachnoid space. However, in the presence of moderately severe cerebral edema, a small piece of brain tissue may be driven into and occlude the proximal end of the screw, rendering it useless. The hollow *subdural bolt* is threaded into the subdural space and then connected to an external transducer. If the seal is not watertight, the bolt may become plugged with brain tissue, which can obliterate or dampen the recording of the ICP. The *IVC* is introduced into a CSF-containing ventricle via a twist-drill burr hole and is connected to an external transducer that converts the hydrostatic pressure force into a graph and numeric readout. The advantages of the IVC are that it provides a direct ICP reading and is more easily kept patent, and CSF can be drained through the catheter to treat ICP elevations. In this way it may serve as a temporary artificial extension of the CSF-shunting compensatory mechanism. Intracranial compliance can also be tested by injecting fluid into the cranium and reading the responding pressure increase. If an abrupt and steep rise in ICP occurs, it can be assumed that compliance no longer exists and that the volume-pressure curve is a steep one. When the patient's arterial pressure is being monitored simultaneously, exact CPP can be calculated at any time. The ventricular catheter also has the advantage of allowing instillation of contrast media or air to study the size and patency of the ventricle. The principal disadvantage of the IVC is that the technique is associated with a 5 to 10 percent incidence of central nervous system infection. The intracranially implanted *ICP transducers* are placed into the epidural space. These systems for monitoring ICP have had significant technical problems associated with calibration and stability of measurements over prolonged periods of use.

ICP monitoring is a valuable tool in assessing the efficacy of nursing interventions that are intended to decrease ICP and is essential in determining accurate assessments of the pressure state within the cranium and in treating elevations in ICP before disastrous consequences occur.

Pressure Waves in Increased Intracranial Pressure

Pressures waves are abnormal, spontaneous variations in ICP. Three patterns have been identified. The first and most significant type is the *A wave*, more commonly called a *plateau wave* (Fig. 29–8A). These waves are associated with increases in ICP between 50 and 100 torr lasting for 5 to 20 minutes. They are seen only in advanced stages of increased ICP (the last phase of the volume-pressure curve) and superimpose themselves when the baseline ICP is elevated and exceeds 20 torr. Early increases in mean systemic arterial pressure do not accompany plateau waves, and autoregulation is impaired. Thus, plateau waves signal hypoxia of brain cells and a decrease in CPP. They may cause both transient and irreversible damage to the brain and may be premonitory signs of acute incidents. The cause of plateau waves is not fully understood, but they probably result from a combination of transient blood volume alterations and CSF obstruction. Hypoventilation (by accumulating carbon dioxide and increasing intracranial blood volume) may be the cause, and the high ICP causes ischemia of the respiratory centers, resulting in irregular breathing.

The second type of pressure wave pattern is called the *B wave*. These waves are sharp, rhythmic oscillations with a sawtooth pattern occurring every 30 seconds to 2 minutes (Fig. 29–8B). These may increase ICP as much as 50 torr and are more commonly seen in patients with unstable increases.

The third type of pattern is the *C wave* (Fig. 29–8C). These waves are smaller rhythmic oscillations in ICP, which occur every 4 to 8 minutes, and they increase ICP as much as 20 torr. They are associated with respiratory influence on the blood pressure, but their significance is questionable.

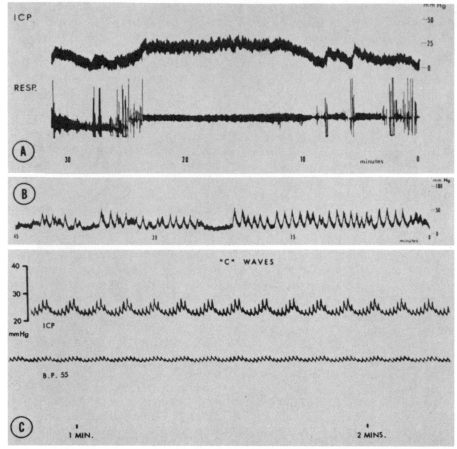

FIGURE 29–8. *A*, plateau (A) wave shown with associated respiratory changes. *B*, B waves: sharp, rhythmic oscillations with a characteristic sawtooth pattern. *C*, C waves: smaller, rhythmic oscillations of intracranial pressure shown for comparison with the Traube-Hering waves of blood pressure. (*A* through *C* from Hanlon, K.: Description and uses of intracranial pressure monitoring. Heart Lung, 5:277, 1976.)

Assessment

Continuous ICP monitoring is the only accurate method of assessing ICP at any given time. This method has two advantages: (1) it provides an ongoing record of the ICP, and (2) it provides a means of assessing intracranial dynamics. The clinical signs of increased ICP are numerous. The early signs are often vague and overlooked, and research has demonstrated the unreliability of these signs in determining or recognizing increased ICP.

Early signs of increased ICP are increasing restlessness, confusion, and severe headache. Nausea, vomiting, paralysis, visual field deficits, conjugate deviation of the eyes, sensory loss, and nuchal rigidity are also early signs. Their presence may or may not confirm a diagnosis of increased ICP.

The late signs of increased ICP are decreasing responsiveness and LOC; pupillary changes; increased systolic blood pressure; bradycardia; widening pulse pressure; alteration in respiratory pattern; decorticate or decerebrate posturing; and absence of or decrease in cough, gag, corneal, and deep tendon reflexes. A positive Babinski reflex is normal in infants younger than 18 months of age but indicates increased ICP in those older than 18 months.

Most of these signs are manifestations of brain shift, with resultant dysfunction of the reticular-activating system, brain stem, and medulla. Pressure would either have to elevate quite rapidly or be sustained at high levels to affect these structures so dramatically. Also to be considered is the fact that primary injury to these structures may elicit the same signs without appreciable increases in ICP. In this situation, they may well indicate the level of brain function and the gravity of the situation but not reflect the pressure dynamics existing at that moment.

Just as these signs may be present without increase in ICP, it is also true that ICP may be dangerously high with few, if any, signs present. Classic brain stem signs (reflecting changes in cardiac, respiratory, or vasomotor function) usually occur late, after the onset of intracranial hypertension, if at all. The most important factor in determining the degree of secondary brain damage incurred by elevated ICP is the effect of altered CPP on the brain. Clinical research has shown that the level of CPP is the best indicator of outcome from severe head injuries. CPP lower than 40 torr has been associated with poor outcomes. CPP needs to be maintained no lower than 50 to 60 torr to provide a minimally adequate blood supply to the brain.

Most hospitals with the capacity for cranial surgery also have the capacity for continuous ICP monitoring. It is not unusual, however, for a patient with multiple trauma to be treated at a smaller community hospital that lacks this capability. This patient may have received a concomitant closed head injury that does not require neurosurgery but nevertheless may require frequent nursing assessments of neurologic status.

With this in mind, the traditional signs and symptoms of increased ICP are discussed here. These are not precise or infallible as indicators of increased ICP. At the very least, they indicate that something is not right and that constant vigilance and further investigation are necessary. Even the transient appearances of these pressure signs are important. They indicate development of a highly delicate and unstable intracranial situation, a sign that the patient may be experiencing plateau waves.

On the patient's arrival in the PACU, airway patency is verified and electrocardiogram monitor electrodes are attached. Vital signs, including temperature, are taken and recorded. If the patient's ICP is being monitored, correct calibration of the monitor must be ensured, ICP value recorded, and waveform described. The same approach is used for arterial pressure recording. Reports should be taken from both the anesthesiologist and the surgeon. Of particular importance are preexistent medical problems, allergies, anesthetics used, and any problems that occurred during surgery. The specific procedure performed, special positioning orders or restrictions, the presence of drains, and known CSF leaks must be noted. The dressing is described, including any visible drainage. LOC and responsiveness, motor activity, pupillary equality, size, and reactivity and the quality and pattern of respirations are also docu-mented. Continued patency of the airway is ensured, and the type of airway or mechanical ventilation used is noted. Urinary catheter drainage must be measured and described. Finally, the written physician orders must be reviewed with the physician and any questions or uncertainties clarified. Figure 29–9 is a sample form for documenting vital signs, LOC, and ICP, in addition to the admitting history. The reverse side should contain a description of the Glasgow coma scale (GCS) (Table 29–1). The GCS is a widely used neurologic assessment tool, because of its simplicity, consistency, and reliability between raters using the scale. However, the GCS cannot assess subtle changes in the patient's neurologic status. When the GCS is used, the patient's responses are scored on a scale of 3 to 15. A score of 3 indicates coma, and a score of 15 indicates a fully alert, oriented person with all neurologic functions intact.

Four major areas of assessment are required in PACU care of the cranial surgical patient: vital signs, LOC, motor and sensory functioning, and pupillary signs. These should be routinely assessed at least every 15 minutes for the first 2 hours postoperatively. Then, if they are within normal limits or unchanged since surgery, they should be assessed every 30 minutes. If the patient's condition is unstable or deteriorating, or if the surgeon specifies, assessments should be made more frequently.

Vital Signs. Assessment of vital signs includes blood pressure, pulse, respirations, and ICP (if monitored). Changes in vital signs may be indicative of increasing ICP, shock, hemorrhage, electrolyte imbalance, or other disturbances. The post anesthesia nurse should keep

Table 29–1. GLASGOW COMA SCALE

Category	Response	Score
Eye opening	Spontaneous	4
	To speech	3
	To pain	2
	None	1
Best verbal response	Oriented to person, place, and time	5
	Confused	4
	Inappropriate words	3
	Incomprehensible sounds	2
	No response	1
Best motor response	Obeys commands	6
	Localizes to pain	5
	Withdrawal from pain	4
	Abnormal flexion	3
	Abnormal extension	2
	Flaccid	1

NEUROSURGERY POST ANESTHESIA RECORD

Name		Age	Received in PACU at:

Procedure Performed	Surgeon(s)

Pt Appearance and Response on Admission	Airway Devices NO YES

V.S. on Admission T BP P R LOC*	Anesthetic(s) Used

EBL	Urine output	Fluids Received in O.R.	Blood Prod.

Pertinent History and Comments

Time ... ICP

LOC*

BP ∨∧ 300 ... 62
290 ... 60
P O 280 ... 58 / 56
270 ... 54
T · 260 ... 52
ICP X 250 ... 50
240 ... 48
230 ... 46
220 ... 44
210 ... 42
200 ... 40
106 190 ... 38
105 180 ... 36
104 170 ... 34
103 160 ... 32
102 150 ... 30
101 140 ... 28
100 130 ... 26
99 120 ... 24
98 110 ... 22
97 100 ... 20
96 90 ... 18
95 80 ... 16
94 70 ... 14
93 60 ... 12
92 50 ... 10
91 40 ... 8
90 30 ... 6
89 20 ... 4
88 10 ... 2

RESP

Patient Identification	Register number	Unit

*Level of consciousness legend on reverse

FIGURE 29–9. Sample neurosurgery post anesthesia record.

in mind that the injured patient may have other pathophysiologic processes occurring unrelated to his or her head injury. Comparisons should be made with the preoperative and intraoperative values. The character of the pulse as well as the rate and rhythm should be noted. Blood pressure and ICP readings may be used to calculate the CPP. Temperature is always taken, and an elevation usually represents an infectious process, most often in the respiratory or urinary tract. Infrequently, elevations are at-

tributable to direct damage to the temperature-regulating center in the hypothalamus. Temperature elevation also increases the metabolic rate of the brain, which may further increase ICP.

Airway patency is ensured, and the rate, depth, and rhythm are noted. Do not be deceived by apparent excursions of the thorax. Movement of the chest may occur without the exchange of air. The patient may exhibit substernal retractions; in this event, there is a probability that the airway is obstructed. Place your hand in front of the patient's mouth and nose or airway to ascertain movement of air. If the rhythm is irregular, try to determine its pattern. Changes in the respiratory pattern may indicate injury to the respiratory center of the brain and the severity of the neurologic injury (Table 29–2). If no irregularity is evident, that should be noted. If the patient is on a ventilator, check the machine for proper functioning and settings. It should be noted, however, that mechanical ventilation may mask changes in the respiratory pattern.

For many years the nursing literature has documented a relation between changes in blood pressure and pulse and increases in ICP. These changes are often referred to as *Cushing's reflex* and *Cushing's triad*. Cushing's reflex is described as an elevated systolic blood pressure, bradycardia, and widening pulse pressure. Further increases in ICP may lead to Cushing's triad, which is described as bradycardia, hypertension, and bradypnea. Cushing's reflex and triad are late clinical signs of increased ICP and may indicate brain stem herniation. Patients with head injury often have a higher than normal blood pressure and heart rate. This maybe the result of pain, hypoxia, and agitation or the release of endogenous catecholamines.

Level of Consciousness. The most important indicator of brain function is the LOC, but it is not necessarily indicative of altered ICP. A decreased LOC in the PACU may be caused by the lingering effects of the anesthesia or by neuromuscular-blocking agents sometimes used with patients on mandatory controlled ventilation. A change in LOC may also be the result of hypoxia, hypoglycemia, vitamin deficiency, and fluid and electrolyte imbalances. Other underlying pathologic changes may cause alterations in LOC; when one is assessing the patient in the PACU, the medical history will be an important factor in determining the cause of a change in LOC. When assessing LOC, it is best to describe the patient's response instead of using vague terms such as *stuporous, semiconscious,* or *unconscious.* A standard assessment form such as the GCS (see Table 29–1) should be available for assessing the LOC. A change in LOC may also be indicative of deterioration or improvement in the patient's condition.

Motor and Sensory Functioning. Assessment of motor and sensory function is part of an ongoing neurologic assessment and is performed to note changes from the baseline assessment. It can also provide clues to extending hemorrhage or expanding edema. Focal changes, such as decreased hand strength unilaterally or an inability to move one side of the body, often accompany these events. Sensations may be decreased owing to brain involvement, not just to spinal cord injury (SCI). Observe whether the patient can move all four extremities. Check both hand grasps simultaneously. Are they weak or strong, equal or unequal? Foot strength can be tested by having the patient push or pull against your hands. (Be sure the patient uses only the foot and an-

Table 29–2. RESPIRATORY PATTERNS		
Pattern	**Description**	**Location of Injury and Other Causes**
Cheyne-Stokes respirations	Regular increase in the rate and depth of breathing that peaks and is followed by a decreasing rate and depth of breathing, which progresses to apnea and then the cycle repeats itself	Bilateral dysfunction of cerebral hemispheres Midbrain and upper pons
Central neurogenic hyperventilation	Deep, rapid, and regular pattern of breathing	Low midbrain and upper pons Increased ICP with head trauma
Apneusis breathing	A pause at full inspiration occurs; may see prolonged inspiratory pause alternating with a prolonged expiratory pause	Mid and low pons Hypoglycemia, anoxia, and meningitis
Cluster breathing	Periodic breathing with frequent apneic episodes	Low pons and high medulla
Ataxic breathing	Irregular breathing with shallow, deep respirations and irregular apneic episodes; usually slow in rate	Medulla

kle, not the entire leg.) If the patient does not respond to simple commands, test to see if a painful stimulus such as a pin prick or pinch will induce movement. (Test both sides to determine sensory impairment.) If the patient does not respond to pain, test for motor function by raising both arms or both legs and let them fall together. A paralyzed limb will fall to the bed more quickly than an unaffected one. To further check leg motor ability, flex both of the patient's knees with the feet flat on the bed; release them at the same time. The normal leg will maintain its position momentarily and then resume the original position. The affected limb will abduct while falling and will maintain knee flexion.

Facial muscle movement should also be tested. If possible, ask patients to wrinkle their foreheads, shut their eyes tightly, smile, and show you their teeth. Any asymmetry should be noted. If the patient is not responsive to verbal commands, pressure on both supraorbital ridges may elicit a grimace or other facial movement. The presence of a Babinski reflex is pathologic and indicative of pyramidal tract dysfunction in any person older than 18 months of age. Starting at the heel and using a moderately sharp object, such as the rounded tip of a bandage scissors or the tip of a retracted pen, stroke the lateral sole and proceed to the ball of the foot. Firm pressure is necessary to elicit an accurate response. The Babinski reflex is present when the great toe dorsiflexes (bends toward the head) and the remaining toes "fan out." The Babinski reflex is not present when the stimulus elicits a plantar or downward flexion of the great toe.

Motor response to a painful stimulus may be one of decerebrate or decorticate rigidity, or these postures may exist in the absence of any stimulation. Decerebrate posturing is characterized by rigidity and contraction of all the extensor muscles. The legs are stiffly extended with the feet plantar flexed. The arms are extended and hyperpronated. Decerebrate rigidity is usually the result of upper brain stem damage; this means that the cerebral hemispheres are functionally cut off. Decorticate posturing indicates that function has been cut off at a lower level and that the entire cortex is cut off physiologically. In this instance, the legs are extended and internally rotated and the feet are plantar flexed. The arms are flexed at all joints, and the hands are frequently held beneath the chin.

Pupillary Activity. Pupillary reactions are controlled by the third cranial nerve. When assessing the pupils, the post anesthesia nurse should examine both simultaneously for shape, size, and equality. Normal pupils are round and, at a midpoint diameter, within the range of 1 to 9 mm. Instead of using terms like *constricted* or *dilated,* it is more precise to measure their diameters directly with a pocket millimeter ruler. Test the direct light reflex of each pupil with a small bright flashlight. Normally, the pupil will constrict briskly. If it reacts sluggishly or not at all, it is abnormal. To test the consensual light reflex, hold both eyelids open, shine the light in one eye, and observe the other pupil. The opposite pupil should constrict simultaneously with the lighted one, although perhaps not to the same degree.

Normal pupillary size and reactivity can be altered by some medical situations and by certain drugs. Previous surgery or direct injury to the eye may alter or abolish reactivity. Blindness abolishes reactivity to light because the sensory part of the reflex pathway is absent.

Unusual eye movements should be noted. Normal gaze in a person who is awake and alert is straight ahead, with no involuntary movements. This is generally true of unresponsive patients, although their eyes may rove slowly and in random fashion. (When detecting this movement, do not be misled into thinking that the patients are actually following you or your movements.) Their eyes should move together in the same direction (conjugate gaze). If the eyes are dysconjugate, they move in a jerky, oscillatory fashion (nystagmus) or the gaze deviates from the midline. These ocular movements are abnormal and should be detailed in the nursing notes.

Nursing Care

The PACU nurse has three primary responsibilities in the care of the neurosurgical patient: (1) to institute measures of care to sustain optimal physiologic function in the post anesthesia patient; (2) to recognize and prevent conditions that increase ICP beyond normal limits; and (3) to detect and communicate signs and symptoms of the patient's condition to the physician.

A patient's condition can change dramatically in as short a time as 15 minutes. Impairment in protective reflexes may occur, and he or she may be unable to perceive or communicate problems such as an obstructed airway or a distended bladder. Vigilant surveillance and high-quality care by the nurse may determine the eventual outcome for the patient.

When caring for the cranial surgical patient,

the PACU nurse should look for drainage from the suture line, the nose, or the ears. CSF may leak from any of these locations and, despite its benign appearance, may threaten the patient's life. The patient must be prevented from blowing or picking his or her nose. Suctioning through the nose is absolutely contraindicated, because CSF may leak through a fracture in the cribriform plate and drain from the nose. This is particularly applicable in patients whose surgery was performed transnasally. If drainage is present, it may be wiped from the nares, or a mustache-type dressing may be applied. If drainage is from the ear, cover it with sterile 4 × 4 gauze. Do not pack the ear or the nose. When the origin of rhinorrhea is unknown, the drainage may be tested with a dextrose stick. If positive for sugar, the drainage is probably CSF, because mucus does not contain sugar but CSF does. Examine the dressings and linen for the "halo sign," a central blood-tinged spot surrounded by a ring of a lighter color (reminiscent of serous fluid). Save any such material for the physician's examination. The patient should be kept at absolute bedrest and as quiet as possible, with the head of the bed raised 30 degrees. This position is most conducive to the spontaneous healing of the source of the leak.

Respiratory Status. Meticulous pulmonary care is essential in all patients. Morbidity and mortality in the neurosurgical patient are most frequently attributed to pulmonary complications and urinary tract infections. Airway patency is of primary importance. If there is no artificial airway, patients may obstruct their airways as their tongues fall into the posterior pharynx. This is less likely to occur if patients are prevented from assuming a supine position. If signs of airway obstruction occur, the jaw should be pulled forward and downward to relieve the obstruction and prevent cerebral hypoxia. Patients can be positioned on their sides with their heads elevated 30 to 45 degrees and their necks maintained in body alignment to prevent airway obstruction. Endotracheal tubes must be kept free of secretions. Mucus plugs occur as readily in a plastic tube as they do in the trachea, and the patients will be unable to cough or expel them.

Suctioning may be necessary, but it has been proved to increase ICP. Therefore, it should be done as needed rather than according to a fixed schedule. To minimize pressure increases, hypercapnia and Valsalva effects must also be minimized. This is best accomplished by preoxygenating with 100 percent oxygen for 1 minute before suctioning and limiting suctioning to 15 seconds, with one to two passes down the

endotracheal tube. Ventilation is then repeated with 100 percent oxygen for 1 minute before previous ventilator settings are resumed.

Cranial surgical patients are frequently maintained on mandatory ventilation into the first postoperative day, or longer, to prevent hypoventilation and to ensure low $PaCO_2$ levels (to aid in keeping ICP within acceptable limits). Positive end-expiratory pressure (PEEP) is often used to help maintain adequate tissue oxygenation. Research indicates that PEEP increases intrathoracic pressures and decreases venous return from the cranium, thereby increasing ICP. Recent studies have suggested using high-frequency jet ventilation. If the use of PEEP is necessary, ICP needs to be monitored closely and PEEP reduced if neurologic deterioration occurs. All settings on the ventilator must be checked for accuracy at least every hour. The cascade must also be checked for proper functioning and an adequate water level. In addition, serial arterial blood gas levels should be determined to detect and correct respiratory acidosis and to verify low $PaCO_2$ levels.

Adult respiratory distress syndrome and neurogenic pulmonary edema (NPE) can develop in the postoperative period. NPE is caused from a sudden and massive increase in ICP. The signs of NPE are dyspnea, restlessness, tachycardia, rapid and frothy respirations, rales, and gray or bluish (cyanotic) skin color. These signs are the same for pulmonary edema except that the patient does not have a history of cardiac disease. Pneumonia, atelectasis, and pulmonary emboli are also potential pulmonary complications of neurosurgery.

Fluid and Electrolyte Balance. Prevention of fluid and electrolyte abnormalities is important. Oral or nasogastric feedings are prohibited during the acute phase because of the danger of regurgitation and aspiration. Intravenous fluids are severely restricted but are maintained at a rate sufficient to ensure an adequate urinary output of 30 ml per hr. A delicate balance exists between overhydration and dehydration in these patients. Overhydration produces or accentuates cerebral edema and causes hyponatremia. It may also decrease the level of responsiveness. Dehydration may follow profuse diaphoresis or inadequate intravenous fluid therapy. If dehydration is allowed to persist, electrolyte disturbances and renal failure will result. Serial blood urea nitrogen, electrolyte, and pH determinations of the blood, hourly urine output, and specific gravity of the urine are the most valuable indices in determining fluid and electrolyte imbalances.

Diabetes insipidus exists in some patients following trauma, surgery, or anoxia of the brain, most particularly to the posterior lobe of the pituitary gland. Antidiuretic hormone (vasopressin) production is markedly reduced and urinary output increases, reaching as much as 2 L per hr, and low urine specific gravity. In diabetes insipidus, restricting fluid intake not only does nothing to alleviate urinary losses but it actually worsens dehydration. Diabetes insipidus is usually transient and subsides when cerebral edema subsides. However, if anoxia is severe and generalized, diabetes insipidus may occur irreversibly. Treatment consists of preventing dehydration and electrolyte disturbances. Vasopressin (Pitressin) may be administered intramuscularly to correct and stabilize water metabolism.

The cranial surgical patient has an indwelling urinary catheter during the acute phase of care. Its main advantage is that it allows accurate determination of hourly urine output. Three-way tidal drainage systems rarely are used in the PACU. In fact, catheters are removed as soon as possible to prevent urinary tract infection. The integrity of the closed-drainage system must not be broken, and urinary catheter care helps prevent urinary tract infections.

Temperature. Significant temperature elevations are rarely seen in the cranial surgical patient in the PACU, because they are most frequently caused by respiratory or urinary tract infections, which usually appear after the second or third postoperative day. When temperature elevations do occur in the acute phase, they may indicate damage to the hypothalamus and may exceed measurable values. If aggressive attempts at lowering the temperature fail, the increased metabolic demands of the body may cause increased ICP, and the patient's condition may deteriorate, causing death. Because this hyperthermia is the result of injury to the hypothalamus or pons rather than an infectious process, conventional measures such as antibiotic and acetaminophen therapy may fail to reduce the temperature. The most effective means of lowering this patient's temperature is by the use of hypothermia blankets and the removal of the primary disorder, if possible.

When hypothermia blankets are used, they should be set no cooler than 1°F below the patient's current body temperature; this prevents shivering or thermal crisis. A constant rectal temperature probe is essential. Many sets are available in which the temperature probe relays its information to, and automatically adjusts, the blanket temperature regulator. Do not allow the patient to shiver. Cold burns may be prevented by placing a bath blanket between the patient and the hypothermia blanket.

Position. Positioning of the patient depends on the type of surgery, monitoring equipment, central lines, endotracheal tubes, and specific orders from the physician.

For supratentorial craniotomy, the head of the bed is elevated 30 to 45 degrees. This position decreases the chance of hemorrhage and promotes venous drainage from the brain. The patient can be turned from side to side, but the neck alignment must be maintained to prevent increased ICP. If a large tumor has been removed, the patient should not be placed on the operative side. If the patient has received a shunt, care must be taken to prevent obstruction of the shunt with repositioning.

For infratentorial craniotomy, the position of the head is usually flat with a small pillow under the back of the neck. The patient must not be allowed to flex the neck, because of the potential of tearing the suture line. The patient may be turned from side to side and neck alignment must be maintained. In the PACU, patients should be placed on their side to help provide for an adequate airway and drainage of oral secretions.

For transphenoidal surgery, the position after surgery is usually in a high-Fowler's position. This position promotes venous return from the brain to prevent increased ICP and hemorrhage at the operative site. Frequent mouth care is important, but do not permit the patient to use a toothbrush because of potential damage to the suture line. After packings are removed from the nose, patients should be instructed not to blow their noses or sneeze for at least 1 month.

Patients must never be placed flat on their backs. Other positioning restrictions may be prescribed by the surgeon, depending on the nature and location of the surgery. The nurse should clearly understand these restrictions before the surgeon leaves the PACU. Frequently, positioning is somewhat limited by the monitoring devices in use. Whether or not the patient is being ventilated or has other injuries also enters into positioning considerations.

Generally, the surgeon specifies that the head of the bed be elevated 30 degrees, which helps keep ICP within normal limits. If hemorrhagic shock occurs, the foot of the bed may be elevated and the arms raised above the patient's head to return blood to the heart without increasing ICP. Positioning should always allow proper drainage of secretions from the mouth and airway. Patients who have had a suboccipital craniectomy are sometimes dressed with a cervical collar and adhesive stripping to restrict movement of the head and neck. When these patients are being turned, it is important to support the head and turn it in unison with the body to prevent strain on the wound or suture line. To gain proper access to the head, remove the headboard from the bed and stand behind the patient.

Patients who are unresponsive or paralyzed are unable to move their limbs from uncomfortable or dangerous positions. Muscle tone is insufficient to prevent dislocation of the shoulder should the arm fall from the side of the bed. If patients can move spontaneously and respond to uncomfortable stimuli, it may be advantageous to place them in a safe but slightly uncomfortable position. This encourages active movement and exercise of the limbs and joints. This is contraindicated if the patient is agitated or if the physician objects.

Skin Care. Although the patient may be in the PACU less than 24 hours, it is necessary to initiate joint and skin care measures as soon as possible. It takes only 48 to 72 hours for a joint to begin to ankylose, and it is not unusual for decubiti to begin forming while the patient is on the operating table. The skin over bony prominences may already be broken by the time the patient comes into the PACU. This is particularly true of elderly, very young, and dehydrated patients. Cover any broken areas with a sterile dressing, and try to prevent further irritation. Prevention is the best treatment. This requires turning the patient at least once every 2 hours and protecting susceptible areas by frequent massage and the use of air mattresses and sheepskin pads. Footdrop and external hip rotation may be prevented by using a footboard and trochanter rolls, respectively. Hand deformities may be avoided through the use of hand rolls or contoured splints placed so that the hands appear to be grasping them.

If the corneal or blink reflex is absent, the eyes must be irrigated with sterile saline and lubricated with mineral oil. In no event should the eyes be taped shut, because a lid may open under the tape and allow an abrasion of the cornea. The patient may have significant periocular edema and ecchymosis following cranial surgery or trauma. Cold compresses may be used if care is taken to avoid contact with the cornea.

The lips and mucosa of the mouth must be kept moist and free of encrustations. Hyperplastic, sensitive gum tissue may be found in any person who has been receiving phenytoin (Dilantin) longer than 6 months. Normal saline or lemon-glycerine swabs may be used to keep the mouth moist. Petrolatum should be applied to the lips. Patients should never be given water by mouth until it has been established that their cough and swallow reflexes are intact and until the surgeon permits oral fluids.

Seizures. Electrical disturbances in the brain or seizures can be a complication of neurosurgery. These disturbances may be the result of the operative lesion, trauma, anoxia, or hematoma. The seizure itself may be a focal, grand mal, Jacksonian, petit mal, psychomotor, or autonomic type.

The patient must be observed constantly during a seizure. The nurse's responsibility is twofold: (1) patients must be prevented from injuring themselves and (2) the seizure activity must be described in detail from beginning to end. At no time should the patient be left alone. Side rails should be padded to protect the limbs. No attempt should be made physically to restrict motion because that would only injure the patient further. Instead, try to protect the head and limbs from sharp or unyielding objects. Also try to protect arterial, intravenous, and intracranial lines from being pulled out. Do not attempt to insert any sort of airway or tongue blades into the mouth after the seizure has begun. If the patient is being ventilated, remove him or her from the ventilator, and try to protect the endotracheal tube. Begin manual inflation of the lungs as soon as the seizure subsides sufficiently. Use 100 percent oxygen to overcome hypoxia and hypercapnia induced by the seizure.

In describing the seizure, state if the patient reported an aura beforehand. If responsive and capable, he or she may have said only, "My hand is tingling," "I smell bacon," or something similar. The statement may have seemed totally insignificant at the time but may aid the physician in localizing the causative lesion. Also describe the actual seizure. Did it begin in one area of the body and "march" to another? Was it simply a persistent twitch in a facial muscle? Was the patient incontinent of stool or urine? How long did tonoclonic movements persist? Describe the postictal state, and monitor the patient closely after a seizure. A grand mal seizure may be the precipitating factor of a sudden deterioration in the patient with cerebral anoxia or increased ICP.

Frequently, patients are placed on prophylactic anticonvulsants postoperatively. These may be combined with a barbiturate, such as phenobarbital. Surgeons sometimes order intravenous diazepam for patients if a seizure occurs. This approach controls muscle activity, but the causative electrical disturbance in the brain will persist, nonetheless.

If hyperactivity or agitation occurs in neurosurgical patients, investigate all possible causes. They may have an obstructed airway, distended bladder, or overlooked bleeding or fracture. They may be too cold or too warm, disoriented or fearful, or experiencing slowly developing hypoxia.

If the cause of the patient's agitation cannot be identified, meningeal irritation must be considered. Personality and behavior can be markedly affected by organic lesions of the brain. Temporal lobe problems commonly cause resentment of interference, hostility, or aggressiveness. Repetition of words or phrases (perseveration) indicates damage to the speech area, as do aphasia and dysarthria. Always remember that the patient's behavior and reactions are beyond his or her control.

Every attempt should be made to calm and reassure the patient. Hyperactivity increases metabolic rate and the release of metabolic wastes within the body that cause increases in ICP. Try to avoid restraining the patient, because this usually evokes rebellion and worsened agitation, which may lead to self-injury and dangerous increases in ICP. However, it will be necessary to protect monitoring lines and endotracheal tubes.

Mild sedation may be prescribed by the surgeon. The most effective approach is small dosages of agents such as chloral hydrate, paraldehyde, or ataractics. Because of their respiratory depressant action and effect on pupillary response, and the potential for difficulty in assessing LOC, narcotics are usually not given.

Intracranial Pressure. Prevention of increased ICP requires identification of its causes. Increased ICP may be detected most accurately through objective ICP monitoring systems. Relations between various internal and external stimuli and ICP variations have been delineated by this method. Several factors are known to precipitate sustained pressure increases as evidenced by plateau waves. These are inhalation anesthetics, hypercapnia (PaCO$_2$ greater than 40 torr), hypoxia (PaO$_2$ less than 50 torr), suctioning, and Valsalva maneuvers. The ICP can be increased by turning, painful stimulation, manipulation, arousal from sleep, agitation, neck flexion or hyperflexion, extreme hip flexion, or the supine position.

Hypoxia may or may not accompany hypercapnia. Both states can increase ICP. Hypercapnia may occur during normal sleep as a result of hypoventilation. It may also occur as a compensatory mechanism in response to metabolic alkalosis, or it may be the prevailing condition in the patient with severe pulmonary emphysema. In addition, it may be the result of sedation or an improperly set ventilator.

Hypoxia sufficient to cause sustained pressure peaks has been reported during intubation, inadequate ventilation, or suctioning. Suctioning should be done only when indicated by chest sounds or arterial blood gas values, not on a fixed schedule.

The Valsalva maneuver increases ICP by increasing intrathoracic pressure. The increased pressure within the thorax impedes venous return and increases cerebral blood volume and ICP. The patient may perform this maneuver during turning, painful manipulation, or suctioning or when agitated. If patients are responsive and cooperative, Valsalva effects can be minimized by instructing them to exhale during turning and not to hold their breaths during painful manipulation. Neck flexion and hyperextension and hip flexion increase ICP by obstructing venous return to the heart. Extreme hip flexion impedes venous return from the leg to the heart. As a result, arterial blood volume and pressure increase within the thorax and increase ICP much like the Valsalva maneuver does.

If ICP is measured continuously, identification and treatment of increasing ICP are made easier. Treatment can be instituted before the signs of transtentorial herniation appear.

The PACU nurse can correlate and document particular activities that prompt pressure increases in the patient. The effectiveness of nursing measures designed to decrease ICP can also be evaluated and documented.

If the baseline pressure is rising gradually but persistently, the surgeon should be notified. He or she may order hyperventilation, controlled drainage of CSF, or administration of osmotic diuretics or corticosteroids to decrease pressure.

Calling the Physician. The physician should be called whenever the patient's condition appears to be deteriorating. The earliest indicators of unstable pressure are often benign in appearance but must be recognized immediately. Any patient who exhibits a slight change in alertness, an increased restlessness, or a slight asymmetry in motor function must be watched closely for other signs of deterioration. Other events that should be brought to the attention of the physician include decreased responsiveness; elevated baseline pressures or sustained peak pressures on the ICP monitor; CSF leaks; copious drainage on dressings; initial seizure activity; new focal deficit, restlessness or agitation, or asymmetric motor function unknown to the surgeon; projectile vomiting; pupillary changes in one or both eyes; severe headache (note onset and location); and changes in vital signs, such as temperature greater than 38.5°C rectally, systolic pressure increase of 30 torr or more, pulse decrease of 20 beats per min or more, respiratory rate of 12 breaths per min or less, and irregular respirations or change in respiratory pattern. The progression of any signs or symptoms should also be noted, because this is frequently important diagnostically. If the nurse has any doubt about the circumstances in which the physician is to be notified, it is probably better to consult him or her.

SPINAL SURGERY

The goal of surgical intervention is to minimize complications related to SCIs, spinal cord tumors, or developmental abnormalities. Complete or incomplete SCI, bony fragments in the canal, unstable dislocation, and evidence of cord compression are some indications for immediate surgical intervention.

Diagnostic Tools

Several methods are used in diagnosing injury or disease involving the spine or spinal canal.

Conventional radiography and *fluoroscopy* identify fractures and fracture-dislocations (Fig. 29–10). Narrowing of an intervertebral space is sometimes evident as a result of a herniated nucleus pulposus, or "slipped disk." Fluoroscopy is used to demonstrate instability of the injured part on manipulation. Splintered or displaced bone fragments and radiopaque foreign bodies (such as bullets or other metal fragments) are also seen on radiograph. Radiographs also demonstrate abnormalities such as scoliosis and osteoporotic and arthritic changes. Tumors may be evidenced by erosion, calcium deposits within the mass, increased interpediculate distance, enlargement of an intervertebral foramen, or collapse of a vertebra.

CT scanning is used to delineate mass lesions

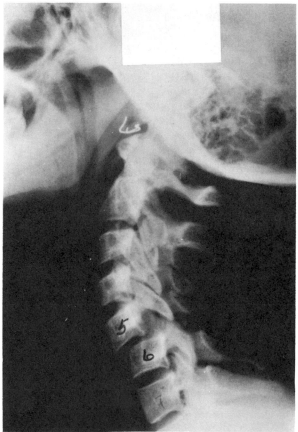

FIGURE 29–10. Radiograph showing a dislocation of the cervical spine. This injury may or may not produce spinal cord or nerve root damage. Reduction is usually achieved by relaxation and skull traction with tongs. Surgery is sometimes necessary to achieve reduction and stabilization. (From Sabiston, D. C., Jr. [ed.]: Davis-Christopher Textbook of Surgery: The Biological Basis of Modern Surgical Practice. 11th ed. Philadelphia, W. B. Saunders, 1977, p. 1528.)

existing in the same plane as the spine and spinal cord. Large blood clots may also be localized with this method.

MRI is being used increasingly to accurately detect and assess space-occupying lesions of the spine, such as herniated nucleus pulposus and tumors.

Electromyography is employed in evaluating muscle function as a means of detecting the nature and location of motor unit lesions. Tumors and herniated nucleus pulposus compressing the cord or motor nerve roots affect the function of the muscle groups they innervate.

Myelography is one of the most valuable tools available in diagnosing compression of the spinal cord due to tumor, fracture-dislocation, or herniated nucleus pulposus. A lumbar puncture is performed, at which time a Queckenstedt test may also be done.* The myelogram consists of the injection of a radiopaque dye into the CSF canal and the fluoroscopic observation of its flow in the suspected area. Cord compression is evidenced by an interruption in the contour of the spinal cord (Fig. 29–11). Disruption of the contours of the spinal nerve roots may also be found.

Injuries of the Spine

The spine protects the spinal cord and the terminal nerve roots. Injuries to the spine and spinal cord occur as a result of acceleration-deceleration accidents, torsion injuries, penetrating wounds, or blunt trauma. Frequently, head injuries accompany injuries to the spine and vice versa. The cervical spine is extremely mobile and therefore particularly susceptible to acceleration-deceleration and torsion injuries that hyperflex or hyperextend the neck. Propulsion may occur anteroposteriorly or laterally. The spinal cord is relatively large in the cervical area and sustains damage fairly easily after injury to the spine. This area is unique in that the superior portion of C2 lacks a vertebral body. Instead, the neck has a dens, or projection, called the *odontoid.* Many injuries to the

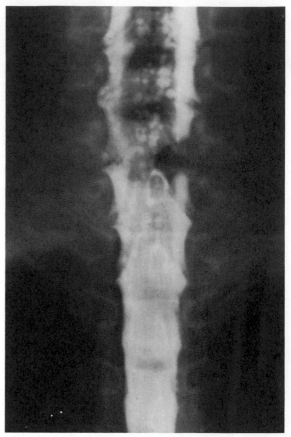

FIGURE 29–11. Pantopaque cervical myelogram with filling defect due to a unilateral ruptured intervertebral disk between C6 and C7 on the right. (From Sabiston, D. C., Jr. [ed.]: Davis-Christopher Textbook of Surgery: The Biological Basis of Modern Surgical Practice. 11th ed. Philadelphia, W. B. Saunders, 1977, p. 1495.)

odontoid extend into C1, or atlas, which has no vertebral body at all.

The thoracic spine is fixed by the ribs, but the lumbar spine is not, so there is an increased incidence of fracture-dislocations of T12, L1, and L2. These fracture-dislocations are found particularly in patients who have been involved in motor vehicle accidents and who wore lap seatbelts without shoulder restraints.

Consequences of injury to the spine are many and varied. The seriousness of the injury depends on the extent and level of involvement of the cord or spinal nerves rather than on the degree of bony destruction alone. Injuries to the bones of the spine include subluxation, dislocation, and simple and compression fractures.

Subluxation is the complete or partial dislocation of a vertebra from its normal alignment. It is caused by a fracture of the articulating facets.

---

*In the Queckenstedt test, the veins of the neck are compressed on one or both sides. In a healthy person, the CSF pressure rises rapidly and then quickly returns to normal when the pressure is taken off the neck. In a patient whose spinal cord is obstructed, little or no increase in pressure is found. This test is diagnostically accurate for most cord compressions; however, false-negative results may be obtained if the lesion is located high in the cervical spine area. The Queckenstedt test is not performed in patients with known or suspected increased ICP.

Compression fractures are fractures of the vertebral body without subluxation. The articulating facets are intact unless the fracture is comminuted.

Fracture-dislocations are displaced fractures of the vertebral bodies. Any of the other vertebral elements may also be fractured.

The spinal cord may experience *concussion,* much as the brain does. This results in transient paralysis and loss of sensation without anatomically demonstrable changes. Concussions are usually the result of blunt trauma. Loss of function can last 24 to 48 hours, depending on the severity of the concussion.

Contusion of the cord is a bruise associated with swelling and hemorrhage that results in some degree of permanent injury. Fracture-dislocations and trauma can cause contusions of the spine. More serious is a contusion that results in *spinal shock.* This may result in partial or complete physiologic transection of the cord.

Lacerations are usually the result of fracture-dislocations that cause a tear in the spinal cord. The neurologic damage is permanent because no method of restoring axonal continuity is currently available.

Pathologic conditions affecting the cord manifest themselves according to the portion of the cord involved. Neurologic loss in trauma to the spine may be partial, or it may be complete, permanent, or transient. With incomplete SCI, there are some sensory and motor functions below the level of the lesion. Incomplete SCIs are classified according to the area that is damaged. The classifications are referred to as syndromes.

Anterior cord syndrome usually occurs as the result of compression of the anterior portion of the cord and loss of blood supply from the anterior spinal artery. Clinical signs are loss of motor function, pain, temperature, and sensation below the level of injury. Touch, position, and vibration sensation are still intact. Anterior cord syndrome is usually caused by flexion injuries in the cervical area.

Central cord syndrome occurs as a result of cellular damage to the central portion of the spinal cord. The cellular damage is precipitated by edema and hemorrhage in this area. Clinical signs are greater motor loss in the upper extremities than in the lower extremities and varying levels of sensory function. Central cord syndrome is usually caused by hyperextension injuries and is seen in elderly patients with cervical arthritis.

Posterior cord syndrome results in loss of sensory function, with motor function remaining intact.

Brown-Sequard syndrome (hemisection of the cord) is the result of disruption on one side of the spinal cord. Clinical signs are ipsilateral loss of motor, touch, pressure, and vibration below the lesion and contralateral loss of pain and temperature below the lesion. Brown-Sequard syndrome can occur as the result of penetrating injuries.

Complete transection results in loss of all sensation with complete paralysis at and below the level of the lesion. This occurs after anatomic severance of the cord or as a physiologic result of cord edema. All SCI signs and symptoms are found at and below the level of the lesion. Motor and sensory functions are unimpaired above the level of the lesion. Clinical findings during the acute phase after total cord transection include the following:

1. Immediate loss of all sensory, motor, autonomic, and reflex functions below the level of the injury owing to spinal shock. Spinal shock may persist for days or weeks, depending on the injury and the patient's general state of health. It usually lasts 4 to 8 weeks.
2. Urinary retention due to bladder sphincter paralysis.
3. Paralytic ileus with progressive abdominal distention.
4. Respiratory insult or cessation. Injury to the lower cervical or upper thoracic spine results in cessation of intercostal function. In this event, respiration is under the sole stimulus of the phrenic nerve, and breathing is diaphragmatic. Injury to the cord at the levels of C3 through C5 injures the phrenic nucleus, paralyzing the diaphragm and causing respiratory failure.
5. Loss of sweating below the level of the lesion.
6. Point tenderness over the injured part. Gibbus or crepitus may or may not be present.

Initial therapeutic efforts are directed at preserving life and residual function (which may develop more fully with later rehabilitation). Mechanical stability, protection of nervous tissue, and freedom from pain are long-term therapeutic goals.

Surgery is indicated immediately after injury in the following instances:

1. When the signs and symptoms of an incomplete transection of the spinal cord are observed to worsen. Myelography usually precedes surgery.
2. When a fracture-dislocation cannot be com-

pletely reduced by skeletal traction alone. If the injury is to the thoracic or lumbar spine, surgery is indicated if the reduction is inadequate after immobilization on the Stryker or Foster frame and the administration of muscle relaxants.

3. When myelography indicates complete obstruction of the cord due to bony compression, hematoma, or protruded disk.
4. When a fragment of bone or foreign body lies in a position where it could cause further cord injury or will later cause chronic myelopathy or radiculopathy.
5. When surgical fusion will prevent a marked kyphotic deformity, which may follow skeletal traction and natural fusion. This kyphotic deformity might later produce chronic myelopathy or radiculopathy.
6. When there are open penetrating injuries requiring surgical débridement.
7. When there is an acutely herniated nucleus pulposus.

Neurosurgeons differ in their opinions as to whether or not emergency surgery is indicated in those patients with complete transection injuries. Although there is at present no hope of restoring function, some surgeons believe exploratory surgery is justified to reassure themselves, the patient, and the patient's family that everything possible is being done to fully assess and correct the injury.

General contraindications to surgery are the existence of associated life-threatening injuries, depressed respiratory function caused by high cervical injuries, lack of skilled personnel and necessary equipment, and a patient with improved neurologic status. Cord edema, which worsens during the first 48 to 72 hours, may extend the degree of respiratory difficulty. Such a patient is usually intubated and placed on assisted ventilation prophylactically. In these situations, immediate treatment of the SCI consists of stabilizing the fracture by immobilizing the neck with skeletal traction and medical management.

Exploration, débridement, or laminectomy may be performed through an anterior or posterior approach, depending on the cord lesion. Fusion is accomplished by the placement of a bone graft fashioned from tibial or iliac bone into the involved interspace or of a fixation device.

The anterior operative approach to the cervical spine allows direct visualization of and access to the lesion responsible for cord compression—this is its major advantage. Anterior fusion generally provides greater stability than

does posterior fusion, and skeletal traction and Stryker frame immobilization are sometimes unnecessary postoperatively.

Nursing Care and Considerations in the Patient with Spinal Cord Injury

In the United States alone, more than 10,000 people annually experience SCIs. Of these people, 50 percent sustain injuries to their spinal cords in motor vehicle accidents, and 82 percent are male. With increased use of motorcycle helmets, many people injured in motorcycle accidents survive what would otherwise have been fatal head injuries, only to be left to deal with cervical cord injuries. Permanent injuries of this nature are devastating to the patient and the patient's family. The nursing responsibilities are great during the acute, rehabilitative, and chronic phases. Patients with SCI may be sent to the PACU in any of these phases, and their care requires special consideration and knowledge of pathophysiology.

The initial assessment of the patient with SCI in the PACU needs to focus on airway patency, adequate respiration, and circulation. Vital signs should be assessed every 15 minutes until stable. Neurologic evaluation should be done along with the initial assessment because of the incidence of head injuries that accompany SCI.

Post anesthesia care of lumbar surgical patients should include keeping the head of the bed flat and log rolling the patient to help maintain proper body alignment, promote skin integrity, and minimize discomfort. The surgical site should be inspected for drainage and hematoma, and if spinal fusion was performed, the donor site should also be inspected. Assessment of the patient's comfort should be performed frequently because of muscle spasms that are often associated with lumbar surgery. The neurologic examination should include assessment of sensation in the lower extremities, noting the presence of tingling, numbness, or paralysis. The pedal pulses, color, temperature, and capillary refill of the lower extremities also should be assessed.

Neurogenic Shock

In neurogenic shock the vascular tone is decreased, resulting in generalized vasodilation. Blood pools in the capillaries of the voluntary muscles and the gastrointestinal system, prohibiting adequate circulating volume to the vital centers. The large voluntary muscles lose their tone and no longer assist the heart in pumping blood throughout the body.

Clinically, the blood pressure falls, the pulse increases, and the respirations become deep with frequent sighs. The skin becomes cool and moist, pallor and cyanosis are evident, and the patient may complain of extreme fatigue. Conditions for thrombus formation are optimal. This is not hemorrhagic shock; therefore, the patient must not be overloaded with intravenous fluids in a misguided attempt to overcome it.

Treatment consists of combating hemostasis; oxygen is given to combat hypoxia. Emergency aid may require the use of a shock suit (applied only after the fracture has been stabilized). Once stabilization of shock has been achieved, antiembolism stockings and passive range of motion exercises are used to combat hemostasis and thrombus formation.

Intramuscular medications should never be administered below the level of the lesion, because they will only cause local inflammation and tissue breakdown, and absorption will be negligible or nil.

Spinal Cord Edema

Spinal cord edema is most pronounced within the first 48 to 72 hours after injury or trauma. Profound danger lies in the ability of the edema to advance to the brain, to physiologically extend injury, or to anatomically promote the possibility of shearing the cord on bone fragments or fracture edges. If edema extends to the level of the phrenic nucleus, respiratory function is threatened. Astute observation of the respiratory pattern may reveal shallow and rapid respirations or flaring of the nares before complete respiratory failure ensues.

Vital capacity should be measured with a Wright respirometer every 2 hours during the acute phase. A downward trend in the values obtained indicates development of respiratory distress and should be reported to the physician immediately. Articles necessary for emergency intubation or tracheostomy and mechanical ventilation must be readily available. Some physicians place the patient on mechanical ventilation prophylactically when the risk of developing respiratory distress is high.

Concomitant Head Injury

Every patient with acute injury to the spine must be observed for signs and symptoms indicative of head injury. Evaluation of cranial status should be done at the same intervals as the vital sign measurements. An abnormal cranial "check" should be reported to the physician immediately, because it may indicate injury to the brain or increased ICP resulting from the upward expansion of cord edema.

Respiratory Complications

Respiratory insufficiency or failure is the most serious complication of SCI. Respiratory complications can be independent of the level of injury. C4 and higher injuries require mechanical ventilation because of the direct involvement of the phrenic nerves. Assessment of a patient's ventilation should include the following parameters: status, rate, depth, and pattern. Evaluation of pulmonary function should include tidal volume, inspiratory force, and vital capacity. Changes in pulmonary function are early indicators of a deterioration in respiratory status and may necessitate ventilator support. Intubation of the patients may depend on their ability to clear secretions and to maintain adequate arterial blood gas values—an inability to create appropriate expiratory flow rates owing to muscle weakness prevents patients from clearing their airways with an effective cough. Auscultation of lung sounds should also be performed routinely to assess the presence of rhonchi or crackles. Chest radiographic examinations and arterial blood gas determinations should be monitored routinely and ordered immediately if signs of deterioration occur. Potential respiratory complications resulting from SCI include pneumonia, aspiration, pulmonary edema, and pulmonary embolism. Because of the rapid onset of pulmonary complications, the PACU nurse must be aggressive in the care of the patient with SCI.

Cardiovascular Complications

Cardiovascular complications can result from the loss of sympathetic function in the patient with SCI. Patients with an injury at or higher than T6 may experience bradycardia and hypotension because of vasodilatation, decreased venous return, and decreased cardiac output. Orthostatic hypotension is also a complication owing to decreased venous return.

Deep vein thrombosis is a potential complication of SCI. Patients with SCI should wear antiembolism stockings, and post anesthesia nursing care should include measurement of leg circumference, passive range of motion of the lower extremities, and foot dorsiflexion.

Anticoagulation therapy may be ordered by the attending physician.

Skeletal Tong Traction

Skeletal tong traction is used in the treatment of subluxations or fracture-dislocations of the cervical spine. It is also used after some posterior fusions of the cervical vertebrae. The tongs grasp the skull firmly on both sides, and traction is applied by weighting the tongs so that a pulling force is exerted in the superior direction. The weight of the body serves as the countertraction. Extreme care must be taken so that the traction weight is continuous and even. Ropes must be free from snags and frays and lie in the proper grooves of the pulley system; knots must be tied securely. The patient's body must be aligned with the long axis of the cervical spine. Any defect in the traction system may result in the sudden release of traction, leading to further injury of the spine or cord.

Several varieties of tongs are currently in use. Crutchfield tongs are frequently used (Fig. 29–12). Vinke tongs are not used as widely. Gardner tongs have grown in popularity because they have a safety bolt that prevents them from slipping out of the skull or penetrating the brain. In some instances, skeletal immobility is obtained by the use of a halo cast (Fig. 29–13). A metal band is anchored by the use of skeletal pins to the head at a level just above the eyebrows. Rigid metal rods attach to the halo and are anchored to a plaster cast or plastic and metal jacket that encases the shoulders and the chest. This approach alone offers sufficient immobilization after some anterior cervical spine fusions. It has the advantages of dispensing with the need for Foster or Stryker frame immobilization and allowing early ambulation.

The area surrounding skeletal pins is generally shaved to prevent contamination. Some surgeons prefer to have the entire head shaved. Pin care should be given immediately after tong insertion and at 6- to 8-hour intervals thereafter. The area surrounding the pins is cleansed of any dried blood or encrustations using sterile saline or equal parts of sterile saline and hydrogen peroxide. A bactericidal ointment is then applied to the sites, which should be covered with sterile 2 × 2 sponges. Sterile technique is always used when pin care is being administered.

Stryker and Foster Frame Precautions

The patient with acute SCI will arrive in the PACU on a Stryker frame (Fig. 29–14) or a Roto Rest bed (Fig. 29–15). These are the two most

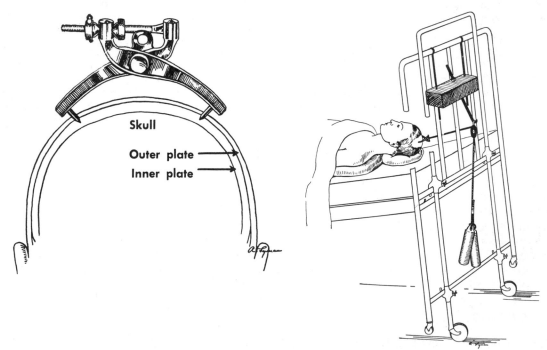

FIGURE 29–12. Crutchfield tongs. (From Larson, C. B., and Gould, M.: Orthopedic Nursing. 7th ed. St. Louis, C. V. Mosby, 1970.)

Skull

Outer plate
Inner plate

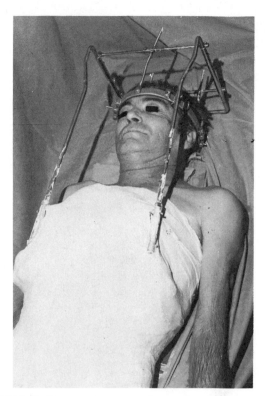

FIGURE 29–13. Halo cast. The halo, which has four screws inserted in the outer table of the skull, provides for rigid fixation of the cervical spine. The halo may be used for cervical traction in the recumbent position or attached to a cast. The patient may be ambulatory in the halo cast. (From Sabiston, D. C., Jr. [ed.]: Davis-Christopher Textbook of Surgery: The Biological Basis of Modern Surgical Practice. 11th ed. Philadelphia, W. B. Saunders, 1977, p. 1526.)

commonly used alternative beds to help manage patients with SCI.

The Stryker frame allows the patient to be turned from the supine to the prone position by manual manipulation of the frame. The frame is designed to allow for maintenance of body alignment and for traction on the spinal column, if used, while turning the patient.

The Roto Rest bed rotates automatically a maximum of 62 degrees to each side constantly. This bed is also designed to maintain body alignment of the patient and is equipped for use of spinal column traction. When using either the Stryker frame or Roto Rest bed, the PACU nurse must take care to ensure that the patient is properly positioned and secured. Extremities must be properly positioned and padded and not allowed to swing free with movement of the beds. Rotation or turning of the patient with SCI should not be started until alignment of the spinal column has been verified radiographically.

Skin Care

As with the cranial surgical patient, skin care for the patient with SCI is an important aspect of PACU nursing care. Skin breakdown or decubiti formation is one of the most obvious, costly, and detrimental complications that a patient with SCI can experience. The patient must be turned and repositioned at least every 2 hours to prevent pressure breakdown of the skin and underlying body tissues. PACU care needs to include frequent massaging of the body prominences and protecting them with proper padding.

Contractures

Contractures result from disuse atrophy and improper positioning of the limbs. They may be minimized by the use of regular passive range-of-motion exercises, footboards, trochanter rolls, and hand rolls or specially fabricated splints.

Bone Demineralization

Long-term immobility causes demineralization of bone tissue. Calcium is freed into the circulation, resulting in osteoporosis, or "silent fractures," and renal calculi.

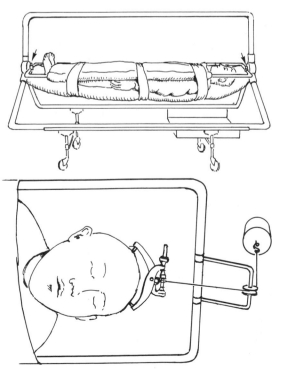

FIGURE 29–14. Stryker frame bed.

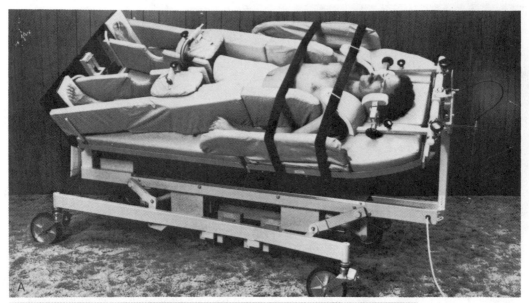

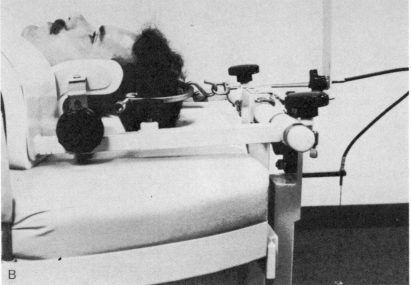

FIGURE 29–15. *A*, Roto Rest® Kinetic Treatment Table Mark 1-C. *B*, cervical traction with tongs used with Roto Rest® Table Mark 1-C. (Roto Rest—KCI's registered trademark for its oscilllating support surfaces. *A* and *B* courtesty of KCI, San Antonio, TX.)

Sensory Loss

The patient with a spinal cord transection experiences an abrupt cessation of all tactile and proprioceptive stimulation below the level of the lesion. Particularly in the patient with a cervical cord injury, visual stimuli are limited to those received from the small patch of floor below or the area of ceiling within his or her limited view. Hearing is intact, but much of the auditory stimuli that is perceived by the patient is foreign and not meaningful. The patient experiences a true isolation from his or her en-

vironment and a psychological loss of body image. This is often compounded by feelings of guilt and fear, creating an environment that fosters emotional withdrawal, reality distortion, and the development of stress ulcers.

When you approach the patient, always situate yourself so that you are in his or her visual field. Speak to the patient, even one who is unable to answer because of endotracheal intubation or tracheostomy. The patient will answer with the eyes or form silent words with the lips. Orient the patient to time and place, and give tactile stimulation to those areas above the level of injury. These measures may allay fears and help prevent or alleviate the devastating isolation that can result from sensory deprivation.

Gastrointestinal Complications

Generalized atony and loss of motility render the stomach and intestine distended and highly susceptible to fecal impactions and obstructions. Distention is relieved by intermittent nasogastric suction. Programs of bowel training are initiated on the parent unit.

There is a high incidence of stress ulcers among these patients, especially in quadriplegics. Here, parasympathetic vagal action is unopposed because of sympathetic block from the ascending and descending visceral nerve paths, and gastric acid secretion by the parietal cells of the stomach is increased. This stressful situation is further compounded by the administration of corticosteroids used to reduce cord edema that are singularly capable of inducing hyperacidity of gastric juices. Antacids or a histamine$_2$ antagonist such as cimetidine (Tagamet) or ranitidine (Zantac), or both, are given prophylactically to prevent stress ulcers. If gastric juices are accessible through a nasogastric tube, gastric pH can be monitored as a guide to treatment. Serial hematocrit determinations establish a baseline and may be the first indicator of a "silent" gastrointestinal hemorrhage.

Urologic Complications

After transection of the spinal cord, the bladder sphincter becomes paralyzed and urinary stasis develops. Indwelling urinary catheterization is necessary to prevent bladder distention during the acute phase. Catheters made of inert material are preferred over those made of rubber, which is irritating to the bladder and urethra. The catheter balloon should not be inflated with more than 5 ml of fluid. Inflation in excess of this amount aggravates bladder spasticity. A three-way tidal drainage system may be instituted as a means of irrigating the bladder with an antibiotic solution. Care should be taken that the amount of irrigation solution instilled does not overdistend the bladder

Long-term catheterization, osteoporosis, decreased muscle tone, fluid and electrolyte abnormalities, alterations in cardiovascular dynamics, anemia, and catabolism contribute to urologic complications. Stasis, calculi and fistula formation, and chronic urinary tract complications leading to septicemia make urologic complications the leading cause of death in the paraplegic and quadriplegic populations.

Temperature Elevations

Temperature elevations after SCI may be the result of any infectious process, the most common being urinary tract and respiratory infections. If this is the case, treatment consists of the administration of antipyretics and appropriate antibiotics.

Unique to paraplegic and quadriplegic patients is the loss of sweating below the level of the lesion. In the absence of this important body-cooling mechanism, alarmingly high temperature elevations may occur. Treatment in this situation consists of tepid water spongings, administration of antipyretics, and removal of blankets and as much clothing as possible. These methods are usually quite effective in reducing fever, but occasionally a cooling blanket is also required.

Autonomic Hyperreflexia

Autonomic hyperreflexia is a condition or syndrome that may occur at any time after SCI but generally is not seen until the period of spinal shock has elapsed and spinal cord reflexes have returned. About 85 percent of patients with spinal cord transections higher than T6 experience this syndrome, whereas those with transections lower than T10 are unlikely to have symptoms of this reflex. Autonomic hyperreflexia most often occurs if the spinal cord is completely transected. It is seldom seen if the SCI is incomplete.

The stimulus that triggers autonomic hyperreflexia usually arises from cutaneous, mucosal, or visceral tissue below the level of the spinal cord lesion. Stimulation below the level of transection is transmitted to the spinal cord via afferent pathways where they enter the cord below the level of injury, resulting in reflex stimulation of the sympathetic nervous system. The sympathetic response causes intense arterial vasoconstriction below the levels of spinal cord transection, which results in systemic hypertension. Normally, this sympathetic activity is countered by parasympathetic activity initiated at higher neurologic centers. Because of the transection of the spinal cord, impulses from the brain to stimulate the parasympathetic system are unable to travel down the cord past the level of transection, leaving the sympathetic system unopposed below this level. Therefore, compensatory vasodilatation can occur only above the level of transection and is often insufficient to counteract the hypertension resulting from the intense vasoconstriction below the transection.

Clinical signs and symptoms of autonomic hyperreflexia are progressive, although somewhat variable. The patient complains of headache and blotching of the skin, and gooseflesh appears. Diaphoresis of the face occurs, and the patient may complain of nasal congestion or obstruction. Severe blood pressure elevations are found and may exceed 300 torr. The patient is bradycardic and restless; headache becomes severe. Seizure, loss of consciousness, stroke, and death may ensue.

Autonomic hyperreflexia may be triggered by a variety of stimuli. The most common offenders are bladder distention (due to a plugged catheter or excessive irrigation solution), fecal impaction, or decubiti. However, reflexive overresponse may also be triggered by conditions as seemingly innocuous as an ingrown toenail, a jarred bed, or even a draft of air.

PACU care centers around the routine prevention of known precipitants of autonomic hyperreflexia. For example, the bladder must not be allowed to become distended, and decubiti must be prevented. If signs and symptoms appear, the stimulus must be sought and removed as rapidly as possible. If the symptoms cannot be alleviated, the nurse should notify the physician, elevate the head of the bed (if not contraindicated), and monitor the blood pressure every 5 minutes. Severe cases can require treatment by spinal anesthesia and the administration of ganglionic blocking agents. For chronic problems, subarachnoid blocks or rhizotomy may be necessary.

Anesthetic Considerations

The most influential factors in the anesthetic management of patients with SCI are the duration of the injury (acute or chronic), fluid and electrolyte status, airway management, and autonomic hyperreflexia.

The use of a depolarizing muscle relaxant (succinylcholine) for intubation purposes in the patient with SCI is conservatively contraindicated owing to the release of potassium. The succinylcholine-induced release of potassium is the result of proliferation of cholinergic receptors in muscle tissue below the level of transection. The resultant hyperkalemia, often as high as 14 mEq per L, can lead to ventricular fibrillation and cardiac arrest. The release of potassium due to succinylcholine administration can be seen as early as 1 day after injury and as long as 9 months later. The degree of muscle involvement, not the dosage of succinylcholine, is the determining factor in the amount of potassium released.

Patients with SCI may experience some degree of hypotension owing to a relative hypovolemia as a result of sympathetic nervous system depression. The degree of the hypotension is dependent on the level of transection and the duration of the injury with regard to whether or not the patient is still experiencing spinal shock. The patient must be adequately resuscitated with fluids, and measures must be taken to monitor fluid status and to ensure adequate organ perfusion.

Airway management is a significant problem in patients with SCI whose injury involves the cervical spine. Endotracheal intubation must be performed without manipulation of the cervical spine so as to avoid further irreversible damage. Intubation may be accomplished by awake, blind oral or nasal approach, fiberoptics, or retrograde intubation. When the airway obstruction is severe, tracheostomy or cricothyrotomy may be necessary. Patients may arrive in the PACU with the endotracheal tube in place and not be extubated until it is ensured that they can adequately manage their airway and ventilation.

Herniated Nucleus Pulposus

Herniated nucleus pulposus (Fig. 29–16) may occur in any of the intervertebral disks but is most commonly found in one of the last two lumbar interspaces. Pain and some degree of compromise in sensory or motor function along the distribution of the involved nerve are common findings preoperatively. Before surgical intervention is undertaken, diagnostic confirmation is sought, and the suspected herniated nucleus pulposus is differentiated from tumor, subluxation of the facets, or rheumatoid spondylitis.

Surgery consists of partial hemilaminectomy and removal of the diseased disk. If fusion is necessary to prevent recurrence of pain or deformity, a bone graft is removed from the iliac crest or tibia and placed as a bridge over the defective space. Spinal fusion lengthens the operative procedure and requires a second operative wound site. Therefore, a greater potential for postoperative complications exists, and the recuperative phase may be lengthened. The threat of shock is also greater owing to increased blood loss and pain.

Movement restrictions in the PACU are de-

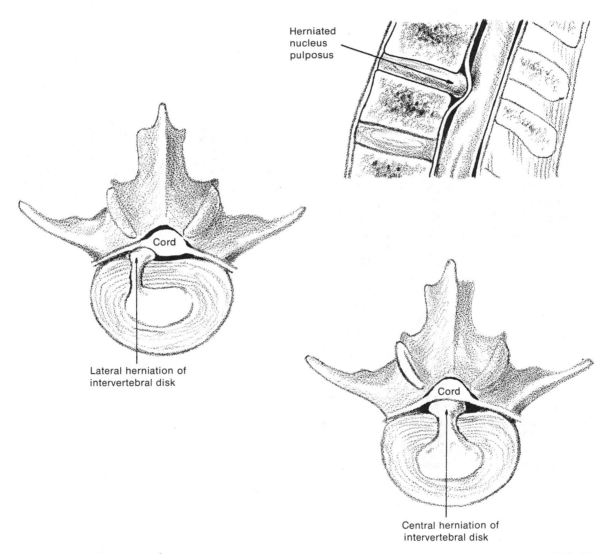

Herniated
nucleus
pulposus

Cord

Lateral herniation of
intervertebral disk

Cord

Central herniation of
intervertebral disk

FIGURE 29–16. Forms of vertebral herniation. (From Luckmann, J., and Sorenson, K. C.: Medical-Surgical Nursing. Philadelphia, W. B. Saunders, 1973, p. 523.)

termined by the surgeon and depend on the extent of the surgery and whether or not a fusion was done. If fusion was not done, the patient is often allowed to stand at the bedside, and ambulation is allowed as soon as the effects of the anesthetic have subsided. If the spine is fused, mobility restrictions are more severe. Usually, turning is allowed if done in the log-rolling fashion.

As in all spinal procedures, sensory function and motor strength of the extremities should be assessed along with the vital signs in the PACU. Evidence of CSF leaks must be sought on dressings and bed linens.

Intraspinal Neoplasms

Intraspinal neoplasms may occur at any level of the cord from the foramen magnum to the sacral canal. Most of the tumors are found in the thoracic region, because this is the longest subdivision of the spine. Cord compression and neurologic deficit produce symptoms similar to those produced by displaced fracture of the spine, but they usually develop and progress at a slower pace. The exact location of the lesion is determined by neurologic examination, myelography, and tomography.

Intraspinal tumors may arise from the cord or its coverings, from fibrous tissue, or as a result of metastatic disease. For descriptive purposes they are placed in the following subdivisions:

Intramedullary tumors: those arising solely from the substance of the cord.

Extradural-extramedullary tumors: those arising outside the dura, either in the epidural space, vertebrae, or surrounding tissues.

Intradural-extramedullary tumors: those arising within or under the dura but not invading the cord (Fig. 29–17).

Dumbbell tumors: those arising within the spinal canal and extending extraspinally along the nerve through the intervertebral foramen.

Early diagnosis and treatment are essential to prevent irreversible damage to the spinal cord. Eighty-five percent of intraspinal neoplasms are benign. The remainder are either primarily malignant or secondary to metastasis. The decision to intervene surgically is made after considering the patient's general condition and life expectancy. Also considered are other metastases and the type and location of the primary tumor.

Treatment consists of laminectomy, surgical

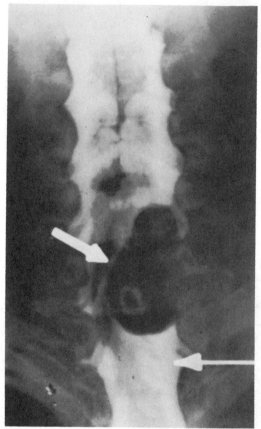

FIGURE 29–17. Myelogram showing an intradural-extramedullary meningioma at C7. The *thin arrow* shows a broad dye column on that side of the spinal canal with the halftone shadow of the cord displaced toward the opposite side. The *broad (upper) arrow* shows the medial border of the tumor mass itself. (From Sabiston, D. C., Jr. [ed.]: Davis-Christopher Textbook of Surgery: The Biological Basis of Modern Surgical Practice. 11th ed. Philadelphia, W. B. Saunders, 1977, p. 1490.)

exploration, and excision of the mass. Most benign tumors can be excised completely. Prognosis depends on the location of the tumor, the severity and duration of the preoperative neurologic deficit, and whether or not the tumor is completely removable. Intramedullary tumors are associated with a more guarded prognosis, because they can rarely be excised without increasing the neurologic deficit.

References

1. Allen, A. (ed.): ASPAN: Core Curriculum for Post Anesthesia Nursing Practice. 2nd ed. Philadelphia, W. B. Saunders, 1991.
2. Alspach, J.: AACN: Core Curriculum for Critical Care Nursing. 4th ed. Philadelphia, W. B. Saunders, 1991.
3. Aumick, J.: Head trauma: Guidelines for care. RN, 54(4):27–31, 1991.

4. Barash, P., Cullen, B., and Stoelting, R. (eds.): Clinical Anesthesia. 2nd ed. Philadelphia, J. B. Lippincott, 1992.
5. Barker, E.: Brain tumor: Frightening diagnosis, nursing challenge. RN, 53(9):46–52, 1990.
6. Benumof, J., and Saidman, L.: Anesthesia and Perioperative Complications. St. Louis, Mosby-Year Book, 1992.
7. Boortz-Marx, R.: Factors affecting intracranial pressure: A descriptive study. J. Neurosurg. Nurs., 17(2):89–94, 1985.
8. Brown, S.: Practical points in the post anesthetic assessment and care of the patient with increased intracranial pressure. J. Post Anesth. Nurs., 1(1):37–40, 1986.
9. Crosby, L., and Parsons, L.: Clinical neurologic assessment tool: Development and testing of an instrument to index neurologic status. Heart Lung, 18(2):121–129, 1989.
10. Dillingham, T.: Prevention of complications during acute management of the spinal cord–injured patient: First step in the rehabilitation process. Crit. Care Nurs. Q., 11(2):71–77, 1988.
11. Drummond, B.: Preventing increased intracranial pressure: Nursing care can make the difference. Focus Crit. Care, 17(2):116–122, 1990.
12. Finocchiaro, D., and Herzfeld, S.: Understanding autonomic dysreflexia. Am. J. Nurs., 90:56–59, 1990.
13. Grimes, C.: Cerebral balloon angioplasty for treatment of vasospasm after subarachnoid hemorrhage. Heart Lung, 20(5):431–435, 1991.
14. Guyton, A.: Textbook of Medical Physiology. 8th ed. Philadelphia, W. B. Saunders, 1991.
15. Hall-Craggs, E.: Anatomy as a Basis for Clinical Medicine. Baltimore, Urban and Schwarzenberg, 1985.
16. Hanowell, L., and Rose, D.: Perioperative care for spinal cord injury. Curr. Rev. Nurse Anesth., 13(12):90–96, 1990.
17. Harper, J.: Use of steroids in cerebral edema: Therapeutic implications. Heart Lung, 17(1):70–73, 1988.
18. Hickey, J.: The Clinical Practice of Neurological and Neurosurgical Nursing. 2nd ed. Philadelphia, J. B. Lippincott, 1986.
19. Hickman, K., Mayer, B., and Muwaswes, M.: Intracranial pressure monitoring: Review of risk factors associated with infection. Heart Lung, 19(1):84–90, 1990.
20. Hilton, G., and Frei, J.: High-dose methylprednisolone in the treatment of spinal cord injuries. Heart Lung, 20(6):675–680, 1991.
21. Howard, R., and Matjasko, J.: The management of intracranial hypertension. Curr. Rev. Nurse Anesth., 13(26):206–212, 1991.
22. Hugo, M.: Alleviating the effects of care on the intracranial pressure (ICP) of head-injured patients by manipulating nursing care activities. Intensive Care Nurs., 3(2):78–82, 1987.
23. ICI Americas, Inc.–Stuart Pharmaceuticals: Diprivan injection: Propofol [Technical brochure]. Wilmington, DE: Stuart Pharmaceuticals, 1989.
24. Jackson, L.: Cerebral vasospasm after an intracranial aneurysmal subarachnoid hemorrhage: A nursing perspective. Heart Lung, 15(1):14–20, 1986.
25. Johnson, S. (ed.): Case Studies in Neuroscience Critical Care Nursing. Gaithersburg, MD, Aspen, 1991.
26. Kane, D.: Practical points in the postoperative management of a craniotomy patient. J. Post Anesth. Nurs., 6(2):121–124, 1991.
27. Katz, J., Benumof, J., and Kadis, L. (eds.): Anesthesia and Uncommon Diseases. 3rd ed. Philadelphia: W. B. Saunders, 1990.
28. Kinney, M., Packa, D., and Dunbar, S. (eds.): AACN's Clinical Reference for Critical Care Nursing. 2nd ed. New York: McGraw-Hill, 1988.
29. Lee, S.: Intracranial pressure changes during positioning of patients with severe head injury. Heart Lung, 18(4):411–414, 1989.
30. Luchka, S.: Working with ICP monitors. RN, 54(4):34–37, 1991.
31. Manifold, S.: Craniocerebral trauma: A review of primary and secondary injury and therapeutic modalities. Focus Crit. Care, 13(2):22–35, 1986.
32. McCance, K., and Huether, S.: Pathophysiology: The Biologic Basis for Disease in Adults and Children. St. Louis, C. V. Mosby, 1990.
33. Miller, R. (ed.): Anesthesia. 3rd ed. New York, Churchill Livingstone, 1990.
34. Motton, C., and Litwick, K.: Practical points in the care of patients following transsphenoidal surgery. J. Post Anesth. Nurs., 4(2):109–111, 1989.
35. Murray, S.: Patient assessment in the post anesthesia care unit: A critical care approach. J. Post Anesth. Nurs., 4(4):232–238, 1989.
36. Nemeth, L., and Kiljanczyk, H.: Intensive care of the spinal cord–injured patient: Focus on early rehabilitation. Crit. Care Nurs. Q., 11(2):79–84, 1988.
37. Partyka, M.: Practical points in the care of the post–lumbar spine surgery patient. J. Post Anesth. Nurs., 6(3):185–187, 1991.
38. Porter, S., and Aker, J.: Electroencephalography for intraoperative assessment of the central nervous system. AANA J., 57(4):356–363, 1989.
39. Richmond, T.: A critical care challenge: The patient with a cervical spinal cord injury. Focus Crit. Care, 12(2):23–33, 1985.
40. Rudy, E., Baun, M., Stone, K., et al.: The relationship between endotracheal suctioning and changes in intracranial pressure: A review of the literature. Heart Lung, 15(5):488–494, 1986.
41. Rudy, E., Turner, B., Baun, M., et al.: Endotracheal suctioning in adults with head injury. Heart Lung, 20(6):667–674, 1991.
42. Sisson, R.: Effects of auditory stimuli on comatose patients with head injury. Heart Lung, 19(4):373–378, 1990.
43. Stewart-Amidei, C.: Hypervolemic hemodilution: A new approach to subarachnoid hemorrhage. Heart Lung, 18(6):590–598, 1989.
44. Stewart-Amidei, C.: Meningioma: Nursing care considerations. J. Post Anesth. Nurs., 6(4):269–278, 1991.
45. Stoelting, R.: Pharmacology and Physiology in Anesthetic Practice. 2nd ed. Philadelphia, J. B. Lippincott, 1991.
46. Stoelting, R., Dierdorf, S., and McCammon, R.: Anesthesia and Co-Existing Disease. 2nd ed. New York, Churchill Livingstone, 1988.
47. Waugaman, W., Foster, S., and Rigor, B.: Principles and Practice of Nurse Anesthesia. 2nd ed. Norwalk, CT, Appleton & Lange, 1992.
48. Wheeler, H.: Magnetic resonance imaging. AANA J., 57(6):515–520, 1989.
49. Wicks, T., and Collins, P.: Excision of an arteriovenous malformation. AANA J., 59(3):260–262, 1991.
50. Wisinger, D., and Mest-Beck, L.: Ventriculostomy: A guide to nursing management. J. Neurosci. Nurs., 22(6):365–369, 1990.
51. Wood, W.: A perioperative case study of frontal lobe meningioma. J. Post Anesth. Nurs., 6(4):265–268, 1991.
52. Wood, M., and Wood, A.: Drugs and Anesthesia: Pharmacology for Anesthesiologists. 2nd ed. Baltimore, Williams & Wilkins, 1990.

Post Anesthesia Care of the Thyroid and Parathyroid Surgical Patient

CHAPTER 30

Susan B. Christoph, D.N.Sc., R.N.

Surgery of the thyroid gland has been performed since the early 1800s and perfected to the degree that postoperative complications are rare. Preoperative preparation of the patient for thyroid or parathyroid surgery is extremely important and includes ensuring that the patient is euthyroid, well rested, at optimum weight, and in good health.

Definitions

Euthyroid: having normal thyroid secretion and function.

Parathyroidectomy: excision of one or more diseased, hypertrophied parathyroid glands.

Thyroidectomy: total excision of the thyroid gland. Total thyroidectomy is normally performed only in patients with thyroid malignancy.

Thyroglossal duct cystectomy: complete excision of all portions of the pretracheal cystic pouch sac and a portion of the hyoid bone to avoid recurrent cystic formation and to prevent infections.

Thyroid lobectomy (partial thyroidectomy): removal of a lobe of the thyroid gland. The objective in the patient with hyperthyroidism is to resect enough of the gland (subtotal thyroidectomy) to reduce the level of circulating hormones to normal levels yet leave sufficient amount of the gland to secrete a supply of the hormone. Patients who undergo total thyroidectomy must receive thyroid hormone replacement therapy.

ANESTHESIA

Surgery on the thyroid and parathyroid glands is most commonly performed under general endotracheal anesthesia. Therefore, all postoperative care indicated for a general anesthesia patient is instituted. A transverse neck incision is used during the surgical process.

NURSING CARE

Positioning

On admission to the PACU, the patient should be placed in the side-lying position if unconscious. He or she should be placed in a semi-Fowler's position to promote venous return as soon as condition permits. The patient should be moved carefully, with support to the head so that no tension is placed on the suture line. Firm support of the head should be continued and can usually be accomplished by placing a firm pillow under the shoulders and head. The patient should be taught to support the head when moving by placing the hands at the back of the neck.

Cardiorespiratory Assessment and Care

Immediate postoperative observations should include close attention to respiratory function, which may be compromised by hemorrhage, venous oozing, laryngeal edema, and spinal cord paralysis. Discourage the patient's talking to excess. A tracheostomy set should be immediately available at the bedside of any patient undergoing thyroid or parathyroid surgery.

Signs and symptoms of respiratory obstruction, such as stridor, air hunger, laryngeal spasm, and inability to speak, should be reported immediately to the anesthesiologist or the surgeon and appropriate measures instituted. A cool-mist humidifier at the bedside is routinely ordered postoperatively to ease the sore throat expected after endotracheal intubation and to promote general respiratory well-being.

The patient should also be checked for the development of subcutaneous emphysema, which may indicate pneumothorax or rupture of the trachea.

Pain Management

Pain should be minimal following thyroidectomy and parathyroidectomy, but small doses of narcotic such as meperidine or morphine may be required during the first 24 hours. Severe pain should be reported to the physician.

Dressings

Postoperative dressings are no longer bulky, and drains are generally not required. A simple thyroid collar including a gauze square over the incision secured with a sterile surgical towel crossed over the gauze is usually used. Drainage should be minimal and should not visibly soak through the dressing. The usual signs and symptoms of hemorrhage should be assessed, and the nurse should watch for swelling of the neck and feel the back of the neck for drainage. Any excess bleeding should be reported immediately.

Intake and Output

Intake and output measures should be carefully assessed. The postoperative patient can be expected to retain some fluid, and this will be manifested as a low urinary output. Caution must be exerted, therefore, to avoid overhydration. Oral fluid can usually be tolerated as soon as the patient regains consciousness and nausea has subsided. Ice chips may be offered to soothe the throat. Warm saline gargles may be comforting.

Complications

Complications are infrequent but may include obstruction of the airway, postoperative bleeding, pneumomediastinum, and pneumo-thorax. Although rare with current advanced surgical techniques, damage to the recurrent laryngeal nerve may occur. Hoarseness or a whispery voice may indicate unilateral damage that is usually temporary. Hoarseness and bilateral flaccid paralysis may indicate bilateral nerve injury and should be reported immediately, because serious airway obstruction could develop rapidly. Following assessment of the voice, the patient should be discouraged from excessive talking, because this aggravates the hoarseness.

Tetany

Although tetany due to hypoparathyroidism is rare, the patient should be evaluated for signs and symptoms that may indicate its development. The signs and symptoms of tetany include tingling of the toes, fingers, and the area around the mouth; apprehension; positive *Chvostek's sign* (tapping the cheek over the facial nerve causes a twitch of the lip or facial muscle); and positive *Trousseau's sign* (carpopedal spasm induced by occluding circulation in the arm with a blood pressure cuff or tourniquet). Calcium lactate or calcium gluconate should be readily available for use if signs of tetany develop. Calcium is administered slowly intravenously, and the patient should be monitored by electrocardiogram continuously before, during, and after the infusion.

Thyroid Storm

In thyroid crisis, or storm, a rare complication, all the symptoms of hyperthyroidism are exaggerated. An increase in pulse, blood pressure, pulse pressure, and temperature, plus air hunger and restlessness, may indicate its development. Treatment includes the intravenous administration of sodium iodide, corticosteroids, and reserpine, as well as supplementary oxygen and cooling with a hypothermia unit. Lithium is the drug of choice for patients who are sensitive to iodine.

References

1. Barash, P., Cullen, B., and Stoelting, R.: Clinical Anesthesia. 2nd ed. Philadelphia, J. B. Lippincott, 1992.
2. Benumof, J., and Saidman, L.: Anesthesia and Perioperative Complications. St. Louis, Mosby-Year Book, 1992.
3. LiVolsi, V. A., and Merino, M. J.: Pathology of thyroid tumors. *In* Thawley, E. E., Panje, W. R., Batsakis, J. G., et al. (eds.): Comprehensive Management of Head and Neck Tumors. Vol. II. Philadelphia, W. B. Saunders, 1987, pp. 1599–1610.

4. Perry, H. A.: The postoperative care of patients after thyroid, parathyroid, and adrenal operations. Curr. Rev. Recov. Room Nurses, 4(8):59–63, 1982.
5. Sarsany, S. L.: Thyroid storm. RN, 51(7):46–48, 1988.
6. Sawin, C. T.: Hypothyroidism. Med. Clin. North Am., 69(5):989, 1985.

7. Sherwood, L. M.: Diagnosis and management of primary hyperparathyroidism. Hosp. Pract., 23(3):9–13, 1988.
8. Stoelting, R., and Dierdorf, S.: Anesthesia and Co-Existing Disease. 3rd ed. New York, Churchill Livingstone, 1993.

Post Anesthesia Care of the Gastrointestinal, Abdominal, and Anorectal Surgical Patient

CHAPTER 31

Denise O'Brien, B.S.N., R.N., C.P.A.N.

Care of the patient following abdominal surgery or surgery on the gastrointestinal tract is an extremely broad subject. This chapter discusses the care involved after surgery on the gastrointestinal tract, including the esophagus and the anus, as well as the accessory organs—the liver, gallbladder, pancreas, and spleen (Fig. 31–1). Surgery on the female reproductive organs, which are also contained within the abdominal cavity, is reviewed in Chapter 33. The care common to all patients undergoing abdominal surgery is discussed, and only the most important variations related to specific procedures are included.

Surgical intervention within the abdominal cavity is generally directed toward restoring normal function and therefore involves repair of congenital abnormalities, reconstruction of deformities, removal of obstructions to restore patency of the gastrointestinal tract and the biliary tract, treatment of malignancies, and maintenance of the integrity of related organs, such as the liver, pancreas, and spleen.

Definitions

Antrectomy: removal of the lower part of the stomach.

Appendectomy: removal of the vermiform appendix.

Cecostomy: creation of an opening for insertion of a tube into the cecum to decompress the bowel by removing air and accumulations of digestive juices.

Cholecystectomy: removal of the gallbladder; the procedure may be performed with an open or a laparoscopic approach with laser or electrosurgical cautery.

Cholecystostomy: establishment of an opening into the gallbladder to permit drainage of the organ and the removal of stones. This is performed infrequently except to provide relief in an extremely debilitated and unstable patient.

Colostomy: opening of the colon onto the abdomen; may be permanent or temporary, single or double lumen. May be performed with either an open procedure or a laparoscopic approach.

Diverticulum: a pouch opening from a hollow viscus, most commonly in the sigmoid colon.

Endoscopic retrograde cholangiopancreatography (ERCP): a side-viewing fiberoptic endoscope is used to cannulate pancreatic, biliary, and hepatic ducts through the ampulla of Vater for cholangiography, pancreatography, stone removal, and invasive manipulation such as sphincterotomy.

Endoscopy: visualization of a body cavity with a lighted tube or scope.

Esophagogastroduodenoscopy (EGD): passage of a fiberoptic gastroscope, usually under topical anesthesia and intravenous sedation, to view the esophagus, stomach, and duodenum.

Esophagoscopy: direct visualization of the esophagus and cardia of the stomach by means of a lighted instrument (esophagoscope). Esophagoscopy may be used to obtain a tissue biopsy or secretions for study to aid in diagnosis.

Gastrectomy: removal of the stomach. Usually a subtotal gastrectomy is done, in which part of the stomach is removed, expressed as a percentage (usually 60 to 80 percent but can be much as 95 percent); also called *gastric resection* (Fig. 31–2A).

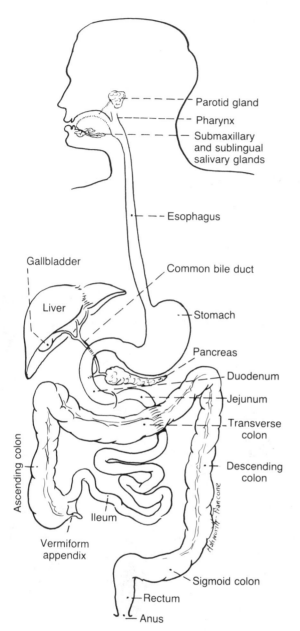

FIGURE 31–1. The digestive system and its associated structures. (From Jacob, S., and Francone, C.: Elements of Anatomy and Physiology. 2nd ed. Philadelphia, W. B. Saunders, 1989, p. 243.)

Gastroenterostomy: creation of an anastomosis between the posterior wall of the stomach near the antrum and the jejunum; used to treat pyloric obstruction (Fig. 31–2B).

Gastroscopy: direct inspection of the stomach and removal of a tissue specimen, if necessary, by means of a lighted instrument (gastroscope).

Hemorrhoidectomy: surgical excision of dilated veins of the rectum.

Hernia: the displacement of any viscus (usually bowel) or tissue through a congenital or acquired opening or defect in the wall of its natural cavity. Usually this term is applied to protrusion of abdominal viscera; however, it is actually the defect itself through which abdominal contents have protruded.

Herniorrhaphy: correction of a hernia, also termed *hernioplasty*. Hernias and herniorrhaphies are classified according to their anatomic sites and the condition of the viscus that has protruded. Reducible hernias are those in which the bowel or contents of the hernial sac can be replaced into their normal cavity. An irreducible, or incarcerated, hernia is one in which the contents cannot be replaced. A strangulated hernia is one in which the blood supply to the protruding segment of bowel is obstructed. When a segment of bowel becomes strangulated, it rapidly becomes necrotic. A strangulated hernia constitutes a surgical emergency.

Herniorrhaphy, diaphragmatic: replacement of abdominal contents that have entered the thorax through a defect in the diaphragm, and repair of the diaphragmatic defect.

Herniorrhaphy, epigastric and hypogastric: ligation of the peritoneal fat or hernial sac, with repair and closure of the abdominal wall.

Herniorrhaphy, femoral: removal and replacement of peritoneum that has protruded through the femoral ring, which is located just below Poupart's (inguinal) ligament and medial to the femoral vein, and repair of the defect in the transverse fascia at the exit of the femoral vessels. Femoral hernias are seldom found in children and occur most frequently in women.

Herniorrhaphy, hiatal: repair of herniation of a portion of the stomach through the esophageal hiatus of the diaphragm. Repair involves reduction through an abdominal or thoracic incision or via laparoscope (Fig. 31–3).

Herniorrhaphy, incisional: reunion in layers of the abdominal wall that may also involve placement of prosthetic (synthetic) mesh (e.g., Marlex, Gore-Tex).

Herniorrhaphy, inguinal: direct or indirect reconstruction of a weakened area in the abdominal wall, after reduction or repair of the opening through which tissue had been protruding.

Herniorrhaphy, sliding: the freeing and reducing of sliding viscus, and the repair of abdominal tissues surrounding and overlying the inguinal canal.

Herniorrhaphy, umbilical: closure of the peritoneal

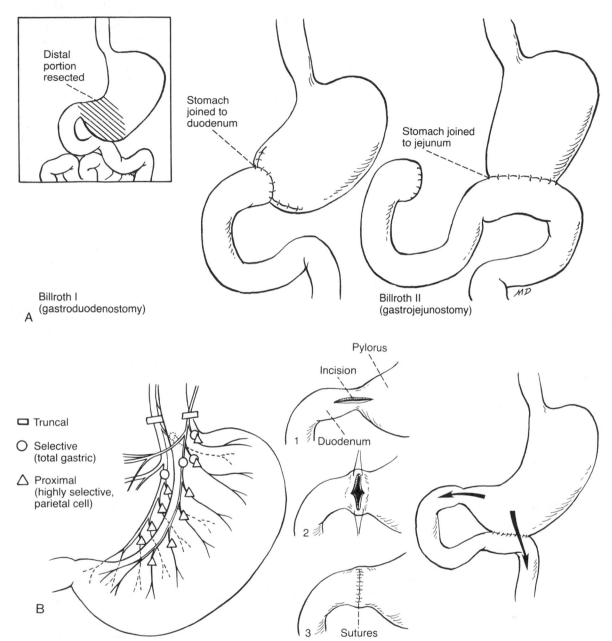

FIGURE 31–2. *A,* gastric surgical procedures: *Left,* vagotomy. *Middle,* pyloroplasty. *Right,* gastroenterostomy. *B,* gastric surgical procedures: Billroth I, Billroth II. (*A* and *B* from Black, J. M., and Matassarin-Jacobs, E.: Luckmann and Sorensen's Medical-Surgical Nursing: A Psychophysiologic Approach. 4th ed. Philadelphia, W. B. Saunders, 1993, p. 1619.)

opening and reconstruction of the abdominal wall surrounding the umbilicus (umbilical ring); usually occurs in pediatric patients and is most common in black infants.

Ileostomy: opening of the ileum to the surface of the abdomen. Used to treat inflammatory conditions of the bowel, such as ulcerative colitis and regional enteritis, and to provide a permanent or temporary stoma after emergency surgery for obstruction or cancer; usually a permanent surgical construction.

Intussusception: telescoping of the bowel into itself.

Laparoscopy (peritoneoscopy): direct visualization of the peritoneal cavity by means of a lighted instrument (often connected to a color video monitor) inserted through the abdominal wall via a stab wound. An increasing number of abdominal procedures are performed assisted by laparoscopy (lap assisted). Gastrointestinal or abdominal procedures currently performed via laparoscope include

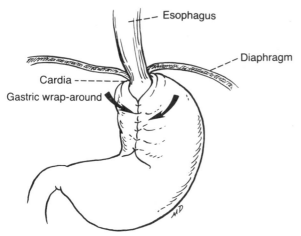

FIGURE 31–3. Hiatal hernia repair with gastric wrap (Nissen fundoplication). (From Black, J. M., and Matassarin-Jacobs, E.: Luckmann and Sorensen's Medical-Surgical Nursing: A Psychophysiologic Approach. 4th ed. Philadelphia, W. B. Saunders, 1993, p. 1590.)

cholecystectomy, truncal vagotomy and gastrojejunostomy, Nissen fundoplication, inguinal herniorrhaphy, appendectomy, colotomy with polypectomy, jejunostomy, colostomy, and ileocolectomy.

Laparotomy (celiotomy): an opening made through the abdominal wall into the peritoneal cavity, usually for exploratory purposes. If an abnormality is found, the operation is usually named according to the procedure or procedures carried out.

Pancreaticoduodenectomy (Whipple procedure): removal of the head of the pancreas, the entire duodenum, a portion of the jejunum, the distal third of the stomach, the lower half of the common bile duct, and a portion of the pancreatic duct, with re-establishment of continuity of the biliary, pancreatic, and gastrointestinal systems. The procedure, which is used primarily for the treatment of malignancy of the pancreas and duodenum, is associated with a 2 to 5 percent risk of mortality. Although this procedure was named for Whipple, who first described it, surgeons modify the operation as needed and rarely perform it in the original manner. The surgeon should explain to the post anesthesia care unit (PACU) nursing staff exactly what procedures were performed.

Percutaneous endoscopic gastrostomy (PEG): endoscopic procedure for the insertion of a gastrostomy tube, performed under local anesthesia and intravenous sedation, for patients who are poor risks for laparotomy or general anesthesia.

Pyloromyotomy (Fredet-Ramstedt operation): enlarging the lumen of the pylorus by longitudinally splitting the hypertrophied circular muscle without severing the mucosa; used as treatment for pyloric stenosis. Pyloric stenosis is most common in first-born male infants.

Pyloroplasty: a longitudinal incision made in the pylorus and closed transversely to permit the muscle to relax and establish an enlarged outlet. Heineke-Mikulicz is the most common type of procedure (see Fig. 31–2B).

Splenectomy: removal of the spleen.

Transduodenal sphincterotomy: partial division of the sphincter of Oddi and exploration of the common duct to treat recurrent attacks of acute pancreatitis due to formation of calculi in the pancreatic duct or blockage of the sphincter of Oddi. Pancreatic division may also be used for treatment.

Vagotomy: division (usually with frozen section) of branches of the vagus nerve that innervate the stomach to reduce secretions and movements (see Fig. 31–2B).

Volvulus: intestinal obstruction due to twisting of the bowel.

GENERAL CARE FOLLOWING ABDOMINAL SURGERY

Abdominal or gastrointestinal surgery may be performed with local, regional, or general anesthesia. The choice of anesthesia varies with the type of procedure, the patient's cardiac and pulmonary status, together with the surgeon's need for muscle relaxation. Usually, only the simpler procedures are performed under local or regional (spinal or epidural) anesthesia. Diagnostic procedures such as endoscopy, biopsy, and percutaneous gastrostomy are frequently performed under local anesthesia with appropriate sedation. Inguinal or femoral herniorrhaphies are often performed with local, spinal or epidural, or general anesthesia and sedation. Most other abdominal surgical and laparoscopic procedures are performed under general anesthesia.

A number of abdominopelvic incisions have been developed and are commonly used (Fig. 31–4). An ideal incision ensures ease of entrance, maximal exposure of the operative site, and minimal trauma. It should also provide good primary wound healing with maximal wound strength.

The reader should review Chapters 19 through 21 for general care following surgery.

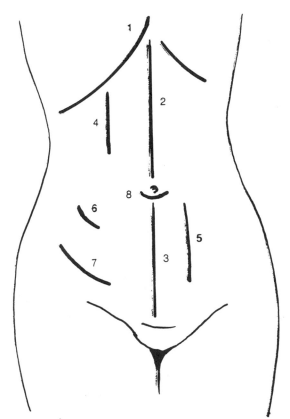

FIGURE 31–4. Commonly used abdominal incisions: 1. Kocher's incision: right side, gallbladder and biliary tract surgery; left side, splenectomy. 2. Upper abdominal midline incision: rapid entry to control bleeding ulcer. 3. Lower abdominal midline incision: female reproductive system. 4. Upper paramedian incision: right side, biliary tract surgery, cholecystectomy; left side, splenectomy, gastrectomy, vagotomy, hiatal hernia repair. 5. Lower paramedian incision: right side, appendectomy, small bowel resection; left side, sigmoid colon resection. 6. McBurney's incision: appendectomy. 7. Inguinal incision: inguinal herniorrhaphy. 8. Infraumbilical: umbilical herniorrhaphy.

PACU Care

As with any procedure, the surgeon and anesthesia care provider should give the PACU nurse a full report on the anesthesia used and the procedure performed. With complicated abdominal procedures, especially those that involve extensive resection or rerouting of the gastrointestinal tract, or both, the surgeon may draw a diagram of the procedure performed, along with the incisions and drainage tubes present. This assists those caring for the patient in an assessment of the wounds, dressings, and expected drainage. The surgeon can draw this diagram on the nursing care plan, which should be initiated on the patient's admission to the PACU, so that continuity of information is ensured.

Positioning

Following abdominal surgery, patients are often positioned on their sides until laryngeal reflexes have started to return. They are then placed in a semi-Fowler's position to ease the tension on suture lines and to promote respiratory effort. Following some procedures on the esophagus, however, patients should be kept flat to avoid tension on the suture line. Following hemorrhoidectomy, patients may assume any position of comfort, which will most likely be on their sides.

Dressings and Drains

All dressings should be checked. It is important for the nurse to know what kind of incision was used and whether any drains are in place. If drains are in place, considerably more drainage can be expected than if there are none. Drains are discussed in more detail under the specific procedures. Drainage should be assessed for character, volume, and odor. The nurse should determine who can or should remove the dressing if needed. Some surgeons reinforce the abdominal incision and dressing with a binder. They believe that this gives the incision valuable support. Others, however, believe that binders restrict respiratory effort and that this disadvantage outweighs the limited advantage of incisional support.

Because drainage is often copious after gastrointestinal surgery, frequent reinforcement of dressings may be necessary. Ask the surgeon for anticipated or expected amounts of drainage for this patient and his or her procedure. If drainage becomes excessive (more than expected from the particular procedure), the surgeon should be notified and the incision directly inspected.

All tubes should be connected to the appropriate drainage device, usually straight-gravity or suction drainage, as the surgeon specifies. Maintenance of the patency of these tubes is one of the most important nursing functions following gastrointestinal surgery. Irrigation of nasogastric tubes after esophageal or gastric surgery should be directed by the surgeon's orders.

Respiratory Function

The promotion of good respiratory function is a nursing priority for the patient who has had abdominal surgery. Painful abdominal incisions cause the patient to restrict chest expansion voluntarily. This is especially true with high abdominal incisions. The patient must be coached frequently in doing sustained maximal inspirations, coughing, and changing position to prevent respiratory complications. Assisting the patient by the splinting of the incision and judiciously using pain medications aid in deep breathing and coughing and prevent the development of atelectasis. Coughing and incentive spirometry in the PACU setting are valuable in promoting respiratory function.

Frequent assessment of breath sounds during the postoperative period can alert the nurse to impending respiratory problems. An accidental nick into the diaphragm during upper abdominal surgery is possible, and breath sounds must be monitored closely to check for pneumothorax.

Fluid and Electrolyte Balance

Fluid and electrolyte shifts or losses can be substantial during gastrointestinal surgery. Losses continue postoperatively through gastrointestinal tubes or other drains. For this reason, accurate intake and output records are mandatory. This begins with the intake and output report from the anesthesia care provider, which should be the first PACU entry. All drainage from incisions should be included in the assessment of electrolyte balance. Frequent serum electrolyte determinations may be necessary if losses are great. Intravenous fluids are used for replacement for at least the first 24 hours postoperatively and until the nasogastric tubes are removed. The reader is referred to Chapter 9 to review the specific problems in electrolyte loss from the gastrointestinal tract.

Urinary retention may become a problem following abdominal surgery, owing to incisional pain, opioid analgesics, anesthetics, and physiologic splinting. Urine output should be checked frequently and accurate records kept. The nurse should also check for bladder distention and document the findings. (The patient may not recognize the need to void, especially following spinal or epidural anesthesia.) The patient should void within 6 to 8 hours postoperatively. If the patient has not voided by the time of discharge from the PACU, notify the receiving unit to check specifically for urinary retention. If permissible, it may help the male patient to stand to void. If urinary retention causes pain, distends the abdomen, or becomes prolonged, urinary catheterization may become necessary. Patients who have had extensive surgery often return to the PACU with a urinary catheter in place. Accurate output records should be maintained.

Care of the Patient with Nasogastric or Intestinal Tubes

Anesthesia and manipulation of the viscera during surgery cause gastric and colonic peristalsis to diminish or disappear completely for 24 to 72 hours afterward. Nasogastrointestinal or nasogastric tubes are commonly used postoperatively to prevent the sequelae of this hypomotility. Edema at the operative site also can result in obstruction. Decompression of the stomach, with removal of accumulated fluid and air, not only prevents vomiting and eases tension on the abdominal suture line but also increases the area's vascularity and so improves its nutrition and reduces the risk of gastric anastomotic leak.

Both short and long tubes can be used, depending on the operative site. Short tubes used include the Levin, the Rehfuss, and the plastic Salem sump, which is a double-lumen nasogastric tube and is the most commonly used tube. The double lumen prevents excessive negative pressure from developing when the tube is connected to suction. Long tubes that may be used to decompress the intestine preoperatively include the Harris, Cantor, Miller-Abbott, and Abbott-Rawson. Baker tubes are often passed during reoperative procedures for severe adhesive obstruction.

When the patient returns from the operating suite with a nasogastric tube in place, the nurse must ascertain why the tube was placed, where it was placed, and whether it should be connected to suction or to straight-gravity drainage. Frequently, the physician will order the tube to be connected to low-pressure, intermittent suction (20 to 80 mm Hg). Usually, only low-pressure, intermittent suction is used because excessive negative pressure in either the stomach or the bowel pulls the mucosa into the lumen of the tube and can cause traumatic ulcers. For double-lumen nasogastric tubes, continuous suction at 40 to 60 mm Hg is usually ordered and necessary for the tube to function properly.

Tube Patency

Patency of the tube must be ensured. The nurse should observe for drainage from the tube. All characteristics of the drainage must be noted: consistency, color, odor, quantity, and any deviations from the expected drainage. After gastrointestinal surgery, initial drainage is bright red in small volumes, but it should become dark after 24 hours. Bloody drainage should not be expected from a nasogastric tube placed only for decompression of the stomach after biliary tract, liver, or splenic surgery. If no drainage is present, if the patient's abdomen becomes distended, or if the patient vomits around the nasogastric tube or complains of nausea, the tube may be clogged or the suction apparatus may be malfunctioning; check both. To maintain the patency of the nasogastric tube, irrigation with 20 to 30 ml of normal saline may be done every hour or more frequently if necessary. Plain water in 20-ml amounts may be used to irrigate the tube without creating electrolyte abnormalities. Larger amounts of plain water should not be used when irrigating for gastric bleeding because of the large volume and the risk of electrolyte alterations. Before any type of irrigation, check with the surgeon, especially after esophageal or gastric procedures. Frequent irrigations increase the loss of electrolytes from the gastrointestinal system. Some surgeons advocate the use of air to irrigate the nasogastric tube to maintain patency.

Irrigation

The amount of irrigating solution instilled should be recorded as such, unless its equivalent is aspirated by syringe. All gastrointestinal drainage should be accurately measured and recorded. The long gastrointestinal tubes can be irrigated in the same way as nasogastric tubes; however, because the tube is so much longer, the irrigating fluid rarely fully returns, so how much irrigating fluid was instilled should always be noted on the intake and output record. If irrigations do not increase drainage, the tubing should be checked for clogs by milking it toward the suction container to dislodge any obstruction. The suction apparatus is checked by disconnecting the nasogastric tube at the junction of the nasogastric tube and the drainage tube leading to the container. With the suction turned on, the end of the drainage tube is placed in a glass of water; if the water is sucked up, the suction device is functioning. If these measures fail, gastric mucosa may be occluding the lumen of the tube or the tube may be kinked. In this instance, the patient or the tube may need to be repositioned. If the patient has had gastric, pancreatic, or esophageal surgery, the tube should not be manipulated; the surgeon should be notified of its malfunctioning.

Patient Comfort

The presence of a nasogastric or long gastrointestinal tube is a most uncomfortable experience for the patient. However, appropriate nursing care can relieve sore throat, dry mouth, hoarseness, earache, sore nose, and dry lips. Ensure that the tube is taped securely and properly (hypoallergenic tape is best) in a position to prevent pressure on the naris. The tube may be secured to the upper lip or nose in the position it naturally assumes. The tube should not be taped to the patient's nose and then to the forehead. This causes pressure on the underside of the nostril and can cause tissue necrosis. To lessen the pressure and pull on the patient's nose, either tape or pin the tube to the gown.

Apply petrolatum ointment to the tube where it enters the nose and around the naris. The outside portion of the tube is kept free of mucus or other drainage. This prevents encrustations from forming and reduces irritation of the nostril. Petrolatum ointment, cream, or Chap Stick is applied to the lips to keep them soft and prevent cracking. Good, frequent mouth care is essential for the comfort of the patient and to prevent parotitis. Lemon-glycerine swabs, mouthwash, or even a toothbrush may be used to provide mouth care for the patient. Simply ensure that the patient understands not to swallow any of the material used. This, of course, would not be fatal but could be detrimental to fluid and electrolyte balance.

Gargles with warm tap water or warm saline, or with viscous lidocaine (Xylocaine), or applications of a local anesthetic spray relieve the patient's sore throat. A physician's order should be provided for these measures. Some surgeons allow their patients to suck on isotonic ice chips or hard candy or to chew gum. Anesthetic throat lozenges, if allowed, are comforting to the patient. All patients with a gastrointestinal tube in place are given essentially nothing by mouth until the tube is removed. The only exception may be certain medications, given orally or through the tube or ice chips, less than 200 ml every 8 hours.

DIAGNOSTIC STUDIES

Invasive diagnostic procedures are occasionally done at the patient's bedside on the nursing unit, but they are more frequently done in a special procedures room, often located within the surgical suite. They require local anesthesia and appropriate sedation or sometimes general anesthesia. Patients may be sent to the PACU for a brief observation period. Care after endoscopy includes all the general care afforded a post anesthesia patient. After esophagoscopy and gastroscopy, the nurse should be alert for the return of the gag reflex. When pharyngeal reflexes have returned, unless contraindicated by the diagnosis or in anticipation of further surgery, the patient may be started on liquids and may progress to a regular diet as tolerated. Rest is the most important treatment for this patient. There may be bleeding, swelling, or dysfunction of the involved area, indicating complications from the procedure.

Patients who have had laparoscopy (peritoneoscopy) have only small bandages or tape strip closures (Steri-Strips) over the stab wounds used for entry of the scope and its accessories. These bandages should remain clean and dry. These patients are probably apprehensive about what was discovered about their conditions during the diagnostic procedure and should be given accurate information by the surgeon following the procedure. The nurse should be familiar with what the patients have been told to interpret or repeat the information for them, if necessary.

CARE FOLLOWING SURGERY ON THE GASTROINTESTINAL TRACT

Esophagus

Surgery on the esophagus includes repair of hiatal hernia and various forms of tracheoesophageal fistulas, excision of esophageal diverticula, treatment of stenosis of the lower end of the esophagus, esophagomyotomy, esophagectomy, and cardiomyotomy.

Postoperative care depends on the kind of incision used to expose the operative site: abdominal or thoracic. Surgery on the esophagus frequently involves a thoracic incision. Care for the patient following a thoracic incision is discussed in Chapter 25. Procedures on the esophagus are performed under general anesthesia. Frequently, a tracheostomy is performed (see Chapter 23 for care of the patient following tracheostomy).

On arrival to the PACU, the patient should be placed in a semi-Fowler's position. This aids in the drainage of blood from the pleural space and prevents tension from impinging on the suture lines. The incision is generally long (from the tip of the scapula to the seventh or eighth rib area) and painful. Analgesics must be given in adequate doses to promote rest and adequate respiratory effort. An interpleural or epidural catheter often is in place for postoperative analgesia. Patient-controlled analgesia may be used. Transcutaneous electrical nerve stimulation (TENS) may also provide incisional pain relief.

A nasogastric tube will be in place and should be cared for as previously discussed. It should not be manipulated by the nurse. Chest tubes should be managed as discussed in Chapter 25. A large sterile dressing should be in place, and it should be checked frequently for drainage and reinforced as necessary. Excessive bloody drainage should be reported to the surgeon.

Stomach

Surgery on the stomach involves procedures to treat ulcers (antrectomy and vagotomy, gastric resection, gastrectomy); removal of portions of the stomach, for malignancy; and rerouting of the gastrointestinal system at this point to treat pyloric obstruction. All postoperative care of the patient is generally the same, and anesthesia is general. The patient should be placed in a semi-Fowler's position postoperatively to relieve tension on the suture line and to promote drainage. The abdominal incisions are fairly high, long, and painful, and particular attention must be paid to pulmonary toilet. This type of patient must be encouraged more frequently than any other to expand the lungs and to cough and must generally have assistance to change position. Assistance in splinting the wound with the hands or with a firm pillow is most appreciated by the patient. These procedures generally produce considerable postoperative pain, and analgesics should be used generously but judiciously. Patient-controlled or epidural analgesia may be effective for upper abdominal incisional and visceral pain.

A nasogastric tube will be in place and should be cared for as previously discussed. Small volumes of bright, bloody drainage from the nasogastric tube can be expected for the first 2 to 3 hours, because it is not uncommon to have bleeding at the anastomotic site in these procedures. However, bright bleeding that does not decrease after this period or bleeding that becomes excessive (more than 75 ml/hr) should be reported immediately to the surgeon. Observe the nasogastric tube and its drainage closely because blood easily clots and clogs the tube; notify the surgeon immediately if the tube stops draining or appears obstructed with blood. Because blood loss may be highly significant in this patient, cardiovascular status must receive careful scrutiny. Vital signs are checked frequently, and a certain amount of hypotension and tachycardia is to be expected. If hypotension and tachycardia persist or maintain a downward trend, the surgeon should be notified.

Blood replacement may have to be instituted. Hemoglobin and hematocrit levels should be determined 4 to 6 hours postoperatively and the surgeon notified if they are significantly lower than previous determinations. Little or no drainage should be expected from the incision unless drains are in place. If drainage does appear, the dressing should be reinforced, and the surgeon notified. The initial dressing should not be replaced by the nurse in the PACU unless so directed by the surgeon. Drains with copious output may need a drainage device applied over them to protect the patient's skin and allow for accurate measurement of drainage.

Urinary retention is commonly a problem, and many surgeons prefer to insert a Foley catheter while the patient is in the operating room. Accurate measurements of output should be ascertained. If a urinary catheter is not in place, the patient should be checked frequently for bladder distention, which may indicate an overfull bladder and urinary retention. If the patient is unable to void, a catheterization order should be obtained.

Perforated Ulcer. Perforation of an ulcer is usually a surgical emergency, and neither the patient nor the family members will be adequately prepared, either physically or emotionally, for the surgery. This is of concern to the PACU nurse because complications, especially hypovolemia and shock, may more readily occur in this patient.

Pyloric Stenosis. Specific care for infants following surgery for pyloric stenosis is detailed in pediatric texts. However, the PACU nurse should be aware of their general care. Position is important. The infant should be kept either on the right side or on the abdomen until the danger of vomiting and aspiration has subsided, then should be placed in an upright position. Careful placement of the diaper is important to avoid contamination of the wound. It may also be helpful to apply a pediatric urine collector not only to prevent contamination of the wound with urine but also to determine accurate output. Feedings are usually begun for these infants 4 to 6 hours postoperatively, but the surgeon's instructions should be explicitly followed.

Small Bowel

Operations on the small bowel include exploratory laparotomy with lysis of adhesions and resection for obstruction or perforation. Care following these procedures is essentially the same as that already mentioned. The patient may have a long gastrointestinal tube in place that should be cared for as noted earlier. No excessive drainage from incisions should be noted, unless drains have been placed. Fluid and electrolyte balance must be monitored carefully. Remember that the loss of sodium and bicarbonate ions will be great, resulting in imbalance, and that fluid losses during surgery may be significant, but fluid overload must be avoided.

The patient with an ileostomy will enter the PACU with a bag in place over the stoma, and returns may be expected almost at once; these should be recorded. Particular attention must be paid to this stoma, the drainage, and the collection device; no leakage onto the skin should be allowed, because this causes significant skin damage. Under the collection device, the peristomal skin is protected with a skin barrier that includes pectin-based and karaya-based wafers or paste.

Large Bowel

Surgery on the large bowel includes appendectomy, colostomy (for obstruction), sigmoid colon resection, herniorrhaphy, removal of tumors or correction of deformities, total proctocolectomy with ileoanal anastomosis (Fig. 31–5), and abdominoperineal resection (Fig. 31–6). Herniorrhaphy is frequently done under spinal anesthesia with appropriate sedation. All other surgical procedures are usually performed under general anesthesia. On return to the PACU, patients are kept flat and on one side until the reflexes have returned; they may then assume a position of comfort unless otherwise specified by the surgeon. Postoperative care is essentially the same as for small bowel surgery.

If the patient returns from surgery with a colostomy, some special care is required. It is unusual for the colostomy to start functioning immediately postoperatively; however, spillage must be prevented from contaminating the incision or excoriating the skin. A pouch or collection device may be in place over the colostomy. The skin around the stoma should be protected with an appropriate skin barrier if drainage is present. Check the color of the stoma—it should be bright red and moist—and document its appearance in the nursing record.

Fluid and electrolyte balance must be monitored carefully. If diverticula were resected, the

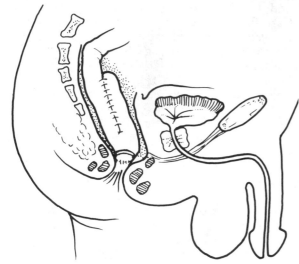

FIGURE 31–5. Ileoanal anastomosis with J-pouch for treatment of ulcerative colitis. (From Black, J. M., and Matassarin-Jacobs, E.: Luckmann and Sorensen's Medical-Surgical Nursing: A Psychophysiologic Approach. 4th ed. Philadelphia, W. B. Saunders, 1993, p. 1645.)

nurse must watch carefully for blood in the urine. Some blood-tinged urine may be expected after colectomy, because retractors used in surgery may have caused contusions of the bladder; however, gross blood may indicate that the bladder was more severely injured. Dressings should remain dry, unless drains were placed in the wound. If drains were placed, some bloody drainage may be expected, and dressings should be reinforced as necessary. If dressings soak through, the drainage should be considered excessive and must be reported to the surgeon.

Incisions may be left open to heal with delayed primary closure. Abdominal wounds for bowel surgery may be contaminated (e.g., traumatic penetrating injuries, colostomies) with an increased risk of infection. The wound is left open, protected with moist gauze, and when clean and red, closed with sutures that were placed during the original surgery and left slack. The cleanliness of the wound and the health of the granulation tissue in the wound generally determine the best time for closure.

Abdominoperineal Resection. Abdominoperineal resection for cancer of the rectum is a most traumatic procedure. Vital signs are monitored carefully, and any adverse trend reported. Shock is one of the frequent complications encountered following this procedure. Blood loss may exceed 2000 ml, and fluid replacement and transfusion during surgery may be inadequate owing to inaccurate loss estimates. Perineal drains will be in place and should be noted on the patient's chart and nursing care plan. The perineal dressings frequently become saturated with bloody drainage and must be reinforced. If drainage remains bright and obviously new bleeding is occurring, and if frequent dressing changes are required, the surgeon should be notified. If sump catheters are used to drain the perineal wound, they may be attached to a grenade or bulb (Jackson-Pratt) device and an accurate measurement of drainage may be obtained.

The patient who has undergone abdominoperineal surgery will have a colostomy. Check the blood supply to the stoma frequently, because impaired blood supply is an early and serious complication. Pain may be severe and should be relieved with adequate doses of

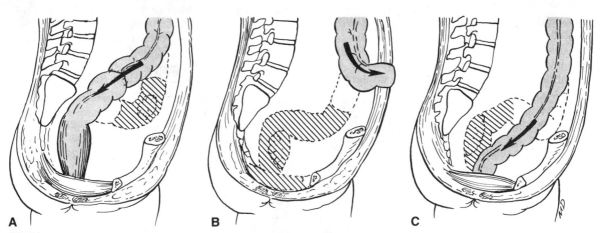

FIGURE 31–6. Large bowel procedures for resection of malignancy: *A,* anterior resection with primary anastomosis. *B,* abdominoperineal (anteroposterior) resection with permanent colostomy. *C,* proctosigmoidectomy with "pull through." (*A* to *C* from Black, J. M., and Matassarin-Jacobs, E.: Luckmann and Sorensen's Medical-Surgical Nursing: A Psychophysiologic Approach. 4th ed. Philadelphia, W. B. Saunders, 1993, p. 1653.)

opioid analgesics or use of an epidural catheter for analgesia to ensure comfort of the patient and promote respiratory sufficiency.

Appendectomy and Herniorrhaphy. Patients who have undergone surgery for appendectomy or herniorrhaphy usually return to the PACU almost fully awake and without serious postoperative complications. No nasogastric tube, Foley catheter, or drain will be in place, and recovery is generally uneventful. However, patients who have large ventral hernia repairs with mesh will have nasogastric tubes and drains in place. Patients may assume a position of comfort as soon as pharyngeal reflexes have returned, and they may start on a progressive diet as tolerated. All the postoperative care outlined in Chapters 19 and 20 is applicable. When the laparoscopic approach is used, general anesthesia usually is given. Patients may complain of shoulder pain or bloating owing to the insufflation of air and of sore throat from intubation and the neuromuscular blocking agents. Monitor fluid intake, and replace fluid losses appropriately. Dressings should remain dry and intact, and any postoperative incisional bleeding or drainage should be reported to the surgeon. The most important postoperative complication is bleeding. The nurse should also watch for urinary retention. If the patient has undergone inguinal hernia repair, the nurse should watch for development of scrotal edema or hematoma, which may indicate slow bleeding from the operative site.

Lower Rectum and Anus

Surgery on the lower rectum and anus includes excision of pilonidal cysts, rectal fissures, fistulas, rectal abscesses, tumors, and hemorrhoids. Post anesthesia nursing care is the same as for any patient undergoing anesthesia, which may be local, regional, or general. Dressings should be checked frequently for excessive drainage and bleeding. The incisions may be closed but frequently are packed to facilitate drainage of infected material and aid in healing. Urinary retention may be a problem, because the proximity of the bladder and operative site may make urination difficult. Pain can be exquisite, but patients are often embarrassed by the location of the operative site and may not ask for analgesia. The nurse should be alert to signs and symptoms of pain and discomfort and administer analgesia as necessary for relief.

SURGERY ON RELATED ORGANS WITHIN THE ABDOMINAL CAVITY

Liver

Surgery on the liver includes biopsy, small wedge biopsy, excision of tumors, major resection, repair of traumatic lacerations, and hepatic transplant.

Liver biopsy is a common procedure, usually performed in the endoscopy suite, although the patient may be taken to the operating suite and may return to the PACU for a short period of observation. Postoperative care depends on the type of anesthesia used; it is usually local but may involve other types if the patient cannot or will not cooperate. The patient should remain positioned on the right side for at least 2 hours after the procedure. Vital signs should be determined frequently: every 10 to 15 minutes for the first hour and every 30 minutes for the second hour. Complications include hemorrhage due to penetration of a blood vessel and peritonitis due to accidental puncture of the bile duct. If the patient's vital signs begin a downward trend, and if he or she reports severe abdominal pain or becomes febrile, the surgeon should be notified immediately.

Open surgery on the liver for the excision of tumors or the repair of lacerations is done under general anesthesia and involves a fairly long upper abdominal vertical or bilateral subcostal oblique (chevron) incision. All care previously discussed for patients following general anesthesia and upper abdominal incisions applies. Respiratory care is of paramount importance. The liver is an extremely vascular and friable organ. It is difficult to suture, and gross bleeding is common and frequently involves large blood losses, especially when surgery is necessitated by traumatic injury or massive resection. Large drains of the Penrose or suction (grenade or bulb [Jackson-Pratt]) type are placed in the region of the laceration or excision of the tumor and are brought through separate sites to the skin surface. For the first 8 hours, expect approximately 250 to 500 ml of sanguinous drainage from the drains.

Coagulation studies must be performed frequently and monitored closely, because many patients develop coagulation abnormalities during and after liver surgery. Specific coagulation factors may be administered, according to the results of the coagulation tests. Hypoglycemia must be avoided. Patients will soon start on peripheral intravenous dextrose 10 percent solutions, total parenteral nutrition, or feeding jejunostomy infusions.

Vital signs must be determined frequently, and any downward trend reported to the surgeon at once. Blood replacement or hemostasis may be inadequate. Frequently, this patient will also have a T-tube in place in the common bile duct (Fig. 31–7). This tube should be attached to straight-gravity drainage, and accurate measurements of the output should be made. A nasogastric tube will be in place and should be cared for as discussed previously. Pain is usually severe, and opioid analgesics or epidural analgesia are necessary to promote rest and respiratory effort.

Spleen

Surgery on the spleen involves general anesthesia and removal of the organ. The spleen is removed because of rupture from trauma; accidental trauma from associated surgery; diseases that cause damage, such as mononucleosis and malaria; and hypersplenism. A midline or left subcostal incision is used. Postoperative care for the patient after splenectomy is the same as that for the patient following repair of a lacerated liver. Dressings should remain dry and intact. A drain may be placed in the subdiaphragmatic space to prevent the collection of blood under the diaphragm and to detect unrecognized injury that may have occurred to the pancreas.

The PACU nurse should be knowledgeable of the circumstances leading to the patient's splenectomy. If it was necessitated by trauma, the nurse must be particularly alert for signs indicating that unrecognized complications from the accident may have developed. Vital signs should be determined frequently and trends watched, especially those indicating progressive bleeding. Neurologic signs should be checked, and the patient should be assessed carefully for any signs of injury to the extremities. Any arrhythmia should be reported, because this may indicate cardiac injury.

Pancreas

Surgery on the pancreas is precarious. It involves general anesthesia, and care for these patients is the same as for other postoperative patients. If the operative procedure done is to remove malignant tumors, a mortality rate of 2 to 7 percent is not unreasonable owing to extensive resection and poor general condition of the patient.

Postoperative care of the patient following a pancreaticoduodenectomy (Whipple or modified Whipple procedure) is one of the greatest nursing challenges. All postoperative care for

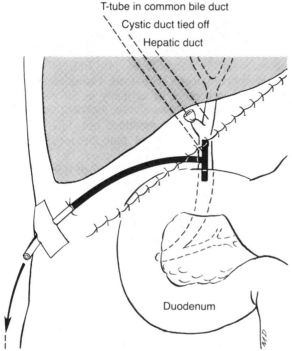

T-tube in common bile duct
Cystic duct tied off
Hepatic duct

Duodenum

To drainage collection

FIGURE 31–7. T-tube placement in common bile duct. (From Black, J. M., and Matassarin-Jacobs, E.: Luckmann and Sorensen's Medical-Surgical Nursing: A Psychophysiologic Approach. 4th ed. Philadelphia, W. B. Saunders, 1993, p. 1742.)

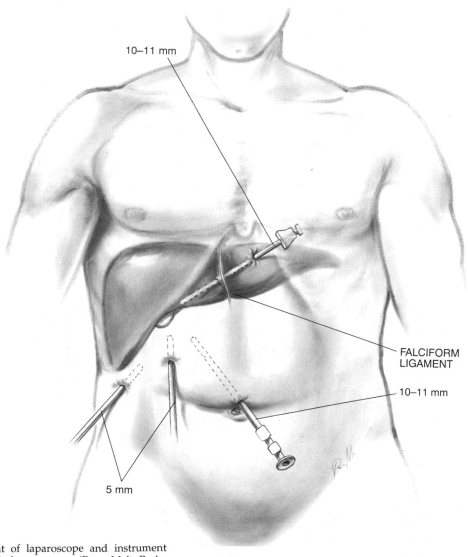

FIGURE 31–8. Placement of laparoscope and instrument ports for laparoscopic cholecystectomy. (From Malt, R. A.: The Practice of Surgery. Philadelphia, W. B. Saunders, 1993, p. 299.)

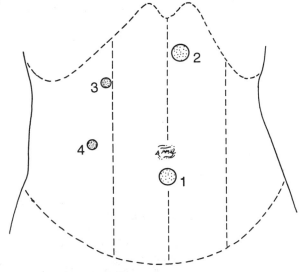

the abdominal surgery patient applies. Particular attention must be paid to drains and catheters. Surgeons should augment their reports to the nurse by explaining exactly what procedure was performed, where drains or wound catheters were placed, and how to care for them. Surgeons should brief the nurse on expected drainage and what should be considered excessive. As with all abdominal surgical patients, intravenous lines and intravenous therapy will already have been initiated. Because of the generally poor nutritional status of these patients, hyperalimentation may be started almost immediately postoperatively.

All respiratory, cardiac, and renal functioning must be monitored carefully and the surgeon notified of any untoward signs. Frequently, assisted ventilation is required for at least 24 hours following this procedure (this type of care is discussed in Chapter 19). Arterial blood gas analysis should be performed frequently for this patient, and an arterial line should be in place for this purpose. Blood gas analysis yields valuable information about the patient's respiratory acid-base status, which may be precarious. Urine output should be determined hourly, and at least 0.5 to 1 ml per kg per hr should be expected.

Frequent assays of blood glucose levels should be ordered on all patients following pancreatic surgery. Most of these patients need to receive intravenous insulin during the postoperative period. Insulin doses are titrated to maintain the blood glucose levels between 180 and 250 mg per dl. This aids in the prevention of hypoglycemia and hyperglycemia.

Large fluctuations in serum glucose levels or acid-base balance can precipitate electrolyte abnormalities in these patients. Potassium and calcium levels, in particular, should be monitored closely.

Biliary Tract

Surgery on the biliary tract includes exploration for removal of stones from the gallbladder and the ducts and removal of the gallbladder. Anesthesia is general, regional, or a combination of both. Currently, the standard is for laparoscopic cholecystectomy that may have been preceded by ERCP. Performed with a laparoscope, the patient has an umbilical incision and three or four abdominal stab wounds for instruments (Fig. 31–8). The open incision is either a right subcostal or a midline incision. On return to the PACU, the patient is placed in a semi-Fowler's position. All tubes must be cared for appropriately. A nasogastric tube will be placed intraoperatively and is often removed when the operative procedure ends. A T-tube will have been placed in the common bile duct if the common duct was opened during surgery. This tube is usually connected to straight-gravity drainage to a bile bag. Careful attention must be paid to maintaining the patency of this tube and its attachment to the patient; the surgeon needs to be called immediately if the tube is dislodged.

Bile drainage should be carefully measured and accurately reported. Between 200 and 500 ml of bile drainage can be expected within a 24-hour period. If more than 25 ml per hr of bile is drained, the surgeon should be notified, because this may indicate severance of the common bile duct, obstruction, or biliary fistula. Dressings should remain dry and intact, unless Penrose drains have been placed. If drains are placed, blood-bile drainage may be expected, and dressings should be reinforced as necessary to keep the surrounding skin dry.

As with all upper abdominal incisions, pain is a problem, and analgesics (intermittent, continuous, or patient controlled), epidural analgesia, TENS, and relaxation exercises should be used to promote rest and respiratory effort. Morphine sulfate should not be used for analgesia, because it may cause biliary spasm. Any downward trend in vital signs, excessive bleeding from the incision, or bleeding noted in the bile drainage from the T-tube should be reported to the surgeon. Bleeding from the cystic artery is a serious complication and can lead to rapid deterioration in the patient's status.

Following laparoscopic cholecystectomy, the patient may be one of the most stable of any seen in the PACU. Any patient with unexplained pain, oliguria, or hypotension should be immediately discussed with the surgeon. Complications of gas embolism, deep vein thrombophlebitis, subcutaneous emphysema, injuries to major vessels and intestine, and bile leakage all have been reported following laparoscopic procedures.

References

1. Acute Pain Management Guideline Panel: Acute Pain Management: Operative or Medical Procedures and Trauma: Clinical Practice Guideline (AHCPR Publication No. 92-0032). Rockville, MD, Agency for Health Care Policy and Research, Public Health Service, US Department of Health and Human Services, February 1992.
2. Amato, E. J.: A nursing reference: Gastrointestinal tubes and drains: I. Crit. Care Nurs., 2(6):50–57, 1982.
3. Amato, E. J.: A nursing reference: Gastrointestinal tubes and drains: II. Crit. Care Nurs., 3(1):46–48, 1983.

4. Beckermann, S., and Galloway, S.: Elective resection of the liver: Nursing care. Crit. Care Nurs., *9*(10):40–49, 1989.

5. Black, J. M., and Matassarin-Jacobs, E.: Luckmann and Sorensen's Medical-Surgical Nursing: A Psychophysiologic Approach. 4th ed. Philadelphia, W. B. Saunders, 1993.

6. Braasch, J. W.: Laparoscopic cholecystectomy. *In* Atlas of Abdominal Surgery. Philadelphia, W. B. Saunders, 1991, pp 309–318.

7. Brozenec, S. A.: Caring for the postoperative patient with an abdominal drain. Nursing 85, *15*:55–57, 1985.

8. Clochesy, J. M., Breu, C., Cardin, S., et al (eds): Critical Care Nursing. Philadelphia, W. B. Saunders, 1993.

9. Gadacz, T. R., Talamini, M. A., Lillemoe, K. D., et al: Laparoscopic cholecystectomy. Surg. Clin. North Am., *70*(6):1249–1262, 1990.

10. Given, B., and Simmons, S.: Gastroenterology in Clinical Nursing. 4th ed. St. Louis, C. V. Mosby, 1984.

11. Jackson, D. C., Martin, T., Evans, M. M., et al: Endoscopic laser cholecystectomy. AORN J., *51*(6):1546–1552, 1990.

12. Kemp, D., and Tabaka, N.: Postoperative urinary retention: II. A retrospective study. J. Post Anesth. Nurs., *5*(6):397–400, 1990.

13. Moody, F. G., Carey, L., Jones, S., et al (eds): Surgical Treatment of Digestive Disease. 2nd ed. Chicago, Year Book, 1990.

14. Nora, P. F. (ed): Operative Surgery: Principles and Techniques. 3rd ed. Philadelphia, W. B. Saunders, 1990.

15. O'Brien, D. D.: The gastrointestinal surgical patient. *In* Litwack, K. (ed): Core Curriculum for Post Anesthesia Nursing Practice. Philadelphia, W. B. Saunders, 1994.

16. O'Brien, D. D., and Burden, N.: The ASC as a special procedures unit. *In* Burden, N. (ed): Ambulatory Surgical Nursing. Philadelphia, W. B. Saunders, 1993, pp 556–583.

17. O'Toole, M. T.: Advanced assessment of the abdomen and gastrointestinal problems. Nurs. Clin. North Am. *25*(4):771–776, 1990.

18. Phippen, M. L., and Wells, M. P.: Perioperative Nursing Practice. Philadelphia, W. B. Saunders, 1994.

19. Sabiston, D. C.: Atlas of General Surgery. Philadelphia, W. B. Saunders, 1994.

20. Sabiston, D. C. (ed): Textbook of Surgery. 14th ed. Philadelphia, W. B. Saunders, 1991.

21. Stillman, A.: Laparoscopic cholecystectomy. AORN J., *57*(2):429–436, 1993.

22. Surratt, S., Ryan, A. B., Hallenbeck, P., et al: Troubleshooting a sump tube. Am. J. Nurs., *93*(1):42–47, 1993.

23. Thompson, J., McFarland, G., Hirsch, J., et al: Mosby's Manual of Clinical Nursing. 3rd ed. St. Louis, C. V. Mosby, 1993.

24. Urban, M.: Endoscopic retrograde cholangiopancreatography: A diagnostic outpatient procedure. AORN J., *50*:572–581, 1989.

Post Anesthesia Care of the Genitourinary Surgical Patient

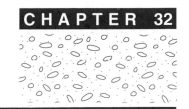

CHAPTER 32

Kathleen Millican Miller, M.S.N., R.N., C.P.A.N.

Genitourinary surgery involves procedures performed on the kidney, ureters, bladder, urethra, and male genitalia. Problems may be congenital or acquired. Adrenalectomy is included in this chapter for convenience and because of the proximity of the adrenal glands to the kidneys.

Definitions

Cystoscopy: direct visualization of the urethra, prostatic urethra, and bladder by means of a tubular lighted telescopic lens.

Renal and Ureteral Surgery

Extracorporeal shock wave lithotripsy: use of shock waves through a liquid medium into the body to disintegrate stones.
Heminephrectomy: partial excision of the kidney.
Kidney transplant: removal of a donor kidney by means of a nephrectomy and ureterectomy, followed by transplantation of the donor kidney into the recipient's iliac fossa.
Nephrectomy: removal of a kidney; used to treat some congenital unilateral abnormalities causing renal obstruction or hydronephrosis; sometimes necessitated by the presence of tumors and following severe injuries.
Nephrostomy: an opening into the kidney to maintain temporary or permanent drainage.
Nephrotomy: an incision into the kidney.
Nephroureterectomy: removal of a kidney and the entire ureter that drains it.
Percutaneous nephrolithotomy: removal or disintegration of renal stones by passage of a nephroscope through a percutaneous nephrostomy tract.
Pyeloplasty: revision or reconstruction of the renal pelvis.
Pyelostomy: an incision into the renal pelvis to establish drainage or to permit irrigation of the renal pelvis.
Pyelotomy: incision into the renal pelvis.
Ureterectomy: complete removal of one or both of the ureters.
Ureterolithotomy: incision into the ureter and removal of stones.
Ureteroneocystostomy (ureterovesical anastomosis; vesicopsoas hitch procedure): division of the ureter from the urinary bladder and reimplantation of the ureter into the bladder at another site.
Ureteroplasty: reconstruction of the ureter.
Ureterostomy, cutaneous (anastomosis of transplant; Bricker operation; ureteroileostomy): diversion of the urinary stream by anastomosing the ureters into an isolated loop of ileum that is brought out through the abdominal wall as an ileostomy (Fig. 32–1).

Bladder Surgery

Bladder neck operation (Y-V plasty): a plastic repair of the bladder neck done to correct stricture.
Cystectomy: excision of the bladder and adjacent structures; may be partial, to excise a lesion, or total, to excise a malignant tumor. This operation usually involves the additional procedure of ureterostomy.
Cystolithotomy: opening of the bladder to remove stones.
Cystotomy: an incision into the bladder.
Vesicourethral suspension (Marshall-Marchetti operation): suspension of the bladder neck to the posterior surface of the pubis in women to treat stress incontinence.

Prostatic Surgery

Prostatectomy: enucleation of prostatic adenomas or hypertrophied masses.

Scrotal Surgery

Epididymectomy: excision of the epididymis from the testis. This procedure is rarely done but

463

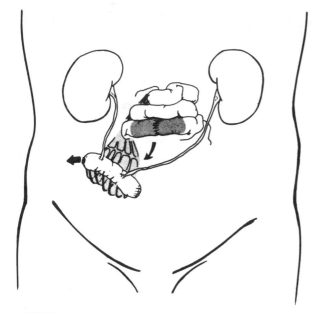

FIGURE 32–1. Ileal conduit, showing ileal segment with anastomosed ureters. (From LeMaitre, G. D., and Finnegan, J. A.: The Patient in Surgery: A Guide for Nurses. 4th ed. Philadelphia, W. B. Saunders, 1980, p. 395.)

may occasionally be indicated to treat persistent infection.

Hydrocelectomy: excision of the tunica vaginalis of the testis to remove a hydrocele (a fluid-filled sac).

Orchiectomy: removal of the testis or testes. This procedure renders the patient sterile.

Orchiopexy: suspension of the testis within the scrotum. This procedure is used to treat an undescended or cryptorchid testis to bring it into the normal intrascrotal position.

Spermatocelectomy: the removal of a spermatocele, which usually appears as a cystic mass within the scrotum, attached to the upper pole of the epididymis. A spermatocele is usually caused by an obstruction of the tubular system that conveys the sperm.

Varicocelectomy: ligation and partial excision of dilated veins in the scrotum.

Vasectomy: excision of a section of the vas deferens. This procedure is carried out electively for birth control or prior to prostatectomy to prevent the spread of infection from the urethra to the epididymis.

Vasoepididymostomy: anastomosis of the vas deferens to the epididymis.

Vasovasostomy: anastomosis of two separate segments of the vas deferens to reverse a vasectomy.

Penile and Urethral Disorders and Surgery

Chordee: downward bowing of the penis due to congenital malformation or to hypospadias with fibrous bands.

Circumcision: excision of the foreskin (prepuce) of the glans penis.

Epispadias: urethral meatus situated in an abnormal position on the upper side of the penis. Surgical correction involves plastic repair.

Hypospadias: a deformity of the penis and malformation of the urethral wall in which the urinary meatus is located on the underside of the penis, either short of its normal position at the tip of the glans or on the perineum or scrotum. This condition is often associated with chordee. Surgical correction involves plastic repair; penile straightening and urethral reconstruction (urethroplasty) are usually done in two or more stages.

Penile implant: a penile prosthesis implanted for treatment of organic sexual impotence.

Phimosis: tightness of the foreskin, so that it cannot be drawn back from over the glans; also, the analogous condition in the clitoris.

Transurethral surgery: piecemeal resection of the prostate gland and of tumors of the bladder and bladder neck, and fulguration of bleeding vessels and of tumors by means of a resectoscope passed into the bladder via the urethra.

Urethral dilatation and internal urethrotomy: gradual dilatation of the urethra and lysis of a urethral stricture.

Urethral meatotomy: incisional enlargement of the external urethral meatus to relieve stenosis or stricture.

Urethroplasty: reconstructive surgery of the urethra.

Adrenal Gland Surgery

Adrenalectomy: partial or total excision of one or both of the adrenal glands.

NURSING CARE AFTER DIAGNOSTIC PROCEDURES

Several invasive diagnostic procedures are used for patients with genitourinary disease. If patients require general anesthesia, they are usually admitted to the PACU for observation.

Renal Angiography

For a renal angiographic examination, a small catheter is threaded through the femoral artery into the aorta or renal artery, radiopaque dye is instilled, and radiographs are made. Local anesthesia is usually all that is needed; however, general anesthesia may be used for children or patients who cannot cooperate during the procedure. When the patient is admitted to the post anesthesia care unit (PACU), check the groin area for bleeding. A pressure type of dressing usually is present and may be replaced by a simple bandage after a few hours. Pedal pulses should be checked to ensure that no interruption of blood supply to the extremities has occurred. If possible, the leg should be kept straight. Fluids should be encouraged to facilitate excretion of the dye.

Renal Biopsy

Renal biopsy is usually performed at the bedside with only local anesthesia, although general anesthesia may be used for children. The patient should be kept at bedrest in a flat, supine position for as long as 4 hours. A small pillow may be positioned under the head for comfort. Vital signs are monitored, and the site of biopsy is checked for bleeding. Coughing and other activities that increase abdominal venous pressure should be avoided. Fluids should be increased to 3000 ml daily, and the urine should be observed for occult blood.

Cystoscopy

Cystoscopy may be performed in a special procedures room with only local anesthesia and appropriate sedation. Children and patients who cannot or will not cooperate during the procedure may need general anesthesia. This procedure may also be performed under spinal anesthesia. It may be performed simply for diagnostic purposes, or it may be used for treatment, such as resection of tumors, removal of stones and foreign bodies, and dilatation of the ureters.

On admission to the PACU, the patient is placed in a side-lying position if general anesthesia was used or flat on his or her back if spinal anesthesia was used. After the effects of anesthesia have been eliminated, the patient may assume a position of comfort. The patient may complain of back pain, a feeling of bladder fullness, and bladder spasms. These symptoms may become severe enough to require analgesia. Belladonna and opium suppositories or intravenous narcotics may be administered to relieve patient discomfort.

Fluid administration should be increased and started as soon as the effects of anesthesia

are gone. Urine output should be monitored carefully. The patient can expect frequency of urination and a burning sensation owing to trauma to the mucous membranes from the procedure, which may inadvertently cause voluntary retention. The urine may be pink tinged for several voidings—this is to be expected. Bright blood or clots in the urine, however, should be reported to the surgeon. If the patient complains of severe abdominal pain, this should be reported, because it may indicate accidental ureteral or bladder perforation or internal hemorrhage.

The patient should be observed for signs of sepsis. The spread of infection throughout the urinary tract or into the blood stream may occur following a cystoscopy. If symptoms of sepsis are noted, such as chills, tachycardia, tachypnea, flushing, and temperature elevation, the surgeon should be notified.

GENERAL POSTOPERATIVE CARE

Assessment of the patient following genitourinary surgery involves particular attention to fluid and electrolyte balance. Intake and output records are especially important and must be accurately maintained. Postoperative care is directed primarily at maintenance of urinary tract function, which is second in importance only to cardiorespiratory function. Maintenance of patency of the urinary tract is often dependent on the use of catheters, which come in a variety of shapes and sizes (Fig. 32–2).

Urethral catheters are used to drain urine from the bladder to keep it decompressed and to measure urine output accurately. A retention catheter is used postoperatively and left in place until the patient's status is stable and the surgeon orders its removal. The catheter is attached to a sterile, closed gravitational-drainage collection system. The urine collection reservoir may be a large (usually 2000-ml) container or a small calibrated chamber that can be emptied into a large reservoir after timed urine output volumes have been determined and recorded (Fig. 32–3).

The catheter should be anchored securely to the patient's thigh with tape and the tubing brought over the leg. Loop the catheter over once before taping to prevent undue tension on the urinary meatus. Attach the connecting tubing to the bed linens so that no proximal loops of tubing lie below the distal tubing—this is a straight gravity drainage system. Check frequently for kinks—the tubing should never be under the patient, because compression of the

A

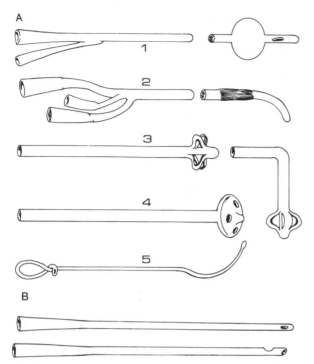

B

FIGURE 32–2. *A,* self-retaining catheters: *1.* Foley catheter; *2.* three-way Foley catheter; *3.* Malecot catheter; and *4.* Pezzer catheter. The self-retaining protuberance at the tip of the Malecot and Pezzer catheters must be elongated with a stylet (*5*), which is passive through the lumen before insertion. After insertion, the stylet is removed and the protuberance secures the catheter in place. *B,* straight catheters. The straight catheter may have a single eye or many eyes; it may have a round tip or a whistle tip. These catheters are not self-retaining and must be secured with adhesive tape when being used as indwelling tubes. (From Whitehead, S.: Nursing Care of the Adult Urology Patient. New York, Appleton-Century-Crofts, 1970.)

tubing obstructs the flow of urine. The urine receptacle should always be kept below the bladder level to prevent urine reflux up the tubing. Particular attention must be paid to this principle during the transfer of patients, because attendants typically pick up the receptacle to transfer it to the new setting.

Mucus or blood, or both, can clog the tubing and prevent urine flow. Irrigations should be carried out only according to the surgeon's orders. All irrigations are sterile procedures. A large sterile Toomey syringe and sterile irrigating solution (usually normal saline or normal saline with a selected antibiotic) are used. Care must be taken to keep all parts of the drainage system sterile. This may be accomplished by placing a small sterile plastic cover on the drainage tubing while the irrigation is performed. Irrigations should never be given under pressure, and when the bladder is irrigated, no more than 30 ml should be instilled

at one time, unless ordered otherwise by the surgeon.

To obtain a urine specimen from the closed system, use a sterile syringe and needle. Some catheters have a small, specially constructed spot from which to draw specimens. On those that do not, use the distal part of the catheter, close to the drainage tubing. Cleanse the area with alcohol or povidone-iodine (Betadine), insert the needle, and withdraw a specimen.

Suprapubic Catheters

Suprapubic catheters are used to drain residual urine from the bladder. The catheter is introduced into the urinary bladder via a stab wound through the lower abdomen and into the anterior bladder wall. The catheter is sutured in place, and a dressing is applied. (Usually a type of dressing that allows direct observation of the puncture site is used.) The catheter is connected to a straight gravitational drainage system. Care of the suprapubic catheter is similar to that of the Foley catheter. The catheter should be securely taped with a loop made to prevent tension on the bladder wall or the abdomen. The skin around the puncture site should be kept clean and dry. The catheter tubing should be checked periodically for kinks and to ensure that the stopcock valve is open to allow the urine to drain from the bladder.

Ureteral Catheters

Ureteral catheters are used to drain urine or to splint the ureters while they heal. They may be placed through the urethra or through abdominal or flank incisions. Care of these catheters is essentially the same as that for urethral catheters. Attention to patency must be especially scrupulous, because the renal pelvis can hold only 5 ml without becoming overdistended and causing damage to the kidneys.

Sterile irrigations are undertaken only as ordered by the physician. Only 5 ml of fluid should be used for the irrigation via gravitational flow. Irrigations should never be given under pressure, such as with a syringe and plunger. The nurse must be sure that situations that may cause dislodgment or displacement of these catheters are avoided, because this could be disastrous to the outcome of the surgery. Special care must be taken during patient transfer to ensure that these catheters stay in place. One person should be assigned this responsibility during the transfer. If the catheters

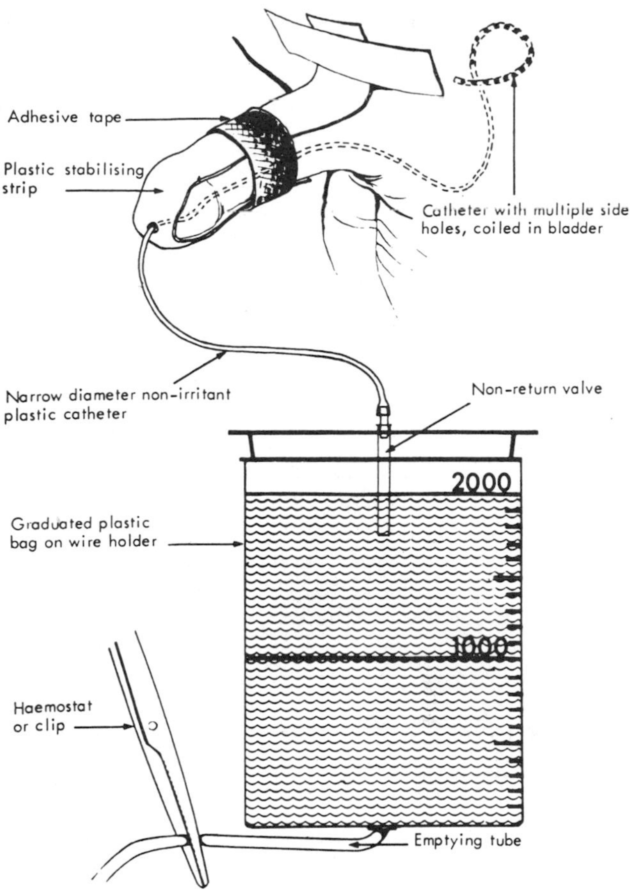

FIGURE 32–3. Closed drainage of the bladder. (From Douglas, A. P., and Kerr, D. S.: A Short Textbook of Kidney Disease. London, Pitman Medical, 1968.)

should become dislodged in spite of all the precautions taken, the surgeon must be notified immediately.

Intake

Optimal fluid intake is exceptionally important for this patient postoperatively; increased fluids are the general rule. If the patient can tolerate oral fluids, they should be given by this preferred route, and intake should be increased to total 3000 ml in a 24-hour period. Parenteral fluid therapy is indicated for a short time until the effects of anesthesia have passed, and it is continued only if the oral route of intake is inadequate.

Dressings

Care of dressings varies according to the procedure. Dressings applied following urinary tract surgery often become soaked with blood and urine. They should be reinforced as necessary, and the surrounding skin should be kept clean and dry to prevent unnecessary excoriation and breakdown. (If excessive staining is unexpected for a particular procedure and indicates a complication, it will be so indicated in the discussion of the specific procedure later in this chapter.) Excessive bleeding and hemorrhage are ever-present dangers of this surgery, because the kidneys and prostatic bed are extremely vascular. Vital signs must be monitored closely, and all avenues of output, especially the incisions and drainage tubes, should be evaluated frequently for bleeding.

Abdominal Distention

All patients should be assessed for abdominal distention following surgery involving abdominal and flank incisions (refer to Chapter 31 for care of the patient following an abdominal incision, because the same care applies following genitourinary surgery). Frequently, these patients arrive with a nasogastric tube, which is cared for as discussed in Chapter 31. In addition, the patient should be assessed for distention due to overfilling of the bladder because of an inability to void or a malfunction of the catheters.

Management of Discomfort and Pain

Discomfort following genitourinary surgery may be relieved with the administration of narcotics, including intravenous meperidine and belladonna and opium suppositories. The physiology of the "need to void" should be explained to the patient preoperatively. The patient should be instructed not to attempt to void around the catheter because exerting pressure causes the bladder muscles to contract and results in painful bladder spasms. The avoidance of straining around the catheter and the intake of excessive fluids decrease bladder irritability and spasms. As the nerve endings become fatigued, the frequency and severity of the spasms diminish.

NURSING CARE AFTER SPECIFIC PROCEDURES

Renal and Ureteral Surgery

Procedures involving the kidneys and ureters include excision of tumors and obstructions to urine flow (such as stones), reconstruction of urine outflow tracts, repair of lacerations, correction of deformities, excision of a kidney, and total organ transplant.

Anesthesia is almost always general for surgery on the kidneys and ureters. The kidneys are usually approached posteriorly through an incision that requires resection of the 11th or 12th rib. The surgical approach to the ureters is usually made through muscle-splitting flank incisions (Fig. 32–4). The post anesthesia course for these patients is usually smooth and involves general care for the post anesthesia patient and maintenance of urinary tract function. The patient should be placed in a position that avoids tension on suture lines or as indicated by the surgeon.

Exceptionally accurate intake and output records must be maintained. Low urine output should be reported to the surgeon.

Dressings should remain dry and intact unless drains are used, in which case dressings should be weighed when they are removed to determine output via this route. When determining output from the dressings, weigh the dressings before applying and then when removing, and subtract the difference.* Patients with drains or stomas may require the use of a small plastic bag over the area for collection of drainage that will consist primarily of urine. Drainage bags should be emptied frequently; if the bags are allowed to fill to capacity, the continual flow of urine will be interrupted.

Skin care for these patients is important. Urine should not be allowed to remain on the skin. Plain water should be used to cleanse the skin, and it should be carefully dried. No powders, lotions, or harsh skin preparations should be applied to the skin. If a ureteroileostomy has been performed, the stoma must be inspected frequently to ensure adequate vascularization. If it turns a bluish hue, the surgeon should be notified immediately.

A Foley catheter is generally in place and is cared for as previously discussed. Fluid intake is increased both orally and parenterally to keep blood clots from forming in the ureters or bladder. Intestinal decompression may be necessary and is accomplished by nasogastric tube (see Chapter 31). This is essential when an ileal conduit procedure (ureterostomy) is performed to allow healing of the intestinal anastomosis. Any evidence of abdominal distention should be reported to the surgeon immediately.

Extracorporeal Shock Wave Lithotripsy

Following extracorporeal shock wave lithotripsy the patient may be admitted to the PACU for a brief period of observation. Vital signs should be monitored as with any renal or ureteral surgery. Fluids should be increased and intake and output monitored carefully. Initially, the color of the urine may be cherry red to pink owing to trauma from surgery; this may take several hours to clear. Petechiae, redness, and bruising may be seen on the skin at the site of lithotripsy. The patient may experience pain from the force of the shock waves. This pain is usually localized to the skin and may be relieved with ice packs. Renal colic pain may also be experienced as the fragments of pulverized stones pass through the lower urinary tract.

Kidney Transplantation

The kidney is the most frequently transplanted organ and the only one that can be preserved in a viable state for some time (Fig. 32–5). The kidney is relatively easy to remove and implant. Most people have two function-

*One gram equals 1 ml of output.

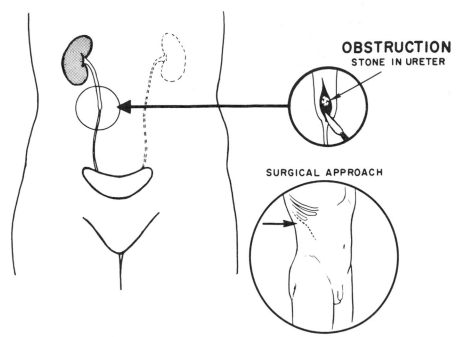

FIGURE 32–4. Right hydroureter due to obstructing calculus. *Inset* shows incision in ureter for removal of stone. (From LeMaitre, G. D., and Finnegan, J. A.: The Patient in Surgery: A Guide for Nurses. 4th ed. Philadelphia, W. B. Saunders, 1980, p. 380.)

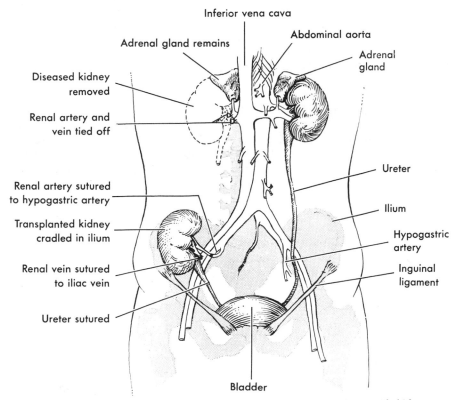

FIGURE 32–5. Transplanted kidney in place. (From Bergersen, B. S., et al (eds): Patients with kidney transplants. Curr. Concepts Clin. Nurs., *1*:1967.)

ing kidneys and need only one to sustain life; therefore, kidney transplantation is done only for patients who need the organ to replace a diseased or nonfunctioning solitary kidney. Transplantation can be accomplished two, three, or even more times in the same patient, with the use of hemodialysis when a functioning kidney is not in place.

Many kidney grafts come from cadaver donors. Some grafts, however, come from live donors, usually a blood relative of the recipient. The closer the recipient and donor in blood line, the better the chances for survival of the kidney graft. Postoperatively, the donor is usually the forgotten member. His or her care is essentially the same as for the patient who has had a single kidney removed. All care considered previously for the urologic patient applies, as does care for the patient following abdominal incision. Because postoperative care is routine, this patient often feels a lack of self-esteem. Before surgery he or she was considered heroic and got a generous helping of attention and glory, whereas postoperatively, attention is directed primarily to the organ recipient. The donor patient feels this, even in the PACU. For this reason, it is extremely important that the PACU nurse be aware of the needs of the postoperative donor and demonstrate concern for his or her physical and psychological well-being. The care of these patients should be assigned to separate teams, if possible. In addition to normal self-concern, the donor will be concerned about the recipient and should receive factual information.

General anesthesia is used for both the donor and the recipient in renal transplantation. If possible, these patients should be placed in a reverse or protective isolation room with all protective isolation measures instituted. Many PACUs do not have protective isolation capabilities; therefore, these patients are returned directly from the operating suite to the surgical intensive care unit, where protective isolation can be instituted.

Protective isolation is necessary because these patients are placed on immunosuppressive therapy, which reduces the white blood cell count. The commonly used immunosuppressive agents, including azathioprine (Imuran), cyclophosphamide (Cytoxan), and cyclosporine (Sandimmune), are nonspecific and suppress the entire immune system. It is therefore imperative that meticulous aseptic technique be used when handling these patients to prevent the introduction of infection.

On admission to the PACU, the recipient should be kept in a flat position for 12 hours to allow the kidney to set. The head of the bed may be elevated 30 degrees to provide comfort and respiratory care. After 12 hours, the patient may turn to the side of the transplant. Turning to the opposite side may dislodge the graft.

All vital signs are monitored continuously. A Foley catheter will be in place, and all urine should be carefully monitored for volume and specific gravity. During the immediate postoperative period, the renal allograft is extremely sensitive to hypovolemia, and even a transient period of poor renal perfusion may result in oliguric renal failure. The kidney from a living donor may start to function almost immediately after transplantation, and diuresis will occur. The volume of urine output may be great enough to warrant measurement every 15 minutes. The cadaver kidney, on the other hand, reacts more slowly, depending on the cold ischemic time spent during transportation.

Urine samples are generally collected hourly to ascertain electrolyte content, creatinine level, and osmolarity. Once daily, the total 24-hour urine collection (minus the small samples sent hourly) is sent to the laboratory for creatinine clearance test and culture. Urine output less than 1 ml per kg per hr should be reported to the surgeon, because any decrease in urine output may be a sign of early rejection. Likewise, any gross hematuria should be reported immediately. A baseline weight postoperatively should be ascertained as soon as feasible.

A nasogastric tube provides intestinal decompression and is cared for as previously discussed.

A central venous pressure line is present to further assess the patient's cardiovascular status. Monitoring of these systems is imperative to ensure adequate renal perfusion.

Dressings over the incision site should evidence a minimal amount of drainage. The recipient may have a stenting catheter from the renal pelvis out through the urethra along with the Foley catheter for the first 36 to 48 hours to ensure ureteral patency.

Intravenous fluids provide most of the intake for these patients until the nasogastric tube can be removed. Intravenous replacement fluid composition is determined by the serum and urine electrolyte content, the hematocrit, and the clinical course of the patient. Volume is determined from necessary fluid requirements of the patient in normal status plus replacement on a volume-to-volume basis of drainage from the Foley catheter, nasogastric tube, ureterostomy, and cystostomy. For the first 72 hours after operation, the major source of output is from the ureterostomy. Meticulous handling of the closed urinary drainage system is mandatory to prevent the introduction of infection.

Vigorous pulmonary toilet should be instituted immediately to prevent atelectasis. The patient may be turned to the side of the kidney graft and back every 30 minutes to provide for change of position. The painful flank incision can be splinted either with the nurse's hands or with a firm pillow or a rolled blanket to assist the patient with coughing.

The threat of graft rejection is ever present, and it must be observed for closely. Hyperacute allograft rejection can occur within minutes of the completion of the vascular anastomosis or in the first few hours postoperatively. Signs and symptoms of hyperacute rejection are noted in Table 32–1. It is of the utmost importance to treat a threatened rejection as soon as it appears to prevent irreversible damage to the kidney.

The patient may experience a strong fear of rejection while still in the PACU. Many patients view this surgery as the last chance to live a normal life, having had to deal with numerous physical, psychological, and socioeconomic stressors. The PACU nurse may need to frequently reassure the patient that the kidney is functioning.

The postoperative kidney transplant patient is usually transferred to the surgical intensive care unit for several days following surgery for close observation and intensive care.

Bladder Surgery

The bladder is a smooth muscle storage tank that holds urine until a reflex, normally under voluntary control, releases the urine to pass

through the urethra to be eliminated. Surgical procedures on the bladder include the removal of stones, foreign bodies, and tumors; the repair of strictures at the bladder neck and of injuries, such as lacerations; and the removal of the bladder itself.

Anesthesia for these procedures may be either spinal or general. On admission to the PACU, the patient is placed in a supine position. The head of the bed may be raised 30 degrees as soon as feasible. The removal of stones or foreign bodies and the resection of selected tumors may be accomplished via cystoscopy, which was discussed earlier. After the repair of lacerations or after cystotomy to remove stones, the patient will be admitted to the PACU with a Foley catheter in place, and a urinary diversion such as a suprapubic cystostomy will usually be in place. Urine from these drainage systems is pink tinged but should not become grossly bloody. Dressings should remain dry and intact, fluids should be increased, and oral fluids should be started as soon as the effects of anesthesia have passed.

Lacerations or ruptures of the bladder are often the result of accidental trauma. They require emergency surgery, and the postoperative patient should be assessed carefully for any unrecognized associated injuries. Pain should be minimal for these patients and easily controlled with mild analgesics. If severe pain is present, it may represent a complication, such as internal hemorrhage and damage to a ureter, and should be reported to the surgeon.

Cystectomy requires the construction of an ileal conduit. Care for an ileal conduit was discussed in the section on ureteral surgery.

Prostatic Surgery

The prostate gland is a small, walnut-sized male reproductive organ. Its sole function is to manufacture a secretion that becomes part of the semen; it is a nonessential organ. Surgical procedures performed on the prostate gland include the excision of tumors and the resection or total removal of the gland.

The preferred anesthesia is spinal, although general anesthesia may be used. Several different approaches are common in surgery on the prostate. Most frequently, the *transurethral approach* is used, especially if only minor obstructive lesions or small portions of the gland are to be removed. A resectoscope is introduced through the urethra, and the surgeon excises the tissue with a moveable tungsten wire that

---

Table 32–1. SIGNS AND SYMPTOMS OF ALLOGRAFT REJECTION

Irritability on the part of the patient
Anxiousness
Restlessness
Lethargy
Swollen, tender kidney
Decreased urine output
Fever; may be low grade
Increased blood pressure
Weight gain
Anorexia
Increased blood urea nitrogen and serum creatinine levels
Decreased creatinine clearance
Increased urine protein and lysozyme activity
Lymphocytes in the urine

operates on high-frequency current controlled with a foot pedal.

When the patient is admitted to the PACU after transurethral resection of the prostate (TURP), a three-way Foley catheter will be in place (see Fig. 32–2A). One lumen allows filling of the retention balloon, one lumen allows outflow of the urine and irrigation fluid from the bladder, and one lumen is attached to the irrigation fluid system. Irrigation fluid, which is usually normal saline at room temperature, is available in 3000 ml plastic bags, and it may be regulated like intravenous solutions. Because of the potential of creating a hypothermic state by irrigating the bladder with this solution, the saline should be warmed prior to administration and the patient's temperature monitored. The triple-lumen catheter is advantageous in that blood clots do not regularly form and block the system when the flow is continuous. The irrigation rate should be regulated so that drainage remains a light-pink, watermelon color. If drainage becomes bright red, speed up the irrigation; if the returning fluid is clear, slow the irrigation down. Some institutions use a Y-connecting system with one arm of the Y connected to the irrigating fluid and the other to straight-gravitational drainage from the bladder. In either instance, a fair amount of bleeding can be expected following TURP, because the prostatic bed is so highly vascular. This bleeding may also increase as the spinal anesthesia wears off and may require frequent irrigation to prevent clogging of the drainage tube.

If the catheter becomes clogged, it may be necessary to irrigate it with a piston syringe using the same normal saline irrigating solution. If patency of the catheter cannot be reestablished, the surgeon must be notified.

The patient's vital signs should be monitored closely. Observe for signs and symptoms of post-TURP syndrome (water intoxication) that may occur as a result of venous absorption of the irrigation fluid through the venous sinuses. Serum sodium and potassium levels should be checked during the postoperative period, because changes in fluid balance may affect these electrolytes. Signs and symptoms of water intoxication include a low serum sodium level, tachypnea, shortness of breath, nausea, vomiting, hypertension, bradycardia, increased pulse pressure, restlessness, apprehension, and mental disorientation. If this syndrome occurs, the PACU nurse should administer oxygen to the patient; monitor blood loss and electrocardiographic and fluid and electrolyte status; and administer intravenous fluid (hypertonic saline

3 or 5 percent in 100 ml per hr increments until the serum sodium level is satisfactory) and diuretics to mobilize the edema.

Oral fluids should be started and increased as tolerated as soon as possible. Diet may be progressed as tolerated.

Pain should be minimal and easily controlled with mild analgesics. Analgesics or tranquilizers may be administered to control the discomfort of bladder spasms and of the presence of the catheter, which makes the patient feel an urgency to void even though the bladder is being emptied. Complaints of abdominal pain, abdominal rigidity, an increase in pulse rate, and other signs of shock should alert the nurse to the possibility that the bladder wall or the capsule of the prostate was accidentally perforated during surgery; these symptoms should be reported to the surgeon immediately.

Other approaches to prostatic surgery include the retrograde or suprapubic, perineal, and retropubic incisions. When the *suprapubic approach* is used, a midline vertical incision is made in the lowest part of the abdomen, then the bladder is incised, and the tumors are removed. This is the procedure of choice when 60 g or more of tissue is to be removed. The patient is admitted to the PACU with a Foley catheter in place that may or may not be attached to an irrigation system. If not connected to an irrigation system, the catheter will have to be irrigated frequently with a syringe to prevent clots from clogging the drainage system. The patient will also have a suprapubic catheter in place that should be connected to straight-gravitational drainage, and output should be measured carefully (Fig. 32–6). In addition, a small Penrose drain will have been inserted in the suprapubic space and brought out through a separate stab wound. A dressing of several layers of 4 × 4 sponges should cover the incision and the drain. A moderate amount of serosanguineous drainage can be expected owing to the presence of the drain. This dressing should be reinforced as necessary to keep the skin clean and dry. If excessive bright-red bleeding occurs, the surgeon must be notified.

The surgeon may apply traction to the Foley catheter by taping the catheter to the inner thigh. Because the traction puts tension against the vesical outlet and promotes hemostasis, it may produce painful bladder spasms that may be relieved by the use of intravenous narcotics such as meperidine, or belladonna and opium suppositories. After the traction is removed, a small increase in bleeding may be expected for a short time.

The *perineal approach*, used for removal of

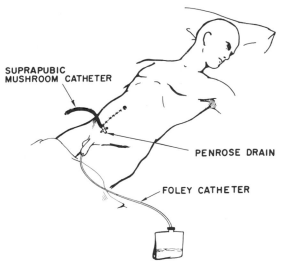

SUPRAPUBIC
MUSHROOM CATHETER

PENROSE DRAIN

FOLEY CATHETER

FIGURE 32–6. Postoperative positions of drainage tubes following suprapubic prostatectomy. (From LeMaitre, G. D., and Finnegan, J. A.: The Patient in Surgery: A Guide for Nurses. 4th ed. Philadelphia, W. B. Saunders, 1980, p. 385.)

blood pressure and increasing pulse rate, which may indicate impending shock.

One of the most frequently occurring postoperative complications following the nerve-sparing radical prostatectomy is pulmonary embolism. For this reason, the surgeon may order low-dose heparin. Care in the PACU should include deep-breathing exercises and position changes along with passive or active movement of the extremities. Some type of antiembolism stocking should be used.

Scrotal Surgery

The scrotum is a sac separated into two pouches, externally by the median raphe and internally by the dartos tunic. Each pouch contains a testis, an epididymis, and a spermatic cord. The vas deferens, which is continuous with the epididymis at the lower end of the testis, together with the arteries, veins, nerves, and lymphatic vessels held together by spermatic fascia, forms the spermatic cord. Operations on the scrotum include excision of masses and tumors, correction of deformities, and excision of diseased or abnormal structures that interfere with normal function.

Anesthesia for scrotal surgery may be local, general, or spinal. Spinal anesthesia is commonly used for adult patients, whereas general anesthesia is usually preferred for children younger than 12 years of age. Local anesthesia is often used for simple procedures such as vasectomy and epididymectomy.

The PACU course following surgery on the scrotal structures is usually uneventful. Care is dictated primarily by the agent of anesthesia and its method of administration.

Postoperatively, the patient may assume a position of comfort. Any dressings present should remain dry and intact. Oral food and fluids may be reinstituted as soon as tolerated by the patient. Commonly, a Bellevue bridge is applied to provide scrotal support and elevation (Fig. 32–7). This device is suspended from thigh to thigh with a tight sling across the expanse, upon which the scrotum is supported. A T-binder may also be used (Fig. 32–8).

The application of a *light* crushed-ice bag helps relieve scrotal edema, enhances hemostasis, and promotes comfort. Scrotal enlargement with apparent tension should be reported to the surgeon immediately. Progressive inguinal swelling may denote lymphatic obstruction following a varicocelectomy, and the surgeon must be notified. Pain should be minimal following these procedures and easily controlled

large amounts of tissue, is the approach of choice for prostatic cancer. A V-shaped incision is made above the rectum in this approach. The patient will be admitted to the PACU with a Foley catheter and a perineal drain in place. Because of the perineal drain, a moderate amount of serosanguineous drainage can be expected, and the dressing should be reinforced as necessary. No instrumentation, including thermometers, should be placed in the rectum during the immediate postoperative period.

When a *retropubic approach* is used, a small incision is made above the pubis, and a capsular incision is made into the upper surface of the prostate. A Foley catheter will be in place, and a small drain will have been inserted in the incision or brought out through a stab wound lateral to the incision.

As with all urologic patients, accurate intake and output records must be maintained following prostatic surgery. The PACU nurse must be sure to indicate whether or not irrigation solution is included in the output data.

Most prostatic surgery is performed on adult men older than 50 years of age, because prostatic hypertrophy most commonly occurs after 40 years of age. Therefore, assessment of cardiorespiratory status should be performed frequently. Oxygen should be administered and weaned using pulse oximetry. All patients should be placed on a cardiac monitor to assess changes. Astute observation of vital signs is imperative to monitor cardiovascular function, because it may be impaired by postoperative bleeding. Observe carefully for decreasing

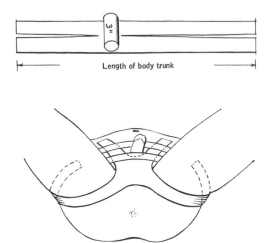

FIGURE 32–7. Bellevue bridge for scrotal support. (From Sutton, A. L.: Bedside Nursing Techniques in Medicine and Surgery. 2nd ed. Philadelphia, W. B. Saunders, 1969, p. 278.)

by mild analgesics. Complaints of severe pain not controlled with mild analgesia should be reported to the surgeon.

As with any genital surgery, the patient's body image concerns and questions of fertility in particular may be of paramount importance. These concerns are not usually addressed in the PACU, but the nurse must be sensitive to them and prepared to assist the patient with factual information and reassurance, should they arise. Often, these patients feel an urgency to inspect the operative site and should be assisted, if necessary, to do so.

The patient may be embarrassed by this type of surgery and reluctant to ask the nurse for assistance or to complain of pain, and he may hesitate to allow the nurse to inspect the incision area. A matter-of-fact attitude on the part of the nurse and efficient care promote a sense of well-being for the patient and may help alleviate these feelings. The nurse should keep in mind that preadolescent and adolescent boys are especially sensitive about the genital area. If at all possible, a male nurse should be assigned to these patients to alleviate their anxiety.

Penile and Urethral Surgery

Surgery on the penis and urethra involves removal of tumors or obstructions to urinary flow, plastic repair of deformities, and circumcision or excision of the foreskin. Rarely, partial or total amputation of the penis is necessary for malignancy, which is essentially skin can-

cer. Laser technique is generally effective for the treatment of condyloma acuminata and squamous cell carcinoma of the penis.

Anesthesia for these procedures may be local, general, or spinal. The PACU course is usually smooth, and care is determined primarily by the type of anesthesia used. Physical care of the patient who has had a plastic repair of hypospadias or epispadias is dictated by the surgeon. Care for the patient following cystoscopy was discussed at the beginning of this chapter; the same care applies for patients undergoing cystoscopy for the resection of tumors.

Following circumcision, which may be performed for correction of phimosis or for elective reasons, the nurse should check for bleeding. Usually, only a small band of petrolatum-impregnated gauze is applied as a dressing around the glans and changed as directed. Bleeding that soaks this dressing is excessive and should be reported.

Patients who have undergone surgery on the penis should avoid erection during the PACU phase and at least a week postoperatively. Patients with penile prostheses should be admitted to the PACU with the penis in a flaccid

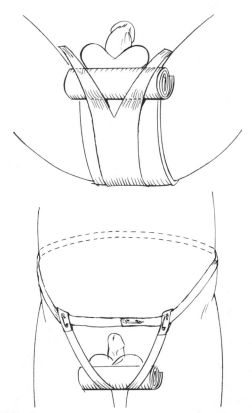

FIGURE 32–8. T-binder for scrotal support. (From Sutton, A. L.: Bedside Nursing Techniques in Medicine and Surgery. 2nd ed. Philadelphia, W. B. Saunders, 1969, p. 277.)

state, and the prosthesis should remain deflated. Inflation of the prosthesis should be avoided until after the first postoperative visit to the surgeon.

Pain may be significant but should not be severe. Scrotal and penile support with a Bellevue bridge and the application of a light ice pack provide some relief; however, analgesia with small doses of narcotics may be necessary. Food and fluids may be restarted as soon as tolerated by the patient. Urine output should be checked and recorded. Palpate for low abdominal distention, which may be caused by voluntary retention. This is not uncommon, owing to fear that micturition will create pain.

Adrenalectomy

Adrenalectomy involves the removal of one or both of the adrenal glands, which are situated on top of the kidneys. Adrenalectomy, which is an extensive and shock-producing procedure, may be performed for several reasons, including metastasized cancer from the reproductive organs, hyperfunction due to hyperplasia of the organ, and adrenal tumors. Two adrenal tumors are of major consequence: pheochromocytoma, a usually benign tumor that causes hyperfunction resulting in severe symptoms, and neuroblastoma, a malignant tumor that is a leading cause of death in childhood.

General anesthesia is used for adrenalectomy and may include the use of cortisone titrated to maintain catecholamine levels and blood pressure. Cortisone is usually necessary only when bilateral adrenalectomy is performed or when the uninvolved adrenal gland has poor function. The administration of cortisone, which is continued in the PACU, is an extremely important nursing procedure. Specific instructions should be given by the anesthesiologist and surgeon as to titration of the solution. Failure to maintain postoperative levels of cortisone leads to hypovolemic and hyponatremic shock. Post anesthesia care of these patients is a nursing challenge—observations must be especially astute.

The surgical approach for adrenalectomy may be lateral, anterior, or posterior. On admission to the PACU, the patient is placed in the side-lying position until reactive from anesthesia, at which time he or she is placed in a semi-Fowler's position. The surgeon may prefer the patient be positioned on the operative side so that the perinephric space is obliterated to discourage bleeding. Assessment is aimed

primarily at the cardiovascular status of the patient, because hemorrhage and shock are the two most common and most disastrous complications. Profound shock may develop, owing to the reduction of circulating catecholamines precipitated by removal of the glands as well as to the effects of the drugs used preoperatively for the control of hypertension. The effects of these drugs usually last for a few hours after surgery. Because most of these drugs produce vasodilatation, they are usually a factor in postoperative hypotension. Therefore, a fluid challenge usually is given in an attempt to treat hypotension. If fluid is not successful in increasing the blood pressure, then vasopressor drugs will be used. Epinephrine or norepinephrine in an intravenous solution may be titrated to maintain blood pressure, according to the surgeon's instructions.

Shock may also result from hemorrhage. The adrenal glands are extremely vascular. Intravenous fluids, including hypertonic saline solutions, blood, plasma, dextran, and glucose in water, may be used to maintain blood volume and prevent shock. Dressings over the bilateral incisions should remain relatively dry even though drains are placed. If these dressings become soaked, the surgeon should be notified, because this represents excessive bleeding. If the patient complains of abdominal pain, abdominal distention, nausea, or vomiting, development of an abdominal hematoma may be indicated; these signs should be reported to the surgeon.

Other parameters of the patient's status that may give clues to the development of shock should also be assessed. Dehydration (increased urine specific gravity) and restlessness may indicate developing shock. Central venous pressure should be checked. A Foley catheter will be in place, and urine output should be monitored hourly. The development of oliguria or output of less than 1 ml per kg per hr may indicate shock and subsequent renal shutdown. Serum and urine electrolyte levels, especially sodium, should be determined hourly.

All care outlined for the patient following high abdominal incisions in Chapter 31 is applicable to this patient. Good pulmonary toilet should be instituted immediately in the PACU. A nasogastric tube is frequently required until normal intestinal peristalsis returns. Incisional pain may require the use of narcotic analgesics. Because many narcotics have a hypotensive effect, they should be titrated judiciously, and blood pressure must be monitored continuously for at least 30 minutes after their administration.

The patient is frequently placed in protective isolation to avoid the introduction of infection. Meticulous sterile technique must be used when changing or reinforcing dressings. Because of their extreme lability, which lasts for approximately 48 hours, these patients should be transferred to the surgical intensive care unit for continuous monitoring.

References

1. Belker, A. M., and Bennett, A. H.: Applications of microsurgery in urology. Surg. Clin. North Am., 65(5):1157–1178, 1988.
2. Chambers, J. K.: Fluid and electrolyte problems in renal and urologic disorders. Nurs. Clin. North Am., 22:815–825, 1987.
3. Gharbieh, P. A.: Renal transplant: Surgical and psychologic hazards. Crit. Care Nurse, 8(6):58–71, 1988.
4. Glenn, J. F. (ed.): Urologic Surgery. 4th ed. Philadelphia, J. B. Lippincott, 1991.
5. Gruendemann, B. J., and Meeker, M. H.: Alexander's Care of the Patient in Surgery. 8th ed. St. Louis, C. V. Mosby, 1987.
6. Keating, M. A., Cartwright, P. C., and Duckett, J. W.: Bladder mucosa in urethral reconstructions. J. Urol., 144(4):827–834, 1990.
7. Kelly, M. J., Zimmern, P. E., and Leach, G. E.: Complications of bladder neck suspension procedures. Urol. Clin. North Am., 18(2):339–347, 1991.
8. Long, B. C., and Phipps, W. J. (eds.): Medical-Surgical Nursing: A Nursing Process Approach. 2nd ed. St. Louis, C. V. Mosby, 1989.
9. Rauscher, J., and Parra, R. O.: Vesico-psoas hitch procedure. AORN J., 52(6):1177–1186, 1990.
10. Schaeffer, A. J.: Use of the CO_2 laser in urology. Urol. Clin. North Am., 13(3):393–403, 1986.
11. Schick, L.: The patient with post-transurethral resection of the prostrate syndrome. J. Post Anesth. Nurs., 6(2):136–142, 1991.
12. Walsh, P. C.: Radical prostatectomy, preservation of sexual function, cancer control. Urol. Clin. North Am., 14(4):663–673, 1987.

Post Anesthesia Care of the Obstetric and Gynecologic Surgical Patient

CHAPTER 33

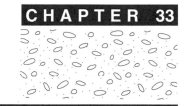

Kathleen Millican Miller, M.S.N., R.N., C.P.A.N.

Surgery on organs of reproduction most commonly involves an adult patient. The post anesthesia care unit (PACU) nurse, however, may encounter pediatric or adolescent female patients undergoing gynecologic surgery for repair or correction of congenital or traumatic deformities. Surgery on the female genitalia may be conveniently divided into three major categories: (1) obstetric, (2) lower genital and vaginal, and (3) abdominal gynecologic.

Definitions

Obstetric Surgery

Cerclage procedure: procedure for the treatment of incompetent cervix. The McDonald procedure involves the placement of a pursestring suture on the cervix at the level of the internal os; the Shirodkar procedure involves placement of a fascia lata (from the thigh) or a surgical band at the level of the internal os.

Cesarean hysterectomy: incision of the abdomen and the uterus, extraction of the infant and the placenta, and performance of a hysterectomy.

Cesarean section (C-section): delivery of an infant through an incision made in the abdominal and uterine walls.

C-section, classic: a midline incision between the umbilicus and the symphysis pubis and an anterior incision through the uterine wall.

C-section, low segment: an incision in the lower part of the uterus made after an abdominal incision.

Ectopic pregnancy: implantation of the fertilized ovum in any site other than the upper half of the uterus (Fig. 33–1).

Uterine aspiration (suction curettage): dilatation of the cervix and the vacuum removal of the uterine contents.

Lower Genital and Vaginal Surgery

Bartholin duct cyst: a cyst that results from chronic inflammation of one of the major vestibular glands at the vaginal introitus (Fig. 33–2).

Bartholinectomy: removal of a Bartholin duct cyst.

Cervical conization: removal of abnormal cervical tissue by scalpel, electrosurgical current, or laser.

Colporrhaphy: repair of the vaginal wall. May be anterior, as for cystocele repair, or posterior, as for rectocele repair.

Culdoscopy: an operative diagnostic procedure in which an incision is made into the posterior vaginal cul-de-sac, through which a tubular instrument similar to a cystoscope is inserted for the purpose of visualizing the pelvic structures, including the uterus, fallopian tubes, broad ligaments, uterosacral ligaments, rectal wall, sigmoid colon, and, sometimes, the small intestine.

Cystocele: prolapse of the bladder into the anterior vaginal wall.

Dilatation of the cervix and curettage of the uterus (D&C): introduction of instruments (dilators) through the vagina into the cervical canal and scraping of the uterus to remove substances, including blood. This procedure is used for diagnostic purposes, as well as for treating conditions such as incomplete abortion, abnormal uterine bleeding, and primary dysmenorrhea.

Enterocele: prolapse of intestine into the pouch of Douglas.

Hysterectomy, vaginal: removal of the uterus using a vaginal approach.

Hysteroscopy: direct visualization of the canal of the uterine cervix and cavity of the uterus using an endoscope.

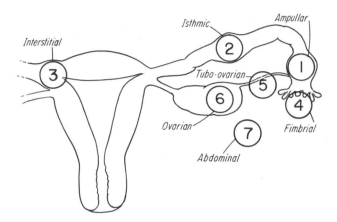

FIGURE 33–1. Ectopic pregnancy. Diagram shows the various implantation sites, numbered in order of decreasing frequency of occurrence. (From Sabiston, D. C., Jr. [ed.]: Textbook of Surgery: The Biological Basis of Modern Surgical Practice. 14th ed. Philadelphia, W. B. Saunders, 1991, p. 1427.)

Procidentia: herniation of the uterus beyond the introitus.

Prolapse of the uterus: downward displacement of the uterus. Vaginal hysterectomy is often recommended for a prolapsed uterus when childbearing is no longer desired or when marked prolapse is present.

Rectocele: prolapse of the rectum into the posterior vaginal wall.

Trachelorrhaphy: removal of torn surfaces of the

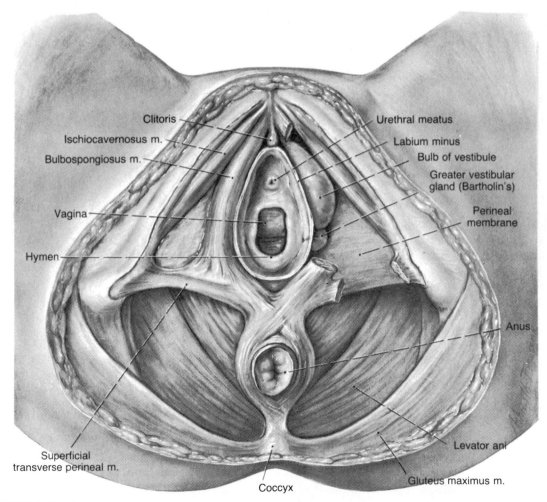

FIGURE 33–2. Female perineum with skin and superficial fascia removed. (From Jacob, S. W., Francone, C. A., and Lossow, W. J.: Structure and Function in Man. 5th ed. Philadelphia, W. B. Saunders, 1982, p. 604.)

anterior and posterior cervical lips and re-construction of the cervical canal.

Urethrocele: prolapse of the urethra into the anterior vaginal wall.

Vaginal plastic operation (anterior and posterior [A&P] repair): reconstruction of the vaginal walls (colporrhaphy), the pelvic floor, and the muscles and fascia of the rectum, urethra, bladder, and perineum. Used to correct a cystocele or rectocele, restore the bladder to its normal position, and strengthen the vagina and the pelvic floor.

Abdominal Gynecologic Surgery

Abdominal myomectomy: removal of fibromyomas.

Laparoscopy (peritoneoscopy, celioscopy): endoscopic visualization of the peritoneal cavity through a small incision in the anterior abdominal wall after the establishment of a pneumoperitoneum.

Oophorectomy: removal of an ovary.

Oophorocystectomy: removal of a cyst on the ovary.

Radical hysterectomy: removal of the uterus, the uterosacral and uterovesical ligaments, the upper third of the vagina, and all the parametrium.

Salpingectomy: excision of all portions of the fallopian tube.

Salpingo-oophorectomy: removal of the fallopian tube and all or part of the associated ovary.

Salpingostomy (tubal plasty): removal of the obstructed portion of the fallopian tube, and suspension of the remaining portion from the side of the pelvic wall or placement of it into the uterine cavity.

Total abdominal hysterectomy: removal of the uterus, including the corpus and the cervix, with or without the adnexa, through an abdominal incision.

Tubal ligation: interruption of fallopian tube continuity resulting in sterilization. The most commonly used technique is the *Pomeroy procedure,* which is done through a laparoscope. A segment of the fallopian tube is ligated and excised. Reversal procedures are now being performed with microsurgery.

OBSTETRIC SURGERY

Obstetric surgery involves procedures on pregnant women to promote full-term pregnancy, to provide an alternative means of delivery when normal vaginal delivery is not feasible for reasons of either fetal or maternal well-being, and to interrupt pregnancy.

Care After Specific Procedures

Cesarean Section

Cesarean sections are performed both on an emergency and on an elective basis. These patients have special physical and psychological needs. A selection of articles is included in the reference list at the end of this chapter to assist the reader who provides care for families experiencing cesarean birth.

Cesarean sections are indicated for dystocia (usually due to cephalopelvic disproportion); antepartum bleeding; some toxemic conditions; certain medical complications, especially diabetes mellitus; and previous cesarean section. The low-segment cesarean section is usually the procedure of choice. Anesthesia may be general inhalation, spinal, or local infiltration of the operative field.

Postoperative care following cesarean section includes all care rendered to a patient undergoing abdominal surgery as well as post-partum care.

On admission to the PACU, the patient should be placed in the side-lying position until reactive to prevent aspiration of stomach contents. As soon as her condition permits, she can assume any position of comfort. Oxygen should be delivered and monitored with the use of pulse oximetry.

Parenteral fluids are usually administered during the first 24 hours postoperatively, but oral fluids can usually be resumed as soon as bowel sounds are audible and the patient desires. Intravenous fluids often contain oxytocin to increase uterine muscle tone and stop excessive blood flow. Usually 10 to 20 units of oxytocin are added to 1000 ml of Ringer's lactate and infused at 125 ml per hr. The main side effect of oxytocin is an antidiuretic effect, and intake and output should be monitored accurately. A progressive diet is advised, pending the return of bowel sounds.

The patient will have an abdominal dressing as well as a perineal pad; both should be inspected for drainage. The abdominal dressing should remain dry and intact. A moderate amount of lochia rubra is normal, but saturation of two or more perineal pads with blood during the first hour is considered excessive. The area underneath the buttocks should be checked for pooling of blood.

The fundus should be checked frequently to ensure that it is firmly contracted. Checking the fundus is an uncomfortable procedure for the patient; therefore, careful explanation should be provided before it is carried out, as follows:

The patient should be encouraged to relax her abdominal muscles as much as possible. Instructing her to take slow, deep breaths with her mouth open facilitates relaxation of those muscles. If the uterus is firmly contracted, it need not be massaged, and in fact should not be, because this may cause uterine muscle fatigue and subsequent relaxation and bleeding. If the uterus is soft and "boggy," it should be gently but firmly massaged through the abdominal wall to stimulate contraction. The patient may be instructed to do this herself under supervision, which may allay anxiety and be less uncomfortable for her. Frequently, oxytocin is administered intravenously and titrated to maintain the uterus in a state of contraction. If oxytocin is employed, the uterus should be checked for firmness but usually does not require frequent massage.

A full bladder is one cause of uterine atony. An indwelling urethral catheter is commonly left in place for the first 12 hours postoperatively. A fundus palpated above the umbilicus or to the side of the abdomen (usually the right side) may indicate a nonfunctioning catheter. The catheter should be positioned for gravitational drainage and avoidance of kinks. The urine should be monitored for volume and color.

Many patients experience transient trembling or shivering after delivery. Several theories have been proposed concerning this sense of chilling, although the actual cause remains unknown. This trembling is generally not associated with an elevation of temperature. Warmed blankets or warm-air therapy should be available as a comfort measure to the mother.

Many hospitals have separate PACUs for post-partum patients, so the special considerations for the cesarean section patient pose no significant problems. The nurse caring for the cesarean section patient within the general PACU must be judicious and often be innovative to meet the needs of not only the mother but also the new family. The mother, the neonate, and the father should be together as soon as possible to allow for the bonding experience. This may be accomplished by using a quiet corner of the unit (if such a place exists), by drawing curtains around the family, or by expediting the discharge process to transfer the patient to the post-partum unit. The mother and father will be anxious to review the details of the birth together, and the PACU nurse should be prepared to answer their questions. Consistent communication between the surgical nurse and the PACU staff makes answering these questions much easier.

Ectopic Pregnancy

Faulty implantation of the ovum may take place in the fallopian tube (in approximately 98 percent of all ectopic pregnancies), in the ovary, in any part of the abdominal cavity, or in the uterine cervix. The treatment of choice for this is laparoscopy (or laparotomy), with removal of the ectopic pregnancy. Preferably, the ovary is not resected or removed, but this may be necessary if the ovary is involved. If implantation occurs in the cervix, a hysterectomy is usually indicated to control hemorrhage. If abdominal implantation has occurred, the fetus is removed, and often the placenta is left within the cavity to be reabsorbed.

Laparoscopy (or laparotomy) is usually performed under general anesthesia; however, spinal anesthesia may be used. Postoperative care is the same as that for the patient undergoing abdominal surgery. The PACU nurse should be especially observant for signs of intra-abdominal hemorrhage and shock, because these are not uncommon complications of ectopic pregnancy, especially one that has ruptured preoperatively. All patients with ectopic pregnancy should have complete typing and crossmatching done for whole blood, which should be kept available in the laboratory for 24 hours. Rh-negative women should receive RhoGAM to prevent sensitization.

Cerclage Procedures

The McDonald or Shirodkar procedure is used to treat an incompetent cervix and is fairly successful in maintaining pregnancy. The suture is usually placed between the 14th and 18th week of gestation. These procedures may be accomplished under general, spinal, or regional anesthesia.

On admission to the PACU, the patient is placed in the side-lying position until reactive. Oxygen should be administered and weaned using pulse oximetry. Food and fluids may be resumed as soon as the patient is conscious and the laryngeal reflexes have returned. A perineal pad should be kept in place. Only a minimal amount of bloody spotting should be considered normal. Pain should be minimal and easily controlled with a simple analgesic such as acetaminophen. Any gross vaginal bleeding or abdominal cramping should be reported to the surgeon, because this procedure may induce labor and expulsion of the uterine contents. The surgeon may order an external fetal monitor to assess the presence of uterine contractions and fetal heart tones. If labor begins, the suture must be removed immediately.

Uterine Aspiration

Uterine aspiration is used to terminate early pregnancy (i.e., first trimester) or to treat incomplete spontaneous abortion. It is a type of dilatation of the cervix and curettage of the uterus (D&C). A general anesthetic may be used, but the trend has been toward the use of a paracervical block and sedation only. Nursing care in the PACU is essentially the same as after D&C by conventional means. The woman who is Rh negative should receive RhoGam to prevent sensitization. Complications from this procedure include incomplete evacuation and hemorrhage, which may be treated with oxytocin. Uterine perforation may occur and must be treated surgically.

GYNECOLOGIC SURGERY

Certain problems are inherent in gynecologic disease processes and the surgical procedures that deal with them. The patient is frequently more chronically anemic than even the peripheral blood indices may indicate because of prolonged or heavy menstrual periods. In addition, large amounts of blood may have accumulated within the pelvic organs at the time of operation and may not be reflected in the external blood loss. Consequently, shock out of proportion to the estimated or measured blood loss may ensue. Many gynecologic operations, although elective procedures, are associated with significant hemorrhage owing to their location, to the large vascular pedicles with their increased blood supply because of the menstrual cycles, and to the large capillary bleeding that complicates hemostasis.

Because of the proximity of the female genitalia to the urinary tract, great care must be taken during surgery and in the observation period afterward to ensure the integrity of this system. Therefore, in addition to overall assessment and general care of these patients, the PACU nurse should direct specific attention toward the patient's cardiovascular status, renal function, and fluid balance.

Laparoscopy

Laparoscopy is commonly performed as outpatient surgery to diagnose and treat gynecologic problems. It also is being used in major gynecologic surgical procedures. A small incision (approximately 1 cm) is made over the umbilicus to allow for insertion of the laparoscopic needle. After a pneumoperitoneum is established, the surgeon can visualize all the organs within the peritoneum. In this instance, the surgeon can examine the ovaries, fallopian tubes, and uterus. A second and third incision may be made suprapubically in the right or left lower quadrant of the abdomen for further instrumentation. Using this procedure, the surgeon may differentially diagnose pelvic inflammatory disease or perform simple procedures, such as aspiration of cysts, adhesiolysis, tissue biopsy, and tubal ligation. Closure of the skin wound involves only a few sutures or staples, and the dressing is an adhesive bandage. There should be minimal or no drainage or bleeding. Pain should be minimal and easily controlled with acetaminophen or mild narcotics. Severe pain may indicate inadvertent intestinal perforation and, if such pain is present, the surgeon should be notified. Postoperative care instructions, including an explanation of the possibility of referred chest or shoulder pain, should be discussed with the patient and a significant other. Instructions should be written and given to the patient for review as necessary after discharge. Special care of the patient undergoing outpatient surgery is outlined in Chapter 37.

Lower Genital and Vaginal Surgery

The conditions that require this type of surgery occur most commonly in parous and older women. Primarily, they are caused by an exaggeration of the normal relaxation of the pelvic ligaments and support, which occurs during childbirth and after menopause. A number of specific procedures, named after their developers, may be encountered, including the following:

Baldy-Webster procedure: shortening the round ligaments and changing the direction of their pull by attaching them to the back of the uterus.

Fothergill-Hunter procedure: complete repair of the vaginal walls, from above downward toward the vulva, to correct faulty supportive structures of the pelvic floor.

Gilliam procedure: shortening the round ligaments by attaching them to the abdominal wall.

LeFort operation (colpocleisis): closure of the vagina by approximation of the anterior and posterior vaginal walls, with or without attendant vaginal hysterectomy.

Radical vulvectomy: abdominal and perineal dissection of the superficial and deep inguinal nodes and portions of the saphenous veins, reconstruction of the vaginal walls and pelvic floor, and closure of the abdominal wounds.

Vulvectomy: removal of the labia majora, labia minora, and possibly the clitoris and perianal area, with a Z-plasty closure. Used to treat leukoplakia vulvae, carcinoma in situ of the vulva, and Paget's disease of the vulva.

Other vaginal surgical procedures include fistula repairs, those to correct urinary stress incontinence, excision of fibromas and tumors, and vaginal reconstruction to repair congenital or acquired defects.

General Postoperative Care

Anesthesia for lower genital and vaginal surgery may be local, general, or regional, depending on the amount of pelvic relaxation necessary to perform these procedures. On admission to the PACU, the patient should be placed in the side-lying position until the laryngopharyngeal reflexes have returned. She may then assume a position of comfort and be encouraged to move about frequently as part of antiembolism care. After making a general assessment of the patient's condition, check all dressings carefully. Frequently, a vaginal packing is in place, with a perineal pad as the only dressing. Saturation of the vaginal packing may be expected after any vaginal surgery; however, saturation of the perineal pad when vaginal packing is in place should be considered excessive bleeding and should be reported. Vaginal and groin wounds frequently have drains, and care must be exercised to avoid dislodging them. If drains are in place, a moderate amount of drainage may be expected.

Food and fluids may be safely resumed after the minor procedures, such as D&C and bartholinectomy, once the pharyngeal reflexes have returned. After more extensive procedures, the patient is usually not given anything by mouth until peristalsis is re-established; intake is supplied by intravenous fluids. Urine output should be monitored carefully for amount and for the presence of blood. If a Foley or suprapubic catheter is in place, care must be taken to ensure its patency.

Pain must be carefully evaluated and may be alleviated by appropriate analgesics. Abdominal cramping is common after gynecologic surgery. For these patients, relaxation exercises are often helpful if they have been learned preoperatively. Warm blankets over the abdomen may also aid in relaxation. Because the patient is often drowsy owing to the anesthesia, she will need coaching, especially during the first hour. If cramping is not relieved by relaxation exercises, analgesics ordered, or other comfort measures, the surgeon should be notified, because this may indicate a perforated uterus. After removal of tumors or cysts from the vaginal area, ice may be applied to reduce edema and provide comfort.

ABDOMINAL GYNECOLOGIC SURGERY

Abdominal gynecologic surgery may be performed alone or in conjunction with vaginal surgery.

General Postoperative Care

Postoperative care after abdominal gynecologic surgery involves all the care and considerations rendered to the patient undergoing any type of abdominal surgery. Anesthesia is most often general.

Overall assessment of the patient, with special emphasis on the cardiovascular status, should be undertaken as soon as the patient is admitted to the PACU.

The most common and dangerous complications of any obstetric or gynecologic surgery are excessive hemorrhage and shock. Therefore, the PACU nurse should direct assessment to a complete evaluation of the patient's circulatory status at frequent intervals. All dressings should be checked for drainage. Pain should be evaluated, and appropriate comfort measures and analgesics should be administered.

Following hysterectomy and other major abdominal procedures, the patient is usually not given anything orally until peristalsis has returned and nausea has subsided. Intake is supplied by intravenous fluids. Occasionally, the patient is admitted to the PACU with a nasogastric tube in place to prevent abdominal distention. If abdominal distention develops, nasogastric and rectal tubes may be used to relieve it.

Frequently, a Foley catheter is in place, and its patency must be ensured. The PACU nurse should accurately document the amount of urinary output as well as the presence of blood. A not uncommon complication of hysterectomy is accidental perforation or ligation of a ureter. Inadvertent injury to the bladder wall or the bowel may also occur.

To help prevent vascular disorders, especially in the lower extremities, the patient's position should be changed frequently, high-Fowler's position should be avoided, and active and passive range-of-motion exercises of the lower extremities should be instituted in the PACU as soon as possible.

References

1. Berger, P. H., and Saul, H. M.: Radical hysterectomy: Treatment for advanced cervical carcinoma. AORN J., 52(6):1212–1222, 1990.
2. Clark-Pearson, D. L., and Dawood, M. Y.: Green's Gynecology: Essentials of Clinical Practice. 4th ed. Boston, Little, Brown, 1990.
3. Combs, C. A., Murphy, E. L., and Laros, R. K.: Factors associated with hemorrhage in cesarean deliveries. Obstet. Gynecol., 77(1):77–82, 1991.
4. Dickason, E. J., Schult, M. O., and Silverman, B. L.: Maternal-Infant Nursing Care. St. Louis, C. V. Mosby, 1990.
5. Edwards, J.: Lasers in gynecology. Nurs. Clin. North Am., 25(3):673–683, 1990.
6. Frieden, F. J., Ordorica, S. A., Hoskins, I. A., et al.: The Shirodkar operation: A reappraisal. Am. J. Obstet. Gynecol., 163(3):830–833, 1990.
7. Harris, A. P.: The obstetric recovery room. Anesthesiol. Clin. North Am., 8(2):311–323, 1990.
8. Iams, J. D., and Zuspan, F. P. (eds.): Zuspan & Quilligan's Manual of Obstetrics and Gynecology. St. Louis, C. V. Mosby, 1990.
9. Janke, J. R.: Prenatal cocaine use: Effects on perinatal outcome. J. Nurse Midwifery, 35(2):74–77, 1990.
10. Jones, W. B.: Surgical approaches for advanced or recurrent cancer of the cervix. Cancer, 60(8):2094–2103, 1987.
11. Lamb, M. A., and Chu, J.: Invasive cancer of the vulva. AORN J., 47(4):928–936, 1988.
12. Litwack, K.: Practical points in the care of obstetrical surgical patients. J. Post Anesth. Nurs., 5(3):182–185, 1990.
13. Long, B. C., and Glazer, G.: The patient with reproductive problems. In Long, B. C., and Phipps, W. J. (eds.): Medical-Surgical Nursing. St. Louis, C. V. Mosby, 1990.
14. Matthews, N. C., and Greer, G.: Embolism during caesarean section. Anesthesia, 45:964–965, 1990.
15. McLucas, B.: Intrauterine applications of the resectoscope. Surg. Gynecol. Obstet., 172(6):425–431, 1991.
16. Peterfreund, D. O.: Outpatient laparoscopy. J. Post Anesth. Nurs., 3(3):185–188, 1988.
17. Rostad, M. E.: The radical vulvectomy patient: Preventing complications. DCCN, 7(5):289–294, 1988.
18. Stanley, M. E., Seaton, P., and Trobaugh, M.: Post anesthesia care for the patient who has had a spontaneous abortion. J. Post Anesth. Nurs., 3(5):317–320, 1988.

Post Anesthesia Care of the Breast Surgical Patient*

CHAPTER 34

Carole A. Mussler, M.S., R.N.

The American public is not well educated about breast surgery, even though numerous articles appear in newspapers and magazines, programs are presented on television, and health seminars and health fairs are commonly held. Breast surgery is most commonly performed on women; however, procedures are occasionally performed on males and children.

Breast surgery is performed for physical and psychological reasons. Nondisease breast procedures may be performed for cosmetic purposes.

The incidence of breast cancer continues to increase. One in nine American women is expected to develop breast cancer during her lifetime, whereas 1 in 100 men is expected to develop breast cancer in his. Cancer of the breast continues to be one of the leading causes of cancer-related deaths in women.

As the patient's advocate, the post anesthesia care unit (PACU) nurse must be supportive, caring, and reassuring to the patient having breast surgery. Positive support is the start of the patient's rehabilitation process.

Definitions

Augmentation mammoplasty: surgery to enlarge or augment the size of the female breast using a breast implant. This is the most popular cosmetic procedure.

Breast biopsy: excision of breast tissue. The specimen is sent to pathology for frozen section. Also, a needle localization can be performed when a suspected lesion is identified on mammogram. The procedure involves placing a thin needle or guide into the breast under mammographic visualization. The lesion is then excised and taken to pathology for a frozen section to determine a diagnosis.

Breast reconstruction (mammoplasty): the breast is reconstructed after mastectomy.

Lumpectomy: only the tumor and surrounding tissue of a "breast lump" are excised. The rest of the breast remains intact. The procedure includes dissection of the axillary lymph nodes. The lump is generally smaller than 4 cm in diameter.

Mastopexy (breast lift): reshaping (uplifting) the sagging breasts by surgically tightening the skin (Figs. 34–1 and 34–2).

Modified radical mastectomy: removal of the entire breast and axillary lymph nodes; the pectoralis major muscle is left intact. In some instances, the pectoralis minor muscle is excised.

Radical mastectomy: removal of the entire breast,

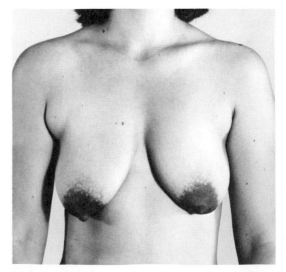

FIGURE 34–1. Mastopexy (breast lift). Before surgery, this patient complained of sagging (ptosis) of the breasts.

*The author gratefully acknowledges the contribution of illustrations and the review of this chapter by Colonel Alan Seyfer, M.C., Chief, Division of Plastic and Reconstructive Surgery, Walter Reed Army Medical Center, Washington, D. C.

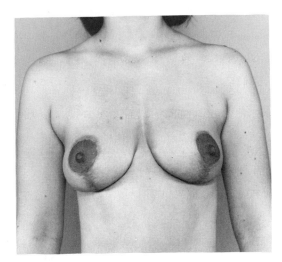

FIGURE 34-2. Mastopexy—same patient as in Fig. 34-1, several weeks postoperatively. The scars are beginning to fade.

skin, nipple, areolar complex, and pectoralis major and minor muscles with axillary node dissection (Figs. 34–3 and 34–4).

POST ANESTHESIA CARE FOLLOWING SPECIFIC PROCEDURES

Breast Biopsy

Lumps in the breast are frequently discovered during monthly self-examination or by routine mammograms. Lumps are aspirated or excised and sent for definitive diagnoses.

In approximately 50 percent of all female patients who undergo a biopsy, the diagnosis is fibrocystic disease. Fibrocystic disease describes a variety of benign and localized tumors or swelling within the breast tissues. Other nonfibrocystic conditions also may cause breast lumps. Inflammatory conditions, such as breast abscesses, fat necrosis, and lipomas of the skin (e.g., sebaceous cysts), may cause breast lumps.

A breast biopsy can be a one-step (biopsy and mastectomy, if needed) or two-step procedure. Two-step procedures are now the most common practice. The two-step procedure allows the patient to be educated about the choices and the opportunity to make an informed decision regarding the type of surgery to be performed in the event of a positive biopsy finding.

Frequently, the patient is admitted as a same-day surgical patient. Owing to natural apprehension, the patient may receive intravenous sedation along with local anesthesia. (See the position statement on intravenous sedation in Chapter 3.)

The patient is usually awake on arrival in the PACU but drowsy owing to the sedation. Routine admission procedures are accomplished. The head of the bed may be elevated 45 degrees.

The dressing is usually a 4 x 4 sponge held in place by the patient's bra. It should be inspected for excessive drainage, but this occurs rarely. The patient can resume fluid and food intake as soon as the cough and gag reflexes have fully returned and nausea has subsided. Pain should be minimal, if any, and easily controlled with minor analgesics.

If the patient has received midazolam (Versed), she may repeatedly ask the same questions. The PACU nurse must patiently repeat the answers and also ensure that home care instructions are understood by the person who will accompany the patient at discharge.

Surgical Choices for the Treatment of Cancer

Advances in early diagnosis and modifications in surgical techniques have increased the number of surgical choices in the treatment of breast cancer (see Fig. 34–3).

Lumpectomy

Lumpectomy is the surgical treatment of choice when the breast tumor is well defined and less than 5 cm in diameter. In clinical trials reported in 1988, the National Surgical Adjuvant Breast Cancer Project reported that lumpectomy followed by radiation therapy produced 8-year disease-free survival rates equal to those of modified radical mastectomy.

Lumpectomy is usually performed under general anesthesia. The tumor is removed along with a margin of surrounding tissue. An axillary node dissection is performed through a separate incision. Axillary dissection involves taking a sample of 10 to 15 lymph nodes lateral and inferior to the pectoralis minor muscles.

When the patient is admitted to the PACU, all the initial assessment measures should be accomplished. The blood pressure cuff should be placed on the arm opposite the operative side. The arm on the operative side should be elevated on a pillow because the removal of lymph nodes increases the risk of lymphedema. The operative-side arm should be as-

SURGICAL MANAGEMENT OF BREAST CANCER

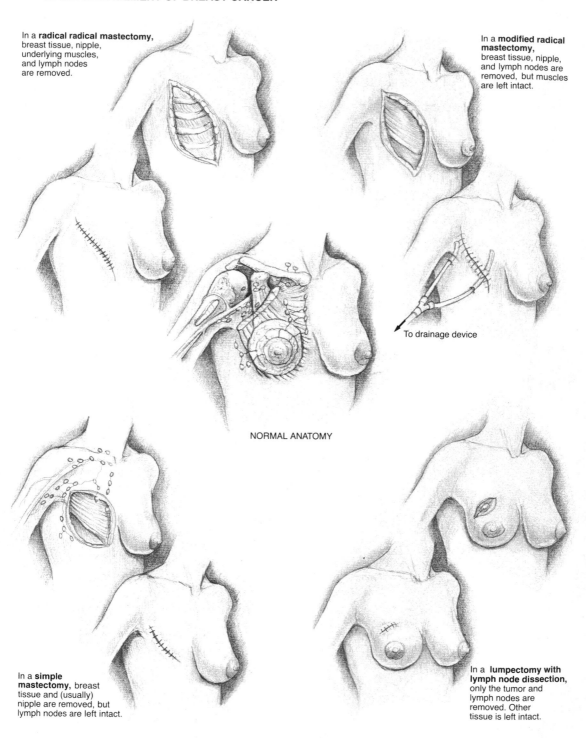

In a **radical radical mastectomy,** breast tissue, nipple, underlying muscles, and lymph nodes are removed.

In a **modified radical mastectomy,** breast tissue, nipple, and lymph nodes are removed, but muscles are left intact.

To drainage device

NORMAL ANATOMY

In a **simple mastectomy,** breast tissue and (usually) nipple are removed, but lymph nodes are left intact.

In a **lumpectomy with lymph node dissection,** only the tumor and lymph nodes are removed. Other tissue is left intact.

FIGURE 34–3. Surgical choices for the treatment of breast cancer. (From Ignatavicius, D. D., and Bayne, M. V.: Medical-Surgical Nursing: A Nursing Process Approach. Philadelphia, W. B. Saunders, 1991, p. 1675.)

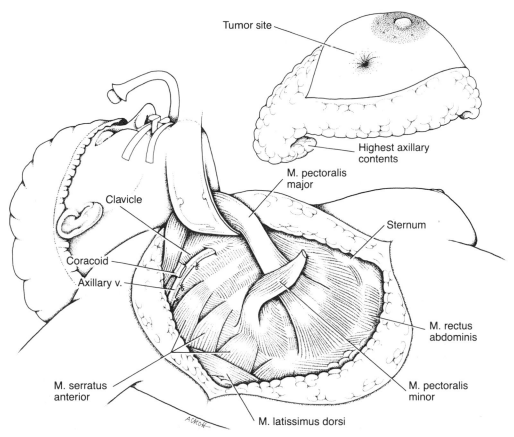

FIGURE 34–4. Mastectomy.

sessed frequently for circulatory adequacy by monitoring color, temperature, capillary refill, and the presence and strength of the radial pulse. Venipunctures and injections should not be performed on the operative-side arm.

Dressings should be small, and bleeding or drainage should be minimal. A Hemovac or Jackson-Pratt closed-drainage system may be connected to drains placed at the incision site.

Nursing personnel should be aware that although this procedure allows the patient to keep her breast, it does not eliminate her fear of the cancer diagnosis or concerns about whether the procedure was successful, and she must be provided factual reassurance.

Mastectomy

Modified Radical Mastectomy. The modified radical mastectomy is the most commonly performed surgery to eliminate breast cancer. The entire breast and axillary nodes are removed. This procedure differs from the Halsted radical mastectomy in that the pectoralis major muscle is left intact.

Radical Mastectomy. The radical mastectomy is seldom performed in the United States. Refined techniques for diagnosis and surgery, radiation therapy, and chemotherapy have made it unnecessary in most instances. Radical mastectomy may be performed in women (primarily elderly women) who do not desire adjuvant therapy (radiation or chemotherapy).

Nursing care after either modified radical or radical mastectomy is essentially the same, except that, of course, the radical mastectomy involves more gross excision of tissue and demands more detailed observation of viability of remaining tissue.

Mastectomy is performed under general inhalation anesthesia. The patient will be admitted to the PACU with the head of her bed elevated 30 to 45 degrees. All admission assessments should be made, oxygen administered, and respiratory sufficiency determined by pulse oximetry.

Dressings are usually bulky and should be checked frequently for excessive serosanguineous drainage and for constriction. The most important postoperative complication is hematoma occurring below the skin flaps. Attention to the drains and the maintenance of free drainage within the vacuum system prevent this. Drains are usually placed under the skin flaps to remove excess blood and serum that would ordinarily collect under the wound site, causing edema, infection, and sloughing of the skin graft. The drains may be connected to Hemovac or Jackson-Pratt devices. Generally, additional vacuum is needed the first 8 hours postoperatively, and the Hemovac is connected to vacuum pressure of 20 to 30 mm Hg. These should be monitored for excessive bleeding, which must be reported to the surgeon. Dressings are necessarily snug but should not impair respiration or circulation to the upper extremity. The arm on the operative side should be supported and elevated on a pillow; it must be checked frequently for cyanosis or pallor, and the pulse palpated for intensity. If signs of respiratory distress or impaired circulation arise, the surgeon should be notified to rearrange the dressing. Unless an emergency arises, the PACU nurse should not attempt to loosen the dressing, because skin grafts may inadvertently be disrupted.

When a radical mastectomy is performed, there is extensive excision, and skin grafting is usually required (see Chapter 35). Donor sites (usually the thigh) should be checked for drainage and treated according to hospital policy.

The patient should be advised to avoid excessive motion in the immediate postoperative period. She should not strain the pectoral girdle by levering herself on the bed with her arms to change position. These patients usually need intravenous fluid augmentation for the first 24 hours postoperatively. There is no reason to refrain from oral feeding after cough and gag reflexes have returned and if there is no nausea. Small sips of fluids may be offered and taken as desired and diet resumed as tolerated. Postoperative pain is moderate to severe and can usually be controlled with narcotics such as meperidine (Demerol) and morphine. Hypothermia may be a problem owing to prolonged exposure in the operating room, and rewarming should be accomplished with additional warmed blankets or a Bair-Hugger.

Postoperative instructions for patients having axillary node dissections should include hand and arm care instructions. Consistent education and support are required. Emotional support may be obtained with support groups such as the "Reach to Recovery" program.*

*Reach to Recovery Program, c/o American Cancer Society, 1599 Clifton Road, NE, Atlanta, GA 30329.

Breast Reconstruction

One of the advances made in breast surgery during recent years is the availability of effective means of reconstructing the breast after removal for cancer. This can be done by a variety of methods in which the surgeon in collaboration with a plastic surgeon, tailors the operation to the patient's deformity. Breast reconstruction may be accomplished in conjunction with mastectomy or at a later time.

For reconstructive augmentation mammoplasty, a pocket is made under the remaining tissues into which a soft silicone bag is made to simulate the natural contour (Figs. 34–5 and 34–6). The pocket can be made at the time of surgery or before the surgery by means of an inflatable tissue extender. The expander method requires the administration of several injections of gradually increasing volumes of saline over a period of weeks. The expander is then replaced surgically with a soft silicone bag prosthesis.

Muscle-skin flap reconstruction (Figs. 34–7 and 34–8) involves moving nearby muscle and skin into the area of the mastectomy to replace the lost volume. Commonly used muscle and skin flaps include the latissimus dorsi and rectus abdominis muscles with attached skin. Nipple-areola reconstruction may be accomplished by using small portions of the labia and grafting to the selected location.

Postoperative care is generally the same as for the patient experiencing other types of

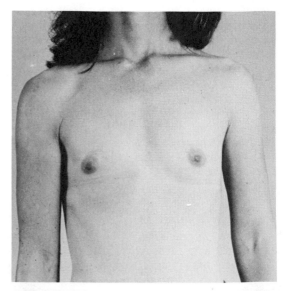

FIGURE 34–5. Appearance of patient before breast augmentation.

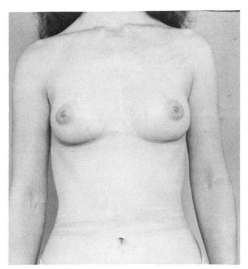

FIGURE 34–6. Postoperative appearance of patient after breast augmentation with silicone bag prostheses.

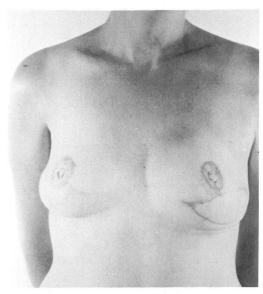

FIGURE 34–8. Appearance of same patient as in Fig. 34–7 after muscle-skin flap (latissimus) and nipple reconstructions. The patient has gained much weight, and later she delivered a healthy baby. She is free of disease 6 years after the mastectomy.

breast surgery, with attention to graft and flap donor sites.

These operations have served to provide a measure of comfort to patients whose body image has been significantly disrupted by mastectomy. They report a return of their sense of femininity and confidence. Many women do not choose to undergo additional surgery after mastectomy, but knowing that the operation is available is reassuring to them.

Mastopexy (Breast Lift)

Breast ptosis (sagging) is defined by the position of the nipple areolar complex related to the inframammary crease. The reshaping process differs from reduction mammoplasty in the amount of tissue removed. Generally less than 300 g of tissue removed is to be considered a mastopexy procedure.

Mastopexy is commonly being performed as a same-day procedure, and postoperative care following mastopexy is generally not demanding. General anesthesia is most commonly used, and only minor adjustments in breast tissue are made.

Postoperatively, the patient is positioned on her back and may assume a semi-Fowler's to high-Fowler's position for comfort as soon as she awakens. The motion of the arms is restricted to below shoulder level.

Postoperative dressings are minimal, and drains are rarely required, because the entire procedure, with the exception of nipple release, is at the level of the dermis. Drainage should be minimal, and if frank bleeding occurs, the surgeon should be notified. Pain is usually not a problem, and discomfort can be controlled with the mild analgesics. Food and fluids may be resumed as tolerated after nausea has disappeared.

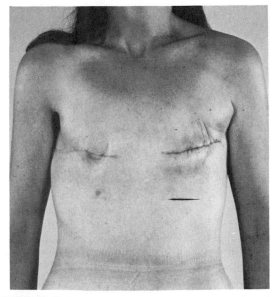

FIGURE 34–7. Appearance of patient after healing from bilateral mastectomies for cancer.

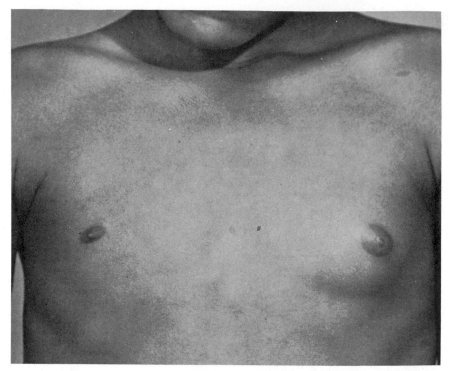

FIGURE 34–9. Gynecomastia (idiopathic hypertrophy of the breast) in an 8-year-old boy. (From Haagensen, C. D.: Diseases of the Breast. 3rd ed. Philadelphia, W. B. Saunders, 1986, p. 69.)

Mammoplasty

Nursing care for reduction and augmentation mammoplasties is essentially the same for both procedures.

Reduction mammoplasty is the surgical method of correcting mammary hypertrophy. Women who experience mammary hypertrophy often complain of shoulder strap discomfort, breast pain, back and neck pain, and an inability to participate in physical activities such as jogging, aerobics, and horseback riding.

A new method in reduction mammoplasty is the laser de-epithelialization technique. When the carbon dioxide laser is used to remove the epidermis from the inferior pedicle, reduction mammoplasty can be performed with little blood loss. The inferior pedicle technique is a frequently used approach to reduction mammoplasty. When the inferior pedicle technique is used, the laser simplifies skin removal. The laser is preferred for pedicle de-epithelialization in all patients, but especially in patients having large ptotic breasts, because rigid stabilization is not necessary.

Anesthesia may be local, in combination with appropriate sedation, or general for breast augmentation. Breast reduction is usually carried out under general anesthesia and may require more extensive manipulation of tissue. Regional anesthesia with intercostal block may be used for either procedure if the patient is not fearful of being conscious during the operation.

On admission to the PACU, the patient is positioned on her back, and as soon as her condition warrants, placed in a low-Fowler's position. Dressings may be of any variety, but most commonly wide strips of Elastoplast, which readily conform to the patient's new skin contours, is used. A Velpeau bandage should be in place to restrain the patient from raising her arms, and she should be advised of this. Drains are rarely required, and drainage should be minimal. If drains are present, they should be connected to a vacuum source, such as the Hemovac. As after mastectomy, the patient should be advised to do nothing that puts strain on the pectoral girdle.

Pain after augmentation is generally minimal and can be relieved with mild analgesics. Light ice packs may be used to relieve discomfort and to minimize tissue swelling. Pain after reduction may be more significant and usually requires the use of narcotic analgesia for the first 24 hours.

Surgery in Gynecomastia

Gynecomastia, or benign hypertrophy of one or both breasts in boys and men, is relatively common (Fig. 34–9). It may be bilateral or unilateral. The causes may be hormonal, systemic disease oriented, drug related, or idiopathic.

In extreme instances, or when it causes problems in psychological adjustment, this excess tissue can be excised or removed with suction lipectomy. Suction lipectomy is useful when the gynecomastia is primarily caused by fat. Good cosmetic results are obtained. The surgical procedure is similar to that of breast reduction in women. A periareolar incision is made and tissue removed. Suction drainage of the incision site is usually necessary and may be conveniently accomplished by use of a Hemovac.

Postoperative care is essentially the same as that for women undergoing breast surgery. If no drains are required, the patient can be discharged the day of surgery once reflexes have returned, nausea has subsided, and food and fluids can be taken.

References

1. American Cancer Society: Cancer Facts and Figures. Atlanta, American Cancer Society, 1989.
2. Becker, D. W., and Bunn, J. C.: Laser de-epithelialization: An adjunct to reduction mammoplasty. Plast. Reconstr. Surg., 79(5):754–760, 1979.
3. Cawley, M., Kostic, J., and Cappello, C.: Information and psychological needs of women choosing conservative surgery. Cancer Nurs., 13(2):90–94, 1990.
4. Fisher, B., Redmond, C., Poisson, R., et al.: Eight-year results of a randomized clinical trial comparing mastectomy and lumpectomy with or without radiation in the treatment of breast cancer. New Engl. J. Med., 320:822–828, 1989.
5. Georgiade, G. S.: Reconstructive and aesthetic breast surgery. In Sabiston, D. C., Jr. (ed.): Textbook of Surgery: The Biological Basis of Modern Surgical Practice. 14th ed. Philadelphia, W. B. Saunders, 1991, pp. 551–555.
6. Harris, J. R., Helman, S., Henderson, I. C., et al.: Breast Diseases. 2nd ed. Philadelphia, J. B. Lippincott, 1991.
7. Iglehart, J. D.: The breast. In Sabiston, D. C., Jr. (ed.): Textbook of Surgery: The Biological Basis of Modern Surgical Practice. 14th ed. Philadelphia, W. B. Saunders, 1991, pp. 510–550.
8. Nielson, B. B., and East, D.: Advances in breast cancer. Nurs. Clin. North Am., 25(2):365–375, 1990.
9. Patrick, M.: Medical-Surgical Nursing. 2nd ed. Philadelphia, J. B. Lippincott, 1991.
10. Stein, P., and Zera, R. T.: Breast cancer. AORN J., 53(4):938–963, 1991.

Post Anesthesia Care of the Plastic Surgical Patient

CHAPTER 35

Carole A. Mussler, M.S., R.N.

The field of plastic surgery continues to grow and expand daily, presenting numerous challenges to the surgeon performing plastic and reconstructive surgery. This discipline has changed profoundly during the past 10 years, especially in the area of reconstructive surgery.

Plastic surgery derives its name from the Greek word *plastikos,* which means to mold or give shape. Plastic and reconstructive procedures correct acquired and congenital deformities. Corrective procedures deal with the body in its entirety, striving to restore normal appearance as well as function.

A deformity can be devastating not only to physical well-being but to spiritual and psychological well-being as well. Each of us desires to be whole. The parents of a child with a congenital malformation often have a profound sense of guilt.

There are few absolutes in plastic surgical techniques and in the associated preoperative or postoperative care. Therefore, only the basic aspects of postoperative care for the plastic surgery patient are presented here. Some elements of care related to specific body parts are discussed in related chapters, and the reader is referred to them.

The most basic techniques of plastic surgery relate to excision of skin lesions, to closure of skin wounds, and to placement of skin grafts and skin flaps. Minor plastic surgical procedures are often performed using local anesthesia. Postoperative nursing care is minimal, primarily involving observation of the surgical site for untoward symptoms. When the patient must undergo general anesthesia, postoperative care includes all the considerations discussed under general care of the postoperative patient, in addition to attention to the surgical site. Postoperative vital signs, including accurate temperature measurement, are especially important in the care of the post anesthesia plastic surgical patient, because these signs provide baselines from which to judge the possible later complications of an immunologic reaction.

SKIN GRAFTS

Skin grafting is the most common method for covering open areas rapidly and permanently. A skin graft is a layer of epidermis with attached dermis of variable thickness that is completely isolated from its blood supply from the donor site. It is transferred to a recipient site elsewhere on the body without formal surgical revascularization.

The types of skin grafts are defined as follows:

1. A *full-thickness graft* includes all underlying dermis.
2. A *split-thickness graft* includes a portion of the underlying dermis. It may be thin, medium, or thick, depending on the amount of dermis that is included.
3. A *composite graft* comprises two or more tissue components, often skin and subcutaneous tissue, cartilage, or mucosa.
4. *Autograft* indicates that the donor and the recipient are the same person.
5. *Isograft* signifies that the donor and the recipient are genetically identical.
6. *Allograft or homograft* means that the donor and the recipient are of the same species.
7. *Xenograft* indicates that the donor and the recipient are of different species.

The most important factor in the success of a skin graft is adherence. The graft must have good contact with healthy tissue that has adequate vascularity. When the graft is properly placed on the recipient site, a fibrin layer forms that binds the graft to the recipient bed. A plasmalike fluid (extravasated from blood vessels in the area) collects at the graft site. This fluid contains sufficient nourishment for the graft to survive until new vascularization has been established.

For cosmetically pleasing results, the color, texture, thickness, and hair-bearing nature of the skin used for grafting must be chosen to match the recipient site. As a rule, the nearer the donor skin is to the recipient area, the better the match will be.

It is important to check during the first 24 hours postoperatively that there is serum or blood present. Too much fluid may cause the graft to lift from its bed. Excess fluid must be removed. The donor site should be kept clean and will heal with a new layer of skin. Because of the variations in surgeons' preferences in the method of dressing wounds, positioning of the patient, use of ice or antibiotic ointments, and handling of donor sites, it is essential that the post anesthesia care unit (PACU) have established policies related to the care of the plastic surgical patient as established by the individual plastic surgeon (see Chapter 36 for additional discussion of care for grafts and donor sites).

Generally, the grafted area should be elevated, if possible, and protected from both pressure and motion. The patient should be positioned to prevent pressure on, or other trauma to, either the graft or the donor site. The physician may order cold packs to reduce the metabolic requirements of the graft and enhance its survival. These can be made by partially filling a rubber glove with cracked ice and cool water or saline, which makes a light, moldable cold pack. Dressings over grafts should be observed closely for drainage, and any excess should be reported to the physician.

Full-thickness donor sites may be sutured closed and treated as a surgical wound if the donor site is small. If a large area is used for full-thickness grafting, it may be necessary to graft the donor site with split-thickness grafts (Fig. 35–1).

FLAPS

The term *flap* commonly refers to a skin flap; however, because of the advances in reconstructive surgery, flaps are not limited to skin tissue. Flaps are classified by their anatomic composition: skin with muscle fascia or bone, or both; skin alone; omentum; or a composite of these tissues.

Local Flaps

Flaps (Fig. 35–2) are the preferred treatment for covering wounds with vascularity inade-

quate to support a skin graft; reconstructing full-thickness defects of specialized body parts such as ears, eyelids, nose and lips; and covering over gliding tendons. Reconstructions requiring tissue bulk, such as decubitus closure, are also done with flaps.

Microvascular Tissue Transfer

Microvascular tissue transfer is one of the most important advances in the field of reconstructive surgery. The surgeon who performs microvascular tissue transfer harvests tissue from one part of the body and transfers it to virtually any other part of the body to replace missing tissue or heal problem wounds.

Microvascular tissue transfer is possible only when the surgeon has access to a sophisticated operative microscope with high magnification. Whichever type of flap is used, the newly positioned flap is kept under constant observation by PACU personnel. The most serious complication in the microvascular tissue transfer procedure is necrosis of the tissue. Tissue death occurs when either the artery or the vein supplying the flap develops a thrombus. Arterial thrombosis can result in complete flap failure within 4 hours of onset. Arterial occlusion is characterized by a pale, cool flap that does not bleed when stuck with a needle.

Venous thrombosis is more common, but it is not an immediate threat. It is identified by a congested, warm, mottled flap that continuously oozes dark blood. Objective assessment of the flap is possible through the use of fluorometry, laser Doppler, temperature monitoring, buried Doppler probe, and a photoplethysmograph (PPG) disk. The PPG disk monitors the blood flow. The PACU nurse should notify the surgeon when the monitoring indicates occlusion is occurring.

Pain at the sites of skin grafting or flaps is usually minimal; donor sites ordinarily generate the more painful stimuli. Management includes mild analgesics and attention to comfort measures.

BONE GRAFTS

When bone grafts have been performed, the graft site must be immobilized and excessive movement of the patient avoided. The patient may experience considerable pain at the donor site and must be moved carefully. Pain can be managed with narcotic analgesics after an assessment of the patient's overall condition is

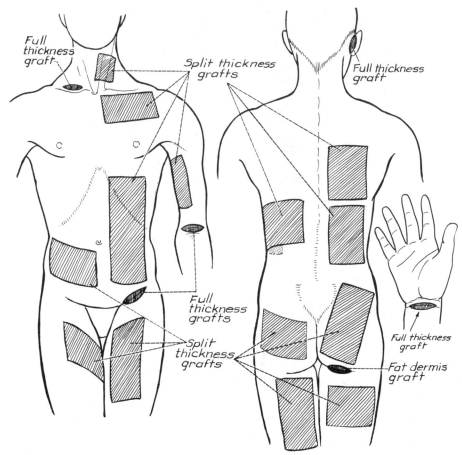

FIGURE 35-1. Available donor sites of skin grafts. (From Converse, J. M.: Reconstructive Plastic Surgery. Vol. 1, 2nd ed. Philadelphia, W. B. Saunders, 1977, p. 176.)

made. If split-rib grafts are used, the patient should be placed in a low-Fowler's position; respiratory status should be checked frequently; and signs of possible pneumothorax, such as tachycardia and tachypnea, should be reported to the surgeon immediately. Graft sites may require elevation, and ice is frequently used for pain management and reduction of swelling.

COSMETIC SURGERY

Physical appearance affects self-image and can be extremely important psychologically. Cosmetic surgery is sought by people striving to enhance their physical appearance, and it has become commonplace. In the United States, this may be the result, in part, of the national preoccupation with youth and the desire to remain forever youthful in appearance.

Whatever the reasons, one must recognize that such surgery does take place, and that,

because it is a surgical procedure, it cannot be taken lightly. These patients have been screened by their surgeon and found to be acceptable in terms of risk, psychological testing, and "anatomic deformity." The patients place an enormous importance (and often expense) on their surgery and should not be looked down on or made the object of insensitive remarks about their vanity. Those associated with postoperative care of the cosmetic surgery patient should give the same professional care to that patient as the care provided any other. If the nurse has significant biases against these procedures, reassignment should be considered.

Dermabrasion

Dermabrasion is the surgical planing of the skin, with removal of the epidermis and portions of the superficial dermis, to remove high spots or other irregularities in an uneven skin

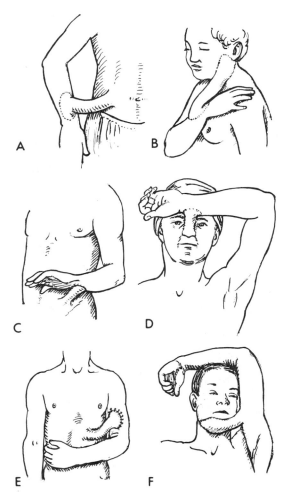

FIGURE 35-2. Various methods of transfer of tubed pedicle flaps. *A* and *B,* transfer via the wrist; *C* and *D,* the "salute" position of Kilner; *E* and *F,* transfer via the arm (Schuchardt). (From Converse, J. M.: Reconstructive Plastic Surgery. Vol. 1, 2nd ed. Philadelphia, W. B. Saunders, 1977, p. 211.)

surface. Enough of the dermal and epidermal elements are preserved to allow re-epithelialization, and the result is smooth healing and blending of the scarred areas with the surrounding skin surface.

Usually the dermabraded areas are treated by the open method, and post anesthesia care includes protection of those areas from abrasion caused by rubbing on pillows or bed clothing. Facial edema, especially of the eyelids, may be expected, and the patient must be reassured that this will subside rapidly. The dermabraded area should be observed closely for the development of moisture. If moisture develops, it should be dried with a heat lamp or a warm hair dryer. This procedure may produce an uncomfortable burning sensation for the patient that may be minimized by holding the lamp or dryer a considerable distance from the area to be dried. Analgesics should be administered as necessary to manage burning-type pain sensations.

Blepharoplasty

Blepharoplasty is a procedure to correct deformities of the upper or lower eyelid by excising redundant skin or protruding fat. The procedure is most frequently performed under local anesthesia with supplemental intravenous sedation. Swelling and bleeding are minimized by using iced compresses. The patient may resume a regular diet postoperatively; however, hot liquids are contraindicated for 24 hours to prevent vasodilatation and bleeding. Activities such as bending and heavy lifting should be avoided. Pain is usually minimal and can be managed with mild analgesics. Aspirin should be avoided. Antibiotic ointment may be used for lubrication (see also Chapter 24).

Rhytidoplasty (Face-Lift)

The face-lift operation is usually done under local anesthesia with supplementary sedation. Although some "lift" is accomplished around the cheek areas, the most important and long-lasting change is in the loose skin of the neck. The facial-neck skin is freed from the underlying tissues and pulled upward and backward toward the postauricular scalp. Excess skin is trimmed off, and meticulous suturing is performed. The procedure takes from 2 to 5 hours, and the patient comes to the PACU with a large, fluffy bandage about the neck and cheeks. Surprisingly, such extensive surgery is not usually associated with significant pain. Pain, especially on one side, is *unusual* and may be the first sign of a complication. It may mean that the skin is being tightened by active bleeding—the most common serious complication of face-lift. The surgeon should be notified at once, and he or she may decide to open the dressing to assess the situation. Bleeding is more common in patients with hypertension. Sedation, a quiet atmosphere, and continued elevation of the head of the bed are important measures in the prevention of complications.

Rhinoplasty

Rhinoplasty is performed to reshape or reconstruct the nose when its shape has been altered as a result of trauma or when the patient is unhappy with its form. Rhinoplasty may be performed under local anesthesia with supplemental narcotics and intravenous sedation or general anesthesia. On admission to the PACU, the patient's head is elevated 30 to 45 degrees. Humidified oxygen is administered. In addition to routine assessment, the nasal area is assessed for swelling and bleeding. Drip pads (2×2s) may be lightly taped under the nostrils.

Otoplasty

Otoplasty is performed to reduce prominence of the ears. The patient has a head dressing for support. Generally, there is only minimal discomfort that lasts no longer than 12 hours postoperatively. Pain that lasts longer suggests a hematoma or other complication and should be reported to the surgeon.

Liposuction

Suction lipectomy (liposuction) is a technique for removing subcutaneous fat to improve facial or body contours. It may be used in conjunction with other techniques. Anesthesia may be local or general. Liposuction is commonly performed in the same-day surgical arena; however, if more than 2500 ml of fat is removed, an overnight stay and fluid replacement may be necessary.

Pain should be minimal. However, if large areas are treated, analgesia with meperidine may be required. Drugs containing aspirin should be avoided so as not to increase bleeding time. If large areas are suctioned, the patient needs intravenous fluid replacement. The patient can usually start oral fluids and a progressive diet as soon as pharyngeal reflexes have returned.

Relatively few complications of this procedure have been reported; however, postoperative bleeding and infection are possible.

SURGICAL REPAIR OF INJURIES TO THE FACIAL BONES

Because of their protrusion and prominence, the facial bones are frequently broken in motor vehicle accidents, fights, and sporting events. Fractures vary in their location and complexity, and the repair may vary from closed reduction to the use of internal fixation with plates and

screws, interosseous wiring, and bone grafting. Repair of injuries to the facial bones often requires general anesthesia. If the damage is extensive and airway obstruction or concomitant cranial or intrathoracic injury is present, a tracheostomy must be performed. All patients who have facial, jaw, or neck surgery should have a tracheostomy set kept at the bedside in the PACU, in the event that an airway emergency should occur. If a tracheostomy is not performed, the endotracheal tube or nasotracheal tube should be left in place until the laryngopharyngeal reflexes have fully returned. Because the apparatus may be most uncomfortable, the nurse must explain the need for it to the patient and enlist his or her cooperation (see Chapters 12 and 21 for the essential procedures).

On admission to the PACU, the patient who has undergone repair of the facial bones is placed in a low-Fowler's position as soon as his or her condition warrants. This aids in minimizing the development of head and neck edema. Careful monitoring of the airway is mandatory.

If interdental wire fixation was performed, a pair of wire clippers should be affixed to the head of the bed (clearly visible to all personnel) in the event that rapid opening of the jaws is needed. Opening of the jaws may become necessary if an airway emergency develops (see Chapter 23 for care of the patient with interdental fixation).

Good oral hygiene is a priority for these patients and may be accomplished with lemon-glycerin swabs and a weak solution of hydrogen peroxide. Petrolatum ointment should be applied to the lips to prevent drying and cracking. Frequent suctioning of secretions may be necessary during the first postoperative hours. Once nausea has subsided and the gag reflex has fully returned, the patient may be allowed small sips of fluids.

SURGICAL REPAIR OF CLEFT LIP AND PALATE

Cleft lips and palates are common congenital defects that have many associated problems, including facial growth abnormalities, dental irregularities, speech difficulties, ear diseases, psychological disorders, and cosmetic problems. A cleft palate creates difficult nursing and swallowing for the infant.

Repair of the cleft lip (Figs. 35–3 and 35–4) is usually accomplished when the child is about 3 months old. He or she should weigh at

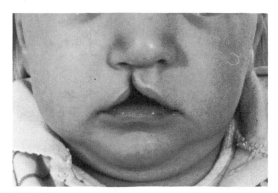

FIGURE 35-3. Preoperative appearance of a unilateral cleft lip.

least 10 lb and have a hemoglobin level of at least 10 g per dl. Repair is accomplished under general anesthesia. On admission to the PACU, the infant is placed in a semiprone position. The infant's arms should be restrained to avoid disruption of the newly repaired lip, and the infant should not be allowed to cry, because crying puts excessive tension on the newly repaired lip. If possible, the mother or father should be allowed in the PACU to hold the child, because this often prevents crying. A rocking chair may prove invaluable in comforting the child, who may be sedated, if necessary.

The most important nursing activity, in addition to preventing trauma to the lip, is airway management. A mist humidifier at the bedside (or rocking-chair side) should be used

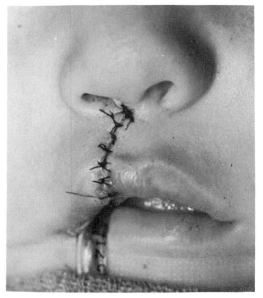

FIGURE 35-4. Postoperative appearance of unilateral cleft lip. The incision is covered with an antibiotic ointment to prevent crusting.

at least 12 hours postoperatively to aid in clearing of secretions and general respiratory well-being. Hemorrhage may occur as a complication but is rare; however, the loss of even a few milliliters of blood in an infant may be significant, and any bleeding requires definitive control. Once the child has fully awakened from anesthesia, small sips of clear fluids may be given.

Pain is usually minimal. Iced normal saline–soaked gauze may be applied to the suture areas to reduce swelling and promote comfort. Analgesia may be provided with the milder oral analgesics.

Repair of a cleft palate is usually completed when the child is 12 to 18 months of age, preferably before the beginning of speech. It is advantageous, again, to have a parent accompany the child in the PACU if possible. On admission to the PACU, the child is placed in the semiprone or "tonsil" position, and careful attention should be given to airway maintenance. As in cleft lip repair, the child's arms should be restrained and crying avoided. The head should not be flexed, because this tends to occlude the airway.

Suctioning of secretions may be necessary but must be performed gently and only if the nurse's view is unobstructed. The catheter, plastic dental suction tip, or Yankauer suction tip should be passed over the dorsum of the tongue, and only minimal vacuum pressure should be used. A mist tent or cold-mist humidifier should be used for at least 12 hours postoperatively to aid in the elimination of tenacious secretions.

Hemorrhage may occur as a complication and requires control. Any bleeding should be recorded and reported to the surgeon. Pain may be managed with mild analgesics, such as acetaminophen elixir. Rarely, a stronger analgesic is needed.

MICROSURGERY

Microsurgery is performed with the aid of the dissecting microscope, which greatly improves visualization of the detail of small structures. Its greatest value in plastic surgery has been in the repair of small blood vessels and nerves. Post anesthesia care for the patient who has undergone microsurgery is the same as that for the principal procedure, with emphasis on notation of color changes in the skin at the operative site. *White* indicates that no blood is entering the area, owing to probable arterial blockage. *Pink* is normal. Check for a blanch reflex—momentary pressure on the skin should produce white blanching, which should return to normal pink color within seconds after release of pressure. *Blue* indicates the presence of blood that is low in oxygen and suggests a problem. *Dark blue to black with swelling* indicates impending death of tissue caused by venous obstruction. Any color change from the normal pink should be reported to the surgeon immediately.

References

1. Arnet, G. F., and Basehore, L. M.: Dentofacial reconstruction. Am. J. Nurs., *84*(12):1488–1490, 1984.
2. Baj, P. A.: Liposuction: "New wave" plastic surgery. Am. J. Nurs., *84*(7):892–893, 1984.
3. Fraulini, K. E.: Nursing care of the plastic/reconstructive surgery patient. Curr. Rev. Recov. Room Nurses, *2*(6):11–15, 1984.
4. Goodman, R.: Grafts and flaps in plastic surgery. AORN J., *48*(4):650–663, 1988.
5. Grossman, J. A.: Body contouring. AORN J., *48*(4):713–714, 1988.
6. Jrukuwicz, M. J., Drezek, T. J., Mathes, S. G., et al.: Plastic Surgery: Principles and Practices. Vol. 1. St. Louis, C. V. Mosby, 1990.
7. Mulliken, J. B.: Principles and techniques of bilateral cleft lip repair. Plast. Reconstr. Surg., *75*:477–487, 1985.
8. Sauter, S. K.: Cleft lips and palates. AORN J., *50*(4):813–823, 1989.
9. Swain, D., and Shell, D. H.: Microvascular tissue transfer. AORN J., *49*(4):1032–1043, 1989.

Post Anesthesia Care of the Thermally Injured Patient

CHAPTER 36

Dennis M. Driscoll, Major, A.N., M.S., R.N., C.C.R.N., C.E.N.

A serious burn is one of the most devastating injuries that a human can sustain. It affects the skin and every organ system of the body, with the magnitude of the effect proportionate to the extent of burn. As the third most common cause of accidental death in the United States, thermal injury is a major health problem in that an estimated 2 million people seek medical attention annually for thermal injuries. Approximately 75,000 are hospitalized, and an estimated 7000 die of the direct effects or complications associated with these injuries.[17] Nursing care for the thermally injured patient requires collaboration between members of a multidisciplinary health care team. Knowledge of the local and systemic manifestations of thermal injury is required to ensure a thorough assessment of the patient's condition and an evaluation of the patient's response.[17]

INTEGUMENTARY SYSTEM

To understand the physiologic reactions to a thermal injury, it is important to review the anatomy of the skin (Chapter 10). The skin is more than a simple hide that covers the body. It is a combination of tissues that form the largest organ of the body that provides a buffer between the internal and external environments. The skin is the first line of defense for protection against infection, prevention of loss of body fluids, regulation of body temperature, and provision of sensory input through the sense of touch.

The anatomic layers of the skin are the epi-

dermis and the dermis. The epidermis is the outermost layer and is composed of stratified squamous epithelial tissue varying in depth from 0.07 to 0.12 mm, with the deepest areas being on the palms of the hands and the soles of the feet.[2] Histologically, the epidermis can be subdivided into five layers, the most important of which are the stratum corneum and the stratum germinativum. The *stratum corneum,* which is constantly shed, is composed of densely packed dead cells, keratin, and surface lipids. The major function of this layer is to provide a barrier to prevent the loss of body fluids or the invasion of microbes or noxious agents from the environment. The *stratum germinativum* is constantly undergoing subdivision to form new cells that replace those shed from surface layers. It is only in the germinativum layer that cells undergo mitosis leading to new epithelium.

The dermis ranges in thickness from 1 to 2 mm and lies below the epidermis. This layer is composed of collagen, connective tissues, smooth muscle, blood vessels, nerves, lymphatics, and glandular structures. Within the dermal layer, the sweat glands and hair follicles are lined with epithelial cells that generate epithelium to assist in the closure of partial-thickness wounds. The dermis provides nutrients and structure for the epidermis. Under the dermis lies the hypodermis, which contains fat, smooth muscle, and areolar tissue. This layer acts as a heat insulator and shock absorber.

THERMAL INJURY CLASSIFICATION

The classification of thermal injuries is based on the depth of the injury, which is directly related to the temperature and duration of exposure to the thermal energy.[12] The longer the tissue is in contact with a high temperature

The opinions or assertions contained herein are the private views of the author and are not to be construed as official or as reflecting the views of the U.S. Army Institute of Surgical Research, the Department of the Army, or the Department of Defense.

499

source, the deeper the tissue destruction. Formerly, the depth of injury was identified as first, second, and third degree. Currently, the preferred nomenclature for reporting depth of injury is *superficial, partial-thickness, and full-thickness injury*. Superficial injury involves the outermost layer of the epidermis and is usually caused by prolonged exposure to the sun. On presentation, the skin appears dry, erythematous, and usually without blisters; is painful; and has a rapid capillary refill. Systemic involvement is limited, with complete healing occurring in 5 to 7 days. The magnitude of the physiologic derangement from edema formation and alteration of the evaporative barrier is minor. The major disability is pain. Patients with superficial injury usually do not require hospitalization.

Partial-thickness injury can be further subdivided into superficial partial-thickness and deep-dermal partial-thickness types. These injuries are characterized by damage involving the epidermis and varying depths of the dermis. The *superficial partial-thickness injury* involves the epidermis with sparing of most dermal appendages. On presentation, the skin is pink or mottled red, may have formed blisters, or is wet with serous exudate. There is a decreased rate of capillary refill, and the wound is extremely painful. The margin of the wound is raised with respect to adjacent unburned tissue owing to the edema within the wound. This level of partial-thickness injury usually heals without skin grafting. *Deep-dermal partial-thickness injury* destroys the entire epidermis and most of the dermis, leaving only the epithelial lining of the hair follicles and sweat glands intact. On examination, the skin appears wet with serous exudate, is dark red or waxy white in color, and has a decreased sensitivity to touch. Because of the structures involved and the compromised perfusion that occurs in deep-dermal injury, mechanical trauma or infection may convert this injury to a full-thickness level.

Full-thickness injury involves the destruction of both layers of the skin to the level of hypodermis or subcutaneous tissue and may involve fat, fascia, muscle, and bone. All epithelial elements are destroyed. These wounds present as dry, charred, or pearly white and have a leathery texture. The wound is depressed relative to unburned tissue or adjacent partial-thickness injury owing to the lack of circulation, loss of elasticity, and coagulation necrosis. With the destruction of the dermal elements, these wounds are anesthetic and require autografting to close the wound.

EXTENT OF INJURY

There are two methods used to estimate the body surface area (extent) of thermal injury. The most commonly used tool for rapid estimation in an adult patient is the Rule of Nines. This guideline reflects the fact that various regions represent 9 percent or multiples of 9 percent of the total body surface area. The head and neck area represents 9 percent; the anterior and posterior trunk each represents 18 percent; each upper extremity represents 9 percent; each lower extremity represents 18 percent; and the perineum and genitalia represent 1 percent (Fig. 36–1). By determining the portion of each region involved, one can quickly estimate the percentage of body surface area injured. Because the percentage of the various regions differs with age, a different tool is needed for infants and children. A more precise prediction is accomplished using the Lund and Browder chart, which is an age-adjusted surface area chart (Fig. 36–2).

TYPES OF THERMAL INJURY

Thermal injury may result from contact with heat, cold, chemicals, or electricity. Most ther-

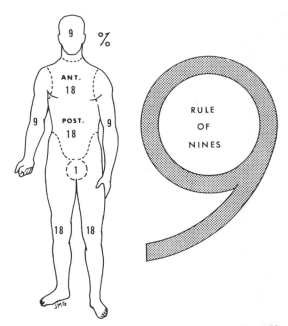

FIGURE 36–1. Schematic outline of the Rule of Nines. Use of the rule provides a rapid method to determine the percentage of body surface burned, but it is of limted accuracy. (From Sabiston, D. C., Jr. [ed.]: Davis-Christopher Textbook of Surgery: The Biological Basis of Modern Surgical Practice. 11th ed. Philadelphia, W. B. Saunders, 1977, p. 298.)

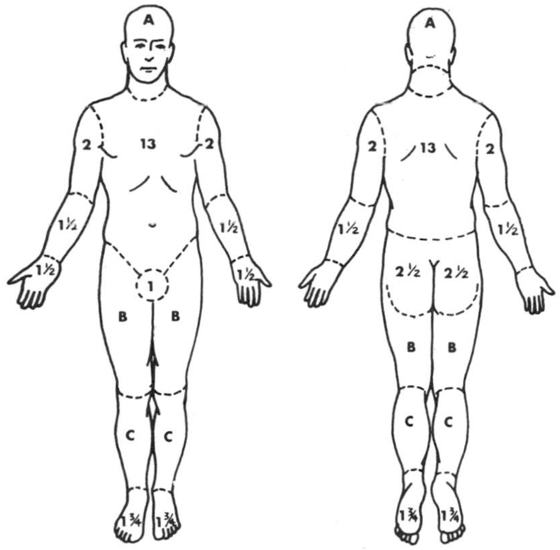

FIGURE 36–2. Classic Lund and Browder chart. The best method to determine the percentage of body surface burn is to mark the areas of injury on a chart and then compute the total percentage according to the patient's age. Every emergency department should have such a chart for plotting the burned area soon after the patient is admitted. (From Sabiston, D. C., Jr. [ed.]: Davis-Christopher Textbook of Surgery: The Biological Basis of Modern Surgical Practice. 11th ed. Philadelphia, W. B. Saunders, 1977, p. 298.)

Relative Percentages of Areas Affected by Growth
(AGE IN YEARS)

	0	1	5	10	15	ADULT
A: 1/2 of head	9 1/2	8 1/2	6 1/2	5 1/2	4 1/2	3 1/2
B: 1/2 of thigh	2 3/4	3 1/4	4	4 1/4	4 1/2	4 3/4
C: 1/2 of leg	2 1/2	2 1/2	2 3/4	3	3 1/4	3 1/2

Total Per Cent Burned _____ 2° + _____ 3° = _____

mal injuries are caused by flames, hot liquids, heated metals, or steam. Cold injuries may occur with immobility of body parts, even at temperatures above freezing when the humidity is high. Frostbite is characterized by the formation of intracellular fluid crystals. In patients with severe frostbite, there is regional ischemia with necrosis of the epidermis, the dermis, or the underlying structures. Because the nursing management and wound care for frostbite are similar to the treatment for heat-related injuries, these patients may be treated in burn centers.

Chemical injury is caused by exposure to acids, alkali, or organic compounds. Acids and alkali are used in industry for cleansing, curing, extracting, and preserving purposes. In the home, they are commonly found in drain cleaners and cleaning solvents that, when used, may cause damage to the extremities. Most exposures to organic compounds are associated with use of fertilizers, pesticides, or petroleum products. The depth of chemical injury is the result of the concentration and quantity of the chemical and the duration of exposure. The proper use of protective clothing decreases the exposure risk. The neutralization of acids or alkali compounds is contraindicated because of the delay in treatment and risk of an exother-

mic reaction when acids and bases are combined.[11] Initial treatment should be irrigation with lots of water immediately to dilute and remove the agent. Patients exposed to chemical agents should be monitored for systemic toxicity, such as pulmonary insufficiency and hepatic or renal failure.[12]

Electric injuries are routinely subdivided into low-voltage (less than 1000 V) and high-voltage (more than 1000 V) types. Electric injury is caused by the passage of electric current through the body, with the conversion of electric current to heat.[16] The current follows the path of least resistance, with the extent of injury related to the intensity of the current and the duration of contact time. The specific tissue resistance is irrelevant with high-voltage electric injury; the body acts as a volume conductor.[12] The contact points may be the only visible wounds, yet deep tissue damage is often sustained. The extent of injury is often difficult to assess immediately after injury and requires sequential assessment to appreciate the amount of tissue involved. Surgical exploration may be required if there is any indication of deep tissue damage as assessed by palpation of the muscle compartments. Associated injuries such as fractures; cardiac dysrhythmias; soft tissue, vascular, and head injuries; cataracts; and neuropathies may occur secondary to electric current passage or associated falls.[18]

PATHOPHYSIOLOGY OF THERMAL INJURY

During the first 48 hours after thermal injury, there are systemic consequences associated with a hypodynamic stage followed by a hyperdynamic stage.[15, 16, 18] Organ system involvement, magnitude, and duration are proportional to the extent of the burn and reach a plateau when the injury is approximately 50 to 60 percent of the total body surface area.[15, 16] Patients with an injury involving more than 25 percent of total body surface area have immense fluid shifts from their intravascular space into the surrounding tissue because of changes in capillary permeability.[13] The initial changes in capillary integrity permit even large protein molecules to pass freely into the interstitium. For this reason, colloid-containing fluids are usually withheld until capillary integrity is restored at 24 hours after injury. Tissue edema occurs in both burned and unburned tissue because of the changes in capillary permeability and hypoproteinemia and of the volume and pressure effects of fluid resuscitation.

The redistribution of body water, electrolytes, and protein due to the increased capillary permeability creates a decrease in the circulating blood volume. This intravascular depletion is accompanied by a sudden, abrupt decrease in cardiac output that does not correlate with the gradual reduction in blood volume.

Peripheral vascular resistance increases as a result of the neurohormonal stress response following injury. This increase in afterload contributes to the decreased cardiac output curtailing perfusion to major organ systems.

Cardiac output and organ perfusion improve with adequate fluid resuscitation. Within 36 hours after injury, cardiac function becomes supranormal. This hyperdynamic phase lasts until the burn wound is closed.[2, 13]

Fluid management of the thermally injured patient requires attention to detail to prevent the potential morbidity associated with either underresuscitation or overresuscitation. Failure to deliver enough fluid may result in inadequate organ perfusion. Overresuscitation may lead to pulmonary or wound edema. Wound edema in a circumferentially burned extremity may decease perfusion of unburned tissue in the distal portion of that extremity.

During the early postinjury period, the patient may present symptoms of modest pulmonary hypertension. Even a patient without inhalation injury may have decreased lung compliance.[1] In the early stages of resuscitation, the minute ventilation may be decreased in a hypovolemic patient but commonly increases in proportion to the extent of burn as the resuscitative phase progresses.[16]

The kidneys experience a similar hypodynamic-hyperdynamic pattern. The consequences of diminished intravascular volume, plasma flow, and glomerular filtration rate result in decreased urine output. Acute renal failure, although rare, may result if fluid resuscitation is delayed. Approximately 24 hours after injury, vascular integrity is restored and fluid requirements decrease. This period is followed by the shift of interstitial fluid to the intravascular compartment, with an ensuing diuresis occurring 48 to 72 hours after injury.[15]

The gastrointestinal tract exhibits decreased activity in patients with injuries involving more than 25 percent of total body surface area.[12] A nasogastric tube should be inserted to decrease the risk of gastric dilatation, emesis, and aspiration. After adequate fluid resuscitation, normal functioning of the gastrointestinal system returns. Endoscopic studies have demonstrated that gastrointestinal ulcerations occur in 80 percent of critically ill patients with thermal injury if some form of prophylactic therapy is not employed. Because of the potential risk of acute stress ulcers, preventive modalities are employed for all thermally injured patients with total body surface area involvement of 35 percent or more.[13] Gastric pH is maintained between 3.5 and 4.5 with antacid or histamine blocker therapy.

There are several hematologic changes that follow a thermal injury. Although the number of red blood cells decreases after injury, the hematocrit level is usually elevated owing to hemoconcentration secondary to the fluid shifts occurring immediately after the injury. Some red blood cells are lysed because of direct thermal injury; however, there may be continued hemolysis for several days. Blood loss related to wound débridement, phlebotomy, or alterations in the coagulation system, such as thrombocytopenia, thrombocytosis, and disseminated intravascular coagulation, should be monitored closely.

The thermally injured patient is highly susceptible to infection because of alterations in host-defense mechanisms. The primary and secondary lines of defense against infection are limited with the loss of integument. There is a depressed responsiveness of lymphocytes in thermally injured patients, and immunosuppressive substances can be isolated in the sera.[19] These changes occur immediately after injury and continue until the wound is closed. The immune response at the cellular level is unclear, and it can only be hypothesized whether changes are caused by the introduction of organisms or a deficiency in components. What have been described are alterations in T-cell function, the humoral B-cell system, and nonspecific host defenses.[1, 19] The immunologic responses result from complex interactions of multiple factors, including the thermal injury, nutritional deficits, stress, microbial products, and treatment.

Extensive thermal injury results in catabolism characterized by a significant elevation of the metabolic rate and loss of lean body mass.[16] Thermally injured patients manifest a negative nitrogen balance in response to the injury. The rate of catabolism may be further increased with infection. Aggressive nutritional support is needed to meet energy requirements, replace the protein losses, and promote wound healing.[3] Blood glucose levels increase in response to a stressful critical injury or illness. Wilmore reported that increased gluconeogenesis accounts for this hyperglycemia.[21] The gastrointestinal tract is the preferred route for feeding the thermally injured patient. If facial injury, altered levels of consciousness, or gastric ileus limit oral intake, initiation of tube feedings should be considered.[18] Total parenteral nutrition should be considered when enteral feeding is contraindicated.

WOUND MANAGEMENT

Twenty-five years ago, patients with extensive thermal injuries had a limited chance of survival. Those who survived the resuscitative phase often succumbed to overwhelming infection. Although wound treatment modalities are initiated at the time of admission, they become the focus of care during the acute phase. The goals of wound management are the prevention of infection, the preservation of tissue, timely wound closure, and the maintenance and restoration of function. Nursing care rendered in the post anesthesia care unit (PACU) is important in the attainment of these goals.

All the energies invested in the care of the thermally injured patient are directed at a single outcome: the transformation of a contaminated open wound to a clean closed wound. The open wound is associated with the hypermetabolic and physiologic stress responses that

do not become corrected until the wound is closed.[16] Current wound management following resuscitation involves excision of the necrotic tissue and coverage of the wound.[9] Advantages of early excision include early mobilization, reduction of pain, early wound closure, reduced risk of infection, and reduced length of hospital stay. Disadvantages include exposure to surgical stress in the early postresuscitation period and the risk of excising viable tissue that might heal.[5, 7, 16]

The necrotic tissue, foreign material, and cellular debris are mechanically removed from the burn wound by either a tangential or full-thickness excision. Tangential excision is the sequential removal of thin layers of necrotic tissue until viable tissue with an adequate blood supply is reached. This débridement technique may be used for both superficial and deep-dermal partial-thickness injury.[5, 7, 16]

Full-thickness excision involves the removal of nonviable tissue to the level of viable tissue, usually down to subcutaneous fat or fascia, using scalpel or electrocautery techniques. Excision of an area of thermal injury exceeding 20 percent of the total body surface at one time is not recommended because of surgical stress and the magnitude of blood loss. Each operative procedure is limited to 20 percent of the total body surface area or 2 hours of operative time. Time between procedures allows for recovery and re-epithelialization of donor sites.[5, 9]

After the excision is complete, hemostasis must be achieved. Topical thrombin may be sprayed onto the excised bed, followed by the placement of warm, moist laparotomy pads. An alternative method is the application of gauze sponges soaked in 1:10,000 epinephrine solution to the wound bed.[7] Pressure is then applied by application of a circumferential gauze dressing. After approximately 10 minutes, the pressure dressing is gently removed. Specific sites of bleeding are identified and cauterized or ligated.

There are many skin grafting techniques available to the surgeon managing the care of the thermally injured patient. For the purposes of this chapter, only the definitive closure of the wound is addressed. Once the necrotic tissue is removed, the exposed underlying tissues must be covered to provide protection and prevent infection. The definitive covering is autograft skin. A portion of the patient's epidermis with a partial layer of dermis is removed from a region of unburned tissue using a dermatome. This tissue is referred to as a *split-thickness skin graft* and can be applied as an intact sheet or an expanded meshed sheet to the wound bed. A *full-thickness skin graft* is one in which a segment of full dermis and epidermis is transplanted to a recipient site.[7, 20] The skin graft is secured in place by fibrin glue, staples, sutures, an immobilizing dressing and splints, or a combination of these methods.

Split-thickness grafts typically vary in thickness from 0.01 to 0.035 inches. Sheet grafts are preferred when the wound location has cosmetic or functional importance, such as the face, neck, hands, and feet. In the post anesthesia period, nurses must assess the healing grafts for the presence of hematoma or seromas, which may prevent graft adherence.

Meshed autograft skin is indicated for patients with extensive thermal injury, because meshing allows for maximum coverage of wounds from limited donor sites. The mesh graft's interstices allow the escape of blood and plasma, thus decreasing the risk of interference with graft vascularization. The meshed autografts are usually expanded one and one half to four times their normal size. A layer of fine-mesh and course-mesh gauze soaked in an antimicrobial or saline solution is applied directly over the grafts and is secured with roller gauze. This dressing prevents the desiccation of the exposed wound bed until the interstices are closed by epithelial migration.

The donor site selection may be limited owing to the extent of the injury, but cosmetic or functional outcomes should be considered, if possible. After the harvesting of the skin grafts, the newly created partial-thickness wound at the donor site must be protected against maceration and infection. Management of these wounds includes the application of various types of dressings or temporary coverings.[5, 7, 20] Fine-mesh gauze is often applied directly over the donor site. Blood is evacuated from beneath the gauze by using a straight edge such as scissors or scalpel handle, and the dressing is allowed to dry. Donor site care in the PACU requires the application of radiant heat to begin drying this dressing. Any insult, such as mechanical trauma, heat or cold injury, and infection, may convert this surgically created partial-thickness wound to a full-thickness injury.

Most operative procedures on thermally injured patients are performed with the patient under general anesthesia. Ketamine may be administered to the thermally injured patient for anesthesia or analgesia. The advantages of ketamine induction include the production of intense analgesia and maintenance of normal pharyngeal and laryngeal reflexes.

Regional anesthesia may be used for local débridement. If grafting is to be completed following the excision, regional anesthesia may not be adequate to allow harvest of donor sites from areas remote from the excision. For additional information on anesthetics, see Section III.

POST ANESTHESIA NURSING CARE

In health care facilities that have a specialty care unit for the treatment of thermally injured patients, post anesthesia care is typically provided in that unit. If a thermally injured patient must be cared for in a PACU, selected factors in addition to standard post anesthesia care must be considered. Ambient room temperature should be maintained at 85°F to prevent hypothermia. Infection control policies, including isolation procedures, handwashing techniques, and a strict dress code, should be developed for the PACU considering this unique patient population.

Post anesthesia nursing care for thermally injured patients includes recovery from anesthesia, proper positioning, immobilization to prevent autograft disruption, use of restraints as appropriate, prevention of hypothermia, inspection of dressings for signs of hemorrhage, and adequate pain management. Assessment and documentation are critical components of nursing management during the post anesthesia period. Assessment must be directed primarily toward the maintenance of a patent airway and adequate respiration and circulation. Standard procedures for the management of patients recovering from anesthesia should be used. The secondary assessment focuses on the donor and graft sites. Documentation should include a review of systems plus the location of graft and donor sites, the appearance of the dressings, patient position, and all medications administered.

Specific wound care depends on the type of operative procedure and the location of the operative site. The most frequent cause of graft loss is mechanical shear from movement of the grafted body part. It is necessary to immobilize the joint above and below the grafted region. Most split-thickness mesh grafts are dressed with a nonadherent material, covered by course-mesh gauze, and secured with roller gauze. Immobilization is accomplished by the application of splints over the dressings. Although hemostasis is achieved intraoperatively, postoperative increases in blood pressure and movement may cause bleeding at the operative sites. If bleeding occurs, the surgeon should be notified.

Sheet skin grafts are generally not dressed to allow direct visualization. Sheet grafts must be assessed for the accumulation of blood or serum under the graft. Formation of hematomas or serous blebs between a graft and the wound bed requires evacuation to prevent graft loss. Fluid accumulations beneath the graft may be aspirated using a small syringe and needle. The surgeon may make a small incision near a bleb to allow the fluid to be expelled or use a cotton-tipped applicator to "roll" the fluid to the edges of the graft.[5]

In the immediate post anesthesia period, the donor sites should receive heat and aeration to promote drying. The nurse must ensure that donor sites remain clean, dry, and free from pressure. With proper care, multiple skin grafts can be harvested from the same location.[5]

Thermal injuries are one of the most painful forms of trauma that one can experience, and pain management provides a major challenge for the PACU nurse. Astute nursing assessment and evaluation are required to differentiate restlessness due to pain from other causes such as hypoxia and bladder or gastric distention. Pain can be reduced by frequent intravenous administration of small doses of morphine sulfate (3 to 5 mg in adults).[10, 15] Intramuscular injections should be avoided during the postoperative period because the normal fluid shifts may impair soft-tissue circulation, rendering analgesia ineffective. As circulatory integrity is restored, narcotics previously deposited in the muscles and subcutaneous tissue may be mobilized, possibly leading to an overdosage. Continuous infusion of intravenous narcotics may be an effective technique to produce a constant level of analgesia but requires careful monitoring for undesirable physiologic effects.[5, 23]

SUMMARY

The nursing care of the thermally injured patient provides an exciting challenge for the PACU nurse. With the advent of successful resuscitation formulas, new surgical techniques, improved nutritional delivery systems, and innovative wound management interventions, the survival rate of patients with major thermal injury has greatly improved. However, the nurse must continue to understand the rationale for intervention to provide optimal monitoring and evaluation of these patients in the post anesthesia period. Outcomes are enhanced when all members of the health care team provide collaborative care for the severely injured patient.

References

1. Arturson, M. G.: The pathophysiology of severe thermal injury. J. Burn Care Rehabil., 6:129, 1985.
2. Burgess, M. C.: Initial management of a patient with extensive burn injury. Crit. Care Nurs. Clin. North Am., 3:165, 1991.
3. Carlson, D. E., and Jordan, B. S.: Implementing nutritional therapy in the thermally injured patient. Crit. Care Nurs. Clin. North Am., 3:221, 1991.
4. DeSantis, D., Phillips, P., Spath, M. A., et al.: Delayed appearance of a circulating myocardial depressant factor in burn patients. Ann. Emerg. Med., 10:22–24, 1981.
5. Duncan, D. J., and Driscoll, D. M.: Burn wound management. Crit. Care Nurs. Clin. North Am., 3:199, 1991.
6. Gruendemann, B. J., and Meeker, M. H.: Alexander's Care of the Patient in Surgery. 8th ed. St Louis, C. V. Mosby, 1987.
7. Heimbach, D. M.: Early burn wound excision and grafting. In Boswick, J. A. (ed.): The Art and Science of Burn Care. Rockville, MD, Aspen, 1987, p. 65.
8. Heimbach, D. M.: Early excision and grafting: Clinical implications. Boots Pharmaceutical Burn Management Report. Vol. 1, No. 4. Lincolnshire, IL, Boots Pharmaceutical Company, 1992.
9. Kravitz, M.: Thermal injuries. In Cardona, V. D., Hurn, P. D., Bastnagel Mason, P. J., et al. (eds.): Trauma Nursing: From Resuscitation Through Rehabilitation. Philadelphia, W. B. Saunders, 1988, p. 707.
10. Molter, N. C.: Pain in the burn patient. In Punctillo, K. A. (ed.): Pain in the Critically Ill: Assessment and Management. Rockville MD, Aspen, 1991, p. 193.
11. Mozingo, D. W., Smith, A. A., McManus, W. F., et al.: Chemical burns. J. Trauma, 28:216, 1988.
12. National Burn Institute: Advanced Burn Life Support Course Manual. Lincoln, NE, National Burn Institute, 1990.
13. Pruitt, B. A., Jr.: Prognosis in Burn Care: Introduction. World J. Surg., 16:1, 1992.
14. Pruitt, B. A., Jr.: The burn patient: Initial care. In Ravitch, M. M. (ed.): Current Problems in Surgery. Chicago, Year Book, 1979, p. 1.
15. Pruitt, B. A., Jr., and Goodwin, C. W., Jr.: Burn injury. In Moore, E. E. (ed.): Early Care of the Injured Patient. Philadelphia, B. C. Decker, 1990, p. 286.
16. Pruitt, B. A., Jr., and Goodwin, C. W., Jr.: Thermal injuries. In Davis, J. H., Drucker, W. R., Foster, R. S., et al. (eds.): Clinical Surgery. St. Louis, C. V. Mosby, 1987.
17. Pruitt, B. A., Jr., Mason, A. D., Jr., and Goodwin, C. W., Jr.: Epidemiology of Burn Injury and Demography of Burn Care Facilities. Prob. Gen. Surg., 7:235, 1990.
18. Pruitt, B. A., Jr., and Treat, R. G.: The burn patient. In Dudrick, S. J., Bave, A. E., Eiseman, B., et al. (eds.): Manual of Preoperative and Postoperative Care. Philadelphia, W. B. Saunders, 1983, p. 697.
19. Warden, G. D.: Immunologic response to burn injury. In Boswick, J. A. (ed.): The Art and Science of Burn Care. Rockville, MD, Aspen, 1987, p. 113.
20. Waymack, J. P., and Pruitt, B. A., Jr.: Burn wound care. Adv. Surg. 23:261, 1990.
21. Wilmore, D. W.: Metabolic changes after thermal injury. In Boswick, J. A. (ed.): The Art and Science of Burn Care. Rockville, MD, Aspen, 1987, p. 137.
22. Wolman, R., and Luterman, A.: The continuous infusion of morphine sulfate for analgesia in burn patients: Extending the use of an established technique [Abstract 150]. In Proceedings of the American Burn Association, Seattle, 1988.

Post Anesthesia Care of the Ambulatory Surgical Patient

CHAPTER 37

Nancy Burden, B.S., R.N., C.P.A.N.

Ambulatory surgery is an area of exciting growth and continually advancing knowledge and technology. In 1990, an American Hospital Association report confirmed that, for the first time, more than 50 percent of all hospital-based surgical procedures were done on an outpatient basis. The total number of surgical procedures performed in the United States in 1990 was 22 million. Of that number, 13.3 million outpatient surgical procedures were done in hospitals, whereas 2.3 million were performed in other types of facilities.[21] It is universally projected that the percentage of outpatient surgical procedures will continue to increase. For example, in 1991, more than 80 percent of surgical procedures performed in one hospital in Tampa, Florida, were performed on outpatients or on patients admitted on the day of surgery.[10] Another solid indication is that the number of outpatient procedures approved for payment under Medicare has already increased from 450 in 1982 to more than 2500 now.

This trend toward the use of the ambulatory surgical process is driven by a variety of factors. Foremost, third-party payers, such as insurance companies, health maintenance organizations, and the federal government, generally mandate that surgical procedures be performed in the lowest cost setting to be eligible for payment.

In addition to such economic pressures, other factors have contributed to the trend of same-day admission and early postoperative discharge. Exciting technologic advances allow more complex procedures to be done with less trauma to the patient's body. For instance, laparoscopic and endoscopic procedures are increasing both in numbers and in the types and complexity of applications.[6] The pharmacologic industry has developed shorter-acting anesthetic agents and adjunctive drugs that allow quicker return to alertness and self-care and have fewer unpleasant side effects. Also, consumers are more sophisticated than in past generations, and our current fast-paced lifestyles lend themselves to "in and out" care.

In response to the special needs of patients who require nursing care in a much shortened time span, a new subspecialty of post anesthesia nursing has emerged. Ambulatory surgical nursing care addresses patient needs related to both anesthesia and surgery. Specific emphasis is placed on providing comprehensive patient and family education. Ambulatory surgical nurses encourage the patient's self-care and self-responsibility for preadmission and post discharge compliance with the planned medical and nursing care. In addition, these nurses emphasize the patient's early ambulation and return to normal life activities, patient teaching, and family involvement in the patient's care.

Because the patient returns home so quickly after surgery, involvement of the family or another responsible adult is integral to the overall plan of care. Postoperative complications such as nausea and vomiting might otherwise be considered minor or merely unpleasant for hospitalized patients who have nursing support. For ambulatory surgical patients, however, these problems become serious deterrents to discharge and can lead to costly, prolonged hospital stays, unplanned hospitalizations, or unpleasant home recuperations.

The basic tenet of nursing care in this setting is the promotion of wellness as a philosophy of care. Patients should be allowed to provide as much self-care as possible and should be continually encouraged to think positively. The concept of self-fulfilling prophecy is an important tool that nurses can employ to help patients expect success and comfort rather than the opposite. According to this concept, an outcome is more likely to happen just because that is what the patient expects. The outcome is "preprogrammed" by the patient's outlook.

Whether the patient has surgery in a hospital setting, in a freestanding ambulatory surgical center (ASC), or in the physician's office, basic nursing needs remain the same. That care combines both critical assessment and monitoring during periods of high dependence, such as immediately after general anesthesia or sedation, with periods when the patient is encouraged and taught how to assume responsibility for self-care. This dual atmosphere is frequently provided through a two-phase recovery plan: the initial post anesthesia care unit (PACU) and a less care-intensive second-phase unit from which the patient is eventually discharged.

The ambulatory surgical patient population has changed drastically during the past 20 years. More complex procedures are now being performed on sicker and older patients. In some communities, the development of post discharge services, such as 23-hour admission units and recovery care centers, has provided the safety net of lengthier postoperative nursing care after more complex procedures, such as anterior cruciate ligament repair, operative laparoscopic procedures, mastectomy, and laparoscopically assisted vaginal hysterectomy. Some physicians are already discharging patients in a few hours or more after even these types of advanced procedures. It is likely that the trend toward early discharge will encompass even more complex procedures as we become more familiar with patient outcomes, the frequency and extent of complications, and the level of patient acceptance based on experience and research.

Because there is not the luxury of several shifts of nurses to prepare and educate patients and families prior to ambulatory surgery or to tend to the patient's postoperative needs, it is important that ambulatory surgical nurses have certain characteristics. Foremost, clinical assessment skills must be accurate and rapid. Ambulatory surgical nurses should be self-motivated and able to communicate in professional terms with their peers and in lay terms with patients. The nurse's documentation skills, as well as the forms used in the facility, should allow for precise documentation of findings in the least amount of time. Probably most important from the patient's viewpoint, the nurse working in ambulatory surgery should present a positive, pleasant demeanor and show genuine concern for and interest in the patient. In fact, managers look for the "ambulatory surgery personality" when hiring nurses. Yozzo describes this type of nurse as one who can establish instant rapport with others and who is "public relations oriented, friendly, dynamic, and adaptable to changing situations," as well as being "goal oriented, an independent thinker, ambitious, organized, able to set priorities, self-confident, a positive thinker, accountable, flexible, team spirited, and able to make quick and accurate assessments."[23]

PREPARATION OF THE PATIENT

Careful preoperative selection and preparation of patients for outpatient surgery are important in reducing the risks of perioperative complications. However, because the primary stimulus moving many patients into the outpatient setting is economic, many patients who are not ideal candidates physically, emotionally, or socially are forced to return home soon after surgery or other procedures. In addition to systemic illnesses that limit their ability to care for themselves and possibly increase the risk of perioperative complications, many people have limited social or family support. Nurses are especially challenged to prepare these more complicated patients for an early transition to home.

The ultimate goals of complication-free recovery and early discharge are supported by what occurs preoperatively. Proper patient selection, preparation, and education all contribute significantly to eventual patient outcome. Patient and procedure selection are primarily the function of the surgeon and anesthesiologist, but the nurse who assesses the patient preoperatively should provide valuable information to the physicians involved in the patient's care.

Nursing preparation of patients for surgery and for other invasive procedures must be comprehensive. Physical assessment, history taking, and evaluation of the patient's social, emotional, and cognitive status are all essential to that care. The challenge for the ambulatory surgical nurse, however, is completing all those evaluations in a much briefer time than was previously available when inpatient status was routine prior to surgery.

Nursing care also must reach beyond the walls of the facility and into the patient's home setting. This includes providing preoperative education that the patient can understand and that helps encourage preparation of a safe home setting for postoperative recuperation. Although nurses cannot be responsible for the actions of patients outside the facility, nurses do provide education, coaching, and suggestions for the patient's preoperative and postoperative care at home. The need to gain the patient's confidence and cooperation as well as to ensure the involvement of a responsible adult cannot be overstated.

Before surgery, an on-site preadmission assessment is ideal. Having the patient come to the hospital or ASC before the day of surgery allows time for the nurse to establish a rapport with the patient. It also provides the nurse with time to secure the patient's history, complete a physical assessment, help reduce patient anxiety, provide comprehensive preoperative instructions, identify potential risk factors, and take steps to reduce those risk factors on or before the day of surgery. Some of these goals can be met by a telephone contact before surgery, although completing the physical assessment process and allowing the patient to become familiar with the facility cannot occur by telephone.

Some institutions may prefer to provide strictly day-of-surgery preparations because of their cost effectiveness and convenience for patients,[20] but these preadmission preparations are not merely nice things to do. When evaluating the cost versus the benefit of seeing patients before the day of surgery, many intangible, yet important, benefits that justify the costs of staffing and allocation of space and equipment can be identified. Details of the patient's financial obligations can be discussed and completed with a business office representative. Early completion of paperwork, diagnostic tests, consent forms, and instructions significantly reduces the time of preparation on the day of surgery, which, in turn, helps avoid delays in surgery. Identifying risk factors early allows time to correct any deficiencies or, if necessary, to cancel the surgery before the day it is scheduled. This is much preferred to day-of-surgery cancellations or unexpected postoperative admissions that are more costly to the institution, upsetting to the patient and physician, and generally time consuming and disruptive for the staff.[13]

Having certain information before the day of surgery allows the ambulatory surgical patient to better prepare for surgery as well as later discharge. Patients should be instructed about what arrangements to make for transportation and adult support, the projected length of stay, and, in general, what to expect on the day of surgery. They should be instructed in the proper clothing to wear for ease of dressing after surgery, how to prepare the home environment, what physical restrictions they may encounter postoperatively, and any equipment or supplies that they should purchase or secure prior to their arrival for surgery.

Patients taking routine medications should be given instructions by the anesthesia provider about which medications can and should be taken on the morning of surgery, usually with a small sip of water. Medications most often continued until the time of surgery include antihypertensives, antiarrhythmics, coronary artery dilators, and bronchodilators. Patients are also encouraged to continue any respiratory inhalants according to their usual protocol. Precise instructions for diabetic patients should be given regarding insulin and diet on the day of surgery. Although these instructions are the responsibility of the physician, they are often reinforced and explained by nursing personnel.

Patients should be encouraged to fill any prescriptions for postoperative medications before the day of surgery, if possible. Many patients are reluctant to fill prescriptions for analgesics ahead of time because they believe they may not actually need the medication after surgery. This may be true for some patients, although the nurse may want to point out the fact that a pharmacy may not be available in the middle of the night should pain be unrelieved by other means. If patients have not yet received any prescriptions, they should know to bring money or insurance cards to obtain medications if it is likely that prescriptions will be given on the day of surgery.

Parents of small children are asked to have two adults accompany the child, one to drive and the other to attend to the child in transit going home. In some institutions, supporting adults are instructed that they must remain at the facility throughout the patient's stay. In others, only parents of minors are required to remain on site. Whatever the policy, patients and families should be told about the expectations ahead of time.

The preparation of patients immediately before surgery is essentially the same as for all surgical patients. Physical assessment includes at least vital signs, breath sounds, peripheral pulses as indicated, baseline oxygen saturation levels, skin condition at the site of surgery or regional anesthetic injection, and other appropriate assessments. Careful preoperative identification of the operative site; assurance of a valid, correct, and signed consent form; and verification of the fasting period are essential.

Fasting Before Surgery

In the ambulatory surgical population, assurance of the required fasting period can be particularly challenging because the nurse has decidedly less opportunity to teach and less ability to control the patient who is not admitted to a hospital bed overnight. Adult patients and parents of pediatric patients must be thoroughly educated about the specifics of the fasting period. They should know that in addition to food and beverages, they must specifically avoid water, gum, candy, coffee, and cough drops. It may be helpful to explain in lay terms that although gum and hard candy are not swallowed, they stimulate the stomach to produce acids that may be harmful if aspirated. Although "scare tactics" are not appropriate, all patients must understand the seriousness of breaking the fasting period and of accurate reporting of noncompliance.

Parents must be enjoined to carefully monitor their children at home and in the automobile so that the child does not eat or drink without the parent's knowledge. Adolescents also may be at particular risk because of their tendency to resist authority or misplaced sense of immortality. On the day of surgery, the nurse must strive to elicit truthful and accurate verification of the patient's actual compliance.

Diagnostic Testing

Diagnostic tests required preoperatively vary widely from one institution to another and are a matter both of clinical judgment by individual physicians and the policies set by the medical board administering the ambulatory surgical program. Current trends are toward performing none or only essential diagnostic tests aimed at providing the basic information necessary for safe anesthesia and surgical interventions. Hemoglobin and hematocrit determinations may be all that are ordered for a healthy patient prior to a relatively minor procedure. Conversely, some health care providers still prefer to use screening measures such as a chest radiograph, serum chemistry analysis, and an electrocardiogram. Economic pressure to reduce the cost of health care supports eliminating any unnecessary testing. The policy in a particular institution remains a matter of choice and philosophy.

One area of controversy concerns whether all women of childbearing age should be screened for pregnancy. Some physicians believe that a careful history taking and query of the patient is sufficient and the most cost-effective approach. Others believe that testing offers greater diagnostic accuracy and reduces both

the danger to the patient and the liability to the institution and the care providers.[17]

Nurses responsible for preparing patients for surgery should carry out the policies of the facility for all diagnostic testing. They should also ensure that results of any tests ordered are included in the medical record and that abnormal results are brought to the attention of the physician before the patient is medicated or transferred to surgery. Hopefully, test results are secured and physician notification is done before the day of surgery.

Preoperative Medications

Some providers prefer to avoid all premedications in the ambulatory surgical patient and may even encourage patients to walk to surgery to promote their sense of normalcy and self-control. Others believe that certain goals can and should be met pharmacologically to smooth the anesthetic course. Preoperative medications may be given for a number of reasons: to decrease salivation; to reduce anxiety; to promote calmness prior to induction of general anesthesia; and, for children, to reduce the fear and stress of separation from their parents. Antiemetic and gastrokinetic medications may be used to reduce the risk of vomiting and subsequent aspiration. Occasionally, opioids may be added to the regimen prior to painful procedures, although their penchant to promote nausea and vomiting often precludes their use preoperatively.

When premedications are given, intravenous (IV) administration is certainly the trend. This route spares the patient from the pain of intramuscular injections and helps avoid prolonged sedative effects that can delay eventual postoperative discharge. Children particularly dread and fear "shots" and for many years may recall an injection more negatively than the surgical procedure. Also, many patients do not arrive at the surgical facility long enough before surgery to be given intramuscular medications and obtain the most effective results.

After the administration of any preoperative medications, patients should be monitored for allergic, atypical, or untoward drug reactions, such as respiratory or cardiac depression. Appropriate interventions to correct such situations should be initiated immediately and concurrently with notification of the physician. Specifically, the sedated patient who vomits should be quickly placed in a side-lying, head-down position. Vomitus should be cleared mechanically from the upper airway, oxygen should be administered at 100 percent, and the anesthesiologist should be notified immediately.

Emotional Support and Positive Thinking

Emotional support also helps reduce patient anxiety and, hopefully, associated complications such as hypertension, tachycardia, vomiting, aspiration, and increased postoperative pain related to fear. The significance of the emotional component of nursing care while the patient is being prepared for surgery cannot be overstressed. All words spoken to the patient should be positive. Questions or statements should imply the positive aspects of recovery, particularly being able to go to a familiar and comfortable home soon after the surgery. The nurse also teaches the family directly and by example to speak in similar positive terms to encourage the patient's confident attitude. This approach supports a climate of wellness and positive outcome.

Preoperative Goals

The primary goals when preparing patients for ambulatory surgery must be focused on identifying and reducing the potential risks related to surgery and anesthesia and promoting each patient's quick return to self-care. This includes a significant shift of responsibility to the patient and family by way of educating them and then encouraging and evaluating their actions. Although patient preparations may not necessarily be identical for inpatients and outpatients, those preparations should meet the same standards of quality of care. Nurses who admit and prepare patients for surgery must be thorough in their assessments and instructions and must be prepared personally and with adequate equipment to intercede effectively in emergency situations.

INTRAOPERATIVE PERIOD

The supportive nursing care of the patient begun prior to admission continues when that patient goes to the operating room (OR). Because of the trend to reduce or eliminate preoperative sedative medications, and because a significant number of ambulatory surgical patients are given regional or local anesthesia, the OR nurse cares for many awake and alert patients who require emotional support throughout the surgical procedure. These same patients are more aware of their surroundings than those under general anesthesia, so the OR nurse also monitors and controls the appropriateness of any discussions taking place near the patient. It should be noted that many patients undergoing general anesthesia have later reported recall of conversations and events intraoperatively, so all conversations should be appropriate near all patients, not just near those who are obviously awake.[19]

Other intraoperative care of the ambulatory surgical patient parallels that of all surgical patients. Specific nursing responsibilities include maintaining asepsis; properly preparing the operative site; providing for patient safety in identification, transfer and positioning; assisting the anesthesia team; maintaining confidentiality; protecting the patient's dignity; handling specimens; and documenting and reporting the intraoperative care and events.

Anesthesia Considerations

Anesthesia for the ambulatory surgical patient incorporates the traditional goals of adequate analgesia, muscle relaxation, amnesia, and, in the event of general anesthesia, loss of consciousness to accomplish the intended procedure. Because the ambulatory surgical patient is discharged soon after the procedure, there is also concern that the anesthesia is as free as possible from postoperative hangover and complications. Both general and regional anesthesia are used. Regional and local techniques are favored by many clinicians because the patient does not lose consciousness, can usually be discharged soon after the procedure, and often has the advantage of prolonged pain relief in the operative site or extremity. The ongoing development of new and shorter-acting general anesthetic agents has significantly reduced complications such as postoperative nausea and vomiting and has encouraged rapid return to alertness, making general anesthesia as likely to be used as other techniques.

Intravenous Conscious Sedation

For many years, OR nurses have been the primary monitors of patients having local anesthesia. Today, more complex procedures are being done under local anesthesia on patients in all stages of wellness, and many patients are now being given IV conscious sedation to aid them through their procedures. Nurses have assumed the responsibility of administering IV conscious sedation under the direction of the physician who is performing the patient's procedure.

Before nurses assume this duty in any institution, specific guidelines should be developed regarding the registered nurse's role in administering IV sedation and monitoring of those patients. Such policies should address at least the following parameters[18]:

Appropriate patients, procedures, and medications
Guidelines for patient monitoring and assessment, including recognition of complications
Emergency preparedness parameters

Policies are best developed by a multidisciplinary group drawing from the expertise of nursing, medicine, pharmacy, and anesthesia disciplines.

Defining IV conscious sedation is the first step and one that has been deliberated about extensively. In 1991 a group of nursing organizations (including the American Nurses Association, the American Society of Post Anesthesia Nurses, and the Association of Operating Room Nurses) developed a position statement about the role of the registered nurse in the management of IV conscious sedation. The definition contained within this document is that under IV conscious sedation, a person "has a depressed level of consciousness but retains the ability to independently and continuously maintain a patent airway and respond appropriately to physical stimulation and/or verbal command."[2] The implication is that if the patient requires mechanical airway maintenance or cannot be aroused, the line has been crossed from IV conscious sedation to general anesthesia. That patient requires particularly attentive monitoring and no further medications until the sedation level has sufficiently reversed. Of particular importance in this position statement is the declaration that the nurse responsible for managing the patient "shall have no other responsibilities that would leave the patient unattended or compromise continuous monitoring."[2]

Nurses should be thoroughly knowledgeable about their associated responsibilities before caring for patients under IV conscious sedation. Again, based on the position statement, that knowledge should include the following:

1. Related cardiac and respiratory anatomy and physiology

2. Pharmacology and potential side effects of medications used, including effective reversal agents
3. Detection of arrhythmias and other complications
4. Principles of oxygen transport and delivery
5. Airway management
6. Resuscitative techniques

The availability of emergency supplies and support personnel must be ensured before the procedure begins. In particular, flumazenil (Romazicon) and naloxone (Narcan), specific reversal agents for benzodiazepines and opioids, respectively, should be immediately available to treat serious respiratory or cardiac depression related to the sedative drugs.

POST ANESTHESIA PERIOD

Recovery of ambulatory surgical patients may occur in one or two stages. After general or major regional anesthesia or after intraoperative complications in any patient, a two-phase recovery is typical. Phase I begins when the patient arrives in a fully equipped and staffed PACU. Once the patient regains consciousness, lucidity, and physiologic stability, transfer to a less-intensive care unit is appropriate. Phase II of recovery is usually completed in a department equipped with lounge chairs and more homelike surroundings where families reunite and where the patient's self-care is encouraged. After local or regional anesthesia, which has a limited effect on physiologic stability, the patient is often transferred from the OR directly to the Phase II level of care.

PACU Care

After receiving a report from the OR and anesthesia personnel, the PACU nurse applies all the usual parameters of PACU care to the ambulatory surgical patient. Airway and respiratory management are paramount. The patient is closely observed for untoward cardiac, respiratory, or other effects from anesthetic agents. The operative site and any related areas are monitored for bleeding, and any existing parenteral fluids are maintained. Further nursing duties include oxygen delivery, monitoring of vital signs and oxygen saturation, and periodic stir-up of the patient to move and deep breathe every 5 to 10 minutes. Observation for any complications of surgery or anesthesia is coupled with rapid and appropriate nursing interventions should problems be identified.

These parameters are essential to the care of all PACU patients, but certain specific needs of ambulatory surgical patients must be met as well. Nursing care should be planned in a manner that not only identifies, reports, and treats complications in their early stages but that actually reduces the risk of unpleasant complications that would delay the patient's discharge to home. For instance, the speed of progressive head elevation should be paced to the individual patient's responses. Faintness, lightheadedness, hypotension, pallor, nausea, or vomiting implies the need to lower the patient's head and begin the process again. Adequate parenteral hydration prior to having the patient sit upright may reduce the patient's risk of developing gastrointestinal symptoms related to hypovolemia or hypotension. Oral fluids are given slowly, with adequate time between drinks, to assess the patient's tolerance.

Pain should be managed aggressively and immediately not only because it is humane and kind to do so but because preventing severe pain is easier than treating it.[1] Again, intramuscular injections may be unpleasant and, for some patients, can interfere with the goal of imminent discharge. Patients having more complex procedures may benefit from the long action of an intramuscular injection, but for most patients, the IV route is the first choice because of its immediate effects and the shortened observation time for related complications such as respiratory depression. Provision of adequate analgesia with oral medications and general comfort measures is usually attained before the patient is transferred to the Phase II post anesthesia area.

The goal of adequate patient comfort is supported when the patient knows, before surgery, that the nurse is concerned about and eager to provide adequate pain relief. Patients should be encouraged to discuss their usual levels of pain tolerance and should not be judged in that regard based on the attitudes and prior experiences of the staff. They should also know that although total absence of postoperative discomfort may not be a realistic goal, acute pain should be reported and will be treated. Patient comfort, supported by positive thinking, general comfort measures, and oral analgesics, is one of the criteria by which eventual discharge readiness is measured, and this goal must be addressed even in the early stages of recovery.

In pediatric patients, some potential postoperative problems include bleeding, croup, nausea and vomiting, and fever of unknown origin, any of which can result in unplanned hospitalization. Postintubation croup generally manifests itself within 3 hours of the extubation, but symptoms that require treatment occur in the PACU within the first hour.[14] Children also need gentle care and emotional support. The presence of a parent can be quite reassuring. Many facilities allow one or both parents to be in the PACU with their child.

Emergence delirium is more common in children than in adults. The child who is agitated and thrashing should be gently restrained to protect him or her from self-injury. Physostigmine (Antilirium) given slowly IV is usually quickly effective in reversing the agitation of emergence delirium. The infrequent side effects of physostigmine are bradycardia, ventricular arrhythmias, abdominal cramps, nausea, and increased bronchial secretions. Atropine is used to reverse some of these untoward effects.[22] In both children and adults, it is essential to accurately differentiate the restlessness associated with emergence delirium from other physiologic complications, such as hypoxia, bladder distention, and pain, that must be treated by other means.

Progressive or Phase II Care

Patients who do not or who no longer require the intensity of PACU care are transferred to the Phase II unit of the ambulatory surgical facility. This area is generally furnished with lounge chairs, although provisions to recline should be available for patients who have had more complex procedures or who experience complications. The decor is more homelike than the PACU to encourage a sense of wellness and normalcy. The Phase II area should include a nourishment center, patient bathrooms and changing areas, and ready access to an outside door for patient discharge. As in all acute health care settings, emergency equipment and support personnel must be readily available.

The goals of nursing care in this setting address the patient's physical, emotional, social, educational, and spiritual needs. These are summarized in Table 37–1. The comprehensive goals also include meeting the needs of the family or other responsible adult. Close nursing observation for potential complications is ongoing during the patient's stay. Expediting a safe discharge with a complication-free recuperation is the ultimate objective of all nursing and medical interventions.

Specific areas of concern in the Phase II unit

Table 37–1. TYPICAL PHASE II UNIT GOALS

To provide close assessment of and attention to the patient's physical, emotional, and educational needs in the postoperative period

To provide an environment and personnel who are prepared for emergency interventions at all times

To provide family-oriented care that stresses the concept of wellness and acknowledges the integral relationship of the patient and family or other supporting adult

To encourage the patient toward as much self-sufficiency as possible, given the type of surgery and anesthesia performed

To respect the patient's right to confidentiality, privacy, and respectful, compassionate nursing care

To maintain accurate records of patient-related care and environmental preparedness

To interact with physicians and other health care providers in a professional manner that results in high-quality patient care

To provide patients and families with a resource for questions, comments, and nursing information during their stay and in the immediate period after discharge

To offer an environment that encourages the professional growth of nursing personnel

---

From Burden, N.: Ambulatory Surgical Nursing. Philadelphia, W. B. Saunders, 1993, p. 325.

include observation of cardiorespiratory status and other vital signs to ensure stability in relation to the patient's preoperative normal levels. Other goals are to ensure adequate nutrition and fluid status, provide effective pain management, avoid unpleasant gastrointestinal symptoms, observe the operative site and associated symptoms, and encourage ambulation.[5] The nurse observes the patients first sitting up in a lounge chair and then walking to ensure that they experience no orthostatic hypotension, faintness, or dizziness and to ascertain if they will be able to maneuver in a similar manner at home. Patients should be able to demonstrate proper use and care of ambulatory aids such as walkers, crutches, and casts. Existing parenteral fluids or IV access ports should be maintained until the patient is able to ambulate without faintness and discharge readiness is ensured.

The tradition of requiring a certain level of oral intake prior to discharge has come under scrutiny. Certainly the patient's level of hydration must be considered, but forcing oral intake on someone who has no desire or interest can be self-defeating, resulting in poor tolerance. The patient's appetite and desire to eat or drink are often considered the best indicators of readiness.[4] In deciding whether to delay discharge until the patient can tolerate oral fluids, the physician considers the patient's overall condition, including gastrointestinal status, the

amount of IV fluid replacement given, and the patient's likeliness to report and to handle any inability to tolerate food or fluids at home. Certainly, extensive nausea or vomiting should be effectively treated before the patient is discharged.

It is most often in the Phase II unit that patients reunite with family members or the responsible adult who will accompany and care for them at home. Early reunion should be encouraged, and nurses in this setting must purposefully involve such support people. The responsible adult may need to learn how to care for the patient's physical needs, such as changing a dressing, observing extremity circulation, or emptying drains. Encouraging a return demonstration of manual skills or having the caretaker repeat information is a good way to reinforce learning and to evaluate the person's ability to provide support. The nurse also helps the responsible adult understand that the patient should perform self-care to the extent of his or her ability and that encouraging that behavior is in the best interest of the patient for both a speedy recuperation and a positive mental outlook.

Discharging patients to home after anesthesia and invasive procedures is a serious responsibility. Planning for that discharge should begin well before the actual time of discharge, hopefully at the time the patient is scheduled for surgery. Still, it is the discharging nurse who ensures that all those plans come together. Ensuring patient safety at home and in transit may require the nurse to discuss problems with the physician and to enlist the assistance of home health agencies or transportation sources. Whatever is necessary, the nurse is ethically obliged to intervene for the patient's safety prior to discharging that patient.

Specific written criteria that patients must attain before discharge should be included in the policies of the institution. In most facilities, it is now within the scope of the nurse's job description to apply those criteria when discharging patients, although any special concern about the patient's actual condition or ability to safely recuperate at home should prompt the nurse to solicit direct physician involvement in the discharge process. The physician is ultimately responsible for the decision to discharge a patient; however, the nurse's application of written discharge criteria that have been previously approved by the physician staff does meet the standards of the Joint Commission on Accreditation of Healthcare Organizations.[12] Table 37–2 lists various areas of concern typically included in such discharge criteria.

Table 37–2. VARIOUS AREAS OF CONCERN TYPICALLY INCLUDED IN DISCHARGE CRITERIA

Discharge Parameter	Typical Criteria	Comments
Vital signs	Stable for 30–60 min prior to discharge; no respiratory distress	Requires that more than one set of vital signs is taken and compared with the patient's preoperative normal vital signs
Level of consciousness	Conscious, oriented to surroundings	Level of sedation more difficult to identify—often depends on the quality of adult supervision the patient will have at home
Nourishment and hydration	Able to tolerate and maintain oral fluids	Whether this is actually necessary for healthy adults is controversial; of special concern if patient is elderly, young, or debilitated or if patient has had extensive procedure
Comfort	Comfortable with use of oral analgesics or none; minimal nausea or vomiting	Total freedom from discomfort is not realistic, but the patient should not be discharged with acute symptoms; concern for comfort related to length of ride home and ability to obtain prescription medications
Activity	Able to walk and dress self	If appropriate to patient's preoperative status and to the type of procedure; ensure ability to use crutches, walker prn; assess patient walking prior to discharge to identify problems such as hypotension or fainting
Surgical site	No untoward symptoms or bleeding, drainage appropriate for procedure; dressing secure; extremity circulation adequate	Patient should understand normal and abnormal parameters and how to check circulation
Instructions	Patient and family or responsible adult should be given verbal and written instructions	Have both sign copy to retain on medical record; individualize for each patient
Responsible adult supervision	Patient to be discharged with responsible adult to drive and remain with patient for 24 hr	Facility should set policies of what is minimum acceptable adult companionship (taxi driver? hospital van driver? minor?) and what actions nurse should take if patient desires to leave against medical advice
	After local anesthesia without sedation, physician may discharge patient without supervision	

Any patient who does not meet the facility's predetermined discharge criteria requires a specific physician's order for discharge. The nurse's notes should reflect why or how the patient did not meet existing criteria and what was done about it. For example, the criteria may require that all patients void prior to discharge, but a certain patient is eager to leave, cannot void after several hours of recovery, and has been discharged by the physician without having to meet the criterion of having to void. The nurse should be sure to note the involvement of the physician, having informed the responsible adult about the problem area, an assessment of the patient's abdomen, the specific guidelines and instructions given to the patient about what symptoms might indicate a full bladder, the importance of avoiding overdistention of the bladder, how long to wait at home without voiding before seeking care, telephone numbers given to the patient for obtaining medical assistance, and any other instructions given. The eventual closure of documentation also should include a nursing notation regarding the patient's urinary status on the following day or later that day as ascertained by telephone contact. This last portion of comprehensive care and documentation is possible only if the person making the telephone call is aware of such an issue. Therefore, it is essential that a mechanism be in place for communication of information from one nurse to the next or that discharging nurses are personally responsible for the eventual post discharge follow-up of patients in their care.

Before discharge, instructions for home care should be provided both in writing and verbally. Anxiety, discomfort, and the amnesic effects of many medications given to patients can result in poor or absent recall of information from the day of surgery, so whenever possible, instructions should be given both to the patient and to the adult assuming responsibility for the patient after discharge.[3]

Most facilities have developed preprinted discharge instruction sheets with carbon copies that remain on the chart after being signed by the patient or the accompanying adult, or both, as proof that the instructions were given. In addition to the usual instructions about eating, hygiene, wound care, ambulation, return physician visit, and telephone numbers for assistance, the patient should receive a description of what symptoms may be usual and what should be reported to the physician. For instance, knowing that a slight sore throat or generalized sore muscles may follow general anesthesia helps the patient avoid worry. When those same discharge instructions have been followed by suggestions for alleviating minor symptoms that may occur, the patient is given an even greater chance of having a comfortable recuperation.

The individual patient's specific needs must be addressed as well. The nurse should ensure that the physician's discharge instructions have included areas such as the following: when should the diabetic patient resume taking insulin and how much? when should oral medications be resumed? when can the patient drive, watch television, have a glass of wine? Although it may not be verbalized by the patient or partner, most patients also want to know if sexual intercourse should be avoided and for how long and why. Providing comprehensive discharge instructions means individualizing information for each patient.

Post Discharge Follow-Up

Mechanisms should exist for assessing patient outcomes as well as patient and family satisfaction with the care provided by the ambulatory surgical unit. Telephone calls and written surveys that can be returned by mail are two means of providing that follow-up. Written surveys most often address satisfaction issues, but evaluating the patient's recuperation from anesthesia and surgery requires a more aggressive and timely approach.

In many communities it has become a standard of care that patients are telephoned on the day following surgery to ascertain their clinical condition and comfort and for the other reasons identified in Table 37–3. Such a contact often serves as a valuable resource for patients who may have symptoms that should be evaluated by their physicians or questions that they are embarrassed or reluctant to telephone and ask their physicians. Not only is the patient's safety and medical condition supported, but the nursing staff is able to identify the effectiveness of current modes of care. Documentation of patient contacts via telephone should become a permanent part of the medical record. This level of follow-up after the patient's discharge is the final evaluation phase of the nursing process.

References

1. Acute Pain Management Guideline Panel: Acute pain management—operative or medical procedures and trauma: Clinical practice guideline. (AHCPR Pub. no. 92-0032.) Rockville, MD, Agency for Health Care Policy and Research, Public Health Service, US Department of Health and Human Services, February 1992.
2. American Nurses Association: Position Statement on the Role of the Registered Nurse (RN) in the Management of Patients Receiving IV Conscious Sedation for Short-Term Therapeutic, Diagnostic, or Surgical Procedures. Washington, DC, American Nurses Association, 1991.
3. American Society of Post Anesthesia Nurses: Standards of Post Anesthesia Nursing Practice 1992. Richmond, ASPAN, 1992.
4. Berry, F.: Pediatric outpatient anesthesia. ASA Refresher Courses in Anesthesiology, 10:17, 1982.
5. Burden, N.: Ambulatory Surgical Nursing. Philadelphia, W. B. Saunders, 1993.
6. Endoscopy to account for half of all surgeries by 1995. Hosp. Purchas. News, 16(6):47, 1992.
7. Fallo, P.: Developing a program to monitor patient satisfaction and outcome in the ambulatory surgery setting. J. Post Anesth. Nurs., 6:176–180, 1991.
8. Fetzer-Fowler, S., and Huot, S.: The use of temperature as a discharge criterion for ambulatory surgery patients. J. Post Anesth. Nurs., 7:398–403, 1992.
9. Figley, E., and Burden, N.: Preparing for the unexpected in the ambulatory surgery unit. J. Post Anesth. Nurs., 6:117–120, 1991.
10. Heinen, C. and Paul, M.: "Operation information" for ambulatory surgical patients. Nurs. Manage. [OR/Ambulatory Surgery Edition], 23(8):64Q, T, 1992.
11. Jaques, J., Gillies, D., and Biordi, D.: Outpatient surgery: A case study. Nurs. Manage. [OR/Ambulatory Surgery Edition], 21(10):88I–K, 1990.

Table 37–3. GOALS OF THE FOLLOW-UP CONTACTS MADE WITH PATIENTS AFTER DISCHARGE

The nurse may identify areas of health-related problems and help the patient address or solve problems.
   Information obtained, advice given, and actions taken by the nurse are a reflection of the quality of care provided by the ambulatory surgical center
The patient is afforded one more example of the caring atmosphere that was established during the surgical experience
Follow-up contacts can have positive marketing effects for the ambulatory surgical facility
The nurse gains a sense of job completion and satisfaction
Follow-up contacts address compliance with community, accrediting body, and association standards
Today's medicolegal climate suggests that an ambulatory surgical facility would want to identify and address any potential liabilities as soon as possible.

From Burden, N.: Ambulatory Surgical Nursing. Philadelphia, W. B. Saunders, 1993, p. 373.

12. Joint Commission on Accreditation of Healthcare Organizations: AHC/92 Ambulatory Health Care Standards Manual. Chicago, JCAHO, 1992, SA 1.17, pp. 37–38.
13. Jones, M.: Verbal presentation. Springfield, MO, Cox Medical Center, August 1, 1992.
14. Kallar, S., and Jones, G.: Postoperative complications. *In* White, P. (ed.): Outpatient Anesthesia. New York, Churchill Livingstone, 1990, pp. 397–415.
15. Laurent, C.: Day surgery: All in a day's work. Nurs. Times, *87*(11):26–30, 1991.
16. Laurent, C.: Time to go home? Nurs. Times, *87*(11):30–32, 1991.
17. Manley, S.: Is routine pregnancy testing necessary [Abstract]? Anesthesiology, *77*:A41, 1992.
18. Murphy, E.: OR nursing law: Legal considerations in RN monitoring of intravenous sedation. AORN J., *48*:1184–1187, 1988.
19. On being aware [Editorial]. Br. J Anaesth., *51*(8):711–712, 1979.
20. On-site preregistration: An idea whose time has gone? Same Day Surg., *17*(1):8–10, 1993.
21. Same-day surgeries surpass inpatient rate. Hosp. Purchas. News, *16*(6):1, 16, 1992.
22. Wetchler, B.: Anesthesia for Ambulatory Surgery. Philadelphia, J. B. Lippincott, 1985.
23. Yozzo, J.: Nursing management in the ambulatory surgery center. *In* Burden, N. (ed.): Ambulatory Surgical Nursing. Philadelphia, W. B. Saunders, 1993, pp. 671–685.

Special Considerations

Post Anesthesia Care of the Patient with Chronic Disorders

CHAPTER 38

CHRONIC OBSTRUCTIVE PULMONARY DISEASE

Chronic obstructive pulmonary disease (COPD) is a term that describes the bronchial obstructive type of respiratory diseases. It is characterized by dyspnea, with or without cough and sputum. The two major clinical manifestations of COPD are airway obstruction and airway destruction. The magnitude of the various disease entities that the term *COPD* includes is great. Therefore, it is difficult to elaborate individually on the diseases, because each deserves separate attention. Rather, this chapter briefly describes the overall characteristics of COPD and general care required in the post anesthesia care unit (PACU). Variations exist among patients diagnosed as having COPD. It is important for the PACU nurse to consult with the physician about the specific nursing care to be administered to the patient with COPD. For discussion of specific COPD diseases, see the references listed at the end of the chapter.

Description of COPD

Three major diseases are part of COPD: asthma, emphysema, and chronic bronchitis. All are characterized by airway obstruction. These diseases may have medically reversible components, such as bronchospasm, or they may have irreversible components, such as alveolar septal destruction. Some of the reversible components of *asthma*, such as retained secretions, bronchospasms, and infections, can be corrected by the interaction of the physician, nurse, physical therapist, and respiratory therapist. The treatment of asthma may include oxygen therapy, bronchodilators, chest physiotherapy, and proper hydration.

Chronic bronchitis is associated with chronic cigarette smoking. The nurse can contribute greatly to the patient's future health by strongly influencing him or her to refrain from smoking. Other therapy for the reversible components may include the use of bronchodilators, chest physiotherapy, and oxygen.

The patient with *emphysema* usually has airway destruction that is irreversible. As the alveolar septa are destroyed, insufficient alveolar ventilation ensues and eventually leads to hypercarbia. As the disease progresses, carbon dioxide cannot be expelled from the lungs and is retained there. The patient usually increases minute ventilation to try to compensate for the hypercarbia. Respiratory acidosis develops slowly as the various acid-base buffer systems try to neutralize the accumulated acid. In this compensated state, the patient usually has a near-normal pH; high plasma bicarbonate, low chloride concentrations; and a high total carbon dioxide level. The $PaCO_2$ usually is low, because some inspired oxygen is unable to cross into the blood from the lungs, owing to the decrease in respiratory diffusion membrane surface area in the lungs. Pulmonary hypertension usually appears as the disease progresses. Cor pulmonale may develop, and because of the pulmonary venous engorgement, the right heart may begin to fail. The patient with emphysema who has irreversible destruction may be treated with chest physiotherapy, bronchodilators, and steroids.

Surgical Considerations

The incidence of pulmonary complications in patients who have undergone abdominal or thoracic surgery is high. Changes occur in the pulmonary status of the patient who undergoes anesthesia and surgery. In the postoperative phase, these changes are characterized by gradual or abrupt alveolar collapse. The patient with COPD, when subjected to surgery, then represents an even higher risk for postoperative complications. It is important that these patients be given meticulous preoperative care so that they may be in the best possible health when they enter surgery. This preoperative medical treatment usually includes hydration, nutrition, chest physiotherapy, bronchodilators, and prophylactic antibiotics if an infection is present. Serial pulmonary function tests and arterial blood gas determinations are used to monitor the progression of the preoperative treatment.

When the patient's pulmonary function reaches a peak preoperatively, that is, when the pulmonary function tests and arterial blood gas test results no longer show continued improvement, surgery is considered, because the patient has reached his or her optimal pulmonary status.

PACU Care

PACU care of the COPD patient centers on prevention of complications. The modified stir-up regimen should include frequent cascade coughing, sustained maximal inspirations (SMIs), and repositioning of the patient (see Chapters 6 and 20). An appropriately implemented modified stir-up regimen is of great importance, especially in patients recovering from upper abdominal or thoracic operations. Surgery at these sites can cause decreased ventilatory effort and a complete absence of sighs by the patient. Given that the patient already has compromised respiratory function, the possibility of retained secretions and atelectasis is magnified. Hence, these patients represent a significant challenge to the PACU nurse.

When the patient is completely reactive, the use of the incentive spirometer may be helpful in reducing the incidence of atelectasis. Consequently, the PACU nurse who is responsible for supportive measures should assist and encourage the patient in using the SMI with or without the incentive spirometer. Based on subjective research findings, it is believed that if the PACU nurse explains the rationale of the SMI maneuver and properly instructs the patient in the use of the technique *preoperatively*, the patient is more likely to correctly use the SMI maneuver postoperatively with or without coaching. The performance of the SMI maneuver, with or without mechanical devices, should be monitored by the nurse to ensure proper production of a sustained inspiration with a 3-second inspiratory hold. The PACU nurse should also encourage and monitor the patient's performance of the cascade cough to facilitate early secretion clearance.

Patients with COPD have some component of reactive airways disease. Consequently, their airways become compliant and can become compressed during a forced expiratory maneuver. This dynamic compression of the airways is a function of the equal pressure point theory as discussed in Chapter 6. To reduce the amount of dynamic compression of the airway during exhalation, the patient should be encouraged to use pursed-lip breathing. Breathing through pursed lips during exhalation can be the same as adding 5 to 10 cm H_2O of positive end-expiratory pressure. Increasing the pressure inside the airway during exhalation reduces the amount of dynamic compression of the airways and decreases the amount of air trapping that commonly occurs in patients with COPD.

The cardiac status should be monitored meticulously because of the frequent involvement of the heart in the pathologic disorders of these patients. Kidney function should also be monitored because it may be altered, especially in patients who exhibit fluid retention and edema of the extremities.

The patient with severe COPD who has marked hypercarbia can present difficulties in the PACU. Patients who have severe emphysema usually fit into this category. Their ventilatory effort is stimulated by the hypoxic drive, in which lack of oxygen serves as the stimulus to ventilation. Hypoxia indirectly stimulates the respiratory center by means of chemoreceptors in the carotid bodies located at the bifurcation of the carotid artery. When oxygen tensions rise in the inspired gas, owing to the patient's being given 100 percent oxygen to breathe in the PACU, the carotid and aortic chemoreceptors will cease to function and the patient will quickly become apneic. The patient's respiratory status should be assessed carefully and the physician consulted before 100 percent oxygen is administered. Mist therapy postoperatively aids in liquefying the secretions and helps in the all-important maintenance of a patent tracheobronchial tree. If excessive bronchial drainage is not removed, it will provide a convenient avenue for bacteria and it might also obstruct the airways, leading to insufficient alveolar ventilation and hypoxia.

The patient with COPD should be under constant surveillance for signs of cardiopulmonary decompensation, including shallow, rapid, gasping respirations; severe dyspnea; substernal retraction; and disorientation. Blood pressure may be elevated or low, but the patient usually has tachycardia, fever, and muscle rigidity. Cyanosis may or may not be present.

Respiratory depressant drugs, such as narcotics, should be given in low dosages, or if the

COPD is severe, they should be avoided completely. Repositioning of the patient and splinting of the incision site, along with reducing the anxiety usually seen in these patients, reduces the need for narcotic drugs. Some form of regional analgesia may be extremely beneficial for these patients.

MYASTHENIA GRAVIS

The patient with myasthenia gravis (MG) deserves special consideration in the PACU because of the respiratory dysfunction and possible pharmacologic ramifications of the disease. MG is a chronic disease characterized by progressive muscle weakness and easy fatigability. Most patients with MG have developed antibodies to muscle acetylcholine receptors. The antibody does not bind exactly on the site that binds the acetylcholine, but it does bind close to it. The acetylcholine receptors are steadily destroyed, with a resulting reduction in the binding of acetylcholine at the postsynaptic myoneural junction. The myasthenic patient will sometimes have a lesion in the myocardium that is a spotty, focal necrosis accompanied by an inflammatory reaction. An alteration in the S-T segment and T wave is sometimes seen in these patients.

The incidence of MG has been estimated to be between 1 in 15,000 and 1 in 40,000. It occurs twice as frequently in females as in males and at an earlier age. The main symptom is weakness involving one or more of the muscle groups, with ptosis of the eyelid the most frequent sign of the disease.

Ptosis is usually accompanied by diplopia, blurred vision, or nystagmus. Ocular signs and symptoms are frequently worsened by bright light. The patient may also have "myasthenic facies," which is caused by weakness of the facial muscles. This can progress to dysphagia and difficulties in speech.

Respiration is often affected in the myasthenic patient. Dyspnea can be either inspiratory, if the diaphragm is involved, or expiratory, if the intercostal and abdominal muscles are affected. The patient may also have emotional disturbances caused by anxiety and depression.

Diagnosis of MG is made on the clinical symptoms and the characteristic electromyogram. The clinical symptoms can be assessed by the neostigmine test or by the edrophonium test, both of which involve anticholinesterases that produce an increase in the strength of the myasthenic muscle. Muscle relaxants, such as *d*-tubocurarine chloride (curare) or gallamine triethiodide (Flaxedil), given in very small dosages, cause an exaggeration of MG symptoms and can be used in the diagnostic workup of the patient.

Treatment for this disease consists of various pharmacologic interventions designed to enhance neuromuscular transmission and slow the progression of the disease. Anticholinesterase drugs, which slow down the enzymatic destruction of acetylcholine at the neuromuscular junction, are commonly used. Oral pyridostigmine and the shorter-acting neostigmine are the anticholinesterases of choice. Myasthenic patients seem to favor pyridostigmine over neostigmine because of its length of action and its less unpleasant side effects. Steroids and other immunosuppressive agents may be used in some patients to reduce antibody production responsible for the disease.

Thymectomy seems to be an appropriate therapeutic mode, because the thymus gland appears to be intimately involved in the disease process. About 67 percent of the myasthenic patients who do not have thymoma experience improvement after thymectomy. On the other hand, about 25 percent of the myasthenic patients with thymoma have improvement in the disease process after thymectomy.

Because thymectomy has been used as a therapeutic intervention in the treatment of MG, the PACU nurse will probably render nursing care to many patients with MG. Because of the location of the incision, the myasthenic patient does not usually receive any intraoperative skeletal muscle relaxants. These myasthenic patients can experience an exacerbation of symptoms in the PACU. Hence, critical monitoring of the patient's ventilatory status should be the primary focus of the PACU nursing care. Myasthenic patients who are recovering from any type of surgical procedure and who have been administered any form of anesthesia (general, inhalation, or regional) can develop an exacerbation of symptoms, as well as myasthenic crisis, in the PACU. Consequently, respiratory support should always be available for these patients.

PACU Care

The patient with MG can present various difficulties because of an impaired respiratory system, possible poor nutrition, susceptibility to infection, altered psychiatric status, and possible altered response to drugs used during anesthesia. The patient should be placed in a quiet area, where no direct light will shine in his or her eyes. The patient's respiratory effort and exchange should be monitored continuously. Oxygen should be administered with humidification, and secretions should be removed by frequent suctioning and postural drainage. Oxygen saturation levels for these patients should be maintained above 96 percent. Any change in respiratory status should be reported to the physician immediately.

Cardiac monitoring should be instituted for every myasthenic patient in the PACU, because cardiac mechanisms may be responsible for some sudden deaths encountered in these patients. It is also important to monitor the fluids administered to myasthenic patients. Hypovolemia and hypervolemia must be avoided because of their deleterious effects on the already compromised heart and lungs.

The patient should be kept as pain free as possible to facilitate good respiratory exchange. Morphine and other narcotics are often potentiated by anticholinesterases. Therefore, the initial narcotic dose should be reduced to half the normal dose and then increased if required. If the patient is receiving continuous mechanical ventilation, the normal amount of medication can be given without compromising the patient's respiratory status.

The emotional status of the myasthenic patient is of considerable importance. As few clinicians as possible should be responsible for the myasthenic patient throughout the emergent phase because the patient is likely to be distrustful of anyone he or she does not know. Communication is important, and the patient should be informed about any nursing procedure to be performed. If the myasthenic patient has a tracheostomy, paper and pencil should be used to facilitate communication between nurse and patient.

DIABETES MELLITUS

Diabetes mellitus is a chronic metabolic disease associated with insulin deficiency or insensitivity, hyperglycemia, and glycosuria. It occurs in about 2 to 3 percent of the general population. One important aspect of this disease is an associated degeneration of the small blood vessels (microangiopathy) that is most marked in the retina, kidneys, and nervous system.

The focus of the physiologic activity of insulin is to "open the door" of the cell to let glucose enter. In the diabetic state, the patient has an elevated blood glucose level because of a defect in the cellular response to insulin and the "door" remains closed. Sources of the excess glucose are dietary carbohydrate, liver glycogen, and glucose formed by the fatty acids metabolized to acetone, or beta-hydroxybutyric acid. These three products are known as ketone bodies. The degree of insulin deficiency is reflected by hyperglycemia, glycosuria, and ketoacidosis exhibited by the patient.

Anesthesia and Diabetes

The goal of anesthetic management of the diabetic patient is the prevention of diabetic acidosis, hypoglycemia, and severe fluid loss. Clinicians differ regarding the specific method to be used to achieve this goal. One method is to withhold the usual dose of long-acting or intermediate-acting insulin. Two liters of 5 percent dextrose, with 10 to 15 units of crystalline regular insulin added to each liter, is given to the patient during surgery. In another method, the patient is administered 5 percent dextrose in Ringer's lactate at 125 ml per hour. Regular insulin, in 5-unit increments, is administered as needed to keep the patient's blood glucose level at or above 200 mg per dl. A more widely used method consists of giving half the daily dose of insulin on the morning of surgery or one third of the daily dose if the surgery is scheduled later in the day. The patient is given 500 to 1000 ml of 5 percent dextrose and water before surgery and at least 1000 ml of 5 percent dextrose and water during surgery. This method avoids hypoglycemia during surgery but increases the need for careful nursing attention in the PACU.

These methods are used in the patient who is undergoing elective surgery. Emergency surgery for the uncontrolled diabetic patient is an entirely different situation. Before the patient undergoes anesthesia and surgery, treatment of the diabetes should be instituted, if possible. Blood glucose levels are frequently determined along with blood urea nitrogen levels to indicate the proper amount of regular insulin to be administered on a sliding scale intraoperatively. Intravenous solutions are given to treat dehydration.

PACU Care

The patient should be monitored for fluid and electrolyte balance and degree of glycosuria. Most authors agree that mild glycosuria is more desirable than glucose-free urine. Hypoglycemia should be avoided. Patients who have had a stressful problem relieved (e.g., the removal of an intra-abdominal abscess) may have a reduced insulin requirement postoperatively. This may be as much as a 50 percent reduction in the first 24 hours. However, because of the stress of surgery, insulin requirements postoperatively are usually increased.

Urine glucose levels can be monitored by the Clinitest method. This method does not monitor the blood glucose level directly but does provide a rough indicator of insulin requirements. Consequently, because the urinary glucose concentration is considered to be a late indicator of blood glucose levels, it should not be used in patients with significant insulin-dependent diabetes. Blood glucose levels can be monitored closely in the PACU by using a Dextrostix (glucose oxidase) with blood from a finger stick. Blood glucose laboratory determinations should be done at least twice daily for 2 to 3 days postoperatively. A sliding scale that is usually used for the Clinitest method is shown in Table 38–1. If the Dextrostix method is being used to monitor the glucose level, the objective during the PACU period is to prevent hypoglycemia and to accept mild hyperglycemia with the aim of maintaining the blood glucose concentration between 150 and 200 mg per dl.

Respiratory acidosis should be prevented by aiding the patient to cough and breathe deeply to promote adequate pulmonary ventilation and carbon dioxide elimination. Metabolic acidosis must be prevented by the administration of fluid and electrolytes. Therefore, strict monitoring of intake and output measurements should be instituted on every diabetic patient admitted to the PACU.

There is a strong possibility that the diabetic patient will receive an insulin preparation in the PACU. The types of insulin, along with times of onset, peak effects, and duration of action, are summarized in Table 38–2.

Observation of the diabetic patient for possible diabetic coma (hyperglycemia) or insulin

Table 38–2. TIME OF ACTION OF VARIOUS INSULIN PREPARATIONS

Types of Insulin	Time of Onset (Minutes)	Peak Effects (Minutes)	Duration of Action (Hours)
Insulin injection, U.S.P. (regular)	0.50	2–4	6
Crystalline zinc insulin	1	2–4	8
Globin zinc insulin	2–4	8	18–24
Isophane insulin injection (N.P.N.)	2	8–20	20–30
Protamine zinc injection (P.Z.I.)	6–8	12–24	24–36
Lente insulin (insulin zinc suspension)	2–4	8–20	20–28

reaction ensures his or her proper emergence from anesthesia. The symptoms of each complication are summarized in Table 38–3. It is sometimes difficult to detect hyperglycemia or hypoglycemia by symptoms when a patient is recovering from an anesthetic. Therefore, frequent tests of blood and urine glucose are most helpful in determining the patient's state. It is also important to keep in mind that any patient who arrives in the PACU, especially in the older age groups, may have undiagnosed diabetes.

RHEUMATOID ARTHRITIS

Rheumatoid arthritis is a relatively common disease that affects the connective tissue of the body. The clinical course varies, but it tends to be progressive, leading to characteristic deformities. A large proportion of the patients become incapacitated over time. The disease affects more women than men, and its incidence in temperate climates is about 3 percent. The cause is not completely understood, but it is thought to be an autoimmune phenomenon. The outstanding clinical feature of this disease is proliferative inflammation. The patient often appears chronically ill, undernourished, and anemic.

These patients often undergo surgery to correct restrictive deformities caused by the disease process (Table 38–4). On arrival in the PACU, they require comprehensive nursing management. Some of the hazards to be aware of in patients with rheumatoid arthritis are listed in Table 38–5.

PACU Care

Airway. Extubation is often deferred in these patients until they are unquestionably able to

Table 38–1. SLIDING SCALE OF INSULIN DETERMINATIONS

Urine Glucose (Trace %)	Regular Insulin Dose (Units)
0.25	5
0.50	8
1	10
2	15

Table 38–3. CHARACTERISTICS OF DIABETIC COMPLICATIONS

Category	Diabetic Coma	Insulin Reaction
Onset	Slow	Sudden
Skin	Flushed, dry, hot	Pale, moist
Behavior	Drowsy	Excited
Breath	Acetone (sweet)	Normal
Respirations	Kussmaul's (air hunger)	Normal—rapid, shallow
Pulse	Rapid, weak	Normal—slow, full bounding
Blood pressure	Low	Normal
Vomiting	Present	Absent
Hunger	Absent	Present
Thirst	Present	Absent
Urine glucose level	Large amount	Absent

maintain their own airways. This is of prime importance, because these patients are often extremely difficult to intubate and are prone to airway obstruction.

Lungs. The patient with rheumatoid arthritis usually has pulmonary dysfunction such as diffuse interstitial fibrosis, granulomatous lesions, or large silicotic nodules. These pulmonary dysfunctions lead to what is termed *stiff lungs*, and these patients are prone to atelectasis, hypoxemia, and hypercarbia in the PACU (see Chapter 6). Postoperative blood gas analysis and good pulmonary support are therefore important. Respiratory depressant narcotics should be given with caution, if at all. Deaths in rheumatoid arthritic patients have resulted from drug-induced respiratory failure during this period.

Heart. Disease of the pericardium, myocardium, endocardium, and coronary vessels is usually associated with rheumatoid arthritis. Therefore, cardiovascular status should be monitored continuously in the PACU. Hypo-

tension should be avoided, because it may lead to left ventricular decompensation and acute heart failure.

Blood. The arthritic patient usually exhibits anemia, most commonly of the hypochromic microcytic variety. In most instances, this type of anemia can be treated with blood transfusion. Postoperative hematocrit and hemoglobin levels should be determined when the patient arrives in the PACU. Blood loss should be extensively monitored, including observation of the stools for blood. The contents recovered from the nasogastric tube (if present) should be checked for blood, because these patients may

Table 38–5. PACU HAZARDS IN PATIENTS WITH RHEUMATOID ARTHRITIS

Area of Concern	Complication
Respiratory system	
Airway	Hypoplastic mandible restriction, cervical spine motion, atlantoaxial subluxation, laryngeal tissue damage
Ventilation	Rheumatoid nodules in lung, chronic diffuse interstitial fibrosis, costovertebral joint disorder that inhibits ventilation, thoracic vertebrae flexion deformity that inhibits ventilation, tuberculous lung
Cardiovascular system	Pericardial, myocardial, coronary artery disorders, aortic valve regurgitation, arrhythmias
Hemopoietic, hepatic and renal systems	Anemia, leukopenia, bleeding tendency (decreased platelets), renal amyloidosis
Miscellaneous	Skin fragility; postoperative chest complications, such as atelectasis, hypercarbia, and hypoxia; multiple joint disease

Table 38–4. CORRECTIVE SURGERY FOR RHEUMATOID ARTHRITIS

Operative Site	Common Operative Procedure
Neck	Atlantoaxial arthrodesis
Shoulder	Synovectomy and partial excision of acromion
Elbow	Synovectomy and radial head excision; resection arthroplasty
Wrist	Synovectomy and excision of distal ulna
Hand	Metacarpal phalangeal arthroplasty and flexor and extensor tenosynovectomy
Hip	Cup or total replacement arthroplasty
Knee	Synovectomy (often bilateral), arthroplasty
Foot	Resection arthroplasty (often bilateral)

From Jenkins, L. C., and McGraw, R. W.: Anaesthetic management of the patient with rheumatoid arthritis. Can. Anaesth. Soc. J., 16:408, 1969.

Modified from Jenkins, L. C., and McGraw, R. W.: Anaesthetic management of the patient with rheumatoid arthritis. Can. Anaesth. Soc. J., 16:408, 1969.

have a bleeding peptic ulcer secondary to long-term aspirin and steroid therapy.

Fluid Balance. Renal function is usually impaired in the patient with chronic rheumatoid arthritis. Therefore, drugs that are primarily excreted by the kidneys should be avoided, and urinary output should be monitored at regular, perhaps hourly, intervals.

OBESITY

Obesity, the most common nutritional disorder in the world today, presents many difficulties to the PACU nurse. Many definitions of obesity can be found in the literature. The American Life Insurance Company states that a person is obese if he or she exceeds the expected or ideal weight, corrected by age and sex, by more than 10 percent. *Morbid obesity* is a term that denotes a weight twice as much as that predicted for age, sex, body build, and height. Morbidly obese patients can be divided into two groups. Obesity with normal levels of arterial carbon dioxide tension is referred to as *simple obesity* and includes 90 to 95 percent of morbidly obese patients. The other group, which represents 5 to 10 percent of obese patients, is referred to as having the *obesity-hypoventilation (pickwickian) syndrome*. This is characterized by extreme obesity and episodic somnolence, and by hypoventilation (increased $PaCO_2$ level) with twitching, plethora, edema, periodic respiration, secondary polycythemia, right ventricular hypertrophy, and right ventricular failure.

The most useful anthropometric index for determining obesity is the *body mass index* (BMI). This measurement employs the person's weight (in kilograms) divided by height squared (in meters):

$$BMI = \frac{weight\ (kg)}{height\ (m)^2}$$

The patient with a BMI of 27 (25 to 30 percent overweight) usually presents minimal risks in the perioperative period. A BMI higher than 30 is associated with an increased perioperative mortality.

Physiologic Considerations in Obesity

Respiratory System. Preoperative evaluation of obese patients reveals that 85 percent of them have exertional dyspnea and some degree of orthopnea. Periodic breathing, especially when sleeping, may also be present.

Obese patients tend to develop some degree of thoracic kyphosis and lumbar lordosis owing to a protuberant abdomen. In addition, the layers of fat on the chest and abdomen reduce the bellows action of the thoracic cage. The overall lung-thorax compliance is reduced, leading to an increased elastic resistance of the system. Usually the diaphragm is elevated, and the total work of breathing is increased as a result of the deposition of abdominal fat. Because of these factors, the oxygen cost of breathing is three or more times that of normal, even at rest.

The primary respiratory defect of obese patients is a marked reduction in the expiratory reserve volume. The reason for the decrease in expiratory reserve volume and other lung volumes is that the obese patient is unable to expand his or her chest in a normal fashion. Therefore, diaphragmatic movement must account for the changes in lung volume to a much greater extent than does thoracic expansion. As previously discussed, the diaphragmatic movement is moderately limited owing to the anatomic changes of obesity that account for the decreased lung volumes.

In the obese patient, the functional residual capacity may be below the closing capacity in the sitting and supine positions. Therefore, the dependent lung zones may be effectively closed throughout the respiratory cycle (see Chapter 6). Consequently, inspired gas is distributed mainly to the upper or nondependent lung zones. The resulting mismatch of ventilation to perfusion produces systemic arterial hypoxemia (Fig. 38–1).

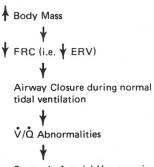

FIGURE 38–1. The relationship of body mass to systemic arterial hypoxemia. FRC = functional residual capacity; ERV = expiratory reserve volume; $\dot{V}/\dot{Q}$ = ventilation/perfusion. (From Drain, C., and Vaughan, R.: Anesthetic Considerations of Morbid Obesity. AANA J. 47[5]:556–565, 1979, p. 558.)

The hypoventilation and ventilation-perfusion abnormalities that contribute to systemic arterial hypoxemia also contribute to retained carbon dioxide, resulting in hypercarbia, which can be observed in the pickwickian syndrome.

Cardiovascular System. It has been estimated that 30 pounds of fat contain 25 miles of blood vessels and that the increased body mass in obesity leads to an increased oxygen consumption and carbon dioxide production. It is not surprising that the cardiac output and the total blood volume are increased in the obese state. This increase in cardiac output is a result of an increase in stroke volume rather than an increase in heart rate, as the latter usually remains normal.

The transverse cardiac diameter has been shown to be greater than normal in approximately two thirds of obese patients. There seems to be a linear relationship between cardiac diameter and body weight.

It has been suggested that obesity predisposes to electrocardiographic changes. The Q-T interval is often prolonged and the QRS voltage is reduced (owing to the increased distance between the heart and the electrodes). Finally, there is an increased likelihood that ventricular arrhythmias can occur in the obese patient.

There is a positive correlation between an increase in body weight and increased arterial pressure. A weight gain of 28 pounds can increase the systolic and diastolic blood pressure by 10 and 7 mm Hg, respectively. The increase in blood pressure is probably due to the increased cardiac output.

Chronic heart failure, although uncommon, does occur in persons with long-standing morbid obesity with or without hypertension. It is usually characterized by high output and biventricular dysfunction, with the left ventricle predominating. Clinically, heart failure may be difficult to diagnose because pedal edema may be chronically present.

Cerebral blood flow in obese persons does not differ significantly from that in normal persons. Oxygen uptake of the brain remains normal in the obese person. However, the fraction of the total body oxygen accounted for in the cerebral metabolism is less than normal because the total body oxygen requirement is increased. Although the kidneys of obese subjects weigh more than those of their normal counterparts, renal blood flow is the same or slightly lower than that found in patients of normal weight.

Pregnancy. Problems associated with obesity in pregnancy occur relatively frequently. Studies indicate that patients weighing at least 250 pounds have a 35 percent chance of operative obstetrics. In fact, some form of obstetric complication may be observed in 63 percent of obese patients. There is seven times more toxemia, five times more pyelonephritis, and ten times more diabetes mellitus than in similar groups of nonobese pregnant patients.

Other Disorders. Diabetes mellitus has been associated with obesity. It is the third most prevalent preoperative pathologic condition found in obese patients. Adult diabetic patients are often obese, and an improved glucose tolerance test follows weight reduction. Other associated problems that may be clinically present include abnormal liver function tests, fatty infiltration of the liver, gallstones, hiatal hernia, and varicose veins.

PACU Care

Respiratory. Significant problems arise in the PACU phase of the perioperative care of the obese patient. In fact, the problems associated with obesity are becoming more apparent to all PACU nurses since the advent of the jejunoileal bypass and gastric stapling procedures for the treatment of morbid obesity. There is a direct correlation between the incidence of postoperative pulmonary complications and the degree of obesity. The mortality rate after upper abdominal operations in obese patients is 2.5 times that of their nonobese counterparts.

Positioning can be a valuable therapeutic tool to improve arterial oxygenation. It has been demonstrated that position significantly affects PaO_2 levels for 48 hours postoperatively. The obese patient should be cared for in a semi-Fowler's position unless cardiovascular instability exists. *Routine use of the supine position should be avoided*, because the functional residual capacity can decrease below the closing capacity and thus reduce the number of ventilated alveoli, which will ultimately lead to hypoxemia. Moreover, early ambulation in the PACU is of great value in enhancing lung volumes of the obese patient.

In the postoperative period, the position of the operative incision is a factor, because it has been demonstrated that obese patients with a vertical incision have a more marked postoperative hypoxemia than obese patients who receive a transverse incision. Therefore, supplemental inspired oxygen may be necessary for 3 to 4 days postoperatively in patients with a vertical incision. Serial arterial blood gas determinations can serve as a guide to supplemental oxygen administration. Along with this, when the patient arrives in the PACU and an arterial line is in place, arterial blood gas determinations should be done to provide a baseline guide for proper ventilation. If the patient arrives in the PACU with the endotracheal tube in place, the patient should be started on a ventilator. The nurse should then auscultate for bilateral breath sounds to ensure proper placement of the endotracheal tube. Because of the many technical difficulties associated with tracheal intubation of the obese patient, the PACU nurse should constantly monitor the patient for proper placement of the tube. If it becomes displaced, the patient should be ventilated with a bag-valve-mask system, and the anesthesia personnel should be summoned immediately.

Cardiovascular pathophysiology may reduce cardiac reserve, especially in the older obese patient. A reduction in arterial oxygen tension due to incision site or postoperative position causes an increase in cardiac output to facilitate tissue oxygen delivery. This could lead to cardiac decompensation in an already compromised cardiovascular system. Arterial hypoxemia should be avoided, because many obese patients cannot compensate for the increased cardiac output demand and the concomitant pulmonary vasoconstriction caused by the reduced arterial oxygen tension.

Early postoperative ambulation is important not only in enhancing lung volumes but also in helping reduce the incidence of venous thrombosis. Indeed, relatively immobile obese persons are particularly susceptible to the development of pulmonary emboli.

Cardiovascular. The obese patient has a higher incidence of hypertension, coronary artery disease, myocardial infarction, and cardiomegaly. Therefore, careful electrocardiographic monitoring should be employed. If an arterial line was not used intraoperatively, a blood pressure cuff that covers one third to one half the length of the upper arm should be employed. A baseline blood pressure measurement when the patient arrives in the PACU will prove valuable when compared with the intraoperative measurements to assess the accuracy of the blood pressure reading.

Fluid Dynamics. Because fatty tissue is 6 to 10 percent water as compared with lean tissue, which is composed of 70 to 80 percent water, alteration in fluid requirements is likely to occur in the obese patient. In the normal person, the percentage of body water is 65; in the obese person, the body water is about 40 percent of total weight. Calculations of fluid requirements must be adjusted to compensate for this reduction in total body water.

Psychological Aspects. Psychological support of the obese patient should not be overlooked when PACU care is administered. Many of these patients have become obese because of repeated episodes of emotional stress. Body image, along with the ability to interact with others, may be a problem for obese patients; they may appear to be demanding and aloof from others. It is important for the PACU personnel to establish a positive rapport with the obese patient preoperatively. Along with this, it is important that the PACU staff not express any negative feelings about the patient or about morbid obesity in general. Hence, the added psychological support will serve to minimize fear and anxiety and ultimately improve the outcome of the obese patient.

CIGARETTE SMOKING

Cigarette smoking affects the manner in which a patient recovers from an anesthetic. The PACU nurse should be aware of the diverse reactions that smoking can have on the patient who is emerging from an inhalation anesthetic.

Although studies on the relationship between smoking and its effects on anesthesia are meager, they do indicate an increase in the risk factor when a patient smokes.

Respiratory Effects

A growing body of convincing scientific literature suggests that almost all pulmonary disease is related in some way to the inhalation of infectious or irritant particulate material. Cigarette smoke in its gaseous phase contains nitrogen, oxygen, carbon dioxide, carbon monoxide, hydrogen, argon, methane, hydrogen cyanide, ammonia, nitrogen dioxide, and acetone. In the particulate phase, cigarette smoke contains nicotine, tar, acids, alcohol, phenols, and hydrocarbons. Smokers inhaling nicotine from a cigarette into the lungs actually receive 25 to 30 percent of the nicotine contained in the cigarette. Thirty percent is destroyed by combustion, and 40 percent is lost in the side stream. Therefore, if a person inhales the smoke from a cigarette containing 2.5 mg of nicotine, 1 mg of nicotine will actually be absorbed by the lungs. It is also known that filters make little difference in this absorption. Contrary to some opinions, smoking cigars and pipes also presents risk for pulmonary disease.

Carbon monoxide combines with the hemoglobin molecule at the same point as does oxygen. It has an affinity for this receptor point that is 210 times greater than that of oxygen. Therefore, the oxygen-carrying capacity of hemoglobin is reduced, and the end result is that less oxygen is given up to the tissues by the hemoglobin. When carbon monoxide combines with hemoglobin, the compound formed is called *carboxyhemoglobin*. The amount of carboxyhemoglobin in the blood is especially important in the patient who has a diseased myocardium, because myocardial oxygenation is limited by the flow of the blood through the coronary arteries. During stress, such as in surgery and anesthesia, the amount of carboxyhemoglobin saturation could lead to severe myocardial hypoxia in heavy-smoking patients with coronary artery disease, because the diseased coronary arteries cannot increase the flow significantly. The only means of preventing hypoxia is to increase the extraction of oxygen from the hemoglobin. Small amounts of carboxyhemoglobin may hinder the uncoupling of the oxygen, resulting in yet more oxygen retention at any given tension. This effect clearly would be greater when the oxygen tension is further reduced by local ischemia and any additional vasoconstriction associated with smoking.

Smoking is an important causative factor in chronic pulmonary disease, especially the obstructive type. The pulmonary function alterations characteristic of smokers usually include a reduction in vital capacity, an increase in residual volume to total lung capacity, an uneven distribution of inspired gas, a decrease in dynamic compliance, and an increase in nonelastic resistance.

Chronic bronchitis is the disease most often associated with smoking and is seen frequently by the PACU nurse. Hypertrophy of bronchial mucous glands, with production of excessive mucus, is the hallmark of this disease. A vicious cycle develops as this failure to remove the mucus leads to retention of pathogenic organisms and irritants. The resulting distorted alveolar septa and the increased pressure on the alveoli from chronic bronchitis can lead to emphysema.

Cigarette smoke can cause a progression from hyperplasia to metaplasia to neoplasia in the lungs. Sometimes associated with bronchial carcinoma is the *Eaton-Lambert syndrome*, often referred to as the *myasthenic syndrome* because its symptoms resemble those of MG. This syndrome in some way affects neuromuscular transmission, and patients experience the classic symptoms of muscle weakness. These patients are especially sensitive to the skeletal neuromuscular blocking agents used in clinical anesthesia. If the anesthetist is unaware of this syndrome and administers the normal dosage of skeletal muscle relaxants, the patient will probably be unable to ventilate spontaneously on emergence from anesthesia even when pharmacologic reversal of the muscle relaxant is attempted. In this situation, postoperative mechanical ventilation is necessary.

Cardiovascular Effects

The correlation between vascular disease and smoking is strong. Smoking may influence thrombosis, and because thrombi and platelets contribute to the development of arteriosclerosis, smoking can help cause arteriosclerosis and its complications.

Inhalation of nicotine produces a release of catecholamines, activates the carotid and aortic chemoreceptor bodies, and directly stimulates the muscles of the vessel walls. As a result, the immediate effects of smoking even a small number of cigarettes can be fairly marked—producing increases in heart rate, peripheral resistance, cardiac workload, and blood pressure. Each of these actions causes a greater myocardial oxygen demand. Furthermore, as the smoker's hemoglobin can provide less oxygen to the myocardium, it is not surprising that smoking can cause cardiac arrhythmias, either through myocardial anoxia or epinephrine release.

PACU Care

Many investigations have demonstrated that patients who smoke have a significant increase in pulmonary complications as compared with nonsmokers. Patients who smoke more than two packs of cigarettes a day are especially prone to perianesthetic complications. Many of these complications develop when cigarette smokers have a preexisting chronic respiratory disease, usually bronchitis. The major postoperative complications associated with smoking are infection, atelectasis, pleural effusion, pulmonary infarction, and bronchitis.

Complications associated with chronic cigarette smoking revolve around the inability of the patient to clear secretions. The goal of nursing care in the PACU centers on clearing the tracheobronchial tree. This necessitates frequent suctioning, cascade coughing, and the use of the SMI maneuver. If rales and rhonchi are heard on auscultation, percussion and postural drainage should be initiated.

Because cardiovascular disease is associated with a long history of cigarette smoking, the patient should have continuous electrocardiographic monitoring. Arrhythmias, such as premature ventricular contractions, should be sought, because they may be the first sign of decreased myocardial oxygenation in the cigarette smoker.

SICKLE CELL ANEMIA

Sickle cell anemia is an inherited type of hemolytic anemia. It is a chronic disease marked by exacerbations. The clinical manifestations are based entirely on sickling of the red blood cells and its consequences.

More than 100 abnormal hemoglobins have been described in humans. This particular form of hemoglobin, when exposed to low oxygen tensions, causes the red blood cell to distort its shape (sickle) and to cause infarction and other complications. Normal hemoglobin is labeled *hemoglobin A,* whereas this sickling hemoglobin is labeled *hemoglobin S.*

Hemoglobin S is thought to have arisen in Arabia in Neolithic times and from there to have spread eastward and westward; it is found today in parts of India, east and west Africa, the West Indies, and among American blacks.

The common sickle cell disorders are sickle cell trait (SA), homozygous sickle cell disease (SS), sickle cell–hemoglobin C disease, and sickle cell–thalassemia. A combination of thalassemia and sickle cell anemia occurs in sickle cell–beta thalassemia.

Sickle cell trait is found in about 8 to 12 percent of the black population, who are heterozygous for sickling, and represents a combination of sickle hemoglobin (SA) and normal hemoglobin (AA). The red blood cells of such persons contain from 20 to 40 percent hemoglobin S but are not misshapen under normal living conditions. The person may experience sickling if exposed to any conditions that cause hypoxia, such as depressed respiratory function from anesthetics in the PACU.

The most common form of sickle cell disease is the homozygous sickle cell disease. It occurs in about 1 in 400 to 500 blacks in the United States. These persons have inherited sickling genes from both parents, and they usually have 80 to 100 percent hemoglobin S. Sickling is present all the times, and minor reductions in oxygen tension can cause a sickle cell crisis.

The onset of symptoms occurs around the age of 2, and rarely do these persons live past the age of 40.

Sickle cell–hemoglobin C disease is caused by the presence of the gene for sickle hemoglobin and the gene for hemoglobin C. The course of the disease is usually milder than that of the homozygous sickle cell disease, although the person will experience discomfort and occasional sickle cell crises.

Sickle cell–thalassemia, which occurs in persons who have traits for sickle cell–thalassemia and beta-thalassemia, has a less severe course and symptoms in comparison with the other forms of these diseases. The sickle cell crises are not seen as commonly in this disease.

Pathogenesis

To understand the pathogenesis of this disease, it is helpful to know what happens to the red blood cell when sickling occurs. If oxygen tension is lowered, long crystals called *tactoids* are formed within the red blood cells, owing to rearrangement of the amino acid chains or polymers. The cell membrane becomes distorted by the twisting of the polymers. The result is the sickle cell shape for which the disease is named (Fig. 38–2). The process can be reversed if the oxygen tension is increased.

The actual pathologic action of sickling occurs in the microcirculation. Because of increased viscosity and the distortion of the red blood cells with the formation of tactoids, which prevents the cells from molding to the size and structure of the capillaries, the sickled cells are wedged in the capillary bed, occluding normal flow. As the cells aggregate, a thrombus is formed. Symptoms depend on whether the thrombus becomes an embolus, and, if so, on where it becomes lodged; infarctive episodes will be caused in that tissue. Areas of infarctive crisis are the spleen, myocardium, kidney, liver, mesentery, bone marrow, and brain.

Oxygen tension causes sickling, but several other precipitating factors are also involved, such as acidosis, hypotension, regional vasodilatation, dehydration, hemoconcentration, stasis of blood, hypothermia, sepsis, decreased cardiac output, and respiratory impairment.

Sickle Cell Anemia and Anesthesia

It is generally believed that anesthesia is not hazardous to patients with sickle cell trait.

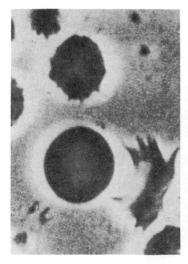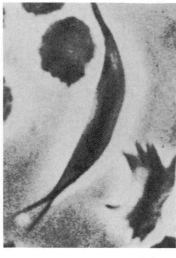

FIGURE 38–2. Comparison of a normal cell *(left)* and a sickle cell *(right)*. (From Sickle cell anemia. Medical World News, December 3, 1971, p. 38.)

Nevertheless, it must be kept in mind that sufficiently adverse hypoxic conditions can precipitate a sickling crisis. Definite hazards arise with anesthesia in patients with sickle cell and sickle cell–hemoglobin C disease. General anesthesia, because of its ability to cause the intravascular sickling syndrome, has been the subject of much research. The most important factor in this syndrome is hypoxemia, which generally occurs during the emergent period rather than intraoperatively. Local anesthesia or nerve block is the technique of choice. Epidural and spinal techniques should be avoided, owing to the possibility of hypotension with these two methods.

PACU Care

Prevention of sickle cell crisis is the main objective in the PACU phase. If diagnostic procedures are not available, or if emergency surgery prevents testing for the sickling trait, all black patients should be treated as possible carriers of the trait, because the incidence of this disease is relatively high among blacks.

In the patient with sickle cell disease, the postoperative period is of crucial importance. This is because incisional pain, analgesics, pulmonary infections, and low arterial oxygen partial pressures all are predisposing factors to the formation of sickle cells. Hence, in the PACU, supplemental humidified oxygen, along with appropriate monitoring of intravascular volume and core temperature, is of utmost importance for ensuring the positive outcomes of the patient.

Temperature regulation is important for the patient with sickle cell disease. Although cold reduces tactoid formation, it also reduces body metabolism, which may lead to crisis. Hyperthermia causes excess sweating, however, and may lead to dehydration, which can also cause sickling. Temperature monitoring and the use of hypothermia and hyperthermia blankets can allow maintenance of body temperature in the optimal range of 36° to 37°C.

Cardiac monitoring is important because the frequency of arrhythmias, such as extrasystole and prolonged P-R interval, in sickling patients is high. Vasodilators or vasoconstrictors should be avoided, if possible, because the dilators may cause hypotension and the vasoconstrictors may cause circulatory stasis.

Respiratory rate and volume should be monitored closely so that hypoxia can be avoided. Oxygen saturation or arterial blood gas monitoring can aid in assessing respiratory status, and postoperative pain should be managed with drugs that do not depress respiratory function.

Kidney function should be monitored because the renal tubules will become blocked by the hemolyzed red blood cells if crisis occurs, and infarcts may occur in some areas of the kidney. Insertion of a urinary catheter to monitor urinary output at regular intervals will prove useful.

SICKLE CELL CRISIS

The types of crisis seen in sickle cell anemia are vaso-occlusive, aplastic, sequestration, and hemolytic. The *vaso-occlusive crisis* is the most common type and is characterized by tissue ischemia, infarction, and necrosis. The bones, tendons, synovia, spleen, liver, and intestine are common sites of occlusion. Infections, dehydration, high altitudes, extreme physical exertion, and emotional upsets can trigger this type of crisis.

The *aplastic crisis* is most grave and constitutes a medical emergency. It is characterized by a sudden drastic decrease in red blood cell production. The patient will initially appear weak and have signs of cardiac decompensation.

The spleen is involved in *sequestration crisis.* A large amount of blood becomes trapped in the spleen, and hypovolemia and shock are the outcome—this constitutes a medical emergency. Clinically, the patient's blood pressure decreases and the pulse rate increases. Palpation and percussion reveal an enlarged mass in the right upper quadrant of the abdomen.

Bacterial infections, poisons, and medications, such as phenothiazines and sulfonamides, aspirin in large quantities, and quinine, are capable of producing *hemolysis* of the red blood cell. The patient also has an enzyme deficiency (glucose-6-phosphodehydrogenase) in this type of sickle cell anemia.

If crisis occurs, the following modes of treatment are recommended: Keep the patient warm, treat infections, and maintain oxygenation, hydration, and alkalinization. Heparin may be administered to reduce the risks of embolus formation, and magnesium sulfate may also be indicated for its vasodilator and anticoagulant properties.

NAUSEA AND VOMITING

One of the most perplexing problems for the PACU nurse is that of the syndrome of postoperative nausea and vomiting. Most often, patients who experience nausea and vomiting have a history of chronic gastrointestinal irritability. Although the incidence of nausea and vomiting has decreased through the years, the problem is still perennial in every PACU. The surgeon hopes that nausea and vomiting will be minimal, because disturbances in electrolyte balance and wound healing are associated with such upsets. The PACU nurse also appreciates a decreased incidence of these upsets because when patients are vomiting, airway management can become most difficult.

Mechanism of Action

The *vomiting center* is located in the medulla near the dorsal nucleus of the vagus nerve (Fig.

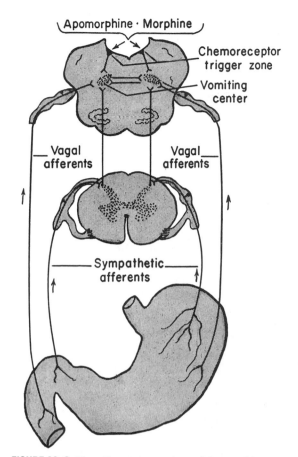

FIGURE 38–3. The afferent connections of the vomiting center. (From Guyton, A. C.: Textbook of Medical Physiology. 7th ed. Philadelphia, W. B. Saunders, 1986, p. 803.)

38–3). It can be excited by reflex impulses arising in the pharynx, stomach, or other portions of the gastrointestinal tract. Foreign materials, such as blood and mucus or irritant gases in the stomach or other portions of the gastrointestinal tract, can produce this syndrome. The vomiting center can be excited by impulses received from cerebral centers. Drugs such as anesthetic agents and narcotics sensitize the vestibular apparatus, the organ of balance. This explains why two of the principal causative factors of nausea and vomiting are rough handling of the patient during transportation and frequent changes of position in the immediate recovery period.

The vomiting center can be excited by chemical materials carried to it in the blood. Drugs such as apomorphine, morphine, and meperidine (Demerol) arrive this way, exciting the vomiting center directly. This is designated as *central vomiting.* The vomiting center can be excited by interference with its blood supply. Severe cerebral anoxia and increased intracranial pressure are examples of this. Finally, the vomiting center can be excited by dehydration and electrolyte imbalance.

Incidence

Studies indicate that the incidence of nausea and vomiting is higher in women than in men. There is a lower incidence in those patients premedicated with morphine than in those who receive meperidine. Of great interest is that patients who receive their anesthetic by mask have a higher incidence of nausea and vomiting than patients who receive their anesthetic by endotracheal tube. Other possible causes of nausea and vomiting of statistical significance are hypotension during surgery, intra-abdominal surgery, increased duration of surgery, obesity, and a history of motion sickness.

Many authors agree that postoperative nausea is related to pain. Opiates of sufficient dosage tend to reduce pain and abate nausea, and they seldom provoke nausea. If the dosage of the analgesic is inadequate, the nausea may persist, and further supplemental doses of analgesic may be required. Other techniques for relief of pain that should be instituted concomitant with the administration of opiate are repositioning the postoperative patient, encouraging the patient to cough and deep breathe, and administering oxygen.

Patients who received a nitrous-narcotic anesthetic and whose state was reversed postoperatively with an excessive dose of naloxone (Narcan) usually exhibit nausea and vomiting in the emergent phase. Naloxone does not possess any emetic properties. Therefore, the analgesic state should be re-established to eliminate the vomiting reaction that is caused by pain when the opiate receptors are occupied by naloxone and not opiates.

PACU Care

If patients complain of nausea, they should be encouraged to perform the SMI and the cascade cough, and oxygen should be administered if there is any suspicion of hypoxemia. A cold washcloth placed on the patient's forehead and words of encouragement sometimes extinguish the nausea. It is mandatory for the nurse to remain with the patient, because the patient can go into the vomiting stage at a moment's notice, and the danger of aspiration of vomitus and obstructed airway is always present.

If the nausea persists or is severe, the patient can be given a pharmacologic remedy as ordered by the physician (Table 38–6).

PACU care of the patient who is vomiting focuses on airway management. The patient should be placed in a head-down position so that the vomitus will drain away from the lungs. Oral suctioning should be instituted if the patient is not able to control his or her airway completely. Oxygen should be administered when there is any question of compromise of the respiratory status. Rapid assessment of the patient's respiratory status should be made during and after the vomiting episode. This is done by auscultation of the chest bilaterally for adventitious sounds. Any possible aspiration of vomitus should be reported to

Table 38–6. DRUGS USED TO CONTROL NAUSEA

Drug	Route of Administration	Action	Side Effects
Prochlorperazine (Compazine)	PO, IM, suppository	Antiemetic, tranquilizer	Drowsiness, dizziness, hypotension, extrapyramidal reactions
Trimethobenzamide (Tigan)	PO, suppository, IM	Antiemetic	Drowsiness, Parkinson-like symptoms, hypotension, blurring of vision
Hydroxyzine (Atarax or Vistaril)	PO, IM	Reduces anxiety, antiemetic	Potentiation of narcotics and barbiturates, and other central nervous system depressants; drowsiness, dry mouth
Droperidol (Inapsine)	IM, IV	Antiemetic, tranquilizer	Drowsiness, hypotension, extrapyramidal reactions
Benzoquinamide (Emete-con)	IM or IV (slowly)	Antiemetic, antihistaminic, mild anticholinergic, sedative	Drowsiness, headache, hypertension, arrhythmias during IV administration, increased temperature, dry mouth, flushing, blurred vision

IM = intramuscular; IV = intravenous; PO = oral.

the physician immediately. If the airway becomes obstructed, place the patient in a head-down position, turn his or her head to one side, and try to remove foreign material by suctioning or with the finger. While performing this maneuver, send another person for a physician or anesthetist. A third person should remain to assist the nurse.

References

1. Anderson, R., and Krogh, K.: Pain as a major cause of postoperative nausea. Can. Anaesth. Soc. J., 23(4):366, 1976.
2. Aronson, R., Weiss, S., Ben, R., and Komaroff, A.: Association between cigarette smoking and acute respiratory tract infections in young adults. JAMA, 248:181–183, 1982.
3. Austin, R.: Cigarette smoking and chronic bronchitis. Br. Med. J., 2(6046):1261, 1976.
4. Ayres, S.: Cigarette smoking and lung diseases: An update. In Basics of Respiratory Disease. New York, American Lung Association, 1975.
5. Barash, P., Cullen, B. and Stoelting, R.: Handbook of Clinical Anesthesia. 2nd ed. Philadelphia, J. B. Lippincott, 1993.
6. Bayes, J.: Asymptomatic smokers: ASA I or II? Anesthesiology, 56:76, 1982.
7. Benumof, J. and Saidman, L.: Anesthesia and Perioperative Complications. St. Louis: Mosby-Year Book, 1992.
8. Berman, L.: Cigarettes, coronary occlusions, and myocardial infarctions. JAMA, 246:871–872, 1981.
9. Biddle, C., and Biddle, W.: A survey of perianesthetic complications in the asymptomatic smoker. AANA J., 51(5):481–484, 1983.
10. Biddle, C., and Hernandez, S.: Perioperative control of diabetes mellitus—revised. AANA J., 51(2):138–141, 1983.
11. Braunwald, E.: Harrison's Principles of Internal Medicine. 12th ed. New York, McGraw-Hill, 1991.
12. Breslow, M., Miller, C., and Rogers, M.: Perioperative Management. St. Louis, C. V. Mosby, 1990.
13. Brown, B. (ed.): Anesthesia and the Obese Patient. Philadelphia, F. A. Davis, 1981.
14. Burrows, B., Knudson, R., Quan, S., et al.: Respiratory Disorders: A Pathophysiologic Approach. 2nd ed. Chicago, Year Book Medical Publishers, 1983.
15. Cameron, L., and Kirsch, J.: Myasthenia gravis pharmacologic management. Crit. Care Rep., 1:157–163, 1989.
16. Drain, C.: Comparison of two inspiratory maneuvers on increasing lung volumes in postoperative upper abdominal surgical patients [Unpublished master's thesis]. Tucson, University of Arizona, 1980.
17. Drain, C., and Vaughan, R.: Anesthetic considerations of morbid obesity. AANA J., 47(5):556–565, 1979.
18. Drain, C.: Cigarette smoking—its effects on anesthesia. AANA J., 42(4):323–325, 1974.
19. Erikssen, J., Hellen, A., and Stormorken, H.: Chronic effect of smoking on platelet count and platelet adhesiveness in presumably healthy middle-aged men. Thromb. Haemost., 38(3):606–611, 1977.
20. Fink, D., and Raymon, R.: Rheumatoid arthritis of the cricoarytenoid joints: An airway hazard. Anesth. Analg., 54(6):742, 1975.
21. Friedman, F.: Mortality in cigarette smokers and quitters: Effects of baseline differences. N. Engl. J. Med., 30:1407–1410, 1981.
22. Frost, E.: Preanesthetic assessment of the patient with respiratory disease. Anesthesiol. Clin. North Am., 8:657–676, 1990.
23. Gibson, J.: Anesthesia for the sickle cell diseases and other hemoglobinopathies. Semin. Anesth., 6(1):27–35, 1987.
24. Gilman, A., Rall, T., Nies, A., et al.: Goodman and Gilman's The Pharmacological Basis of Therapeutics. 8th ed. New York, Pergamon Press, 1990.
25. Guyton, A.: Textbook of Medical Physiology. 8th ed. Philadelphia, W. B. Saunders, 1991.
26. Katz, J., Benumof, J., and Kadis, L.: Anesthesia and Uncommon Diseases. 3rd ed. Philadelphia, W. B. Saunders, 1990.
27. Lynch, J.: Preoperative and intraoperative insulin needs in diabetic patients. AANA J., 52(3):275–279, 1984.
28. Maduska, A.: Sickling dynamics of red blood cells and other physiologic studies during anesthesia. Anesth. Analg., 54(3):361–364, 1975.
29. Miller, R.: Anesthesia. 3rd ed. New York, Churchill Livingstone, 1990.
30. Schenker, M., Samet, J., and Spiezer, E.: Effect of cigarette tar content and smoking habits on respiratory symptoms in women. Am. Rev. Respir. Dis., 125:684–690, 1982.
31. Stoelting, R., Dierdorf, S., and McCammon, R.: Anesthesia and Co-Existing Disease. 2nd ed. New York, Churchill Livingstone, 1989.
32. Vaughan, R., Engelhardt, R. C., and Wise, L.: Postoperative hypoxemia in obese patients. Ann. Surg., 180(6):877, 1974.
33. Wightman, J.: A prospective survey of the incidence of postoperative pulmonary complications. Br. J. Surg., 55:85–91, 1968.

Post Anesthesia Care of the Pediatric Patient

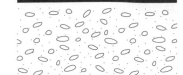

CHAPTER 39

Pediatric anesthesia is a popular subspecialty in the practice of anesthesiology. For clarification, the *newborn* is defined as less than 72 hours old, the *infant* less than 1 month old, and the *child* less than 13 years old. Infants and children cannot be regarded as just small adults, because their immaturity presents various definite physiologic differences. Some of the main differences lie in the endocrine, cardiovascular, and respiratory systems and in the regulation of body temperature.

Anesthetic management of the pediatric patient has been revised in several areas as comprehension of pediatric physiology and pathophysiology has improved. Because of this greater understanding, pediatric anesthesiology and post anesthesia care have become even more challenging and rewarding.

ANATOMIC AND PHYSIOLOGIC DIFFERENCES

Endocrine System

At birth, the infant has a diminished response to surgical trauma because the infant's cortical cellular organization is not as fully functional as that of the adult adrenal cortex. Some physicians may use supplementary cortisone therapy during the postoperative period to improve the response in infants to surgical stress.

Cardiovascular System

Average pulse and blood pressure measurements for newborns, infants, and children are summarized in Tables 39–1 and 39–2. With the advent of more sophisticated blood pressure monitoring devices, measurements in infants can be taken with great accuracy. It is important to monitor the infant's blood pressure because shock can develop rapidly, and the observation of the blood pressure is actually more

important in infants and children than in adults. This is because the pediatric patient does not have the physiologic reservoirs (e.g., blood volume) to rely on in situations in which shock can occur. The author has observed that the pediatric patient ordinarily demonstrates the usual signs of impending shock or airway obstruction, and yet, if the problem is not rectified rapidly, the pediatric patient's physiologic status will deteriorate two or three times faster than that of the adult. Hence, the post anesthesia care unit (PACU) nurse must always monitor the physiologic parameters of the pediatric patient, and if abnormalities arise, prompt interventions are essential.

The heart rate of the pediatric patient is another parameter that should be monitored constantly in the PACU. After the patient's arrival, when the vital signs are obtained, the PACU values should be first compared with the preoperative and intraoperative recordings of vital signs. Changes in the heart rate of the pediatric patient are one of the first clues of impending physiologic dysfunction. In the PACU, the

Table 39–1. AVERAGE BLOOD PRESSURE OF CHILDREN

Age	Systolic (mm Hg)	Diastolic (mm Hg)
Newborn	75–85	40–50
2 wk–4 yr	85	60
5 yr	87	60
6 yr	90	60
7 yr	92	62
8 yr	95	62
9 yr	98	64
10 yr	100	65
11 yr	105	65
12 yr	108	67
13 yr	110	67
14 yr	112	70
15 yr	115	72
16 yr	118	75

From Vaughan, V. C., and McKay, R. J. (eds.): Textbook of Pediatrics. 10th ed. Philadelphia, W. B. Saunders, 1975.

Table 39–2. AVERAGE PULSE RATE AT DIFFERENT AGES

	Pulse Rate (beats per min)		
Age	Lower Limits of Normal	Average	Upper Limits of Normal
Newborn	70	120	170
1–11 mo	80	120	160
2 yr	80	110	130
4 yr	80	100	120
6 yr	75	100	115
8 yr	70	90	110
10 yr	70	90	110

From Vaughan, V. C., and McKay, R. J. (eds.): Textbook of Pediatrics. 10th ed. Philadelphia, W. B. Saunders, 1975.

heart rate of infants and children is influenced by physical activity and by the administration of atropine, glycopyrrolate, and anesthetic agents. Crying, struggling, or pain can increase the heart rate; glycopyrrolate (Robinul), an anticholinergic atropine-like drug, may elevate the heart rate mildly but not as much as atropine does; and anesthetic agents such as halothane, enflurane, and isoflurane cause a decrease in heart rate.

The hemoglobin level and number of blood cells are high at birth. Values then decrease rapidly until age 3 months. The rates then rise slowly to the normal adult value by age 12 years (Fig. 39–1).

Respiratory System

Newborns are usually obligate nose breathers and are prone to airway obstruction. This is because the newborn has small nares, a large tongue, a small mandible, a short neck, and a large amount of upper airway lymphoid tissue. Consequently, when ventilating a newborn by use of a face mask, the nurse should be careful not to apply too much pressure over the soft tissue of the neck, because pressure of this kind can easily obstruct the airway.

The vocal cords of the newborn are situated at about the level of C4, as opposed to the location at C6 in the adult. Normally, in the adult, the opening of the vocal cords is the narrowest portion of the trachea and, in the newborn, the narrowest portion of the trachea is the cricoid cartilage (see Chapter 6). The clinical implications of this anatomic feature are that if edema about the cricoid cartilage occurs because of infection or mechanical irritation from an endotracheal tube, significant narrowing of the airway may occur. Also, because the cricoid ring is the narrowest part of the larynx, this limits the size of the endotracheal tube to

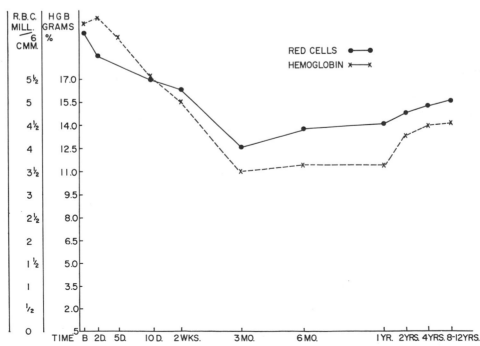

FIGURE 39–1. Normal variation in hemoglobin (HGB) and red blood cell (RBC) count during infancy and childhood. (From Nelson, W. E. [ed.]: Textbook of Pediatrics. 7th ed. Philadelphia, W. B. Saunders, 1959.)

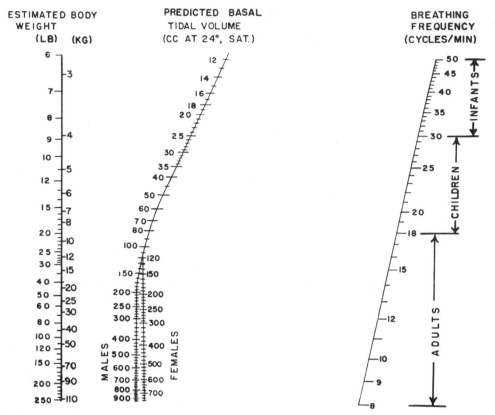

ESTIMATED BODY
WEIGHT
(LB)   (KG)

PREDICTED BASAL
TIDAL VOLUME
(CC AT 24°, SAT.)

BREATHING
FREQUENCY
(CYCLES/MIN)

FIGURE 39–2. Nomogram for predicted basal tidal volume. Corrections to be applied: add 10 percent if subject is awake; add 9 percent for each degree centigrade of fever; add 8 percent for each 1000 m of altitude above sea level; calculate the required tidal volume. If a tracheostomy is in use, subtract the patient's estimated physiologic dead space (i.e., subtract 1 ml/kg body weight). Add the dead space of the anesthetic apparatus. (Reprinted with permission from *The New England Journal of Medicine*, 251:877, 1954.)

be used. The endotracheal tube selected should allow a slight leakage around itself when positive pressure is applied by use of an anesthesia bag. Finally, the epiglottis of the newborn is U-shaped and usually long and narrow, as compared with the flatter epiglottis of the adult.

Newborns are diaphragmatic breathers. This is because the ribs are situated horizontally in a cylindrical thorax, which limits thorax expansion. Consequently, the ventilatory effort is the result almost entirely of the movement of the diaphragm. Because newborns are diaphragmatic breathers, they are susceptible to ventilatory problems, such as hypoventilation when the excursions of the diaphragm are impeded. Hence, gastric distention due to faulty bag and mask ventilation, improper positioning, or bowel obstruction can produce inadequate ventilation. In addition, the sternum and anterior rib cage are compliant, and the intercostal and accessory muscles of respiration are poorly developed. In the premature infant, the sternum may be retracted deeply with each inspiration, causing impaired ventilation.

As in the adult, the newborn's primary drive to ventilation is carbon dioxide (see Chapter 6). However, the secondary drive in the newborn is different from that of the adult. The newborn younger than 1 week of age responds to a reduction in the partial pressure of oxygen by hyperventilation followed by hypoventilation. This secondary drive response is aggravated by hypothermia, a condition that can occur in the PACU.

The respiratory rate is higher and the tidal volume lower in infants and children. When ventilation equipment, such as a mask, is used, dead space is increased. The Radford nomogram can be used to predict basal tidal volume (Fig. 39–2).

The respiratory control center in the infant and child is easily fatigued; therefore, ventilatory reaction to high carbon dioxide tensions or to low percentage of oxygen is not rapid. As a result, the infant may not be able to compensate for rapid changes in arterial blood gas levels. Along with this, infants and small children may breathe irregularly and be unable to respond to oxygen, owing to their lack of a mature respiratory center; periodic breathing is often seen in this age group.

Endotracheal intubation is becoming more widely accepted in pediatric anesthesia. (See Table 39–3 for a guide to proper-sized endotracheal tubes.) The advantages of this technique are decreased dead space, avoidance of laryngospasm and gastric distention, and prevention of aspiration. However, the incidence of post-intubation edema from trauma and infections may be increased.

The Kidney and Fluid Balance

The kidney of the newborn matures rapidly. By the end of the first month, the kidneys reach about 90 percent maturity. However, at about 5 days of age, renal function is characterized by an obligate salt loss, slow clearance of fluid overload, and an inability to conserve fluid. Consequently, newborns who are 5 days or younger in age are intolerant of both dehydration and fluid overload. The blood volume of the newborn varies from 60 to 130 ml per kg, depending on the position of the newborn in relation to the placenta and perineum during delivery and whether the cord was "milked" toward or away from the newborn before its clamping. The blood volume of the infant is about 80 to 85 ml per kg, as compared with 65

ml per kg in the adult female and 70 ml per kg in the adult male.

Water distribution in the various body compartments is markedly different among the premature newborn, the normal newborn, the child, and the adult. Premature and normal newborns have the most water in their extracellular fluid compartment. This condition continues until about the second year, when adult proportions of 20 percent extracellular and 40 percent intracellular water are reached. Table 39–4 summarizes the daily maintenance fluids and normal urine output for the pediatric patient.

Important considerations for fluid management of the pediatric patient include monitoring for hypervolemia or hypovolemia and ensuring proper administration of fluids. Consequently, the monitoring of the pediatric patient should include the following parameters: (1) urine output, specific gravity, and osmolality; (2) temperature; (3) electrocardiographic (ECG) status, pulse, and blood pressure; (4) hydration of the mucosa; and (5) blood loss. It is essential to make an accurate assessment of blood loss intraoperatively and postoperatively, because a miscalculation of just a few milliliters can have a serious impact on the total blood volume of the infant. If the pediatric patient loses 10 percent of blood volume, the possibility of blood replacement is usually considered by the physician. In losses as high as 15 to 20 percent of blood volume, replacement is usually instituted. The usual blood replacement is such that for each 1 ml lost, 1 ml of whole blood is administered to the patient.

During the administration of fluids, the PACU nurse should ensure that the indwelling catheter is patent and not infiltrated and should use a constant infusion pump to facilitate the proper administration of the correct volume and rate of fluids. To prevent inadvertent overhydration, not more than one third of the day's maintenance intravenous fluid volume should be measured into the intravenous bag at any time.

Infants and newborns expend a great amount of energy maintaining alveolar ventilation, cardiac output, muscular activity, and an appropriate temperature. Because of these high-energy metabolic processes, glycogen and fat stores may be mobilized and depleted rapidly. Consequently, in the PACU, cold, stress, pain, and increased muscle activity compound the need for adequate caloric intake. Therefore, one of the cornerstones of fluid replacement in the PACU is the provision of enough glucose intake to maintain the glycogen and fat stores.

Table 39–3. ENDOTRACHEAL TUBE SIZE IN CHILDREN*

Age or Weight	Endotracheal Tube Size			Suction Catheter (French)
	Internal Diameter (mm)	External Diameter (French)	Length (cm)	
Under 1500 gm	2.5 uncuffed	12	8	6
Newborn– 6 mo	3.0 uncuffed	14	10	6
6–18 mo	3.5 uncuffed	16	12	8
18 mo–3 yr	4.0 uncuffed	18	14	8
3–5 yr	4.5 uncuffed	20	16	8
5–6 yr	5.0 uncuffed	22	16	10
6–8 yr	5.5 cuffed	24	18	10
8–10 yr	6.0 cuffed	26	18	10
10–12 yr	6.5 cuffed	28	20	12
12–14 yr	6.5 cuffed	28	20	12
14–16 yr	♂7.0 cuffed	30	22	12
	♀6.5 cuffed	28		
16–21 yr	♂7.5 cuffed	32	22	12
	♀7.0 cuffed	30		

*Endotracheal tube should fit so as to allow full expansion of both lungs on manual inflation but allow a definite leak with pressure of 20–25 cm H$_2$O.
From Smith, R. M.: Anesthesia for Infants and Children. 4th ed. St. Louis, C. V. Mosby, 1980.

Table 39–4. MAINTENANCE FLUIDS AND NORMAL URINE OUTPUT IN PEDIATRIC PATIENTS

Age	Body Weight (kg)	24-Hour Fluid Requirement	Normal Urine Output (ml/kg/hr)
Premature and full-term newborn younger than 5 days	3–3.5	50–70 ml/kg	0.3–0.7
Premature and full-term newborn older than 5 days up to 1 month	3.5–4	150 ml/kg	1–2.7 (5–7 days)
Older than 1 month up to 1 year	4–10	100 ml/kg	3 (over 7 days)
1 to 5 years	10–20	1000 ml, plus 50 ml/kg over 10 kg	2 (over 2 years)
5 years to adult	20–>70	1500 ml, plus 20 ml/kg over 20 kg	1

Adapted from Dripps, R., Eckenhoff, J., and Vandam, L.: Introduction to Anesthesia: The Principles of Safe Practice. 6th ed. Philadelphia, W. B. Saunders, 1982.

One-fourth to one-third strength saline solution in 5 percent dextrose is the most common maintenance fluid used in the PACU care of the pediatric patient.

PEDIATRIC ANESTHESIA TECHNIQUES

Administration of anesthetic drugs to the pediatric patient has progressed from the technique of open-drop ether to the non-rebreathing technique. The Bain circuit is sometimes used in pediatric anesthesia, because it offers the advantages of conserving body heat, of not using valves, and of keeping the patient normocarbic (see Chapter 13).

Many anesthesia practitioners do not use premedication drugs in pediatric patients. Some practitioners still use atropine to protect against the bradycardia that is produced by succinylcholine or halothane intraoperatively. Also, midazolam administered intranasally has become quite popular as a pediatric premedicant.

The most popular inhalation anesthetic agents used for pediatric anesthesia are halothane, isoflurane, and enflurane. All offer rapid induction and rapid emergence. Halothane remains the most popular pediatric inhalation agent; freedom from airway irritation and smooth emergence are especially important characteristics of halothane that make it the anesthetic of choice. The Liverpool technique, which consists of nitrous oxide, oxygen, and curare, can be used for patients younger than 3 years of age. It also offers the advantage of rapid emergence.

Ketamine, a dissociative anesthetic, is sometimes used in pediatrics as an induction agent or for short procedures that do not require muscle relaxation. Emergence time depends on route of administration and whether the drug was repeated during the operation.

PACU CARE OF THE PEDIATRIC PATIENT

When the pediatric patient arrives in the PACU, vital signs, including core temperature, should be obtained and a warmed and humidified air-oxygen mixture (high flow) administered before the report from the anesthetist is given. The patient should be placed in lateral position; however, following an intraoral surgical procedure, the patient should be placed in prone position to facilitate adequate drainage of secretions or blood. During the report, dressings should be checked for drainage and the intravenous infusion line should be checked for patency and for assurance that the line is adequately secured. Also, children's teeth should be checked routinely on admission to the PACU, especially if loose teeth are present, and again before discharge. Because of the improved anesthesia techniques and rapid-acting anesthetic agents, the pediatric patient will usually arrive in the PACU awake and responsive and with good muscle tone. These patients usually respond quickly to the stir-up regimen. However, about 10 to 15 percent of pediatric patients recovering from general anesthesia exhibit hyperactive behavior. They require constant nursing care to prevent injury to themselves, because they are extremely restless and often scream loudly. This agitation or excitement may be related to drug responses, hypoxemia, pain, or awakening in strange surroundings. Therefore, if a pediatric patient is demonstrating hyperactive behavior, the PACU nurse should assess the patient in the aforementioned areas before providing interventions.

Cardiovascular and Fluid Monitoring

If the pediatric patient is moderately to severely ill, monitors for central venous pressure, ECG status, urine output, specific gravity, and an arterial line may be used.

The central venous pressure line is usually inserted via the superior vena cava or the external jugular vein. It provides information on blood volume and serves as an avenue for fluid replacement. The arterial line, which is inserted through the umbilical or radial artery, can measure blood pressure and heart rate and provide for instantaneous blood gas sampling. The ECG provides information on cardiac rate and rhythm. Blood pressure and pulse should be ascertained and recorded every 5 to 10 minutes, depending on the physical status of the patient. Any deviation in the cardiac or pulmonary physiologic parameters should be reported immediately to the attending physician.

Dressings should be watched for excessive bleeding. Such bleeding should be reported at once to the attending physician, because the infant and small child do not have enough blood volume to compensate for losses.

The urine output and specific gravity yield information on kidney function and volume expansion.

Respiratory Monitoring

The rate and depth of ventilation should be monitored in the PACU. Respiratory depression occurs with greater frequency if muscle relaxants are used during anesthesia. Because of the rapid ventilatory changes that can occur in the PACU, the oxygen saturation monitor should be used on all pediatric patients.

Infants and small children usually have a low incidence of postoperative atelectasis, because crying from pain or unhappiness automatically keeps the airway clear. Older children tend to remain in one position and not to move about. They must be encouraged to cough and to perform the sustained maximal inspiration (SMI) maneuver to prevent atelectasis. If the pediatric patient is unable to perform the SMI maneuver, deep breathing should be encouraged.

Temperature Regulation

Newborns, infants, and children are sensitive to heat loss because they have a relatively large surface area, a relatively small amount of subcutaneous fat, and poor vasomotor control, and because they seldom shiver. Ordinarily, to maintain a body temperature within normal limits, they metabolize brown fat, cry, and move about vigorously. Thus, newborns, infants, and children respond to a cold environment by increasing their metabolism, which ultimately leads to an increase in oxygen consumption and to the production of organic acids. If a child in this age group arrives in the PACU with inadvertent hypothermia, the nurse should assess the patient for (1) vital signs (core temperature, pulse, and respiratory rate) and (2) the degree of emergence from anesthesia. The patient should be monitored on a continuous ECG, because dysrhythmias and cardiovascular depression are associated with hypothermia. If the patient is experiencing a delayed emergence from anesthesia, the nurse should protect the patient from aspiration of gastric contents and from hypoventilation by positioning (Fig. 39–3) and stimulation. Finally, to avoid excess oxygen demand and acidosis that are associated with hypothermia, newborns and infants should be maintained in a neutral thermal environment in the PACU by the use of incubators, infrared heating, blankets, or elevated room temperature.

A word of warning is needed here. If a water mattress is to be used to rewarm the patient, the temperature setting should be no higher than 37°C, and four layers of sheets should be used between the mattress and the skin to prevent burns. Whatever rewarming method is used, the temperature of the device should be monitored constantly to prevent overwarming. Records should be kept of core body temperature (rectal, esophageal, or tympanic), room temperature, and device temperature.

Psychosocial Considerations

When the pediatric patient emerges from general inhalation anesthesia, certain emotional needs should be met by the PACU nurse to facilitate positive outcomes of perioperative experience. Infants can become distressed when physical needs are not met. Taking into consideration the type of surgery and the degree of emergence from anesthesia, the primary care giver should hold or rock the patient if age appropriate, or do both. This will usually relax the patient, and infants especially enjoy cuddling, rocking, fondling, and hearing the voice of the nurse. Because the infant mimics facial expressions, the nurse should smile and use facial expressions of happiness when caring for

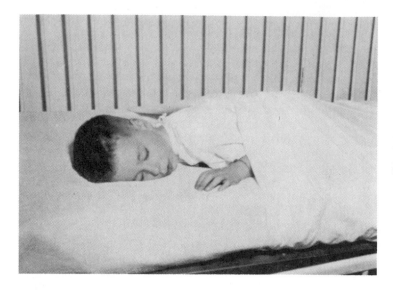

FIGURE 39–3. After surgery, the child lies face down with the shoulder supported and one arm and leg flexed. (From Smith, R. M.: Anesthesia for Infants and Children. 3rd ed. St. Louis, C. V. Mosby, 1968, p. 188.)

the child. Another consideration is that the PACU is a strange environment for the child. Often, dolls, teddy bears, and other familiar objects from home are taken to surgery and will arrive with the patient in the PACU. These special toys should remain with the child, especially during emergence, to help cope with the environmental change.

Children at ages 1 to 3 years are at the stage of autonomy versus self-doubt. They may exhibit independence that alternates with sudden dependence and the need for periodic cuddling and reassurance. Negativism may be the child's means of demonstrating control; thus, "no" may actually mean "yes." Children of this age are prone to temper tantrums, ritualistic behavior, and breath-holding spells. The PACU nurse should be sure to differentiate apnea from breath-holding spells when assessing the respiratory status of the patient. Three-year-old children are certainly special children, lovable but stormy. They are too young to use their own reason and become impatient at times. It is therefore important for the PACU nurse to avoid criticism and provide acceptable behavior alternatives to the patient.

Between the ages of 3 and 6 years, the child begins to become independent. However, in the PACU, dependency can occur because of pain, course of disease, or immobilization. Guilt can occur when the child desires to remain dependent. Consequently, the PACU nurse should provide as much opportunity for independence as possible. This can be done by allowing the child to select alternatives in care.

The ages of 6 to 12 years coincide with school entrance. These children are striving for approval when tasks are completed and usually do not tolerate failure, because it promotes their sense of inferiority and inadequacy. Because children lose control when they are immobilized or ill, the nurse should allow as much individualization and self-care as possible. The nurse should also encourage self-expression and compliment the child on accomplishments during recovery from anesthesia.

The adolescent years of ages 12 to 18 are a transitory time characterized by vacillations between dependence and independence, idealism and realism, confidence and uncertainty. Privacy is of utmost importance to these patients; therefore, the adolescent's body should be covered as much as possible to prevent exposure and resulting embarrassment.

COMPLICATIONS

Because the pediatric patient does not have the physiologic reserves of the adult patient, when complications occur, serious untoward sequelae can and will take place. Hence, the PACU nurse must monitor for and react to any complication in a timely fashion.

Retrolental Fibroplasia

Retrolental fibroplasia is a neovascularization and scarring of the retina due to elevated inspired oxygen tensions. The risk of this retinal disorder is to newborns, especially premature infants who are born before 36 weeks' gestation. The risk of developing retrolental fibroplasia is negligible beyond 44 weeks after conception. Therefore, the preterm neonate who has a gestation of 36 weeks remains at risk until about 8 weeks of age. Current recommendations are that the PaO_2 for the premature infant be between 40 and 60 mm Hg and between 60 and 80 for the normal newborn. The fraction of inspired oxygen (FIO_2) should be kept below 0.4. The exact length of time the patient must be exposed to the hyperoxic environment for retrolental fibroplasia to develop is unknown. In susceptible patients who are exposed to a hyperoxic environment, blood gas tension should be measured and an oxygen analyzer used to confirm the oxygen concentration. The key thought when dealing with this situation is that attempts to prevent arterial hyperoxia must be tempered with the realization that unrecognized arterial hypoxemia can result in irreversible brain damage.

Idiopathic Respiratory Distress Syndrome

Infant respiratory distress syndrome (IRDS), also called *hyaline membrane disease*, is a severe disorder of the lungs of the newborn. The incidence of IRDS increases with maternal diabetes, toxemia, hemorrhage, and prenatal asphyxia. The basis of the pathogenesis of IRDS is insufficient surfactant levels. Surfactant can be described as having the following two functions: (1) reducing surface tension so that less pressure is required to hold the alveoli open, and (2) maintaining alveolar stability by adjusting surface tension to changes in alveolar size. Insufficient surfactant levels increase surface tension at the alveolar air-liquid interface, resulting in alveolar collapse, an inordinate increase in the work of breathing, and impaired gas exchange. This impaired gas exchange results in hypoxemia and hypercarbia. Along with this, the pulmonary vascular resistance is increased, resulting in hypoperfusion of the pulmonary and systemic circulations. This hypoperfusion, along with hypoxemia, causes tissue hypoxia and metabolic acidosis.

More specifically, low surfactant levels produce a high surface tension in the alveoli, which, besides causing alveolar collapse, reverses the gradient for transcapillary fluid movement. Hence, the products derived from the blood, as well as cellular debris, are pulled into the alveoli. This cellular "junk" ends up lining the alveoli and making up what is referred to as the *hyaline membrane*. Profound atelectasis results and the lungs become very stiff, which leads to a severely reduced functional

residual capacity, hypoxemia, and, finally, ventilatory failure.

The cardinal signs of IRDS, which appear soon after birth, are tachypnea, grunting respiration, and chest retraction. Treatment for neonates with IRDS includes oxygen therapy, fluid restriction, temperature regulation, chemical monitoring (glucose, bilirubin, and arterial blood gases), and continuous positive airway pressure (CPAP). If, during CPAP, the infant becomes apneic and develops hypercarbia with a respiratory acidosis (pH <7.2), or if the arterial oxygen tension falls below 50 mm Hg, mechanical ventilation is begun. The mechanical ventilation probably uses high positive end-expiratory pressure to ventilate the exceptionally stiff lungs of these neonates.

Airway Obstruction

In the PACU, each pediatric patient who has been intubated during anesthesia should be monitored for signs of airway obstruction. When laryngeal swelling occurs, the diameter of the airway of the infant or small child can become significantly reduced; in fact, 1 mm of edema in the infant's trachea at the cricoid level decreases the diameter of the airway by 75 percent! The symptoms of laryngeal obstruction, in order of appearance, are croupy cough, hoarseness, inspiratory stridor, and aphonia. These symptoms are accompanied by increasing restlessness, tachypnea, use of accessory muscles of respiration, retraction of the suprasternal notch and intercostal spaces, and drawing in of the upper abdomen. If these symptoms appear, the PACU nurse should act immediately to relieve the obstruction *and* should send someone to notify the anesthesiologist, because the progression of these symptoms can be rapid.

Treatment of postintubation croup involves use of a high-humidity atmosphere that is oxygen-enriched, optimum body hydration, and administration of antibiotics when indicated. Steroids such as dexamethasone (Decadron) are usually prescribed to decrease the laryngeal inflammation. If laryngeal edema is allowed to progress, the patient may require reintubation or a tracheostomy. If tracheostomy is performed, the PACU nurse should observe the patient for pneumothorax, mediastinal emphysema, and bleeding. Auscultation of the chest should be done every 15 minutes for breath sounds to ascertain if the tracheostomy tube is above the bifurcation of the trachea (at the carina). The PACU nurse should also determine during auscultation whether excess secretions are present. If suctioning is required, sterile suction technique should be used. Aspiration of secretions should be done by slow suction to prevent injury to the tissue. Before the tracheostomy suctioning is instituted, the procedure should be explained fully to the child in language that can be readily understood.

A 75 percent atmospheric humidity should be provided to the pediatric patient with a tracheostomy. This helps decrease the viscosity of the sputum. Maintenance of good hydration is also important if an infection is present.

Malignant Hyperthermia

Although malignant hyperthermia (MH) is discussed in detail in Chapter 43, a brief description of the condition is given here, because the incidence of MH is approximately 1 in 14,000 in children, as compared with 1 in 52,000 in adults. This genetically determined condition is triggered by inhalation anesthetic agents, such as halothane and succinylcholine, and by stress. The pathophysiology of the condition centers on the enhanced release and diminished reuptake of calcium in the skeletal muscle. This causes sustained skeletal muscle contraction and, ultimately, profound hyperthermia. The drug dantrolene effectively treats MH by inhibiting further release of calcium in the skeletal muscles. In most instances, the MH occurs in the operating room; however, a patient may first experience the disorder in the PACU, or the successfully treated MH patient may have an exacerbation of MH in that setting.

In most cases of MH, the first clinical clue is tachycardia or other dysrhythmias; tachypnea and a profound increase in tidal volume are then observed in the spontaneously breathing PACU patient. The temperature will begin to rise, sweating will occur, and the patient's skin will become mottled.

Blood chemistry studies reveal an elevated potassium level and an initially elevated calcium level that then decrease to below normal. Arterial blood gas levels demonstrate severe metabolic acidosis with an elevated $PaCO_2$ and a decreased pH. The PaO_2 may be normal, depending on the FiO_2.

To facilitate a reversal of this condition, the PACU nurse must understand the pathophysiology of MH and should know exactly where the MH emergency cart (as described in Chapter 43) is located. If a patient appears to be developing MH, SEND FOR HELP! Start ven-

tilating the patient, using high-flow 100 percent oxygen, and check to be sure the intravenous line is patent. Once the appropriate personnel arrive, have one person mix the dantrolene (20 mg per 60 ml of sterile water).

A note of warning is needed. Be sure that the sterile water does not contain any preservatives, because much sterile water will be used. The usual dose of dantrolene is 1 to 2 mg per kg over 1 to 2 minutes. This can be repeated up to 10 mg per kg or until the patient's temperature is reduced.

SPECIAL CONSIDERATIONS

Gastrointestinal Surgery

Pediatric patients recovering from gastrointestinal surgery should be observed for prolonged paralytic ileus; if it goes longer than 72 hours, the physician should be notified, because complications such as intestinal obstruction, local abscess, or pneumoperitoneum may be present. During the PACU report on the patient, nursing personnel on the surgical unit should be properly warned about the possibility of prolonged paralytic ileus occurring.

Otolaryngologic Surgery

Pediatric patients who have tonsillectomies and other operations on the pharynx, larynx, and esophagus require intensive PACU care, because the airway can become obstructed postoperatively as a result of surgical manipulation and bleeding. When the patient is admitted to the PACU, the laryngeal and pharyngeal reflexes should be present. The patient should be placed in the tonsillectomy position (see Fig. 39–3), prone with the arm and leg flexed and the head turned to the side. This position improves drainage of secretions and blood from the mouth, preventing possible aspiration. The patient should be kept in this position until the gag reflex has returned completely.

References

1. Barash, P., Cullen, B., and Stoelting, R.: Handbook of Clinical Anesthesia. 2nd ed. Philadelphia, J. B. Lippincott, 1993.
2. Berman, S.: Pediatric Decision Making. Philadelphia, B. C. Decker, 1985.
3. Cote, C.: A single-blind study of combined pulse oximetry and capnography in children. Anesthesiology, 74(6):980–988, 1991.
4. Frost, E., and Andrews, I.: Recovery Room Care. Int. Anesthesiol. Clin., 21(1):1, 1983.

5. Gregory, G.: Pediatric Anesthesia. New York, Churchill Livingstone, 1989.
6. Hannallah, R.: Propofol: Effective dose and induction characteristics in unpremedicated children. Anesthesiology, *74*(6):989–993, 1990.
7. Jolin, R.: Neonatal physiology and anesthesia. AANA J., *51*(6):594–603, 1983.
8. Levin, R.: Pediatric Anesthesia Handbook. 3rd ed. New York, Medical Examination Publishing, 1984.
9. Longnecker, D., and Murphy, F.: Dripps/Eckenhoff/Vandam Introduction to Anesthesia. 8th ed. Philadelphia, W. B. Saunders, 1992.
10. Miller, R.: Anesthesia. 3rd ed. New York, Churchill Livingstone, 1990.
11. Motoyama, E., and Davis, P.: Smith's Anesthesia for Infants and Children. 5th ed. St. Louis: C. V. Mosby, 1990.
12. Mubroy, J. Safety and efficacy of alfentanil and halothane in paediatric surgical patients. Can. J. Anaesth., *38*(4):445–449, 1991.
13. Pittet, J.: Neuromuscular effect of pepiuronium bromide in infants and children during nitrous oxide–alfentanil anesthesia. Anesthesiology, *73*(2):432–436, 1991.
14. Stoelting, R., Dierdorf, S., and McCammon, R.: Anesthesia and Co-Existing Disease. 2nd ed. New York, Churchill Livingstone, 1989.
15. Walbergh, E.: Plasma concentrations of midazolam in children following intranasal administration. Anesthesiology, *74*(2):233–236, 1991.
16. Westrin, P.: The induction dose of propofol in infants 1–6 months and children 10–16 years of age. Anesthesiology, *74*(3):455–459, 1991.

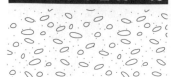

CHAPTER 40

Post Anesthesia Care of the Geriatric Patient

It is difficult to define chronologically when old age begins, because some persons age much more quickly than their chronologic age indicates. Legally, however, old age is defined as 65 years or older. The geriatric population (older than 65 years) constitutes approximately 11 percent of the population, and projections are that they will constitute 13 percent by 2000 and 17 percent by 2030. Because of the refinements in surgical and post anesthesia care, a greater percentage of geriatric patients will undergo anesthesia and surgery in the future. This category of patients presents a challenge to the post anesthesia care unit (PACU) nurse. This is because 80 percent of the patients older than 65 years of age have one or more chronic diseases when they present for anesthesia and surgery.

Care of the geriatric patient is of particular importance in the PACU because of the physiologic changes that usually occur during the later years. These include congestive heart failure, insufficient oxygenation of the blood, improper elimination of carbon dioxide, fluid and electrolyte imbalance, drug toxicity, nerve palsies, and psychological changes. To ensure that the geriatric patient will have a positive surgical outcome, the PACU nurse must have the knowledge of the physiologic alterations caused by aging and the effects of anesthesia on the aged patient.

AGE-RELATED PROBLEMS

Cardiovascular System

When first admitted to the PACU, the geriatric patient often presents many physiologic and psychological problems. With advancing age, the cardiovascular system often undergoes some changes. The aged heart has less reserve and less ability to adjust to stress. Coronary sclerosis is common, and there is usually some atrophy of the myocardial fibers. There is a delay in the recovery from excitability in the

aged heart muscle, and it is more susceptible to dysrhythmias. Cardiac output in the aged is lower than it is in the young, and there is less ability to increase it during periods of stress.

The systolic blood pressure is usually higher in the geriatric patient owing to degenerative arterial disease, which decreases elasticity of the large arteries. This disease makes it difficult for the cardiovascular system to react to stress. Hypotension should be avoided because of the danger of thrombosis and the reduced amount of oxygen that can be transported to the vital organs. Hypertension, on the other hand, must be equally avoided. The most immediate problem of hypertension in the aged is damage from a cerebral vascular hemorrhage. Other areas of concern are hypovolemia, increased susceptibility to hemorrhage, and anemia.

When geriatric patients arrive in the PACU, they may experience some degree of cardiovascular depression because of the anesthetic agents administered intraoperatively. With an age-related decrease in cardiac index, these patients require less inhalation anesthesia and, consequently, usually wake up faster in the PACU. However, because of this, these patients are particularly susceptible to experience hypotension and bradycardia during emergence from anesthesia. Because glycopyrrolate does not cross the blood-brain barrier, the bradycardia should be treated with that drug. With this approach, the confusion that can be produced by atropine is avoided. Also, because the circulation times are decreased in the aged, intravenous agents usually take a longer time to produce their effects. Consequently, drugs such as succinylcholine have a longer onset and duration of action.

Respiratory System

The aging process frequently affects the respiratory system. The thoracic bone structure usually becomes calcified, a condition that decreases the elastic recoil properties of the chest wall, which causes a premature balance in the elastic forces of the lungs and the chest wall. Thus the functional residual capacity, vital capacity, and total lung capacity are decreased (see Chapter 6). As a person ages, the ratio of residual volume to total lung capacity progressively rises, making ventilation less and less adequate. Senile emphysema causes the intrapulmonary mixing of gases to become less effective, leading to hypoxemia and hypercarbia. The upper respiratory tract is also affected by advancing age, leading to increased secretions and airway resistance.

In the PACU, the geriatric patient's ventilation should be constantly assessed. The modified stir-up regimen of reposition, cascade cough, and sustained maximal inspiration (SMI) is mandatory for the geriatric patient (see Chapter 20) to reduce the incidence of postoperative pulmonary complications. Along with this, secretions should be removed by assisting the patient to cough and, if required, by suctioning. Positioning to facilitate good ventilatory excursion may be difficult in the geriatric patient owing to bone deformity or arthritis, or both. Usually, head-up positions promote proper ventilation.

Neuromuscular System

The weight of the brain decreases with advancing age. Along with this, the loss of neurons caused by the aging process is particularly marked in the cerebral cortex. These atrophic changes interfere with the basic neuronal process and are responsible for the increased susceptibility of the elderly to central nervous system side effects of drugs that are seen clinically in the PACU.

In relation to anesthesia, aging is associated with a progressive decrease in the minimum alveolar concentration for general inhalation anesthetic agents (see Chapter 13). Hence, in the PACU, patients of advanced age may experience a prolonged emergence following the administration of an inhalation anesthetic. There seems to be a loss of neurotransmitters and synaptic function, along with a decrease in the number of axons supplying peripheral muscles and muscles innervated by each axon. Consequently, over time, denervation and atrophy of the skeletal muscles become apparent, which lead to a reduction in conduction velocity in peripheral nerves. This is the reason that the dose requirement for regional anesthetics progressively declines with advancing age.

Renal System

As in other organ systems, there is a progressive decrease in renal function and mass with advancing age, which includes a decrease in the glomerular filtration rate and renal blood flow. Thus, with a reduced cardiac and renal function, the geriatric patient is especially susceptible to fluid overload. Along with this, the mechanisms involved in maintaining the constancy and volume in the extracellular fluid are progressively blunted with advancing age. This reduction in functional adaptive renal mechanisms is responsible, in part, for the problems in fluid and electrolyte balance seen in geriatric patients. An electrolyte of particular importance in the context of advancing age is *sodium.* The geriatric patient has a progressively blunted response to sodium deficiency; that is, patients in this age group lose the ability to conserve sodium in response to acute reduction in sodium intake. The geriatric patient, because of this salt-losing tendency, may experience symptoms such as confusion, loss of thirst, and disorientation in the PACU. This is particularly true when a transurethral resection of the prostate is performed or, for that matter, any surgical procedure in which urinary irrigation is used. The geriatric patient who has experienced this type of surgical procedure should be monitored in the PACU for a deficiency in this electrolyte.

The first symptom of sodium deficiency is probably disorientation. Because some patients in the geriatric population may be somewhat disoriented, it is important that the PACU nurse differentiate among the possible types of disorientation. Blood for electrolyte determination should be drawn and analyzed immediately, before any sedation is administered to the patient. If the level of sodium is below normal, intravenous sodium will resolve the clinical picture of disorientation rather rapidly.

Another electrolyte of concern when caring for the geriatric patient is *potassium.* Advancing age is associated with a progressive decrease in plasma renin concentration. Along with this, there is an equal reduction in the concentration of aldosterone, which acts on the distal tubule to increase sodium reabsorption and to enhance the excretion of potassium, thereby protecting against hyperkalemia. With advancing age, the protective mechanism that prevents hyperkalemia during periods of potassium challenge is lost. Given that the glomerular filtration rate is reduced in the geriatric patient, hyperkalemia may result when potassium is administered. Therefore, along with monitoring the electrocardiogram for the peaking of T waves, electrolytes should be monitored particularly when a geriatric patient has received potassium salts intravenously in the perioperative period.

Because of the reduction in physiologic function of the renal system associated with advancing age, kidney function should be monitored in the PACU, including fluid and electrolyte balance. Fluid intake and output measurements should be monitored meticulously to ensure an adequate urinary output of 0.5 to 1 ml per kg per hr, because these patients are subject to oliguria and, in some instances, anuria. Also, drugs dependent on renal excretion for their elimination (such as gallamine) are affected by the decrease in kidney function, leading to a prolonged plasma concentration and, ultimately, to a prolongation of the effect of the drug.

Hepatobiliary System

Advancing age is associated with a progressive reduction in hepatobiliary function. Hepatic blood flow is progressively reduced, and an age-related decrease in the functioning of the hepatic microsomal enzymes has been demonstrated. This ultimately leads to an age-related reduction in the biotransformation actions of the liver, and drugs that are dependent to a major extent on hepatic metabolism usually have a prolonged effect in the elderly population. Because there is considerable danger of hepatic injury from drugs, hypoxia, and blood transfusions in the routine PACU care of the geriatric patient, careful attention should be given to appropriate airway care to enhance oxygenation and to ensure that the appropriate dosage of depressant drugs is given.

Drug Interactions

The physiologic response to a drug occurs in a twofold manner. The first process deals with the drug concentration at the site of action and is termed *pharmacokinetics.* The second process deals with the ability of the drug to react with a specific receptor and to translate that effect on the receptor into a physiologic response, which is called *pharmacodynamics.* Advancing age is associated with progressive alterations in both the pharmacokinetics and the pharmacodynamics of drug therapy. Furthermore, the geriatric patient may experience pharmacologic problems because of the multiple types of

drugs being taken and the adverse drug interactions that may occur. Table 40–1 may be used to determine the possible adverse effects or drug interactions that may take place in the geriatric patient during the perioperative period.

Psychological Aspects

The psychological aspects of PACU care of the geriatric patient center on maintaining the patient's self-esteem. Feelings of uselessness and lack of self-worth promote tension and anxiety, which, in turn, can affect the patient's physiologic status. Geriatric patients are usually set in their ways, and it is important for them to be able to contribute to their own care. Because their hearing and vision may be impaired, these patients tend to isolate themselves and may not be able to understand oral communication well. Therefore, when conversing with a geriatric patient with possible or documented hearing loss, it is important to speak slowly and distinctly and in a loud voice.

Alzheimer's Disease

Senile dementia of the Alzheimer type (SDAT), or Alzheimer's disease, is presently receiving a great deal of attention by medical researchers. This disease consists of a multiplicity of neuronal pathway degenerative processes resulting in impairment of cognition and behavioral changes such as depression, aggression, paranoia, anxiety, agitation, and insomnia. No treatment or identification of risk factors exists for this disease.

General anesthesia is usually administered to the patient with SDAT. This is because SDAT patients lack the cognitive function and cooperative skills necessary for the successful performance of regional anesthesia. These patients are sensitive to the effects of all medications, including the anesthetic agents, and therefore require reduced dosages. Because of this, delayed emergence from anesthesia is not uncommon. SDAT patients usually require a longer time in the PACU. The PACU nurse should take every step to keep the patient normothermic because hypothermia prolongs emergence. Along with this, maintaining adequate hydration optimizes the emergence process and helps reduce the incidence of confusion. Finally, drugs in the anticholinergic category should be avoided in the SDAT patient. This is because drugs such as scopolamine and atro-

Table 40–1. ADVERSE EFFECTS OR DRUG INTERACTIONS ASSOCIATED WITH THE GERIATRIC PATIENT[10,12]

Drug	Adverse Effect or Drug Interaction
Antibiotics	Prolongation of muscle relaxants
Antidysrhythmics	Prolongation of muscle relaxants
Benzodiazepines	
Diazepam	Decreased metabolism
Chlordiazepoxide	Increased CNS effects
Flurazepam	Prolonged drowsiness
Digoxin	Decreased renal excretion with increased CNS disorientation, anorexia, nausea, and cardiotoxicity; blood levels two to three times higher in the elderly with any given dose
Diuretics	Hypokalemia
	Hypovolemia
Halothane	Decreased anesthetic requirement
Lithium	Clearance decreased by 65% and effective dose by 30% compared with age 25
	Increased side effects of tremor, diarrhea, and edema
Meperidine	Markedly elevated plasma levels and decreased red blood cell and plasma binding of drug
	Increased incidence of nausea, respiratory distress, and hypotension
Methyldopa	Enhanced hypotensive effects
Pancuronium	Decreased clearance from plasma
Propranolol	Plasma level approximately three to four times higher in the elderly, owing to decreased metabolism
	Bradycardia, congestive heart failure, bronchospasm, mental confusion, and attenuation of autonomic nervous system activity
Tricyclic antidepressants	Increased anticholinergic effects—confusion, agitation, and disorientation
	Cardiac conduction disturbances
	Increased anesthetic requirements
Warfarin	Enhanced sensitivity

CNS = central nervous system.

pine exacerbate the behavioral symptoms of SDAT.

POST ANESTHESIA CARE

The geriatric patient can be challenging to care for in the PACU. Postoperative pulmonary complications must be monitored for and require positive nursing interventions. Oxygen should be administered by high-flow mask. For the geriatric patient with chronic obstructive pulmonary disease, a Venturi-type mask at a specific low percentage should be administered (see Chapter 20). Oxygen saturation should be monitored closely to detect hypoxemia. If the geriatric patient becomes delirious, hypoxemia should be suspected. If the oxygen saturation is normal and the patient received an anticholinergic drug such as atropine, 1 or 2 mg of physostigmine should be administered to reverse the anticholinergic toxicity. The modified stir-up regimen must be instituted on the patient on arrival in the PACU. More specifically, the cascade cough should be encouraged and tracheal suctioning must be resorted to if the cascade cough is ineffective. Aggressive use of the SMI also helps reduce the chance of the geriatric patient developing atelectasis. Finally,

if possible, early ambulation should be encouraged in these patients, because it prevents clot formation in the lower extremities and enhances lung function.

Hypothermia is a common outcome of the intraoperative surgical procedure. This is because the geriatric patient has a lower metabolic rate and a reduced peripheral circulatory status.

The aged population has an increased sensitivity to the depressant effects of anesthetic drugs. Prolonged emergence from general anesthesia can be expected. Consequently, airway management and rapid institution of the modified stir-up regimen are required. Along with this, the geriatric patient should receive a reduced dosage of postoperative analgesics because the usual dosage can have a profound respiratory depressant effect. It is best to titrate to effect with the intended outcome being a reduction in pain and restlessness with minimal reduction in respiratory status.

A reduced renal function along with an increased output of antidiuretic hormone during and after surgery places the geriatric patient at increased risk of postoperative overhydration. Therefore, urinary output along with the amount of fluid administered to the patient should be monitored closely.

Finally, in an effort to facilitate psychological security, personal items such as dentures, glasses, and hearing aids should be returned to the patient as soon as possible.

References

1. Barash, P., Cullen, B., and Stoelting, R.: Handbook of Clinical Anesthesia. 2nd ed. Philadelphia, J. B. Lippincott, 1993.
2. Benumof, J., and Saidman, L.: Anesthesia and Perioperative Complications. St. Louis: Mosby/Year Book, 1992.
3. Breslow, M., Miller, C., and Rogers, M.: Perioperative Management. St. Louis, C. V. Mosby, 1990.
4. Hazzard, W., Andres, R., Bierman, E., and Blass, J. (eds): Principles of Geriatric Medicine and Gerontology. New York, McGraw-Hill, 1990.
5. Code, W., and Roth, S.: Anesthesia in the geriatric patient. Gerontology, 2(2):11–13, 1987.
6. Cusack, B.: Drug Metabolism in the elderly. J. Clin. Pharmacol., 28(6):571–576, 1988.
7. Del Portzer, M.: Geriatric cardiovascular problems. AANA J., 44(6):609, 1976.
8. Jansen, V.: The TURP syndrome. Can. J. Anaesth., 38(1):90–97, 1991.
9. Katz, J., Benumof, J., and Kadis, L.: Anesthesia and Uncommon Diseases. 3rd ed. Philadelphia, W. B. Saunders, 1990.
10. Krechel, S. (ed.): Anesthesia and the Geriatric Patient. New York, Grune & Stratton, 1984.
11. Lee, E.: Disposition of drugs in the elderly. Ann. Acad. Med., 16(1):128–132, 1987.
12. Miller, R.: Anesthesia. 3rd ed. New York, Churchill Livingstone, 1990.
13. Stoelting, R., Dierdorf, S., and McCammon, R.: Anesthesia and Co-Existing Disease. 2nd ed. New York, Churchill Livingstone, 1989.
14. Waugaman, W.: Preoperative and postoperative considerations for patients with Alzheimer's disease. Geriatr. Nurs., 9:227–230, 1988.
15. Waugaman, W., Foster, S., and Rigor, B.: Principles and Practice of Nurse Anesthesia. 2nd ed. Norwalk, CT, Appleton & Lange, 1992.

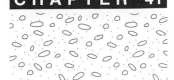

CHAPTER 41

Post Anesthesia Care of the Pregnant Patient

The incidence of surgery performed on pregnant women for reasons unrelated to the pregnancy itself has been reported to be as high as 40,000 to 50,000 cases per year. The most common conditions requiring surgical intervention are acute appendicitis, ovarian cysts, and breast tumors. However, there are reports of more complicated procedures such as craniotomy, open heart surgery, and aneurysm repair that have been performed successfully in pregnant patients.

When caring for the pregnant patient postoperatively, one must remember that there are two patients who require nursing care and assessment: the mother and the fetus. Post anesthesia nursing care should be directed toward providing emotional support for the mother, as well as avoiding uterine stimulation that could produce preterm labor. Also of prime importance is the prevention of respiratory depression in the mother and the maintenance of normal uterine placental blood flow to ensure adequate fetal supply of oxygen and nutrients.

PHYSIOLOGIC CHANGES OF PREGNANCY

Almost every system in the body is affected in some way during pregnancy, either by hormonal changes or because of the increasing size of the uterus. The changes that will impact on post anesthesia nursing care are outlined in Table 41–1 and discussed in the following sections.

Cardiovascular Changes

Hemodynamic Alterations

The cardiovascular system undergoes significant change as pregnancy advances. Cardiac output and heart rate increase progressively during pregnancy until, at 30 to 34 weeks' gestation, the cardiac output is 30 to 50 percent higher than normal and the heart rate is about 15 percent above the nonpregnant normal level, with electrocardiographic changes and heart sounds possibly developing (Table 41–2). The systolic blood pressure decreases to about 20 mm Hg below the nonpregnant level at about 20 weeks' gestation and then increases to about 10 mm Hg below the nonpregnant level at term. The diastolic blood pressure is reduced to about 15 mm Hg below the nonpregnant level at 20 weeks' gestation and then slowly returns to the nonpregnant level at term.

Perhaps the most significant effect on the cardiovascular system for the nurse to consider in routine post anesthesia management is obstruction of the inferior vena cava and the pelvic veins by the enlarging uterus (Figs. 41–1 and 41–2). This condition, known as *aortocaval compression* or *Scott's syndrome,* can develop by the second trimester and cause supine hypotension. It becomes mandatory to avoid the supine position postoperatively, because it can significantly aggravate the obstruction. The side-lying position is the one of choice in the post anesthesia care unit (PACU) (Fig. 41–3).

Collateral circulation for venous return develops through the intervertebral venous plexus and the azygos vein. This condition reduces the volume of the epidural and subarachnoid spaces. Therefore, the amount of drug required during regional anesthesia should be decreased. Keeping this in mind, the PACU nurse should assess the patient on admission for a high block and monitor dermatone levels frequently thereafter (see Chapter 18).

In the nonpregnant patient, the sympathetic nervous system plays a role in promoting venous return to the heart from the lower extremities. This sympathetic stimulation of vasomotor tone is enhanced during pregnancy in an effort to counteract the negative effects of uterine compression of the vena cava. Clinically, this protective mechanism is abolished by spinal or epidural anesthesia because it acts as a pharmacologic sympathectomy. Without an appropriate preload of fluids, the pregnant pa-

Table 41–1. PHYSIOLOGIC CHANGES IN PREGNANCY

Cardiovascular System

Flow and pressure changes
Cardiac output increases from 20% at the end of the first trimester to 40% at term
Heart rate >15% of nonpregnant level
Stroke volume increases
Ejection fraction increases
Pulmonary capillary wedge pressure has no significant change
Central venous pressure has no significant change
Systolic blood pressure decreases to about 10 mm Hg below nonpregnant level at term
Diastolic blood pressure decreases by 10 to 15 mm Hg in early gestation through 30 weeks and then returns to pregestation levels at term

Blood volume and constituents
Total blood volume increases to about 45% above nonpregnant levels
Total plasma volume increases to about 55% above nonpregnant levels
Red blood cell mass increases to about 30% above nonpregnant levels
Hematocrit levels decrease to about 36 mg/dl during gestation
Hemoglobin levels decrease to about 11.6 g/dl
Plasma cholinesterase levels decrease as much as 80% of nonpregnant levels

Coagulation
Prothrombin time and partial thromboplastin time decreases 20%
Platelet count decreases 15%
Bleeding time decreases 10%

Respiratory System

Anatomic changes
Capillary engorgement of the nasal and oropharyngeal mucosa and larynx
Increased circumference of the thoracic cage
Elevated diaphragm
Respiratory system flow, volume, and ventilation changes

No change in FEV_1
No change in flow-volume loop
Total pulmonary resistance decreases
Tidal volume increases from 20% to 45% above nonpregnant levels
Functional residual capacity decreases by 20% to 60% below the nonpregnant level
Alveolar ventilation increases by 30 to 45% above nonpregnant level
Minute ventilation increases by 45% above nonpregnant level

Changes in blood gases
$Paco_2$ decreases to about 30 mm Hg
Pao_2 increases to about 103–105 mm Hg
Arterial pH from 10 weeks' gestation until delivery is about 7.44

Metabolic rate and acid-base status
Metabolic rate is depressed during first 12–16 weeks
Metabolic rate is 15% above nonpregnant level at term
Oxygen consumption is 35% above nonpregnant level at term
Oxygen consumption is 40% above nonpregnant level during first stage of labor
Oxygen consumption is 75% above nonpregnant level during second stage of labor
Respiratory alkalosis with some metabolic compensation is present

Gastrointestinal System

Gastric emptying delays after 34 weeks' gestation
Gastric volume increases
Gastric pH decreases
Pyrosis (heartburn) is present in >50% of pregnant women
Intragastric pressure increases
Hepatic blood flow and function not altered

Renal System

Glomerular filtration rate increases
Urine output increases

FEV_1 = forced expiratory volume in 1 second.

---

tient may experience a 30 to 50 percent decrease in blood pressure during the anesthesia. Therefore, it is extremely important that the pregnant patient receive an appropriate preload of fluids before epidural or spinal anesthe-

Table 41–2. POSSIBLE ALTERATIONS IN CARDIOVASCULAR PARAMETERS

Heart sounds are louder with the development of a split S_2
Short systolic murmur
More forceful apical impulse
Inverted T waves in leads III, V_1, and V_2
Left axis deviation in months 2–6
Flattened T waves
Depressed ST segments

*If findings develop during pregnancy, they usually disappear after delivery.

sia. Hemodynamic stability can be secured by the infusion of 15 ml/kg of colloid solution or 30 ml/kg of crystalloid solution. If the patient is to receive an inhalation anesthetic agent such as enflurane, similar fluid preloading is given. This is because the inhalation anesthetic agents produce peripheral vasodilatation.

This increased fluid requirement has significant implications for the PACU care of the pregnant patient. Consequently, the patient's cardiac and hydration status must be monitored closely throughout the emergence phase of regional anesthesia (see Chapter 18).

Hematologic Alterations

Blood volume increases along with the number of platelets, fibrinogen levels, and the level of activity of several clotting factors. However, there is a smaller rise in the number of circulat-

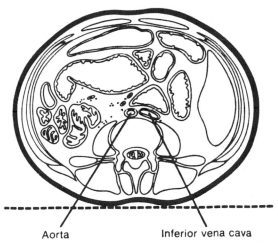

FIGURE 41–1. Cross section of the lower abdomen (nonpregnant). (From Ostheimer, S. W. [ed.]: Regional Anesthesia Techniques in Obstetrics. New York, Breon Laboratories, 1980, pp. 7–9.)

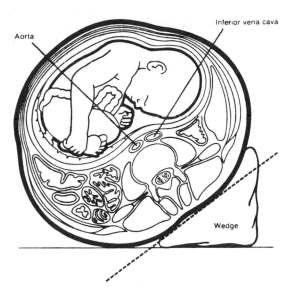

FIGURE 41–3. Uterine displacement with a wedge under the hip to relieve aortocaval compression. (From Ostheimer, S. W. [ed.]: Regional Anesthesia Techniques in Obstetrics. New York, Breon Laboratories, 1980, pp. 7–9.)

ing red blood cells. This difference results in lower hematocrit and hemoglobin levels (see Table 41–1), even though there is an actual increase in red blood cell mass. This condition is known as *physiologic anemia of pregnancy.*

The plasma concentration of the enzyme cholinesterase is decreased during pregnancy, and because plasma cholinesterase is involved in the mechanisms of clotting, the PACU nurse should monitor the pregnant patient for thromboembolism. Plasma cholinesterase is also involved in the destruction of the depolarizing muscle relaxant succinylcholine. The recovery time from succinylcholine is unaltered and in fact may even be somewhat faster in pregnant women. This is explained by the fact that there

is an increase in the volume distribution of succinylcholine during pregnancy because of an elevation in the plasma volume. In the immediate post-partum period, there is a further reduction in the plasma cholinesterase concentration and a reduction in the plasma volume distribution. Consequently, between post-partum days 1 and 2, prolonged paralysis and apnea following the administration of succinylcholine can occur, and the dosage of succinylcholine during this period should be reduced by about 50 percent.

Respiratory Changes

Upper Airway Anatomy

During pregnancy, there is capillary engorgement of the upper respiratory tract to include the nasal and oropharyngeal mucosa and larynx, and pregnant women may complain of nasal stuffiness. Along with this, nose breathing is difficult and nosebleeds can occur.

Lung Mechanics and Ventilation

The diaphragm elevates and the rib cage flares, so that at term 85 percent of respiratory effort is intercostal and 15 percent is diaphragmatic. (Normally, approximately 70 percent is intercostal and 30 percent is diaphragmatic.) Because of the mechanical changes in the lungs and chest wall, the lung volumes and capacities

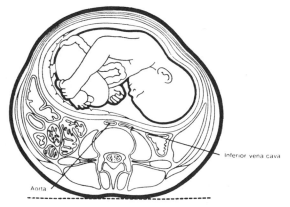

FIGURE 41–2. The pregnant uterus compressing the aorta and the inferior vena cava (aortocaval compression). The patient is in the supine position. (From Ostheimer, S. W. [ed.]: Regional Anesthesia Techniques in Obstetrics. New York, Breon Laboratories, 1980, pp. 7–9.)

do change during pregnancy. Overall, the inspiratory lung volumes and capacities moderately increase and the expiratory lung volumes and capacities decrease. The inspiratory reserve volume and the inspiratory capacity increase by 5 to 15 percent. The functional residual capacity (FRC) decreases by approximately 20 to 60 percent. Also, the residual volume and expiratory reserve volume, which make up the FRC, are also decreased.

The tidal volume also increases about 20 to 45 percent and the respiratory rate does not change, which leads to a 30 to 45 percent increase in the alveolar ventilation and the minute ventilation. Therefore, during pregnancy, the arterial oxygen level ranges from 95 to 105 mm Hg and the arterial carbon dioxide level is approximately 30 mm Hg with an arterial pH of 7.44. Consequently, the pregnant patient has some respiratory alkalosis that is compensated for by the renal excretion of bicarbonate. Hence, the normal bicarbonate level during pregnancy is about 19 mEq per L, and the base excess is reduced by 2 mEq per L.

In regard to flow rate changes, the forced expiratory volume in 1 second and the flow-volume loop remain unchanged. Along with this, the closing capacity (see Chapter 6) does not change during gestation. Consequently, it can be said that the small and large airways conductance and resistance do not change during pregnancy.

Gastrointestinal Changes

Motility and Secretions

Gastric emptying slows during pregnancy because the stomach is displaced as the uterus enlarges. Along with this, the gastric volume increases during hours 1 to 8 in the post-partum period. Therefore, the PACU nurse must be cognizant of the potential for vomiting and aspiration, particularly in patients who have had general anesthesia. Muscle relaxants may have been used, resulting in the patient's normal protective mechanisms being obtunded. Once again, the side-lying position becomes of significant importance.

Hepatic System

Liver function test results are abnormal, but there is no evidence of alteration in liver function, and hepatic blood flow remains constant. Therefore, those anesthetic agents that are me-

tabolized in the liver should have the same duration of effect.

Renal Changes

Early in pregnancy, the kidneys receive an increased blood flow; therefore, glomerular filtration and urine formation rates increase. This is necessary to handle the increased amount of waste products produced. Monitoring of output should reflect this expected increase in volume. Intervention may be required for hypovolemia even though the urine output is within ranges acceptable in a nonpregnant patient.

INTRAOPERATIVE ANESTHESIA CARE OF THE OBSTETRIC PATIENT

Because the effects of anesthesia have such a profound effect on the emergence of the pregnant patient, a complete review of the techniques and procedures of general and regional anesthesia are presented.

Positioning

Because the supine position causes a reduction in uterine blood flow in the pregnant patient, the semi-Fowler's position is used when possible. To prevent aortocaval compression, the patient is placed in the lateral decubitus position, and the right hip is elevated using a pillow or the uterus is displaced to the left using devices on the operating table.

Gastrointestinal Considerations

The pregnant patient has a reduced gastric emptying time and a reduced gastric pH. However, research has demonstrated that gastric volume and acidity in the pregnant patient do not differ significantly from those in the nonpregnant patient. However, many anesthesia clinicians believe strongly that the pregnant patient, especially the patient with pyrosis, is at risk of developing aspiration pneumonitis. Consequently, preoperative pharmacologic interventions are usually taken. Drugs that may be administered include a nonparticulate antacid such as sodium citrate (Bicitra) to increase the gastric pH, cimetidine (Tagamet), or ranitidine (Zantac), which are histamine-2 receptor blockers that reduce gastric acid secretion, and metoclopramide (Reglan), which speeds up gastric emptying time and elevates lower esophageal tone.

General Anesthesia

Induction. Because of the strong full-stomach considerations, the pregnant patient is intubated using a rapid-sequence endotracheal intubation technique (see Chapter 21) using intravenous (IV) thiopental, etomidate, or ketamine followed by succinylcholine. A defasciculation dose of a nondepolarizing muscle relaxant may be given prior to the administration of the succinylcholine to avoid the increase in intragastric pressure. Some clinicians do not administer a defasciculating dose of a nondepolarizing muscle relaxant because it can delay the onset, reduce the intensity, and shorten the duration of action of succinylcholine. Cricoid pressure (Sellick maneuver) is used once the barbiturate is administered and is released after confirmation of appropriate placement of the endotracheal tube.

The endotracheal tube should be a small tube, usually 7 mm in diameter or smaller, because of increased mucosal engorgement in the nasal and oropharyngeal areas. Along with this, nasotracheal intubation is not used because of the high risk of tissue trauma.

Maintenance. Nitrous oxide in 50 percent concentration with oxygen is usually administered. Inhalation agents such as halothane, isoflurane, and enflurane can be used. Analgesic concentrations of 0.5 minimum alveolar concentration (see Chapter 13) or less to avoid significant uterine relaxation can be used safely for these inhalation drugs. However, these inhalation agents, particularly halothane, may be used in high concentrations for a short period to produce uterine relaxation for intrauterine manipulation of the fetus or removal of a retained placenta. The clinical implication in the PACU for the patient who received a high concentration of an inhalation agent, even for a short period (<2 minutes), is to monitor for post-partum hemorrhage and maternal hypotension. Also, the uterine response to oxytocic drugs is reduced when high concentrations of these inhalation agents are used.

In regard to skeletal muscle relaxation, succinylcholine infusion or short-acting nondepolarizing muscle relaxants such as atracurium and vecuronium can be used safely because they lack autonomic side effects and have a low degree of placental transfer. In the immediate post-partum period, the neuromuscular-blocking effects of vecuronium are prolonged.

Emergence. At the end of the surgical procedure, the residual effects of the nondepolarizing muscle relaxants are reversed and the inhalation anesthetic agents are discontinued. When the patient is awake, responsive, and able to ventilate without assistance, she is extubated.

Regional Anesthesia

Regional anesthesia, primarily spinal and epidural, is used extensively for anesthesia in the pregnant patient because it produces analgesia without causing neonatal depression. This technique also reduces the risk of maternal hypoventilation and the need for narcotics and sedatives. Regional anesthesia does not require airway management, preserves airway reflexes, and allows the mother to remain awake during birth. It is contraindicated in patients with severe coagulation problems, severe hypovolemia, sepsis, and infection at the needle insertion site; in situations when immediate delivery is crucial, such as in fetal distress; and when the patient refuses the procedure.

The level of sensory blockade for either spinal or epidural anesthesia for cesarean section is from T4 to S4. The commonly used local anesthetic drugs for spinal anesthesia are lidocaine, bupivacaine, and tetracaine (see Chapter 17). For epidural anesthesia, the commonly used local anesthetic agents are 2-chloroprocaine (Nesacaine), lidocaine with epinephrine, and bupivacaine.

The epidural approach, compared with the spinal approach, is the preferred technique because drugs can be administered throughout the surgical procedure via a continuous epidural catheter. The anesthesia clinician then has the ability to control the onset, distribution, and duration of anesthesia. Along with this, the incidence of postdural puncture is much lower when compared with the spinal technique.

CARE OF THE MOTHER AND THE FETUS IN THE PACU

Studies have not shown one anesthetic technique to be better than another in the gravid patient. As with nonpregnant patients, the choice of technique is determined by the following:

1. Surgery to be performed

2. American Society of Anesthesiologists classification of the patient
3. Anesthetist's preference
4. Patient's preference
5. Underlying disease entities

The care of the pregnant patient postoperatively should be the same as for any patient undergoing that procedure or for one recovering from that particular anesthetic. There are, however, additions to the routine nursing care that must be instituted for all pregnant patients.

Positioning

To alleviate compression of the vena cava, the uterus should be displaced to the left, either by positioning the patient on her left side or by tilting the pelvis using a folded sheet or bath towel under the woman's right iliac crest. Slight elevation of the legs and the use of thigh-high elastic stockings should be standard.

Psychological and Emotional Support

The mother's concern for her unborn child is paramount. Constant reassurance is mandatory. If possible, allow the mother to listen to the fetal heart beat frequently during the recovery phase. Explain all procedures and why they are being done before carrying them out. If your PACU allows visitors, involvement of the father should also be considered.

Fetal Monitoring

The fetal heart rate must be monitored every 15 minutes if the fetus has reached viability (Table 41–3). If available, an indirect fetal monitoring system should be used for constant assessment of fetal stability (Fig. 41–4).

Table 41–3. FETAL HEART RATES

Description	Rate (beats/min)
Normal fetal heart rate	120–160
Moderate tachycardia	160–180
Marked tachycardia	>180
Moderate bradycardia	100–120
Marked bradycardia	<100

The second type of monitoring required is to observe the patient closely for signs of premature labor. These include spontaneous rupture of membranes, increased fetal heart rate, presenting of vaginal mucus plug, uterine palpitations, uterine contractions, and restlessness of the mother.

Initially, the patient may not feel the contractions or be aware of membrane rupture; therefore, palpation of the abdomen and assessment of vaginal discharge must be performed by the nurse. If premature labor begins, transfer of the patient to the labor and delivery area as soon as possible is recommended. A drug may have to be given to stop labor. These drugs should be administered by personnel familiar with proper protocols for administration and their side effects.

Pain Management

The Post Cesarean Section Patient

The post cesarean section patient presents unique challenges in regard to pain management. More specifically, more women desire to care for their newborns within the first 24 hours. Heavy sedation with opioids and IV or epidural catheters inhibit the mother's ability to care for the infant. Also, the infant can be affected through the transfer of the drug in breast milk.

Patient-controlled analgesia (PCA) is becoming quite popular in pain management of the post cesarean section patient (see Chapters 15 and 22). It is well documented that the PCA interrupts the pain cycle, gives the patient a feeling of control, hastens the time to ambulation, and reduces the length of stay in the hospital. Morphine is the preferred drug to be administered by PCA. The usual dose is 1 to 1.5 mg, a lockout of 10 minutes, and a hourly limit of 10 to 12 mg.

Epidural administration of opioids is another option that can be used for the control of pain in the PACU. Morphine is the preferred drug because of its demonstrated safety and prolonged duration of action after a single dose of 5 mg. The primary side effects of epidural morphine are pruritus and nausea. Some clinicians have advocated using the narcotic antagonist naloxone (5 to 10 µg/kg/hr) to treat these side effects. However, problems arise with some reversal of the analgesia. Most clinicians treat the nausea with 0.5 mg of IV droperidol (Inapsine) and the pruritus with 12.5 mg of IV diphenhydramine (Benadryl).

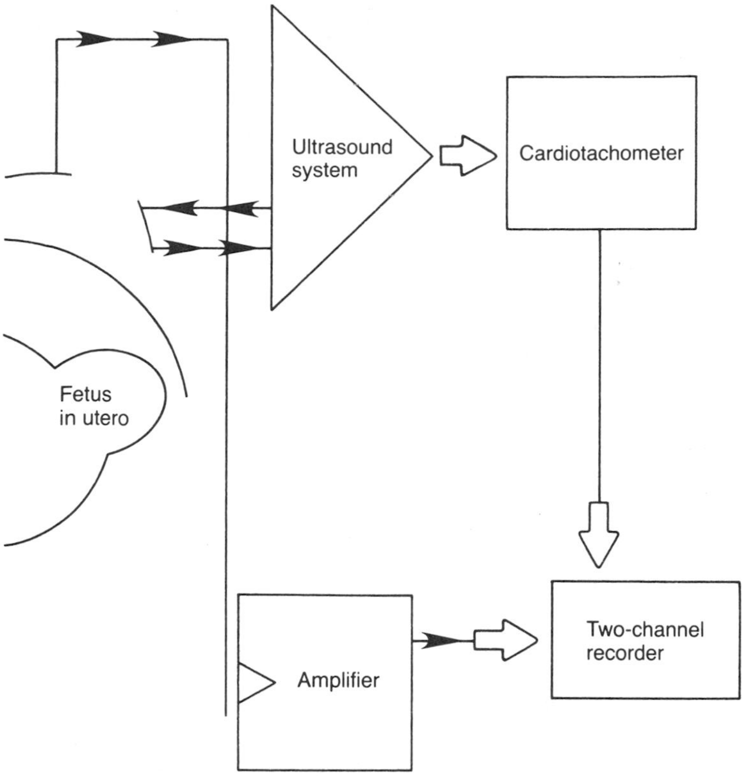

FIGURE 41–4. Indirect fetal monitoring system. A Doppler ultrasound device transmits a beam to determine fetal heart rate. When the beam strikes a moving object within the fetus, such as a mitral valve leaflet, the frequency of the transmitted beam is shifted up or down, depending on which way the leaflet is moving. This valve movement is counted and displayed as a heart rate on the recorder.

Fentanyl is a alternative to morphine for epidural analgesia. The difficulty with fentanyl is that has a duration of action of less than 5 hours and must be administered by continuous infusion or intermittent boluses. The epidural fentanyl technique provides excellent analgesia; however, most women desire to be ambulatory as soon as possible and do not like to be encumbered with the catheter, tape, and pump.

When administered epidurally with opioids, 2-chloroprocaine inhibits the analgesic effects of the opioids. This inhibitory action of 2-chloroprocaine is probably due to the ethylenediaminetetraacetic acid (EDTA) that is used in the solution of the drug. EDTA is an antioxidant that has analgesic antagonism properties because it is a strong chelator of calcium. Therefore, clinically epidural opioids should be avoided for at least 6 to 8 hours after 2-chloroprocaine has been administered.

A variety of receptor specific drugs to include opioids, alpha$_2$-adrenergic agonists, and local anesthetics are being evaluated for use via the intraspinal approach. With the refining of the spinal technique to include the use of small needles and ultrafine catheters, this technique is gaining in popularity for post cesarean section pain relief. Morphine, 0.3 mg administered intrathecally, has a longer duration of action than 4 mg of morphine administered via the epidural route. Some anesthesia clinicians are now adding morphine to bupivacaine intraoperatively, with the outcome being excellent analgesia lasting well into the post anesthesia period.

The Pregnant Patient

Because of the growth in consumer awareness, the administration of medication during pregnancy has become a controversial issue and one that must be dealt with on an individual basis. For pain management in the PACU, when the pregnant patient is in a hypersuggestive state, the use of distraction techniques such as guided imagery and breathing exercises has had favorable results in place of drugs.

If a mild analgesic is required, the drug of choice is acetaminophen (Tylenol) and, for moderate pain management, propoxyphene (Darvon). Both drugs have been evaluated through prospective studies and have been shown to pose minimal risks to the fetus if used appropriately for short-term pain management. Narcotic analgesia may be warranted for severe pain but must be used judiciously, keeping in mind the respiratory depressive effects.

Ketorolac (Toradol), a prostaglandin synthetase inhibitor, is becoming quite popular in postoperative pain therapy. However, because prostaglandins have a profound effect on the neonatal cardiovascular and renal systems, research must be conducted to determine if ketorolac has a negative effect on those systems before its use can be instituted in the post anesthesia period.

The gravid patient in the PACU is a rare occurrence and one that requires the nurse to have a great deal of knowledge and the ability to provide continual support during this stressful situation. The nurse must be able to provide a quiet, calm, reassuring atmosphere for the patient. The objective of the care delivered is an optimum environment for both the mother and the fetus.

References

1. Abboud, T.: Nonobstetric surgery during pregnancy. Semin. Anesth., 11(1):51–54, 1992.
2. Barash, P., Cullen, B., and Stoelting, R.: Clinical Anesthesia. 2nd ed. Philadelphia, J. B. Lippincott, 1992.
3. Conklin, K.: Maternal physiological adaptations during gestation, labor, and the puerperium. Semin. Anesth., 10(4):221–234, 1991.
4. Eisenach, J.: Pain management in the parturient: Theoretical and practical aspects. Semin. Anesth., 11(1):55–65, 1992.
5. Johnson, M., and Ostheimer, G.: Airway management in obstetric patients. Semin. Anesth., 11(1):1–12, 1992.
6. Kelly, M.: Maternal position and blood pressure during pregnancy and delivery. Am. J. Nurs., 82:809–812, 1982.
7. Miller, R.: Anesthesia. 3rd ed. New York, Churchill Livingstone, 1991.
8. Moran, D., and Dewan, D.: Anesthesia for cesarean delivery. Semin. Anesth., 10(4):286–294, 1991.
9. Norris, M. (ed.): Obstetric Anesthesia. Philadelphia, J. B. Lippincott, 1993.
10. Shnider, S., and Levinson, G.: Anesthesia for Obstetrics. 3rd ed. Baltimore, Williams & Wilkins, 1993.
11. Ziadlourad, F., and Conklin, K.: Anesthesia for obstetric emergencies. Semin. Anesth., 8(3):222–231, 1989.

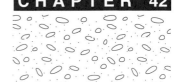

Post Anesthesia Care of the Substance Abuser

T he great increase in the number of persons using narcotics, amphetamines, cocaine, hallucinogens, and barbiturates has created new problems in post anesthesia nursing care.

Drug abuse is the nonmedical use of a drug and consists of the self-administration of any drug in a manner that deviates from the approved medical or social practices within a given culture. *Physical dependence* is an altered physiologic state caused by repeated administration of a drug that necessitates the continued administration of the drug to prevent the appearance of the withdrawal or abstinence syndrome characteristic for that drug. *Psychological dependence* is habituation-compulsive drug use. In this type of abuse, a drug is used to alter mood and feeling, and eventually, dependent people come to believe that the effects of the drug are necessary to maintain an optimal state of well-being. Another term that should be defined when discussing substance abuse is *tolerance*. *Drug tolerance* is a state in which, after repeated administration of a drug, a given dose produces a decreased effect or, on the other hand, increasingly larger doses are needed to obtain the same effect as that of the original dose.

The pharmacologic agents that are most commonly abused can be grouped as follows: (1) *opioid analgesics;* (2) *general central nervous system* (CNS) *depressants,* such as alcohol and the barbiturates; (3) *CNS sympathomimetics,* such as amphetamines and cocaine; (4) *cannabinoids,* such as marihuana; and (5) *psychedelics,* of which lysergic acid diethylamide (LSD) and phencyclidine are the prototypic drugs (Table 42–1).

OPIOID ANALGESICS

Opioid analgesics (narcotics) cause strong psychological dependence. Physical dependence is manifested by the withdrawal syndrome of autonomic storm and CNS irritabil-

ity. Also, there is a strong tolerance for these drugs as well as a cross-tolerance with other drugs of the same classification of opioid analgesics. Studies indicate that in people who are chronically addicted to opioid analgesics such as morphine, the minimum alveolar concentration of halothane (Fluothane) is increased, indicating that a cross-tolerance with general inhalation anesthetics may exist.

Heroin, an opioid analgesic that is derived from morphine, is degraded in the body to morphine about 30 minutes after injection. The most common problem associated with the use of heroin and other opioid analgesics is pulmonary edema; other dysfunctions include superficial bacterial infections, adrenal insufficiency, bacterial endocarditis, liver disease, urinary abnormalities (proteinuria and glycosuria), and false-positive serology. In addition, about 30 percent of the opiate abusers have positive results on Venereal Disease Research Laboratory test for syphilis, but only about 25 percent of these are true-positive when checked by the *Treponema* immobilization test.

Post anesthesia care unit (PACU) care of an opiate abuser, such as the heroin addict, centers around monitoring the patient for complications. Probably foremost is monitoring for the withdrawal (abstinence) syndrome. The abstinence syndrome after opiate abuse occurs in two phases. The acute phase occurs during the first few days. The protracted phase, which is not readily treatable, can persist for as long as 2 to 6 months. The acute opiate abstinence phase is not dangerous to life because it is usually not associated with convulsions and delirium. Instead, the symptoms are anxiety, nervousness, jittery behavior, anorexia, rhinorrhea, hypotension, muscle twitching, insomnia, sweating, pupillary dilation, gooseflesh, and nausea and vomiting. Symptoms during the protracted phase include those of the acute phase, along with convulsions and delirium. Treatment for the acute opiate abstinence phase is accomplished with any narcotic analgesic; reports indicate that clonidine has proved to be most effective in attenuating the symptoms.

Table 42–1. CATEGORIES OF SUBSTANCE ABUSE: EFFECTS AND SIGNS OF ABUSE AND WITHDRAWAL

Category	Possible Effects	Signs of Abuse	Signs of Withdrawal
Opioid Analgesics Opium Morphine Codeine Heroin Meperidine (Demerol) Sublimaze (Fentanyl) Methadone (Dolophine)	Euphoria, "rush" with IV injection, feeling of detachment, drowsiness, miosis, nausea, respiratory depression Tolerance, physical and psychological dependence	Injection scars or needle marks, usually on inner surfaces of arms Thrombophlebitis at injection sites, cellulitis Pinpoint pupils Uncoordinated movements Confusion, disorientation Heavy smoking	Watery eyes, runny nose, scratching, yawning, anorexia, irritability, tremors, panic, chills and sweating, muscle pains and cramps, nausea, vomiting, diarrhea

General CNS Depressants
Alcohol
	Loss of inhibitions
	Impaired judgment
	Carefree mood
	Impaired motor coordination, concentration, memory
	Ataxia, incoherence
	Stupor, coma
	Tolerance and physical dependence
		Reported intake:
		  Heavy drinker*
		  Alcohol addicted†
		  GI disturbances
		  Malnutrition
		  Heavy smoking
		  Trauma
		  Psychological problems
		  Social maladjustment
			8 hours after abstinence:
			Tremors, GI disturbances, anxiety, jittery feeling, and headache
			24–72 hours or longer of withdrawal:
			Increased tremors, hyperactivity, irritability, nervousness, insomnia, delusions, hallucinations, seizures, delirium tremens (DTs), high fever, profuse sweating, tachycardia, hyperventilation, nausea and vomiting

Barbiturates
  Amytal
  Butisol
  Nembutal
  Seconal
  Tuinal
  Phenobarbital
	Euphoria, reduced anxiety, dry intoxication (drunken behavior without odor of alcohol)
	Tolerance, physical and psychological dependence
		Drowsiness, lack of interest, fatigue, irritability
		Changes in personality and behavior
		Possession of pills of varying colors and shapes
			Range from anxiety, weakness, confusion, anorexia, and mild tremors to delirium disorientation, hallucinations, and convulsions

Benzodiazepines
  Valium
  Librium
  Serax
  Ativan
  Verced
	Same as barbiturates	Same as barbiturates	Same as barbiturates

CNS Sympathomimetics Amphetamines	Increased alertness, euphoria, anorexia, insomnia, elevated blood pressure, tachycardia, anxiety Tolerance, psychological dependence	Possession of pills of varying color Injection scars, needle marks Compulsion to talk, extreme activity, chain smoking Frequent nose rubbing or scratching, licking of dry lips, bad breath Changed eating and sleeping habits Projected sense of prowess or capability Possible aggressive or antisocial behavior	"Crashing" (response produced when stimulant effect ends); hunger, extreme lethargy, profound depression, and sleep disturbance

Table 42–1. CATEGORIES OF SUBSTANCE ABUSE: EFFECTS AND SIGNS OF ABUSE AND WITHDRAWAL *Continued*

Category	Possible Effects	Signs of Abuse	Signs of Withdrawal
CNS Sympathomimetics *Continued*			
Cocaine	Same as amphetamines Possible tolerance, no physical dependence, high psychological dependence	Same as amphetamines Inflamed nasal mucosa	Same as amphetamines "Crashing" may be profound
Cannabinoids Marihuana (hashish)	Sense of relaxation and well-being Distorted orientation to time and space Altered sensory perception Occasional excitement and spontaneous (often uncontrolled) laughter Increased appetite Tolerance and psychological dependence, degree of physical dependence unknown	Possession of off-white or brown cigarette papers and coarse brownish-green tobacco Conjunctival congestion, dilated pupils Wearing of dark glasses because of light sensitivity	Reported abstinence symptoms: hyperexcitability, insomnia, decreased appetite
Psychedelics Lysergic acid diethylamide (LSD) Phencyclidine (PCP)	Illusions Distorted perceptions of time, distance, body image, mood, affect Depersonalization and ego dissociation Psychotic behavior Tolerance, degree of psychological dependence unknown	Possession of perforated small squares of blotter paper with colored designs, ampules of clear liquid, or capsules of white or colored powder, or tablets Unusual body odor Marked mood changes Dream-like or trancelike state	None reported

*Heavy drinker: a person who consumes five or more drinks on some occasions and at least 45 drinks a month.
†Alcohol addicted: a person who consumes approximately 20 drinks of beer, wine, or liquor a day and has developed physiologic tolerance.
CNS = central nervous system; IV = intravenous; GI = gastrointestinal.
Adapted from Knor, E.: Substance abuse. *In* Decision Making in Obstetrical Nursing. Toronto, B. C. Decker, 1987, pp. 58–60.

Treatment for the protracted phase centers around protection of the patient and abatement of the symptoms demonstrated by the patient. If a patient is a suspected opiate abuser, narcotic antagonists such as naloxone (Narcan) should not be administered because the withdrawal syndrome can be precipitated. No attempt should be made at withdrawal of the active abuser during the PACU period. Liberal use of morphine or methadone in the PACU appears to be satisfactory. The former abuser should not receive narcotics; analgesics, such as pentazocine (Talwin) and butorphanol (Stadol), should be used in their place.

GENERAL CNS DEPRESSANTS

The *barbiturate addict* may present only as nervous and anxious before surgery. However,

the patient should be monitored postoperatively for anxiety, tremors, and hallucinations. These symptoms usually develop on the second or third postoperative day and can be treated with a barbiturate until acute illness has passed. These patients also appear to have an increased tolerance to anesthesia and therefore have an increased chance of anesthetic toxicity.

The use and abuse of the *benzodiazepine* compounds have increased significantly during the last decade. The benzodiazepine drug is usually taken in combination with marihuana or alcohol to obtain a "high." Chronic intoxication has been reported with the use of these compounds. The most abused benzodiazepine is diazepam (Valium); however, midazolam (Verced) will soon rank at the same level as diazepam. These drugs are becoming popular because of their rapid onset of action coupled with their pleasure-giving effects. The pharmacologic effects of the benzodiazepines are similar to the barbiturates. This classification of drugs is somewhat addicting and includes withdrawal syndromes.

To treat mild to moderate overdosages of benzodiazepines, the drug physostigmine in an adult dosage of 1 to 2 mg given intravenously can be used. A new antagonist with a longer action and fewer side effects has been introduced into clinical practice. This drug, flumazenil (Mazicon) is a true benzodiazepine receptor antagonist. The usual adult dosage is 0.1 to 0.2 mg given intravenously. As with the use of naloxone with narcotic-addicted patients, flumazenil must be used with caution with benzodiazepine-dependent patients. More specifically, reversal of benzodiazepine-dependent patients is associated with precipitating the withdrawal syndrome, including seizures.

Alcoholism has long been widespread, yet it is difficult to define. An *alcoholic,* for purposes of this discussion, is a person who is excessively dependent on alcohol and who has developed a noticeable degree of mental, physical, psychological, or pathologic disorders. Alcohol was the first anesthetic; it can produce anesthesia, respiratory depression, and hypotension.

Alcohol affects many of the body's major systems. It is well known that in the later stages of alcoholism, cirrhosis of the liver is quite common. This is of importance to the PACU nurse because the liver detoxifies many drugs administered during the perioperative period (see Chapter 9). Hepatic cirrhosis may produce significant alterations in pulmonary and cardiovascular functions. Hyperventilation and arterial oxygen desaturation are common findings caused by an increase in shunting of blood away from areas in the lung where diffusion of oxygen takes place. Concomitant with this is an increase in blood volume that may lead to cardiac hypertrophy and, eventually, to congestive heart failure. Fluid balance is affected by the presence of alcohol, because alcohol exhibits antidiuretic effects by inhibiting the release of antidiuretic hormone. Alcoholic cirrhosis (Laennec's cirrhosis) is also associated with portal vein hypertension, renal failure, hypoglycemia, duodenal ulcer, esophageal varices, and hepatic encephalopathy.

The alcoholic, when compared with the nonalcoholic, usually requires a larger amount of sodium thiopental for induction and a higher concentration of anesthetic agents during surgery. It is difficult to predict the time or the character of emergence from anesthesia in the alcoholic patient. This patient may be anxious and may have a stormy emergence and postoperative phase.

During the PACU phase, the alcoholic patient should be monitored for withdrawal symptoms. The *minor alcohol withdrawal syndrome* is characterized by symptoms such as tremulousness, insomnia, and irritability. Because of autonomic nervous system imbalance, signs such as tachycardia, hypertension, and cardiac dysrhythmias are often observed. The minor alcohol withdrawal syndrome can occur within 6 to 8 hours after abstinence by the alcoholic patient. The signs and symptoms of this syndrome usually disappear within 48 hours without treatment.

In about 5 percent of the alcoholic population, when the ingestion of alcohol is abruptly ceased, the *severe alcohol withdrawal syndrome,* or *delirium tremens,* will occur. The mortality rate from this syndrome is about 15 percent, and it is considered a medical emergency. The time of onset of delirium tremens is about 48 to 72 hours after the abrupt discontinuation of alcohol ingestion.

The patient is difficult to manage if withdrawal symptoms are allowed to develop. The severe withdrawal syndrome should be suspected if symptoms occur, such as restlessness, disorientation, tremulousness, and hallucinations. In addition, because of activation of the sympathetic nervous system, symptoms such as diaphoresis, hyperpyrexia, tachycardia, and hypertension are seen. When any of these symptoms is observed, hypoxia should first be ruled out, because the symptoms of withdrawal can be confused with those of hypoxia. The treatment used to control the withdrawal symptoms is sedation with diazepam, along with intravenous fluids and electrolytes, vitamin replacement (i.e., thiamine), and glucose. If deemed necessary by the attending physician, propranolol may be given to suppress the clinical manifestations of the increased sympathetic nervous system activity. Along with this, should cardiac dysrhythmias occur, lidocaine may be administered intravenously.

CNS SYMPATHOMIMETICS

Cocaine has a two-pronged effect—vasoconstriction and mood alteration—because it inhibits the reuptake of catecholamines. The mood-altering effect is similar to the psychological effect produced by amphetamines. Cocaine is steadily becoming one of the most popular drugs among substance abusers. Patients who are known abusers of cocaine should be closely monitored in the PACU for hypertension and cardiac arrhythmias. Also, these patients are quite prone to frequent nosebleeds. Hence, care should be taken when administering nursing care near or directly to the nose and nasal cavity.

CNS stimulants, which include amphetamines, tend to be long-acting vasopressors. The patient will have dilated pupils, tachycardia, palpitations, cardiac arrhythmias, and changes in temperature regulation and will appear to be extremely anxious. If the stimulant is wearing off, the patient will be lethargic and very depressed. Continuous electrocardiographic monitoring for cardiac arrhythmias is necessary, coupled with frequent blood pressure and pulse measurements. The mental sensorium should also be monitored throughout the patient's stay in the PACU.

CANNABINOIDS

The hemp plants, of which cannabis is the generic name, contain about 30 active substances that are called *cannabinoids*. Of these, tetrahydrocannabinol (THC) is the most active. *Marihuana* is the generic term applied to the hemp plants. The marihuana cigarette contains rolled-up or crushed, dried leaves from the hemp plant. Each marihuana cigarette contains about 0.005 g of THC. The cannabinoids are three times more potent when inhaled than when ingested orally. Psychological changes occur minutes after inhalation of marihuana and the effects peak in an hour, with a duration as long as 3 hours.

The peripheral effects of THC on the autonomic nervous system include vagal blockade and beta-adrenergic stimulation. Hence, the abuser of marihuana experiences tachycardia, peripheral vascular dilatation, bronchodilatation, conjunctival congestion, and a dry mouth. The actual effects of THC on the CNS are not known.

Because of the rapid effects of the drug, along with the short duration of action and the absence of physiologic dysfunction or changes, abusers of marihuana do not seem to present any added problems in the PACU. However, because of the chronic irritation produced by the inhalation of smoke from the marihuana cigarette, chronic abusers should be monitored for chronic bronchitis.

PSYCHEDELICS

Phencyclidine is the hallucinogen most commonly used today. This drug is a popular veterinary anesthetic agent (Sernylan) and is related pharmacologically to the drug ketamine. It can be ingested, taken parenterally, or inhaled. The sensory effects have a rapid onset and last approximately 1 to 2 hours, and the CNS effects can last for 1 or more days. The CNS activation usually produces sympathetic nervous system activation.

It is unlikely that the PACU nurse will have much contact with a patient under the influence of this drug. However, if a patient who abuses this drug should require PACU care, the nurse must monitor this patient for sympathetic activation, and symptoms such as dilated pupils, increased pulse, and elevated blood pressure should be reported immediately to the attending physician.

LSD is a hallucinogen that reached its peak of use in the late 1960s and is now becoming a popular drug in the 1990s. This drug is ingested orally, and its major effects occur in a dose-related manner. Moderate dosage of the drug causes euphoria, marked sensory distortion (including heightened awareness of sensory stimuli), and occasional visual hallucinations. Large doses of LSD usually lead to frightening hallucinations and a distorted body image—what is commonly referred to as a "bad trip." This drug also produces some hypertension, dilated pupils, and increased temperature, by virtue of its stimulation of the central hypothalamic area of the brain. The onset of the psychological effects of LSD is after about 40 minutes, and the duration is about 2 hours. Some of the milder effects of LSD have been reported to last as long as 8 hours after ingestion.

The primary focus of PACU nursing care for the patient who is in the hallucinogenic state is to prevent self-injury and sedation. The "bad trip" effects can be managed with chlorpromazine (Thorazine) or diazepam. Other considerations in regard to the patient who has ingested LSD are that the analgesic effects of narcotics are potentiated by LSD and that the plasma cholinesterases are somewhat inhibited by LSD. Hence, narcotic dosage may need to be reduced in these patients, and if succinylcholine is to be administered to the patient, a possibility of prolonged apnea does exist.

References

1. Barash, P., Cullen, B. and Stoelting, R.: Handbook of Clinical Anesthesia. 2nd ed. Philadelphia, J. B. Lippincott, 1993.
2. Frost, E. and Seidel, M.: Preanesthetic assessment of the drug abuse patient. Anesthesiol. Clin. North Am., 8(4):829–842, 1990.

3. Huckabee, M.: Perioperative care of the active substance abuser. J. Post Anesth. Nurs., 3(4):254–259, 1988.
4. Katz, J., Benumof, J., and Kadis, L.: Anesthesia and Uncommon Diseases. 3rd ed. Philadelphia, W. B. Saunders, 1990.
5. Knor, E.: Substance abuse. *In* Knor, E.: Decision Making in Obstetrical Nursing. Toronto: B. C. Decker, 1987.
6. Miller, R.: Anesthesia. 3rd ed. New York, Churchill Livingstone, 1990.
7. Rogers, E.: Post anesthesia care of the cocaine abuser. J. Post Anesth. Nurs., 6(2):102–107, 1991.
8. Stoelting, R., Dierdorf, S., and McCammon, R.: Anesthesia and Co-Existing Disease. 2nd ed. New York, Churchill Livingstone, 1989.
9. Weiss, S.: Anesthesia for the alcoholic and addict. AANA J., 47(3):309–312, 1979.

Post Anesthesia Care of the Patient with Thermal Imbalance

Patients admitted to the post anesthesia care unit (PACU) usually experience some form of thermal imbalance. *Thermal imbalance* is defined as body core temperature that is outside the normothermic rage of 36° to 38°C. Most likely, they experience hypothermia mostly because of the combination of anesthetic drugs and a cold environment intraoperatively. This chapter reviews the current concepts of hypothermia and hyperthermia and how they impact on the care of the PACU patient.

OVERVIEW OF THERMOREGULATION

The body maintains its temperature between the narrow range of 36° and 38°C. This is done by a balance of heat production and heat loss that is controlled by thermoregulatory mechanisms in the central nervous system (CNS). These mechanisms receive input from various thermoreceptors located in the skin, nose, oral cavity, thoracic viscera, and spinal cord. These thermoreceptors send sensory information in hierarchical order: spinal cord, reticular formation, and the primary control in the preoptic hypothalamic region of the brain.

The central temperature controls maintain body temperature by two primary responses: physiologic and behavioral. The *physiologic thermoregulatory* response consists of sweating, shivering, and alterations in the peripheral vasomotor tone. These responses fine-control the regulatory process of body temperature; consequently, there is reduction in heat loss by vasoconstriction and increase in heat loss by vasodilatation and sweating. Also, they work by reducing heat production, lowering the metabolic rate, and increasing muscle tone and shivering to enhance heat production. The *behavioral thermoregulation* is run by subjective feelings of discomfort or comfort. For example, if in a hot environment, a person seeks air conditioning, and in a cold environment the person seeks heat. It is a stronger response mechanism but does not exhibit fine control such as in the physiologic thermoregulatory response system.

Body heat is produced by metabolism, and it has a circadian cycle, with the core temperature being lower in the morning as compared with the afternoon. Body heat is removed by four methods of heat transfer: radiation, conduction, convection, and evaporation (see Chapter 10), of which radiation is the major method of heat transfer.

POSTOPERATIVE HYPOTHERMIA

Hypothermia is defined as a core body temperature lower than 36°C. About 60 percent of the patients who arrive in the PACU experience some degree of hypothermia, and of those hypothermic patients, 18 to 23 percent actively shiver in the PACU. However, the relationship between hypothermia and shivering is not clear. Patients older than 60 years of age usually have lower admission and discharge temperatures in the PACU when compared with younger patients. However, elderly patients appear to have a delayed ability to compensate for the hypothermia. Patients who have general anesthesia experience a more rapid increase in post anesthesia temperature and a shorter duration of hypothermia in the PACU than the patients who are administered intraoperative spinal or epidural anesthetics.

Body temperature is assessed by one of three methods. The thermistor responds to increased heat by emitting a lower voltage. The thermocouple, which has two dissimilar metals, responds to increased heat by sending out an increased voltage. The last sensor is called the *direct-reading liquid crystal colorimetric sensor.* This sensor is placed on the skin, usually the forehead, and the temperature is read directly from the sensor. The colorimetric sensor is not a good estimate of core temperature because of many uncontrollable factors such as vasoconstriction and environmental temperature.

Body temperature varies by the site being monitored (see Chapter 19). For example, the rectal temperature is usually 0.5° to 0.7° higher than the axillary or oral temperature. Axillary monitoring sites are used in many countries but less in the United States, and the tympanic probe is associated with perforation of the tympanic membrane. Consequently, the oral or axillary temperature site is usually the route of choice. For the pediatric age group, the rectal site is the route of choice.

Hypothermia is the most frequent problem for patients recovering from anesthesia in the PACU. Moderate hypothermia in the PACU is generally well tolerated. However, in the medically compromised patient or if the hypothermia is unrecognized, major problems can ensue.

Post anesthesia shivering (PAS) is caused by intraoperative exposure to a cold environment and the CNS depressant and peripheral vasodilatation effects of anesthesia. Muscles of the trunk and extremities can be involved; however, the PAS may be more obvious in the jaw and the shoulders. PAS can increase the metabolic rate 400 to 500 percent. This will cause the minute volume and cardiac output to increase, and if cardiopulmonary compensation does not occur, anaerobic cellular metabolism can result. Consequently, patients with ischemic disease of the myocardium, kidneys, or brain can be at risk during PAS. In fact, PAS has been associated with death in the PACU due to myocardial infarction.

On arrival in the PACU, the patient should be assessed for hypothermia. This is particularly true if the intraoperative procedure lasted longer than 1 hour. Oxygen should be administered by mask, and pulse oximetry monitoring should be instituted to detect possible hypoxemia. After the oral or axillary temperature is obtained, the rewarming therapy should be instituted. The goal is to return the patient to a temperature of 36°C. Various rewarming techniques are available for use in the PACU. Warmed cotton blankets do not increase core body temperature or decrease the duration of hypothermia. Water-circulating warming mattresses have been found to be about as effective as warmed cotton blankets in the treatment of hypothermia. Also, complications such as burns and pressure necrosis have been reported with the use of the water-circulating warming mattress. Infrared heat lamps are effective for the patient who is experiencing PAS. However, the most successful intervention for hypothermia is the use of convective warming (warm air therapy). This therapy is most effec-tive because about 70 percent of the body surface area is exposed to the warm air that is circulating in a blanket.

MALIGNANT HYPERTHERMIA

In the past, there have been reports in the medical literature about young, healthy persons who, after exercise in hot weather, developed "heat stroke" that was followed by death. Clinical reports of this syndrome continued to appear, especially of patients in the operating room developing an accelerated temperature during induction of anesthesia, and by the 1950s, more information had become available. Because of research, the morbidity and mortality from this syndrome have now been reduced. Its cause is a genetically determined condition called *malignant hyperthermia* (MH). MH is precipitated by certain general inhalation anesthetics, depolarizing skeletal muscle relaxants, amide local anesthetics, and stress. The incidence of MH ranges from 1 in 14,000 to 15,000 in children and 1 in 50,000 in adults. The onset of MH usually occurs during induction of anesthesia. Once the acute episode is treated in the operating room, the patient may be admitted to the PACU. There have been reports of MH recurring in the PACU. Because successful management of MH depends on early assessment and prompt intervention, the PACU nurse must be knowledgeable in the pathophysiology and treatment of this syndrome.

Identification of MH-Susceptible Patients

Genetics

Humans probably inherit susceptibility to MH with more than one gene or more than one group of possible mutational forms of a gene. The pattern of inheritance may range from recessive to dominant, with graded variations in between. The ease of initiation of an episode of MH seems to depend on the degree of genetic susceptibility and on environmental factors; this explains why some patients who are known to be susceptible show no signs of MH when exposed to confirmed MH-triggering agents. It is also possible that an MH-susceptible (MHS) patient could be given an anesthetic in the presence of trigger agents; this patient might not experience an acute MH reaction intraoperatively, but it could develop instead in the PACU.

Evaluation of Susceptibility

Identification of patients, before anesthesia, who may be susceptible to MH is of major therapeutic importance. On history and physical examination, MHS patients usually demonstrate some subclinical muscle weakness or abnormality, such as deficient fine motor control. Many MHS patients complain of muscle cramps that occur spontaneously, during an infectious illness, or during or after exercise. When these cramps are present, they may be so severe that they are almost incapacitating. The patient may also describe heat prostration during physical exertion that is associated with environmental heat stress. In addition, there may be a positive patient history or a positive genealogy going back two generations; that is, the patient or immediate relatives may show MH symptoms during an anesthetic experience. Physical examination of the MHS person may reveal myopathies such as wasting of the distal ends of the vastus muscles and hypertrophy of the proximal femoral muscles of the thigh. Other myopathies that are associated with MH susceptibility are cryptorchidism, pectus carinatum, kyphosis, lordosis, ptosis, and hypoplastic mandible. Electromyographic changes are seen in fewer than half of MHS patients. Electrocardiograms of MHS patients may reveal ventricular or atrial hypertrophy, or both, bundle branch block, myocardial ischemia, and ventricular dysrhythmias. Measurements of blood creatine phosphokinase (CPK) are usually about 70 percent reliable in estimating susceptibility to MH.

The most definitive test for detecting MH susceptibility is the biopsy of skeletal muscle. Samples are obtained from the quadriceps muscle and are subjected to isometric contracture testing. The skeletal muscle of the MHS patient has an increased isometric tension when exposed to caffeine or halothane.

Patients at high risk for development of an acute MH crisis have been classified as follows: (1) patients who have an MH-positive muscle biopsy or who have survived an acute MH crisis; (2) patients who have a first-degree relative known to be MHS or to have had a positive muscle biopsy; (3) patients whose family members have a clinically demonstrated muscle abnormality; and (4) patients who are members of a family whose plasma CPK measurements have been found to be elevated in one or more samples (taken on at least three occasions).

Normal Skeletal Muscle Physiology

Although a complete discussion of skeletal muscle contraction can be found in Chapter 16, a brief synopsis is presented here. The events leading to the contraction of a skeletal muscle begin with an electrical impulse that is transmitted down the axon to the motor nerve terminal, where vesicles containing acetylcholine are located. On stimulation, the contents of the vesicles are released. This quantum of acetylcholine crosses the myoneural junction and interacts with its receptor on the postsynaptic membrane. This receptor activation causes a transient increase in the permeability for sodium and potassium ions which ultimately creates an electrical action potential (nerve impulse) that is propagated along the muscle membrane. This action potential electrically excites the sarcolemma and releases into the myoplasm calcium ions that are stored in the sarcoplasmic reticulum. These calcium ions then attach to troponin C, an inhibitory muscle protein that, when stimulated by the calcium, permits the actin and myosin protein filaments to interact and cause muscle contraction. The calcium ions in the myoplasm are then taken up by a reuptake mechanism into the sarcoplasmic reticulum. The process by which the electrically excited sarcolemma is coupled to the calcium released from the sarcoplasmic reticulum is known as *excitation-contraction* (E-C) *coupling*.

Pathophysiology of Malignant Hyperthermia

When a susceptible patient is exposed to a trigger agent, such as halothane, causing MH to occur, the clinical features are produced by an excess of calcium ions in the myoplasm. Although the exact pathophysiology of MH is not known, it appears that in MH the reuptake of calcium from the myoplasm by the sarcoplasmic reticulum is decreased; it has also been suggested that the E-C coupling mechanism is defective. With an elevated calcium ion concentration in the myoplasm, the skeletal muscle contraction will be intense and prolonged, finally leading to a hypermetabolic state of acid and heat production. More specifically, heat is produced by the accelerated and continued synthesis and use of adenosine triphosphate (ATP) during glycolysis. The metabolic by-product of glycolysis, lactic acid, is transported to the liver, where part of it is oxidized to provide the ATP necessary to help make glucose. This glucose, along with glycogen, is released from the liver and transported back to the metabolically active muscle, where the entire cycle repeats. This revolving process liberates much heat and produces a significant amount of metabolic acid. Respiratory and metabolic acidosis develop because of this hypermetabolic state, and symptoms such as tachycardia, tachypnea, ventricular dysrhythmias, and unstable blood pressure appear. Because of intense vasoconstriction, the skin is mottled and cyanotic (Table 43–1). Elevated body temperature can actually be a late sign of MH; for this reason, the nurse should not prolong the assessment of the patient on the assumption that the patient's temperature must be significantly elevated before intervention is attempted. Once the patient's temperature begins to rise, it may increase at a rate of 0.5°C every 15 minutes and may approach levels as high as 46°C.

Muscle rigidity occurs in about 75 percent of the patients who experience MH. This is especially true in MHS patients following the administration of succinylcholine. In fact, the spasm of the masseter muscles following the injection of succinylcholine may be so severe that the nurse cannot open the patient's mouth to insert an airway. The onset of skeletal muscle rigidity following the administration of succinylcholine could be a sign of the impending development of MH.

Triggering of Malignant Hyperthermia

Various environmental stimuli and pharmacologic agents can stimulate an acute episode

---

Table 43–1. SIGNS AND SYMPTOMS* OF MALIGNANT HYPERTHERMIA

Signs (Objective Findings)
Central venous desaturation
Central venous hypercapnia
Metabolic acidosis
Respiratory acidosis
Hyperkalemia
Myoglobinemia
Elevated creatine phosphokinase

Symptoms (Subjective Findings)
Tachycardia
Tachypnea
Ventricular dysrhythmias
Cyanosis
Skin mottling
Fever—hot, flushed skin
Rigidity
Profuse sweating
Unstable blood pressure

*Primary signs and symptoms are italicized.

Table 43–2. ENVIRONMENTAL STIMULI AND PHARMACOLOGIC AGENTS THAT MAY TRIGGER MALIGNANT HYPERTHERMIA

Environmental Stimuli
Extensive skeletal muscle injury
Emotional crisis
Very hot and humid weather
Strenuous and prolonged exercise

Pharmacologic Agents
Halothane
Enflurane
Isoflurane (?)
Succinylcholine
d-Tubocurarine
Gallamine (?)
Amide local anesthetics—lidocaine, mepivacaine, bupivacaine, etidocaine
Caffeine

---

of MH (Table 43–2). Fatigue, emotional upset, or very hot and humid weather can trigger a waking febrile episode. Patients usually respond to dantrolene, surface cooling, and other symptomatic treatment. The anesthetic agents that trigger MH seem to affect the sarcoplasmic reticulum or the E-C coupling mechanism, or both. Because of their wide use, halothane and succinylcholine are the most common trigger agents. Amide local anesthetics, such as lidocaine, are also trigger agents; it has been demonstrated that lidocaine causes the release of calcium ions into the myoplasm in vitro. In MHS patients or in patients who have had an episode of acute MH in the operating room, all possible trigger agents should be stringently avoided. As another precaution, because emotional upsets trigger MH, the PACU nurse should provide a stress-free environment for the MHS patient.

Pharmacologic Agents Associated with Malignant Hyperthermia

Dantrolene Sodium (Dantrium). Dantrolene is a muscle relaxant that is chemically and pharmacologically unrelated to other muscle relaxants. It is the only known pharmacologic agent that is effective in the treatment of MH. The site of action of this drug is distal to the end plate within the muscle fiber. The main pharmacologic action of dantrolene results in a reduction in the release of calcium by the sarcoplasmic reticulum without affecting reuptake. Consequently, the concentration of calcium in the myoplasm is reduced, inhibiting the E-C coupling mechanism and causing muscle contraction to cease. When administered orally, dantrolene has a half-life of 8 hours; when administered intravenously, the half-life is 5 hours. When it is used in the treatment of acute MH, the intravenous dosage is 1 to 2 mg per kg, which can be repeated every 5 to 10 minutes with a maximum dose of 10 mg per kg. If the acute episode of MH occurs in the operating room and the patient is treated successfully, dantrolene therapy will be continued into the recovery (PACU) period to prevent recurrence of MH. After the acute period in the PACU has passed, the patient will be given oral dantrolene in four divided doses. Because dantrolene is poorly soluble, it is supplied in vials in the form of a lyophilized powder. To reconstitute a vial of lyophilized powder, 60 ml of sterile water for injection, USP, is added to the vial, and it is shaken until the solution is clear; many compatibility problems arise when dantrolene is mixed with solutions other than sterile water for injection, USP. Also, the sterile water for injection, USP, that is used to reconstitute the dantrolene should not contain any bacteriostatic agents because it is not unusual to use more than 2000 ml of diluent during the treatment of acute MH in an adult weighing 70 kg.

Procainamide (Procamide, Procapan, Pronestyl). Procainamide once was the main drug in the treatment of MH. The use of procainamide is controversial, particularly since the recommended initial dose is two to five times its cardiotoxic dose. Some authors suggest that if this drug is used in the treatment of MH, isoproterenol should be administered to maintain cardiac function. The recommended dose of procainamide is 0.5 to 1 mg per kg per min, up to a maximum dose of 15 to 30 mg per kg. The dosage should be lowered when there is a reduction in the heart rate or dysrhythmias. At a lower dose range, procainamide may be useful in the treatment of the dysrhythmias during the acute episode of MH.

Perioperative Management of the MH-Susceptible Patient

Preoperatively, the MHS patient may be given oral dantrolene in four divided doses of 4 to 7 mg per kg daily for 1 to 3 days before the administration of the anesthetic. The patient is usually well premedicated; however, anticholinergics, such as atropine, should be avoided because they interfere with the normal heat loss mechanisms and, in the case of atropine, can cause tachycardia that may cause

Table 43–3. DRUGS THAT ARE CONSIDERED SAFE TO ADMINISTER TO A MALIGNANT HYPERTHERMIA–SUSCEPTIBLE PATIENT

Nitrous oxide
Diazepam
Droperidol
Pancuronium
Thiopental
Ketamine
Fentanyl
Morphine
Ester local anesthetics—procaine, tetracaine, 2-chloroprocaine

confusion in the diagnosis of acute MH. Also, phenothiazines should be avoided in the perioperative period, because they may cause a release of calcium from the sarcoplasmic reticulum. Intraoperative anesthesia requires the use of agents that will not trigger an episode of MH (Table 43–3). Although regional anesthesia avoids the use of the general inhalation anesthetic agents and skeletal muscle relaxants, elevated temperatures in MHS patients have been reported with its use. If local anesthetic agents are to be used, amides such as lidocaine and mepivacaine should be avoided.

Intraoperative monitoring of the MHS patient includes the electrocardiographic, temperature, arterial blood gas (including acid-base), and precordial stethoscope determinations. These monitoring parameters should be continued into the PACU period (Table 43–4). Because some MHS patients have had MH triggered in the postoperative period, they should be followed for a minimum of 24 hours postoperatively and should not be subjected to anxiety or stress. These patients should be reassured that physicians and nurses have reliable instruments to monitor for MH and

Table 43–4. SUGGESTED COMPONENTS OF MONITORING OF THE PATIENT WITH ACUTE MALIGNANT HYPERTHERMIA

Continuous ECG (consider 12-lead ECG and EEG after acute phase)
Core and axillary temperature
Urine output
Arterial pressure line
Pulse and blood pressure
Central venous pressure*
Swan-Ganz catheters*

*Should be considered; however, do not delay treatment if the insertion of these monitors is physically or technically difficult.
ECG = electrocardiogram; EEG = electroencephalogram.

that prompt and effective treatment will be provided if it develops.

Treatment of Acute Malignant Hyperthermia in the PACU

The cornerstone of the successful treatment of MH is early detection (see Table 43–1). Table 43–5 lists the suggested equipment and drugs that should be kept in the PACU to be used in the treatment of acute MH. If the assessment indicates that the patient is developing acute MH, the following steps should be taken[11]:

1. Discontinue the use of any trigger agent (see Table 43–3), and SEND FOR HELP!
2. Rapidly ventilate the patient with large tidal volumes, using a bag-valve-mask system and oxygen (total oxygen flow should exceed 15 L per min). Oral endotracheal intubation should be performed if the patient's airway is compromised.
3. Insert arterial and central venous lines, and send venous and arterial blood samples to the laboratory for immediate results on electrolyte and arterial blood gas analysis.
4. Start reconstituting the dantrolene as soon as possible.
5. Administer the intravenous dantrolene—1 to 2 mg per kg over 1 to 2 minutes, up to 10 mg per kg or until the patient's temperature starts to decrease.
6. *Cool the patient.* Cover all exposed surfaces with towels soaked in water. Cover the wet towels with ice. Use cooling blankets and fans if possible. Use cold gastric lavage and hydrate with iced intravenous fluids. To avoid hypothermia, discontinue all the cooling interventions when body temperature decreases to 38°C.
7. Administer sodium bicarbonate intravenously at a dosage of 1 to 2 mEq per kg. When results of the arterial blood gas analysis are available, correct the base deficit using sodium bicarbonate according to the following formula[13]:

$$\text{base deficit} = 0.3 \times \text{weight (kg)} \times \text{base excess (mEq/L)}$$

If the $PaCO_2$ is elevated, increase the tidal ventilation of the patient. Do not administer sodium bicarbonate to correct respiratory acidosis, because the $PaCO_2$ will only increase, which may lead to ventricular fibrillation.
8. Constantly monitor the patient's core temperature, blood pressure, pulse, cardiac rhythm, and pupil size and reactivity, and watch for cyanosis (see Table 43–4).
9. The hyperkalemia can be treated with intravenous insulin and glucose (0.25 to 0.5 U per kg of insulin to 0.25 to 0.5 g per kg of glucose).
10. If possible, catheterize the bladder and monitor urinary output and appearance. To secure a high urinary output, furosemide (1 mg per kg) or mannitol (1 g per kg) may be given.
11. *Do NOT treat dysrhythmias with LIDOCAINE because it is a trigger agent.* Do not give intravenous calcium because it may also cause dysrhythmias.
12. Hypotension can be treated by the infusion of cold crystalloid solution.
13. Continue to send arterial and venous blood samples to the laboratory for prompt determination of arterial blood gases and electrolytes.
14. Look for such hopeful prognostic signs as a lessening coma, hyperactive tendon reflexes, and a stabilization of the tempera-

---

Table 43–5. SUGGESTED EQUIPMENT AND DRUGS TO BE USED IN THE TREATMENT OF ACUTE MALIGNANT HYPERTHERMIA

Equipment Needed
Intravenous lines with assorted cannula gauges
Central venous pressure sets (2)
Sterile venous and arterial strain gauge
Swan-Ganz catheter
Laboratory test tubes for blood chemistry analysis
Crystalloid solution (10 1000-ml bottles)—labeled **FOR HYPERTHERMIA ONLY** and stored in the PACU refrigerator
Bucket of cracked ice—labeled **FOR HYPERTHERMIA ONLY** and stored in freezer of the PACU refrigerator
Cooling blanket
Fan

Drugs Needed
Sodium bicarbonate (12 ampules of 8.4% strength)
Mannitol (4 ampules—12.4 g/50 ml)
Furosemide (4 vials)
Calcium gluconate (2 ampules—100 mg/10 ml)
Potassium chloride (2 ampules)
Glucose (2 bottles of 50% strength)
Iced intravenous saline (10 1000-ml bottles in refrigerator)
Procainamide (2000 mg)
Regular insulin (1 ampule of 100 units)
Dantrolene (Dantrium) intravenous—36 vials of lyophilized powder with at least 2200 ml of sterile water for injection, USP (*without a bacteriostatic agent*) to reconstitute the dantrolene

---

Note: All the above equipment and drugs should be stored in a box or cart in the PACU. The box or cart should be labeled **HYPERTHERMIA.**

ture. Once the temperature returns to normal, continue constant observation of the patient.

Complications Following Acute Malignant Hyperthermia

Renal failure can occur because of myoglobinuria or hypotension. Consumption coagulopathies, such as disseminated intravascular coagulation, have been reported along with acute heart failure and pulmonary edema. Brain deterioration can occur in patients who are not promptly diagnosed and treated for MH.

References

1. Augustine, S.: Hypothermia therapy in the post anesthesia care unit: A review. J. Post Anesth. Nurs., 5(4):254–263, 1990.
2. Barash, P., Cullen, B. and Stoelting, R.: Handbook of Clinical Anesthesia. 2nd ed. Philadelphia, J. B. Lippincott, 1993.
3. Burns, S., and Bostek, C.: Avoiding unintentional hypothermia: Anesthesia implications. Nurse Anesth., 1(3):128–133, 1990.
4. Feldman, M.: Inadvertent hypothermia: A threat to homeostasis in the post anesthetic patient. J. Post Anesth. Nurs., 3(2):82–87, 1988.
5. Flacke, J. and Flacke, W.: Inadvertent hypothermia: Frequent, insidious, and often serious. Semin. Anesth., 2(3):183–196, 1983.
6. Gronert, G.: Malignant hyperthermia. Anesthesiology, 53:395–423, 1980.
7. Hardy, F., Cirillo, B. and Gutzeit, N.: Rewarming patients in the PACU: Can we make a difference? J. Post Anesth. Nurs., 3(5):313–316, 1988.
8. Katz, J., Benumof, J., and Kadis, L.: Anesthesia and Uncommon Diseases. 3rd ed. Philadelphia, W. B. Saunders, 1990.
9. Lipton, J., and Giesecke, A.: Body temperature and shivering in the perioperative patient. Semin. Anesth., 7(1):3–10, 1988.
10. Litwack, K.: Practical points in the management of hypothermia. J. Post Anesth. Nurs., 3(5):339–341, 1988.
11. Miller, R.: Anesthesia. 3rd ed. New York, Churchill Livingstone, 1990.
12. Morrison, R.: Hypothermia in the elderly. Int. Anesthesiol. Clin., 26(2):124–133, 1988.
13. Stoelting, R., Dierdorf, S., and McCammon, R.: Anesthesia and Co-Existing Disease. 2nd ed. New York, Churchill Livingstone, 1989.
14. Vaughan, M., Vaughan, R., and Cork, R.: Postoperative hypothermia in adults: Relationship of age, anesthesia, and shivering to rewarming. Anesth. Analg., 60(10):746–751, 1981.
15. Yarborough, J.: Malignant hyperthermia. AANA J., 52(1):58–64, 1984.

Post Anesthesia Care of the Shock Trauma Patient

CHAPTER 44

Myrna E. Mamaril, M.S., R.N., C.P.A.N.

In the United States, trauma continues to impact the lives of more than 70 million people each year and results in about 100,000 deaths. Swiftly and without warning, traumatic injuries span all ages, cultures, and races, reaching epidemic proportions. Furthermore, trauma accounts for more deaths in the United States during the first four decades of life than any other disease and is the fourth leading cause of death among the entire U.S. population.[24]

Although 80 percent of all deaths attributed to trauma occur within minutes to hours after the injury, the remaining 20 percent of deaths occur as a result of complications.[12] Overwhelming infection and sepsis result from these traumatic injuries, and trauma patients are at risk for respiratory, circulatory, and renal failure. Numerous pathologic conditions may contribute to this high incidence of late mortality due to sepsis.

PREHOSPITAL PHASE

During the past 20 years, the ultimate goal of emergency medical services has been to improve the field stabilization, resuscitation, and subsequent transportation of the multitrauma patient to the appropriate-level trauma center.[2] The concept of the "golden hour," which was introduced by R. Adams Cowley, M.D., emphasizes the importance of the time in which resuscitation of severely injured patients must begin so as to achieve maximal survival.[24]

During the prehospital phase, vital information regarding the trauma patients' condition at the scene of the injury reveals important clues to how the patients later will present. For example, if the patients experienced a prolonged extrication period at the scene, their airways may have been compromised; they may have had active or uncontrolled bleeding; or they may have been exposed to environmental elements, decreasing core temperature.

Other conditions at the scene that may influence the trauma patient's outcome include such considerations as (1) whether seat belts were used; (2) whether the passenger was ejected from the car; (3) what position the patient was found in; (4) whether the car rolled over; (5) whether the windshield was broken; (6) whether the patient wore a motorcycle helmet; and (7) whether there were other fatalities at the scene. All these observations by the first providers help piece each part of the trauma puzzle together to ensure a comprehensive approach to the management of the trauma patient.

Mechanisms of Injury

To accurately assess the trauma patient in the post anesthesia care unit (PACU), the nurse needs to have a basic understanding of the different mechanisms of injury. Because the mechanisms of injury are related to the type of injuring force and subsequent tissue response, a thorough understanding of these aspects of injury helps in determining the extent and nature of the damage.[27] The major factors that influence injury are the velocity of the objects and the force in terms of physical motion of moving or stationary bodies.[4] (Force is the mass of an object times acceleration.) Numerous studies conclude that mechanism of injury helps identify common injury combinations, predict eventual outcomes, and explain the type of injury.[24, 27]

Various forms of traumatic injuries are blunt (high velocity); penetrating, such as gunshot and stab wounds; falls from great heights; and chemical, electrical, and thermal burns. Motor vehicle accidents create forces that fracture extremities, crush organs, and lead to massive blood loss and soft-tissue damage.[8] Finally, forces are depicted in relation to acceleration, deceleration, shearing, and compression.[4, 14, 27]

Blunt Trauma

Blunt trauma may best be described as a wounding force that does not communicate to the outside of the body. High-velocity motor vehicle accidents and falls from great heights cause blunt-trauma injuries that are associated with direct impact, deceleration, continuous pressure, and shearing and rotary forces.[24] These blunt-trauma injuries are usually more serious and life threatening than other types of trauma because the extent of the injuries is less obvious and diagnosis is more difficult.[27] Because blunt injuries leave little outward evidence of the extent of internal damage, the nurse must be extremely thorough in making observations and assessments.

When the body decelerates, the organs continue to move forward at the original speed. As the body's organs move in the forward direction, they are torn from their attachments by rotary and shearing forces.[24] Furthermore, blunt forces disrupt blood vessels and nerves. This mechanism of injury to the microcirculation causes widespread epithelial and endothelial damage, stimulating cells to release their constituents and further activating the complement, the arachidonic acid, and the coagulation cascades. Finally, blunt trauma may mask more serious complications related to the pathophysiology of the injury.

Penetrating Trauma

Penetrating wounds, such as stab and gunshot wounds, are produced by a foreign body. The mechanism of injury causes the crushing of underlying tissues. Tissue damage inflicted by bullets is dependent on the bullet's velocity, range, mass, and trajectory. These penetrating wounds cause disruption of tissues and cellular function, resulting in the introduction of debris and foreign bodies into the wound.[4, 26] Finally, the insult to the body may occur as local ischemia, or it may extend to a fulminant hemorrhage resulting from these penetrating injuries.

Contusion of Tissues

When blunt trauma is significant enough to produce capillary injury and destruction, contusion of tissues occurs. Consequently, the extravasation of blood causes discoloration, pain, and swelling.[5] If a large vessel ruptures, a hematoma may occur, producing a distinct, palpable lesion. With a massive contusion or hematoma, an increase in myofascial pressures often results in sequelae known as *compartment syndrome*.[5] A compartment is a section of muscle enclosed in a confined, supportive membrane called *fascia*, and compartment syndrome is a condition in which increased pressure inside an osteofascial compartment impedes circulation, resulting in an alteration in neurovascular function. Damaged vessels in the ischemic muscle dilate in response to histamine and other vasoactive chemical substances, such as the arachidonic cascade and oxygen free radicals. This dilatation, with resultant leakage of fluid into the tissues causing loss of capillary integrity, impedes the microvascular perfusion and results in increased edema and tissue pressure.[5] These pathologic changes cause a repetitive cycle within the confined tissues, increasing swelling and leading to increased compartment pressures.

STABILIZATION PHASE

The initial assessment, resuscitation, and stabilization processes that are initiated in the admitting area (Fig. 44–1) extend into the operating room (OR), the PACU (Fig. 44–2), and the critical care unit. Because the most common cause of shock in the trauma patient is hypovolemia resulting from acute blood loss, the ultimate goal in fluid resuscitation is prompt restoration of blood volume through replacement of fluids so that tissue perfusion and delivery of oxygen to the tissues are maintained.[11, 22] Rapid-volume infusors, such as the Bard 37 and the level 1 fluid warmer (Fig. 44–3) are able to deliver warmed intravenous fluids at a rate of 500 to 700 ml per min.[3, 22] (The fluids should be warmed to prevent hypothermia.) Crystalloids, colloids, or blood products may be used effectively to reverse hypovolemia.

Crystalloids are electrolyte solutions that diffuse through the capillary endothelium and can be distributed evenly throughout the extracellular compartment. Examples of crystalloid solutions are lactated Ringer's injection, Plasma-Lyte, and normal saline solution. Although controversy exists between crystalloid versus colloid fluid resuscitation in multiple trauma, the American College of Surgeons' Committee on Trauma recommends that isotonic crystalloid solutions of lactated Ringer's or normal saline be used for that purpose.[23]

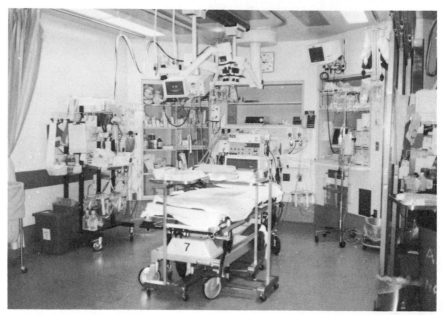

FIGURE 44–1. Trauma Resuscitation Unit in the Admitting Area at the R. Adams Cowley Shock Trauma Center at the Maryland Institute of Emergency Medical Services Systems, Baltimore, Maryland.

Furthermore, crystalloids are much cheaper than colloids.

Colloid solutions contain protein or starch molecules or aggregates of molecules that remain uniformly distributed in fluid and fail to form a true solution.[22, 23] When colloid solutions are administered, the molecules remain in the intravascular space, thereby increasing the os-motic pressure gradient within the vascular compartment. Volume for volume, the half-life of colloids is much longer than that of crystalloids. Colloid solutions commonly used are plasma protein fraction, dextran, normal human serum albumin, and hetastarch.

Although crystalloid and colloid solutions serve as primary resuscitation fluids for vol-

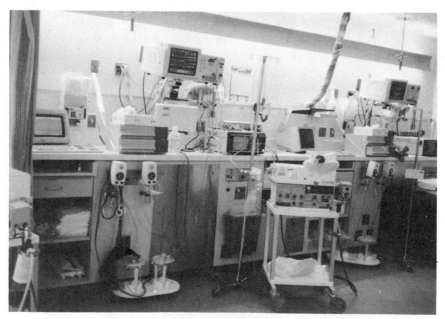

FIGURE 44–2. Patient unit in the Post Anesthesia Care Unit at the R. Adams Cowley Shock Trauma Center at the Maryland Institute of Emergency Medical Services Systems, Baltimore, Maryland.

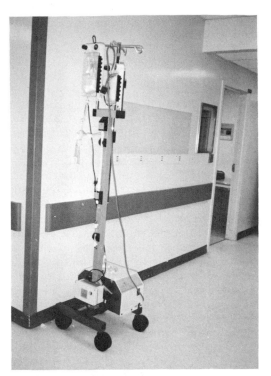

FIGURE 44-3. Level 1 high-efficiency fluid warmer with rapid-pressure infusion devices. Photograph was taken at the R. Adams Cowley Shock Trauma Center at the Maryland Institute of Emergency Medical Services Systems, Baltimore, Maryland.

ume depletion, blood transfusions are necessary to restore the capacity of the blood to carry adequate amounts of oxygen. Furthermore, blood component therapy is considered after the trauma patient's response to the initial resuscitative fluids is evaluated.[22] Because type-specific whole blood is often administered to trauma victims during the first hours of the resuscitation period, this blood product may be administered more rapidly with less likelihood of transfusion reactions. Other blood products may be given to the trauma patient, such as platelets and fresh frozen plasma owing to a consumption coagulopathy. Finally, the therapeutic goal of all blood component therapy is to restore the circulating blood volume, to give back other needed blood with red blood cells, and to correct coagulation deficiencies.[23]

In summary, fluid resuscitation of the trauma patient must be administered early and rapidly to ensure that adequate circulating volume, as well as vital oxygen and nutrients, is delivered to the tissues.

Diagnostic Studies and Protocols

Diagnostic tests and laboratory studies play a vital role in establishing the patient's baseline as well as current status. The results of these tests predicate the treatment protocols that will be initiated.

Comprehensive diagnostic studies are required to establish an accurate diagnosis and to plan effective treatment of the patient with multiple injuries. The initial routine studies may be arterial blood gas determinations, diagnostic peritoneal lavage, urinalysis, complete blood count, electrolyte levels, prothrombin and partial thromboplastin times, and type and crossmatch. Other diagnostic studies that may be ordered for suspected injuries include lateral cervical spine, upright anteroposterior chest, and anteroposterior pelvic radiographs, computed tomography (CT) scan, 12-lead electrocardiogram, ultrasound, and toxicology laboratory studies. Pregnancy tests should be performed on all women of childbearing age.

Collaborative Approach

Collaborative practice is essential in the care of the trauma patient. During the initial prehospital phase, vital communication with the trauma team is initiated at the trauma center. Subsequently, when the patient is first admitted, a comprehensive approach to patient care is initiated. Together, the nurse, anesthesiologist, respiratory therapist, surgeon, and radiology technician form a collaborative environment so that care becomes focused and directed.[2] This collaborative practice continues through the intraoperative as well as the post anesthesia periods.

The OR nurse communicates a comprehensive systems report to the PACU nurse and verbally reviews any definitive findings of the CT scan, including whether there is generalized edema or a lesion. Vital nursing information is communicated to the appropriate OR and PACU nurses caring for the trauma patient.

POST ANESTHESIA PHASE

Anesthesia Report

The anesthesiologist's report provides valuable information to the PACU nurse concerning the trauma patient's presenting status. This report includes significant facts pertaining to the mechanism of injury, prehospital phase, admitting and stabilization period, operative report, intubation, anesthetic agents, estimated blood loss, fluid resuscitation, cardiopulmonary status, and treatment abnormalities.

When reviewing the anesthesia report, the nurse should note if there was difficulty intubating the patient. The nurse should be suspicious if the secretions are pink tinged or bloody, which may otherwise indicate an infectious process, pulmonary edema, or uncontrolled hemorrhage.

A detailed operative report reveals the surgical insult to the patient. It also presents a comprehensive review of all anesthetic agents that reflects a rapid sequence of induction, balanced analgesia, and heavy use of narcotics, including the time these agents were given as well as the amount and type of muscle relaxants and reversal agents used.

The anesthesia report should reveal any untoward events that occurred during surgery, such as hypothermic or hypotensive events and significant dysrhythmias, including ischemic changes.

Another important aspect of the anesthesia report is the estimated blood loss and fluid replacement, which are carefully monitored through the hemodynamic status of the trauma patient. With the use of arterial lines and Swan-Ganz catheters, the anesthesiologist can closely monitor the patient's hemodynamic status. In severe chest injuries, Thora-Drain chest drainage units as well as autotransfusions or Cell Saver blood recovery systems may be used to conserve the vital, life-sustaining resource—blood. Because the goal of treatment is to keep the patient in a hyperdynamic state, the intraoperative trending should reveal that the patient is volume supported. This is because the body responds hypermetabolically to trauma, and achieving that state ensures the delivery of oxygen and other nutrients to essential tissues in the body. End-organ perfusion is monitored and measured by the urinary output.

Nursing Assessment

Nursing assessment of the shock trauma patient in the PACU begins with evaluating the patency of the airway. This may begin by proper positioning of the patient's head, always maintaining the cervical spine protection if injury is suspected. Also, the patient may need to have the airway cleared by suctioning and removal of secretions. Finally, the use of airway adjuncts, such as oropharyngeal and nasopharyngeal airways, may be needed.

Next, the nurse evaluates the patient's breathing. Recalling the mechanism of injury, such as blunt or penetrating trauma to the chest, the nurse should be highly suspicious of pulmonary contusions, fractured ribs, or shearing forces. By observation, the nurse assesses spontaneous respirations, respiratory excursion, chest wall integrity, symmetry, depth, respiratory rate, use of accessory muscles, and the work of breathing. By auscultation, the nurse assesses the lungs for bilateral breath sounds as well as evaluates for adventitious breath sounds. In addition, the use of pulse oximetry and end-tidal CO_2 monitoring augments the complete respiratory assessment of the trauma patient.

After thoroughly evaluating the airway and breathing, the nurse begins the circulatory assessment. With the use of palpation, the nurse evaluates the circulation, checking the quality, location, and rate of the pulses. If the nurse can palpate a radial pulse, the arterial pressure is at least 80 mm Hg. If no radial pulse is palpable, the nurse then palpates the femoral pulse (a situation indicating a pressure of 70 mm Hg). If only a carotid pulse is palpable, then the arterial pressure is approximately 60 mm Hg. The patient's blood pressure and pulse (rate and rhythm) should be monitored via the cardiac monitor.

Simultaneously, during the palpation of pulses, the nurse assesses the patient's skin temperature, color, and capillary refill.

Another aspect of assessment is circulatory access. The nurse should inspect the peripheral, central, and arterial lines, ensuring the patency of the lines and healthy intravenous sites. Each line should be identified and labeled to distinguish the type of parenteral fluid and medication administration in use.

The operative site and all dressings and drains should be assessed and described. Furthermore, all drains should be labeled, drainage of fluid measured, and color and consistency described. Precise documentation of all fluid output is essential for accurate fluid replacement.

After completing the initial primary survey, the PACU nurse begins the secondary comprehensive survey with a high degree of suspicion concerning the trauma patient's mechanism of injury for specific post anesthesia problems. Frequently, the initial surgery is directed at repairing the major life-threatening injuries. During the comprehensive secondary survey, head-to-toe assessment is performed as the trauma patient is emerging from anesthesia. The PACU nurse may discover other injuries, such as pulmonary, cardiac, or renal contusions and compartment syndrome of different extremities.

The head-to-toe assessment begins with a neurologic assessment, including the patient's level of consciousness; the appropriateness of verbal response; pupillary reactivity, size, and shape; equality of pupillary response to light and accommodation; movement; sensation; and pain response in the extremities. Each aspect is carefully evaluated and documented. Next, the head and face are inspected for abrasions, lacerations, puncture wounds, ecchymoses, and edema. These structures are palpated for subcutaneous emphysema or tenderness. The eyes are assessed for gross vision by asking the patient to identify the number of fingers the nurse is holding up. Furthermore, the eyes are evaluated for ecchymosis, "raccoon's eyes," and possible conjunctival hemorrhage. Extraocular movements are also evaluated.

The ears are inspected for Battle's sign (ecchymosis behind the ears). The nose is examined for drainage of blood or clear fluid. Clear fluid draining from the nose or ears should be checked for the presence of cerebrospinal fluid.

The neck should be evaluated for edema, ecchymosis, tracheal deviation, pulsating or distended neck veins, and subcutaneous emphysema. As the PACU nurse continues the assessment of the chest, the anterior as well as the lateral thorax and axilla are inspected for lacerations, abrasions, contusions, puncture wounds, ecchymosis, and edema. The nurse carefully palpates the chest for tenderness and subcutaneous emphysema. The chest wall is observed for symmetry, depth, and equality of expansion and excursion. Again, breathing is observed for rate, degree of effort, use of accessory muscles, or paradoxic chest wall movements. Breath and heart sounds are auscultated, noting adventitious lung sounds (such as wheezing, rales, and friction rubs) or murmurs, bruits, and muffled heart sounds. The PACU nurse carefully notes the patient's facial expressions or body reactions that may suggest possible cardiac contusions or rib fractures.

The next areas to be inspected are the abdomen, pelvis, and genitalia. Again, all abrasions, contusions, edema, and ecchymoses are noted. The abdomen is auscultated for bowel sounds and palpated for tenderness and rigidity. The nasogastric tube, jejunostomy, or T-tube drainage is examined for color, consistency, and amount of fluid. In suspected internal hemorrhage, abdominal girth measurements should be assessed. The pelvis is palpated for stability and tenderness, especially over the crests and the pubis. (Priapism may be noted. In addition, preexisting herpes may also be present.) The urinary catheter is inspected for color and amount of drainage. Hematuria may indicate kidney or bladder trauma. Furthermore, urinary output must be vigilantly monitored to ensure a minimum of 30 ml per hr in adults so that the patient does not develop acute renal failure. The vagina and rectum are checked carefully for neurologic function and bloody drainage.

All extremities are examined for circulatory, sensory, and motor functions. Frequently, because the trauma patient is rushed to the OR to correct life-threatening injuries, minor soft-tissue injuries may be missed. Later, however, in the PACU, these soft-tissue and musculoskeletal injuries may develop into compartment syndrome. Again, each extremity must be thoroughly examined for abrasions, contusions, puncture wounds, ecchymoses, and edema. If there is neurovascular compromise, an arteriogram or venogram may be performed as a conclusive diagnostic study.

The patient is then log-rolled onto his or her side, maintaining cervical spine integrity, to assess the back, flanks, and buttocks for abrasions, contusions, and tenderness. Posterior chest assessment is completed as a last step in the head-to-toe assessment. Finally, a detailed, succinct description of the primary and secondary assessment is documented.

Pain

Assessment and management of pain are important parts of the scope of care provided to the trauma patient in the PACU. The trauma patient experiences severe musculoskeletal injuries or even ruptured organs, causing severe pain. The PACU nurse needs to recognize that because pain is subjective, verbal, nonverbal, and hemodynamic changes that indicate the patient may be exhibiting signs of pain should be noted. Pain scales should be used to augment the nursing assessment of pain.

According to Mlynczak, optimal management of acute pain may employ the following techniques: (1) patient-controlled analgesia and intravenous, subcutaneous, or epidural infusions; (2) intravenous conscious sedation using alfentanil; (3) major plexus blocks; and (4) fentanyl patches.[17] There is a higher incidence of substance abuse in the trauma patient population that may require higher doses of narcotics or analgesics.[3] Other relaxation techniques, such as music therapy and guided imagery, may be initiated and used as adjuncts when the trauma patient returns for subsequent surgical procedures or wound débridement. Finally, continual pain assessment is vital to the patient's optimal care.

Psychological Assessment

Often, the psychological and emotional condition of the trauma patient is not considered a priority because the initial events are life threatening. However, when the patient regains consciousness in the PACU, this aspect of the patient's care may prove to be the most challenging.

As the patient emerges from anesthesia, the PACU nurse orients him or her to place and time. Because the patient may not even remember or recall the event that caused the accident, the nurse orients the patient to the hospital. Fear of death, mutilation, or change in body image may increase the patient's anxiety. The trauma patient may regain consciousness only to find that his or her extremities are in a Hoffmann apparatus or even amputated. Because a high incidence of injuries is related to alcohol or substance abuse, the patient may have no memory of events before, during, or after the injury. The patient may experience alterations in visual and auditory functions. If the patient was alert at the scene and remembers that loved ones were severely injured or killed, the patient may become upset or hysterical, often reliving the tragic event. Consequently, the patient not only experiences loss of body integrity and control but also the loss of loved ones.

The PACU nurse needs to be supportive but also focused on maintaining the patient's integrity and coping skills. The nurse needs to speak to the patient calmly, slowly, and clearly, using simple language that is easily understood. The practitioner should be honest with the patient.

Infectious Risk

Because trauma patients represent the unknown population, infectious or communicable diseases, such as human immunodeficiency viral infection, hepatitis, venereal diseases, measles, chickenpox, and mumps, may be transmitted by these patients. The nurse needs to use universal precautions to decrease the risk of exposure to pathogens. The use of gloves, protective eyewear, masks, impervious gowns, and frequent handwashing is important in reducing the risk of exposure to blood and body fluids. The trauma nurse should also consider being immunized with hepatitis B

vaccine as an additional precaution because of the high risk of exposure to blood and body fluids.

Nursing Diagnosis

Nursing diagnoses are identified, such as ineffective airway clearance, ineffective gas exchange, alteration in cardiac output, alteration in tissue perfusion, high risk for fluid volume deficit, high risk for hypothermia, high risk for injury, altered comfort, altered thought processes, communication, high risk for anxiety, ineffective coping, disturbance in self-concept, and posttraumatic stress disorder. After nursing diagnoses are formulated, a plan of care is developed and implemented, and patient outcomes are evaluated.

The focus of the nursing care of the trauma patient is on vigilant, continuous reassessment. Consequently, treatment priorities are established on the basis of presenting signs and symptoms as well as abnormal laboratory values and diagnostic studies. The PACU nurse must be cognizant of the complex pathophysiologic responses to the traumatic injury and should always anticipate that the trauma patient might exhibit subtle or overt signs of shock. Furthermore, if shock progresses, the PACU nurse should be aware of other complications, such as adult respiratory distress syndrome, acute renal failure, and multisystem organ failure. Nursing care of the trauma patient provides a special challenge because of the unique physiologic responses.

SHOCK AS A COMPLICATION IN THE MULTITRAUMA PATIENT

The most common complication associated with traumatic injuries is shock. Although there may be different types of shock, all exhibit a profound problem with inadequate delivery of oxygen and nutrients to the cells, resulting in inadequate tissue perfusion.[10, 19] A measure of the body's overall metabolism is expressed as oxygen consumption ($\dot{V}O_2$).[25] When $\dot{V}O_2$ is inadequate, cellular hypoxia evolves. The magnitude of oxygen debt correlates with the lactic acid levels; indeed, this measure quantifies the severity and prognosis in different shock states.[10] Consequently, this complex syndrome of disequilibrium between oxygen supply and demand causes a functional impairment in cells, tissues, organs, and, eventually, body systems.[19] Important tissues such as the heart, brain, liver, kidneys, and lungs require large amounts of oxygen to support their specialized functions. Furthermore, these functions can be maintained only by energy derived from aerobic metabolism, and they cease when oxygen is in short supply.

Unfortunately, ischemia rapidly initiates a complex series of events that affect every organelle and subcellular system in the body. As cells become anoxic, adenosine triphosphate stores are depleted and virtually all energy-dependent functions cease. Protein synthesis is depleted. There are changes in ion transport and glycolysis, resulting in the loss of intracellular potassium and the production of lactic acid. This may result in lethal complications for the ischemic heart. Finally, irreversible anoxic cellular injury kills vital tissues.

Clinical manifestations of shock include signs and symptoms of decreased end-organ perfusion: cool, clammy skin; cyanosis; restlessness; altered level of consciousness; altered skin temperature; tachycardia; dysrhythmias; tachypnea; pulmonary edema; decreased urinary output; increased platelet, leukocyte, and erythrocyte counts; sludging of blood; and metabolic acidosis.[10]

Types of Shock

There are three major types of shock: (1) hypovolemic; (2) cardiogenic; and (3) distributive (Table 44–1). The first and most common type of shock, hypovolemic, results from an acute hemorrhagic loss in circulating blood volume that decreases vascular filling pressure.[24] The second type of shock is cardiogenic, which results from an impaired ability of the heart to pump, causing inadequate cardiac output. In the trauma patient, this may be secondary to cardiac tamponade, direct cardiac injury, or myocardial infarction (MI). The third type of shock is distributive, which causes an abnormality in the vascular system, producing a maldistribution of blood volume.[19] Distributive shock include neurogenic, anaphylactic, and septic types.

Hypovolemic Shock

Hypovolemic shock may be defined as a decrease in intravascular volume, resulting in the fluid volume ineffectively filling the intravascular compartment.[19] Consequently, hypovolemic shock may evolve from many causes, such as internal and external hemorrhage,

plasma volume loss, third spacing of fluids, and decreased venous return.[25]

Classifications of Hemorrhage. As hemorrhage progresses, the cardiovascular system produces characteristic clinical manifestations that are classified according to approximate blood loss.[24] The following hemorrhagic classifications are described in the conceptual framework of the Committee on Trauma of the American College of Surgeons' Advanced Trauma Life Support Course.[6]

Class I hemorrhage, or the early phase, may be defined as a loss of as much as 750 ml of blood, or approximately 1 to 15 percent of the body's total blood volume. Minimal physiologic changes occur in heart rate, blood pressure, capillary refill, respiratory rate, and urinary output. However, the patient may experience mild anxiety in response to the sympathetic nervous system.

Class II hemorrhage, or the moderate phase, may be described as a loss of 750 to 1500 ml of blood, or approximately 15 to 30 percent of blood volume. In this phase, multiple, incremental physiologic changes occur. The patient may experience increased anxiety and restlessness as a result of cerebral stimulation by the sympathetic nervous system and subsequent catecholamine release.[7, 15] The heart rate may be higher than 100 beats per min. Although minimal changes in blood pressure occur, peripheral vasoconstriction does develop, and a rise in diastolic blood pressure results, decreasing pulse pressure. Capillary refill is delayed slightly, and the skin is cool and pale. Finally, urinary output may be slightly depressed.

Class III hemorrhage, or the progressive phase, may be described as a loss of 1500 to 2000 ml of blood, or a 30 to 40 percent loss of blood volume. These patients exhibit signs of cerebral hypoperfusion, hypoxia, and acidosis that create a progressive reduction in the level of consciousness. The patient may be confused, agitated, and anxious, and the heart rate may be higher than 120 beats per min. The patient may experience systolic as well as diastolic hypotension. Capillary refill time may be delayed more than 2 seconds. Deep, rapid respirations result from the ensuing metabolic acidosis. As renal perfusion decreases, urinary output may be 5 to 15 ml per hr.

Class IV hemorrhage is described as a blood loss of more than 2000 ml of blood, or approximately 40 percent of the body's blood volume. This significant blood loss profoundly impacts the trauma patient. The patient's level of consciousness may be lethargic, stuporous, or unresponsive. The heart rate may be 140 beats per

Table 44–1. TYPES OF SHOCK

Type	Definition	Causes	Symptoms
Hypovolemic	Caused by a decrease in the intravascular volume relative to the vascular capacity and is generally associated with a blood volume deficit	Hemorrhage Excessive vomiting Excessive diarrhea Severe dehydration	Hypotension Tachycardia Cool, clammy skin Low central venous pressure Decreased urine output
Cardiogenic	Caused by impaired function of the heart as a pump	Acute myocardial infarction Pulmonary embolus Tamponade	Hypotension Bradycardia or tachycardia Increased central venous pressure
Distributive Neurogenic	Caused by damage to or pharmacologic blockage of the sympathetic nervous system, producing vasodilatation of the arterioles in the affected portion of the body and increased vascular capacity	Deep general anesthesia High spinal anesthesia Disease or damage of the spinal cord Brain damage	Hypotension (high spinal anesthesia and spinal cord damage) Bradycardia (high spinal anesthesia and spinal cord damage) Hypertension (early), then hypotension (late), in the patient with brain damage Tachycardia (early), then bradycardia (late), in the patient with brain damage
Septic	Associated with severe sepsis. It can be divided into *hyperdynamic*, associated with impaired cell metabolism with normal or increased cardiac output, or *hypodynamic*, which has relative or absolute hypovolemia due to increased capillary leakage and low cardiac output	The effects of various noxious chemicals and vasoactive substances liberated from damaged, ischemic, or infected tissues	High fever Marked vasodilation Sludging of the blood Hypotension Tachycardia
Anaphylactic	An exaggerated hypersensitivity reaction to a drug or other substance	Administration or contact with some type of antigen	Bronchospasm Hypotension Arrhythmia Cardiac arrest

min or higher, and the peripheral pulses may be weak and difficult to palpate. The capillary refill time may be more than 10 seconds. The patient may experience severe hypotension, and the blood pressure may be difficult to obtain. The skin may be cold, clammy, diaphoretic, and even cyanotic. The respiratory rate is shallow, irregular and higher than 35 breaths per min. Finally, there is no renal end-organ perfusion, resulting in anuria.

According to Stene and associates, the treatment of patients experiencing classes I and II hemorrhage is rapid infusion of 1 or 2 L of balanced salt solution, thus maintaining a renal output of more than 0.5 ml per kg per hr.[24] Patients with class III hemorrhage may tolerate a low hematocrit (20 to 25 percent) and not require blood transfusions. However, patients with class IV hemorrhage require not only 2 L of crystalloids but also blood transfusions (packed red blood cells or whole blood) maintaining 0.5 ml per kg per hr.

Treatment. The primary goal of treating patients with hypovolemic shock is fluid replacement. By filling the vascular "tank," the heart is able to generate adequate cardiac output and produce enough hydrostatic pressure to allow perfusion of the tissues.[28]

Cardiogenic Shock

Cardiogenic shock induced by inadequate cardiac output usually occurs in the trauma patient secondary to pericardial tamponade, direct injury to the heart muscle (e.g., cardiac lacerations, contusions, and ruptured heart or injury to heart valves or septa), or, occasionally, MI.[24] MIs, however, may either precipitate or precede the traumatic event. Consequently, the patient with a history of heart disease or age-related cardiac reserve limitations or who requires myocardial depressants, such as anesthesia, has a high propensity for cardiogenic shock.[15] Finally, this trauma patient population is also at greater risk for developing cardiac failure owing to the rapid fluid resuscitation.

Cardiogenic shock is circulatory failure caused by a consequence of impairment of cardiac pumping, not by a loss of intravascular fluid volume. This impaired pumping ability of the heart may result from destruction of contractility of the ventricles, as in MI. Another cause of pump failure occurs from the disruption of normal conduction sequence, as in heart blocks or dysrhythmias. Myocardial depression, resulting from the release of vasoactive substances like myocardial depressant factor during septic shock, causes dysfunction and decreased myocardial contractility. Cardiogenic shock may also be caused by an obstructive source, such as acute pulmonary embolism, dissecting aortic aneurysm, vena cava obstruction, and cardiac tamponade. These conditions, however, differ from the other causes in that the myocardium is normal. Finally, the result of all these pathologic mechanisms is decreased cardiac output, which is the basic physiologic defect in cardiogenic shock.[28]

Another method of classifying causes of cardiogenic shock is to identify the shock as either coronary or noncoronary. Rice described coronary cardiogenic shock as an obstructive coronary artery disease process that interrupts blood flow and oxygen delivery to heart muscle cells, resulting in ischemia and death.[19] The infarcted area of heart muscle is necrotic and dead, thus providing no function. Because the area of infarction and the surrounding area of ischemic heart muscle do not contract normally, the heart's ability to pump blood is compromised.

Patients with acute MIs are at greatest risk of developing cardiogenic shock, especially when a significant portion (more than 40 percent) of the left ventricle is involved. This loss of contractility reveals a low cardiac output, elevated left-ventricular filling pressure, peripheral vasoconstriction, and arterial hypotension. Another problem involves the volume of blood accumulating in the left ventricle after systolic ejection, increasing the left-ventricular filling pressure. This back-pressure mechanism causes the following sequence of events: (1) an increased left-atrial pressure; (2) an increased pulmonary venous pressure; and (3) an increased pulmonary capillary pressure, resulting in pulmonary interstitial edema and intra-alveolar edema.[19] A small percentage of MIs, however, do involve the damaged right ventricle, which does not propel sufficient blood forward through the lungs into the left heart.[19] Again, cardiac output decreases, and systemic circulation is not sufficient to maintain the body's needs.

As discussed previously, noncoronary cardiogenic shock may develop in the absence of coronary artery disease and heart muscle damage, such as cardiomyopathies, valvular heart abnormalities, cardiac tamponade, and dysrhythmias.[19]

Cardiogenic shock may be defined as shock secondary to acute myocardial dysfunction, including the following clinical and diagnostic criteria: systolic blood pressure less than 80 mm Hg, or less than 30 mm Hg of baseline in the hypertensive patient; cardiac index less than 2.1 L per min per m^2; urinary output less than 20 ml per hr; diminished cerebral perfusion evidenced by confusion or obtundation; and cold, clammy, cyanotic skin characteristic of a low cardiac output state.[28] However, classic signs and symptoms of cardiogenic shock, such as pulmonary congestion, edema, neck vein distention, and hepatic congestion, may not be seen in the trauma patient with co-existing acute hypovolemia.[15]

Other clinical indicators may be obtained through hemodynamic monitoring. Cardiac, stroke, and left-ventricular stroke work indexes are decreased because of pump failure. Pulmonary artery and pulmonary capillary wedge pressures are increased, indicating an increased left-ventricular end-diastolic pressure. Systemic vascular resistance is increased, reflecting vasoconstriction. Systemic venous oxygen saturation is decreased because of decreased cardiac output and increased oxygen extraction from the capillary bed. Arterial blood gas determinations reveal respiratory and metabolic acidosis that is associated with hypoxemia. Consequently, cardiogenic shock is the most lethal, resulting in mortality rates ranging from 80 to 100 percent.

Treatment. The importance of early recognition and treatment of cardiogenic shock cannot be overemphasized. Prompt improvement of myocardial oxygen supply and tissue perfusion, thus decreasing myocardial oxygen demand, is vital not only to minimizing heart damage but also to increasing the trauma patient's chance of survival. The goals of treatment for cardiogenic shock are to establish an airway, maintain ventilation and oxygenation, provide proper positioning, relieve pain, correct acidosis, monitor urinary output, and deliver pharmacologic support to improve or correct cardiac rhythm. Furthermore, increasing cardiac output may be achieved by judiciously increasing intravascular volume to improve preload. The heart rate and myocardial contractility may be increased with the inotropic and vasoactive drugs such as epinephrine, dopamine, and dobutamine. Another goal of therapy is to decrease afterload, which may be accomplished by lowering peripheral vascular resistance. Other important pharmacologic agents that may be employed in cardiogenic shock are vasopressors, vasodilators, adrenergic blocking agents, corticosteroids, digitalis, and thrombolytic agents.

When pharmacologic support fails to improve the oxygen supply and demand balance, alternative methods such as the intra-aortic balloon pump and the right-ventricular and left-ventricular assist devices help increase myocardial oxygen supply, decrease myocardial $\dot{V}O_2$, relieve pulmonary congestion, and improve organ perfusion.[21]

Distributive Shock

Distributive, or vasogenic, shock is an abnormal placement or a maldistribution of the vascular volume.[19] Indeed, the heart's ability to pump blood, as well as the body's blood volume, is normal. Therefore, this category of shock describes a unique pathologic condition existing within the vascular circulatory network that causes an alteration in blood vessels. The three types of distributive shock are neurogenic, anaphylactic, and septic.

Neurogenic shock

Neurogenic shock is described as a tremendous increase in the vascular capacity such that even the normal amount of blood becomes incapable of adequately filling the circulatory system.[9] When the body experiences an increase in vascular capacity, the mean systemic pressure decreases, causing a decreased venous return to the heart. Because the sympathetic nervous system causes vasoconstriction to maintain vascular tone, the loss of sympathetic innervation results in domination of the parasympathetic nerves, causing vascular dilatation, or "venous pooling." This massive vasodilatation of veins occurs as a result of the loss of sympathetic vasomotor tone. Neurogenic shock, however, is frequently transitory and does not commonly occur.

Although neurogenic shock may be caused by deep general or spinal anesthesia, loss of sympathetic vasomotor tone in the trauma patient may occur directly from a brain concussion or contusion of the basal regions of the brain or secondary to spinal cord injury above the level of T6.

Because massive, unopposed vasodilatation induces arterioles to dilate, decreasing peripheral vascular resistance, venules and veins also dilate, causing blood to pool in the venous vasculature and decreasing venous return to the right heart.[19] Consequently, the following series of events occurs: (1) decreased ventricular filling pressure; (2) decreased stroke volume; (3) decreased cardiac output; (4) decreased blood pressure; (5) decreased peripheral vascular resistance; and (6) decreased tissue perfusion.

The clinical presentation in neurogenic shock is quite different from that in hypovolemic shock, even though the blood pressure is low. The patient is frequently bradycardic, and the skin is warm, dry, and even flushed. Hemodynamic monitoring reveals a decrease in cardiac output, secondary to a decrease in resistance in arteriolar vasculature, and also a decrease in venous tone.

Treatment. The treatment of neurogenic shock may require extensive volume expansion as well as the use of vasopressors, such as ephedrine. In the case of spinal anesthesia, the PACU nurse should place the patient in a supine position and, if possible, elevate the legs. Finally, the goal of treatment in neurogenic shock is to balance volume expansion with the titration of vasopressor administration.[18]

Anaphylactic shock

Anaphylactic shock results from a severe antigen-antibody reaction. Although this type of shock is not commonly seen in the trauma patient, the condition may occur as an iatrogenic complication during resuscitation.[15] Other causes of anaphylactic shock are reactions to antibiotics, contrast media, and blood transfusions.

The pathophysiologic response of anaphylaxis relates to the inflammatory process and the activation of the complement and arachidonic cascades. The sequence of events involved in the development of anaphylactic shock may be divided into three phases, as follows[1]:

1. The sensitization phase, in which immunoglobulin E antibody is produced in response to an antigen and binds to mast cells and basophils.
2. The activation phase, in which re-exposure to the specific antigen triggers mast cells to release their vasoactive contents.
3. The effector phase, in which the complex response of anaphylaxis occurs as a result of

the histamine and vasoactive mediators released by the mast cells and basophils.

These vasoactive mediators act on blood vessels, causing massive vasodilatation and increased capillary permeability, which allows fluid to leak from the intravascular space to the interstitial space.[19]

Clinical symptoms of anaphylactic shock include conjunctivitis, angioedema, hypotension, laryngeal edema, urticaria, bronchoconstriction, dysrhythmias, and cardiac arrest. One or all of these symptoms may occur. Therefore, immediate and effective life-saving treatment must be initiated.

Treatment. The initial treatment of the patient in anaphylactic shock is identification and removal of the specific antigen that has caused the allergic reaction. Furthermore, if the patient is receiving an infusion of blood or blood products, the PACU nurse should immediately discontinue the transfusion and initiate an intravenous infusion with normal saline. Administration of oxygen by face mask should be started. The initial pharmacologic agent of choice is epinephrine, a bronchodilator that helps restore vascular tone as well as increase arterial blood pressure. Aminophylline may be administered to reduce bronchial constriction and wheezing and to minimize respiratory distress.[20] Diphenhydramine (Benadryl), an antihistamine, is another drug of choice. Finally, corticosteroids may be used to decrease the inflammatory response.

Septic shock

Septic shock, the most common type of distributive shock, results from an acute systemic response to invading blood-borne microorganisms.[27] The sepsis may be caused by gram-positive bacteria; however, the most common cause is gram-negative bacteria. Other pathogens that may cause septic shock are viruses, fungi, parasites, or rickettsiae. The trauma patient is predisposed to the following determinants that affect the outcome of septic shock: infection as a result of contaminated wounds, poor nutritional status, preexisting disease state, and altered integrity of the body's defense mechanisms.[20] Furthermore, sepsis-associated tissue damage is a major complication and remains the principal cause of death in the trauma patient surviving the first 3 days after the injury.[15]

Septic shock may be defined as a clinical syndrome that, on a continuum, begins with sepsis and ends with multisystem organ failure. Septic shock is primarily a complex cellular disease that results in a loss of autoregulation and tissue dysfunction occurring early and persisting despite increased cardiac output. Interactions between bacterial toxins and the body's cellular, humoral, and immunologic systems are considered to activate the kinins and complement, arachidonic, and coagulation cascades, which generate other endogenous mediators that only intensify regional malperfusion.[12]

The profound hemodynamic instability of septic shock is revealed in the body's biphasic response. The first phase, or the hyperdynamic response, is characterized by a high cardiac output and a low systemic vascular resistance, whereas the second phase, the hypodynamic response, reflects the classic shock picture with a low cardiac output and an extremely high systemic vascular resistance.[13] These phases may also be referred to as *early shock*, or a warm, hyperdynamic phase, and *late shock*, or a cold, hypodynamic phase. During early shock, the patient's skin is pink, warm, and dry because of the increased cardiac output and peripheral vasodilatation. With progressing shock, fluid leaks from the vascular compartment, and the patient develops relative hypovolemia, decreasing cardiac output, and increasing peripheral vasoconstriction.[19] The clinical manifestations of late shock are cold, clammy skin; decreased cardiac output; severe hypotension; and extreme vasoconstriction.[12, 19]

In septic shock, the degree of myocardial depression is directly related to the severity of sepsis. Decreased force of contractions may be due to the release of vasoactive chemical mediators, such as myocardial depressant factor, endotoxins, tumor necrosis factor, complement, leukotrienes, and endorphins.[13, 19] Furthermore, decreased ventricular preload resulting from increased capillary permeability augments the myocardial depression.

Rice describes alterations in peripheral circulation as massive vasodilatation, occurring secondary to mediator activation of the bradykinins, histamines, endorphins, complement split products, platelet-activating factor, and prostaglandins.[13] Another aspect of altered circulation is observed in the maldistribution of blood volume that occurs when some tissues receive more blood flow than is needed and other tissues are deprived of needed oxygen and nutrients. Finally, increased capillary permeability causes reduced circulating blood volume, increased blood viscosity, hypoalbuminemia, and interstitial edema.[19]

One of the first target organs to be affected in septic shock is the lung.[13] Endotoxin stimulates the production of complement split products, producing bronchoconstriction, and the release of other vasoactive mediators that cause neutrophil and platelet aggregation to the lungs increases capillary permeability. Consequently, fluid collects in the interstitium, increasing diffusion distance, decreasing compliance, and thereby causing hypoxemia. Pulmonary vasoconstriction may be caused by thromboxane A_2, augmenting capillary permeability and leading to adult respiratory distress syndrome.

Septic shock also causes a profound alteration in metabolism. This metabolic dysfunction is attributed to the following: (1) increasing oxygen debt and rising blood lactate levels; (2) sustained proteolysis; (3) altered gluconeogenesis with concurrent insulin resistance; and (4) liberation of free fatty acids.[13]

Treatment. The treatment of septic shock consists of identifying and eliminating the focus of infection. With culturing of the blood, urine, sputum, wound drainage, and invasive lines, the organism can be identified, and the proper definitive antimicrobial therapy can be initiated. Hemodynamic monitoring ensures an accurate means to assess the patient's circulatory status as well as the patient's response to therapeutic interventions. Initially, the PACU nurse may elect to use supplemental oxygen and encourage the patient to breathe deeply. However, as the shock state progresses, the patient's respiratory status becomes compromised. Aggressive ventilator support must be established to maintain adequate oxygenation and tissue perfusion. Proper selection of parenteral fluid administration is important not only in correcting the cause of shock but also in supporting tissue perfusion.[20] Pharmacologic support, including the use of positive inotropes, vasodilators, and vasopressors, may be indicated to augment contractility, preload, and afterload.[20]

SUMMARY

The PACU nurse must be cognizant of the complex pathophysiologic responses in the trauma patient. The focus of nursing care is on vigilant, continuous assessment. The PACU nurse must anticipate and identify the patient at risk of developing shock. Furthermore, prevention of shock must be the primary goal in caring for the trauma patient. Consequently, the challenge of caring for the critically ill trauma patient demands that the PACU nurse be familiar with current research concerning the pathophysiology and clinical manifestations of the condition as well as with new therapeutic regimens.[13]

References

1. Benjamini, E., and Leskowitz, S.: Immunology: A Short Course. 2nd ed. New York, Wiley-Liss, 1991.
2. Cardona, V. D.: Nursing practice through the cycles of trauma. In Cardona, V. D., Hurn, P. D., Mason, P. J. B., et al. (eds.): Trauma Nursing: From Resuscitation Through Rehabilitation. Philadelphia, W. B. Saunders, 1988, pp. 71–80.
3. Casey, M. F.: Hypovolemic shock. In Sommers, M. S. (eds.): Difficult Diagnoses in Critical Care. Rockville, MD, Aspen, 1989, pp. 1–25.
4. Childs, S. A.: Musculoskeletal injury in the trauma patient: The role of free oxygen radicals [Unpublished master's thesis]. Baltimore, MD, University of Maryland, 1990, pp. 11–25.
5. Childs, S. A.: Nailgun injury. Orthop. Nurs., 10:60–66, 1991.
6. Committee on Trauma of the American College of Surgeons: Advanced Trauma Life Support Course [Student manual]. Chicago, American College of Surgeons, 1985.
7. De Angelis, R.: The cardiovascular system. In Alspach, J. G., and Williams, S. M. (eds.): Core Curriculum for Critical Care Nursing. 3rd ed. Philadelphia, W. B. Saunders, 1985, pp. 115–123.
8. Fontaine, D. K.: Physical, personal, and cognitive responses to trauma. Crit. Care Clin. North Am., 1:11–22, 1989.
9. Guyton, A. C.: Textbook of Medical Physiology. 7th ed. Philadelphia, W. B. Saunders, 1986, pp. 330–333.
10. Houston, M. C.: Pathophysiology of shock. Crit. Care Nurs. Clin. North Am., 2:143–149, 1990.
11. Kruskall, M. S., Mintz, P. D., Bergin, J. J., et al.: Transfusion therapy in emergency medicine. Ann. Emerg. Med., 17:876–879, 1988.
12. Littleton, M. T.: Complications of multiple trauma. Crit. Care Clin. North Am., 1:75–84, 1989.
13. Littleton, M. T.: Pathophysiology and assessment of sepsis and septic shock. Crit. Care Nurs. Q., 11:30–47, 1988.
14. Magnusson, A., and Schriver, J.: Mechanisms of injury: Pathophysiology of blunt, blast, and penetrating injury to the chest. Top. Emerg. Med., 10:1–10, 1988.
15. McQuillan, H. A., and Wiles, C. E.: Initial management of traumatic shock. In Cardona, V. D. (eds.): Trauma Nursing: From Resuscitation Through Rehabilitation. Philadelphia, W. B. Saunders, 1988, pp. 160–183.
16. Miller, S. E., Miller, C. L., and Trunkey, D. D.: The immune consequences of trauma. Surg. Clin. North Am., 62:167–181, 1982.
17. Mlynczak, B.: Assessment and management of the trauma patient in pain. Crit. Care Nurs. Clin. North Am., 1:55–65, 1989.
18. Peitzman, A. B.: Shock. In Simmons, R. L., and Steed, D. L. (eds.): Basic Science Review for Surgeons. Philadelphia, W. B. Saunders, 1990, pp. 130–139.

19. Rice, V.: Shock, a clinical syndrome: An update: I. An overview of shock. Crit. Care Nurse, *11*:20–27, 1991.
20. Rice, V.: Shock, a clinical syndrome: An update: III. Therapeutic management. Crit. Care Nurse, *11*:34–39, 1991.
21. Rice, V.: Shock, a clinical syndrome: An update: IV. Nursing care of the shock patient. Crit. Care Nurse, *11*:40–51, 1991.
22. Roberts, M. K.: Fluid resuscitation in the adult trauma patient. Orthop. Nurs., *8*:41–46, 1989.
23. Sommers, M. S.: Fluid resuscitation following multiple trauma. Crit. Care Nurse, *10*:74–81, 1990.
24. Stene, J. K., and Grande, C. M.: Trauma Anesthesia. Baltimore, Williams & Wilkins, 1991.
25. Summers, G.: The clinical and hemodynamic presenta-
tion of the shock patient. Crit. Care Nurse, *11*:161–166, 1991.
26. Tikka, S.: The contamination of missile wounds with special reference to early microbial therapy. Acta Chir. Scand., *508*:281–287, 1982.
27. Weigelt, J. A., and McCormack, A. F.: Mechanism of injury. *In* Cardona, V. D., Hurn, P. D., Mason, P. J. B., et al. (eds.): Trauma Nursing: From Resuscitation Through Rehabilitation. Philadelphia, W. B. Saunders, 1988, pp. 127–159.
28. Wilkins, E. W.: MGH Textbook of Emergency Medicine. Baltimore, Williams & Wilkins, 1978.

Cardiopulmonary Resuscitation in the Post Anesthesia Care Unit

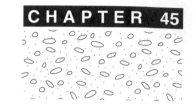

Many advances have been made in cardiopulmonary resuscitation. The morbidity and mortality rates have been substantially reduced after cardiac arrest because of these new techniques. In the post anesthesia care unit (PACU), there is a high probability that the nurse will be confronted with a patient who requires cardiopulmonary resuscitation. To best understand the process of cardiopulmonary resuscitation, the pathophysiology and treatment of shock must be understood.

PATHOPHYSIOLOGY OF SHOCK

Shock may be considered a severe pathophysiologic syndrome associated with abnormal cellular metabolism, which in most instances is due to poor tissue perfusion. Shock also may be due to other factors, such as sepsis. Shock can be divided into three stages: a nonprogressive or compensated stage, a progressive stage, and an irreversible stage. In the nonprogressive stage, the tissue perfusion is decreased, but not enough to cause the vicious circle of cardiovascular deterioration. When the patient enters the progressive stage, cardiac deterioration has reached the point at which, if shock is not treated, death will ensue. The hallmark of the irreversible stage is that all forms of treatment prove inadequate to save the life of the patient.

Types of Shock

The types of shock are hypovolemic or hemorrhagic shock, neurogenic shock, anaphylactic shock, septic shock, and cardiogenic shock (Table 45–1).

Hypovolemic Shock

Hypovolemic shock is the most common type of shock encountered in the PACU. A di-

minished blood volume leads to a decreased systemic filling pressure, which will have as a consequence decreased return. The cardiac output decreases and shock ensues.

A patient can lose approximately 10 percent of blood volume without any appreciable loss in arterial pressure or cardiac output. As the patient approaches 15 to 18 percent blood loss, the arterial pressure and cardiac output begin to fall. Both decrease to zero when the blood loss is 35 to 45 percent of the total blood volume (Fig. 45–1).

As blood volume is lost, sympathetic reflexes become activated and cause peripheral vasoconstriction and reflex tachycardia; blood flow is allowed to decrease; and cardiac depression, vasomotor failure, and vascular failure ensue.

Treatment. Treatment for hypovolemic shock involves improving the blood volume status by the administration of blood products appropriate to the patient's condition.

Neurogenic Shock

Neurogenic shock results from loss of vasomotor tone without any loss of blood volume.

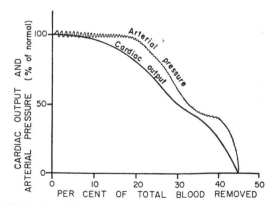

FIGURE 45–1. Effect of hemorrhage on cardiac output and arterial pressure. (From Guyton, A. C.: Textbook of Medical Physiology. 5th ed. Philadelphia, W. B. Saunders Co., 1976, p. 358.)

Table 45–1. TYPES OF SHOCK

Type of Shock	Definition	Causes	Symptoms
Hypovolemic	Caused by a decrease in the intravascular volume relative to the vascular capacity; is generally associated with a blood volume deficit	Hemorrhage Excessive vomiting Excessive diarrhea Severe dehydration	Hypotension Tachycardia Cool, clammy skin Low central venous pressure Decreased urine output
Neurogenic	Caused by damage to or pharmacologic blockage of the sympathetic nervous system, producing vasodilatation of the arterioles in the affected portion of the body and increased vascular capacity	Deep general anesthesia High spinal anesthesia Disease or damage of the spinal cord Brain damage	Hypotension (high spinal anesthesia and spinal cord damage) Bradycardia (high spinal anesthesia and spinal cord damage) Hypertension (early), then hypotension (late) in the patient with brain damage Tachycardia (early), then bradycardia (late) in the patient with brain damage
Anaphylactic	An exaggerated hypersensitivity reaction to a drug or other substance	Administration or contact with some type of antigen	Bronchospasm Hypotension Arrhythmia Cardiac arrest
Septic	Associated with severe sepsis. Can be divided into *hyperdynamic,* associated with impaired cell metabolism with normal or increased cardiac output, or *hypodynamic,* which has relative or absolute hypovolemia due to increased capillary leakage and low cardiac output	The effects of various noxious chemicals and vasoactive substances liberated from damaged, ischemic, or infected tissues	High fever Marked vasodilatation Sludging of the blood Hypotension Tachycardia
Cardiogenic	Caused by impaired function of the heart as a pump	Acute myocardial infarction Pulmonary embolus Tamponade	Hypotension Bradycardia or tachycardia Increased central venous pressure

Some of the causes of neurogenic shock are deep general anesthesia, spinal anesthesia, and spinal cord disease or damage. In the PACU, this type of shock may be seen after spinal anesthetics that reach above T4 dermatome.

Treatment. Treatment of neurogenic shock uses the Trendelenburg position and the administration of oxygen. If blood pressure does not improve, alpha-adrenergic vasopressors can be used to cause peripheral vasoconstriction to get more blood to the heart to improve the cardiac output. Administration of fluids also contributes to the restoration of normal hemodynamics in these patients.

Anaphylactic Shock

Anaphylaxis is an exaggerated hypersensitivity reaction to a drug or other substance. The theoretical basis for anaphylaxis is that when a person is exposed to a specific antigen, antigen-specific immunoglobuin E (IgE) antibodies are formed that interact only with that particular antigen. Subsequent exposure causes a series of intramembrane and intracellular events that culminate in the release of histamine and of the slow-acting substance of anaphylaxis (SRS-A) from the cell. These mediators, in turn, may directly elicit local and systemic pharmacologic effects, may cause the release of other mediators, or may activate reflexes that ultimately produce the clinical picture of anaphylaxis. Histamine is believed to be the major mediator of anaphylaxis. It is found in mast cells and in basophils. It can cause bronchial constriction, increased capillary constriction, and vasodilatation.

The onset of anaphylaxis following the administration of the antigen is usually seen within 30 minutes. This time can be delayed up to an hour or more, depending on how rapidly the antigen is taken up by the circulation. The symptoms of anaphylaxis include conjunctivitis, vasomotor rhinitis, pilomotor erection, pruritic urticaria, angioedema, various gastrointestinal disturbances, laryngeal edema, bronchospasm, hypotension, arrhythmias, cardiac arrest, coma, and death. These symptoms are highly variable and unpredictable. Fatal anaphylaxis may be limited to one symptom, or it may manifest with a wide spectrum of symptoms. Because of the high degree of variability of responses, any systemic manifestation must be considered as the beginning of a severe anaphylactic reaction and be treated vigorously.

Treatment. Five classes of drugs can be used in the treatment of an anaphylactic reaction: adrenergic agonists, methylxanthines, antihistamines, anticholinergics, and corticosteroids. The first line of treatment is epinephrine, usually in a dose of 0.3 ml of 1:1000 intramuscularly or intravenously. The rationale for the selection of epinephrine is that it produces both alpha and beta effects. It also reverses rhinitis, urticaria, bronchoconstriction, and hypotension during anaphylaxis.

The methylxanthines are used when bronchial relaxation and an increase in cardiac output are desired. Aminophylline is the drug of choice in this group. Anticholinergics such as atropine, scopolamine, or glycopyrrolate (Robinul) can be used to help relax bronchiolar smooth muscle and block further cholinergic stimuli. Antihistamines such as diphenhydramine (Benadryl) help block the actions of histamines. Corticosteroids can be used, because evidence suggests that they have some potential benefits, especially when the anaphylactic reaction is not improved by other forms of treatment, and persistent bronchospasm or hypotension is present.

The anaphylactic reaction is a medical emergency. It is important for the PACU nurse to recognize and respond when a patient exhibits any one of the symptoms of anaphylaxis. The drugs mentioned should be available in the PACU at all times. Oxygen should be administered immediately to the patient, because the pathophysiology of this reaction appears to affect the pulmonary structures to a high degree. The blood pressure and pulse should be continuously monitored. The respirations should also be monitored for rate, depth, and rhythm. The larynx should be observed for edema, which is characterized by "crowing" respirations. A physician should be called immediately to institute further treatment of the patient if this occurs.

Septic Shock

Septic shock results from a widely disseminated infection in the body. Some causes of septic shock are peritonitis, generalized infection resulting from a localized infection, and a generalized gangrenous infection caused by gas gangrene bacilli.

The early clinical features of septic shock include high fever, marked vasodilatation, and sledging of the blood. As the septic shock progresses, its end stages resemble those of hypovolemic shock.

Septic shock can be divided into two types: hyperdynamic and hypodynamic. The hyperdynamic type is associated with a normal or increased cardiac output. It is associated with impaired cell metabolism, which prevents the tissues from properly utilizing nutrients such as glucose and oxygen. Increased arteriovenous shunting or improper distribution of blood aggravates this tendency.

Hypodynamic septic shock is associated with a low cardiac output. These patients have a relative or absolute hypovolemia, which is due to an increased capillary leak throughout the body, particularly in the inflamed or infected area.

Treatment. Once septic shock has occurred, the patient must be given *definitive therapy*, such as early surgical débridement or drainage of the wound and appropriate antibiotics. Other recommended measures, including fluid replacement, steroid administration, pulmonary therapy, and the use of vasoactive drugs, represent *adjunctive therapy*, which is useful when preparing the patient for surgical intervention or to support the patient until the infectious process is controlled.

Cardiogenic Shock

Cardiogenic shock is caused by an impaired function of the heart as a pump. The heart begins to fail, usually owing to an acute myocardial infarction or rupture of the ventricular septum, or to the development of significant mitral incompetence. With this type of cardiogenic shock the patient exhibits problems such as peripheral vascular resistance, increased pulse rate, and cool, clammy skin. As many as 10 to 15 percent of these patients may exhibit symptoms of significant hypotension and bradycardia, and they may not have cold, clammy skin.

Because of the increased peripheral vascular resistance, the central venous pressure usually rises. Because the heart is unable to pump blood in significant amounts to all parts of the body, the urine output falls, as does the arterial oxygen content, and the arterial carbon dioxide content rises. The arterial blood lactate rises, leading to metabolic acidosis.

Treatment. It is suggested that cardiogenic shock treatment can be divided into three main categories: (1) medical treatment, (2) circulatory assists, and (3) surgery. Medical treatment is centered around a pharmacologic reversal of the causative factors of the cardiogenic shock. Oxygen should be administered, as should bicarbonate, after a base deficit has been determined. The drugs used in treatment should contribute to increasing the performance of the heart without increasing the myocardial oxygen demand and returning the peripheral vascular resistance to a more normal level. Drugs such as dopamine may prove effective for this condition because of their positive inotropic effect and minimal effect on peripheral vascular resistance. Dopamine also increases renal and mesenteric blood flow. Hypovolemia and electrolyte imbalance should also be corrected.

Circulatory assists use the balloon counter pulsator, which helps mechanically to decrease the work of the heart and increase coronary perfusion. Surgical correction of cardiogenic shock can help a small number of patients, depending on whether the medical facility has the capability to perform open heart surgery. Other factors involved are the selection of the patient and the timing of surgery.

PATHOPHYSIOLOGY OF DEATH

When the blood flow ceases, generalized tissue anoxia takes place. In the brain, the anoxia causes a reversible loss of function. Owing to this anoxia, the patient loses consciousness and, if ventilation is not restored, becomes completely apneic because the control center for respiration is blocked. At this point, the patient is clinically dead and, if cardiopulmonary resuscitation is not instituted within 3 to 6 minutes, irreversible brain damage occurs and the patient is biologically dead. It is critical that the PACU nurse recognize and react quickly and efficiently in this medical emergency. Along with this, it is of utmost importance that the PACU nurse be completely familiar with all facets of cardiopulmonary resuscitation and that essential equipment be readily available (Table 45–2).

Indications for Resuscitation

The precipitating factors in cardiac arrest are hypoxia, an excess of anesthetic agents, and hypotension. All these factors occur in the PACU.

Hypoxia is difficult to recognize. It is suspected when the patient has tachycardia and is restless, sweating, and cyanotic. Absence of cyanosis is not proof of adequate oxygenation, because anemia or cutaneous vasodilatation may give a pink color in spite of profound hypoxia, of which cyanosis is a late sign. Hypercarbia should be considered if the patient becomes progressively somnolent. Another symptom to be considered is loss of muscle tone, although a brief tonic seizure can occur in the first few seconds after cardiac arrest, and the pupils will begin to dilate bilaterally and symmetrically immediately after the arrest. Dilation of the pupils will be complete within 2 minutes after arrest.

Assessment of these patients is for airway obstruction and apnea. The nurse should look for movements of the chest and abdomen and listen and feel for the movement of air in the lungs. In complete obstruction, no respiratory movements are seen and the breath sounds are absent. If a partial obstruction exists, there may be a crowing sound, which usually indicates laryngospasm; gurgling, which usually indicates foreign matter; or wheezing, which indicates bronchial obstruction.

Rapid assessment of the heart by auscultation may reveal cardiac standstill or bradycardia. If a stethoscope is unavailable, the carotid pulse can be checked. The carotid artery is large and lies just anterior to the sternocleidomastoid muscle in the neck. Use of the carotid pulse also reduces time in assessing the patient, because the nurse can check the airway, pupils, chest, and pulse simultaneously. If the patient is connected to an electrocardiograph (ECG), the following dysrhythmias may be observable:

1. Ventricular asystole
2. Bradycardia
3. Premature ventricular contractions, more than 6 per minute, multifocal, or R-on-T phenomena
4. Ventricular tachycardia
5. Ventricular fibrillation
6. Atrioventricular blocks of all degrees
7. Atrial fibrillation and flutter

In essence, the indications for cardiopulmonary resuscitation are either respiratory arrest or cardiac arrest, or both. Nursing assessment should be conducted in seconds, and cardiopulmonary resuscitation should be instituted rapidly.

As cardiopulmonary resuscitation is begun, another nurse should be called. Optimally, there should be two attendants, one to assist in

Table 45–2. ESSENTIAL EQUIPMENT AND DRUGS FOR CARDIOPULMONARY RESUSCITATION

Respiratory Management

Oxygen supply (two E cylinders) with reducing valves capable of delivering 15 L/min with masks and reservoir bag
Oropharyngeal airways (Guidel type—pediatric; small, medium, and large)
Laryngoscope with blades (curved and straight, for adult, child, and infant) and extra batteries and bulbs
Assorted adult-sized (cuffed) and child-sized (uncuffed) endotracheal tubes with stylet and 15 mm/22 mm adapters
Syringe (10 ml) with clamp for inflating endotracheal tube cuff
Bag-valve-mask unit, with provision for 100 percent oxygen ventilation
Suction (preferably portable), with catheters, sizes 6–18 French
Yankauer suction tips
Tracheotomy set and tubes

Circulatory Management

Portable defibrillator-monitor with ECG electrode-fibrillator paddles or portable direct-current defibrillator and portable ECG monitor
Portable electrocardiogram machine, direct-writing, with connection to monitor
Venous infusion sets (micro and regular)
Indwelling venous catheters, catheter outside needle (14–22 gauge), catheter inside needle (14–22 gauge), central venous pressure catheters
Intravenous solutions (5 percent dextrose in water and lactated Ringer's solution)
Cutdown set
Sterile gloves
Urinary catheters
Assorted syringes and needles, stopcocks, venous extension tubing
Intracardiac needles
Tourniquets, adhesive tape, alcohol sponges
Thoracotomy tray
Essential drugs as listed in Table 45–3
Useful drugs
    Aminophylline
    Dexamethasone (Decadron)
    Dextrose 50 percent (Ion-trate Dextrose 50 percent)
    Digoxin (Lanoxin)
    Diphenhydramine hydrochloride (Benadryl)
    Ethacrynic acid
    Furosemide (Lasix)
    Isoproterenol hydrochloride (Isuprel)
    Lanatoside C (Cedilanid)
    Levarterenol bitartrate (Levophed)
    Metaraminol bitartrate (Aramine)
    Methylprednisolone sodium succinate (Solu-Medrol)
    Morphine
    Naloxone (Narcan)
    Nitroglycerine
    Pancuronium bromide (Pavulon)
    Phenylephrine hydrochloride (Neo-Synephrine)
    Potassium chloride
    Procainamide (Pronestyl)
    Propranolol hydrochloride (Inderal)
    Quinidine
    Sodium Nitroprusside (Nipride)
    Succinylcholine chloride (Anectine)
    Tubocurarine chloride
    Verapamil

ECG = electrocardiograph.

the administration of resuscitation and the other to summon emergency aid.

STEPS IN CARDIOPULMONARY RESUSCITATION

The A-B-C steps in cardiopulmonary resuscitation are *airway*, *breathing*, and *circulation*.

Airway

If it has been determined that some degree of airway obstruction exists, patency of the airway should be immediately re-established. Therefore, the PACU nurse should place the patient in a supine position, with the head tilted backward and the neck hyperextended. Then the nurse should lift the angle of the lower jaw upward using moderate pressure. Many times this maneuver is all that is required for spontaneous respirations to occur.

If the patient's airway remains obstructed, an oral airway should then be inserted, as described in Chapter 21.

Breathing

If spontaneous ventilation does not occur, a bag-valve-mask unit (i.e., Ambu bag), connected to an oxygen source should be used to ventilate the patient. Chapter 21 describes in detail the method of ventilating the obtuned or apneic patient.

During the initial ventilation of the patient, an assistant should assess the adequacy of the ventilation by auscultation of the chest. If an assistant is not present, the nurse should check to see if the chest rises and falls or if air escapes during expiration. If the ventilation is considered inadequate, an oral airway should be inserted (see Chapter 21).

If a bag-valve-mask system is not available, mouth-to-mouth ventilation should be instituted until appropriate support materials and personnel become available. The technique involves hyperextending the neck and lifting up the jaw with one hand and holding the nose shut with the other (Fig. 45–2). An airtight seal is formed with the nurse's mouth over the patient's mouth. The patient is ventilated 15 to 20 times per minute. The patient is observed to see if the chest rises and falls or if air escapes on expiration. For infants and small children, the nurse can cover the mouth and nose simultaneously to provide a good seal. The infant

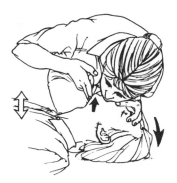

FIGURE 45–2. Mouth-to-mouth resuscitation. (Reproduced with permission. © *Basic Life Support Heartsaver Guide*, 1993; Copyright American Heart Association.)

has a very pliable neck, so that forceful flexing of the head may in itself cause obstruction; therefore, the nurse must not exaggerate the flexed position in infants.

If the PACU nurse is unable to ventilate the patient by either the bag-valve-mask system or mouth-to-mouth, oral endotracheal intubation should be performed as described in Chapter 21.

Ventilation of the Patient

The adult patient should be ventilated approximately 14 to 18 times per minute at a tidal volume of 8 to 10 ml per kg. Infants should be ventilated at approximately 26 to 30 times per minute at a volume large enough to raise their chests on inspiration. However, when time permits, a tidal volume of 7 ml per kg should be used. Children should be ventilated at a rate of 18 to 24 breaths per minute. The tidal volume to be delivered can be determined in the same manner for infants.

Circulation

Assessment should be done to see if a carotid pulse is present or, if a stethoscope is available, whether an apical heart sound is present. In infants and small children, the hand can be placed over the precordium to feel the apical beat. Absence or questionable presence of the pulse is the indication for instituting external cardiac compression.

External Cardiac Compression

External cardiac compression (Fig. 45–3) should be performed with the patient in a horizontal position on a firm surface, and the

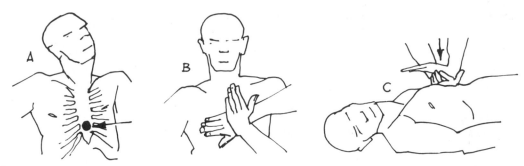

FIGURE 45-3. External cardiac compression. *A*, point of lower hand placement at the sternum. *B*, two-hand placement with the heel of one hand on top of the other, with the fingers straight. *C*, sternal compression, about 4 to 5 cm toward spine. (*A* to *C* from Dripps, R., Eckenhoff, J., and Vandam, L.: Introduction to Anesthesia: The Principles of Safe Practice. 6th ed. Philadelphia, W. B. Saunders, 1982, p. 404.)

lower extremities elevated to promote venous return. Stand at the patient's side and place the heel of one hand over the lower half of the sternum, about 1.5 to 2 inches above the tip of the xiphoid process. Place the other hand on top of the first one. Keeping the arms straight and the shoulders over the patient's sternum, depress the lower sternum a minimum of 1.5 to 2 inches. The sternum should be held down for 0.5 second, then released rapidly. Pressure is reapplied every second or at a slightly faster rate. Rates slower than 60 compressions per minute do not provide sufficient blood flow. In children, the sternum is compressed with one hand only; in infants, it is compressed with the tips of two fingers. In infants and children a rate of 100 to 120 compressions per minute is recommended.

The compressions must be regular, smooth, and uninterrupted. If the external cardiac compression is done correctly, the systolic blood pressure will approach 100 mm Hg, the diastolic pressure will be zero, and the mean pressure will be 40 mm Hg. The amount of circulation is only 20 to 40 percent of normal, so the rhythmic compressions should not be interrupted for more than a few seconds.

External cardiac compression must be combined with ventilation of the lungs. If only one nurse is administering the cardiopulmonary resuscitation, a ratio of 2 ventilations to every 15 sternal compressions at 1-second intervals should be used. The patient's head should be hyperextended while ventilating. A rolled towel or blanket placed under the shoulders maintains this position. Both the ventilation and the compressions should be performed at the patient's side to decrease the time interval in going from one maneuver to the other (Fig. 45-4).

If two persons are administering cardiopul-

monary resuscitation, the ratio of ventilation to compression should be 1:5. One person compresses the sternum at 1-second intervals, and the second person interposes one deep lung inflation after every fifth sternal compression. If ventilation of the lung is difficult in the non-intubated patient, use the 2:15 ratio even when two persons are conducting the resuscitation.

Sternal compressions should be interrupted every 2 minutes to check for the return of spontaneous pulses. If there is no return, continue the sternal compressions; if spontaneous ventilation occurs, ventilate the lungs when the patient inspires to assist ventilation. Once the patient's spontaneous ventilation is determined to be adequate, the positive pressure ventilation can be discontinued, although the nurse should continue to administer oxygen to the patient.

MEDICAL THERAPY

Other resuscitative efforts to be instituted by another nurse, when possible, include starting

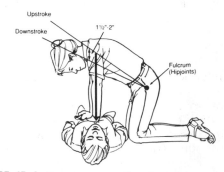

FIGURE 45-4. One-person cardiopulmonary resuscitation includes 15 chest compressions (rate of 80 per minute) and two quick lung inflations. (Reproduced with permission. © *Basic Life Support Heartsaver Guide*, 1993; Copyright American Heart Association.)

an intravenous solution of 5 percent dextrose in Ringer's lactate solution with a 16- or 18-gauge needle. The patient should be connected to an ECG and monitored on lead II. The cardiac arrest cart should be brought to the patient's bedside and medications prepared for administration. The essential and useful drugs should be readily available (Table 45–3).

Atropine Sulfate

Atropine sulfate, an anticholinergic agent, reduces vagal tone, enhances atrioventricular conduction, and accelerates the cardiac rate. It is especially useful in preventing cardiac arrest in patients with profound bradycardia due to myocardial infarction, especially when hypotension is present. The initial dose of this drug is 0.5 mg intravenously, and it may be repeated until the pulse rate is higher than 60 beats per minute. The total dose should not exceed 2 mg except in cases of third-degree atrioventricular block, when larger doses of this drug may be required.

Sodium Bicarbonate

Sodium bicarbonate is used to combat acidosis. The initial dose of this drug is 1 mEq per kg of body weight intravenously. When blood gas determinations are not accessible, half the initial dose can be administered at 10-minute intervals. Once effective spontaneous respirations are restored, administration of the so-

---

Table 45–3. DRUGS FOR CARDIOPULMONARY RESUSCITATION

Essential
Sodium bicarbonate
Epinephrine
Atropine sulfate
Lidocaine
Calcium chloride
Dopamine (Intropin)
Dobutamine

Useful
Vasoactive drugs
Bretylium tosylate (Bretylol)
Levarterenol
Metaraminol
Isoproterenol
Procainamide (Pronestyl)
Propranolol
Corticosteroids
   Methylprednisolone sodium succinate
   Dexamethasone phosphate

---

dium bicarbonate should be discontinued. This drug and epinephrine should not be administered intravenously in the same infusion, because sodium bicarbonate can inactivate epinephrine.

Bretylium Tosylate

Bretylium (Bretylol) has postganglionic adrenergic-blocking properties, antidysrhythmic actions, and a positive inotropic effect. Use of bretylium should be considered when ventricular fibrillation and ventricular tachycardia are refractory to therapy with lidocaine or procainamide and to repeated countershocks. If the patient is experiencing ventricular fibrillation, 5 mg per kg of undiluted bretylium should be given rapidly. After injection, electrical defibrillation should be administered to the patient, because bretylium's ability to terminate ventricular fibrillation resides in its synergistic actions with direct-current (DC) countershock. If the ventricular fibrillation continues after the initial dose of bretylium and DC countershock, the dose can be increased to 10 mg per kg and repeated as necessary. The dosage of bretylium for refractory or recurrent ventricular tachycardia is 5 to 10 mg per kg. Bretylium is injected intravenously over a period of 10 minutes.

Calcium Chloride

Calcium chloride increases myocardial contractility, prolongs systole, and enhances ventricular excitability. It is useful in cardiovascular collapse and may enhance electrical defibrillation. The usual dose of this drug is 2.5 to 5 ml of a 10 percent solution. It should be injected intravenously at 10-minute intervals. It should not be administered together with sodium bicarbonate, because a precipitate will form. Calcium chloride should be administered continuously to a patient receiving digitalis therapy or to patients who have atrioventricular block.

Corticosteroids

Corticosteroids are indicated in the treatment of cardiogenic shock or lung shock, which may be a complication of cardiac arrest. The dosage forms are 5 mg per kg of methylprednisolone sodium succinate or 1 mg per kg of dexamethasone phosphate. Table 45–4 describes drugs commonly used for infants and children.

Table 45–4. COMMONLY USED DRUGS FOR INFANTS AND CHILDREN		
Drug	**Suggested Dose**	**Remarks**
Epinephrine	Intracardiac: 0.3 to 2 ml diluted 1:10,000 (0.1 ml/kg) IV: 10 µg/kg	
Calcium chloride (10%)	IV: maximum dose of 1 ml/5 kg; intracardiac: 1 ml/5 kg diluted 1:1 with saline	Use caution in digitalized children
Sodium bicarbonate	IV: 1 ml (0.9 mEq/kg diluted 1:1 with sterile water	Repeat dosage after pH obtained and base deficit calculated
Levarterenol bitartrate (Levophed)	*Infants*–IV: 1 mg/500 ml of 5% D/W *Children*–IV: 2 mg/500 ml of 5% D/W	Titrate to desired effect. Not to be used in endotoxic shock or renal shutdown
Metaraminol bitartrate (Aramine)	IV: 25 mg/100 ml 5% D/W	Titrate to desired effect
Mephentermine sulfate (Wyamine)	IV: 0.05 mg	
Lidocaine (Xylocaine)	*Infants*–IV: 0.5 mg/kg *Children*–IV: 5 mg and repeat until desired effect obtained IV drip: 6 mg/kg/4 hr (100 mg/500 ml of 5% D/W)	Not to exceed 100 mg/hr
Isoproterenol hydrochloride (Isuprel)	IV drip: 1–5 mg/500 ml of 5% D/W	Titrate to desired effect

IV = intravenous; D/W = dextrose in water.

Dobutamine

Dobutamine is a synthetic derivative of isoproterenol (Isuprel) that acts directly on the beta$_1$ receptors in the heart. Its principal action is to increase myocardial contractility without greatly changing peripheral resistance or heart rate. Dobutamine is useful in the treatment of congestive heart failure and for the patient who is emerging from cardiopulmonary bypass surgery. The dosage for dobutamine via continuous intravenous infusion is 2 to 10 µg per kg per min. This direct-acting beta$_1$ adrenergic receptor–stimulating agent can cause tachycardia, dysrhythmias, nausea, headache, angina, palpitations, and dyspnea, especially when blood levels are in excess of 20 µg per kg per min.

Dopamine

Dopamine (Intropin) is a naturally occurring biochemical catecholamine precursor of norepinephrine. Dopamine exerts a positive inotropic effect (change in contractile force) and a minimal chronotropic effect (change in contractile rate) on the heart. Therefore, the contractility of the heart is increased without changing the afterload (total peripheral resistance), which leads to an increase in cardiac output. The increase is in the systolic and pulse pressures, with virtually no effect on diastolic pressure. Dopamine is not associated with tachyarrhythmias and produces less of an increase in myocardial oxygen consumption than does isoproterenol. Blood flow to peripheral vascular beds may decrease, whereas mesenteric flow increases. One of the major reasons for the increased use of dopamine clinically is its action on the renal vasculature, that is, that of dilatation. This action is secondary to the inotropic effect and decreased peripheral resistance produced by dopamine. Therefore, the glomerular filtration rate is increased with the renal blood flow and sodium excretion.

The usual dose of dopamine is 0.4 to 1.6 mg per min until adequate blood pressure is attained. The dopamine infusion is made by adding 200 mg of dopamine to 250 ml of 5 percent dextrose and water. The resulting solution will be 0.8 mg per ml of dopamine. The dopamine should not be given through an infusion with sodium bicarbonate, because dopamine is inactivated in an alkaline solution.

In the intubated patient in whom an intravenous route cannot be established, epinephrine or lidocaine can be instilled into the trachea via the endotracheal tube to produce the pharmacologic effects. The epinephrine can be diluted with sterile distilled water as a 1 to 2 mg per 10 ml solution. Lidocaine is diluted with sterile distilled water to a 50- to 100-ml solution.

The intramuscular route can be used only when adequate spontaneous circulation is present. Atropine sulfate in a dose of 2 mg or lidocaine in a dose of 300 mg will be effective if given by this route.

Epinephrine

Epinephrine increases myocardial contractility, elevates perfusion pressure, and, in some instances, restores myocardial contractility. The dosage is 0.5 to 1.0 mg intravenously or via the endotracheal tube and can be repeated every 5 minutes during the resuscitative effort. Intracardiac injection of this drug should be done by a physician trained in this technique.

Isoproterenol

In patients who have complete heart block in which profound bradycardia is present, isoproterenol is an effective immediate treatment. It is also effective in profound bradycardia that does not respond to atropine sulfate. The dose of this drug is 2 to 20 μg per min. This solution can be made by adding 1 mg of isoproterenol to a 500-ml solution of 5 percent dextrose in water. This will yield a concentration of 2 μg per ml.

Levarterenol Bitartrate

Vasoactive drugs may be effective in the resuscitation period. If the patient has peripheral vascular collapse, with hypotension and absence of peripheral vasoconstriction, levarterenol bitartrate (Levophed) in a dose of 16 mg per ml or metaraminol bitartrate (Aramine) in a dose of 0.4 mg per ml of dextrose in water can be titrated intravenously to support the blood pressure.

Before levarterenol bitartrate is administered, it should be ascertained that the intravenous cannula is correctly positioned inside the vein. Any extravasation of this drug produces tissue necrosis. Metaraminol can also be administered intravenously in a 2- to 5-mg bolus.

Lidocaine

Lidocaine, also a local anesthetic agent, is useful as an antiarrhythmic agent. It is administered slowly intravenously at a dose rate of 50 to 100 mg and can be repeated as necessary. Lidocaine can be administered in a continuous infusion at 1 to 3 mg per min, usually not exceeding 4 mg per min.

Intravenous Nitroglycerin

Nitroglycerin dilates the large coronary arteries, increases coronary collateral blood flow, and can improve perfusion of ischemic myocardium. This drug relaxes all smooth muscle, particularly vascular smooth muscle. The ventricular systolic and diastolic volumes fall, resulting in a reduced myocardial wall tension, which leads to a decreased myocardial oxygen demand. Intravenous nitroglycerin is indicated for unstable angina pectoris, acute myocardial infarction, and congestive heart failure. This drug should be administered via an automated infusion pump. The dose is about 10 to 20 μg per min. The dosage, which can be increased by 5 to 10 μg per min every 5 to 10 minutes, is usually titrated to achieve the desired clinical effect.

Sodium Nitroprusside

Sodium nitroprusside (Nipride) is a rapid-acting, potent peripheral vasodilator. Because it will cause an immediate reduction of peripheral arterial resistance, sodium nitroprusside is especially useful in the treatment of hypertensive crisis. It is also useful in the treatment of patients with left ventricular failure and pulmonary edema. For dosage and precautions associated with sodium nitroprusside, the reader is encouraged to review Chapter 5.

Procainamide

Procainamide (Pronestyl) may be useful in suppressing premature ventricular complexes and recurrent ventricular tachycardia that do not resolve after treatment with lidocaine. If ventricular ectopy has not been resolved by at least 225 mg of lidocaine administered by intermittent bolus injection and an intravenous lidocaine infusion of 4 mg per min after each bolus, procainamide should be administered. The intravenous dosage of procainamide is 100 mg every 5 minutes (20 mg per min). The bolus administration of procainamide should be stopped when the dysrhythmia is suppressed, or the QRS complex is widened by 50 percent, or hypotension occurs, or the total dose of the procainamide reaches 1 g. The maintenance rate of procainamide is 4 mg per min, and the therapeutic blood level for this drug is 4 to 8 μg per ml.

Intravenous procainamide should be administered cautiously in the PACU, especially to those patients with an acute myocardial infarction. Severe hypotension can result from rapid injection. Hence, arterial blood pressure and ECG monitoring are essential during the ad-

Table 45–5. RECOMMENDED ENERGIES FOR COUNTERSHOCK

Arrhythmia	Amount of Shock (watt-seconds or joules)
Atrial tachycardia	50
Atrial flutter	50
Atrial fibrillation	200
Ventricular tachycardia	200
Ventricular flutter	200
Ventricular fibrillation	200 (advance quickly to 400 if unsuccessful)

ministration of the drug. The warning signs of impending hypotension are a widening of the QRS complex and a lengthening of the PR or the QT interval.

Propranolol

In patients with ventricular fibrillation who do not respond well to lidocaine, the beta blocker propranolol (Inderal) may be administered. The usual dose is 1 mg slowly infused intravenously. The dose can be repeated up to a total dose of 3 mg and should be given when the patient is being monitored by ECG. Because this drug is a beta-blocking drug, it should be used with extreme caution in patients who have pulmonary disease or cardiac failure.

Verapamil

Verapamil, a slow channel blocker, is primarily useful in emergency cardiac situations as an antidysrhythmic agent. More specifically, the drug is highly effective in the treatment of paroxysmal supraventricular tachycardia. The dosage of verapamil is 0.075 to 0.15 mg per kg, which is administered via intravenous bolus over a 1-minute period. Not more than 10 mg of the drug should be administered at any one time. After 30 minutes, if the initial response is inadequate, a dose of 0.15 mg per kg can be repeated. Again, this dose should not be more

than 10 mg, and the total cumulative dose of verapamil within the 30-minute period should not be more than 15 mg.

ELECTRICAL CARDIOVERSION

Cardioversion depolarizes all cardiac cells, restoring synchrony and allowing the predominant pacemaker to regain control of the rhythm. DC countershocks should be administered as soon as possible if the heart is known to be in ventricular fibrillation. It is also indicated in ventricular tachycardia and ventricular asystole (Table 45–5).

The electrode position should be kept standard, one electrode just to the right of the upper sternum below the clavicle and the other electrode just to the left of the cardiac apex or left nipple. Standard electrode paste or 4 × 4 gauze pads saturated with normal saline provide conduction of the electrical impulse.

References

1. Barash, P., Cullen, B., and Stoelting, R.: Handbook of Clinical Anesthesia. 2nd ed. Philadelphia, J. B. Lippincott, 1993.
2. Butterworth, J.: Atlas of Procedures in Anesthesia and Critical Care. Philadelphia, W. B. Saunders, 1992.
3 Guyton, A.: Textbook of Medical Physiology. 8th ed. Philadelphia, W. B. Saunders, 1991.
4. Longnecker, D., and Murphy, F. (eds.): Dripps/Eckenhoff/Vandam Introduction to Anesthesia. Principles of Safe Practice. 8th ed. Philadelphia, W. B. Saunders, 1992.
5. McIntyre, K., and Lewis, A.: Textbook of Advanced Cardiac Life Support. New York, American Heart Association, 1981.
6. Miller, R.: Anesthesia. 3rd ed. New York, Churchill Livingstone, 1990.
7. Morrow, D., and Luther, R.: Anaphylaxis: Etiology and guidelines for management. Anesth. Analg., 55(4):493, 1976.
8. Otto, C.: Current concepts in cardiopulmonary resuscitation. Semin. Anesth., 9(3):169–181, 1990.
9. Standards for cardiopulmonary resuscitation and emergency cardiac care. JAMA, 244(5):453–509, 1980.
10. Stoelting, R., Dierdorf, S., and McCammon, R.: Anesthesia and Co-Existing Disease. 2nd ed. New York, Churchill Livingstone, 1989.
11. Wood, M., and Wood, A.: Drugs and Anesthesia: Pharmacology for Anesthesiologists. 2nd ed. Baltimore, Williams & Wilkins, 1990.

Index

Note: Page numbers in *italics* refer to illustrations; page numbers followed by t refer to tables.

A

A fibers, of afferent nerve, 246
A wave(s), 83, *84*
   in intracranial pressure, 421, *422*
A-alpha fibers, of afferent nerve, 246
AAMI (Association for the Advancement of Medical
      Instrumentation), 13t
A-B-C steps, in cardiopulmonary resuscitation, 589–590, *590*
Abdominal distention, after genitourinary surgery, 467–468
Abdominal myomectomy, definition of, 479
Abdominal surgery, care after, 450–453, *451*
   diagnostic, 453–454
   dressings and drains after, 451
   fluid and electrolyte balance after, 452
   incisions in, types of, 450, *451*
   nasogastric or intestinal intubation after, 452–453
   patient positioning after, 451
   respiratory function after, 451–452
Abdominoperineal resection, care after, 456–457
Abducens nerve, function of, 63t
A-beta fibers, of afferent nerve, 246
Absorption, in pharmacokinetic interactions, 184
Abuse, drug, 557–561. See also *Drug abuse.*
Acceleration-deceleration injury, contusion due to, 412
Access, routine, to PACU, 5–6
Acetonuria, definition of, 138
Acetylcholine, 226–227
   as mediator, 92, 92t
   in coronary circulation, 88
   pharmacologic and physiologic actions of, 94, 95t
   synthesis of, 92, 93t
Acetylcholinesterase, 227, *227–228*
Achalasia, definition of, 156
   esophageal, 156–157
Acid-base balance, metabolic disorders of, 126, 126t
   respiratory disorders of, 125t, 125–126
   role of kidney in, 143–144
Acid-base relationships, 125t, 125–126, 126t
Acidemia, definition of, 104
Acidity, 125
Acidosis, definition of, 104
   metabolic, 126, 143
      causes of, 126t
   renal correction of, 144
   respiratory, 125, 143

Acidosis *(Continued)*
   causes of, 125t
ACLS (advanced cardiac life support), certification in, 19
Acoustic nerve, function of, 63t
Acquired immunity, 172–175
   cellular type of, 174–175
   definition of, 171
   humoral type of, 172–174, *173*
Acquired immunodeficiency syndrome (AIDS), virus causing,
      transmission of, 34
Acromegaly, 151
ACTH. See *Adrenocorticotropin (ACTH).*
Actin filaments, 86
Active acquired immunity, definition of, 171
Activity, in post anesthesia recovery score, 33t
Adalat. See *Nifedipine (Procardia, Adalat).*
Adam's apple, anatomy of, 106
Addisonian crisis, 154
Additive effect, definition of, 181
A-delta fibers, of afferent nerve, 246
Adenohypophysis, 150
   hormones of, 150–151
Adenoidectomy, definition of, 331
   tonsillectomy and. See *Tonsillectomy and adenoidectomy.*
ADH. See *Antidiuretic hormone (ADH).*
Adrenal gland, anatomy and physiology of, 152–153
   cholinergic stimulation of, 95t
   insufficiency of, acute, 154
Adrenalectomy, 475–476
   definition of, 464
Adrenergic, definition of, 82
Adrenergic nerve(s), functional anatomy of, 92, 92t
Adrenergic neurotransmitter, biochemistry of, 92–94, 93t
Adrenergic receptor(s), 94–97, *95*, 96t, *97*
   types of, 95
Adrenocorticotropin (ACTH), 151
   deficiency of, 154
Adult respiratory distress syndrome, after cranial surgery, 427
Advanced cardiac life support (ACLS), certification in, 19
Adventitious sounds, definition of, 104
Afferent, definition of, 53
Afterload, definition of, 82
A-gamma fibers, of afferent nerve, 246
Age, advanced. See also *Geriatric patient.*
   health problems associated with, 544–548
   postoperative complications of, 134

Age (Continued)
  considerations of, analgesic agents and, 319–320
  old, definition of, 544
Agglutination, antibody, 174
AIDS (acquired immunodeficiency syndrome), virus causing,
    transmission of, 34
Air conditioning, in PACU, 8
Air embolization, associated with invasive hemodynamic
    monitoring, 282t
Airway(s), artificial, removal of, 263
    types of, 263
  closure of, concept in, 113, 114
  for cardiopulmonary resuscitation, 589
  in chronic obstructive pulmonary disease, 520
  oropharyngeal, insertion of, 305–306, 307
    vs. nasopharyngeal, 306
  patent, maintenance of, 361
  postoperative care of, 305–306, 306t, 306–307
    in rheumatoid arthritic patient, 523–524
  upper, anatomy of, during pregnancy, 551
Airway obstruction, in pediatric patient, 541–542
  indications of, 305
  postoperative, 262–263
  soft-tissue, technique of overcoming, 305, 306
Airway receptors, in regulation of breathing, 131
Akathisia, 58
Alarm(s), vital sign monitor, disabling, 14
Alarm reaction, in Selye's adaptation syndrome, 23
Albumin, for transfusion, 295
Albuminuria, definition of, 138
Alcohol, abuse of, 558t, 560
Alcohol withdrawal syndrome, 560
Alcoholic, definition of, 560
Alcoholism, 560
Alcuronium chloride (Alloferin), action and dosage of, 233
Aldomet. See Methyldopa (Aldomet).
Aldosterone, 142, 153
Aldosterone antagonists, 145
Alfentanil (Alfenta), 218–219
Alkalemia, definition of, 104
Alkalinity, 125
Alkaloid(s), belladonna, 94
Alkalosis, definition of, 104
  metabolic, 126, 143
    blood gas discrepancies in, 126t
    renal correction of, 144
  respiratory, 125–126, 143
    causes of, 125t
Allen test, 85
Allergic response, of immune system. See Hypersensitivity
    reaction(s).
  to blood transfusion, 293–294
  to local anesthetic agents, 249–250
Allograft(s), definition of, 492
  rejection of, as delayed hypersensitivity reaction, 176
    signs of, 471t
Alpha receptor(s), 95, 95–96
Althesin, 213
Alveolar dead space, 128, 129
Alveolar sac, 109, 110
Alveolus(i), anatomy of, 109, 110
  movement of inhalant anesthetic from anesthesia machine to,
    192
Alzheimer's disease, 546–547
Ambulatory surgery, 506–515
  anesthesia for, 510
  day-of-surgery assessment for, 508
  diagnostic testing for, 509
  discharge of patient after, 513
    areas of concern in, 514t
    preprinted discharge instruction sheets and, 514–515

Ambulatory surgery (Continued)
  emotional support for, 510
  fasting period before, 508–509
  history of, 506
  intraoperative period of, 510–511
  intravenous conscious sedation in, 510–511
  nursing care and, 506–507
  on-site preadmission assessment for, 508
  PACU care in, 511–512
  patient preparation for, 507–510
    primary goals of, 510
  positive thinking and, 510
  post anesthesia period of, 511–515
    post discharge follow-up in, 515, 515t
    progressive or phase II care in, 512–515, 513t, 514t
  preoperative medication for, 509–510
    intravenous administration of, 509
  trend toward, 506
American National Standards Institute (ANSI), 13t
American Society for Testing and Materials (ASTM), 13t
American Society of Post Anesthesia Nurses (ASPAN), Scope
    of Practice document published by, 15, 16t–18t
Amines, sympathomimetic, interaction of, in PACU patient, 188
Amphetamine abuse, effects and signs of, 558t
Amputation, cineplastic (kineplastic), definition of, 399
  limb, post anesthesia care after, 407
  Syme, definition of, 399
Amygdala, 54, 57
Amyotrophic lateral sclerosis, muscle relaxant response in, 243t
Analgesia, basal infusion rate in, 224, 224t
  epidural, patient-controlled, 223t, 223–224, 224t
  for post cesarean section pain, 554
  for postoperative pain, 320, 321
  lockout interval in, 224
  minimum effective analgesic concentration in, 223–224
  stage of, in anesthesia, 190
Analgesic agent(s), for postoperative pain, 319–322
  age considerations in, 319–320
  commonly used, 319t
  intrathecal and epidural administration of, 320–322
  intravenous administration of, 320
  patient-controlled, 320, 321
  side effects of, 319t, 322–323
Anaphylaxis, 175, 175t, 578t, 580–581, 585–586
  definition of, 181
  slow-reacting substance of, 175
  treatment of, 581, 586
Anatomic dead space, 128, 129
Anatomic shunt, 128
Androgen(s), adrenal secretion of, 153
Anemia, hemolytic, as cytotoxic hypersensitivity reaction, 175–
    176
  in rheumatoid arthritic patient, 524–525
  sickle cell, anesthesia and, 529–530
    PACU care and, 530
    pathogenesis of, 529, 530
Anesthesia, axillary nerve block, 256
  PACU care after, 256
  brachial plexus nerve block, 256
    PACU care after, 256
  components of, 190
  conduction, 245
  definition of, 399
  diabetes mellitus and, 522
  effects of, on heart, 88
    on renal function, 145–146
  emergence from, 291
    postoperative assessment of, 283
  epidural, 255–256
    administration of, 255
    mechanism of action of, 255

Anesthesia *(Continued)*
    PACU care after, 255–256
    field block, 245
    for ambulatory surgery, 510
    for bronchoscopy, 352
    for cardiac surgery, 380
    for kidney transplantation, 470
    for large vessel surgery, 394, 396
    for ophthalmic surgery, 344–345
    for pediatric patient, 538
    for pregnant patient, general, 553
        regional, 553
    for spinal surgery, 440
    for thyroid surgery, 444
    for vascular surgery, 389
    infiltration, 245
    inhalation, 239
        administration techniques for, 194–196, *195–197*
            circle systems as, 194–195
            insufflation methods as, 195
            open systems as, 195
            semiopen systems as, 195–196, *196–197*
        basic concepts of, 190–194
        emergence phase of, 194
        hyperthermia and hypothermia following, 203
        pharmacokinetics of, 192–193, 193t
        signs and stages of, evolution of, 190–192, *191*
        stage I, 190
        stage II, 190
        stage III, 190–191
        stage IV, 191
        water and electrolyte balance affected by, 203
    intravenous, nonopioid, 205–213
        barbiturates as, 205–206
        dissociatives as, 212–213
        mechanism of action of, 205
        nonbarbiturates as, 206–208
        other agents as, 213
        tranquilizers as, 208–212
    opioid, 215–224
        administration of, 222–224
        comparisons of, 220t
        concepts of, 215
        intrathecal and epidural administration of, 222–223
        patient-controlled administration of, 223t, 223–224, 224t
    local, 245–250
        agents used in, 246–250, 248t
        complications of, 249–250
        intermediate-duration, 247–249
        long-duration, 249
        physiology of nerve and nerve conduction and, 245–246, 246t
        short-duration, 247
    nerve block, 256
    regional, 245, 251–257
        intravenous, 256–257
            PACU care after, 257
        types of, 252–257
    regurgitation after, 159
    sickle cell anemia and, 529–530
    spinal, 252–255
        administration of, 252–253, *253*
        complications of, 253–255
        mechanism of action of, 253
        PACU care after, 255–256
    steroid, 213
    technique of, postoperative pain and, 315–316
    topical, 245
Anesthesia machine, 194, *195*
    movement of inhalant anesthetic from, to alveoli, 192
Anesthesia machine circuit, *196*

Anesthesia report, on shock trauma patient, 573–574
Anesthetic agent(s), dissociative, 212–213
    for postoperative pain, 315
    inhalant, 196–202. See also specific agent, e.g., *Halothane (Fluothane)*.
        assessing effect of, in PACU, 202–203
        gaseous, 196–197
        intracranial pressure and, 418–419
        modern, 198–202
        movement of, from alveoli to arterial blood, 192–193, 193t
            from anesthetic machine to alveoli, 192
            from arterial blood to brain, 193, 193t
        potency of, 194
        properties of, 193t
        traditional, 197–198
        volatile, 196
    intracranial pressure and, 418–419
    intravenous, intracranial pressure and, 419
    local, 246–250
        allergic reactions to, 249–250
        complications of, 249–250
        definition of, 245
        intermediate-duration, 247–249
        long-duration, 249
        overdosage of, 250, 250t
        properties of, 246
        short-duration, 247
        uses of, 248t
    triggering malignant hyperthermia, 566, 566t
Aneurysm(s), cerebral, 415
    definition of, 387
    of distal aorta, *394*
    ventricular, *378*
        repair of, 378
Angina pectoris, definition of, 82
Angiography, definition of, 387
    renal, care after, 464–465
Angioplasty, percutaneous transluminal. See *Percutaneous transluminal angioplasty*.
Angioscopy, definition of, 387
Angiotensin I, 153
Angiotensin II, 142, 153
Ankyloglossia, definition of, 330
Annuloplasty, definition of, 368
ANSI (American National Standards Institute), 13t
Antagonist(s), aldosterone, 145
Antibiotic(s), adverse effects of, in geriatric patient, 547t
    interaction of, in PACU patient, 187
    neuromuscular blocking properties of, 238t
Antibody(ies). See also *Immunoglobulin* entries.
    definition of, 171
    protective function of, 174
    reaginic, 175
Anticholinesterase drug(s), 234
Antidepressants, adverse effects of, in geriatric patient, 547t
Antidiuretic hormone (ADH), 151
    in renal function, 140, 142, 146
Antidysrhythmic agent(s), adverse effects of, in geriatric patient, 547t
    cardiac, 238
Antigen(s), definition of, 171
Antigen-antibody complex, 174
Antihypertensive(s), interaction of, in PACU patient, 188
Antilirium. See *Physostigmine (Antilirium)*.
Antral window, definition of, 329
Antrectomy, definition of, 447
Antrostomy, intranasal, definition of, 329
    radical, definition of, 329
Antrum, pyloric, 157
Anus, anatomy and physiology of, 160
    surgery of, care after, 457

Anxiety, postoperative, signs and symptoms of, 287t
Aorta, coarctation of, *372*
    definition of, 371
    distal, aneurysm of, *394*
Aortic insufficiency, 368
Aortic regurgitation, definition of, 368
Aortic stenosis, *370*
    definition of, 368–369
Aortic valve disease, definition of, 369
Aortocaval compression, during pregnancy, 549, *551*
Aortocoronary grafting, 374
Aortoiliac Dacron bypass graft, *395*
Apnea, definition of, 104
Apneustic breathing, 425t
    definition of, 104
Apneustic center, of brainstem, 132
Appendectomy, care after, 457
    definition of, 447
Apresoline. See *Hydralazine (Apresoline)*.
Aqueduct of Sylvius, 68
Arachnoid mater, *66, 67, 68*
    spinal, 74
Aramine. See *Metaraminol bitartrate (Aramine)*.
Arciform (arcuate) artery(ies), 138–139, *140*
Arduan. See *Pipecuronium bromide (Arduan)*.
Arfonad. See *Trimethaphan camsylate (Arfonad)*.
Arm surgery, post anesthesia care after, 403–404
Arrhythmia(s), after thoracic surgery, 367
    definition of, 82
    sinus, postoperative monitoring of, 274–275, *274–275*
    supraventricular, postoperative monitoring of, 275–276, *275–276*
    ventricular, postoperative monitoring of, 276–277, *276–278*
Arterial pressure, mean, postoperative monitoring of, 278
Arterial spasm(s), associated with invasive hemodynamic monitoring, 281t
Arteriography, care following, 389–390
    definition of, 387
    for cranial surgery, 410–411, *411*
Arteriole(s), anatomy of, 91
Arteriosclerosis, definition of, 82
Arteriovenous malformation(s), 415–416
Artery(ies). See also named artery, e.g., *Carotid artery(ies)*.
    great, transposition of, 376
    of head and neck, *72*
    peripheral, palpation for pulse in, 391, *391*
Artery banding, pulmonary, definition of, 375
Arthritis, rheumatoid. See *Rheumatoid arthritis*.
Arthrodesis, definition of, 399
Arthroplasty, definition of, 399
Arthroscopy, definition of, 399
Arthrotomy, definition of, 399
Arthus hypersensitivity reaction(s), 175t, 176
Articular process, of vertebrae, 74
Articulation, definition of, 399
Arytenoid cartilages, 106, *107*
Aseptic technique(s), cutaneous importance of, 167, 167t, 168t, 169–170
ASPAN (American Society of Post Anesthesia Nurses), Scope of Practice document published by, 15, 16t–18t
Aspiration, of gastrointestinal contents, after tracheal intubation, 313
    uterine, care after, 481
Aspiration pneumonia, 159
Aspiration reflex, 131
Association areas, of brain, 58
Association for the Advancement of Medical Instrumentation (AAMI), 13t
Asthma, 519
ASTM (American Society for Testing and Materials), 13t
Atarax. See *Hydroxyzine (Atarax, Vistaril)*.

Ataxic breathing, 425t
Atelectasis, after thoracic surgery, 365–366
    definition of, 104, 350
    in postoperative period, 135
Ativan. See *Lorazepam (Ativan)*.
Atlas (C1), 74, *75*
Atracurium besylate (Tracrium), action and dosage of, 232
    pharmacology of, 229t
Atrial contraction, premature. See *Premature atrial contraction*.
Atrial fibrillation, postoperative monitoring of, 276, *276*
Atrial flutter, postoperative monitoring of, 276, *276*
Atrial pressure, postoperative monitoring of, 278, 279t
Atrial septal defect, definition of, 369
Atrial standstill, postoperative monitoring of, 275
Atrial syncytium, 86
Atrial tachycardia, postoperative monitoring of, 275–276, *276*
Atrioventricular canal defects, 369
Atrioventricular (AV) node, 86–87
Atrioventricular (AV) valves, 83, 85
Atrioventricularis communis, definition of, 369
Atrium (atria), of heart, 83
Atropine sulfate, for cardiopulmonary resuscitation, 591
Auditory area, of brain, 58
Augmentation mammoplasty, definition of, 484
Auscultation, of chest, postoperative, 263–264
Autograft(s), definition of, 492
Autologous blood transfusion, 292
Automatic blood pressure monitor(s), 271–272, *272*
Automatic implantable cardioverter-defibrillator, 369–371
    activation of, 370–371
    candidates for, 369–370
    two-patch technique in, 370
Automaticity, definition of, 82
Autonomic drug(s), site of action of, 97–98, 98t
Autonomic hyperreflexia, after spinal injuries, 439–440
    clinical signs and symptoms of, 440
Autonomic nervous system, 80–81
Autoregulation, definition of, 53
    in renal function, 140
Autotransfusion, in hip surgery, 404–405
    in knee surgery, 406
    in orthopedic surgery, 402, *402*
Axillary nerve block, 256
Axis (C2), 74, *75*
Ayre T-piece, of anesthesia machine, 195, *196*
Azotemia, definition of, 138

B

B fibers, of afferent nerve, 246
B lymphocyte(s), definition of, 171
    in humoral immunity, 172, *173*
B wave, in intracranial pressure, 421, *422*
Babinski sign, 415
    positive, 422
Bag-valve-mask unit, for cardiopulmonary resuscitation, 589
    in airway management, 305–306, *306*
    requirements for, 306t
Bain anesthesia circuit, 195–196, *197*
Baldy-Webster procedure, 481
Barbiturate(s). See also specific agent, e.g., *Thiopental (Pentothal)*.
    abuse of, 558t, 559
    as nonopioid intravenous anesthetic, 205–206
    intracranial pressure and, 419
Baroreceptor(s), 85
    definition of, 409
    in ADH secretion, 151
    in regulation of breathing, 132
Bartholin duct cyst, definition of, 477
Bartholinectomy, definition of, 477

Basal ganglia (cerebral nuclei), anatomy of, 54, *57*
Basal tidal volume, Radford nomogram for, 536, *536*
Base excess, 125
Basic cardiac life support (BCLS), certification in, 19
Basilar artery, 71, *72–73*
Bathmotropic, definition of, 82
BCLS (basic cardiac life support), certification in, 19
Bed(s), in PACU, 5
Behavior, as indicator of pain, 318
Behavioral symptoms, of stress, 24, 24t
Behavioral thermoregulatory response, 563
Belladonna alkaloid(s), 94
Bellevue bridge, for scrotal support, 473, *474*
Benadryl. See *Diphenhydramine (Benadryl)*.
Benzodiazepine(s), abuse of, 558t, 559–560
    adverse effects of, in geriatric patient, 547t
    as nonopioid intravenous anesthetic, 208–209
    intracranial pressure and, 419
Benzodiazepine antagonist(s), as nonopioid intravenous
        anesthetic, 209–210
Benzquinamide (Emete-con), for nausea, 532t
Beta receptor(s), 96, *97*
Bicarbonate, in carbon dioxide transport, 123–124, *124*
Bigeminy, definition of, 82
Bile duct, T-tube placement in, 458, *458*
Bileaflet valve, 376–377, *377*
Biliary, definition of, 156
Biliary lithotripsy, 162
Biliary tract, surgery of, care after, *459*, 460
Bilirubin, metabolism of, 161
Biologic valve(s), 377
Biopsy, breast, 484, 485
    needle, bronchoscopy and, 353
    renal, care after, 465
Biotransformation, pharmacokinetic parameters of, 187
Bladder, drainage of, closed, 465, *467*
    surgery of, 471
Bladder neck operation (Y-V plasty), definition of, 463
Blade(s), insertion of, in oral tracheal intubation, 310
    laryngoscope, 308, *308*
Blankets, hypothermia, 428
Bleeding. See *Hemorrhage*.
Bleeding time, 90
Blepharoplasty, 495
    definition of, 343
Blood, arterial, movement of inhalant anesthetic from alveoli to,
        192–193, 193t
    transfusion of. See *Transfusion(s)*.
Blood flow, detection of, Doppler instrument for, 391, *391*
Blood gas(es). See *Gas(es)*.
Blood loss, after orthopedic surgery, 401–402
Blood pressure, arterial, 85
    in pediatric patient, 534, 534t
    postoperative, measurement of, 271–273
        clinical issues in, 273
        invasive, 272–273
        noninvasive, 271–272, *272*
    systolic, in geriatric patient, 544
Blood supply, to brain, 71, *72–73*
    to head and neck, *72*
    to kidneys, 138–139, *139*
    to nose, 105
    to spinal cord, 80
Blood vessels. See also named vessel, e.g., *Coronary artery*.
    anatomy of, 91
Blood volume, maintenance of, after thoracic surgery, 365
Blood-borne diseases, control of, 34
Blood-brain barrier, 69–71
    site of, 70
Blood-CSF barrier, 69–71
Blood-gas partition coefficient, 192, 202–203

Blow-counterblow injury, contusion due to, 412
Blunt trauma, 571
BMI (body mass index), calculation of, 525
Body fluids, regulation of, role of kidney in, 142, 142t
Body mass index (BMI), calculation of, 525
Body response, to stress, 23
Body temperature. See *Temperature, body*.
Bohr effect, on oxygen transport, 122
Bohr equation, 128–129
Bone demineralization, from spinal injuries, 437
Bone graft(s), 493–494
Boundaries, of post anesthesia nursing practice, 17t
Bowman's capsule, 139, *140*
Brachial plexus, 79
Brachial plexus nerve block, 256
Bracket systems, in PACU, 7
Bradycardia, definition of, 82
    muscle relaxants and, 244
    sinus, postoperative monitoring of, 274, *274*
Bradypnea, definition of, 104
Brain. See also specific part, e.g., *Cerebrum*.
    anatomy of, 53–72
    arterial blood supply to, 71, *72–73*
    basal view of, *56*
    cerebrospinal fluid circulation in, *66*
    coronal section of, *68*
    injuries to, consequences of, 413–415, *414*
        types of, 412
    lateral ventricles of, 54, *57*
    lateral view of, *55*
    lobes of, 54, *55*
    movement of inhalant anesthetic from arterial blood to, 193,
        193t
    pathologic conditions of, types of, 415–416
    protection of, 63, *64*, 65, *66–70*, 67–71
    venous drainage of, *67*
Brain scanning, 411
Brain stem, anatomy of, 62–63
    in breathing regulation, 235–236
Breast, sagging of, 489
Breast augmentation, 488, *488–489*
Breast biopsy, 485
    definition of, 484
Breast cancer, surgical choices for, 485–491, *486–487*
Breast lift (mastopexy), *484–485*, 489
    definition of, 484
Breast reconstruction, 488–489, *488–489*
    definition of, 484
    muscle-skin flaps in, 488, *489*
Breast surgery, 484–491
    for gynecomastia, *490*, 491
    post anesthesia care after, 485–491
    procedure(s) in, biopsy as, 485
        lumpectomy as, 485, *486*, 487
        mammoplasty as, 490–491
        mastectomy as, *486–487*, 487–488
        mastopexy as, *484–485*, 489
        reconstruction as, 488–489, *488–489*
Breathing. See also *Respiration*.
    apneustic, definition of, 104
    diaphragmatic, in newborn, 536
    during cardiopulmonary resuscitation, 589, *589*
    regulation of, 129–133
        carbon dioxide response in, 131, *131*
        central chemoreceptors in, 130–131
        controllers in, 132–133
        hypoxic drive in, 130
        lung receptors in, 132
        peripheral chemoreceptors in, 129–130
        secondary drive in, 130
        upper airway receptors in, 131

Breathing pattern, sighless, 134
Bretylium tosylate, for cardiopulmonary resuscitation, 591
Brevibloc (esmolol), for hypertension, 101t, 102–103
Brevital. See *Methohexital (Brevital).*
Broca's area, of brain, *57,* 58
Bronchiectasis, definition of, 104
Bronchiole(s), anatomy of, 109
Bronchitis, chronic, 519
    cigarette smoking and, 528
Bronchoscope, flexible fiber-optic, *352*
    placement of, *351*
    rigid, *351*
Bronchoscopy, 351–353
    anesthesia for, 352
    definition of, 350
    laser therapy used with, 351–352
    needle biopsy and, 353
Bronchospasm, definition of, 104
    postoperative, 263–264
Bronchus(i), anatomy of, 108–109, *110*
    bifurcation of, 109
Brown-Séquard syndrome, 433
Bruising, of brain, 412
Buffer(s), 125
Bupivacaine (Marcaine), for local anesthesia, 248t, 249
Buprenorphine (Buprenex), 221
Burn(s), 499–505
    care of, 169–170
    chemical, 169, 501
    classification of, 499–500
    deep-dermal, 169
    electrical, 169, 501–502
    extent of injury from, 500, *500–501*
    first-degree, 169
    fluid balance after, 502
    fourth-degree, 170
    full-thickness, 169–170, 500
    partial-thickness, 169, 500
    pathophysiology of, 502–503
    post anesthesia care of, 504–505
    second-degree, 169
    superficial, 500
    thermal, 169, 500–501
    third-degree, 169
    types of, 500–502
    wound care for, 503–504
Burnout, of staff, 22–25, 24t
Bursa-dependent cell(s). See *B lymphocyte(s).*
Butorphanol (Stadol), 219–220, 220t
Butyrophenone(s), as nonopioid intravenous anesthetic, 210–212
Bypass, definition of, 387

C

C fibers, of afferent nerve, 246
C wave(s), 83, *84*
    in intracranial pressure, 421, *422*
Caged-ball valve, 376, *377*
Calan. See *Verapamil (Calan, Isoptin).*
Calcitonin, 152
Calcium, deficiency of, muscle relaxants and, 237–238
Calcium channel blockers, 97
Calcium chloride, for cardiopulmonary resuscitation, 591, 592t
Caldwell-Luc operation, definition of, 329
Calices, renal, 138
cAMP (cyclic adenosine monophosphate), 149
Cancer, breast, surgical choices for, 485–491, *486–487*
    of head and neck, reconstruction surgery for, 340–341
Cannabinoid abuse, 561
    effects and signs of, 559t
Cannula, nasal, oxygen administration via, 296, 297t

Capillary(ies), pulmonary, fluid movement from, 119, *119*
Capnogram, changes in, interpretation of, 268–269, *268–270*
    normal, 267, *268*
Capnograph, mainstream, 267
    sidestream, 267
Capnography, changes in, interpretation of, 268–269, *268–270*
    clinical issues in, 269–270
    monitoring ventilation by, 267–270
    normal, 267, *268*
    technical overview of, 267–270, *268–270*
Capnometer, 267
Carbaminohemoglobin, 123
Carbocaine. See *Mepivacaine (Carbocaine).*
Carbon dioxide, end-tidal, exponential decrease in, 268, *269*
    gradual decrease in, 269, *270*
    gradual increase in, 268, *269*
    sudden decrease in, 268, *268*
    vs. arterial, 267–268
    in respiratory gases, monitoring, 267–270, *268–270*
    muscle relaxants and, 238
Carbon dioxide dissociation curve, 123, *124*
Carbon dioxide response curve, 130, *130*
Carbon dioxide transport, 123–125, *124*
    as bicarbonate ions, 123–124, *124*
    as carbaminohemoglobin, 123
    chloride shift in, 124
    Haldane effect on, 123
    in solution, 123
Carbonic anhydrase inhibitors, 145
Carboxyhemoglobin, 528
Cardia, 156
Cardiac. See also *Heart* entries.
Cardiac arrest, definition of, 82
Cardiac catheterization, definition of, 371
Cardiac compression, in cardiopulmonary resuscitation, external, 589–590, *590*
Cardiac cycle, 83–84, *84*
Cardiac defect(s), of atrioventricular canal, 369
    septal, ventricular, 378, *379*
Cardiac index, definition of, 82
    postoperative monitoring of, 279
Cardiac muscle, 86, *86*
    excitability and contractility of, factors affecting, 86t
Cardiac output, 84–85
    definition of, 82
    postoperative monitoring of, 278–279
Cardiac patients, functional classification of, 88t
Cardiac surgery, 368–386
    anesthesia for, 380
    chest tube drainage systems in, 381
    complication(s) of, 382–386
        cardiac tamponade as, 383
        cardiovascular, 382–385
        congestive heart failure as, 382–383
        dysrhythmias as, 383
        gastrointestinal, 385–386
        hemorrhage as, 384
        inadequate volume status as, 384–385
        myocardial infarction as, 382
        nervous system, 385
        peripheral vascular, 386
        peripheral vasoconstriction as, 383–384
        renal, 385
        respiratory, 385
        wound dehiscence and infection as, 384
    ECG recordings in, 380–381
    intraoperative considerations in, 379–380
    intravascular parameters in, 381
    PACU care following, 380–382
Cardiac tamponade, after cardiac surgery, 383
Cardiogenic shock, 578t, 578–580, 586

Cardiogenic shock *(Continued)*
    definition of, 579
    treatment of, 579–580, 587
Cardiomyopathy, hypertrophic obstructive, 369
Cardioplegia, definition of, 371
Cardiopulmonary bypass, *372*
    definition of, 371
    physiologic changes associated with, 379–380
Cardiopulmonary resuscitation (CPR), A-B-C steps in, 589–590, *590*
    airway for, 589
    bag-valve-mask unit for, 589
    breathing during, 589, *589*
    cardiac compression in, external, 589–590, *590*
    circulation during, 589
    electrical cardioversion in, 594, 594t
    equipment for, 588t
    in PACU, 584–594
    indications for, 587, 589
    medical treatment for, 588t, 590–594, 591t
    mouth-to-mouth ventilation in, 589, *589*
    one-person, 590, *590*
    ventilation of patient in, 589
Cardiopulmonary status, after large vessel surgery, 396
Cardiovascular disease, effect of, on pharmacologic action, 184
Cardiovascular function, postoperative, 270–273
        blood pressure measurement and, 271–273
            clinical issues in, 273
            invasive, 272–273
            noninvasive, 271–272, *272*
        clinical assessment of, 270
        pulse pressure monitoring and, 273
Cardiovascular system, age-related problems of, 544
    anatomy and physiology of, 82–103
    changes in, during pregnancy, 549–551, 550t, *551*
    circulation in, 90–91
    complications of, after cardiac surgery, 382–385
        after spinal injuries, 435–436
    effect of adrenergic and cholinergic receptors on, 91–103
    effect of cigarette smoking on, 528
    heart in, 83–90
    in obese patient, 526
        postoperative, 527
    in pediatric patient, 534t, 534–535, *535*, 535t
        monitoring of, 539
Cardioversion, electrical, during cardiopulmonary resuscitation, 594, 594t
Cardizem. See *Diltiazem (Cardizem)*.
Carina, 108, *109*
Carotid artery(ies), 71, *72–73*
Carotid blowout, as complication of radical neck surgery, 339–340
Carotid endarterectomy, 393
    cranial nerve assessment in, 394t
Catabolism, after burns, 503
Cataract, definition of, 343
Catecholamines, muscle relaxants and, 238
Catheter(s), pulmonary artery, 89–90
    suprapubic, 466
    types of, *466*
    ureteral, 466–467
    urethral, 465–466
Catheterization, cardiac, 371
Cauda equina, 77
Caudate nucleus, of brain, 54, *57*
CBF. See *Cerebral blood flow (CBF)*.
CC (closing capacity), 113
CDC (Centers for Disease Control and Prevention),
        recommendations by, for blood-borne diseases, 34
    for tuberculous patient, 34
Cecostomy, definition of, 447

Celioscopy, definition of, 479
Celiotomy, definition of, 450
Cellular (cell-mediated) immunity, 174–175
    definition of, 171
Centers for Disease Control and Prevention (CDC),
        recommendations by, for blood-borne diseases, 34
    for tuberculous patient, 34
Central nervous system. See also specific part, e.g., *Brain*.
    anatomy and physiology of, 53–80
    blood-brain and blood-CSF barriers of, 69–71
    depression of, compromised renal function and, 146
    oxygen toxicity in, 136
    postoperative assessment of, 283
Central nervous system depressants, abuse of, 559–560
    effects and signs in, 558t
Central nervous system sympathomimetics, abuse of, 560–561
    effects and signs in, 558t–559t
Central neurogenic hyperventilation, 425t
Central venous pressure, monitoring of, 89
Cerclage procedure(s), care after, 480–481
    definition of, 477
Cerebellum, anatomy of, *61*, 62
    relationship of, to brain stem, *61*
Cerebral aneurysm, 415
Cerebral aqueduct, 61, *61*
Cerebral artery(ies), 71, *72–73*
Cerebral blood flow (CBF), autoregulation of, 417
        lower limit of, 417–418
    critical, 417
    factors affecting, 416–417
    metabolic regulation of, 417
Cerebral cortex, anatomy of, 54, *55–56*
Cerebral nuclei (basal ganglia), anatomy of, 54, *57*
Cerebral peduncles, 61
Cerebral perfusion pressure, 417
    autoregulation of, 71, *73*
Cerebrospinal fluid (CSF), 68–69, *69–70*
    carbon dioxide levels in, breathing regulation and, 130
    circulation of, 68
        in brain and spinal cord, *66*
    pressure system of, 71
    reabsorption of, 68–69
Cerebrum, anatomy of, 54, *55*
    association areas of, 58
    auditory area of, 58
    coronal section of, *57*
    coronal view of, *60*
    functional aspects of, 54–56, *57*, 58–59
    gustatory area of, 58
    motor speech area of, *57*, 58
    olfactory area of, 58
    prefrontal area of, 58
    premotor area of, 55–56, *57*, 58
        extrapyramidal tracts in, 56
    primary motor area of, 55, *57*
    sensory areas of, 58
    visual area of, 58
Certification in post anesthesia nursing (CPAN), 18, 19
Cervical conization, definition of, 477
Cervical plexus, 79
Cervicodorsal sympathectomy, 392
Cesarean hysterectomy, definition of, 477
Cesarean section, care after, 479–480
    definition of, 477
    pain management after, 554–555
Chalazion, definition of, 343
Chemical(s), as immunological defense barrier, 172
Chemical burn(s), 169, 501
Chemoreceptor(s), in regulation of breathing, central, 130–131
    peripheral, 129–130
Chemotactic factor, 175

Chemotactic factor *(Continued)*
  of lymphokines, 174
Chest. See also *Thoracic* entries.
  flail, 361, *362*
  funnel, 350
  postoperative inspection of, 262–263
  postoperative listening and auscultation of, 263–264
  postoperative palpation of, 263
  postoperative percussion of, 263
Chest cavity, surgical approach to, 353, *354*
Chest drainage, 353–360
  after cardiac surgery, 381
  Heimlich valve for, *355*, 355–356
  indications for, 353–354
  PACU care for, 356–360
    ensuring patency of tubing in, 357–359, *358*
    maintaining proper function in, 359–360
    monitoring volume of drainage in, 357, *357–358*
  suction for, 356, *356*
  tubes for, insertion of, 353–354, *354*
  types of, *355*, 355–356
  volume in, 361
Chest tube(s), milking of, *358*, 358–359
  patency of, 357–358
  placement of, 353–354, *354*
  stripping of, 359, *359*
Chest wall, mechanical features of, *115*, 115–116
Cheyne-Stokes respiration, 425t
  definition of, 104
Chilblains, 169
Child, 534. See also *Pediatric patient.*
Chloride shift, in carbon dioxide transport, 124
Chloroform (Trichlormethane), 197
Chloroprocaine (Nesacaine), for local anesthesia, 247, 248t
Cholecystectomy, definition of, 447
  laparoscopic, *459*, 460
Cholecystostomy, definition of, 447
Cholelithiasis, 162
  definition of, 156
Cholinergic, definition of, 82
Cholinergic nerve(s), functional anatomy of, 92, 92t
Cholinergic neurotransmitter, biochemistry of, 92, 93t
Cholinergic receptor(s), 94, 95t
Chordae tendineae, 85, *86*
Chordee, definition of, 464
Christoph's conceptual model, of postoperative pain relationships, *315*
Chronic obstructive pulmonary disease (COPD), 519–521
  airways and, 520
  description of, 519
  drug interactions and, 520–521
  PACU care and, 520–521
  surgical considerations of, 519–520
Chronotropic, definition of, 82
Chvostek's sign, 445
Chylothorax, definition of, 350
Chyme, definition of, 156
Cigarette smoking, 527–529
  cardiovascular effects of, 528
  PACU care and, 528–529
  postoperative complications associated with, 133–134, 528–529
  pulmonary diseases associated with, 528
  respiratory effects of, 527–528
Cilia, nasal, 105, *106*
Cimetidine (Tagamet), for gastric hypersecretory states, 159
Cineplastic (kineplastic) amputation, definition of, 399
Circle of Willis, 71, *72–73*
Circle system, of administration of inhalation anesthesia, 194–195
Circulation, 90–91

Circulation *(Continued)*
  coronary, 87–88, *88*
  during cardiopulmonary resuscitation, 589
  in post anesthesia recovery score, 33t
  micro-, 91
  platelets in, 90–91
  pulmonary. See *Pulmonary circulation.*
  red blood cells in, 90
  systemic, 91
    removal of drugs from, 183–184
  white blood cells in, 90
Circulatory function, after thoracic surgery, 364–365
Circulatory overload, as delayed reaction to transfusions, 294
Circulatory status, after carotid endarterectomy, 393
  after large vessel surgery, 396–397
  after peripheral vascular surgery, 391, *391*
Circumcision, definition of, 464
Circumflex artery, 87
Circus movement (re-entry), definition of, 83
Cirrhosis, alcoholic, 560
Cistern, definition of, 53
Cisterna magna, 68
Citanest. See *Prilocaine (Citanest).*
Citrate intoxication, as delayed reaction to transfusions, 294
Claustrum, 54, *57*
Cleft lip and palate, surgical repair of, 496–497, *497*
Clinical nurse specialist (CNS), in PACU, 19–20
Clone(s), definition of, 171
  in humoral immunity, 172
Clonidine withdrawal syndrome, 95
Closing capacity (CC), 113
Closing volume (CV), 113
Cluster breathing, 425t
CNS (clinical nurse specialist), in PACU, 19–20
Coarctation of aorta, *372*
  definition of, 371
Cocaine, abuse of, 559t, 560–561
  for local anesthesia, 247, 248t
Coccyx, 74
Cochlear implant, 328
  definition of, 325
Cold injury, 169, 501
Colliculum, of brain stem, 61
Colloids, for shock, 572
Colon, anatomy and physiology of, 160
Color, in post anesthesia recovery score, 33t
Colostomy, definition of, 447
Colpocleisis (Le Fort operation), 481–482
Colporrhaphy, definition of, 477
Comfort, of patient, in PACU, 302
Commissure, definition of, 53
Commissurotomy, definition of, 371
Communicating hydrocephalus, 416
Compartment syndrome, after orthopedic surgery, 403
Compazine. See *Prochlorperazine (Compazine).*
Complement, activation of, antigen-antibody complex in, 174
Compliance, definition of, 409
  lung, definition of, 104
Composite graft, 492
Compressed Gas Association, Inc., 13t
Compression, aortocaval, during pregnancy, 549, *551*
Compression fracture, of spine, 433
Computed tomography (CT), in cranial surgery, 411, *411*
  in spinal surgery, 431–432
Concentration effect, in inhalation anesthesia, 192
Concussion, 412
  of spinal cord, 433
Conduction, definition of, 82
Conduction anesthesia, 245
Condyle(s), femoral and tibial, 406
Congestive heart failure, after cardiac surgery, 382–383

Conscious sedation, intravenous, definition of, 511
   in ambulatory surgery, 510–511
Consciousness, level of, assessment of, 423t, 425
Contact dermatitis, as delayed hypersensitivity reaction, 176
Continuous positive airway pressure (CPAP), following cardiac surgery, 380
   mechanical ventilation and, 296–297
Continuous quality improvement (CQI), in PACU, 35, 35–36
Contracture(s), from spinal injuries, 437
   Volkmann, definition of, 399
Controller(s), in regulation of breathing, 132–133
Contusion, of brain, 412
   of spinal cord, 433
   of tissues, in trauma, 571
Conus medullaris, 76
COPD. See Chronic obstructive pulmonary disease (COPD).
Cor pulmonale, definition of, 82
Core, of post anesthesia nursing practice, 16t
Corneal transplant surgery, 346
Corniculate cartilages, 106, 107
Coronary artery, 87
Coronary artery bypass, 374
Coronary artery steal, 87
Coronary circulation, 87–88, 88
Corpora quadrigemina, 61
Corpus callosum, 54
Corpus striatum, 54
Cortex, adrenal, 153
   cerebral, 54, 55–56
   renal, 138, 139
Corticobulbar tract(s), of pons, 62
Corticospinal tract(s), of cerebrum, 55
   of pons, 62
Corticosteroid(s), for anaphylactic shock, 586
   for cardiopulmonary resuscitation, 591, 592t
   intracranial pressure reduced by, 420
Corticosterone, 153
Corticotropin-releasing hormone (CRH), 151
Cortisol. See Hydrocortisone.
Cortisone, 153
Cosmetic surgery, 494–496
Coughing, in stir-up regimen, 290
Countershock, direct-current, emergency administration of, 277, 277–278
   recommended energies for, 594t
Coup-contrecoup injury, contusion due to, 412
CPAN (certification in post anesthesia nursing), 18, 19
CPAP (continuous positive airway pressure), following cardiac surgery, 380
   mechanical ventilation and, 296–297
CPR. See Cardiopulmonary resuscitation (CPR).
CQI (continuous quality improvement), in PACU, 35, 35–36
Cranial bone(s), 63, 64, 65
Cranial cavity, interior of, 64
Cranial nerve(s). See also specific nerve, e.g., Olfactory nerve.
   assessment of, following carotid endarterectomy, 394t
   functions of, 63t
Cranial surgery, 410–431
   body temperature following, 428
   diagnostic tools used in, 410–412
   fluid and electrolyte balance following, 427–428
   intracranial pressure following, 430. See also Intracranial pressure (ICP).
   invasive technique(s) in, 410–412
      arteriography as, 410–411, 411
      brain scanning as, 411
      CT scanning as, 411, 411
      magnetic resonance imaging as, 411–412
      pneumoencephalography as, 410
      positron emission tomography as, 412
      ventriculography as, 410

Cranial surgery (Continued)
   level of consciousness following, 423t, 425
   motor and sensory functioning following, 425–426
   noninvasive technique(s) in, 412, 413
   nursing care following, 426–431
   patient positioning following, 428–429
   post anesthesia record following, 423, 424
   pupillary activity following, 426
   respiratory status following, 427
   seizures following, 429–430
   skin care following, 429
   vital signs following, 423–425, 425t
Cranial venous sinus(es), 65, 66
Cranium, 65
Creatine phosphokinase, serum, in malignant hyperthermia, 565
Creatinine, in urine, 143, 143t
Creatinine clearance, in renal failure, 147
Crepitus, definition of, 409
CRH (corticotropin-releasing hormone), 151
Cross-tolerance, definition of, 181
Croup, postintubation, treatment of, 541–542
Crutchfield tongs, for spinal injuries, 436, 436
CryoCuff system, in knee surgery, 405, 405
Cryoprecipitate, in transfusions, 295
Crystalloids, for shock, 571–572
CT. See Computed tomography (CT).
Cuff, of tracheal tube, 308–309, 309
Culdoscopy, definition of, 477
Cushing's reflex, 425
Cushing's triad, 425
CV (closing volume), 113
Cyanosis, definition of, 82, 104
Cyclic adenosine monophosphate (cAMP), 149
Cyclopropane, 197
Cystectomy, definition of, 463
Cystitis, definition of, 138
Cystocele, definition of, 477
Cystolithotomy, definition of, 463
Cystoscopy, care after, 465
   definition of, 463
Cystostomy, definition of, 463
Cytotoxic hypersensitivity reaction(s), 175t, 175–176

D

Dacron graft, 394
   aortoiliac, 395
Dacryocystitis, definition of, 343
Dacryocystorhinostomy, definition of, 343
Dalgan. See Dezocine (Dalgan).
Dalton's law of partial pressure, 120
Dantrium. See Dantrolene (Dantrium).
Dantrolene (Dantrium), for malignant hyperthermia, 542, 566–567, 568t
D&C (dilation and curettage), definition of, 477
Dead space, anatomic, 128, 129
   physiologic, 128, 129
Death, pathophysiology of, 587, 588t, 589
Decamethonium bromide (Syncurine), as depolarizing neuromuscular agent, 237
Decompensation, definition of, 409
Decortication (of lung), definition of, 350
Decussate, definition of, 53
Deep vein thrombosis, after orthopedic surgery, 402
Deep-breathing exercises, 289
Deep-dermal burn, 169
Deglutition, definition of, 156
Delayed hypersensitivity reaction(s), 175t, 176
Delayed-onset respiratory depression, caused by fentanyl, 217
Delirium, emergence, 291
   postanesthesia, 314

Delirium *(Continued)*
  stage of, in anesthesia, 190
Delirium tremens, 560
Delta opioid receptor(s), 215
Demerol. See *Meperidine (Demerol).*
Dens, of axis, 74
Depolarization, of presynaptic membrane, 227
Depressants, CNS, abuse of, 558t, 559–560
Dermabrasion, 494–495
Dermatitis, contact, as delayed hypersensitivity reaction, 176
Dermatochalasis, definition of, 343
Dermatome(s), arrangement of, 253, *253*
Dermis, 499. See also *Skin.*
  anatomy of, 165
Desflurane, 201
  properties of, 193t
Desquamation, of skin, 165
Dexamethasone, for Addisonian crisis, 154
  for cardiopulmonary resuscitation, 591
Dextran, in transfusions, 295
Dezocine (Dalgan), 220t, 220–221
  intravenous dose of, 221
Diabetes insipidus, definition of, 409
  in cranial surgical patient, 428
Diabetes mellitus, ADH deficiency and, 151
  anesthesia and, 522
  complications of, characteristics of, 524t
  obesity associated with, 526
  PACU care and, 522–523, 523t, 524t
Diagnostic testing, for ambulatory surgery, 509
Diaphragmatic herniorrhaphy, definition of, 448
Diarrhea, definition of, 156
Diastasis, 83
Diastole, 85
  definition of, 82
Diazepam (Valium), 208
  intracranial pressure and, 419
Diazoxide (Hyperstat), for hypertension, 100, 101t
Dibucaine (Nuperaine), for local anesthesia, 248t
Diencephalon, anatomy of, 59–60
Diethyl ether, 197–198
Digoxin, adverse effects of, in geriatric patient, 547t
Dilation and curettage (D&C), definition of, 477
Diltiazem (Cardizem), 97
Dimensions, of post anesthesia nursing practice, 16t–17t
Diphenhydramine (Benadryl), for post cesarean section pain, 554
Diprivan. See *Propofol (Diprivan).*
Direct-current countershock, emergency administration of, *277,* 277–278
Disarticulation, cineplastic (kineplastic), definition of, 399
Discharge criteria, in ambulatory surgery, areas of concern and, 513–514, 514t
Discharge instruction sheets, preprinted, ambulatory surgery and, 514–515
Discharged patient, follow-up contacts made with, goals of, 515t
Discomfort, following genitourinary surgery, 468
Diskectomy (discectomy), definition of, 399
Dissociation curve, carbon dioxide, 123, *124*
Dissociative anesthetic(s), 212–213
Distribution, in pharmacokinetic interactions, 184, 187
Distributive (vasogenic) shock, 578t, 580–582
Diuretic(s), 144–145
  adverse effects of, in geriatric patient, 547t
  intracranial pressure reduced by, 419–420
  loop, 145
  osmotic, 144
  potassium-sparing, 145
  thiazide, 144–145
Diverticulum, definition of, 447
Dobutamine (Dobutrex), 98

Dobutamine (Dobutrex) *(Continued)*
  for cardiopulmonary resuscitation, 592
Donor site(s), of skin grafts, *494*
  care of, 505
Dopamine (Inotropin), 97–98
  for cardiopulmonary resuscitation, 592
Dopaminergic receptor(s), 95
Doppler instrument, for detection of blood flow, 391, *391*
Dorsal, definition of, 53
Dose-response relationship(s), of pharmacologic agents, 182
Doxacurium, action and dosage of, 231
  pharmacology of, 229t
Drainage, after abdominal surgery, 451
  after prostatectomy, 472, *473*
  after radical mastectomy, 488
Dressing(s), after abdominal surgery, 451
  after breast biopsy, 485
  after eye surgery, 348–349, *348–349*
  after genitourinary surgery, 467
  after large vessel surgery, 397
  after peripheral vascular surgery, 392
  after radical mastectomy, 487
  after renal and ureteral surgery, 468
  after thyroid surgery, 445
  mustache, after nasal surgery, *329*
Dromotropic, definition of, 82
Droperidol (Inapsine), 210–212
  antiemetic dose of, 211
  as neuroleptic, 211
  emergence from, PACU care during, 211–212
  for post cesarean section pain, 554
  mechanism of action of, 211
  negative effects of, 211
Drug(s). See also named drug.
  biotransformation of, in liver, 161–162
  distribution of, physiologic and compartmental models in, 182, *183*
  effects of, in patients with compromised renal function, 146
  efficacy of, definition of, 181
  elimination of, from body, 182–183
  for cardiopulmonary resuscitation, 588t, 590–594, 591t
  for hypertension, 100–103, 101t
  graded response of, 182
  loading dose of, 182
  potency of, definition of, 181
  preoperative, intravenous administration of, 509
  quantal response of, 182
  removal of, from circulation, 183–184
  routes of administration of, systemic absorption by, 183
  tolerance to, 557. See also *Drug abuse.*
  used in nausea control, 532t
Drug abuse, 557–561
  effects and signs of, 558t–559t
  of cannabinoids, 559t, 561
  of CNS depressants, 558t, 559–560
  of CNS sympathomimetics, 558t–559t, 560–561
  of opioid analgesics, 557, 558t, 559
  of psychedelics, 559t, 561
  physical dependence in, 557
  psychological dependence in, 557
  tolerance in, 557
Drug abuser, PACU care of, 557, 559–561
Drug interaction(s), associated with geriatric patient, 546, 547t
Drug response(s), 182–184
  dose-response relationships in, 182
  effects of physiologic dysfunction on, 184
  in removal from systemic circulation, 183–184
  pharmacokinetic actions in, 182–183, *183*
  routes of administration and, systemic absorption by, 183
Drug-drug interaction(s), 184, 185t–186t, 187
  and PACU, 187–188

Drug-drug interaction(s) *(Continued)*
  pharmacodynamic, 187
  pharmacokinetic, 184, 187
Drug-induced parkinsonism, 56, 58
Ducts of Bellini, 139–140
Dumbbell tumor(s), 442
Duodenum, anatomy and physiology of, 160
Dura mater, 65, *66*, 66, *68*
  folds of, 65
  spinal, 74, 251
Dwarfism, 150
Dyskinesia, tardive, 58
Dyspnea, definition of, 104
Dysrhythmia(s), after cardiac surgery, 383
  as delayed reaction to transfusions, 294
  associated with invasive hemodynamic monitoring, 282t
Dystonic reactions, acute, 58
Dysuria, definition of, 138

E

Ear, divisions of, *326*
  frontal section through, *326*
  surgery of, 325–328. See also specific procedure, e.g., *Stapedectomy.*
    complications following, 328
    special considerations in, 328
Ectopic, definition of, 82
Ectopic pacemaker, definition of, 82
Ectopic pregnancy, *478*
  care after, 480
  definition of, 477
Ectropion, definition of, 343
Edema, pulmonary. See *Pulmonary edema.*
  spinal cord, 435
Effective dose, of drug, concept of, 194
Effector T lymphocyte(s), in cellular immunity, 174
Efferent, definition of, 53
Efficacy of drug, definition of, 181
Elastic recoil, of lung, 114
Elderly. See *Geriatric patient.*
Electrical burn(s), 169, 501–502
Electrocardiogram (ECG), after cardiac surgery, 380–381
Electrocardiographic monitoring, postoperative, 273–278
    lead placement in, 274, *274*
    of sinus arrhythmias, 274–275, *274–275*
    of supraventricular arrhythmias, 275–276, *275–276*
    of ventricular arrhythmias, 276–277, *276–278*
Electrode(s), placement of, in postoperative electrocardiographic monitoring, 274, *274*
Electroencephalography, 412
Electrolyte(s), definition of, 82
  loss of, prevention of, 167
Electrolyte balance, after abdominal surgery, 452
  after cranial surgery, 427–428
  clinical states affecting, 284t
  effect of inhalation anesthesia on, 203
  postoperative evaluation of, 284–286
Electrolyte imbalance, symptoms of, 287t
Electromagnetic interference scanning. See *Computed tomography (CT).*
Electromyography, in spinal surgery, 432
Elimination, in pharmacokinetic interactions, 187
Embolectomy, definition of, 387
Embolism, definition of, 82
  fat, after orthopedic surgery, 402–403
  pulmonary, after orthopedic surgery, 402
Embolization, associated with invasive hemodynamic monitoring, 281t–282t
Embolus, definition of, 387
Emergence, delayed, 291

Emergence delirium, 291
  postanesthesia, 314
Emergency evacuation, from PACU, 5–6
Emcte-con. See *Benzquinamide (Emete-con).*
Emotional support, for ambulatory surgical patient, 510
  of pregnant patient, 554
Emphysema, 519
  senile, 545
  subcutaneous, after tracheostomy, 338
Encephalon. See *Brain.*
End plate, of muscle, 226, *227*
Endarterectomy, carotid, 393
    cranial nerve assessment in, 394t
  definition of, 387
Endocardial cushion defects, 369
Endocarditis, associated with invasive hemodynamic monitoring, 282t
Endocrine gland, definition of, 149
Endocrine system. See also specific gland, e.g., *Thyroid gland.*
  in pediatric patient, 534
  mediators of, 149–150
  physiology of, 150–154
  syndromes and diseases associated with, 154–155
Endoscopic retrograde cholangiopancreatography (ERCP), definition of, 447
Endoscopy, definition of, 329, 447
Endotracheal intubation, of pediatric patient, 535–536
  tube size in, 537t
  oral. See *Tracheal intubation, oral.*
Endotracheal tray(s), adult and pediatric, equipment for, 307t
Endotracheal tube(s), placement of, 310–311
  recommended sizes for, 307t
  used in intubation, 308–309, *309*
Enflurane (Ethrane), 198–199
  advantages of, 199
  hemodynamic effects of, 198
  intracranial pressure and, 418–419
  properties of, 193t
Engineering, design of PACU based on, 3–4
Enteric system, definition of, 156
Enterocele, definition of, 477
Entropion, definition of, 343
Enucleation, definition of, 343
Enuresis, definition of, 138
Environmental stimulus(i), triggering malignant hyperthermia, 566, 566t
Enzyme(s), induction of, in liver, 161–162
  lysosomal, 175
Epidermis, 499. See also *Skin.*
  anatomy of, 165, *166*
Epididymectomy, definition of, 463–464
Epidural analgesia, for postoperative pain, 320–322
  patient-controlled, 224, 224t
Epidural anesthesia. See *Anesthesia, epidural.*
Epidural blood patch procedure, for postspinal headache, 255
Epidural hematoma, from brain injury, 413–414
Epidural route of administration, of opioids, 222–223
    advantages and disadvantages of, 223
Epidural space, 74
Epigastric herniorrhaphy, definition of, 448
Epiglottis, 106, *107*
  raising, in oral tracheal intubation, 310, *311*
Epinephrine, for anaphylactic shock, 586
  for cardiopulmonary resuscitation, 592t, 593
  metabolism of, 93, *93*
Epiphora, definition of, 343
Epispadias, definition of, 464
Epistaxis, 105–106
  definition of, 104
Epithalamus, 60
Epithelium, as immunologic defense barrier, 171–172

ERCP (endoscopic retrograde cholangiopancreatography), definition of, 447
Ergonomics, design of PACU based on, 4
Error messages, vital sign monitors and, 14
ERV (expiratory reserve volume), 111
    definition of, 111t
Erythroblastosis fetalis, prevention of, 176
Esmolol (Brevibloc), for hypertension, 101t, 102–103
Esophagogastroduodenoscopy, definition of, 447
Esophagoscopy, definition of, 447
Esophagus, anatomy of, 156, *157*
    disorders of, 156–157
    surgery of, care after, 454
Estrogen, 154
Estrus, definition of, 53
Ether(s), as inhalant anesthetic agent, 196. See also specific agent, e.g., *Diethyl ether.*
Ethmoid bone, of cranium, 65
Ethrane. See *Enflurane (Ethrane).*
Ethylene, 198
Etidocaine, for local anesthesia, 248t, 249
Etomidate (Duranest), 206–207
    induction doses of, 207
    inhibition of steroid synthesis by, 207
    intracranial pressure and, 419
Euthyroid, definition of, 444
Evisceration (of eye), definition of, 343
Excitability, definition of, 82
Excitation-contraction (E-C) coupling, in muscle cell, 227
    in muscle physiology, 565
Excitation-secretion coupling, 92
Excitement, emergence, 291
Excretion, pharmacokinetic parameters of, 187
Exenteration (of eye), definition of, 343
Exercise(s), deep-breathing, 289
    desaturation of gases on, 118
    range-of-motion, after orthopedic surgery, 402
Exhaustion, in Selye's adaptation syndrome, 24
Expertise, nursing, development of, 22, *23*
Expiratory reserve volume (ERV), 111
    definition of, 111t
External fixators, definition of, 399
Extracorporeal shock wave lithotripsy, care after, 468
    definition of, 463
Extradural-extramedullary tumor(s), 442
Extrapyramidal tract(s), 56
Extubation, of intubated patient, 312
Eye(s), anatomy of, *344*
    cholinergic stimulation of, 95t
    oxygen toxicity in, 136
    surgery of, 343–349
        anesthesia for, 344–345
        cardiopulmonary assessment after, 347–348
        dressings for, 348–349, *348–349*
        PACU care following, 345, 347–349
        pain management in, 348
        patient positioning after, 345, 347
        psychologic assessment after, 349
    tumors of, iodine plaque irradiation for, 348, *348*
Eye care, after cranial surgery, 429
Eye shield, plastic, 349, *349*

F

Face mask(s), oxygen administration via, 296, 297t
Face tent, oxygen administration via, 297t
Face-lift (rhytidoplasty), 495
Facial bones, trauma to, surgical repair of, 496
Facial nerve, function of, 63t
"Facies," myasthenic, 521
Falx cerebelli, 65

Falx cerebri, 65
Fasciotomy, definition of, 399
Fasting period, before ambulatory surgery, 508–509
Fat embolism syndrome, after orthopedic surgery, 402–403
Febrile reaction(s), to blood transfusion, 293
Femoral herniorrhaphy, definition of, 448
Femoral surgery, post anesthesia care after, 404–405
Fenestration, 328
    definition of, 325
Fentanyl (Sublimaze), 217–218
    administration of, protocol for, in post cesarean section patients, 224t
    delayed-onset respiratory depression caused by, 217
    dose range of, 218
    for post cesarean section pain, 555
    therapeutic index of, 219
Fetal monitoring, 554, 554t, *555*
Fiberoptic laryngoscopy, 11
Fibrillation, atrial, postoperative monitoring of, 276, *276*
    definition of, 82
    ventricular, postoperative monitoring of, *277*, 277–278
Fibrinolytic therapy, definition of, 387
    for vascular disease, 388–389
Fibroplasia, retrolental, 136
    in pediatric patient, 540–541
Fick technique, cardiac output calculation by, 84
Field block anesthesia, 245
Filtration, renal, 140, 141t
Filum terminale, 76
Fink phenomenon, 202
FIO$_2$ (fractional inspired concentration of oxygen), definition of, 104
Fire extinguishers, in PACU, 7
First-degree burn, 169
Fissure(s), of cerebral hemispheres, 54, *55–56*
    of Sylvius, of cerebral hemispheres, 54, *55*
Fixation, internal, definition of, 399
Fixator(s), external, definition of, 399
Fixed chest syndrome, 218
Flail chest, 361, *362*
Flange, of laryngoscope blade, 308
Flap(s), 493
    pedicle, methods of transfer of, *495*
Flaxedil. See *Gallamine (Flaxedil).*
Flooring materials, in PACU, 7
Fluid(s), input and output of, after large vessel surgery, 397
    after peripheral vascular surgery, 392
    intravenous, postoperative, 284–285
    oral intake of, 285
    postoperative intake of, 284–285
    postoperative output of, 285–286, 286t
Fluid balance, after abdominal surgery, 452
    after burns, 502
    after cranial surgery, 427–428
    after thyroid surgery, 445
    clinical states affecting, 284t
    in pediatric patient, maintenance of, 537–538, 538t
        monitoring of, 539
    in rheumatoid arthritic patient, 525
    maintenance of, after thoracic surgery, 364
    muscle relaxants and, 237
    postoperative evaluation of, 284–286
Fluid dynamics, in obese patient, 527
Fluid imbalance, symptoms of, 287t
Fluid intake, after genitourinary surgery, 467
Fluid overload, in geriatric patient, 545
Fluid warmer, with rapid-pressure infusion device, 571, *573*
Flumazenil (Mazicon, Romazicon), 210
    for benzodiazepine overdose, 560
    reversal dose for, 210
Flunitrazepam, 209

Fluoroscopy, in spinal surgery, 431
Fluothane. See *Halothane (Fluothane)*.
Fluroxene (Trifluoroethyl vinyl ether, Fluoromar), 198
Flutter, atrial, postoperative monitoring of, 276, *276*
  definition of, 82
Flutter valve closure, of esophagus, 156
Focal deficit, definition of, 409
Foley catheter, *466*
  in renal and ureteral surgery, 468
Follicle-stimulating hormone (FSH), 151
Foot surgery, post anesthesia care after, 406
Foramen magnum, 65
Foramen of Magendie, 68
Foramen of Monro, 68
Foramina of Luschka, 68
Forane. See *Isoflurane (Forane)*.
Forearm surgery, post anesthesia care after, 403–404
Forebrain, anatomy of, 54–60, *55–57, 59–60*
Fortral. See *Pentazocine (Fortral, Talwin)*.
Fothergill-Hunter procedure, 481
Fourth-degree burn, 170
Fractional inspired concentration of oxygen (FIO_2), definition of, 104
Fracture(s), compression, of spine, 433
  skull, radiograph of, 412, *413*
Fracture-dislocation, of vertebral bodies, 433
Frank-Starling law, 84
FRC (functional residual capacity), 112
  definition of, 111t
  in postoperative period, 134–135, *135*
Fredet-Ramstedt operation, definition of, 450
Frontal bone, of cranium, 65
Frontal lobe, of brain, 54, *55–56*
Frostbite, 169, 501
FSH (follicle-stimulating hormone), 151
Full-thickness burn, 169–170
Full-thickness skin graft, 492
  for burns, 504
Functional residual capacity (FRC), 112
  definition of, 111t
  in postoperative period, *135*, 234–135
Fundus, examination of, after cesarean section, 479–480
  gastric, 157
Funnel chest, 350
Furosemide (Lasix), for hypertension, 100
  intracranial pressure reduced by, 419–420
Fusion, spinal, definition of, 399

G

GABA (gamma-aminobutyric acid), nonopioid drug interaction with, 205
Gallamine (Flaxedil), action of, 231
Gallbladder, anatomy of, 162, *162*
Gallstones, 162
Gamma-aminobutyric acid (GABA), nonopioid drug interaction with, 205
Ganglion, autonomic, cholinergic stimulation of, 95t
Gardner tongs, for spinal injuries, 436
Gas(es), desaturation of, on exercise, 118
  exchange of, in pulmonary circulation, 116–118
  transport of, 120–125
    carbon dioxide in, 123–125, *124*
    oxygen in, 121–123, *122*
Gaseous anesthetic agent(s), 196–197. See also specific agent, e.g., *Nitrous oxide*.
Gastrectomy, definition of, 447
Gastric resection, definition of, 447
Gastritis, definition of, 156
Gastroenterostomy, definition of, 448, *449*

Gastrointestinal contents, aspiration of, after tracheal intubation, 313
Gastrointestinal surgery, care following, 454–457
  in pediatric patient, 542
Gastrointestinal tract. See also specific part, e.g., *Esophagus*.
  anatomy and physiology of, 156–164, *157*
  complications of, after cardiac surgery, 385–386
    after spinal injuries, 439
  decreased activity of, after burns, 502
  during pregnancy, changes in, 550t, 552
    intraoperative considerations of, 552–553
Gastroscopy, definition of, 448
Gaze, conjugate, 426
GCS (Glasgow Coma Scale), 423, 423t
Genital surgery, terms used in, 477–479
Genitourinary surgery, abdominal distention after, 467–468
  care after, 463–475
    general, 465–468
    diagnostic, 464–465
    dressings for, 467
    fluid intake after, 467
    pain and discomfort after, 468
    postoperative use of catheters after, 465–467, *466–467*
    terms used in, 463–464
Geriatric patient, 544–548
  age-related problem(s) in, 544–547
    Alzheimer's disease as, 546–547
    cardiovascular, 544
    drug-interactions as, 546, 547t
    hepatobiliary, 546
    neuromuscular, 545
    psychological, 546
    renal, 545–546
    respiratory, 544–545
  post anesthesia care of, 547–548
Giantism, 150–151
Gibbus, definition of, 409
Gilliam procedure, 481
Glasgow Coma Scale (GCS), 423, 423t
Glaucoma, definition of, 343
Glomerulus, 139, *140*
Glossectomy, definition of, 330
Glossopharyngeal nerve, function of, 63t
Glottis (rima glottidis), anatomy of, 106–107
Glucagon, 153, 163
Glucocorticoid(s), 153
Gluconeogenesis, definition of, 149
Glycogenesis, definition of, 149
Glycopyrolate, dosage of, 234
Glycosuria, definition of, 138
Gonad(s), physiology of, 154
Gonadotropic hormone(s), 151
Gonadotropin-releasing hormone, 151
Goniotomy, definition of, 343
Governance, shared, in PACU, 28
Graded response, of drugs, 182
Graft(s), bone, 493–494
  Dacron, *394*
    aortoiliac, *395*
  kidney, donor of, 470
  rejection of, after kidney transplantation, 471, 471t
  skin, 492–493, *494*
    for burns, 503–504
Gray matter, of brain, 55
  of spinal cord, 79, *80*
Great artery(ies), transposition of, 376
Growth hormone, 150
Growth hormone-inhibiting hormone, 150
Guanethidine, 97, 98t
Gustatory area, of brain, 58
Gynecologic surgery, 481–483

Gynecologic surgery *(Continued)*
  abdominal, care after, 482–483
    terms used in, 479
  laparoscopy in, 481
Gynecomastia, surgery for, *490*, 491

H

H_2 receptor-blocking drugs, for gastric hypersecretory states, 159
Haldane effect, on carbon dioxide transport, 123
Hallucinogens, abuse of, 559t, 561
Halo cast, for spinal injuries, 436, *437*
Halogenated hydrocarbon(s), as inhalant anesthetic agent, 196. See also specific agent, e.g., *Halothane (Fluothane)*.
Halothane (Fluothane), 199–200
  adverse effects of, in geriatric patient, 547t
  hepatitis and, 199
  intracranial pressure and, 418
  MAC of, 194
  oil-gas partition coefficient of, 193
  potency of, 194
  properties of, 193t
  recovery phase of, 200
Hand surgery, post anesthesia care after, 403
Hapten, definition of, 171
Harrington rods, definition of, 399
Head, arterial blood supply to, *72*
  cancer of, reconstruction surgery for, 340–341
  venous drainage of, *67*
Head injury, concomitant, and spinal injuries, 435
Head position, for oral tracheal intubation, 310, *310*
Headache, dural, from epidural analgesia, 322
  oxygen toxicity and, 136
  postspinal, 254–255
Headwall system, built-in, in PACU, 5, *5*
Heart. See also *Cardiac* entries.
  anatomy of, 83–90
  cholinergic stimulation of, 95t
  circulation of, 87–88, *88*
  effect of anesthesia on, 88
  impulses of, conduction of, 86–87
  valves of, 85, *86*
Heart block, definition of, 82
Heart disease, in rheumatoid arthritic patient, 524
Heart failure, congestive, after cardiac surgery, 382–383
Heart rate, in pediatric patient, 534
Heat loss, mechanisms of, 165–166, *166*
"Heat stroke," 564
Heimlich chest drainage valve, *355*, 355–356
Helper T lymphocyte(s), in cellular immunity, 174
Hematocrit, 90
Hematologic alterations, after burns, 502
  during pregnancy, 550–551
Hematoma(s), from brain injury, epidural, 413–414
  intracerebral, 415
  subdural, 414–415
Hematuria, definition of, 138
Hemiarthroplasty, definition of, 399
Hemilaminectomy, partial, for herniated nucleus pulposus, 440, 442
Heminephrectomy, definition of, 463
Hemiplegia, muscle relaxant response in, 243t
Hemodynamic alterations, during pregnancy, 549–550, 550t, *551*
Hemodynamic parameters, postoperative monitoring of, 278–283
  in cardiac output and cardiac index, 278–279
  in left-atrial pressure, 278
  in mean arterial pressure, 278
  in pulmonary artery pressure, 278

Hemodynamic parameters *(Continued)*
    in pulmonary capillary wedge pressure, 278
    in pulmonary vascular resistance, 280, 283
    in right-atrial pressure, 278
    in systemic vascular resistance, 279–280
    invasive methods in, 279t
    line placement in, 278, *280*
    potential problems associated with, 281t–282t
Hemoglobin, 90
  reduced, definition of, 105
Hemoglobin level, in pediatric patient, 535, *535*
Hemolysis, of red blood cells, 531
Hemolytic anemia, as cytotoxic hypersensitivity reaction, 175–176
Hemolytic jaundice, 161
Hemolytic reaction(s), to blood transfusion, 293
Hemorrhage, after adrenalectomy, 475
  after cardiac surgery, 384
  after radical neck surgery, 339
  after thoracic surgery, 366
  after tonsillectomy and adenoidectomy, 332
  associated with invasive hemodynamic monitoring, 282t
  classifications of, 577–578
  from dilution of coagulation factors and platelets, as delayed reaction to transfusions, 294
Hemorrhoidectomy, definition of, 448
Hemothorax, *353*
  after cardiac surgery, 385
  definition of, 350
Hemovac drainage device, use of, after laryngectomy, 339, *340*
Hepatic system. See also *Liver*.
  changes in, during pregnancy, 552
Hepatitis B virus, transmission of, 34
Hepatitis C virus, transmission of, 34
Hepatobiliary system, age-related problems of, 546
Hering-Breuer reflex, 132
Hernia, definition of, 448
  from brain injury, supratentorial, 415
    uncal, 415
  hiatal, 157
Herniated nucleus pulposus, spinal injury and, 440, *441*, 442
Hernioplasty, definition of, 448
Herniorrhaphy, care after, 457
  definition of, 448
Heroin, abuse of, 557, 558t
Hetastarch, in transfusions, 295
Hexafluorenium bromide (Mylaxen), as depolarizing neuromuscular agent, 237
Hiatal hernia, 157
Hiatal herniorrhaphy, definition of, 448, *450*
Hilum, renal, 138, *139*
Hindbrain, anatomy of, *61*, 61–62
Hip surgery, post anesthesia care after, 404–405
Histamine(s), 175
HIV (human immunodeficiency virus), transmission of, 34
Hoarseness, after tracheal intubation, 312–313
Homeostasis, role of kidney in, 142, 142t
Homograft(s), 377
  definition of, 492
Homozygous sickle cell disease, 529
Hormone(s). See also specific hormone.
  definition of, 149
  endocrine, 149–150
  gonadotropic, 151
  in renal function, 140, 142, *142*
  lactogenic, 151
  of adenohypophysis, 150–151
  of neurohypophysis, 151
Horner's syndrome, from brachial plexus nerve block, 256
Human factor, design of PACU based on, 3–4
Human immunodeficiency virus (HIV), transmission of, 34

Humidification, after thoracic surgery, 364
Humidifier(s), 296
Humidity, respiratory function and, 296
Humoral immunity, 172–174, *173*
  definition of, 171
Hyaline membrane disease, 541
Hydralazine (Apresoline), for hypertension, 100, 101t, 102
Hydration, maintenance of, after thoracic surgery, 364
Hydrocarbon(s), halogenated, as inhalant anesthetic agent, 196.
    See also specific agent, e.g., *Halothane (Fluothane).*
Hydrocelectomy, definition of, 464
Hydrocephalus, 416
Hydrocortisone, 153
  for Addisonian crisis, 154
Hydroxyzine (Atarax, Vistaril), for nausea, 532t
Hyperactivity, definition of, 181
Hypercapnia, definition of, 104
  intracranial pressure and, 430
Hyperdynamic left-ventricle syndrome, 377
Hyperdynamic response, to septic shock, 581, 586
Hyperemia, postischemic, 85
Hyperglycemic factor, 153, 163
Hyperkalemia, in renal failure, 148, *148*
Hyperoxemia, definition of, 104
Hyperpnea, definition of, 104
Hyperreflexia, autonomic, after spinal injuries, 439–440
    clinical signs and symptoms of, 440
Hypersensitivity, definition of, 181
Hypersensitivity reaction(s), 175–176
  categories of, 175t
  type I (anaphylactic), 175, 175t. See also *Anaphylaxis.*
  type II (cytotoxic), 175t, 175–176
  type III (arthus), 175t, 176
  type IV (delayed), 175t, 176
Hyperstat. See *Diazoxide (Hyperstat).*
Hypertension, 99
  definition of, 82
  in geriatric patient, 544
  treatment of, 99–103, 101t
Hyperthermia, during cardiac surgery, 380
  malignant, 564–569
    complications following, 569
    dantrolene for, 566–567, 568t
    genetics and, 564–565
    in pediatric patient, 542
    monitoring of, 567, 567t
    pathophysiology of, 565–567, 566t
    perioperative management of, 567t, 567–568
    procainamide for, 567, 568t
    signs and symptoms of, 566t
    skeletal muscle physiology and, 565
    susceptibility to, evaluation of, 565
      patient identification in, 564–565
    treatment of, 568t, 568–569
      pharmacologic agents in, 566–567
    triggering of, 566, 566t
  physiologic alterations associated with, 284t
  post-anesthesia, 203
Hypertrophic obstructive cardiomyopathy, 369
Hyperventilation, 125t
  definition of, 104
  neurogenic, central, 425t
Hypervolemia, after cardiac surgery, 385
  definition of, 82
Hypoadrenocorticism, 154
Hypocapnia, definition of, 104
Hypocarbia, hypothermia-related, 379
Hypochlorhydria (achlorhydria), definition of, 156
Hypodermis, anatomy of, 165
Hypodynamic response, to septic shock, 581, 586
Hypogastric herniorrhaphy, definition of, 448

Hypoglossal nerve, function of, 63t
Hyporeactivity, definition of, 181
Hypospadias, definition of, 464
Hypotension, 98
  due to spinal anesthesia, 254
  in geriatric patient, 544
  neurogenic, after thoracic surgery, 367
  treatment of, 98–99, 99t
Hypothalamus, 60
Hypothermia, definition of, 372, 563
  during cardiac surgery, 379
  management of, 284
  muscle relaxants and, 238
  physiologic alterations associated with, 284t
  post-anesthesia, 203
  postoperative, 563–564
Hypothermia blankets, 428
Hypoventilation, 125t, 127
  definition of, 104
Hypovolemia, after cardiac surgery, 384–385
  after thoracic surgery, 366
Hypovolemic shock, 577–578, 578t, 584, *584*
  definition of, 577
  treatment of, 578, 584
Hypoxemia, after thoracic surgery, 365, *365*
  causes of, 127–129, *128–129*
  definition of, 104
Hypoxia, definition of, 104
  diffusion, following nitrous oxide anesthesia, 202
  intracranial pressure and, 430
Hysterectomy, cesarean, definition of, 477
  radical, definition of, 479
  total abdominal, definition of, 479
  vaginal, definition of, 477
Hysteresis, pulmonary, 112–113, *113*
Hysteroscopy, definition of, 477

I

IC (inspiratory capacity), 112
  definition of, 111t
ICP. See *Intracranial pressure (ICP).*
ICP transducer(s), 421
Idiopathic hypertrophic subaortic stenosis, 369, *370*
IEC (International Electrotechnical Commission), 13t
Ileocecal valve, 160
Ileostomy, definition of, 449
Immersion foot, 169
Immobilization device(s), after orthopedic surgery, care of, 401
Immune system, acquired immunity of, 172–175
  allergic response of, 175t, 175–176
  immunosuppression and, 176–177
  innate immunity of, 172
  physical and chemical barriers of, 171–172
  physiology of, 171–177
Immunity, acquired, 172–175
    cellular type of, 174–175
    humoral type of, 172–174, *173*
  definition of, 171
  innate, 172
Immunodeficiency disease, definition of, 171
Immunoglobulin(s). See also *Antibody(ies).*
  in humoral immunity, 172, *173*
Immunoglobulin A (IgA), 173, *173*
Immunoglobulin D (IgD), 173, *173*
Immunoglobulin E (IgE), 173, *173*
Immunoglobulin G (IgG), *173*, 173–174
Immunoglobulin M (IgM), *173*, 174
Immunosuppressed patient, PACU care of, 176–177
Immunosuppression, 176–177
  definition of, 171

Immunosuppression *(Continued)*
  forms of, 176
Immunosuppressive therapy, after kidney transplantation, 470
Implant(s), cochlear, 328
  intraocular lens, *345*
    definition of, 343
IMV (intermittent mandatory ventilation), 297
Inadequate volume status, after cardiac surgery, 384–385
Inapsine. See *Droperidol (Inapsine).*
Incentive spirometry, in PACU patient, 289–290
Incision(s), abdominal, types of, 450, *451*
  in renal and ureteral surgery, 468, *469*
Incisional herniorrhaphy, definition of, 448
Incontinence, urinary, definition of, 138
Inderal. See *Propranolol (Inderal, Ipran).*
Infant, 534. See also *Pediatric patient.*
Infant respiratory distress syndrome, 541
Infarction, definition of, 82
  myocardial. See *Myocardial infarction.*
Infection(s), after burns, 502–503
  after cardiac surgery, 384
  after thoracic surgery, 366
  associated with invasive hemodynamic monitoring, 282t
  control of, in PACU, 301
    postoperative, 33–34, 34t
  risk of, from shock trauma patients, 576
Inferior, definition of, 53
Infrared tympanic membrane thermometry, 284
Infusion device, rapid-pressure, fluid warmer with, 571, *573*
Inguinal herniorrhaphy, definition of, 448
Inhalation anesthesia, 190–203. See also *Anesthesia, inhalation.*
Injury. See *Trauma.*
Innate immunity, definition of, 171
Inotropic, definition of, 83
Inspection, of chest, postoperative, 262–263
Inspiration, sustained maximal. See *Sustained maximal inspiration (SMI).*
Inspiratory capacity (IC), 112
  definition of, 111t
Inspiratory reserve volume (IRV), 112
  definition of, 111t
Instrument(s), in PACU, 10–11, 11t
Insufflation technique, of administration of inhalation anesthesia, 195
Insulin, 153, 163
  after pancreatic surgery, 460
  dosage of, determination of, 523t
  preoperative, for diabetic patient, 522
  time of action of, 523t
Integumentary system. See *Skin* entries.
Intensity, of postoperative pain, 317, *317*
Interferon, 175
Intermittent mandatory ventilation (IMV), 297
Internal fixation, definition of, 399
International Electrotechnical Commission (IEC), 13t
International Organization for Standardization (ISO), 13t
Intersections, of post anesthesia nursing practice, 17t–18t
Interstitial edema, 120
Intervertebral disk, 74
Intervertebral foramina, 73
Intervertebral notches, 73
Intestinal intubation, after abdominal surgery, 452–453
Intoxication, citrate, as delayed reaction to transfusions, 294
Intracerebral hematoma, from brain injury, 415
Intracranial lesion(s), diffuse, muscle relaxant response in, 243t
Intracranial pressure (ICP), 416–426
  anesthetic agents and, 418–419
  assessment of, 422–426
  dynamics of, 71–72, *73*, 416–426, *418*
  increased, post anesthesia care for patients with, 416–418, 430

Intracranial pressure (ICP) *(Continued)*
    pressure waves in, 421, *422*
    signs of, 422–423
  monitoring of, *420*, 420–421
  reduction of, adjunctive drugs used in, 419–420
  vs. intracranial volume, 416, *417*
Intracranial tumor(s), 416
Intradural-extramedullary tumor(s), 442, *442*
Intramedullary tumor(s), 442
Intramuscular route of administration, of drugs, 183
Intranasal antrostomy, definition of, 329
Intraocular lens implant, *345*
  definition of, 343
Intrapulmonary shunt, 128
Intrathecal analgesia, for postoperative pain, 320
Intrathecal route of administration, of opioids, 222–223
Intravenous route of administration, of drugs, 183
Intravenous therapy, postoperative, 291
  sterile technique for, 167, 169
Intubation, endotracheal, of pediatric patient, 535–536
      tube size in, 537t
    nasogastric or intestinal, after abdominal surgery, 452–453
      irrigation of, 453
      patient comfort and, 453
      tube patency in, 452–453
    tracheal. See *Tracheal intubation.*
Intussusception, definition of, 449
Iodine plaque irradiation, for ocular tumors, 348, *348*
Ipran. See *Propranolol (Inderal, Ipran).*
Iridectomy, definition of, 343
  technique of, *346*
Irrigation, tube, in nasogastric or intestinal intubation, 453
Irritant receptors, in regulation of breathing, 132
IRV (inspiratory reserve volume), 112
  definition of, 111t
Ischemia, definition of, 83, 387
Islets of Langerhans, 153, 163
ISO (International Organization for Standardization), 13t
Isoflurane (Forane), 200
  intracranial pressure and, 419
  properties of, 193t
Isograft(s), definition of, 492
Isolation room, in PACU, 6
Isometric contraction, in cardiac cycle, 83, *84*
Isometric relaxation, in cardiac cycle, 83, *84*
Isoproterenol (Isuprel), for cardiopulmonary resuscitation, 592t, 593
Isoptin. See *Verapamil (Calan, Isoptin).*
Isthmus, of thyroid, 152

J

J receptors, in regulation of breathing, 132
Jaundice, 161
Jejunum, anatomy and physiology of, 160
Joint replacement, definition of, 399
Juxtaglomerular apparatus, 142

K

Kappa opioid receptor(s), 215
Keratoplasty, *346*
  definition of, 343
Kerley's B lines, 120
Ketamine, 212–213
  clinical characteristics of, 212
  emergence from, PACU care during, 212–213
  intracranial pressure and, 419
  intramuscular and intravenous dose of, 212
Ketorolac (Toradol), 220t, 221
  dose range of, 221

Kidney(s). See also *Renal* entries.
anatomy of, 138–140, *139–141*
of pediatric patient, 537–538
role of, in acid-base balance, 143–144
in homeostasis, 142, 142t
Kiesselbach's plexus, 105
Knee surgery, post anesthesia care after, 405–406, *405–406*
Korotkoff sounds, 271
Kussmaul respirations, definition of, 104

L

Labetalol (Normodyne, Trandate), for hypertension, 101t, 103
Labyrinthectomy, definition of, 325
Lacerations, of bladder, 471
spinal, 433
Lacrimation, in anesthesia, 192
Lactogenic hormone(s), 151
Laennec's cirrhosis, 560
Laminectomy, definition of, 399, 409
Laparoscopy, after ectopic pregnancy, 480
definition of, 449–450, 479
for gynecologic problems, 481
Laparotomy, after ectopic pregnancy, 480
definition of, 450
Large bowel, surgery of, care after, 455–457, *456*
Laryngeal nerve(s), 107, *108*
Laryngectomy, 332t, 338–339
definition of, 331
partial, 338
supraglottic, 338
total, *331*, 338
use of Hemovac drainage device after, 339, *340*
Laryngofissure, definition of, 331
Laryngoscope(s), commonly used, in PACU, 10–11, 11t
for tracheal intubation, 307–308, *308*
Laryngoscope bulbs, 11
Laryngoscopy, 333–334
definition of, 331
fiberoptic, 11
Laryngospasm, 107–108
after tonsillectomy and adenoidectomy, 333
after tracheal intubation, 313
postoperative, 263
treatment of, 108
Larynx, anatomy of, 106–108, *107*
muscles of, 107
nerve supply to, 107, *108*
Laser dissection, of tonsils and adenoids, 332
Laser-assisted percutaneous transluminal angioplasty, for
vascular disease, 388
Le Fort operation (colpocleisis), 481
Left-ventricular end-diastolic pressure (LVEDP), 89
Lentiform nucleus, of brain, 54, *57*
Leukocyte(s), 90
Leukocytosis, definition of, 83
Leukopenia, definition of, 83
Levallorphan (Lorfan), 222
Levarterenol bitartrate (Levophed), for cardiopulmonary
resuscitation, 592t, 593
Level of consciousness, assessment of, 423t, 425
LH (luteinizing hormone), 151
Licensed practical nurse (LPN), in PACU, 20
Licensed vocational nurse (LVN), in PACU, 20
Lidocaine (Xylocaine), for cardiopulmonary resuscitation, 592t,
593
for local anesthesia, 247–248, 248t
Ligation, *388*
definition of, 387
Lighting, in PACU, 10
Limb amputation, post anesthesia care after, 407

Limbic system, anatomy of, 58–59, *59*
Lip, cleft, surgical repair of, 496–497, *497*
Lip(s), care of, after cranial surgery, 429
Lipolysis, definition of, 149
Liposuction, 496
Liquid crystal colorimetric sensor, direct-reading, 563
LiteLift continuous passive motion machine, after knee surgery,
406, *406*
Lithium, adverse effects of, in geriatric patient, 547t
Lithotripsy, biliary, 162
definition of, 156
Little's area, 105
Liver, anatomy of, 160–161
bilirubin metabolism in, 161
drug biotransformation in, 161–162
physiology of, 161–162
protein synthesis in, 161
surgery of, care after, 457–458, *458*
Liver disease, effect of, on pharmacologic action, 184
Liver failure, acute, 162
Loading dose, of drug, 182
Lobe(s), of brain, 54, *55–56*
Lobectomy, definition of, 350
thyroid, definition of, 444
Local anesthesia. See *Anesthesia, local.*
Location, of postoperative pain, 316–317
Lockout interval, in patient-controlled analgesia, 224
Logrolling, of spinal patient, 407
Loop diuretic(s), 145
Loop of Henle, 139, *140*
Lopressor (metoprolol), for hypertension, 101t, 103
Lorazepam (Ativan), 209
Lordosis, definition of, 399
Lorfan. See *Levallorphan (Lorfan).*
Lower motor neurons, definition of, 53
LPN (licensed practical nurse), in PACU, 20
LSD (lysergic acid diethylamide), abuse of, 559t, 561
Lumbar plexus, 79
Lumbar puncture, 75
Lumbar sympathectomy, 392–393
Lumpectomy, 485, *486*, 487
definition of, 484
Lund and Browder chart, for burn injury, 500, *501*
Lung(s). See also *Pulmonary* entries.
anatomy of, 109–110, *110*
cholinergic stimulation of, 95t
dysfunction of, in rheumatoid arthritic patient, 524
elastic properties of, 113
elastic recoil of, 114
mechanical forces of, 112–113, *113*
oxygen toxicity in, 136
stiff, 524
surface tension phenomenon in, 113–114
unit recruitment in, 113, *114*
water balance in, 118–120, *119*
Lung capacity, 111t, 112
Lung compliance, 114–116, *115*, *117*
alterations in pulmonary force balance and, 115, *117*
chest wall mechanics and, *115*, 115–116, *117*
definition of, 104, 114
normal value for, 114
pulmonary time constant and, 115
Lung disease, chronic, cigarette smoking and, 527–528
obstructive, 133
pre-existing, postoperative complications of, 133
restrictive, 133
Lung mechanics, during pregnancy, 551–552
Lung receptors, in regulation of breathing, 132
Lung volume, 111t, 111–112
in PACU patient, 289
postoperative complications concerning, 133–135

Lung volume *(Continued)*
  preoperative vs. postoperative, 134, *134*
Luque rods, definition of, 399
Luteinizing hormone (LH), 151
LVEDP (left-ventricular end-diastolic pressure), 89
LVN (licensed vocational nurse), in PACU, 20
Lymphocyte(s), 90
Lymphokines, T lymphocyte release of, 174–175
Lymphopenia, definition of, 171
Lymphotoxin, 175
Lysergic acid diethylamide (LSD), abuse of, 559t, 561
Lysosomal enzymes, 175

M

MAC (minimum alveolar concentration), drug potency
    determination with, 194
  modern concept of, 190–191
MAC awake, 194
MAC hours, 194
MAC-BAR, 194
Macintosh blade, of laryngoscope, 308, *308*
Mackintosh laryngoscope, 10
Macrophage(s), immunologic function of, 172
  in cellular immunity, 174
Magill attachment, for anesthesia machine, 195, *197*
Magill forceps, for nasotracheal intubation, 311–312, *312*
Magnesium, muscle relaxants and, 237
Magnetic resonance imaging (MRI), in cranial surgery, 411–412
  in spinal surgery, 432
Malecot catheter, *466*
Malignant hyperthermia, 564–569. See also *Hyperthermia,
    malignant.*
  in pediatric patient, 542
Mammoplasty, augmentation, definition of, 484
Mannitol, intracranial pressure reduced by, 419–420
Manometer tube, 356
MAP (mean arterial pressure), 417
  postoperative monitoring of, 278
Marcaine. See *Bupivacaine (Marcaine).*
Margin of safety, of drugs, 182
Marihuana abuse, 561
  effects and signs of, 559t
Marshall-Marchetti operation (vesicourethral suspension),
    definition of, 463
Mask(s), oxygen administration via, 297t
Mast cell(s), chemical mediators released by, 175
Mastectomy, radical, *486*, 487–488
  definition of, 484–485
  modified, *486*, 487
Mastoidectomy, 328
  definition of, 325
Mastopexy (breast lift), *484–485*, 489
  definition of, 484
Maxillofacial surgery, 341–342
  preoperative preparation for, 341
Mazicon. See *Flumazenil (Mazicon, Romazicon).*
McDonald procedure, care after, 480
MEAC (minimum effective analgesic concentration), in patient-
    controlled analgesia, 223–224
Mean arterial pressure (MAP), 417
  postoperative monitoring of, 278
Mechanical assist devices, definition of, 372–373
Mechanical valve(s), 376–377, *377*
Mechanical ventilation. See *Ventilation, mechanical.*
Median effective dose, of drugs, 182
Mediastinoscopy, 353
  definition of, 350
Medical director, of PACU, 15, 18
Medulla, adrenal, 153
  renal, 138, *139*

Medulla oblongata, anatomy of, *61*, 62
Melanocyte-stimulating hormone, 151
Melatonin, pineal body and, 60
Mendelson's syndrome, 159
Meninges, anatomy of, 65, *66*, 67–68
  coronal section of, *68*
  spinal, 74–75
Meningioma, intradural-extramedullary, 442, *442*
Meniscectomy, definition of, 399
Meperidine (Demerol), 216, 220t
  adverse effects of, in geriatric patient, 547t
Mephentermine sulfate (Wyamine), for cardiopulmonary
    resuscitation, 592t
Mepivacaine (Carbocaine), for local anesthesia, 248t, 248–249
Mesencephalon, anatomy of, 61, *61*
Messenger ribonucleic acid (mRNA), 149
Metabolic acidosis, 126, 143
  causes of, 126t
Metabolic alkalosis, 126, 143
  blood gas discrepancies in, 126t
Metabolic dysfunction, septic shock causing, 582
Metabolic regulation, definition of, 53
Metabolism, of bilirubin, 161
Metaraminol bitartrate (Aramine), for cardiopulmonary
    resuscitation, 592t
Metareactivity, definition of, 181
Methemoglobin, definition of, 104
Methohexital (Brevital), 206
Methoxyflurane (Penthrane), 198
  properties of, 193t
Methyldopa (Aldomet), 97–98, 98t
  adverse effects of, in geriatric patient, 547t
Methylprednisolone, for cardiopulmonary resuscitation, 591
Metoclopramide (Reglan), for gastric hypersecretory states, 159
Metocurine (Metubine), action and dosage of, 231
  pharmacology of, 229t
Metoprolol (Lopressor), for hypertension, 101t, 103
Metubine. See *Metocurine (Metubine).*
Microcirculation, 91
Microphage(s), immunologic function of, 172
Microsomal enzymes, in liver, 161–162
Microsurgery, in plastic surgery, 497–498
Microvascular tissue transfer, 493
Midazolam (Versed), 208–209
  dosage of, 209
  intracranial pressure and, 419
Midbrain, anatomy of, 61, *61*
Migration inhibitory factor, of lymphokines, 174
Miller blade, of laryngoscope, 308, *308*
Miller laryngoscope, 10
Mineralocorticoid(s), 153
Minimum alveolar concentration (MAC), drug potency
    determination with, 194
  modern concept of, 190–191
Minimum effective analgesic concentration (MEAC), in patient-
    controlled analgesia, 223–224
Minute ventilation (V̇E), definition of, 104
Mitral regurgitation, definition of, 373
Mitral stenosis, definition of, 373
Mitral valve(s), 85, *86*
Mivacurium chloride (Mivacron), action and dosage of, 233
  pharmacology of, 229t
Mobilization, stir-up regimen and, 290
Modern care station, in PACU, 5, *6*
Modified radical mastectomy, definition of, 484
Monitor(s), in PACU, 13–14, *14*
Monitoring, hemodynamic, postoperative, 278–283. See also
    Hemodynamic parameters, postoperative monitoring of.
  of central venous pressure, 89
Monocyte(s), immunologic function of, 172
Morbid obesity, 525

INDEX 613

Morphine, 216–217, 220t
advantage of, 217
analgesic effect of, 216
for post cesarean section pain, 554, 555
Motility, gastrointestinal, during pregnancy, 552
Motor area, of brain, 55, 57
Motor function, assessment of, 425–426
Motor neurons, definition of, 53
Motor speech area, of brain, 57, 58
Mouth care, after cranial surgery, 429
of PACU patient, 302
Mouth-to-mouth ventilation, in cardiopulmonary resuscitation, 589, 589
MRI. See Magnetic resonance imaging (MRI).
mRNA (messenger ribonucleic acid), 149
Mu opioid receptor(s), 215
Multiple sclerosis, muscle relaxant response in, 243t
Multitrauma patient, shock as complication in, 576–582
Murmur, definition of, 83
Muscarinic receptors, 226
observable responses to, 234t
Muscarinic response, of cholinergic receptors, 94, 95t
Muscle, cardiac, 86, 86
excitability and contractility of, factors affecting, 86t
skeletal, cholinergic stimulation of, 95t
physiology of, 565
Muscle relaxant(s), 226–244. See also Neuromuscular entries.
calcium deficiency and, 237–238
carbon dioxide and, 238
catecholamines and, 238
depolarizing, 234–237
factors influencing, 237–239, 238t
fluid balance and, 237
hypothermia and, 238
magnesium and, 237
mycins and, 238, 238t
nonpolarizing, 230–234
intermediate-acting, 232–233
long-acting, 230–232
reversal of, 233–234, 234t
short-acting, 233
pH and, 238
phase I block of, 242
phase II block of, 242–243
potassium deficiency and, 237
response of patients with neuromuscular disorders to, 243t
skeletal, pharmacology of, 228, 229t, 230
sodium deficiency and, 237
special problems associated with, 242–244
use of, 226
Muscle-skin flaps, in breast reconstruction, 488, 489
Muscular denervation, muscle relaxant response in, 243t
Muscular dystrophy, muscle relaxant response in, 243t
Mustache dressing, following nasal surgery, 329
Myasthenia gravis, diagnosis of, 521
incidence of, 521
muscle relaxant response in, 243t
PACU care and, 521–522
treatment of, 521
"Myasthenic facies," 521
Myasthenic syndrome, muscle relaxant response in, 243t
Mycins, muscle relaxants and, 238, 238t
Myelography, in spinal surgery, 431, 432
Mylaxen (hexafluorenium bromide), as depolarizing neuromuscular agent, 237
Myocardial infarction, 88–89
after cardiac surgery, 382
assessment of, 88
Myocardial protection technique, definition of, 373
Myocardial revascularization, definition of, 373–374
Myocardium, definition of, 83

Myomectomy, abdominal, definition of, 479
Myoneural junction, application of threshold stimulus to, 227, 228
at resting state, 226, 227
Myosin, 86
Myotonia, muscle relaxant response in, 243t
Myringoplasty (tympanoplasty), 328
definition of, 325
Myringotomy, 328
definition of, 325

N
Nalbuphine (Nubain), 220, 220t
Naloxone (Narcan), 222
for post cesarean section pain, 554
Naltrexone, 222
Narcan. See Naloxone (Narcan).
Narcotic(s). See Opioid(s).
Narcotic antagonist(s), 221–222
Nasal. See also Nose.
Nasal cannula, oxygen administration via, 296, 297t
Nasal suctioning, 298
Nasogastric intubation, after abdominal surgery, 452–453
irrigation of, 453
patient comfort and, 452–453
tube patency in, 452–453
Nasopharynx, anatomy of, 106
Nasotracheal intubation, 311–312, 312. See also Tracheal intubation.
National Fire Protection Association (NFPA), 13t
Nausea. See also Vomiting.
after epidural analgesia, 322
after spinal anesthesia, 254
control of, drugs used in, 532t
definition of, 156
postoperative, 531–533
incidence of, 532
Neck, arterial blood supply to, 72
cancer of, reconstruction surgery for, 340–341
radical surgery of, 339–341, 341
complications of, 339–340
venous drainage of, 67
Needle(s), used, disposal of, 34
Needle biopsy, bronchoscopy and, 353
Neoplasm(s). See Tumor(s).
Neostigmine, dosage of, 234
Nephrectomy, definition of, 463
Nephritis, definition of, 138
Nephrolithotomy, percutaneous, definition of, 463
Nephron, 139, 140
Nephrosis, definition of, 138
Nephrostomy, definition of, 463
Nephrotomy, definition of, 463
Nephroureterectomy, definition of, 463
Nerve(s), abducens, function of, 63t
acoustic, function of, 63t
adrenergic, functional anatomy of, 92, 92t
axillary, anesthesia of, 256
brachial plexus, 79
anesthesia of, 256
cervical plexus, 79
cholinergic, functional anatomy of, 92, 92t
cranial, assessment of, following carotid endarterectomy, 394t
functions of, 63t
facial, function of, 63t
glossopharyngeal, function of, 63t
hypoglossal, function of, 63t
laryngeal, 107, 108
oculomotor, function of, 63t
olfactory, function of, 63t

Nerve(s) *(Continued)*
  optic, function of, 63t
  phrenic, blockage of, 256
  pudendal plexus, 79
  spinal accessory, function of, 63t
  trigeminal, function of, 63t
  trochlear, function of, 63t
  vagus, 157
    function of, 63t
Nerve block, axillary or brachial plexus, 256
  emergence sequence of, 246t
  PACU care after, 256
Nerve conduction, physiology of, local anesthetics and, 245–246, 246t
Nervous system, autonomic, 80–81
  central. See *Central nervous system.*
  complications of, after cardiac surgery, 385
  parasympathetic, 81
  sympathetic, 81
Nesacaine. See *Chloroprocaine (Nesacaine).*
Neuraxial administration, of opioids, 222
Neuroblastoma, 475
Neuroendothelial body(ies), 118
Neurogenic hyperventilation, central, 425t
Neurogenic pulmonary edema, after cranial surgery, 427
Neurogenic shock, 578t, 580, 584–585
  from spinal injuries, 434–435
Neuroglia, definition of, 53
Neurohumoral transmission, 226
Neurohypophysis, 150
  hormones of, 151
Neuroleptanalgesia, 211
Neuroleptanesthesia, 211
Neurologic status, after carotid endarterectomy, 393, 394t
  after large vessel surgery, 397
  in post anesthesia recovery score, 33t
Neuromuscular blockade, assessment of, 239–242, 240–242
  nondepolarizing, criteria for recovery from, 239, 239t
Neuromuscular disorder(s), response of patients with, to muscle relaxants, 243t
Neuromuscular system, age-related problems of, 545
Neuromuscular transmission, physiology of, 226–228, 227–228
Neuron(s), of respiratory group, 132–133
Neurotransmitter(s), adrenergic and cholinergic, biochemistry of, 92–94
  synthesis of, 93t
Neurovascular assessment, after orthopedic surgery, 400–401
Neutralization, antibody, 174
Neutrophil(s), immunologic function of, 172
Newborn. See also *Pediatric patient.*
  definition of, 534
  diaphragmatic breathing of, 536
  vocal cords of, 535
NFPA (National Fire Protection Association), 13t
Nicotine, inhalation of, 527, 528
Nicotinic receptors, 226
  observable responses to, 234t
Nicotinic response, of cholinergic receptors, 94, 95t
Nifedipine (Procardia, Adalat), 97
  for hypertension, 100, 101t
Nipride. See *Sodium nitroprusside (Nipride).*
Nitroglycerin, for hypertension, 101t, 102
Nitrous oxide, 201–202
  administration of, balanced technique in, 201
    diffusion hypoxia following, 202
    pent-nitrous technique in, 201–202
  intracranial pressure and, 419
  potency of, 194
  properties of, 193t
  solubility of, 202
Nitrous oxide washout, 202

Nitrous-narcotic balance technique, of anesthesia, 216
Nonbarbiturate(s). See also specific agent, e.g., *Etomidate (Duranest).*
  as nonopioid intravenous anesthetic, 206–208
Noncommunicating hydrocephalus, 416
Nonopioid intravenous anesthesia, 205–213. See also *Anesthesia, intravenous, nonopioid.*
Non-rebreathing mask, oxygen administration via, 297t
Norcuron. See *Vecuronium (Norcuron).*
Norepinephrine, as mediator, 92, 92t
  in coronary circulation, 88
  metabolism of, 93, *93*
  release of, mechanism of, 92–93
  storage site of, 92
Normodyne. See *Labetalol (Normodyne, Trandate).*
Normotensive, definition of, 83
Nose. See also *Nasal; Naso-* entries.
  anatomy of, 105–106
  bleeding from, 105–106
  cilia of, 105, *106*
  sagittal section of, *105, 329*
  surgery of, 328–330
Novocain. See *Procaine (Novocain).*
Nubain. See *Nalbuphine (Nubain).*
Nucleus, phrenic, definition of, 409
Nucleus pulposus, 74
Nurse manager, of PACU, 15, 18
Nursing expertise, development of, 22, *23*
Nursing personnel, for PACU, assignment of, 19–20
  certification by professional associations of, 19t
  manager of, 18
  selection of, 18–19
  staffing patterns of, 20
Nutrients, in pulmonary circulation, 118
Nystagmus, 426

O

Obesity, 525–527
  considerations of, cardiovascular, 526
    postoperative, 527
    fluid dynamics and, 527
    physiologic, 525–526
    pregnancy and, 526
    psychological, 527
    respiratory, *525*, 525–526
    postoperative, 526–527
  definition of, 525
  diabetes mellitus associated with, 526
  morbid, 525
  PACU care and, 526–527
  postoperative complications of, 134
  simple, 525
Obesity-hypoventilation (pickwickian) syndrome, 525
Obstetric surgery, care after, 479–481
  intraoperative care during, 552–553
  terms used in, 477
Obstruction, of airways. See *Airway obstruction.*
Obstructive jaundice, 161
Obstructive lung disease, postoperative complications of, 133
Occipital bone, of cranium, 65
Occipital lobe, of brain, 54, *55–56*
Occlusion, definition of, 83
Occupational Safety and Health Administration (OSHA), infection control and, 301
  suggested PACU policies based on, 34t
Oculomotor nerve, function of, 63t
Odontoid process, injuries to, 432
  of axis, 74
Oil-gas partition coefficient, 202–203
  definition of, 193

Olfactory area, of brain, 58
Olfactory nerve, function of, 63t
Oliguria, definition of, 138
Oophorectomy, definition of, 479
Oophorocystectomy, definition of, 479
Open drop method, of administration of inhalation anesthesia, 195
Open reduction, definition of, 399
Open system, of administration of inhalation anesthesia, 195
Ophthalmic surgery. See *Eye(s), surgery of.*
Opioid(s), 215, 216–222
    abuse of, 557, 559
        effects and signs in, 558t
    concept of, 215
    epidural administration of, for post cesarean section pain, 554–555
    interaction of, in PACU patient, 188
    intracranial pressure and, 419
    neuraxial administration of, 222
    previous use of, pain control and, 320
    synthetic, 215
    used in nitrous-narcotic balance technique, 216
Opioid intravenous anesthesia, 215–224. See also *Anesthesia, intravenous, opioid.*
Opioid receptor(s), 215
Opium, naturally occurring alkaloids of, 215
Opsonin, in phagocytosis, 172
Optic nerve, function of, 63t
Oral route of administration, of drugs, 183
Oral suctioning, 298
Orchiectomy, definition of, 464
Orchipexy, definition of, 464
Orientation program, for PACU, 20–22
        content of, 21–22
Oropharynx, anatomy of, 106
Orotracheal intubation. See *Tracheal intubation, oral.*
Orthopedic surgery, 399–407
    complications of, observation for, 402–403
    immobilization devices after, care of, 401
    neurovascular assessment after, 400–401
    patient positioning after, 400, *401*
    post anesthesia care in, 400–403
    range-of-motion exercises after, 402
    wound care after, 401–402, *402*
Orthopnea, definition of, 104
Oscillometric technology, in blood pressure measurement, 271–272, *272*
OSHA (Occupational Safety and Health Safety Administration), infection control and, 301
    suggested PACU policies based on, 34t
Osmoreceptor(s), in ADH secretion, 151
Osmotic diuretic(s), 144
Ossiculoplasty, definition of, 325
Osteoporosis, definition of, 399
Osteotomy, definition of, 399
Ostium secundum defect, definition of, 369
Oswald solubility coefficient, definition of, 192
Otolaryngeal surgery, in pediatric patient, *540,* 542
Otoplasty, 496
Oximeter, pulse, 264, *264*
Oximetry, pulse, applications of, 264–265
        clinical issues in, 265–266
        interpretations of measurements in, 265, *265*
        monitoring oxygenation by, *264–265,* 264–266
        technology overview of, 264–266
Oxygen, administration of, in PACU, 129, 135–136
        methods of, 296, 297t
    after thoracic surgery, 362
    for respiratory function, 295–296
    toxicity of, 136
    transport of, 121–123, *122*

Oxygen *(Continued)*
        Bohr effect on, 122
        factors affecting, 122
    wall-supply, 8, 9, *9*
Oxygen dissociation curve, pulse oximetry and, 123
Oxygen flowmeter, 9, *9*
    calibration and maintenance of, 9–10
    misuse of, 9, *10*
Oxygenation, postoperative, monitoring of, *264–265, 264–266*
Oxyhemoglobin, 121
    definition of, 104
Oxyhemoglobin dissociation curve(s), 121, *122,* 265, *265*
Oxyntic glands, definition of, 156
Oxytocin, 151

P

Pacemaker, definition of, 83
    ectopic, definition of, 82
Packed red blood cells, transfusion of, 294–295
PACU. See *Post anesthesia care unit (PACU).*
Pain, following genitourinary surgery, 468
    management of, after thyroid surgery, 445
        in PACU patient, 290–291
        in post cesarean section patient, 554–555
        in pregnant patient, 555–556
        in shock trauma patient, 575–576
    postoperative, 314–323
        analgesics for, 319t, 319–322
            adjuncts to, 322
            age considerations in, 319–320
            intrathecal and epidural administration of, 320–322
            intravenous administration of, 320
            patient-controlled, 320, *321*
            previous narcotic use and, 320
            side effects of, 319t, 322–323
        assessment of, 314–318
        indicator(s) of, 316–318
            behavioral cues as, 318
            physiologic changes as, 317
            verbalization as, 316–317
        influence of anesthetic agents and technique in, 315–316
        influence of nurses' attitude and perceptions on, 318
        intensity of, 317, *317*
        location of, 316–317
        management of, 318–323
            noninvasive interventions in, 322–323
            pharmacologic, 319–322
        physiologic impact of, 314
        prevention of, 318–319
        psychologic impact of, 314, *315*
        quality of, 317
        relaxation for, 323
        transcutaneous electrical nerve stimulation for, *322,* 322–323
        variations in, 317
Pain relief, after eye surgery, 348
    after large vessel surgery, 397
    after peripheral vascular surgery, 392
    after thoracic surgery, 362–364, *363*
Palate, cleft, surgical repair of, 497
Paletouvuloplasty, definition of, 331
Palpation, for pulsations, in peripheral arteries, 391, *391*
    of chest, postoperative, 263
Palpitation, definition of, 83
Palsy, due to spinal anesthesia, 254
Pancreas, anatomy of, 153, 163, *163*
    physiology of, 153–154
    surgery of, care after, 458, 460
Pancreaticoduodenectomy, care after, 458, 460
    definition of, 450

Pancreatitis, 163
   definition of, 156
Pancuronium (Pavulon), action and dosage of, 230–231
   adverse effects of, in geriatric patient, 547t
   as muscle relaxant, 228
   pharmacology of, 229t
Panhypopituitarism, 154
Papillae, renal, 138
Paralysis, due to spinal anesthesia, 254
Paraplegia, muscle relaxant response in, 243t
Parasympathetic nervous system, 81
Parathormone, 152
Parathyroid gland, anatomy and physiology of, 152
   surgery of, 444–445. See also *Thyroid gland, surgery of.*
Parathyroidectomy, definition of, 444
Paresthesia, definition of, 399
Parietal bone(s), of cranium, 65
Parietal lobe, of brain, 54, *55–56*
Parkinsonism, drug-induced, 56, 58
Parkinson's disease, muscle relaxant response in, 243t
Parkinson's syndrome, 54
Paroxysmal nocturnal dyspnea, definition of, 104
Paroxysmal tachycardia, definition of, 83
PARS (post anesthesia recovery score), 33t
Partial pressure, definition of, 105
Partial rebreathing mask, oxygen administration via, 297t
Partial thromboplastin time (PTT), 90
Partial-thickness burn, 169
Passive acquired immunity, definition of, 171
Patency, tube, in nasogastric or intestinal intubation, 452–453
Patent ductus arteriosus, definition of, 374
Patient, comfort of, nasogastric or intestinal intubation and, 453
   geriatric. See *Geriatric patient.*
   immunosuppressed, PACU care of, 176–177
   intubated, extubation of, 312
      PACU care of, 312
   pediatric. See *Pediatric patient.*
   post anesthesia, care of, 289–303
      comfort and safety measures for, 302
      coughing in, 290
      deep-breathing exercises for, 289–290
      delayed emergence in, 291
      emergence excitement in, 291
      humidity and, 296
      infection control and, 301
      intravenous therapy for, 291
      mechanical ventilation of, 296–298, *298–300*
      mobilization of, 290
      oral and nasal suctioning of, 298
      oxygen therapy for, 295–296
         administration of, 296, 297t
      pain management in, 290–291
      positioning of, 290
      respiratory function in, maintenance of, 295–301
      stir-up regimen for, 289–291
         modification of, 291
      tracheal suctioning of, 298–299, *301*
      transfer of, from PACU, 302–303
      transfusion therapy for, blood components in, 294–295
         non-blood volume substitutes in, 295
         reactions to, 293–294
            delayed, 294
         whole blood in, 292–293
   pregnant. See *Pregnant patient.*
   preparation of, for ambulatory surgery, 507–510
   transfer of, from PACU, 302–303
   ventilation of, during oral tracheal intubation, 311
Patient assessment, 261–288
   at PACU admission, 262
   during oral tracheal intubation, 311
   electrocardiographic monitoring in, 273–278

Patient assessment *(Continued)*
   hemodynamic monitoring in, 278–283
   of cardiovascular function and perfusion, 270–273
   of central nervous system, 283
   of fluid and electrolyte balance, 284–286
   of respiratory function, 262–270
   of thermal balance, 283–284
   preoperative, 261–262
   psychosocial, 286–288
Patient classification, in PACU, 28–29, 29t
Patient discharge, from PACU, 30–33, 33t
Patient position, after abdominal surgery, 451
   after carotid endarterectomy, 393
   after cranial surgery, 428
   after eye surgery, 345, 347
   after large vessel surgery, 396
   after orthopedic surgery, 400, *401*
   after peripheral vascular surgery, 390–391
   after thoracic surgery, 360
   after thyroid surgery, 444
   during obstetric surgery, 552
   for oral tracheal intubation, 310
   stir-up regimen and, 290
Patient records, 30, *31–32*
Patient-controlled analgesia (PCA), 223t, 223–224
   basal infusion rate in, 224, 224t
   for post cesarean section pain, 554
   for postoperative pain, 320, *321*
   lockout interval in, 224
   minimum effective analgesic concentration in, 223–224
Patient-controlled epidural analgesia, 224, 224t
Pavulon. See *Pancuronium (Pavulon).*
PCA. See *Patient-controlled analgesia.*
PCP (phencyclidine), abuse of, 559t, 561
Pectus excavatum, definition of, 350
Pediatric patient, anesthesia for, 538
   complication(s) associated with, 540–542
      airway obstruction as, 541–542
      idiopathic respiratory distress syndrome as, 541
      malignant hyperthermia as, 542
      retrolental fibroplasia as, 540–541
   differences in, anatomic and physiologic, 534–538
      cardiovascular, 534t, 534–535, *535*, 535t
      endocrine, 534
      fluid, 537–538, 538t
      renal, 537–538, 538t
      respiratory, 535–537, *536*, 537t
   gastrointestinal surgery in, 542
   monitoring of, cardiovascular, 539
      fluid, 539
      psychosocial, 539–540
      respiratory, 539
   otolaryngeal surgery in, *540*, 542
   PACU care of, 538–540
   post anesthesia care of, 534–542
   temperature regulation of, 539, *540*
PEEP (positive end-expiratory pressure), mechanical ventilation
      and, 296
Pelvis, renal, 138, *139*
Penetrating trauma, 571
Penile implant, definition of, 464
Penile surgery, 474–475
Pentazocine (Fortral, Talwin), 219, 220t
Penthrane. See *Methoxyflurane (Penthrane).*
Pentothal. See *Thiopental (Pentothal).*
Peptic ulcer, definition of, 156
Percussion, of chest, postoperative, 263
Percutaneous endoscopic gastrostomy, definition of, 450
Percutaneous nephrolithotomy, definition of, 463
Percutaneous transluminal angioplasty, definition of, 387
   for vascular disease, 388

Percutaneous transluminal coronary angioplasty, 374–375
  definition of, 374
Perfusion of blood, in lungs, decreased ventilation to, 127–128
    distribution of, 127
      increased ventilation to, 128–129
Pericardiectomy, definition of, 375
Pericarditis, definition of, 83
Perineum, female, 478
Period of ejection, in cardiac cycle, 83
Peripheral resistance, definition of, 83
Peripheral vascular system, complications of, after cardiac
    surgery, 386
Peripheral vasoconstriction, after cardiac surgery, 383–384
Peritoneoscopy, definition of, 449–450, 479
Peritubular capillaries, of kidney, 139, 140
PET (positron emission tomography), in cranial surgery, 412
Pezzer catheter, 466
pH, 125
  kidney regulation of, 143–144
  muscle relaxants and, 238
  of sweat, 166
Phagocytosis, definition of, 171
  in innate immunity, 172
Pharmacodynamics, in geriatric patient, 546
Pharmacokinetics, in geriatric patient, 546
  of drugs, 182–183, 183
  of inhalation anesthesia, 192–193, 193t
Pharmacology. See also Drug entries.
  basic principles of, 181–188
Pharynx, anatomy of, 106
Phencyclidine (PCP), abuse of, 559t, 561
Phentolamine (Regitine), for hypertension, 101, 101t
Pheochromocytoma, 475
Phimosis, definition of, 464
Phrenic nerve, blockage of, 256
Phrenic nucleus, definition of, 409
Physical comfort, of patient, in PACU, 302
Physical dependence, on drugs, 557
Physiologic dead space, 128, 129
Physiologic shunt, 128
Physiologic thermoregulatory response, 563
Physostigmine (Antilirium), 209–210
  dosage of, 210
  for benzodiazepine overdose, 560
Pia mater, 66, 67–68, 68
  spinal, 75, 251
Pickwickian (obesity-hypoventilation) syndrome, 525
Pineal body, melatonin production by, 60
Pineal gland, anatomy and physiology of, 151–152
Pinocytosis, 92
Pipecuronium bromide (Arduan), action dosage of, 232
  pharmacology of, 229t
Pituitary gland, anatomy of, 150
  dysfunction of, 151
  physiology of, 150–151
Plaque, definition of, 343–344
Plasma concentration curve, 182
Plasma protein(s), in transfusions, 295
Plasma protein fraction (PPF), in transfusions, 295
Plastic surgery, blepharoplasty in, 495
  bone grafts in, 493–494
  cosmetic, 494–496
  dermabrasion in, 494–495
  for cleft lip and palate, 496–497, 497
  for facial trauma, 496
  liposuction in, 496
  microsurgery in, 497–498
  otoplasty in, 496
  post anesthesia care after, 492–498
  rhinoplasty in, 495–496
  rhytidoplasty in, 495

Plastic surgery (Continued)
  skin flaps in, 493, 495
  skin grafts in, 492–493, 494
Plateau wave, in intracranial pressure, 421, 422
Platelet(s), 90–91
  transfusion of, 295
Platelet count, 90
Pleura, visceral, 110
Plexus, definition of, 53
Plication, 388
  definition of, 387
Plumbing, in PACU, 8
Pneumoencephalography, 410
Pneumonectomy, definition of, 350
Pneumonia, aspiration, 159
Pneumotaxic center, of brainstem, 132
Pneumothorax, 353
  after cardiac surgery, 385
  definition of, 350
  types of, 116
Policies and procedures, for PACU, 28t
Polycythemia, definition of, 83, 105
Polymorphonuclear leukocyte(s), 90
  immunologic function of, 172
Pons, anatomy of, 61, 61–62
Pontocaine. See Tetracaine (Pontocaine).
Positioning, of patient. See Patient position.
Positive end-expiratory pressure (PEEP), definition of, 105
  for cranial surgical patient, 427
  mechanical ventilation and, 296
Positron emission tomography (PET), in cranial surgery, 412
Post anesthesia care record, 31–32
Post anesthesia care unit (PACU), access to, 5–6
  admission to, 262
  air conditioning in, 8
  design of, 3–5
    based on human factors and ergonomics, 4
    based on human factors engineering, 3–4
    planning objective in, 4–5, 5–6
  emergency evacuation from, 5–6
  fiberoptic laryngoscopy in, 11
  fire extinguishers in, 7
  flooring materials in, 7
  ideal setting for, 3
  infection control in, 33–34, 34t
  instruments in, 10–11, 11t
  isolation room in, 6
  lighting in, 10
  monitors and memory in, 13–14, 14
    disabling alarms in, 14
    error messages in, 14
  organizational structure in, 15, 18
  orientation program for, 20–22
  overall design of, subsystems of, 7
  oxygen administration in, 129, 135–136
  oxygen flowmeters in, calibration and maintenance of, 9–10
    flow rate of, 9
    misuse of, 9, 10
  patient classification system in, 28–29, 29t
  patient discharge from, 30–33, 33t
  patient monitoring in, 11–14, 13t
  patient records in, 30, 31–32
  physical structure of, 3
  plumbing in, 8
  policies of, 27–36, 28t
  power outlets in, 8
  purpose of, 27
  quality improvement in, 35, 35–36
  shared governance in, 28
  shelves and bracket systems in, 7
  space configurations in, 5–11

Post anesthesia care unit (PACU) *(Continued)*
  special considerations in, 6–7
  staffing of, 18–20, 19t, 27–28
  standardization in, 11–12, 13t
    success through, 12–13
  Standards Writing Organizations defining safety and performance in, 13t
  storage space in, 6–7
  stress and burnout in, 22–25, 24t
  utility area in, 6
  visitors in, 29–30
  wall vacuum system in, 10, *10–11*
  wall-supply oxygen in, 8–9, *9*
Post anesthesia nursing, as speciality, 15–26
  development of expertise in, 22, *23*
  self-scheduling in, 28
  standards of care in, 33
Post anesthesia nursing practice, resource 16: ACLS and equivalent testing, 49t
  resource 14: data for initial, ongoing, and discharge assessment, 47t–48t
  resource 10: patient classification, 46t
  resource 5: recommended equipment for phase 1 PACU, 44t–45t
  standard I: patient rights and ethics, 37t
  standard II: environment, 38t
  standard III: personnel management, 39t
  standard IV: continuous quality improvement, 40t
  standard V: research, 40t
  standard VI: interdisciplinary collaboration, 41t
  standard VII: assessment, 41t
  standard VIII: planning and implementation, 42t
  standard IX: evaluation, 42t
  standard X: advanced cardiac life support, 43t
  standard XI: pain management, 43t
Post anesthesia patient, care of, 289–303. See also *Patient, post anesthesia.*
Post anesthesia practice, characteristics of, 16t–17t
Post anesthesia recovery score (PARS), 33t
Post anesthesia shivering, 564
Post-tetanic facilitation, 240–241, *241*
Post-TURP syndrome, 472
Postural reflexes, definition of, 53
Potassium, deficiency of, muscle relaxants and, 237
  monitoring of, in geriatric patient, 545–546
Potassium-sparing diuretic(s), 145
Potency, of drug, definition of, 181
  of inhalant anesthetic agents, 194
Power outlets, in PACU, 8
PPF (plasma protein fraction), in transfusions, 295
Practice acts, 12
Precipitation, antibody, 174
Pre-excitation syndrome, definition of, 83
Prefrontal area, of brain, 58
Pregnancy, changes in, cardiovascular, 549–551, 550t
    hematologic alterations in, 550–551
    hemodynamic alterations in, 549–550, *551*
  gastrointestinal, 550t, 552
  hepatic, 552
  physiologic, 549–555, 550t
  renal, 550t, 552
  respiratory, 550t, 551–552
  ectopic, *478*
    care after, 480
    definition of, 477
  effect of, on gastric motility and secretions, 158
  obesity in, problems associated with, 526
Pregnant patient, 549–556
  fetal monitoring of, 554, 554t, *555*
  intraoperative anesthesia care of, 552–553
  pain management of, 554–556

Pregnant patient *(Continued)*
  positioning of, 554
  postoperative care of, 553–556
  psychological and emotional support of, 554
Preload, definition of, 83
Premature atrial contraction, postoperative monitoring of, 275, *275*
Premature ventricular contraction, postoperative monitoring of, *276*, 276–277
Premotor area, of brain, 55–56, *57*, 58
Preoperative assessment, of surgical patient, 261–262
Press-Mate noninvasive blood pressure monitor, 13, *14*
Pressure-volume curve(s), combined, of lung and chest wall, 116, *117*
  in postoperative period, *117*
  of chest wall, 115, *115*
  of lung, 112–113, *113–114*
Presynaptic membrane, depolarization of, 227
Prilocaine (Citanest), for local anesthesia, 249
Procainamide (Pronestyl), for cardiopulmonary resuscitation, 593–594
  for malignant hyperthermia, 567, 568t
Procaine (Novocain), for local anesthesia, 247, 248t
Procardia. See *Nifedipine (Procardia, Adalat).*
Prochlorperazine (Compazine), for nausea, 532t
Procidentia, definition of, 478
Prolactin, 151
Prolapse, of uterus, definition of, 478
Pronestyl. See *Procainamide (Pronestyl).*
Propanidid, 213
Propofol (Diprivan), 207–208
  advantages of, 208
  emergence from, PACU care during, 207–208
  induction doses of, 207
Propranolol (Inderal, Ipran), adverse effects of, in geriatric patient, 547t
  for cardiopulmonary resuscitation, 594
  for hypertension, 100, 101t, 102
Proprioception, definition of, 53
Prosencephalon, anatomy of, 54–60, *55–57, 59–60*
Prostatectomy, definition of, 463
  drainage after, 472, *473*
Prostatic surgery, 471–473
  perineal approach in, 472–473
  retropubic approach in, 473
  suprapubic approach in, 472
  transurethral approach in, 471–472
Prosthetic valve(s), mechanical, 376–377, *377*
  types of, 376–377, *377*
Protective gear, use of, blood-borne diseases and, 34
Protein(s), loss of, prevention of, 167
  plasma, in transfusions, 295
  synthesis of, in liver, 161
Prothrombin time (PT), 90
Protodiastole, in cardiac cycle, 83, *84*
Pruritus, from epidural analgesia, 322
Psychedelic abuse, 561
  effects and signs of, 559t
Psychologic support, of pregnant patient, 554
Psychological dependence, on drugs, 557
Psychosocial assessment, postoperative, 286–288, 287t
PT (prothrombin time), 90
Pterygium, definition of, 344
Ptosis, breast, 489
  definition of, 344
PTT (partial thromboplastin time), 90
Pudendal plexus, 79
Pulmonary. See also *Lung(s); Lung* entries.
Pulmonary artery banding, definition of, 375
Pulmonary artery catheter, 89–90

Pulmonary artery pressure, postoperative monitoring of, 278, 279t
Pulmonary capillary wedge pressure, postoperative monitoring of, 278, 279t
Pulmonary circulation, 91, 116–118
  gas exchange in, 116–118
  nutrients in, 118
  protective role of, 118
  reservoir for left ventricle in, 118
  vs. systemic circulation, 118
Pulmonary edema, 119–120
  alveolar, 120
  definition of, 119
  interstitial, 120
  neurogenic, after cranial surgery, 427
Pulmonary embolism, after orthopedic surgery, 402
Pulmonary forces, balance of, alterations in, 116, 117
Pulmonary function, abnormal, 133–134
Pulmonary hysteresis, 113–114, 114
Pulmonary nursing care, postoperative, physiology of, 134–135, 134–135
Pulmonary stenosis, definition of, 375
Pulmonary stretch receptors, in regulation of breathing, 132
Pulmonary time constant, 115
Pulmonary vascular resistance, 118
  postoperative monitoring of, 280, 283
Pulse, character of, 273
  palpation for, in peripheral arteries, 391, 391
  radial, obliteration of, 256
Pulse deficit, definition of, 83
Pulse oximeter, 264, 264
Pulse oximetry. See Oximetry, pulse.
  and oxygen dissociation curve, 123
Pulse pressure, postoperative monitoring of, 273
Pulse rate, in pediatric patient, 534, 535t
Pupil(s), constricted, 426
  dilated, 426
Pupillary activity, assessment of, 426
Purkinje system, of heart, 86–87, 87
Pyelitis, definition of, 138
Pyeloplasty, definition of, 463
Pyelostomy, definition of, 463
Pyelotomy, definition of, 463
Pyloric antrum, 157
Pyloric stenosis, surgery for, care after, 455
Pyloromyotomy, definition of, 450
Pyloroplasty, definition of, 450
Pyramidal signs, definition of, 409
Pyramids, renal, 138, 139
Pyridostigmine, dosage of, 234
Pyrosis, definition of, 156

Q

Quadriplegia, muscle relaxant response in, 243t
Quality, of postoperative pain, 317
Quality assurance programs, in PACU, 35, 35–36
Quantal response, of drugs, 182
Queckenstedt test, 432

R

Radford nomogram, 536, 536
Radial pulse, obliteration of, 256
Radical antrostomy, definition of, 329
Radical hysterectomy, definition of, 479
Radical mastectomy, 486, 487–488
  definition of, 484–485
  modified, 486, 487
Radiography, conventional, in cranial surgery, 412, 413
  in spinal surgery, 431, 431

Rales, definition of, 105
Ramus(i), definition of, 53
  spinal, 79
Range-of-motion exercise(s), after orthopedic surgery, 402
Ranitidine (Zantac), for gastric hypersecretory states, 159
Rapid-pressure infusion device, fluid warmer with, 571, 573
RAS (reticular activating system), 63
Ratchet effect, of sliding filament, 227
Reabsorption, renal, 140, 141t
Reagin(s), 175
Receptor(s), adrenergic, 94–97, 95, 96t, 97
  types of, 95
  airway, in regulation of breathing, 131
  alpha, 95, 95–96
  beta, 96, 97
  cholinergic, 94, 95t
  dopaminergic, 95
  irritant, in regulation of breathing, 132
  muscarinic, 226
  nicotinic, 226
    observable responses to, 234t
  opioid, 215
  stretch, in ADH secretion, 151
    in regulation of breathing, 132
  volume, in ADH secretion, 151
Rectocele, definition of, 478
Rectum, anatomy and physiology of, 160
  surgery of, care after, 457
Recurarization, muscle relaxants and, 243–244
Red blood cell(s), 90
  hemolysis of, 531
  packed, transfusion of, 294–295
Reduction, open, definition of, 399
Reduction mammoplasty, 490
Re-entry (circus movement), definition of, 83
Reflex, aspiration, 131
  Babinski, 415, 422
  Cushing's, 425
  Hering-Breuer, 132
  postural, definition of, 53
  righting, definition of, 53
  sniff, 131
Regional anesthesia. See Anesthesia, regional.
Regitine. See Phentolamine (Regitine).
Reglan. See Metoclopramide (Reglan).
Regulatory T lymphocyte(s), in cellular immunity, 174
Regurgitation, after anesthesia, 159
  aortic, 368
  mitral, 373
  of gastric contents, 158–159. See also Vomiting.
  passive, 159
  tricuspid, 376
Relaxant(s), muscle. See Muscle relaxant(s).
Relaxation, for postoperative pain, 323
Releasing factor (RF), definition of, 149
Releasing hormone (RH), definition of, 149
Renal. See also Kidney(s).
Renal angiography, care after, 464–465
Renal artery, 138, 139
Renal biopsy, care after, 465
Renal changes, after burns, 502
Renal disease, effect of, on pharmacologic action, 184
Renal failure, acute, 146–147
    common cause of, 147
  PACU nursing care and, 147–148, 148
Renal function, alterations in, 147, 147
  autoregulation, 140
  compromised, effects of drugs on, 146
  counter-current mechanism in, 140
  effects of anesthesia on, 145–146
  hormone control in, 140, 142, 142

Renal function *(Continued)*
  impaired, in rheumatoid arthritic patient, 525
  regulation of, 140, 142, *142*
Renal pelvis, 138, *139*
Renal physiology, 140, 141t
Renal surgery, care after, 468, *469*, 470–471
Renal system, age-related problems of, 545–546
  changes in, during pregnancy, 550t, 552
  complications of, after cardiac surgery, 385
Renal transplantation, anesthesia for, 470
  care after, 468, *469*, 470–471
  definition of, 463
  donor for, 470
  graft rejection in, 471, 471t
  immunosuppressive therapy after, 470
Renin, 142, 153
Renin-angiotensin system, 153
Renin-angiotensin-vasoconstrictor mechanism, for arterial
    pressure control, 142, *142*
Resection, abdominoperineal, care after, 456–457
  gastric, definition of, 447
Reserpine, 97, 98t
Residual volume (RV), 111–112
  definition of, 111t
Resistance, in Selye's adaptation syndrome, 23–24
  peripheral, definition of, 83
Respiration. See also *Breathing.*
  Cheyne-Stokes, definition of, 104
  complications of, after spinal injuries, 435
  definition of, 105
  in post anesthesia recovery score, 33t
  Kussmaul, definition of, 104
  patterns of, after cranial surgery, 425t
  phases of, 120
  postoperative, 262
Respiratory acidosis, 125, 143
  causes of, 125t
Respiratory alkalosis, 125–126, 143
  causes of, 125t
Respiratory care patient record, 298, *300*
Respiratory depression, delayed-onset, caused by fentanyl, 217
  from epidural analgesia, 322
Respiratory distress syndrome, idiopathic, in pediatric patient,
    541
Respiratory function, after thoracic surgery, 361–364
  assessment of, 361–362, *362*
  anesthetic agents affecting, 104
  humidity and, 296
  in obese patient, *525*, 525–526
    postoperative, 526–527
  maintenance of, 295–301
  mechanical ventilation and, 296–298, 298t, *298–300*
  oxygen therapy and, 295–296
    methods of administration in, 296, 297t
  postoperative, 262–270
    clinical assessment of, 262–264
      inspection in, 262–263
      listening and auscultation in, 263–264
      palpation in, 263
      percussion in, 263
    monitoring oxygenation in, *264–265*, 264–266
    monitoring ventilation in, 267–270, *268–270*
  suctioning and, 298–299, *301*
Respiratory rate, resting, 262
Respiratory status, after abdominal surgery, 451–452
  after cranial surgery, 427
  after thyroid surgery, 444–445
Respiratory system, age-related problems of, 544–545
  anatomy of, 105–110
  changes in, during pregnancy, 550t, 551–552
  complications of, after cardiac surgery, 385

Respiratory system *(Continued)*
  effect of cigarette smoking on, 527–528
  in pediatric patient, 535–537, *536*, 537t
    monitoring of, 539
  physiology of, 110–136
Response curve, carbon dioxide, 130, *130*
Restrictive lung disease, postoperative complications of, 133
Resuscitation, cardiopulmonary. See *Cardiopulmonary
    resuscitation (CPR).*
Retention, urinary, definition of, 138
Reticular activating system (RAS), 63
Reticular formation, of brain stem, 62–63
Retinopexy, definition of, 344
Retrolental fibroplasia, 136
  in pediatric patient, 540–541
Rewarming therapy, for hypothermia, 564
RF (releasing factor), definition of, 149
RH (releasing hormone), definition of, 149
Rheumatoid arthritis, 523
  corrective surgery for, 523, 524t
  PACU care and, 523–525
    airway in, 523–524
    blood in, 524–525
    fluid balance in, 525
    heart in, 524
    lungs in, 524
  PACU hazards in, 524t
Rhinencephalon, 58–59, *59*
Rhinoplasty, 495–496
Rhizotomy, definition of, 409
Rhombencephalon, anatomy of, *61*, 61–62
Rhonchus(i), definition of, 105
Rhytidoplasty (face-lift), 495
Righting reflexes, definition of, 53
Rima glottidis (glottis), anatomy of, 106–107
Rocuronium bromide (Zemuron), action and dosage of, 233
Rolando fissure, of cerebral hemispheres, 54
Romazicon. See *Flumazenil (Mazicon, Romazicon).*
Ropivacaine, for local anesthesia, 249
Roto Rest bed, for spinal injuries, 437, *438*
  precautions with, 436–437
Route of administration, of drugs, 183
Rule of Nines, in burn injury, 500, *500*
RV (residual volume), 111–112
  definition of, 111t

S

Sacral plexus, 79
Sacrum, 74
Safeguards, in blood transfusions, 292
Safety, of drugs, 182
  of patient, in PACU, 302
Salpingectomy, definition of, 479
Salpingo-oophorectomy, definition of, 479
Salpingostomy (tube plasty), definition of, 479
Saphenous femoropopliteal bypass graft, *390*
Saphenous vein bypass graft, *374*
Scleral buckle, definition of, 344
Scoliosis, definition of, 399
Scott's syndrome, 549, *551*
Scrotal surgery, 473–474, *474*
SDAT (senile dementia of Alzheimer's type), 546–547
Second-degree burn, 169
Secretion(s), gastric, during pregnancy, 552
Sedation, conscious, intravenous, definition of, 511
  in ambulatory surgery, 510–511
Segmental resection (of lung), definition of, 350
Seizure(s), after cranial surgery, 429–430
Self-scheduling, of staff, 28
Selye's adaptation syndrome, stress and, 23–24

Semilunar valve(s), 85
Semiopen system, of administration of inhalation anesthesia,
      195–196, *196–197*
Semiprone position, stir-up regimen and, 290
Senile dementia of Alzheimer's type (SDAT), 546–547
Senile emphysema, 545
Sensitized lymphocyte(s), definition of, 171
Sensor(s), in regulation of breathing, 129–132, *131*
Sensory areas, of brain, 58
Sensory function, assessment of, 425–426
Sensory loss, after spinal injuries, 438–439
Septal defect, ventricular, 378, *379*
Septic shock, 578t, 581–582, 586
      definition of, 581
      treatment of, 582, 586
Sequestrectomy, definition of, 399
Serum sickness, as arthus hypersensitivity reaction, 176
Sevoflurane, 200–201
      properties of, 193t
Sex hormone(s), 153
Shelves, in PACU, 7
Shirodkar procedure, care after, 480
Shivering, post anesthesia, 564
Shock, after adrenalectomy, 475
      after orthopedic surgery, 403
      after thoracic surgery, 366
      anaphylactic, 578t, 580–581, 585–586. See also *Anaphylaxis.*
      cardiogenic, 578t, 578–580, 586
            definition of, 579
            treatment of, 579–580, 587
      collaborative approach to, 573
      diagnostic studies and protocols for, 573
      distributive (vasogenic), 578t, 580–582
      early, 581
      hypovolemic, 577–578, 578t, 584, *584*
            definition of, 577
            treatment of, 578, 584
      late, 581
      neurogenic, 434–435, 578t, 580, 584–585
            treatment of, 585
      nursing diagnosis and, 576
      pathophysiology of, *584*, 584–587, 585t
      patient in, anesthesia report on, 573–574
            infectious risk from, 576
            nursing assessment of, 574–575
            pain management of, 575–576
            psychological assessment of, 576
      post anesthesia care for, 570–582
      septic, 578t, 581–582, 586
            definition of, 581
            treatment of, 582, 586
      spinal, definition of, 409
      treatment of, post anesthesia phase in, 573–576
            prehospital phase in, 570–571
            stabilization phase in, 571–573, *572–573*
      types of, 577–582, 578t, 584–587
Shoulder surgery, post anesthesia care after, 404
Shunt(s), in ventilation-perfusion mismatching, 128
SIADH (syndrome of inappropriate secretion of antidiuretic
      hormone), 155
Sickle cell anemia, and anesthesia, 529–530
      PACU care and, 530
      pathogenesis of, 529, *530*
Sickle cell crisis, 530–531
      aplastic, 531
      sequestration, 531
Sickle cell trait, 529
Sickle cell–hemoglobin C disease, 529
Sickle cell–thalassemia, 529
Sigh, 134
Sighless breathing pattern, 134

Sigma opioid receptor(s), 215
Simmonds' disease, 150
Simple pneumothorax, 116
Sinoatrial (SA) node, 86, *87*
Sinus(es), surgery of, 330
Sinus arrest, postoperative monitoring of, 275
Sinus bradycardia, postoperative monitoring of, 274, *274*
Sinus tachycardia, postoperative monitoring of, 275, *275*
Sinusoids, hepatic, 160
Skeletal muscle, cholinergic stimulation of, 95t
      physiology of, 565
Skin, anatomic layers of, 499
      anatomy of, 165, *166*
      aseptic techniques for, importance of, 167, 167t, 168t, 169–
            170
      burn injuries to, 169–170
      function of, 165–167
            protective, 167
            thermoregulation as, 165–167, *166*
      layers of, 165
      thermal injury to. See *Burn(s).*
Skin care, after cranial surgery, 429
      after renal and ureteral surgery, 468
      after spinal injuries, 437
Skin graft(s), 492–493, *494*
      for burns, 503–504
      types of, 492
Skull, coronal section of, *68*
      lateral view of, *64*
Skull fracture, depressed, radiograph of, 412, *413*
Sliding herniorrhaphy, definition of, 448
Small bowel, surgery of, care after, 455
SMI (sustained maximal inspiration), as postoperative breathing
      exercise, 359, 362
Smoking, cigarette. See *Cigarette smoking.*
Sniff reflex, 131
Sniffing position, for oral tracheal intubation, 310, *310*
Sodium, deficiency of, in geriatric patient, 545
            muscle relaxants and, 237
      intestinal absorption of, 160
Sodium bicarbonate, for cardiopulmonary resuscitation, 591,
            592t
Sodium nitroprusside (Nipride), for cardiopulmonary
            resuscitation, 593
      for hypertension, 100–101, 101t
Somatostatin, 153
Somatotropin. See *Growth hormone.*
Sore throat, after tracheal intubation, 312–313
Sounds, adventitious, definition of, 104
Space planning objective(s), in PACU design, 4–5, *5–6*
Spasm(s), arterial and venous, associated with invasive
            hemodynamic monitoring, 281t
Spatula, of laryngoscope blade, 308
Spermatocelectomy, definition of, 464
Sphenoid bone, of cranium, 65
Sphincter, of Oddi, 162
      precapillary, 91
Sphincterotomy, transduodenal, definition of, 450
Sphygmomanometer, types of, 271
Spinal accessory nerve, function of, 63t
Spinal anesthesia. See *Anesthesia, spinal.*
Spinal block, high, due to spinal anesthesia, 253–254
Spinal cord, anatomy of, 72–80, 251–252
      ascending and descending tracts of, 77–78, *78*
      cerebrospinal fluid circulation in, *66*
      concussion and contusion of, 433
      gray matter of, 79, *80*
      meninges of, 74–75
      nerve roots of, 76–79, *77–78*, *80*
      protection of, 72–75
      structure and function of, 75–79, *76–78*, *80*

Spinal cord *(Continued)*
  vascular network of, 80
  white matter of, 78–79, *80*
Spinal cord syndrome, 433
Spinal fusion, definition of, 399
Spinal injuries, 432–434
  anesthetic considerations in, 440
  autonomic hyperreflexia after, 439–440
  bone demineralization from, 437
  complications from, cardiovascular, 435–436
    gastrointestinal, 439
    respiratory, 435
    urologic, 439
  concomitant head injury with, 435
  contractures from, 437
  edema after, 435
  herniated nucleus pulposus and, 440, *441*, 442
  neurogenic shock from, 434–435
  nursing care and considerations in, 434–440
  Roto Rest bed for, 437, *438*
  sensory loss from, 438–439
  skin care after, 437
  Stryker frame bed for, 437, *437*
  temperature elevation after, 439
  tong traction for, 436, *436–437*
Spinal neoplasms, 442, *442*
Spinal nerve(s), anatomy of, 252
Spinal shock, definition of, 409
Spinal surgery, 431–442
  contraindications to, 434
  diagnostic tools used in, 431–432, *431–432*
  indications for, 433–434
  logrolling patient after, 407
  post anesthesia care after, 406–407
Spine, anatomy of, *251*, 251–252
  bones of. See *Vertebra(e)*.
Spinous process, of vertebrae, 74
Spirometry, incentive, in PACU patient, 289–290
Spleen, anatomy and physiology of, 164
  surgery of, care after, 458
Splenectomy, definition of, 450
Split-thickness skin graft, 492
  for burns, 503–504
Stadol. See *Butorphanol (Stadol)*.
Staff orientation program, for PACU, 20–22
    content of, 21–22
Staffing, of PACU, 18–20, 19t, 27–28
    nurse manager in, 18
    nursing personnel in, 19–20
    patterns of, 20
    selection of nurses in, 18–19, 19t
    self-scheduling in, 28
Stage of analgesia, 190
Stage of delirium, in anesthesia, 190
Stage of surgical anesthesia, 190–191
Standard, definition of, 12
Stapedectomy, *327*, 328
  definition of, 325
Starling equation, 119
Stem cells, definition of, 171
  in humoral immunity, 172, *173*
Stenosis, aortic, *370*
    definition of, 368–369
  mitral, definition of, 373
  pulmonary, 375
  pyloric, surgery for, care after, 455
  tricuspid, 376
Sterile technique, for intravenous therapy, 167, 169
Sternotomy, definition of, 350
Steroid(s), adrenal secretion of, 153
  interaction of, in PACU patient, 188

Steroid(s) *(Continued)*
  synthesis of, etomidate inhibition in, 207
Steroid anesthesia, 213
Stewart technique, cardiac output calculation by, 84
Stir-up regimen, 289–291
  deep-breathing exercises in, 289
  modifications of, 291
Stomach. See also *Gastric; Gastro-* entries.
  anatomy of, 157, *158*
  contents of, vomiting and regurgitation of, 158–159
  motility and secretions of, effect of pregnancy on, 158
  physiology of, 157–158
  surgery of, care after, 454–455
Storage space, in PACU, 6–7
Strabismus, definition of, 344
Stratum corneum, 499
  of epidermis, 165
Stratum germinativum, 499
Stratum granulosum, of epidermis, 165
Stratum lucidum, of epidermis, 165
Stratum spinosum, of epidermis, 165
Stress, behavioral symptoms of, 24t
  body's response to, 23
  causes of, 24t
  definition of, 22, 149
  elimination of, approaches to, 24–25
  in PACU, 24t, 24–25
  staff burnout and, 22–25
Stress syndrome, 22–24
Stretch receptor(s), in ADH secretion, 151
  in regulation of breathing, 132
Stricture, definition of, 138
Stryker frame bed, for spinal injuries, 437, *437*
  precautions with, 436–437
Subarachnoid block, definition of, 410
Subarachnoid screw, in ICP transducer, 421
Subarachnoid space, 74
Subcutaneous route of administration, of drugs, 183
Subdigital arteriography, definition of, 387–388
Subdural bolt, in ICP transducer, 421
Subdural hematoma, from brain injury, 414–415
Subdural space, 74
Sublimaze. See *Fentanyl (Sublimaze)*.
Sublingual route of administration, of drugs, 183
Subluxation, definition of, 410
  of vertebra, 432
Submucosal resection, of nose, definition of, 329
Substance abuse. See *Drug abuse*.
Subthalamus, 60
Succinylcholine, advantages of, 235
  as depolarizing neuromuscular agent, 234–237
  as muscle relaxant, 228, 230
  disadvantages of, 235–236
  for laryngospasm, 108
  pharmacology of, 229t
  side effects of, 236–237
  untoward reactions to, 235
  uses of, 235
Suction curettage, definition of, 477
Suction lipectomy, 496
Suctioning, for chest drainage, 356, *356*
  nasal, 298
  oral, 298
  tracheal, 335, 337, *337*
    after thoracic surgery, 364
    in PACU, 298–299, *301*
Sufentanil (Sufenta), 218
  administration of, protocol for, in post-cesarean section patients, 224t
Sulcus, of brain, 54, *55–56*
Suppressor T lymphocyte(s), in cellular immunity, 174

Suprapubic catheter(s), postoperative use of, 466
Supratentorial herniation, from brain injury, 415
Supraventricular arrhythmia(s), postoperative monitoring of, 275–276, *275–276*
Surface tension phenomenon, in lung, 113–114
Surfactant, in lung, 113–114
Sustained maximal inspiration (SMI), as postoperative breathing exercise, 359, 362
Sustained maximal inspiration (SMI) maneuver, 289
Sweat glands, 166–167
Sylvian fissure, of cerebral hemispheres, 54, *55*
Syme amputation, definition of, 399
Sympathectomy, cervicodorsal, 392
    definition of, 388
    lumbar, 392–393
Sympathetic nervous system, 81
Sympathomimetic amines, interaction of, in PACU patient, 188
Sympathomimetics, CNS, abuse of, 558t–559t, 560–561
Syncope, definition of, 83
Syncurine (decamethonium bromide), as depolarizing neuromuscular agent, 237
Syncytium, atrial and ventricular, 86
Syndrome of acute water intoxication, 155
Syndrome of inappropriate secretion of antidiuretic hormone (SIADH), 155
Synergistic effect, definition of, 181
Systemic lupus erythematosus, as arthus hypersensitivity reaction, 176
Systemic vascular pressure, postoperative monitoring of, 279–280
Systole, 85
    definition of, 83

T

T lymphocyte(s), definition of, 171
    in cellular immunity, 174
    in humoral immunity, 172, *173*
    release of lymphokines by, 174–175
T lymphocyte suppressor cell(s), 173, *173*
Tachycardia, atrial, postoperative monitoring of, 275–276, *276*
    paroxysmal, definition of, 83
    sinus, postoperative monitoring of, 275, *275*
    ventricular, postoperative monitoring of, 277, *277*
Tachyphylaxis, definition of, 181
Tactoids, in sickle cell anemia, 529
Tagamet. See *Cimetidine (Tagamet)*.
Talwin. See *Pentazocine (Fortral, Talwin)*.
Tamponade, cardiac, after cardiac surgery, 383
Tardive dyskinesia, 58
Target organ, definition of, 149
T-binder, for scrotal support, 473, *474*
Teflon clip, partially occluding, on vena cava, *395*
Telencephalon. See *Cerebrum*.
Temperature, body, accuracy of, 284
    after large vessel surgery, 397
    after spinal injuries, 439
    assessment of, 563
    changes in, 284t
    factors influencing, 283t
    in pediatric patient, regulation of, 539, *540*
    maintenance of, 563
    normal, 283
    of cranial surgical patient, 428
    postoperative measurement of, 283–284
    variations in, 564
    muscle relaxants and, 238
Temporal bone(s), of cranium, 65
Temporal lobe, of brain, 54, *55–56*
TENS. See *Transcutaneous electrical nerve stimulation (TENS)*.
Tension pneumothorax, 116

Tentorial hiatus, 415
Tentorium cerebelli, 65
Testosterone, 154
Tetanic stimulus, 240, 241
Tetanus, muscle relaxant response in, 243t
Tetany, 445
Tetracaine (Pontocaine), for local anesthesia, 248t, 249
Tetrahydrocannabinol (THC), abuse of, 559t, 561
Tetralogy of Fallot, definition of, 375–376
    features of, 375, *375*
Thalamus, 59–60, *60*
THC (tetrahydrocannabinol), abuse of, 559t, 561
Therapeutic index, 182
    of fentanyl, 219
Thermal balance, postoperative assessment of, 283t, 283–284, 284t
Thermal burn(s), 169
Thermal imbalance, definition of, 563
    post anesthesia care and, 563–569
Thermal injury(ies), 500–501. See also *Burn(s)*.
Thermometry, infrared tympanic membrane, 284
Thermoregulation, 165–166, *166*
    overview of, 563
Thermoregulatory response, behavioral, 563
    physiologic, 563
Thiazide, 144–145
Thinking, positive, of ambulatory surgical patient, 510
Thiopental (Pentothal), administration of, pent-nitrous technique of, 205
    advantages of, 206
    emergence from, PACU care during, 206
    intracranial pressure and, 419
    mode of action of, 205–206
    use of, 205
Third-degree burn, 169
Thoracentesis, 353
    definition of, 350
Thoracic. See also *Chest* entries.
Thoracic cavity, invasive diagnostic procedures involving, 351–353
Thoracic surgery, 350–367
    care after, 361–367
    chest drainage after, 353–360, *354–359*
        volume in, 361
    circulatory functions after, 364–365
    complication(s) of, 365–367
        arrhythmias as, 367
        atelectasis as, 365–366
        hemorrhage as, 366
        hypovolemia as, 366
        hypoxemia as, 365, *365*
        infection as, 366
        neurogenic hypotension as, 367
        shock as, 366
        ventilatory mechanical problems as, 366
    fluid balance after, 364
    general care following, 360–361
    humidification after, 364
    institution of oxygen therapy after, 362
    modified stir-up regimen after, initiation of, 362
    pain relief after, 362–364, *363*
    patent airway maintenance after, 361
    positioning after, 360
    respiratory function after, 361–364
        assessment of, 361–362, *362*
    tracheal suctioning after, 364
    vital signs after, 361
Thoracoplasty, definition of, 350
Thoracotomy, definition of, 350
Threshold, pain, 317
Throat, surgery of, 331–339

Thrombectomy, definition of, 388
Thrombophlebitis, associated with invasive hemodynamic
    monitoring, 281t
Thrombosis, deep vein, after orthopedic surgery, 402
    definition of, 83
Thrombus, definition of, 388
Thymectomy, for myasthenia gravis, 521
Thyrocalcitonin, 152
Thyroglobulin, 152
Thyroglossal duct cystectomy, definition of, 444
Thyroid gland, anatomy and physiology of, 152
    surgery of, 444–445
        anesthesia for, 444
        cardiorespiratory assessment after, 444–445
        complications after, 445
        dressings for, 445
        fluid input and output after, 445
        pain management after, 445
        patient positioning after, 444
        postoperative nursing care in, 444–445
Thyroid lobectomy, definition of, 444
Thyroid storm, 445
Thyroidectomy, definition of, 444
Thyroid-stimulating hormone (TSH), 151
Thyrotropin. See *Thyroid-stimulating hormone (TSH)*.
Thyrotropin-releasing hormone, 151
Thyroxine (T$_4$), 152
Tidal volume (V$_T$), 111t
    definition of, 111t
Tigan. See *Trimethobenzamide (Tigan)*.
Tilting-disk valve, 376, *377*
Tip, of laryngoscope blade, 308
Tissue compartments, groups of, 192–193
Tissue contusion, in trauma, 571
Tissue transfer, microvascular, 493
TLC (total lung capacity), 112
    definition of, 111t
Tolerance, definition of, 182
    to drugs, 557. See also *Drug abuse*.
    to pain, 317
Tong traction, for spinal injuries, 436, *436–437*
Tongue, surgery of, 330
Tongue tied, definition of, 330
Tonoclonic movements, definition of, 410
Tonsil tray, contents of, 332t
Tonsillectomy, definition of, 331
Tonsillectomy and adenoidectomy, 331–333
    complication of, 332
    dissection in, *333*
    equipment tray for, 332t
    laryngospasms after, 333
    laser dissection in, 332
Toomey syringe, 466
Topical anesthesia, 245
Toradol. See *Ketorolac (Toradol)*.
Torr, definition of, 105
Total abdominal hysterectomy, definition of, 479
Total lung capacity (TLC), 112
    definition of, 111t
Toxic jaundice, 161
Toxicity, of oxygen, 136
Trabeculectomy, definition of, 344
Trachea, anatomy of, 108
    bifurcation of, 108, *109*, 109t
Tracheal dilator and hook, *337*
Tracheal intubation, 307–313
    adverse sequelae after, 312–313
    aspiration of gastrointestinal contents after, 313
    equipment for, 307t, 307–309, *308–309*
    hoarseness and sore throat after, 312–313
    laryngoscope in, 307–308, *308*

Tracheal intubation *(Continued)*
    laryngospasm after, 313
    nasotracheal, 311–312, *312*
    oral, 309–311
        blade insertion in, 310
        head position for, 310, *310*
        patient assessment in, 311
        patient position for, 310
        patient ventilation in, 311
        raising epiglottis and visualizing vocal cords in, 310, *311*
        tube placement in, 310–311
    PACU patient care following, 312
    recommended tube sizes for, 307t
    tracheal tube in, 308–309, *309*
    tube removal in, 312
Tracheal suctioning, 335, 337, *337*
    after thoracic surgery, 364
    in PACU, 298–299, *301*
Tracheal tube, placement of, 310–311
    used in intubation, 308–309, *309*
Tracheal tug, in anesthesia, 191
Trachelorrhaphy, definition of, 478–479
Tracheostomy, 334–338
    care of, suctioning and, 335, 337, *337*
    complications of, 337–338, *337–338*
    definition of, 331
    incision for, *334*
    patient with, bedside equipment needed for, 334, 335t
    tubes available for, 334, *336–337*
    wound drainage from, 335, *337*
Tracheostomy tray, contents of, 334t
Tracheostomy tube(s), 334, *336–337*
    care and cleaning of, 335
    positions of, *338*
    securing of, 335, *337*
    types of, 334, *336–337*
Tracrium. See *Atracurium besylate (Tracrium)*.
Train-of-four stimulation, 241–242, *242*
Trandate. See *Labetalol (Normodyne, Trandate)*.
Tranquilizer(s). See also specific agent, e.g., *Diazepam
        (Valium)*.
    as nonopioid intravenous anesthetic, 208–212
Transcutaneous electrical nerve stimulation (TENS), for
        postoperative pain, *322*, 322–323
Transduodenal sphincterotomy, definition of, 450
Transfer factor, of lymphokines, 174
Transfusion(s), 291–295
    administration of, 292
    allergic reactions to, 293–294
    autologous, 292
    febrile reactions to, 293
    for shock, 573
    hemolytic reactions to, 293
    infusion solutions and, 292–293
    of blood components, 294–295
    of non-blood volume substitutes, 295
    of whole blood, 292–293
        indication for, 292
    reactions to, 293–294
        delayed, 294
        treatment of, 294
    safeguards in, 292
Transplantation, corneal, *346*
    definition of, 376
    kidney. See *Renal transplantation*.
Transposition of great arteries, definition of, 376
Transurethral surgery, definition of, 464
Transverse process, of vertebrae, 74
Trauma, blunt, 571
    cranial, 416–418
    mechanisms of injury in, 570–571

Trauma (Continued)
  penetrating, 571
  shock, post anesthesia care for, 570–582. See also Shock.
  spinal, 432–434. See also Spinal injuries.
  tissue contusion in, 571
Trauma resuscitation unit, 572
Treponema immobilization test, 557
Trichlormethane. See Chloroform (Trichlormethane).
Trichloroethylene (Trilene), 198
Tricuspid regurgitation, definition of, 376
Tricuspid stenosis, definition of, 376
Tricuspid valve(s), 85
Trifluoroethyl vinyl ether. See Fluroxene (Trifluoroethyl vinyl ether, Fluoromar).
Trigeminal nerve, function of, 63t
Triiodothyronine (T$_3$), 152
Trilene. See Trichloroethylene (Trilene).
Trimethaphan camsylate (Arfonad), for hypertension, 101t, 102
Trimethobenzamide (Tigan), for nausea, 532t
Trochlear nerve, function of, 63t
Tropic hormone, definition of, 149
Trousseau's sign, 445
True shunt, 128
TSH (thyroid-stimulating hormone), 151
T-tube, placement of, in bile duct, 458, 458
Tubal ligation, definition of, 479
Tuberculin skin test, delayed response in, as hypersensitivity reaction, 176
Tuberculosis, control of, 33–34
d-Tubocurarine, action of, 230
  as muscle relaxant, 228
  pharmacology of, 229t
Tuffier's line, 252
Tumor(s), dumbbell, 442
  intracranial, 416
  intraspinal, 442, 442
  ocular, iodine plaque irradiation for, 348, 348
Tympanoplasty (myringoplasty), 328
  definition of, 325

U

Ulcer(s), peptic, definition of, 156
  perforated, surgery for, care after, 455
Ultrasonography, in cranial surgery, 412
Umbilical herniorrhaphy, definition of, 448–449
Uncal herniation, from brain injury, 415
Underwriter's Laboratories, Inc., 13t
Upper motor neurons, lower, definition of, 53
Urea, in urine, 143, 143t
Uremia, definition of, 138
Ureteral catheter(s), postoperative use, 466–467
Ureteral surgery, care after, 468, 469, 470–471
Ureterectomy, definition of, 463
Ureterolithotomy, definition of, 463
Ureteroneocystostomy, definition of, 463
Ureteroplasty, definition of, 463
Ureterostomy, definition of, 463
Urethral catheter(s), postoperative use of, 465–466, 467
Urethral dilatation, definition of, 464
Urethral meatotomy, definition of, 464
Urethral surgery, 474–475
Urethrocele, definition of, 479
Urethroplasty, definition of, 464
Urethrotomy, internal, definition of, 464
Uric acid, in urine, 143, 143t
Urinary incontinence, definition of, 138
Urinary retention, after orthopedic surgery, 403
  definition of, 138
  due to spinal anesthesia, 254
  from epidural analgesia, 322

Urine, components of, 142–143, 143t
  secretion of, 140, 141t
Urine output, in pediatric patient, 537–538, 538t
Urologic complications, from spinal injuries, 439
Uterine aspiration, care after, 481
  definition of, 477
Uterus, prolapse of, definition of, 478
Utility area, in PACU, 6

V

V waves, 83, 84
Vaginal hysterectomy, definition of, 477
Vaginal plastic operation, definition of, 479
Vaginal surgery, 481–482
  care after, 482
  procedures in, 481–482
  terms used in, 477–479
Vagotomy, definition of, 450
Vagus nerve, 157
  function of, 63t
Valium. See Diazepam (Valium).
Valleculae, 106
Valsalva maneuver, definition of, 410
  intracranial pressure and, 430
Valve(s), atrioventricular, 83, 85
  heart, 85, 86
  ileocecal, 160
  mechanical, 376–377, 377
  mitral, 85, 86
  prosthetic, types of, 376–377, 377
  replacement of, 376–378
    patient undergoing, 378
  semilunar, 85
  tricuspid, 85
Varicocelectomy, definition of, 464
Vasa recta, 140
Vascular disease, noninvasive treatment of, 388–389
Vascular resistance, in cardiac output, 85
  pulmonary, 118
Vascular surgery, 387–397
  anesthesia for, 389
  diagnostic procedures in, 389–390
  general considerations in, 389
  on large vessels, 393–394, 394–395, 396–397
    anesthesia for, 394, 396
    body temperature after, 397
    cardiopulmonary status after, 396
    circulatory status after, 396–397
    dressings for, 397
    fluid input and output after, 397
    neurologic status after, 397
    pain relief following, 397
    positioning after, 396
  peripheral, carotid endarterectomy in, 393, 394t
    circulatory status after, 391, 391
    dressings after, 392
    fluid input and output after, 392
    PACU care following, 390–392
    pain relief after, 392
    positioning after, 390–391
    procedures in, 390–397
    sympathectomy in, 392–393
  postarteriography care in, 389–390
Vascular system, peripheral, complications of, after cardiac surgery, 386
Vasectomy, definition of, 464
Vasoconstriction, peripheral, after cardiac surgery, 383–384
Vasoepididymostomy, definition of, 464
Vasomotion, 91
Vasomotor center, effect of, on blood pressure, 85

Vasopressin. See *Antidiuretic hormone (ADH)*.
Vasovasostomy, definition of, 464
VC (vital capacity), 112
  definition of, 111t
V$_D$/V$_T$ ratio, 128–129
V̇$_E$ (minute ventilation), definition of, 104
Vecuronium (Norcuron), action and dosage of, 232–233
  pharmacology of, 229t
Vena cava, partially occluding Teflon clip on, *395*
Venous sinus(es), cranial, 65, *66*
Venous spasm(s), associated with invasive hemodynamic
    monitoring, 281t
Venous thrombosis, deep, after orthopedic surgery, 402
Ventilation, alveolar, matched to perfusion, 127
  role of, in delivery of anesthetic gas, 192
  definition of, 105
  distribution of, 126–127
  during pregnancy, 551–552
  in cardiopulmonary resuscitation, 589
    mouth-to-mouth, 589, *589*
  mechanical, complications of, after thoracic surgery, 366
    CPAP and, 296–297
    IMV and, 297
    in PACU, 296–298
    nursing responsibilities and, 297–298, *298–300*
    PEEP in, 296
  minute, definition of, 104
  patient, during oral tracheal intubation, 311
  postoperative, monitoring of, 267–270, *268–270*
  terminology in, 298t
  to perfusion of blood, decreased, 127–128
    increased, 128–129
Ventilation-perfusion matching, 126–127
Ventilation-perfusion mismatching, 127–129, *128–129*
Ventral, definition of, 53
Ventricle(s), of brain, fourth, *61*, 62
  lateral, 54, *57*
  lateral and superior views of, *70*
  third, 60, *60*
  of heart, 83
Ventricular aneurysm repair, definition of, 378
Ventricular arrhythmia(s), postoperative monitoring of, *276–*
  277, 276–278
Ventricular contraction, premature. See *Premature ventricular
  contraction*.
Ventricular fibrillation, postoperative monitoring of, 277, *277–*
  278
Ventricular septal defect, 378, *379*
Ventricular syncytium, 86
Ventricular tachycardia, postoperative monitoring of, 277, *277*
Ventriculography, 410
Venturi mask, oxygen administration via, 297t
Venule(s), anatomy of, 91
Verapamil (Calan, Isoptin), 97
  for cardiopulmonary resuscitation, 594
  for hypertension, 101t
Verbalization, patient's, of postoperative pain, 316–317, *317*
Versed. See *Midazolam (Versed)*.
Vertebra(e), 72–74
  cervical, 74, *75*
  herniated, forms of, *441*
  lumbar, 74
  structure of, 73, 75–76, *76*
  subluxation of, 432
  thoracic, 74
Vertebral artery(ies), 71, *72–73*
Vertebral bodies, fracture-dislocation of, 433
Vertebral foramen, 74
Vesicourethral suspension (Marshall-Marchetti operation),
  definition of, 463
Vinke tongs, for spinal injuries, 436

Visceral pleura, 110
Visitor(s), in PACU, 29–30
Vistaril. See *Hydroxyzine (Atarax, Vistaril)*.
Visual area, of brain, 58
Vital capacity (VC), 112
  definition of, 111t
Vital sign monitor(s), 13–14, *14*
Vital signs, after thoracic surgery, 361
  assessment of, 423–425, 425t
Vitrectomy, definition of, 344
Vocal cords, of newborn, 535
  visualizing, in oral tracheal intubation, 310, *311*
Voice box. See *Larynx*.
Volatile anesthetic agent(s), 196. See also specific agent, e.g.,
    Halothane (Fluothane).
Volkmann contracture, definition of, 399
Volume receptor(s), in ADH secretion, 151
Volvulus, definition of, 450
Vomiting, 158–159. See also *Nausea*.
  after epidural analgesia, 322
  after spinal anesthesia, 254
  central, 531
  definition of, 156
  mechanism of action of, 531–532
  postoperative, 531–533
    incidence of, 532
    PACU care in, 532t, 532–533
Vomiting center, 531
  afferent connections of, *531*
V$_T$ (tidal volume), 111
  definition of, 111t

W

Wall vacuum system, for PACU, 10, *10–11*
Wall-supply oxygen, in PACU, 8–9, *9*
Warfarin, adverse effects of, in geriatric patient, 547t
Warm air therapy, for hypothermia, 564
Water balance, effect of inhalation anesthesia on, 203
  in lung, 118–120, *119*
Water intoxication, after prostate surgery, 472
Water loss, prevention of, 167
Water-seal chest drainage system, 355, *355*
Wedge resection, definition of, 350
Wheeze, definition of, 105
Whipple procedure, care after, 458, 460
  definition of, 450
White blood cell(s), 90
White matter, of brain, 54
  of spinal cord, 78–79, *80*
Withdrawal signs. See also *Drug abuse*.
  in drug abuse, 558t–559t
Wound(s), tracheostomy, drainage from, 335, *337*
Wound care, after burns, 503–504
  after orthopedic surgery, 401–402, *402*
Wound dehiscence, after cardiac surgery, 384
Wyamine. See *Mephentermine sulfate (Wyamine)*.

X

Xenograft(s), 377
  definition of, 492
Xylocaine. See *Lidocaine (Xylocaine)*.

Y

Yawn, 134
Yawn maneuver, 113
Y-V plasty (bladder neck operation), definition of, 463

Z

Zantac (ranitidine), for gastric hypersecretory states, 159
Zemuron. See *Rocuronium bromide (Zemuron)*.